Radiographic Atlas of the Genitourinary System

VOLUME II

Charles Ney, M.D.

Assistant Clinical Professor of Urology, Albert Einstein School of Medicine; Assistant Attending Urologist, Montefiore Hospital and Medical Center; Attending Urologist and Chief of Urology, Bronx-Lebanon Hospital Center, New York, New York

Richard M. Friedenberg, M.D.

Professor and Chairman, Department of Radiological Sciences, University of California, Irvine, Orange, California

28 Contributors

SECOND EDITION

Radiographic Atlas of the Genitourinary System

VOLUME II

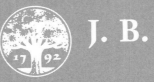

J. B. Lippincott Company
PHILADELPHIA • TORONTO

2nd Edition

Copyright © 1981, by J. B. Lippincott Company.
Copyright © 1966, by J. B. Lippincott Company.
For information address J. B. Lippincott Company, East Washington Square, Philadelphia, Pennsylvania 19105.

1 3 5 6 4 2

Library of Congress Cataloging in Publication Data

Ney, Charles, ed.
    Radiographic atlas of the genitourinary system.

    Includes bibliographies and index.
    1. Genito-urinary organs — Radiography. I. Friedenberg,
Richard.   II. Title.
RC874.N4   1981   616.6'07572   80-25504
ISBN 0-397-50408-X

Printed in the United States of America

Dedicated to our wives, Doris and Gloria,
who maintained
the same patience
during the preparation of the
second edition
that they did during the first

Contents

Contributors

SEYED A.S. BAGHERY, M.D.

Staff Radiologist
Cleveland Clinic Hospital
Cleveland, Ohio

SHELDON BAUM, M.D.

Director of Nuclear Medicine
The Milton S. Hershey Medical Center
The Pennsylvania State University
Hershey, Pennsylvania

JOSHUA A. BECKER, M.D.

Professor and Chairman of the Department of
*   Radiology*
State University of New York
Downstate Medical Center
Brooklyn, New York

PAULA W. BRILL, M.D.

Associate Professor of Radiology
Department of Radiology
The New York Hospital–Cornell Medical Center
New York, New York

GUIDO CURRARINO, M.D.

Professor and Director
Department of Radiology
Children's Medical Center
Dallas, Texas

RICHARD M. FRIEDENBERG, M.D.

Professor and Chairman,
Department of Radiological Sciences,
University of California, Irvine,
Orange, California

LAWRENCE GOULD, M.D.

Chief, Radiology Service
Veterans Administration Medical Center
Lyons, New Jersey;
Clinical Associate Professor of Radiology
College of Medicine and Dentistry of New Jersey
New Jersey Medical School
Newark, New Jersey

MONEER K. HANNA, M.D.

Chief of Pediatric Urology,
Long Island Jewish-Hillside Medical Center,
New Hyde Park, New York;
Director of Pediatric Urology,
Children's Hospital of Newark,
Newark, New Jersey;
Clinical Associate Professor of Surgery,
College of Medicine and Dentistry of New Jersey;
Director, Division of Pediatric Urology,
College of Medicine and Dentistry of New Jersey;
Pediatric Urologist,
Newark Beth Israel Medical Center
Newark, New Jersey

GLEN W. HARTMAN, M.D.

Professor of Radiology
Mayo Medical School
Department of Diagnostic Radiology
Mayo Clinic, Rochester, Minnesota

ROBERT R. HATTERY, M.D.

Associate Professor of Radiology
Mayo Medical School
Department of Diagnostic Radiology
Mayo Clinic, Rochester, Minnesota

FRANK HINMAN, JR., M.D.

Clinical Professor of Urology
School of Medicine
University of California, San Francisco
San Francisco, California

BAO-SHAN JING, M.D.

Professor of Radiology
Department of Diagnostic Radiology
The University of Texas System Cancer Center
M.D. Anderson Hospital and Tumor Institute
Texas Medical Center
Houston, Texas

DONALD L. KING, M.D.

Professor, Department of Radiology
Columbia-Presbyterian Medical Center
New York, New York

RAJENDRA KUMAR, M.D.

Assistant Professor of Radiology
Chief, Genitourinary Section
University of Texas Medical Branch
Galveston, Texas

ROSALYN KUTCHER, M.D.

Assistant Professor of Radiology
Albert Einstein College of Medicine
Montefiore Hospital and Medical Center
Bronx, New York

ERICH K. LANG, M.D.

Professor and Chairman,
Department of Radiology
Louisiana State University Medical Center;
Professor of Radiology,
Louisiana State University Medical Center,
Tulane School of Medicine;
Director of Radiology,
Charity Hospital;
New Orleans, Louisiana

*FILEMON LOPEZ, M.D.

Professor of Radiology
College of Medicine and Dentistry
of New Jersey, Newark, New Jersey

LEON LOVE, M.D.

Professor and Chairman of Radiology
Loyola University Medical Center
Foster G. McGaw Hospital
Maywood, Illinois

THOMAS F. MEANEY, M.D.

Chairman, Division of Radiology
Cleveland Clinic, Cleveland, Ohio

MORTON A. MEYERS, M.D.

Professor and Chairman
Department of Radiology
Health Sciences Center
State University of New York Stony Brook
Stony Brook, New York

ALBERT A. MOSS, M.D.

Professor of Radiology
Chief, CT Body Scanning
University of California, San Francisco
San Francisco, California

CHARLES NEY, M.D.

Assistant Clinical Professor of Urology,
Albert Einstein School of Medicine;
Assistant Attending Urologist,
Montefiore Hospital and Medical Center;
Attending Urologist and Chief of Urology,
Bronx-Lebanon Hospital Center,
New York, New York

* Deceased.

IRWIN SCHLOSSBERG, M.D.

Assistant Professor, Department of Radiology
Albert Einstein College of Medicine
Bronx, New York

SEYMOUR SPRAYREGEN, M.D.

Professor of Radiology
Albert Einstein College of Medicine;
Chief, Section of Angiography,
Montefiore Hospital and Medical Center
Bronx, New York

SIDNEY WALLACE, M.D.

Professor of Radiology
Department of Diagnostic Radiology
The University of Texas System Cancer Center
M.D. Anderson Hospital and Tumor Institute
Texas Medical Center
Houston, Texas

PATRICK C. WALSH, M.D.

Professor and Director
Department of Urology
The Johns Hopkins University School of Medicine;
Director, James Buchanan Brady Urological Institute,
The Johns Hopkins Hospital
Baltimore, Maryland

BYRN WILLIAMSON, JR., M.D.

Assistant Professor of Radiology
Mayo Graduate School of Medicine
Department of Diagnostic Radiology
Mayo Clinic, Rochester, Minnesota

PATRICIA WINCHESTER, M.D.

Associate Professor of Radiology
Department of Radiology
The New York Hospital-Cornell Medical Center
New York, New York

Radiographic Atlas of the Genitourinary System

VOLUME II

Part Three

ADRENAL GLAND

Striking radiologic advances permit precise anatomic localization and often the specific histologic diagnosis in the patient with adrenal disease. Multiple approaches provide accurate parameters of an adrenal lesion. The choice and order of diagnostic roentgenographic studies are best made with appreciation of the clinical findings. Basic to a thorough and accurate radiologic evaluation is a detailed knowledge of the advantages and limitations of each technique.

NORMAL GROSS ANATOMY

Apart from their suprarenal position, the right and left adrenal glands have important differences in gross morphology and relationships.

The right adrenal is roughly triangular in shape. It lies deep to the nonperitonealized (bare) area of the right lobe of the liver laterally and deep to the inferior vena cava medially. Posteromedially the gland is near the diaphragm. Inferiorly, it has only a loose attachment to the upper pole of the kidney.

The left adrenal is closely adjacent to the upper medial border of the kidney, at times extending anteriorly to the level of the renal hilus. It thus presents typically a semilunar contour, concave laterally facing the kidney and convex medially. Anteriorly, the gland is in relationship to the tail of the pancreas and the posterior parietal peritoneum of the lesser sac and posteriorly, to the lumbar insertions of the diaphragm.

The adrenal gland is composed of the cortex (80% of the adult gland by weight) and the medulla. The cortex is derived from mesoderm and the medulla, from neuroectodermal tissue. Cells of the adrenal medulla are composed of ganglion cells and of functioning chromaffin cells (pheochromocytes). There are multiple sites of extra-adrenal chromaffin tissue.

16

The Adrenal Glands: Roentgenologic Techniques

Morton A. Meyers

These are called paraganglia. The largest collection of such cells occurs on either side of the origin of the inferior mesenteric artery, called the organs of Zuckerkandl. Paraganglia are also commonly found in the celiac, hypogastric, adrenal, aortic, and renal plexuses and in relation to other parts of the sympathetic nervous system.

ADRENAL ANOMALIES

ABSENCE

Absence of adrenal glands is extremely rare. Although the adrenal glands arise in intimate anatomic relation to the kidneys, their separate origin means that their development is generally unaffected by common renal anomalies. In congenital renal hypoplasia and crossed renal ectopia, the adrenals mature fully and develop in their normal position (Figs. 16–1 to 16–3).[10] In unilateral renal agenesis, there is ipsilateral absence of the adrenal gland in only 8 per cent.[7] When present the gland may be round rather than triangular.[12]

HETEROTOPIA

If the primordial adrenal does not separate from the coelomic epithelium, it may become partly or wholly incorporated into contiguous organs such as the kidney (Fig. 16–4) or liver.[8, 11] Both cortical and medullary tissue are found.

ACCESSORY ADRENALS

Accessory adrenals are formed from fragments of tissue that split off from the cortical anlage. Accessories at a distance from the adrenal gland have uniformly revealed cortical tissue only, whereas those close to the gland proper are more likely to be composed also of medullary tissue.[9, 13] Cortical rests from 2 to 8 mm. in size are found in over half of all cases with careful dissection. They occur most often in strands of the celiac plexus and less frequently in periadrenal fat or the spermatic cord.

RADIOLOGIC TECHNIQUES

PLAIN FILMS AND INTRAVENOUS UROGRAPHY

Because of the surrounding periadrenal fat, the outline of normal adrenal glands may occasionally be seen on plain films, particularly properly exposed low-kilovolt radiographs.

Adrenal masses may be visualized (1) directly as soft-tissue densities (Fig. 16–5), (2) by their effects of renal displacement (Figs. 16–6 to 16–9), and (3) by their frequent calcification (Figs. 16–10 to 16–14).

Bilateral adrenal hyperplasia is not visualized on the plain film. A rough estimate of the potential vertical diameter of the adrenals or of a suprarenal mass can be determined on 20- to 30-degree oblique abdominal films by measuring the distance between the posterior diaphragmatic sulcus and the upper renal pole. Filling the stomach with gas may enhance visualization of the suprarenal areas, particularly on the left.[16]

The left kidney is normally lower than the right in 5 to 15 per cent of cases. Inferior and lateral displacement of the kidney typically results from a large adrenal tumor. This has been shown in 40 per cent to 50 per cent of proved cases of various adrenal tumors.[15, 18] The upper renal pole is displaced outward and downward, producing the characteristic "drooping water-lily" appearance of its collecting system (Figs. 16–7 to 16–9). Lateral projections document the typical anterior displacement of the upper portion of the kidney (Fig. 16–9B). Erect films may be helpful in distinguishing an adrenal tumor from a renal mass (Fig. 16–10). The kidney may descend sufficiently to be clearly separated from the adrenal, which is fixed superiorly to Gerota's fascia and does not fall. Changes in the ureters and urinary bladder may indicate tumors at extra-adrenal sites.

Calcification plays a significant role in radiographic diagnosis (Figs. 16–11 to 16–14).[4, 17, 18] It may vary from fine, stippled, or curvilinear collections to confluent and dense calcifications. It is seen particularly in neuroblastoma (50%), adrenocortical carcinoma (31%), Addison's disease (25%), Wolman's disease, chronic adrenal hemorrhage, and pseudocysts. Other tumors that may occasionally calcify are pheochromocytomas, adrenal adenomas, and neurofibromas. The calcifications must be distinguished from calcified costal cartilages, mesenteric lymph nodes, calcification in the superior pole of the kidney, the aorta and branches, the liver, a thrombus in the inferior vena cava, meconium peritonitis, paravertebral or perirenal abscesses, or calculi in the kidney, pancreas, or gall bladder.

The abdominal studies are also useful in identifying the bony changes and increased fat in Cushing's syndrome, the skeletal lesions and possible paraspinal extension of neuroblastoma (Fig. 16–15), hepatic and splenic enlargement, the intestinal gas pattern, ascites from disseminated tumor, and metastatic nodules in the lower lung fields.

TOMOGRAPHY

Laminography or tomography eliminates overlying bowel and gas shadows, occasionally separates an adrenal mass from the closely adjacent kidney (see

Fig. 16–19), and better localizes and defines calcifications.[20-22]

NEPHROTOMOGRAPHY

The presence of normal adrenals can be ascertained by nephrotomography (Fig. 16–16). It is important to realize that the adrenal glands lie in different planes (the left is more anterior) so that both are not clearly seen on the same tomographic cut. Small tumors within the body of the gland or projecting from a contour not seen in profile may be missed.

Hartman and associates evaluated nephrotomography in a series of adrenal tumors.[23, 23a] The location of at least 70 per cent of surgically proved tumors was correctly identified. Adenomas were seen if they were 2.5 cm. in diameter (Figs. 16–17, 16–18). Carcinomas were large and all were identified. Aldosteronomas were less than 2.5 cm. in diameter and were not seen. Hyperplastic adrenal glands could be identified in only 2 of 23 patients with Cushing's syndrome. They conclude that nephrotomography can be used to localize the tumor in 85 per cent of patients with Cushing's syndrome caused by adrenal adenoma or carcinoma and is of little value in patients with adrenal hyperplasia or in patients with aldosteronism.

We have found nephrotomography also useful in instances of adrenal enlargement from metastases (Fig. 16–19) and adrenal abscesses (Fig. 16–20).

GASTROINTESTINAL STUDIES

Barium studies are of value in helping to determine an abdominal mass as adrenal in position. They may first suggest the presence of an asymptomatic or nonfunctioning adrenal lesion.

Masses in the right adrenal region may cause anterior displacement of the descending duodenum, particularly its proximal portion (Figs. 16–21, 16–22).[26, 27] We have observed that this is often caused by renal displacement and rotation consequent to the mass. When the adrenal mass is extremely large, displacement of the stomach and duodenum to the left (Fig. 16–23) and depression and anterior displacement of the hepatic flexure of the colon (Figs. 16–7, 16–24) may result.

Large masses in the left adrenal region indent the posterior gastric wall and cause displacement of the stomach anteriorly (Figs. 16–22, 16–25), medially (Fig. 16–26), and superiorly (Fig. 16–27). There may be anterior displacement of the duodenojejunal junction.[24, 25] Depression of the distal transverse colon and splenic flexure may be present (Fig. 16–26).

Extra-adrenal pheochromocytomas (Fig. 16–28), neuroblastomas, and ganglioneuromas (Fig. 16–29) may be revealed by displacement of bowel.

RETROPERITONEAL PNEUMOGRAPHY

Outlining of the adrenal glands by gas can be obtained via a flank perirenal injection or by presacral injection.[31-34, 54, 55] The presacral approach is considered easier, carries less risk of complications, and provides bilateral visualization.

Retroperitoneal pneumography has now been virtually replaced by adrenal arteriography and venography and by computed tomography.

TECHNIQUE

Injection is usually made near the midline through the anococcygeal raphe into the retrorectal presacral space. The transacral and transcoccygeal routes have been used by some.[51, 57] Gas is introduced incrementally in a ratio of approximately 15 cc./kg. of body weight, averaging 1200 to 1500 cc. in the adult and 200 to 500 cc. in children. Room air should not be used because of the danger of air embolism.[40, 49, 52] Carbon dioxide is preferred by many because it is 20 times more soluble than oxygen.[43] However, others cite the technical disadvantage of its rapid absorption and the need for immediate filming. Oxygen is thus preferred by others.[49] After injection, the head of the table is raised or the patient performs flexion movements of the trunk to facilitate symmetric extraperitoneal distribution of the gas. Radiographs and tomograms are obtained in the frontal and oblique positions. Erect films (Fig. 16–30) may be particularly helpful. When oxygen is used, the films are sometimes best obtained several hours later to take advantage of optimal gaseous dissection into the suprarenal areas. The steps of the technique have been individually detailed.[29, 30, 35-38, 43, 48, 49, 58-61]

COMPLICATIONS

There are few serious complications. Abdominal discomfort, pneumomediastinum, shoulder pain, and subcutaneous emphysema extending into the neck or scrotum may occur, but are transient (Fig. 16–31). Oxygen rarely produces gas embolism[52]; carbon dioxide can be utilized with complete safety.[43]

VISUALIZATION OF NORMAL ADRENAL GLANDS

The outline of normal adrenal glands is clearly seen with adequate dissection of the gas through the periadrenal fat (Fig. 16–32). It must be appreciated that each gland can be satisfactorily evaluated only on multiple projections and that both are often not clearly seen on the same frontal tomographic level.

Coursing through the fat are numerous connective tissue fibers that may give a reticulated or granular appearance.[28, 63] The glands are triangular-shaped with gently concave borders, giving the classic "cocked-hat" appearance. The left adrenal, however, is often crescentic or semilunar and frequently extends medially and anteriorly over the upper pole of the kidney. For this reason, the medial contour of the *left* adrenal gland may normally be convex. Tomograms in the left posterior oblique projection are often best for demonstrating the left adrenal gland. Superior attenuated prolongations of the gland are sometimes present (Fig. 16–32D).

Steinbach and Smith have established normal values for the area of the adrenal glands on anteroposterior films or tomograms: right adrenal 2.0 to 7.8 cm.² (average 4.2 cm.²) and left adrenal 2.0 to 8.7 cm.² (average 4.3 cm.²).[61] Adrenal volume is related directly to body weight and surface area, but is disproportionately great in children.[62] Due to the variety in shape, the range of normal measurements is too wide to be practical. A useful rule is that the height of a normal gland does not usually exceed that of an adjacent vertebral body. The contour is a much more reliable index.

However, demonstrable concave margins do not guarantee a normal gland. Hyperplastic glands may become large before losing their concave borders, but other associated findings permit their diagnosis.[31, 45, 49, 61]

VISUALIZATION OF ENLARGED ADRENAL GLANDS

The earliest sign of enlargement is the appearance of a convex margin on one side (Figs. 16–33, 16–34). This is seen in small tumors and, bilaterally, in hyperplasia.

Larger adrenal lesions are outlined usually as spherical masses. Identification of Gerota's fascia itself as a thin radiopaque stripe laterally (Fig. 16–35B) excludes other extraperitoneal masses arising outside of the renal–adrenal axis.

ACCURACY

Meyers evaluated retroperitoneal pneumography in a series of 61 surgically proved adrenal lesions with high diagnostic accuracy in hyperplasia and adenoma.[49] In adrenal carcinoma, the mass may not be directly seen because of poor dissection of the gas. The location of 13 of 29 pheochromocytomas (including extra-adrenal sites) was established.

ARTERIOGRAPHY

The adrenal glands are among the most vascular organs in the body. Adrenal blood flow is estimated at 5 to 8 cc./g./minute. Arteriography has become the most widely employed special radiologic procedure for delineation of adrenal masses.

ANATOMY OF ADRENAL ARTERIES

Three basic arterial pathways supply the adrenal glands (Fig. 16–36).[66, 68, 70, 78, 86, 89] Each originates from different sites and supplies different portions in a zonal distribution.

The *inferior adrenal arteries*, 1 to 4 on each side, arise from the renal arteries, either directly or with the superior renal capsular branch, or occasionally from the aorta. They supply the lower portion of the glands, including the lateral aspect on the left.

The *middle adrenal arteries* arise from the aorta laterally most often above or at the renal artery level.[71] In about one-eighth of cases, they arise below the renal arteries. On each side, they break up into a spray of 4 to 5 twigs just barely visible with contrast opacification.

The middle adrenal artery is present on the right in two-thirds and on the left in three-fourths of cases. Multiple middle adrenal arteries occur in 30 per cent.

The middle adrenal artery supplies the region containing the medulla and main draining veins. On the left, its distribution is often extensive and appears, in many cases, to supply most of the gland.[79]

The *superior adrenal arteries* arise principally from the inferior phrenic arteries, which are anterior or anterolateral branches of the aorta just above the celiac axis or, almost as frequently, branches of the celiac artery itself.[74] Occasionally, the inferior phrenic may arise from the renal artery. The superior adrenal arteries are multiple (12–20) small branches that radiate from the main inferior phrenic artery and its posterior division to supply the upper pole of each gland.

Between 50 and 60 small threadlike twigs pass from the three main arteries into a subcapsular plexus that connects with a widely interconnecting vascular plexus in the zona reticularis, and then drainage occurs into the medullary sinusoids.

AORTOGRAPHY

Because of the multiple branches to the adrenal glands and their segmental distribution, "scout" aortography is performed first. This also permits identification of extra-adrenal tumors in cases of suspected pheochromocytoma.

Performance of the Valsalva maneuver during aortography may enhance visualization of the adrenal glands.[83, 84] Accurate interpretation may be precluded by superimposition of visualized arteries, the dense renal opacification during the nephrographic phase, and the contrast opacification of the stomach, pancreas, small bowel, splenic vein, and inferior vena cava. Lindvall clearly demonstrated both glands in only 33 per cent of cases.[83] He points out that the arrow-shaped right gland described by Ahlback is a sign that only the upper part of the gland has been filled.[64] An indication that the whole organ is seen is visualization of the cortex of the lower portion. On the left side, it is considerably more difficult to decide whether the whole gland has been filled, owing to its more varied position and appearance.

A hypervascular adrenal mass may be readily revealed by aortography, often with a characteristic contour identifiable in the "capillary" phase. Avascular or cystic tumors may displace nearby vessels. A large mass may displace the aorta,[90] or the renal, lumbar, left gastric, splenic, or hepatic arteries. Characteristic of large adrenal masses on the left is downward displacement of the renal artery and elevation of the splenic artery (Figs. 16–37, 16–38). Irregularity of extrinsic vessels may indicate invasion by a malignant adrenal tumor.

In cases of pheochromocytoma, Meany and Buonocore have shown the value of "provocative arteriography" in identifying the presence of the lesion.[85] With injection of contrast medium into the aorta or renal artery, there is a significant rise in blood pressure (50/20 to 80/40 mm. Hg.) in patients with pheochromocytoma. Phentolamine is available for immediate intravenous injection through an intravenous infusion maintained throughout the procedure.

When a pheochromocytoma is strongly suspected clinically and the abdominal aortogram has shown no abnormalities in the region of the adrenals, it is advisable to perform a thoracic aortogram as well as a pelvic arteriogram to detect extra-adrenal location of the tumor.

If, on aortography, there is a suggestion of increased vascularity in the region of the adrenal gland, hypertrophy of an adrenal artery, evidence of tumor stain, or displacement of extrinsic vessels, selective catheterization is then performed. Just as a lesion may appear avascular on aortography and demonstrate irregular tumor vessels on a selective injection, so may a selective arteriogram now show the full extent of a tumor that may be more readily revealed by aortography (Fig. 16–39).

"Combined adrenography," the simultaneous performance of presacral gas studies with aortography, has been cited by some but is arduous and unduly uncomfortable for the patient and should be generally discouraged.[73, 87]

SELECTIVE CATHETERIZATION

Advances in the ability to catheterize selectively the vessels contributing to vascularization of the adrenal glands have greatly refined their roentgenographic diagnosis. A flexible curved catheter with side holes is usually employed. Selective renal artery injection opacifies the inferior adrenal branches and selective celiac artery injection visualizes the superior adrenal branches when the inferior phrenic artery is a celiac tributary. Winkler and Kahn have shown that adrenal visualization is enhanced in both of these sites by the injection of epinephrine (about 10 μg. in the renal artery and 20 μg. in the celiac) a few seconds before the angiogram is taken.[93] Contrast material is then preferentially directed into the adrenal vessels, which do not constrict. It is apparent that epinephrine should not be used in cases of suspected pheochromocytoma. Selective catheterization of the inferior phrenic arteries and middle adrenal arteries is usually possible.[79] Selective injection of lumbar arteries and the inferior mesenteric artery may outline an extra-adrenal pheochromocytoma.

Because selective injection opacifies only a segment of the adrenal gland, multiple injections are required to obtain a complete picture (Fig. 16–40). The adrenal cortex presents as a dense blush, usually about 2 mm. wide when seen in profile. The medulla is relatively less opaque.[78]

ARTERIOGRAPHIC SIGNS OF ADRENAL TUMORS

Adrenal tumors are characterized by dilated and displaced vessels, disorganized and tortuous vascular patterns of varied caliber, arteriovenous shunts, vascular lakes filled with contrast material, tumor stain, and displacement or infiltration of neighboring organs. They show no vascular specificity indicating medullary or cortical origin of a neoplasm. Vascular patterns vary even in tumors of the same origin, mainly secondary to areas of hemorrhage and necrosis.

INFERIOR VENACAVOGRAPHY

Displacement or distortion of the inferior vena cava may help to localize adrenal masses and may be useful in follow-up evaluation after treatment (Fig. 16–41). Large adrenal masses on the right typically displace the inferior vena cava forward and often to the right (Figs. 16–41 to 16–44). Invasion of its wall or infiltration into its lumen (Figs. 16–45, 16–46) represents a definite sign of malignancy. Complete obstruction is uncommon and may be due to spurious factors.[94, 95, 98] Large masses compress the cava against the spine and, particularly in children, crying or an involuntary Valsalva maneuver causes an appearance of obstruction. Cavography in the right posterior oblique or lateral projection is of particular value.

In cases of pheochromocytoma, caval catheterization with analysis of regional venous blood samples for epinephrine and norepinephrine is useful in localizing the tumor.[96] The technique is especially helpful in localizing extra-adrenal tumors in the chest and below the renal veins.

ADRENAL VENOGRAPHY

Masoni described in 1957 the feasibility of adrenal vein catheterization.[114]

ANATOMY OF ADRENAL VEINS

The right adrenal vein (Fig. 16–47) is short and drains directly into the posterolateral side of the inferior vena cava near the level of T-12 a few centimeters above the right renal vein.[105, 110] Hepatic veins normally empty into the posterior aspect of the inferior vena cava close to the adrenal vein. Rarely, the central adrenal vein joins an accessory hepatic vein before entering the vena cava.[110] The glandular tributaries of the adrenal vein present a broomlike or stellate configuration. They have collateral connections with the inferior phrenic, renal capsular, and other retroperitoneal veins.[117, 120]

The left adrenal vein (Fig. 16–48) is larger and drains into the left renal vein on its superior surface near the point at which the renal vein crosses the lateral border of the vertebral body. Before this junction, the central vein usually receives the inferior phrenic vein, which courses just medial to the adrenal gland. No valves are present in the adrenal veins, but a valve in the distal inferior phrenic vein usually prevents retrograde opacification from the adrenal vein. The glandular tributaries present the configuration of veins of an elm leaf.[124] A renal capsular vein also often joins the adrenal vein, and other connections may occur to ascending lumbar, splenic, spermatic or ovarian, and hemizygous veins.

TECHNIQUE

The adrenal veins are individually and selectively catheterized, most often by a percutaneous femoral vein approach. A percutaneous jugular vein puncture has also been recommended particularly for catheterization of the left adrenal vein.[113] For the right side, a flexible double-curved catheter is usually employed.[105, 111, 118] For the left, a coaxial catheter system or preformed catheters are used.[111, 115, 121, 122, 124] Here, the catheter is advanced beyond the inferior phrenic vein junction to avoid dilution of adrenal vein blood.

Adrenal vein blood samples for hormone assay (mainly cortisol, aldosterone, epinephrine, and norepinephrine, as indicated) are withdrawn prior to filming. Cortisol levels are helpful in confirming the accuracy of the adrenal vein sampling site. Samples are also taken from the vena cava below the level of the renal veins. Adrenal vein sampling may permit localization of tumors that are too small to see by any radiographic method.[115]

Injection of 0.5 to 5 cc. of contrast medium, depending upon location of the catheter tip and possible occlusion of the vein by the catheter tip, is gently made to avoid rupture of the gland. The patient is warned to expect some flank discomfort with the injection.

Successful catheterization of the right adrenal vein is more difficult, because of its small size, short course, and proximity to draining hepatic veins. Selective catheterization on the right has beeen generally achieved in 60 to 85 per cent of cases.[104, 124] Mitty and associates, however, have had a success rate of 94 per cent in a large series of patients.[122] On the left, success is achieved in 96 per cent to 98 per cent.[104, 124]

COMPLICATIONS

Adrenal rupture is a specific complication of retrograde injection into the adrenal veins,[125] usually occurring from overdistention beyond a catheter-blocked vessel. In experienced hands, its incidence after successful bilateral adrenal venography is approximately 5 to 10 per cent.[100, 101, 104, 111, 123] Extravasation, usually at the periphery of the gland (Fig. 16–49), is accompanied by severe flank pain. Adrenal function is usually not impaired. However, adrenal insufficiency and remission of primary aldosteronism and of Cushing's syndrome secondary to tumor damage have recently been reported after venography.[104, 106, 107, 108] Intra-adrenal hematomas may also cause difficulty in locating small tumors during subsequent adrenal exploration.[101]

NORMAL FINDINGS

On the right side, the short adrenal vein is seen on end and the branches appear to radiate at the catheter tip. Inadvertent injection into a hepatic vein may be made (Fig. 16–51). On the left, the central adrenal vein is well visualized descending medial to the upper pole of the kidney (Fig. 16–50A). When the injection is made near the junction of the left adrenal vein with the renal vein, the left inferior phrenic vein below its lowest valve is regularly seen. On both sides, several extra-adrenal veins may be opacified (Fig. 16–50). A number of slightly sinuous tributary veins and perhaps a sinusoidal blush lasting only a few seconds are seen. A planimetric area outlined by the major veins of 17 cm.² has been suggested as normal.[124] No distinct filling defects are present.

VENOGRAPHIC SIGNS OF ADRENAL LESIONS

The major finding in tumor is displacement of intra-adrenal veins, often discretely circumscribing a mass (Fig. 16–52). Bilateral hyperplasia may be shown by diffuse spreading of the veins within enlarged glands.

ISOTOPIC VISUALIZATION

The adrenal glands have been visualized using intravenous doses of ^{131}I-19-iodocholesterol and a rectilinear photoscanner of an Anger gamma camera.[128-130] Radioiodinated cholesterol uptake by the adrenal cortex reflects the functioning level of the gland in a manner similar to the uptake of ^{131}I by the thyroid gland. The hyperfunctioning adrenal cortex can thereby be differentiated from the normal.[130]

In Cushing's disease, it appears to be a reliable method of differentiating bilateral hyperplasia from unilateral adrenocortical adenoma.[130] The functioning tumor is seen as a large area of increased radioactivity concentration (Fig. 16–53) with no indication of concentration by the other adrenal gland compatible with functional suppression of that gland.

The adrenal medulla is not visualized by this method, and large tumors of medullary origin may be reflected by no concentration on the involved side. Nonvisualization of one adrenal gland indicates a process of either infiltration or compression of the adrenal cortex or suppression of function.

Preliminary studies also suggest that the primary aldosterone adenoma may be identified by gamma-camera imaging and a differential determination of percentage uptake.[127] Here, the adenoma merely adds counts to the normal adrenal counts.

A new adrenal imaging agent, ^{131}I-6 β-iodomethyl-norcholesterol (NP-59), has been reported to yield enhanced uptake, thereby providing the ability to obtain earlier images. It appears to be particularly useful in evaluating primary aldosteronism and selected cases of Cushing's syndrome.[130a, 130b]

ULTRASONOGRAPHY AND COMPUTED TOMOGRAPHY

In the last few years, clinical application of the noninvasive modalities of ultrasonography and computed tomography (CT) has revolutionized radiologic diagnosis of adrenal lesions. Sample has perfected a precisely designed sonographic approach that can image normal adrenal glands in 85 per cent of cases.[135, 136] This accuracy may be heightened with the use of the decubitus position and an oblique scanning plane for aligning the adrenal gland between kidney and aorta or inferior vena cava. Montagne and co-workers and Reynes and colleagues have visualized the normal adrenal glands by computed tomography in 85 to 97 per cent of cases (Fig. 16–54).[133, 134] The location, size, and shape of the glands on serial CT sections have been meticulously detailed.[130-134]

Most adrenal neoplasms appear as smooth or lobulated solid masses replacing the normal triangular or crescent outline and produce characteristic displacement effects upon neighboring structures. Larger lesions often show central sonolucencies or low densities due to cystic areas of hemorrhage or necrosis.

Computed tomography has become the method of choice for adrenal visualization. A separate section on this topic is included at the end of Chapter 17.

COMMON ADRENAL PSEUDOTUMORS

There are many conditions in the abdomen, both normal and abnormal, which may be radiologically misinterpreted as an adrenal mass.[137-144] Most common among these are the following:

1. A fluid-filled gastric fundus on the left side, particularly in a cascade-type stomach (Fig. 16–55). Erect or prone films and, if necessary, ingestion of carbonated beverages or effervescent powders readily show the true condition.
2. A fluid-filled gastric antrum (Fig. 16–56), duodenal bulb (Fig. 16–57), or descending duodenum on the right side. Similar positional changes may demonstrate the transient nature of such a "mass."

Other densities that may be occasionally mistaken for an adrenal tumor include redundancies of the splenic artery, anomalous projections from the lobes of the liver, lobulations or enlargement of the spleen, accessory spleens (Fig. 16–58), and the tail of the pancreas (Fig. 16–59).

CHAPTER 16 ILLUSTRATIONS

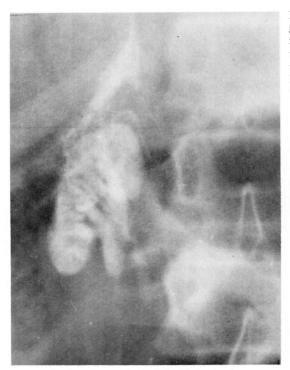

FIG. 16–1. Normal adrenal gland associated with congenital renal hypoplasia. Capillary phase of selective renal arteriogram shows a normal-sized adrenal despite the kidney maturing in size no longer than the height of the adjacent vertebral body. (Meyers, M.A., Friedenberg, R., King, M. et al.: Significance of the renal capsular arteries. Br. J. Radiol., *40*:949, 1967)

FIG. 16–2. Late phase of aortogram demonstrates a normal adrenal gland on the right (*arrows*) in association with congenital renal hypoplasia. Compensatory hypertrophy involves the left kidney.

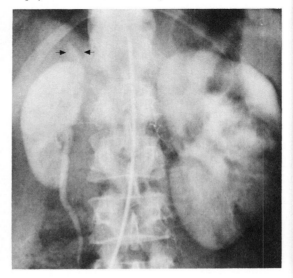

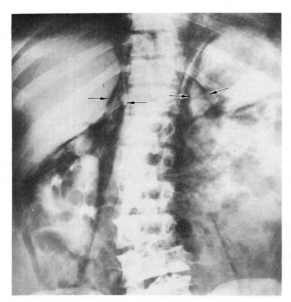

FIG. 16–3. Normal adrenal glands (*arrows*) outlined on retroperitoneal pneumography in presence of crossed fused renal ectopia.

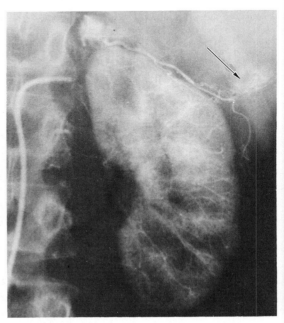

FIG. 16–4. Late phase of selective renal arteriogram. Accessory adrenal tissue (*arrow*) in perirenal fat lateral to the kidney, supplied by the capsular artery. Note the presence of a normal adrenal gland.

FIG. 16–5. Plain film visualization of left pheochromocytoma in a 69-year-old man. Mass (*arrows*) is clearly seen through superimposed gas-distended stomach.

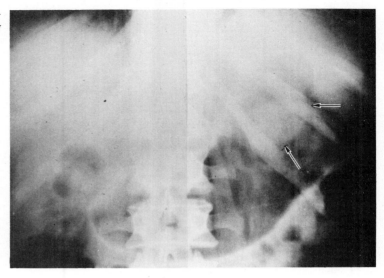

FIG. 16–6. IVP. Large left adrenal pseudocyst is clearly outlined as a round mass depressing the kidney.

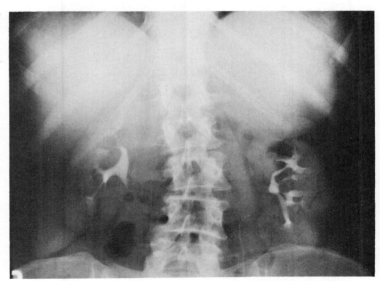

FIG. 16–7. IVP. Metastatic melanoma to the right adrenal gland. The kidney is displaced inferiorly and the upper pole laterally, resulting in the "water-lily" appearance of the renal collecting system. Note that the hepatic flexure of the colon is also depressed.

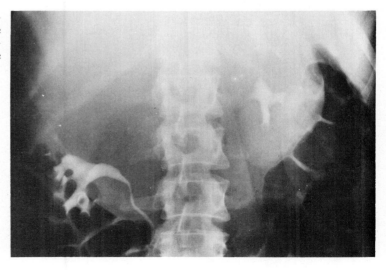

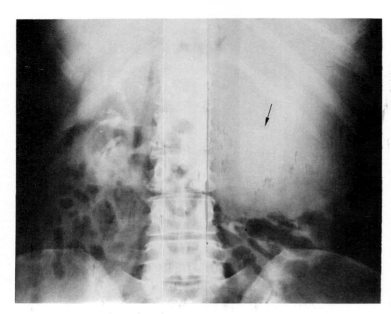

FIG. 16–8. IVP. Large left cystic pheochromocytoma, containing a nidus of calcification (*arrow*), depresses the kidney and compresses it against the spine.

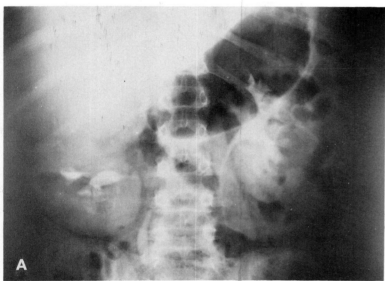

FIG. 16–9. IVP. **(A)** Right adrenal carcinoma in a child causes the characteristic "water-lily" depression of the kidney. **(B)** Lateral projection documents anterior displacement of the upper renal pole.

FIG. 16–10. IVP. Erect projection permits the kidney to fall, clearly outlining a large adrenal mass containing flecks of calcifications. This represents an adrenal carcinoma in a 17-year-old girl with Cushing's syndrome. (Meyers, M.A.: Diseases of the Adrenal Glands: Radiologic Diagnosis. Springfield, Charles C Thomas, 1963)

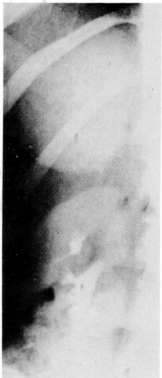

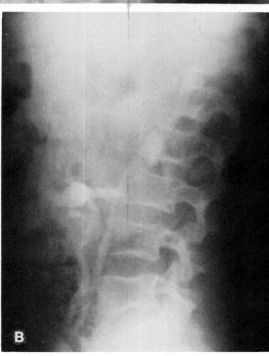

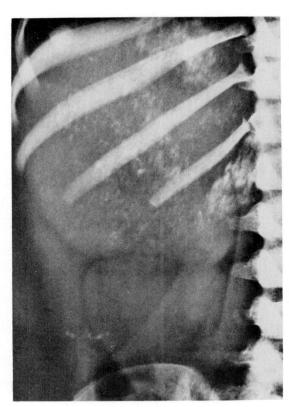

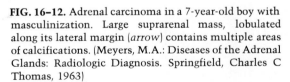

FIG. 16–11. Neuroblastoma. Plain film shows multiple, dense speckled calcifications within a large adrenal mass depressing the kidney. (Meyers, M.A.: Diseases of the Adrenal Glands: Radiologic Diagnosis. Springfield, Charles C Thomas, 1963)

FIG. 16–12. Adrenal carcinoma in a 7-year-old boy with masculinization. Large suprarenal mass, lobulated along its lateral margin (*arrow*) contains multiple areas of calcifications. (Meyers, M.A.: Diseases of the Adrenal Glands: Radiologic Diagnosis. Springfield, Charles C Thomas, 1963)

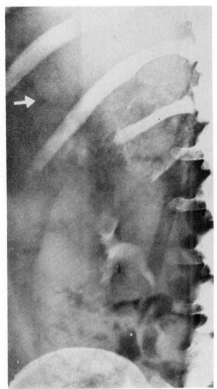

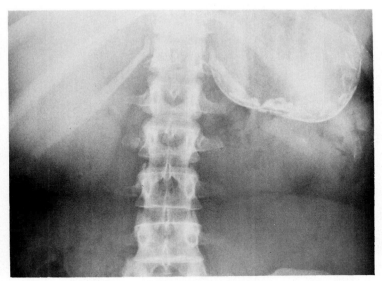

FIG. 16–13. Adrenal hemorrhagic pseudocyst in an adult with a past history of abdominal trauma. Plain film shows dense curvilinear calcifications circumscribing a left upper quadrant mass.

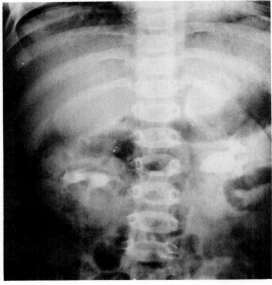

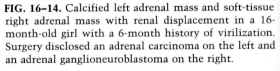

FIG. 16–14. Calcified left adrenal mass and soft-tissue right adrenal mass with renal displacement in a 16-month-old girl with a 6-month history of virilization. Surgery disclosed an adrenal carcinoma on the left and an adrenal ganglioneuroblastoma on the right.

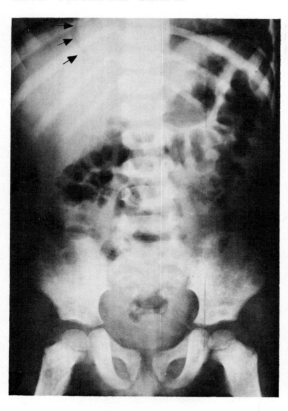

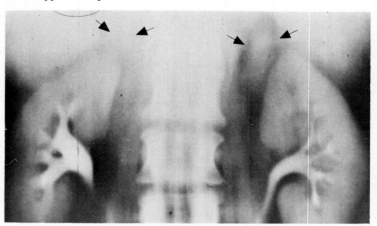

FIG. 16–15. Neuroblastoma. Plain film demonstrates intrathoracic paraspinal extension (*arrows*) of abdominal neuroblastoma. Bony metastases are also evident in the pelvis and femurs.

FIG. 16–16. Nephrotomogram. Normal adrenal glands (*arrows*) can be identified in size, shape, and position. Note that the right is completely suprarenal in position, but the left extends downward along the medial aspect of the upper renal pole.

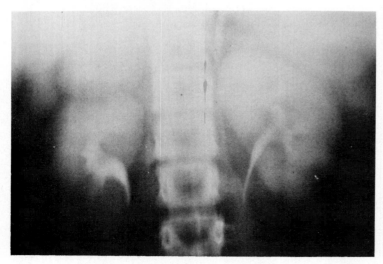

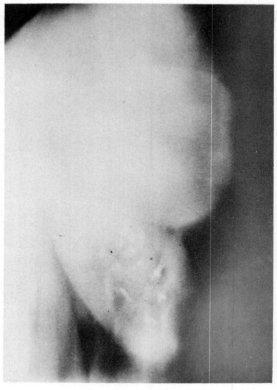

FIG. 16–17. Nephrotomogram demonstrates a vascular tumor of the right adrenal gland in a female patient with mixed symptoms of Cushing's disease and the adrenogenital syndrome. At surgery, this was found to be a cortical adenoma.

FIG. 16-18. Nephrotomography in LPO-projection outlines an unusually large left adrenal adenoma.

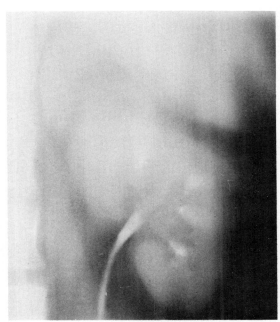

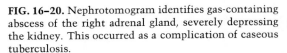

FIG. 16–19. Nephrotomography outlines a left adrenal gland enlarged from metastatic melanoma.

FIG. 16–20. Nephrotomogram identifies gas-containing abscess of the right adrenal gland, severely depressing the kidney. This occurred as a complication of caseous tuberculosis.

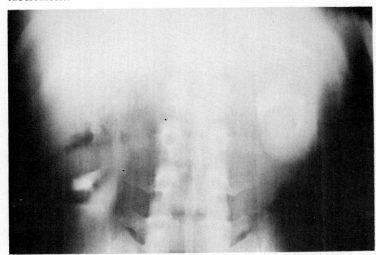

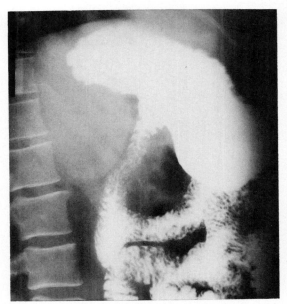

FIG. 16–21. Upper GI series, lateral view. The proximal portion of the descending duodenum is displaced forward by a large right adrenal mass.

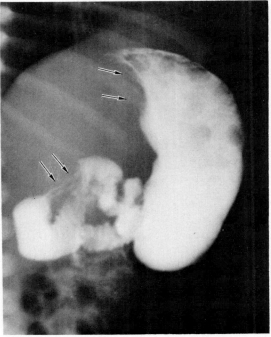

FIG. 16–22. Upper GI series, lateral view. Bilateral neonatal adrenal hemorrhage. The right adrenal mass stretches and displaces the proximal descending duodenum (*upper arrows*), and the left adrenal mass displaces the stomach anteriorly and indents the posterior gastric wall (*lower arrows*). (Rose, J., Berdon, W.E., Sullivan, T., et al.: Radiology, *98*:263–272, 1971)

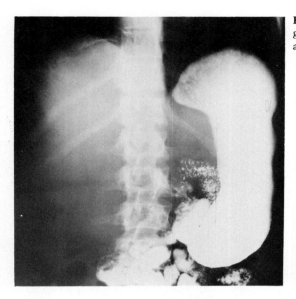

FIG. 16–23. Massive enlargement of the right adrenal gland by metastatic melanoma displaces the stomach and duodenum to the left.

FIG. 16–24. Barium enema, lateral view. A right adrenal carcinoma results in anterior displacement of the hepatic flexure of the colon (*arrows*).

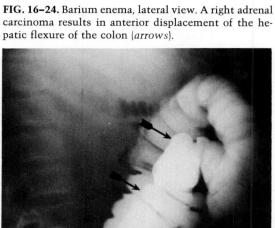

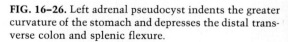

FIG. 16–25. Upper GI series, lateral view. A left adrenal adenoma in a 2-year-old with adrenogenital syndrome causes a mass impression upon the posterior wall of the stomach (*arrow*).

FIG. 16–26. Left adrenal pseudocyst indents the greater curvature of the stomach and depresses the distal transverse colon and splenic flexure.

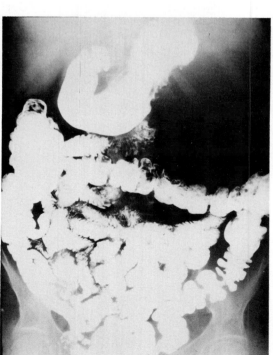

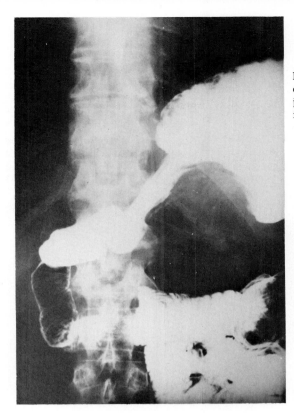

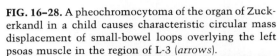

FIG. 16–27. Left adrenal carcinoma elevates the greater curvature of the stomach and depresses proximal jejunal loops. The presence of this nonfunctioning lesion in an elderly man was first revealed by this GI series.

FIG. 16–28. A pheochromocytoma of the organ of Zuckerkandl in a child causes characteristic circular mass displacement of small-bowel loops overlying the left psoas muscle in the region of L-3 (*arrows*).

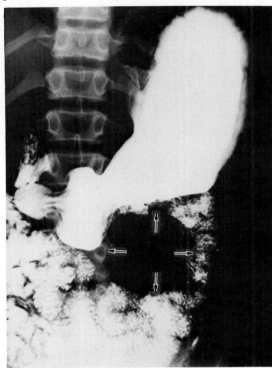

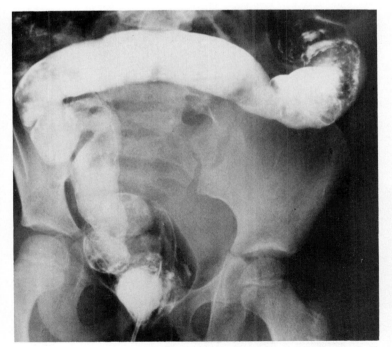

FIG. 16–29. A pelvic ganglioneuroma in a 4-and-a-half-year-old girl elevates the sigmoid colon.

FIG. 16–30. Retroperitoneal pneumography. Pheochromocytoma. Erect film allows the kidney (**K**) to fall, clearly identifying an adrenal mass (**A**). (Meyers, M.A.: Diseases of the Adrenal Glands: Radiologic Diagnosis. Springfield, Charles C Thomas, 1963)

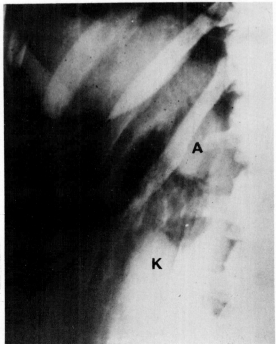

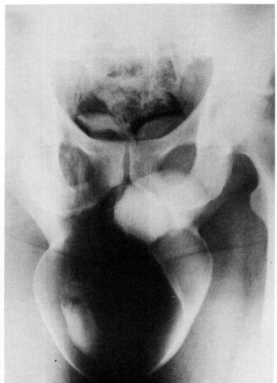

FIG. 16-31. A complication of retroperitoneal pneumography is scrotal emphysema.

FIG. 16-32. Different examples (A–D) of demonstration of normal adrenal glands on presacral retroperitoneal pneumography. (Meyers, M.A.: Diseases of the Adrenal Glands: Radiologic Diagnosis. Springfield, Charles C Thomas, 1963)

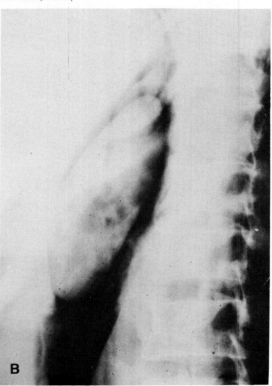

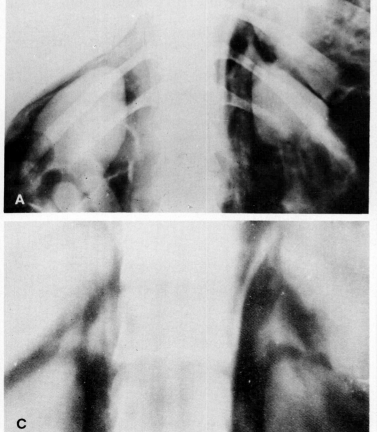

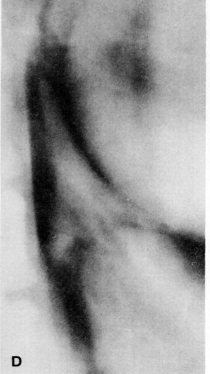

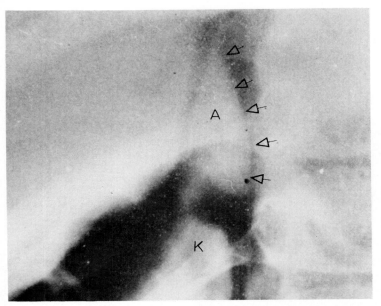

FIG. 16–33. Retroperitoneal pneumogram. Right adrenal adenoma (**A**) demonstrating the earliest changes of neoplasm. Note convex medial margin (*arrows*), **K** = kidney. (Meyers, M.A.: Diseases of the Adrenal Glands: Radiologic Diagnosis. Springfield, Charles C Thomas, 1963)

FIG. 16–35. Right pheochromocytoma. (**A**) IVP shows depression of the kidney by a suprarenal mass. (**B**) Retroperitoneal pneumogram clearly outlines the mass lying within Gerota's fascia (*arrows*). Identification of this structure places all images within it to be of either renal or adrenal origin. (Meyers, M.A.: Diseases of the Adrenal Glands: Radiologic Diagnosis. Springfield, Charles C Thomas, 1963)

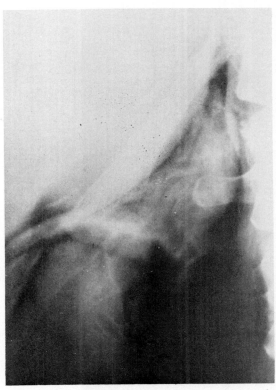

FIG. 16–34. Retroperitoneal pneumogram. Right pheochromocytoma showing the earliest changes of adrenal neoplasm. The gland is enlarged and the medial margin is convex. (Meyers, M.A.: Diseases of the Adrenal Glands: Radiologic Diagnosis. Springfield, Charles C Thomas, 1963)

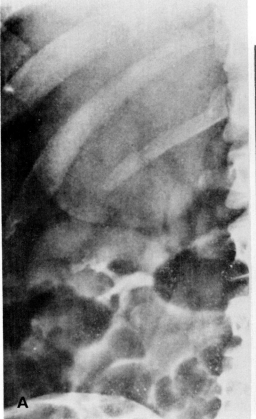

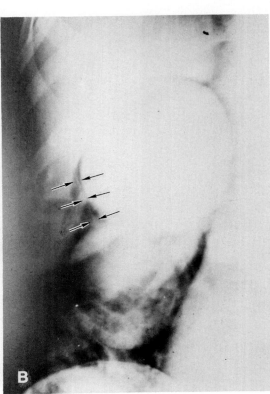

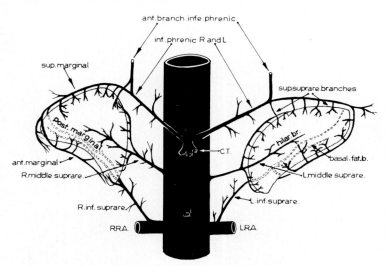

FIG. 16–36. The blood supply to the adrenal glands. (Merklin, R.J., and Michels, M.A. J. Int. Coll. Surg., *29*:41, 1958)

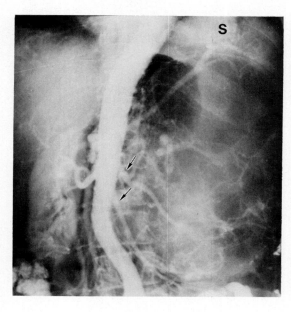

FIG. 16–37. Aortogram. Large cystic pheochromocytoma depresses the renal artery (*lower arrow*) and elevates the splenic artery and spleen (**S**). The tumor is supplied by a hypertrophied middle adrenal artery (*upper arrow*). The aorta is displaced to the right.

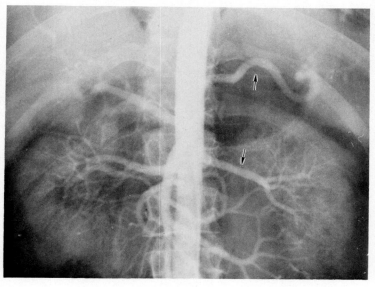

FIG. 16–38. Aortogram. Left adrenal enlargement from metastatic melanoma results in depression of the kidney and renal artery (*lower arrow*) and elevation of the splenic artery (*upper arrow*).

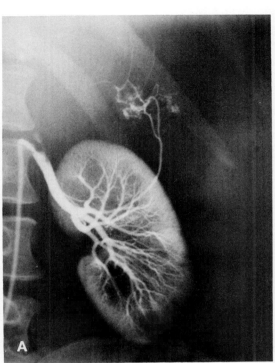

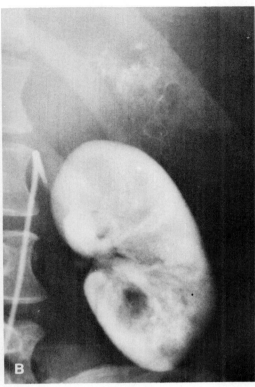

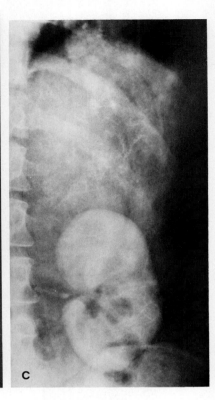

FIG. 16–39. Nonfunctioning adrenal carcinoma in a 55-year-old woman. (**A and B**) Selective renal arteriogram demonstrates a localized focus of tumor hypervascularity with staining within the suprarenal tissues, supplied by a communication of a perforating renal capsular artery. (**C**) Aortography, late phase, demonstrates the full extent of the tumor and its hypervascularity.

FIG. 16–40. Adrenal carcinoma. (**A**) Selective renal artery injection (via percutaneous brachial artery catheterization) shows limited number of tumor vessels from inferior adrenal artery (*arrow*). (**B**) Inferior phrenic artery injection reveals rich neoplastic hypervascularity with areas of tumor staining.

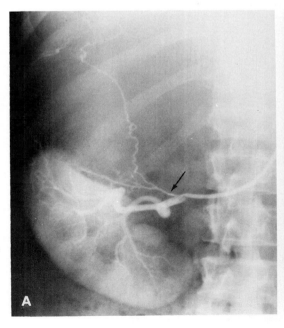

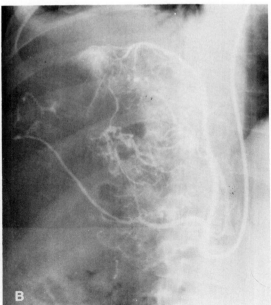

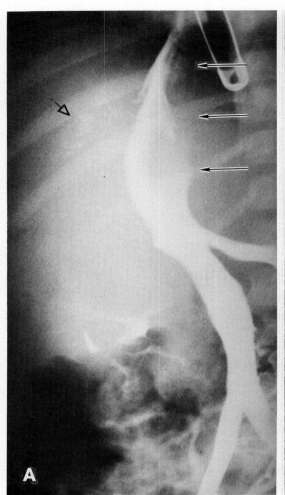
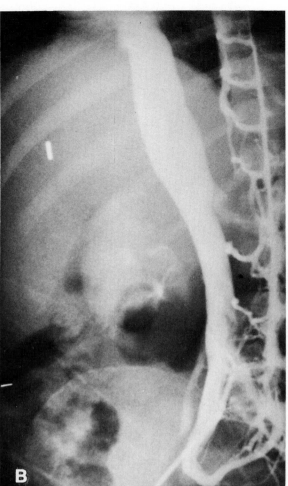

FIG. 16–41. Extensive neuroblastoma containing calcifications (*open arrow*). **(A)** Inferior venacavogram demonstrates retrocaval extension of tumor, displacing the inferior vena cava anteriorly (*black arrows*). The kidney is depressed by the mass. **(B)** Follow-up study 2 months after treatment shows return to normal.

FIG. 16–42. Right adrenal pseudocyst. Inferior venacavogram shows mass pressure on lateral wall of the inferior vena cava.

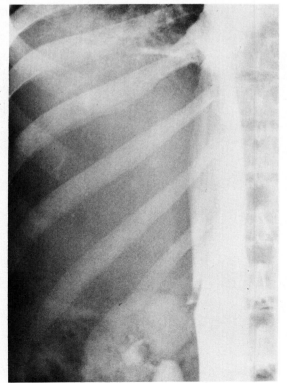

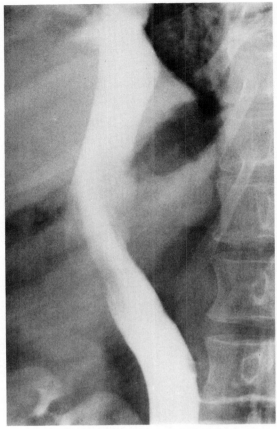

FIG. 16-43. Inferior venacavogram. Nonfunctioning carcinoma of the right adrenal gland displaces the inferior vena cava anteriorly and toward the right.

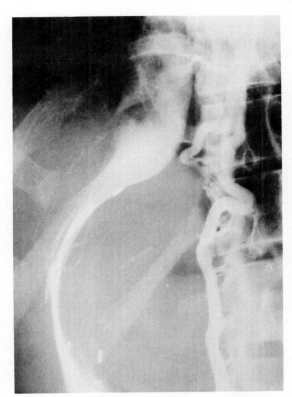

FIG. 16-44. Inferior venacavogram. A postoperative recurrence of a pheochromocytoma of the right adrenal gland is reflected by gross mass displacement of the inferior vena cava to the right, with marked compression of its lumen.

FIG. 16-45. Inferior venacavogram. A nonfunctioning carcinoma of the right adrenal gland has grossly infiltrated into the lumen of the cava (arrows).

FIG. 16-46. Inferior venacavogram. Metastatic breast carcinoma to the right adrenal gland has grown into the lumen of the cava at the site of the adrenal vein (arrow) above the filling defect produced by renal vein blood.

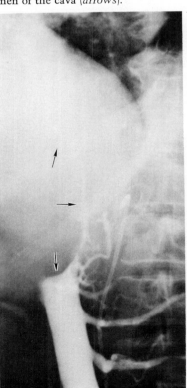

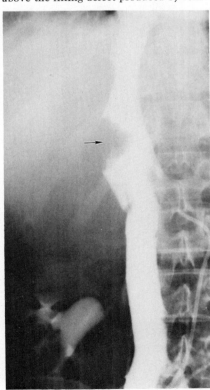

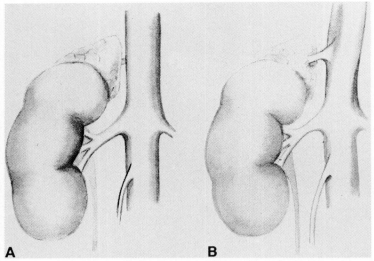

FIG. 16–47. Anatomic relationships of right adrenal vein (**A, B**). The central vein enters the posterior aspect of the inferior vena cava laterally. (O'Neil, L.: Surgery of the Adrenal Glands. St. Louis, C.V. Mosby Co., 1968)

FIG. 16–48. Anatomic relationships of left adrenal vein. It usually is joined by the inferior phrenic vein before its confluence with the renal vein (**A**), but each may enter separately (**B**). (O'Neal, L.: Surgery of the Adrenal Glands, St. Louis, C.V. Mosby Co., 1968)

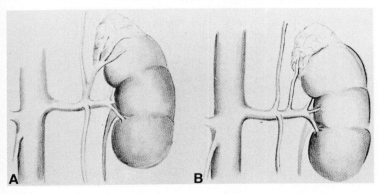

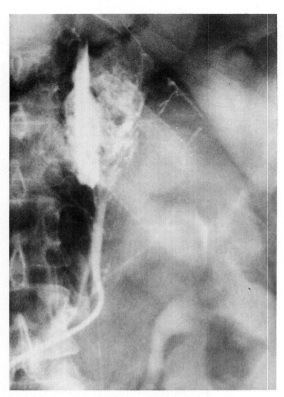

FIG. 16–49. Parenchymal extravasation from venous rupture during attempted left adrenal venography is shown by dense accumulation.

FIG. 16–50. Examples of normal left adrenal venograms (**A–E**). Adrenal tributary veins (*open arrows*) drain into the central vein. Connections to extra-adrenal veins are demonstrated (*black arrows*).

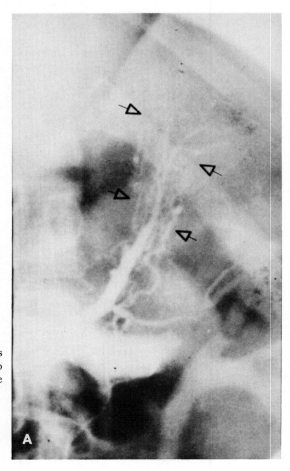

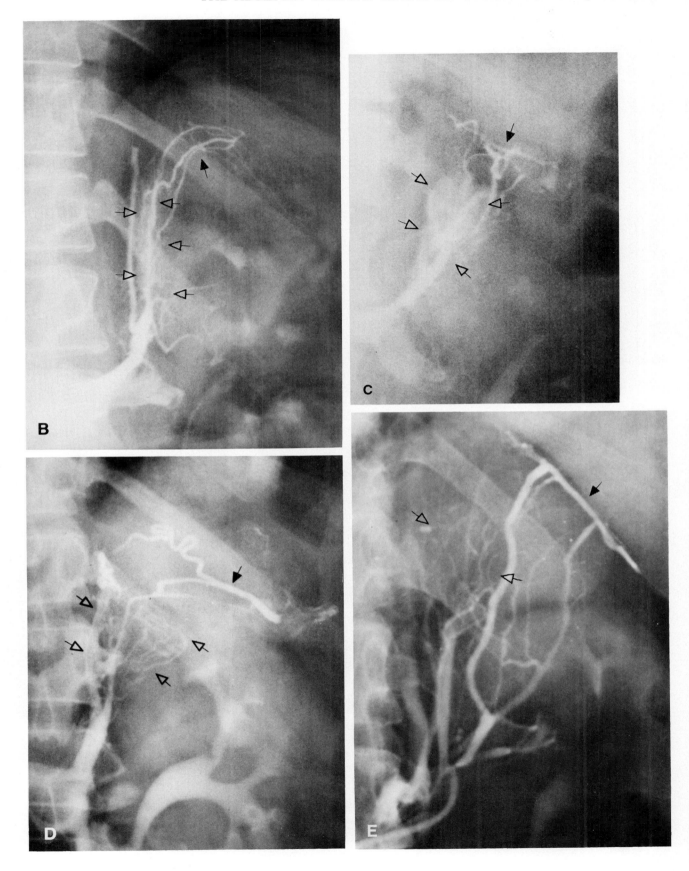

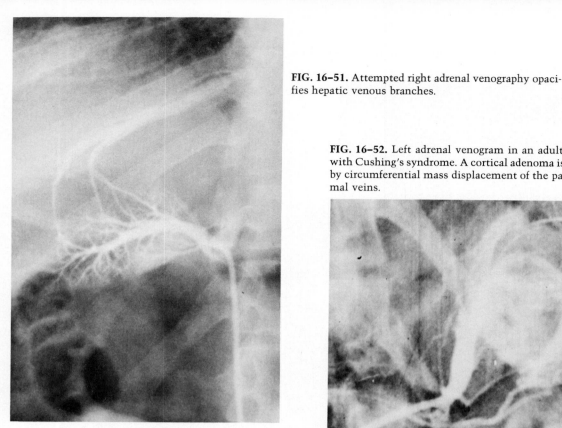

FIG. 16–51. Attempted right adrenal venography opacifies hepatic venous branches.

FIG. 16–52. Left adrenal venogram in an adult female with Cushing's syndrome. A cortical adenoma is shown by circumferential mass displacement of the parenchymal veins.

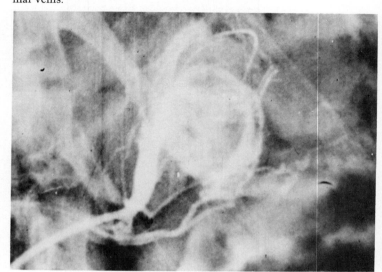

FIG. 16–53. Rectilinear posteroanterior photoscans 3 and 9 days after isotopic dose of ^{131}I-19-iodocholesterol in an 18-year-old woman with Cushing's syndrome demonstrate a 3.5-cm. adenoma of the right adrenal gland and functional suppression on the left. (Lieberman, L.M., Beierwaltes, W.H., Conn, J.W., et al.: N. Engl. J. Med., *285*:1387, 1971)

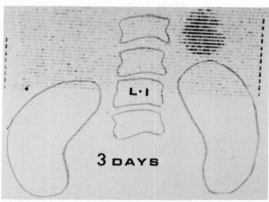

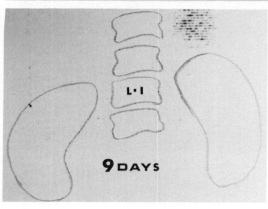

FIG. 16–54. Normal adrenal glands (*arrows*) shown bilaterally by computed tomography, documenting their normal outline, shape, and position anterior to the kidneys (**K**). On the right, the gland lies just behind the inferior vena cava (**C**). (Courtesy of Carlos Reynes, M.D., Loyola University School of Medicine, Maywood, Illinois)

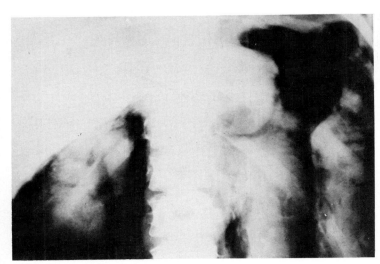

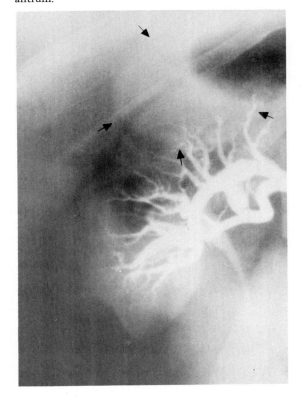

FIG. 16-55. Retroperitoneal pneumogram. Left adrenal pseudotumor produced by a fluid-filled gastric fundus. (Meyers, M.A.: Diseases of the Adrenal Glands: Radiologic Diagnosis. Springfield, Charles C Thomas, 1963)

FIG. 16-56. Selective renal arteriogram. Right adrenal pseudotumor (*arrows*) results from a fluid-filled gastric antrum.

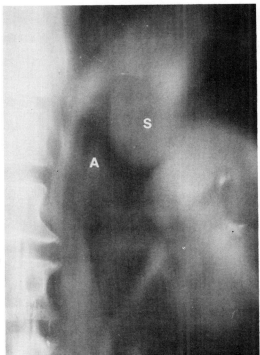

FIG. 16-57. Nephrotomogram. Right adrenal pseudotumor (*arrows*) is produced by fluid-filled gastric antrum or duodenal bulb.

FIG. 16-58. Nephrotomogram. Suprarenal mass (**S**), representing an accessory spleen, displaces the left kidney. The normal adrenal gland (**A**) can be identified. (Courtesy of Andrew Crummy, Jr., M.D., Univ. of Wisconsin Medical Center, Madison, Wisconsin)

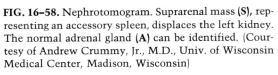

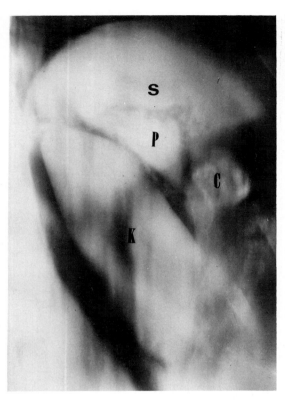

FIG. 16–59. Retroperitoneal pneumogram. The tail of the pancreas (**P**) is seen as a triangular density in the region of the hilus of the spleen (**S**), lateral to the left kidney (**K**), and above the colon (**C**). It should not be mistaken for an adrenal mass. (Meyers, M.A.: Dynamic Radiology of the Abdomen: Normal and Pathologic Anatomy. New York, Springer-Verlag, 1976)

BIBLIOGRAPHY

General References

1. Cope, C.L.: Adrenal Steroids and Disease. Philadelphia, J.B. Lippincott, 1972.
2. Coupland, R.E.: The Natural History of the Chromaffin Cell. Longmans, London, 1965.
3. Christy, N.P.: The Human Adrenal Cortex. Harper & Row, New York, 1971.
4. McAfee, J.G., and Balli, C.E.: Radiological diagnosis of diseases of adrenal origin. Am. J. Med. Sci., 232:572–599, 1956.
5. O'Neal, L.: Surgery of the Adrenal Glands. C.V. Mosby, St. Louis, 1968.
6. Symington, T.: Functional Pathology of the Human Adrenal Gland. Williams & Wilkins, Baltimore, 1969.

Adrenal Anomalies

7. Ashley, D.J., and Mostofi, F.K.: Renal agenesis and dysgenesis. J. Urol., 83:211–230, 1960.
8. Culp, O.S.: Adrenal heterotopia. A survey of the literature and report of a case. J. Urol., 41:303–309, 1959.
9. Graham, L.S.: Celiac accessory adrenal glands. Cancer, 6:149–152, 1953.
10. Meyers, M.A., Friedenberg, R., King, M., et al.: Significance of the renal capsular arteries. Br. J. Radiol., 40:949–956, 1967.
11. O'Crowley, C.R., and Martland, H.S.: Adrenal heterotopia, rests, and the so-called Grawitz tumor. J. Urol., 50:758–768, 1943.
12. Quinan, C., and Berger, A.A.: Observations on human adrenals with especial reference to the relative weight of the normal medulla. Ann. Intern. Med., 6:1180–1192, 1933.
13. Schechter, D.C.: Aberrant adrenal tissue. Ann. Surg., 167:421–426, 1968.

Intravenous Urography

14. Fishback, H.R., Jr.: Renal dystopia due to intra-abdominal masses. Am. J. Roentgenol., 52:521–528, 1944.
15. Kaplan, J.H., and Greene, L.F.: The urographic findings in cases of tumor of the suprarenal gland. Surg. Clin. North Am., 28:1071–1078, 1948.
16. Kraus, S.: Visualization of adrenal gland. J.A.M.A., 143:132, 1950.
17. Martin, J.F.: Suprarenal calcification. Radiol. Clin. North Am., 3:129–138, 1965.
18. Meyers, M.A.: Diseases of the Adrenal Glands: Radiologic Diagnosis, With Emphasis on the Use of Presacral Retroperitoneal Pneumography. Charles C Thomas, Springfield, Ill., 1963.
19. Shambaugh, P.: Displacements of left kidney in diagnosis of tumors of left flank and abdomen. Radiology, 26:335–339, 1936.

Laminography

20. Laws, J.W.: Radiology of the suprarenal glands. Br. J. Radiol., 31:352–360, 1958.
21. Wilhelm, S.F.: Laminography in the visualization of the suprarenal glands. J. Urol., 49:785–788, 1943.
22. Wilhelm, S.F.: Roentgenographic delineation of adrenal glands with the aid of laminography. Br. J. Urol., 19:85–89, 1947.

Nephrotomography

23. Hartman, G.W., Witten, D.M., and Weeks, R.E.: The role of nephrotomography in the diagnosis of adrenal tumors. Radiology, 86:1030–1034, 1966.
23a. Pickering, R.S., Hartman, G.W., Weeks, R.E., et al.: Excretory urographic localization of adrenal cortical tumors and pheochromocytomas. Radiology, 114:345–349, 1975.

Barium Studies

24. Brown, S.: Radiological study of stomach and duodenum, with special reference to value of lateral view. Radiology, 17:85–98, 1931.
25. Capurro, F.G., and Blanco, R.P.: Semilogia Clinica-Radiologica de las Tumoraciones Abdominales. A. Monteverde & Cia, Montevideo, Uruguay, 1946.
26. Ganem, E.J., Wallwork, D.W., and West, G.V.: Anterior displacement of the descending duodenum as an aid in the diagnosis of retroperitoneal tumors: A roentgenographic sign of possible significance in some cases of enlargement of the right adrenal gland. N. Engl. J. Med., 254:552–555, 1956.
27. Messenger, H.M., and Monroe, L.: An unusual case of duodenal deformity in Addison's disease. Gastroenterology, 29:313–317, 1955.

Retroperitoneal Pneumography

28. Andersen, P.E.: Pneumoretroperitoneum in suprarenal disease. Acta. Radiol., 43:289–297, 1955.
29. Biel, L., Jr., and Eliasoph, J.: A technique for retrorectal gas insufflation. J. Urol., 72:1255–1259, 1954.
30. Blackwood, J.: Presacral perirenal pneumography. Br. J. Surg., 39:111–119, 1951.
31. Cahill, G.F.: Tumors of the adrenals and the use of air insufflation in their diagnosis. Radiology, 37:533–543, 1941.
32. Cahill, G.F., and Melicow, M.M.: Tumors of the adrenal gland. J. Urol., 64:1–25, 1950.
33. Carelli, H.H.: Sur le pneumopéritoine et sur une methode personnelle pour voir le rein sans pneumopéritoine. Bull. Soc. Med., Paris, 45:1409–1412, 1921.
34. Carelli, H.H., and Sordelli, E.: Un nuevo procedimiento para explorar el rinon. Rev. Assoc. Med. Argent., 34:424–425, 1921.
35. Cocchi, U.: Retropneumoperitoneum und Pneumomediastinuum. Fortschr. Rontgenstrahl. Erg., 79:1–226, 1957.
36. Duff, J., Kenyon, H.R., and Hyman, R.M.: Pyelography in combination with simultaneous retroperitoneal pneumography. J. Urol., 70:963–968, 1953.
37. Fagerberg, S.: Pneumoretroperitoneum: Technique and results. Acta Radiol., 37:519–530, 1952.
38. Gennes, L. de, May, J.P., and Helie, J.: Le Pneumo-Retro-Peritoine. Masson et Cie., Paris, 1952.
39. Giraud, M., Bret, P., Kuentz, M., and Anjou, A.: Bilan de cent examens après pneumorétroperitoine. J. Radiol. Électrol., 35:838–846, 1954.
40. Glassman, I., Shapiro, R., and Robinson, F.: Air embolism during presacral pneumography: A case report. J. Urol., 75:569–571, 1956.
41. Godlowski, Z.Z.: The value of the perirenal insufflation of air as a diagnostic method of estimating gross anatomical enlargement of the suprarenals and kidneys. J. Fac. Radiologists, 5:148–154, 1953.
42. Harrison, R.H., and Doubleday, L.C.: Roentgenological appearance of normal adrenal glands. J. Urol., 76:16–22, 1956.
43. Landes, R.R., and Ranson, C.L.: Presacral retroperitoneal pneumography utilizing carbon dioxide: Further experiences and improved techniques. J. Urol., 82:670–673, 1959.
44. Lerman, F., Harper, J.G.M., Hertzberg, A.D., et al.: Presacral oxygen injection. J. Urol., 70:312–317, 1953.
45. Lurà, A., Forni, G., and Biavati, C.: Le immagini dei surreni attenute con insufflazione retroperitoneale al controllo operatorio. Ann. Radiol. (Diag.), 27:298–351, 1954.
46. May, J.P., Raguin, M., Grall, Y., et al.: Les Affections de la Surrenale (Radio-diagnostic Clinique). Supplement international des Monographies Médicales et Scientifiques, Paris, 1962.
47. McLachlan, M.S.F., and Beales, J.S.M.: Retroperitoneal pneumography in the investigation of adrenal disease. Clin. Radiol., 22:188–197, 1971.
48. McLlelland, R., Landes, R.R., and Ransom, C.L.: Retroperitoneal pneumography: A safe method using carbon dioxide. Radiol. Clin. North Am., 3:113–128, 1965.
49. Meyers, M.A.: Diseases of the Adrenal Glands: Radiologic Diagnosis, with Emphasis on the Use of Presacral Retroperitoneal Pneumography. Charles C Thomas, Springfield, Ill., 1963.
50. Musgrove, J.E., and MacQuigg, R.E.: Successful treatment of gas embolism. J.A.M.A., 150:28, 1952.
51. Palubinskas, A.J., and Hodson, C.J.: Transvertebral retroperitoneal gas insufflation. Radiology, 70:851–854, 1958.
52. Ranson, C.L., Landes, R.R., and McLelland, R.: Air embolism following retroperitoneal pneumography: A nationwide survey. J. Urol., 76:664–670, 1956.
53. Rothfield, S.H., Hamm, F.C., and Harlin, H.C.: Perirenal air insufflation by paracoccygeal method. J. Urol., 69:721–725, 1953.
54. Ruiz Rivas, M.: Neuva técnica de diagnóstico radiográfico aplicable a órganos y estructuras retroperitoneales, mediastinicas y cervicoles. Rev. Clin. Espan., 25:206–207, 1947.
55. Ruiz Rivas, M.R.: Generalized subserous emphysema through a single puncture. Am. J. Roentgenol., 64:723–734, 1950.
56. Russ, F. II., Glenn, D.L., and Gianturco, C.: Gas embolism during extraperitoneal insufflation. Recovery in the left decubitus position. Radiology, 61:637–638, 1953.
57. Schnur, B.M., and Sakson, J.A.: Trans-sacral retroperitoneal pneumography. J. Urol., 94:701–705, 1966.
58. Smith, D.R., Steinbach, H.L., Lyon, R.R., et al.: Extraperitoneal pneumography. J. Urol., 68:953–959, 1952.
59. Steinbach, H.L., Hinman, F., Jr., and Forsham, P.H.: The diagnosis of adrenal neoplasms by contrast media. Radiology, 69:664–671, 1957.
60. Steinbach, H.L., Lyon, R.P., Smith, D.R., et al.: Extraperitoneal pneumography. Radiology, 59:167–175, 1952.
61. Steinbach, H.L., and Smith, D.L.: Extraperitoneal pneumography in diagnosis of retroperitoneal tumors. A.M.A. Arch. Surg., 70:161–172, 1955.
62. Tähka, H.: On the weight and structure of the adrenal glands

and the factors affecting them, in children of 0–2 years. Acta Pediatr. (Supple.), *40*:1–95, 1951.

63. Vespignani, L.: The roentgen reticular appearance of the perirenal fat tissue in extraperitoneal pneumoabdomen (retroperitoneum) and tomography. Acta Radiol., *36*:509–515, 1951.

Adrenal Arteriography

64. Ahlbäck, S.: The suprarenal glands in aortography. Acta Radiol., *50*:341–350, 1958.
65. Alfidi, R.J., Gill, W.M., Jr., and Klein, H.J.: Arteriography of adrenal neoplasms. Am. J. Roentgenol., *106*:635–641, 1969.
66. Anson, B.J., Cauldwell, E., Pick, J., et al.: The blood supply of the kidney, suprarenal gland, and associated structures. Surg. Gynecol. Obstet., *84*:313–320, 1947.
67. Colapinto, R.F., and Steed, B.L.: Arteriography of adrenal tumors. Radiology, *100*:343–350, 1971.
68. Donnellan, W.L.: Surgical anatomy of the adrenal glands. Ann. Surg. (Suppl.), *154*:298, 1961.
69. Edsman, G.: Angionephrography and suprarenal angiography: A roentgenographic study of the normal kidney. Expansive renal and suprarenal lesions and renal aneurysms. Acta Radiol. (Suppl.), *155*:1–141, 1957.
70. Gagnon, R.: The arterial supply of the human adrenal gland. Rev. Can. Biol., *16*:421–443, 1957.
71. Gagnon, R.: Middle suprarenal arteries in man: "A statistical study of two hundred human adrenal glands." Rev. Can. Biol., *23*:461–467, 1964.
72. Gérard, G.: Contribution à l'étude morphologique des artères des capsules surrénales de l'homme. J. Anat. (Paris), *49*:269–303, 1913.
73. Goodwin, W.E., Moore, E.V., and Pierce, E.C.: Roentgenographic visualization of adrenal glands: Use of aortography and/or retroperitoneal pneumography to visualize adrenal glands: "combined adrenalography." J. Urol., *74*:231–242, 1955.
74. Greig, H.W., Anson, B.J., and Coleman, S.S.: The inferior phrenic artery: Types of origin in 850 body-halves and diaphragmatic relationship. Q. Bull. Northwest. Med. Sch., *25*:345–350, 1951.
75. Ivemark, B., Ekstrom, T., and Lagergren, C.: The vasculature of the developing and mature human adrenal gland. Acta Paediatr. Scand., *56*:601–606, 1967.
76. Kahn, P.C.: The epinephrine effect in selective renal angiography. Radiology, *85*:301–305, 1965.
77. Kahn, P.C.: Selective angiography of the inferior phrenic arteries. Radiology, *88*:1–8, 1967.
78. Kahn, P.C.: Adrenal Arteriography, Chapt. 58. *In* Abrams, H.L.: Angiography, Second Edition, Vol. II (ed.). Little Brown, Boston, 1971.
79. Kahn, P.C., and Nickrosz, L.V.: Selective angiography of the adrenal glands. Am. J. Roentgenol., *101*:739–749, 1967.
80. Köhler, R., and Holsti, L.R.: Angiographic localization of suprarenal tumours. Acta Radiol., *4*:21–32, 1966.
81. Lagergren, C.: Angiographic changes in the adrenal glands. Am. J. Roentegenol., *101*:732–738, 1967.
82. Lang, E.K., Nourse, M., Mertz, J., et al.: The diagnosis of suprarenal mass lesions by retroperitoneal gas studies and arteriography. Am. J. Roentgenol., *98*:215–221, 1966.
83. Lindvall, N., and Slezak, P.: Arteriography of the adrenals. Radiology, *92*:999–1005, 1969.
84. Ludin, H.: Angiographische Nebennierendar-Stellung. Fortschr. Roentgenstr., *99*:654–666, 1963.

85. Meany, T.F., and Buonocore, E.: Selective arteriography as a localizing and provocative test in the diagnosis of pheochromocytoma. Radiology, *87*:309–314, 1966.
86. Merklin, R.J., and Michels, N.A.: The variant renal and suprarenal blood supply with data on the inferior phrenic, ureteral and gonadal arteries: A statistical analysis based on 185 dissections and review of the literature. J. Int. Coll. Surg., *29*:41–76, 1958.
87. Münster, W., Wierny, L., and Portsmann, W.: Angiographie der nebennieren-tumoren. Fortschr. Geb. Roentgenstr., *104*:367–378, 1966.
88. Portsmann, W., Wierny, L., and Münster, W.: Die selektive nebennierenangiographs. Fortschr. Geb. Roentgenstr., *104*:150–157, 1966.
89. Rossi, P.: Arteriography in adrenal tumours. Br. J. Radiol., *41*:81–98, 1968.
90. Roux-Berger, J.L., Naulleau, J., and Contiadès, X.J.: Corticosurrénalome malin. Aortographie. Exerese. Guerison operatoire. Bull. Soc. Nat. de Chir., *60*:791–802, 1934.
91. Susse, H.J., and Radke, H.: Nachweis und Lokalisierung von Nebennierentumoren mittels Aortographie. Fortschr. Geb. Rontgenstrahlen, *86*:599–604, 1957.
92. Walter, R.C., and Goodwin, W.E.: Aortography and pneumography in children. J. Urol., *77*:323–328, 1957.
93. Winkler, S.S., and Kahn, P.C.: Pharmacologic aids in adrenal angiography. J. Invest. Radiol., *2*:48–52, 1967.

Inferior Venacavography

94. Berdon, W.E., Baker, D.H., and Santulli, T.V.: Factors producing spurious obstruction of the inferior vena cava in infants and children with abdominal tumors. Radiology, *88*:111–116, 1967.
95. Doppman, J., Foley, T., and Hammond, W.: Inferior vena caval compression. The pseudo-obstruction syndrome. Am. J. Roentgenol., *100*:411–416, 1967.
96. Harrison, T.S., Seaton, J.F., Cerny, J.C., et al.: Localization of pheochromocytoma by caval catheterization. Arch. Surg., *95*:339–343, 1967.
97. Lund, R.R., Garcia, N.A., III, LeBlang, G.A., et al.: Inferior vena cavography in preoperative localization of pheochromocytoma. J. Urol., *83*:768–773, 1960.
98. Münster, W., Wierny, L., and Portsmann, W.: Angiographie der Nebennieren-Tumoren. Fortschr. Geb. Rontgenstrahlen, *104*:367–378, 1966.

Adrenal Venography

99. Anson, B.J., Cauldwell, E., Pick, J., et al.: The blood supply of the kidney, suprarenal gland, and associated structures. Surg. Gynecol. Obstet., *84*:313–320, 1947.
100. Bayliss, R.I.S., Edwards, O.M., and Starer, F.: Complications of adrenal venography. Br. J. Radiol., *43*:531–533, 1970.
101. Bookstein, J., Conn, J.W., and Reuter, S.R.: Intra-adrenal hemorrhage as a complication of adrenal venography in primary aldosteronism. Radiology, *90*:778–779, 1968.
102. Bucht, H.: Percutaneous catheterization of the left adrenal vein in man. Scand. J. Clin. Lab. Invest. (Suppl.), *14*:27, 1962.
103. Bucht, H., Bergström, J., Lindholmer, B., et al.: Catheterization of the left adrenal vein for contrast injection and steroid analysis in a case of Conn's syndrome. Acta Med. Scand., *176*:233–241, 1964.
104. Cerny, J.C., Nesbit, R.M., Conn, J.W., et al.: Preoperative tumor localization by adrenal venography in patients with

primary aldosteronism: a comparison with operative findings. J. Urol., *103*:521–528, 1970.

105. Cope, C., Isard, H.J., and Wesolowski, W.E.: Selective adrenal phlebography. Radiology, *90*:1105–1112, 1968.
106. Eagan, R.T., and Page, M.I.: Adrenal insufficiency following bilateral adrenal venography. J.A.M.A., *215*:115–116, 1971.
107. Fellerman, H., Dalakos, T.G., and Streeten, D.H.P.: Remission of Cushing's syndrome after unilateral adrenal phlebography. Ann. Intern. Med., *73*:585–589, 1970.
108. Fisher, C.E., Turner, F.A., and Horton, R.: Remission of primary aldosteronism after adrenal venography. N. Engl. J. Med., *20*:334–336, 1971.
109. Gagnon, R.: The venous drainage of the human adrenal gland. Rev. Can. Biol., *14*:350–357, 1956.
110. Johnstone, F.R.C.: The suprarenal veins. Am. J. Surg., *94*:615–620, 1957.
111. Kahn, P.C.: Adrenal Venography, Chap. 59. *In* Abrams, H.L. (ed.): Angiography, 2nd Ed., Vol. II. Little, Brown, Boston, 1971.
112. Kirschner, M.A., and Jacobs, J.B.: Combined ovarian and adrenal vein catheterization to determine the sites of androgen overproduction in hirsute women. J. Clin. Endocrinol. Metab., *33*:199–209, 1971.
113. Lecky, J.W.: Percutaneous transjugular approach to adrenal venography. Am. J. Roentgenol., *104*:380–385, 1968.
114. Masoni, A.: Catheterization of the right adrenal vein in man. Acta. Med. Scand., *159*:225–233, 1957.
115. Melby, J.C., Spark, R.F., Dale, S.L., et al.: Diagnosis and localization of aldosterone-producing adenomas by adrenal-vein catheterization. N. Engl. J. Med., *277*:1050–1056, 1967.
116. Melby, J.C., Spark, R.F., Dale, S.L., et al.: Diagnosis and localization of aldosterone-producing adenomas by percutaneous bilateral adrenal vein catheterization. Prog. Clin. Cancer, *4*:175–184, 1970.
117. Merklin, R., and Eger, S.A.: The adrenal venous system in man. J. Int. Coll. Surg., *35*:572–585, 1961.
118. Mikaelsson, C.G.: Retrograde phlebography of both adrenal veins: Preliminary report. Acta Radiol., *6*:348–354, 1967.
119. Mikaelsson, C.G.: Epinephro-phlebography in two cases of Conn's syndrome. Acta Radiol., *7*:410–416, 1968.
120. Mikaelsson, C.G.: Venous communications of the adrenal glands. Acta Radiol., *10*:369–393, 1970.
121. Mitty, H.A.: Catheterization of left adrenal vein without mechanical catheter or guide-wire manipulator. Radiology, *102*:445–446, 1971.
122. Mitty, H., Nicolis, G.L., and Gabrilove, J.L.: Adrenal venography: Clinical–roentgenographic correlation in 80 patients. Am. J. Roentgenol., *119*:564–575, 1973.
123. Nicolis, G.L., Mitty, H.A., Modlinger, R.S., et al.: Percutaneous adrenal venography. A Clinical Study of 50 Patients. Ann. Intern. Med., *76*:899–909, 1972.
124. Reuter, S.R., Blair, A.J., Schteingart, D.E., et al.: Adrenal venography. Radiology, *89*:805–814, 1967.
125. Starer, F.: Percutaneous suprarenal venography. Br. J. Radiol., *38*:675–681, 1965.
126. Sutton, D.: Diagnosis of Conn's and other adrenal tumours by left adrenal phlebography. Lancet, *1*:453–455, 1968.

Isotopic Visualization

127. Conn, J.W., Beierwaltes, W.H., Lieberman, L.M., et al.: Primary aldosteronism: Preoperative tumor visualization by scintillation scanning. J. Clin. Endocrinol. Metab., *33*:713–716, 1971.
128. Herwig, K.R., Conn, J.W., Schteingart, D.E., et al.: Localization of adrenal tumors by photoscanning. J. Urol., *109*:2–4, 1973.
129. Lieberman, L.M., Beierwaltes, W.H., Conn, J.W., et al.: Diagnosis of adrenal disease by visualization of human adrenal glands with ^{131}I-19-iodocholesterol. N. Engl. J. Med., *285*:1387–1393, 1971.
130. Morita, R., Lieberman, L.M., Beierwaltes, W.H., et al.: Per cent uptake of ^{131}I radioactivity in the adrenal from radioiodinated cholesterol. J. Clin. Endocrinol. Metab., *34*:36–43, 1972.
130a. Ryo, U.Y., Johnston, A.S., Kim, I., et al.: Adrenal scanning and uptake with ^{131}I-6β-iodomethyl-nor-cholesterol. Radiology, *128*:157–161, 1978.
130b. Miles, J.M., Wahner, H.W., Carpenter, P.C., et al.: Adrenal scintiscanning with NP-59, a new radioiodinated cholesterol agent. Mayo Clin. Proc., *54*:321–327, 1979.

Ultrasound Imaging and Computed Tomography

131. Birnholz, J.D.: Ultrasound imaging of adrenal mass lesions. Radiology, *109*:163–166, 1973.
132. Brownlie, K., and Kreel, L.: Computer assisted tomography of normal suprarenal glands. J. Comp. Assisted Tomography, *2*:1–10, 1978.
133. Montague, J.-P., Kressel, H.Y., Korobkin, M., et al.: Computed tomography of the normal adrenal glands. Am. J. Roentgenol., *130*:963–966, 1978.
134. Reynes, C.J., Churchill, R., Moncada, R., et al.: Computed Tomography of Adrenal Glands. Radiol. Clin. North Am., *17*:91–109, 1979.
135. Sample, W.F.: A new technique for the evaluation of the adrenal gland with gray scale ultrasonography. Radiology, *124*:463–469, 1977.
136. Sample, W.F.: Adrenal ultrasonography. Radiology, *127*:461–466, 1978.

Adrenal Pseudotumors

137. Cocchi, U.: Retropneumoperitoneum und Pneumomediastinum. Fortschr. Rontgenstrahl. ERG., *79*:1–226, 1957.
138. Hamm, F.C., and Scordamaglia, L.J.: A diagnostic aid for visualization of the left suprarenal space. J. Urol., *73*:885–887, 1955.
139. Harrow, B.R.: Simplified method for evaluation of left suprarenal and gastric masses. J. Florida M.A., *42*:732–734, 1956.
140. Joelson, J.J., Persky, L., and Rose, F.A.: Radiographic diagnosis of tumors of the adrenal gland. Radiology, *62*:488–494, 1954.
141. May, J.P., Raguin, M., Grall, Y., et al.: Les Affections de la Surrenale (Radio-diagnostic Clinique). Supplement international des monographies Medicales et Scientifiques, Paris, 1962.
142. Meyers, M.A.: Diseases of the Adrenal Glands: Radiologic Diagnosis, with emphasis on the use of presacral retroperitoneal pneumography. Charles C Thomas, Springfield, Ill., 1963.
143. Poutasse, E.F.: Value and limitation of roentgenographic diagnosis of adrenal disease. J. Urol., *73*:891–900, 1955.
144. Scordamagila, L., Hamm, F.C., and Waterhouse, K.: Roentgen diagnosis of suprarenal densities. N.Y. J. Med., *60*:68–78, 1960.

Lesions of the adrenal glands often present a challenging constellation of findings clinically, biochemically, and radiologically. Roentgenographic diagnosis is most specific and accurate when integrated with an understanding of the basic disease processes.

FUNCTIONAL MORPHOLOGY OF THE ADRENAL GLAND AND CLASSIFICATION OF ADRENAL TUMORS

The adrenal cortex is divided into three generally distinct zones (Fig. 17–1):

1. The *zona glomerulosa,* which may be ill-defined and present focally, forms salt-active steroids (aldosterone). Hyperactivity results in primary aldosteronism.
2. The *zona fasciculata,* which constitutes most of the cortex, forms corticosteroids, such as cortisol and corticosterone. Excess secretion results in Cushing's syndrome.
3. The *zona reticularis* is responsible for sex hormone biosynthesis. Hyperfunctioning lesions result in the adrenogenital syndrome.

The adrenal medulla is composed of pheochromocytes in an anastomosing network of cells between which are rich vascular plexuses of capillaries and sinusoids. A tumor of these cells is known as a pheochromocytoma. Sympathetic ganglion cells lie singly or in groups in the medulla. Immature ones may give rise to a neuroblastoma.

A practical classification of adrenal lesions is as follows:

Cortical tumors
    Adenoma

17

Diseases of the Adrenal Glands

MORTON A. MEYERS

1061

Carcinoma
Hyperplasia
Medullary tumors
  Pheochromocytoma
  Neuroblastoma
  Ganglioneuroma
Cysts
  Pseudocysts
  Lymphangiomatous cysts
Connective Tissue Tumors
  Neurofibroma, fibroma, lipoma, hemangioma,
  myelolipoma, and others
Secondary tumors
  Metastatic or direct extension

Cortical adenomas and carcinomas may be either (hyper) functioning or nonfunctioning. Hyperplasia is a bilateral process and is always functional. Extra-adrenal pheochromocytomas (paragangliomas) are included in a discussion of the medullary tumors. Neuroblastoma and ganglioneuroma are related to the sympathetic nerve cells of the adrenal medulla.

Two features are particularly important in an understanding of adrenal lesions:

1. There is absolutely no correlation between the size of a tumor or hyperplasia and the degree of hyperfunction.

2. Histologic criteria that are usually accepted as evidence of malignancy in nonendocrine tissues cannot be applied to endocrine tumors. It may be difficult to determine from either the gross or microscopic findings whether adrenal tumors are malignant or benign. Even in the absence of demonstrable local invasion or distant metastases, recurrence may take place.

CHARACTERISTIC SHAPES OF PHEOCHROMOCYTOMAS AND ADRENOCORTICAL ADENOMAS

Meyers has noted that the shape alone of an adrenal tumor may reliably indicate its nature.[7] Pheochromocytomas and adrenocortical adenomas, in particular, often present a characteristic outline. This outline may be seen on plain films or tomograms but more often is demonstrated on nephrotomograms, retroperitoneal pneumograms, or in the capillary phase of arteriograms. It can also be documented occasionally by computed tomography.

Interpretation of the morphologic basis of these characteristic shapes depends upon an understanding of the corticomedullary relationships in the different parts of the gland (Fig. 17–2). The medulla resides within the base of the gland, and the major portion of the cortex (80–90%) lies in the apex. In fact, the apex of the adrenal gland is composed of cortical tissue only. A specific radiologic diagnosis is thus possible by a geometric appreciation of the alterations in outline produced by a neoplasm developing within either of the gland's two distinct components (Fig. 17–3).

APICAL SIGN OF PHEOCHROMOCYTOMA

Pheochromocytoma, developing within the adrenal medulla, results in mass enlargement of the base of the gland but often permits visualization of the uninvolved apex (Figs. 17–4 to 17–6a). The apex is clearly seen as a small triangular cap at the upper extremity of the mass and represents most of the intact cortex of the gland. The apical sign is not seen in the unusually large pheochromocytomas that distort the outline of the entire adrenal gland nor is it seen in extra-adrenal pheochromocytomas.

WEDGE SIGN OF ADRENOCORTICAL ADENOMA

The width of the adrenal's apex normally represents only a fraction of the width of its base. Cortical adenomas may result in generalized glandular enlargement, but often cause proportionately much greater enlargement of the upper third of the adrenal. The outline thus produced is diamond- or wedge-shaped (Figs. 17–7 to 17–10). It is virtually pathognomonic of cortical adenomas and is identifiable in over 60 per cent of cases associated with Cushing's syndrome or the adrenogenital syndrome. It is not seen in the small adenomas associated with primary aldosteronism. An outline resembling the "wedge sign" has not been seen in cases of adrenal cortical carcinoma.

ADRENAL CORTICAL SYNDROMES

Hyperactivity of the adrenal cortex results in three conditions: (1) Cushing's syndrome, (2) the adrenogenital syndrome, and (3) primary aldosteronism (Conn's syndrome). Each condition can result from hyperplasia or tumor of the adrenal cortex (Table 17–1).

CUSHING'S SYNDROME

Clinical Feature. In 1932, Harvey Cushing first described the syndrome secondary to liberation by the adrenal cortex of increased levels of hydrocortisone and corticosterone that now bears his name.[6] The classic features of Cushing's syndrome are well recognized. These include an insulin-resistant dia-

TABLE 17–1.
Hyperadrenocortical Syndromes

Hormonal Excess	Cortical Zone	Clinical Syndrome	Adrenal Lesions	Per Cent
Aldosterone	Zona glomerulosa	Primary aldosteronism	Adenoma	80–90
			Bilateral nodular hyperplasia	10–20
			Carcinoma	Rare
Corticoids	Zona fasciculata	Cushing's syndrome	<1st year: Carcinoma	40
			Adenoma	40
			Bilateral hyperplasia	20
			<10th year: Usually carcinoma	
			>10th year: Bilateral hyperplasia	60–85
			Adenoma	10–25
			Carcinoma	10–25
Androgens	Zona reticularis	Adrenogenital syndrome		
		Congenital	Bilateral hyperplasia	
		♂ Macrogenitosomia precox		
		♀ Pseudohermaphroditism		
		Postnatal	(Adenoma)	
		♂ Pseudoprecocious puberty	(Carcinoma)	Rare
		♀ Virilism		

betes, muscle weakness, osteoporosis, easy bruisability, cutaneous striae, low resistance to infection, moonface, buffalo hump, amenorrhea, hirsutism without other evidence of virilism, hypertension, and cardiovascular disease.

Etiology and Incidence. The adrenal lesions responsible for Cushing's syndrome relative to age are summarized in Table 17–1. In childhood, tumor predominates. If "pure" Cushing's syndrome is present, the tumor is usually small, but when the mixed form with evidence of hirsutism or virilism occurs, the tumor is more likely to be large and malignant. Irrespective of age, 80 per cent of tumors are seen in females.[2, 15]

In the adult, the majority of the lesions are bilateral hyperplasia. Although this lesion may occur at any age, the prototype of Cushing's syndrome is a 34-year-old woman with symptoms of 4 to 5 years' duration.[4, 33, 42] Sudden onset of signs and symptoms suggests adrenal cortical adenoma or carcinoma.

Neville and Symington pointed out the presence of bilateral "adenomatous" or nodular hyperplasia, which accounts for 15 per cent of hyperplastic adrenals in adults and 31 per cent in children.[37] These are superimposed upon some degree of diffuse cortical hyperplasia of the zona fasciculata but the nodules may not be obvious on roentgenographic examination or to the surgeon during operation. In the past, these lesions were erroneously diagnosed histologically as adenomas rather than as examples of nodular hyperplasia, which is a bilateral condition and requires subtotal or bilateral adrenalectomy.[37]

It is difficult to assess the frequency with which pituitary (usually basophilic) adenomas are involved in Cushing's syndrome. Cope and Raker state that "the minute basophilic adenomas of the pituitary believed by Cushing to be responsible for the disease may have been incidental findings."[4] They are probably present clinically in no more than 10 per cent of cases. Others have concluded that pituitary tumors are present in the great majority of patients with Cushing's disease, even in the absence of demonstrable tomographic changes in the sella turcica and that selective removal corrects hypercortisolism with little morbidity.[47]

Also recognized is the *ectopic-ACTH syndrome* in which functioning adrenal hyperplasia occurs in association with malignant tumors of nonendocrine tissue. It appears that the tumors liberate a trophic hormone that stimulates the adrenal glands to marked hyperplasia and hyperactivity.[27, 28] The tumors most frequently involved are bronchogenic carcinoma (anaplastic or oat-cell type), thymomas, and carcinoma of the pancreas (adenocarcinoma and islet-cell carcinomas, but Cushing's syndrome may dominate the clinical picture, at least initially.[23, 32, 33, 42] The reported incidence varies from 6 to 25 per cent of patients with Cushing's syndrome.[27, 37, 42]

Laboratory Diagnosis. The hallmark is an increase in urinary 17-hydroxycorticosteroids and, in the "mixed" Cushing's syndrome, 17-ketosteroids. Differential diagnosis between hyperplasia and tumor may be supported by laboratory findings.[16, 19, 26] Hyperplasia is indicated by a positive intravenous ACTH response with increase in plasma cortisols and a positive oral dexamethasone test with suppression of urinary 17-OHCS. Negative responses indicate an adrenal tumor that tends to be functionally autonomous. Nodular hyperplasia may be confusing because it may yield a positive ACTH test but negative dexamethasone suppression so the pathologic lesion is usually diagnosed clinically as an adenoma.[37] An increase in the excretion of the beta fraction of ketosteroids is particularly suggestive of adrenal carcinoma.[17]

General Roentgenographic Findings. The systemic effects of Cushing's syndrome are radiologically identifiable chiefly in the bones, muscle, fat, and thymus.

Bone changes include the following conditions:[36, 45, 48]

1. Osteoporosis, most marked in the central skeleton, is characterized by diminished bone density, thought to be secondary to diminished bone formation as well as increased bone resorption.[41] The bony trabeculae are diminished in number and thinned. In a child, retarded bone age with delayed epiphyseal development may be seen.[7]
2. Pathologic fractures most commonly involve the midspine. Multiple vertebral bodies may have a biconcave shape or show asymmetric compression fractures. Fractures may also develop particularly in the anterior ribs and the pubic and ischial rami. Excessive callus formation, although poorly defined, may follow these fractures.
3. Aseptic necrosis, affecting principally the ends of the femora and proximal humeri, occurs as localized destructive lesions with a surrounding sclerotic border.[31, 34]

A striking increase in superficial and deep fat of the entire trunk with, perhaps, the prominent "buffalo hump" may be seen radiologically. In children, the excessive subcutaneous fat also involves the extremities, accompanying some decreased muscle mass. It may be expressed as a "muscle–cylinder ratio." Thus, muscle–cylinder ratio = muscle diameter/total cylinder diameter. In the normal infant, this ratio has a value of 0.64 to 0.72. In infants with Cushing's syndrome, ratios are usually markedly depressed, whereas simple exogenous obesity has little effect on the ratios.[29]

Chest roentgenograms may further demonstrate cardiac enlargement and, at times, increase in the pericardial fat pads. Widening of the superior mediastinum due to accumulation of fat has been reported in patients with prolonged steroid therapy,[22] but not in those with spontaneous Cushing's syndrome. Thymic atrophy may be a striking finding in infants (Fig. 17–11).[7, 30]

Other abnormal roentgenographic findings in Cushing's syndrome include an increased incidence of cholelithiasis, pyelonephritis, renal calculi, and premature vascular calcification.

Hemihypertrophy is a bizarre feature that occasionally accompanies an adrenal carcinoma.[5, 7, 10] Radiologic studies document that unilateral enlargement of viscera is associated with the somatic changes (Fig. 17–12).

Radiology of the Adrenals. Adrenal visualization may be important in differentiating tumor from hyperplasia.

In adrenal hyperplasia, urography and nephrotomography are of little value.[33, 43, 44] Retroperitoneal pneumography demonstrates 90 per cent of hyperplastic glands in Cushing's syndrome.[16, 33, 43] Characteristic findings (Figs. 17–13 and 17–14) include (1) enlargement of the glands, (2) a tendency toward loss of the concave margins, and (3) an exaggerated reticular appearance of the periadrenal fat with relatively poor definition of outline, secondary to fatty edema of the tissues. On aortography, an enlarged capillary blush bilaterally is only occasionally evident. Selective adrenal artery injections may show increased size of the glands by adding the composite blushes. Adrenal venography verifies hyperplasia in about 50 per cent by the demonstration of spreading of veins with, perhaps, increased convexity[35]; planimetry may show an area greater than 17 cm.^{2} (See also Chapter 16.) Hyperfunctioning glands are not necessarily enlarged either roentgenologically or at surgery. Often the only characteristic features are broadening of the cortex and intracortical nodularity. Isotopic imaging, described in Chapter 16, holds promise. Enlarged hyperplastic glands have been clearly demonstrated by ultrasonography and by computed tomography.[8, 40, 50]

Adrenal carcinomas and adenomas resulting in Cushing's syndrome can be localized in 85 to 100 per cent by urography and nephrotomography (see Figs. 16–21, 17–7, 17–8).[33] Most functioning carcinomas of the adrenal gland are larger than 4 cm. and often average 14 cm. in diameter.[16, 33] Adenomas are frequently smaller and consequently more difficult to diagnose. In a patient with Cushing's syndrome, the finding of calcifications in the adrenal region indicates a carcinoma. About 30 per cent of adrenal carcinomas exhibit calcification, varying from small flecks to flocculant areas.[33] Calcification in adrenal adenomas is rare.

An adrenal tumor is outlined on retroperitoneal pneumograms in 70 to 100 per cent of cases.[16, 33, 43] Poor dissection of the gas may be a consequence of malignant infiltration into surrounding tissues.

Arteriography demonstrates adenomas, which may be as small as 3.5 cm. in diameter, as relatively vascular tumors, showing sharply defined borders, a few tumor vessels, and a capillary blush of variable density (Fig. 17–14).[65, 67, 79, 89] This often displays the characteristic wedge sign (see Fig. 17–10). The adrenal arteries may be slightly to moderately enlarged and there is occasionally some early venous filling. Although the hypervascularity of adenomas may not be readily detected on aortograms, it is easily identified on selective angiograms. Adrenal atrophy on the opposite side from suppression by the functioning tumor may be revealed by absence of a cortical blush.[78, 79] Carcinomas are generally vascular and typically demonstrate gross tumor neovascularity, arteriovenous lakes, and early opacifications of adrenal veins in the late arterial or capillary phase (Fig. 17–15).[65, 79, 89] Occasionally they may appear almost completely avascular,[67] secondary to extensive necrosis and hemorrhage. Hepatic metastases may be detected often by celiac arteriography (Fig. 17–15).[65]

Venography demonstrates a tumor as a round mass, usually at least several centimeters in diameter, with a plexus of circumferential veins and a network of vessels within the tumor (Figs. 17–16, 17–17). It is not possible from the displacement of adrenal veins alone to differentiate between adenoma and carcinoma, but invasion of the inferior vena cava on a cavogram (see Fig. 16–45) clearly indicates malignancy.

Both ultrasonography and particularly computed tomography represent remarkable advances in the noninvasive imaging of adrenal adenomas and carcinomas.[3, 8, 40, 50] The preferred method for visualizing the adrenal glands is computerized tomography. Together with ultrasound, it has largely replaced vascular and air studies (see Figs. 17–17a, 17–17b, 17–30a, 17–49a, 17–49b, 17–49c, 17–69a, 17–70a, 17–78a, and Chap. 47.)

NELSON'S SYNDROME

Following adrenalectomy in Cushing's syndrome associated with adrenal hyperplasia, the syndrome of pituitary chromophobe adenoma, visual field defects, hyperpigmentation, and marked elevation of plasma adrenocorticotropic hormone is encountered in about 8% of adults as first described by Nelson and co-workers in 1958.[52, 53] The incidence of the syndrome in children is higher, in the range of 25 per cent.[54] Chromophobe adenoma is the most common pituitary tumor associated with Cushing's syndrome,[55] the tumors appearing 6 months to 16 years after adrenalectomy.[52] Evidence suggests that there is a preexisting tumor in many of these cases. Although the course is usually benign,[52] it is advisable that all such patients be followed indefinitely with periodic radiographs of the sella turcica. These may show enlargement, "ballooning" with a "double" floor appearance in asymmetric masses, or erosion of the clinoid processes and dorsum sellae.[56, 57]

ADRENOGENITAL SYNDROME

This fascinating pathologic condition has been described as a syndrome in which "little girls become little boys and little boys little men. These little men pass through the 'seven ages' of Shakespeare in as many years."[63] In childhood, the adrenogenital syndrome is six times more common than Cushing's syndrome.[64] It affects females in about 80 per cent of cases.[58, 63, 66]

Etiology and Clinical Features. The congenital form is due to a heritable enzyme defect in cortisol production. There is impaired cortisol formation and hyperplasia of adrenal cortex, secondary to increased ACTH through negative feedback. In the virilizing types, there is increased adrenal androgen production.

Adrenocortical activity begins in the fetus about the third month of gestation. In the female, evidence of virilization is present at birth, but may not be recognized in the male for 2 or 3 years. Characteristic changes occur in the female external genitalia and vary from simple clitoral enlargement to a phalloid organ complete with urethra.[60, 67] There may be varying degrees of labioscrotal fusion with perhaps a urogenital sinus. These variable appearances are reviewed by Prader.[76] The internal genitalia are not affected. The congenital adrenogenital syndrome is the most common cause of female pseudohermaphroditism. In the male, there is penile enlargement but the testes remain small. Patients of both sexes grow rapidly during the first years of life and acquire sexual hair, acne, and a deep voice. There is rapid somatic maturation and muscular development resulting in the classic "infant Hercules."

In approximately one-third of the cases, the biosynthetic block is more complete and the patients present with virilism associated with severe urinary salt loss as a neonatal adrenal crisis. There is no sex predilection in the salt-losing syndromes.

When the adrenogenital syndrome is due to a tumor, patients may be seen at any period of life.

A specialized variety of adrenogenital syndrome due to neoplasm occurs in adult males and causes feminization (gynecomastia, testicular and penile atrophy). Most are highly malignant carcinomas.[62, 68, 77]

Laboratory Diagnosis. The hallmark is an increase in urinary 17-ketosteroids (17-KS) and pregnanetriol in the congenital form and 17-ketosteroids in the acquired form. Distinction between hyperplasia and tumor may be indicated by laboratory findings. After adequate replacement therapy with cortisol, the 17-KS and pregnanetriol values in the urine decrease to normal levels in hyperplasia whereas in the presence of a hormone-secreting neoplasm, there is usually little or no change.

General Roentgenographic Findings. As manifestations of adrenal insufficiency in the severe salt-losing variety, chest roentgenograms may show overaerated lungs, a normal to small-sized heart, and a decrease in thickness of the soft tissues of the chest wall.[71] Abdominal radiographic findings may simulate congenital hypertrophic pyloric stenosis or high gastrointestinal obstruction because of the paucity or absence of intestinal gas from persistent vomiting.[71, 80] Care should be used in the administration of hypertonic water-soluble contrast media in these patients because of the danger of increase in dehydration.

Advanced skeletal maturation is seen generally after the first 6 months of life.[60] Radiographs of the extremities show large muscle masses for the chronologic age compared with the standards of Maresh.[71, 73] Premature epiphyseal fusion, however, at the age of 8 or 10 years results in the dwarfed adult. There is also accelerated dental development and premature calcification of the cartilage of the ribs and larynx.[61, 71, 72, 74, 79]

The dimensions of the urogenital sinus and the anatomy of the internal genital organs are easily documented radiographically by the direct injection of contrast medium.[65, 71, 75, 78] On the basis of these anatomic findings alone, a diagnosis of adrenogenital hyperplasia cannot be made because pseudohermaphrodites and true hermaphrodites may present similar changes.

Radiology of the Adrenals. Roentgenographic evaluation of the adrenal glands in the adrenogenital syndrome is essentially analogous to that of Cushing's syndrome (Figs. 17–18 to 17–22). Adrenal hyperplasia in the congenital form requires no specific radiologic documentation.

PRIMARY ALDOSTERONISM

This condition, first described by Conn in 1955, arises from the excess secretion of aldosterone and results in hypertension and renal loss of potassium.[83] Clinical symptoms include weakness, periodic paralysis, polyuria and polydipsia, tetany and paresthesias. These are all secondary to the biochemical imbalance of hypokalemia, hypernatremia, alkalosis, and hyperaldosteronuria. The entity is an increasingly recognized cause of curable hypertension.

An adrenal cortical adenoma accounts for the majority of cases (Table 17–1), usually smaller than 3 cm. in diameter. Many of these lesions are minute, only a few millimeters in size. Most of these tumors escape detection by palpation and inspection of the adrenal gland in situ. Up to 75 per cent occur in women, most often between the ages of 30 and 50. They are significantly more frequent on the left.[86] Bilateral adenomas may be as frequent as 10 per cent. Other cases are caused by bilateral nodular hyperplasia. A malignant tumor is rare.[90]

The major problems in the diagnosis of primary aldosteronism are localization of the lesion and differentiation of an adrenal aldosteronoma from bilateral hyperplasia. Adrenal arteriography is limited because of the small size of the adenomas and their generally avascular nature. The larger tumors may be identified primarily as a negative filling defect in the parenchymal phase of selective injections.[92] Rarely, they may exhibit hypervascularity and a blush. Advances in aldosterone assay of the adrenal venous blood have proved highly successful in localizing an adenoma and in documenting bilateral hyperplasia.[89, 91, 93-97] Subsequent venography through the same catheter may be confirmatory and provide information regarding size (Figs. 17–23 to 17–25). The adenomas appear as rounded masses surrounded by a circumferential vein from which abnormal tributaries may radiate into the lesions. Bilateral hyperplasia is shown by diffuse separation of adrenal veins.

Ultrasonography has shown aldosteronomas 1.3 cm. in size,[99, 100] and computed tomography is currently being used to demonstrate them.[88, 95]

NONFUNCTIONING CORTICAL TUMORS

Most cases that were considered nonfunctioning cortical adenomas in the past are probably instances of intracortical nodular hyperplasia and are now regarded as a response to stress, particularly hypertension and diabetes. True nonhormonal adrenal adenomas are rare.

Nonfunctioning cortical carcinomas, however, are occasionally encountered clinically, usually in older men. They frequently grow to a large size and may be incidentally discovered or made first apparent by their metastases. Radiographic documentation of their nature may be revealed by arteriography that demonstrates their typical neovascularity (Figs. 17–26 to 17–30). If considerable hemorrhage and necrosis develop, they may appear relatively avascular. Ultrasonography and computed tomography may also readily reveal their presence (Fig. 17–30a).

ADDISON'S DISEASE (CHRONIC PRIMARY ADRENOCORTICAL INSUFFICIENCY)

The recognition by Thomas Addison in 1855 of the clinical features of a disease, which now bears his name, secondary to destruction of the adrenal cortex, laid the cornerstone of modern endocrinology.[108]

Clinical Features. Chronic hypocorticalism can occur at any age but is uncommon in infants and children. Symptoms are often nonspecific and include fatigue, muscle weakness, weight loss, anorexia, and gastrointestinal symptoms. Hypotension and pigmentation of the skin and buccal mucous membranes are always present.

Etiology. About 90 per cent of the adrenal cortex must be destroyed before clinical manifestations arise.[111] In the past, the most common cause was tuberculosis.[117] Even so, evidence of extra-adrenal tuberculosis is uncommon and when present the lesions are small and quiescent.[123, 124] The most common cause today is idiopathic atrophy. There is some evidence that this may be of an autoimmune nature.[109, 113] Other unusual causes of adrenal destruction include other granulomatous diseases, leukemic infiltration, primary and metastatic tumors, venous thrombosis, hemorrhage, amyloidosis, hemochromatosis, and operative removal for breast carcinoma and Cushing's syndrome. Adrenal failure may be one manifestation of pituitary insufficiency.

Laboratory Diagnosis. The urinary levels of 17-KS or 17-OHCS are low. There is no increase in plasma cortisol or urinary steroids after ACTH injection.

Roentgenographic Findings. Adrenal calcifications, either on one or both sides, are seen in about 25 per cent of patients.[119] They are usually multiple, discrete deposits (Fig. 17–31) that may outline the entire gland but are occasionally gross or homogeneous. Mild oblique projections of the abdomen may best demonstrate them.[110, 118] Tomography is only rarely helpful in detecting adrenal calcifications not previously demonstrated on the plain abdominal film,[119] but it may rarely demonstrate markedly enlarged glands caused by an infectious agent,[121] metastatic carcinoma, amyloidosis, or hemorrhage. Adrenal atrophy in Addison's disease has been demonstrated by retroperitoneal pneumography,[112, 115, 126] but this is not necessary for the diagnosis.

The size of the heart is invariably small. After institution of therapy, the heart often gradually increases in size, but does not enlarge unless an excessive steroid dosage is given. This has been used as an index to the response to therapy. The lungs may show evidence of chronic granulomatous disease that is occasionally active. An increased incidence and severity of costal cartilage calcification has been observed, but is of no diagnostic value.

Splenomegaly is present in 25 per cent.[119] Evidence of renal or skeletal tuberculosis is rarely seen now. Intermittent paralytic ileus may result from electrolyte disturbances.

Calcification in the pinnae of the ears has been reported. These calcifications are not pathognomonic and can also be found in acromegaly, hypercalcemia, trauma, ochronosis, frostbite, diabetes mellitus, inflammatory lesions of the ear, hyperthyroidism, hypopituitarism, familial cold hypersensitivity, and certain collagen diseases.

PHEOCHROMOCYTOMA

Pheochromocytoma is a tumor of the pheochromocytes, or chromaffin cells, of the adrenal medulla. The lesion derives its name from being "dun" colored whereas the cells themselves store catecholamines in granules that demonstrate an affinity in histologic staining for chrome salts. Chromaffin elements are also found in the celiac, hypogastric, aortic, and renal plexuses and in relation to other parts of the sympathetic nervous system. Throughout the fetal stage, the adrenal medulla is functionally immature. The organs of Zuckerkandl, composed of paired chromaffin tissue on each side of the lower abdominal aorta in relationship to the origin of the inferior mesenteric artery, are the major source of catecholamines, principally norepinephrine.[220] Normally, the organs of Zuckerkandl begin to fibrose soon after birth and are virtually nonfunctioning by the third year of life.[220] During the first year of life, norepinephrine is the principal catecholamine in the adrenal medulla. At 2 years of age, an increase in the epinephrine content occurs so that it becomes the principal hormone in the adult, occurring at a concentration 4 to 5 times the concentration of norepinephrine. The first successful removal of a pheochromocytoma was accomplished by Charles Mayo in 1927 and the earliest correct preoperative diagnosis was established by Pincoffs two years later.[187, 202] The tumor offers a particular diagnostic challenge because of its possible multiplicity and location in extra-adrenal sites, its potential malignancy, and its occasional association with other syndromes.

Signs and Symptoms. The clinical hallmark of pheochromocytoma is hypertension that is typically paroxysmal but may be persistent.[158, 161] The metabolic effects of epinephrine contribute to the characteristic "triad of Hs": hypertension, hypermetabolism, and hyperglycemia.[159] A host of findings may accompany these basic alterations, including headache, palpitations, precordial pain, sweating, flushing, abdominal pain, nausea, vomiting, blurred vision, anxiety, polydypsia, polyuria, and perhaps convulsions and unconsciousness.[161] The episodic nature of such attacks is often mistaken initially for such conditions as thyrotoxicosis or diabetic shock. The episodes often increase in frequency rather than in severity. Gastrointestinal complications include ischemic enterocolitis and megacolon secondary to the effects of catecholamines.[149, 164, 204, 211] About 6 to 14 per cent of pheochromocytomas are clinically palpable.[159, 161, 215, 219]

In about half of the cases of pheochromocytoma of the urinary bladder, distention of the bladder or the act of micturition may initiate hypertension, sweating, palpitation, marked anxiety, and other signs and symptoms.[156, 180]

Incidence. It has been estimated that about 0.6 per cent of all hypertensive patients suffer from pheochromocytoma.[177]

The tumor occurs most frequently between the ages of 20 and 50 years.[161] In children, the peak incidence is between 9 and 14 years of age.[170]

Site. The sites of origin of pheochromocytoma are listed in Table 17–2. In the adult, about 90 per cent arise within the adrenal gland. In children, the incidence of bilateral, multiple, and extra-adrenal tumors is considerably higher. Pheochromocytomas may develop not only within both glands but also in one gland and in other extra-adrenal sites or only in single or multiple extra-adrenal locations.[156] Such paragangliomas form in islands of accessory medullary tissue. The most common of these occur in the organs of Zuckerkandl,[130, 146, 172, 184] followed by the remaining abdominal preaortic regions, thorax (related to the paravertebral sympathetic chains), urinary bladder (from paraganglia in the region of the sympathetic nerve plexus within its muscle wall), and hilum of the kidney.

Malignancy. Benign and malignant pheochromocytomas have similar histologic appearances. The only absolute criterion for diagnosing a malignant pheochromocytoma is the presence of secondary tumor deposits in sites in which chromaffin tissue is not found normally. Close postoperative clinical follow-up is necessary. The true incidence is rare and is generally about 1 to 3 per cent.[170, 194] In the Mayo Clinic series of 117 patients with pheochromocytoma, the incidence of malignancy

TABLE 17–2
Sites of Pheochromocytoma

Site	General Incidence (6) (Per Cent)	Familial Incidence (6) (Per Cent)	Incidence in Children (288) (Per Cent)
Left adrenal	33	22	15
Right adrenal	48	13	33
Bilateral	9	47	20
Extra-adrenal	5	4	13
Multiple	4	10	18
Thoracic	1	—	1
Unknown	—	4	—

was 13.7 per cent.[171] One-third of malignant pheochromocytomas are extra-adrenal, arising primarily from chromaffin tissue associated with the sympathetic ganglia and rarely from the organ of Zuckerkandl.[200] Malignancy can occur at any age and at any site. The most common sites of metastases are the liver, lymph nodes, lung, vertebrae, ribs, and skull.[131, 171] Recurrences are generally apparent within one year and survival is rare after three years. Metastases are usually functioning but may be nonfunctioning.[131, 143, 171, 172]

Familial Pheochromocytoma. Symington (Table 17–2) found 70 examples of pheochromocytoma occurring in 25 unrelated families in a survey of the literature to 1968. The incidence of bilateral tumors is higher (47%) and the lesion occurs at an earlier age (average 27.5 years). Malignancy was evident in 3 per cent. The site of the pheochromocytoma is often the same for each member of the group. Carman and Brashear believe that familial pheochromocytoma results from a genetic defect inherited as a dominant trait with a high degree of penetrance.[140] Other lesions with an underlying genetic defect may be associated with familial pheochromocytoma:

1. Neurocutaneous syndromes. About 5 to 10 per cent of all cases of pheochromocytoma are associated with neurofibromatosis,[147, 160, 170] hemangioblastoma of the cerebellum,[199] or perhaps other aspects of von Hippel-Lindau's disease.[160]

2. Thyroid medullary carcinoma (Sipple's syndrome), with which the incidence of bilateral pheochromocytoma is 68 per cent.[201, 210, 212, 221]

Laboratory Diagnosis. The important metabolic products of epinephrine and norepinephrine are metanephrine, normetanephrine, and 3-methoxy-4-hydroxymandelic acid (VMA). Norepinephrine is the principal hormone in most adrenal pheochromocytomas. Elevated levels of plasma or urinary epinephrine are detected almost exclusively when the pheochromocytoma is of adrenal or organ of Zuckerkandl origin. Other extra-adrenal pheochromocytomas never have a higher concentration of epinephrine than of norepinephrine. Such findings are aids in the preoperative localization of the tumor. The histamine and thyramine stimulation tests may also be used to confirm the clinical diagnosis.[152]

Radiologic Findings. Plain films only occasionally show calcification in the tumor. These generally appear in areas of necrosis or hemorrhage. Meyers and King reviewed 24 cases and noted that the duration of symptoms is often at least 8 years but may be as long as 25 years.[195] X-ray evidence of calcification in pheochromocytomas in children is uncommon.[163, 215] The calcifications are usually plaquelike or ringlike,[148, 151, 155] and they have been referred to as "egg-shell" calcification occurring within the capsule of the pseudocyst.[151, 162] They may be seen in extra-adrenal pheochromocytomas as well (Fig. 17–32).[154, 196] They may also form as a nidus of calcium (Figs. 16–9 and 17–33).[195, 197]

Urography demonstrates a suprarenal mass in 40 to 50 per cent of cases perhaps with some renal displacement.[170, 194] This is dependent on the size of the pheochromocytomas, which range from 1.5 to 35 cm. in diameter. Most average about 7 cm. in diameter when diagnosed.[194] Nephrotomography increases the accuracy of excretory urography. Paragangliomas in the hilus of the kidney may distort the renal pelvis. Pheochromocytomas of the organ of Zuckerkandl may be revealed by lateral mass displacement of the left ureter at the level of L-3 and L-4 (Fig. 17–34);[130, 164, 188, 194, 195] obstructive hydronephrosis (Fig. 17–35) or nonfunction of the kidney is rare.[145, 172, 186] Paragangliomas of the urinary bladder present as filling defects.[137, 154, 198] Even though they most commonly affect the trigone region, they rarely cause hydronephrosis.[180]

Retroperitoneal pneumography identifies the lesion in 60 to 80 per cent of cases.[139, 194] It permits localization of small tumors and often shows the characteristic deformity of tumefaction within the basal medullary portion of the adrenal gland with an intact apex. Although the lesion may be completely outlined by gas to demonstrate a smooth contour, the contour is no assurance of benignancy (Fig. 17–36). Multiple or bilateral adrenal pheochromocytomas have been demonstrated by this method.[173, 176, 217] Paragangliomas of the organ of Zuckerkandl may be outlined by extraperitoneal pneumography as a mass overlying the left psoas muscle (Fig. 17–37) or lumbosacral junction.[130, 194]

Arteriography. If computed tomography is not available, arteriography is now the special procedure of choice for identification of a pheochromocytoma and possesses an extremely high degree of accuracy.

The translumbar approach to aortography should not be employed, because local trauma and hemorrhage may produce fatal hypertensive crises.[142, 176, 182, 209] The percutaneous femoral artery approach is safer and permits abdominal and thoracic aortography and selective catheterization of vessels. It is not without risk, however, and should be performed with monitoring of blood pressure and with an ECG, and with adequate anesthesia and antihypertensive medications immediately available; the elevation of blood pressure following the contrast injection in about 50 per cent of patients has been used as a test, provocative arteriography, to localize a pheochromocytoma.[191]

The typical angiographic pattern shows enlargement of one or more adrenal arteries leading into a tumor composed of a finely reticulated network of small, normal-appearing or irregular vessels (Figs. 16–37, 17–38 to 17–40).[136, 175, 191, 207] A pronounced homogeneous tumor "stain" in the capillary phase outlines the size and shape of the tumor and frequently demonstrates the characteristic "apical" sign (see Figs. 17–5, 17–6). The individual tumor vessels at times enter from the periphery of the mass. If hemorrhagic pseudocyst formation is present, the vascular blush may typically show as an opaque suprarenal halo (Figs. 17–41 and 17–42).[144, 179] This central zone of radiolucency within the tumor stain has been described as a "lemon peel" appearance. Large pheochromocytomas on the left typically result in elevation of the splenic artery and perhaps of the spleen and depression of the renal artery and kidney (Figs. 17–41 and 17–42). Hypertension may be exaggerated by renal artery stenosis from compression by the tumor or intimal hyperplasia, which can result in persistence of hypertension after removal of the pheochromocytoma.[141, 205, 218] A few pheochromocytomas without necrosis or hemorrhage are not hypervascular and may not be demonstrated by angiography.[157] In malignant pheochromocytomas, a pattern of irregular, disorganized vessels in the arterial phase and early venous filling in the capillary phase has been observed by some,[169, 206] but it has not been validated by others.[136]

Extra-adrenal pheochromocytomas are also clearly demonstrable by arteriography. Paragangliomas in the renal hilus (Figs. 17–43 and 17–44) and in association with the lumbar sympathetic chain (Figs. 17–45 and 17–46) derive their blood supply from renal and adjacent lumbar and gonadal arteries.[132, 145, 174] Pheochromocytomas of the organ of Zuckerkandl (Figs. 17–47 and 17–48) are supplied by branches of the inferior mesenteric artery and are shown best by selective catheterization.[174, 188] Pheochromocytomas of the urinary bladder (Fig. 17–49) derive their hypervascularity from the hypogastric arteries.[168, 216] Paraspinal pheochromocytomas in the chest are demonstrated by thoracic aortography.[183]

An association of hibernomas, often in the perirenal area, with pheochromocytomas has been noted.[192] Angiographically, these brown fat tumors can mimic highly vascular neoplasms and be mistaken for a pheochromocytoma, but they can be differentiated by their vascular characteristics of normal glandular structure.[153, 181]

Inferior Venacavography. This modality occasionally shows indentation of the cava by a right adrenal pheochromocytoma.[185] Inferior vena cava catheterization with analysis of regional venous samples for epinephrine and norepinephrine has proved useful for localizing pheochromocytoma and functioning metastases.[166, 190]

Adrenal Venography. This method is not usually used with pheochromocytomas, but can demonstrate large veins draining the tumor. It is possible to identify a residual normal triangular cap of cortical tissue at the superior aspect of these medullary tumors.

Ultrasonography and Computed Tomography. Although ultrasonography may demonstrate a suprarenal mass, computed tomography graphically localizes the lesion and may readily reveal bilateral, extra-adrenal, and multiple tumors and show characteristics such as calcifications, hemorrhage, and cyst formation (Figs. 17–49a, 17–49b, 17–49c).[135, 150, 203, 222, 223]

NEUROBLASTOMA AND GANGLIONEUROMA

Neuroblastoma is a malignant tumor of immature neuroblasts and is second only to leukemia in frequency in childhood. About one-third arise in the first year of life and 60 per cent are manifest before the age of 3 years.[259] It affects males predominantly. The tumor may be found at any site where sympathetic ganglion cells or their precursors are located. About 40 per cent arise within the medulla of the adrenal glands,[234, 244, 259] and about 20 per cent originate in the upper abdominal ganglia of the sympathetic chain. Over 10 per cent of the tumors are intrathoracic, usually arising in the paravertebral gutter in the posterior mediastinum. The remainder are found in the cervical, thoracic, or lower abdominal sympathetic chain or in the visceral ganglia.[234, 244, 256, 259] Metastases are already present in about 65 per cent at the time of hospitalization.[244, 259] They are found in the related lymph nodes, liver, and skeleton. Prognosis in neuroblastoma depends on the age of onset, site, and the presence or absence of metastases. The survival rate is definitely better if the lesions are situated outside the adrenal gland. Adrenal lesions metastasize more frequently than extra-adrenal tumors.[245] Prognosis is also worse if the patient is over 2 years of age and if metastases are present when the tumor is detected.[232]

Ganglioneuroma is a benign tumor of mature ganglion cells and their related fibers, surrounded by a connective tissue capsule. It is much less common than neuroblastoma. All ganglioneuromas must at one time have been neuroblastomas during their growth period but the factors determining whether a neuroblastoma undergoes spontaneous maturation are unknown.[225] Intermediate forms are known as ganglioneuroblastomas, and in a single tumor it may be possible to find all three histologic patterns. Clinical maturation from neuroblastoma to ganglioneuroma spontaneously or following radiotherapy has been observed rarely.[227, 230, 236, 237, 240, 246, 259, 260] Ganglioneuromas are seen usually in young adults with females predominating.[257] Sites of origin correspond closely to those of neuroblastoma; about half arise within the abdomen and about 25 per cent of these within the adrenal glands.[257]

The symptoms of neuroblastoma are protean. Patients often present initially with an abdominal mass or signs and symptoms of metastatic disease. Ganglioneuromas are often symptomless tumors discovered during a routine examination. Occasionally, chronic diarrhea and abdominal distention are associated with neuroblastomas, ganglioneuroblastomas, and ganglioneuromas. This is a consequence of the recently discovered functional endocrine activity of some of these tumors with increased urinary excretions of norepinephrine, VMA, dopamine, and homovanillic acid.[238, 239]

Radiographic Findings. On plain films, a suprarenal mass is evident in 40 per cent to 75 per cent.[244, 256] Calcifications, within areas of hemorrhage and necrosis, are seen in approximately 50 per cent.[234, 252, 256] The calcifications may vary in size, shape, distribution, and amount. They usually present as multiple finely stippled, punctate or flocculant opacities (Figs. 16–13, 17–50 to 17–52) but may be dense and confluent (Fig. 17–53). They may extend across the midline. Calcifications may be found in metastatic foci in regional lymph nodes (Fig. 17–55) or in the liver.[255] Calcifications in the primary neuroblastoma first appearing post-radiotherapy may indicate regression of the tumor (Fig. 17–54). Paravertebral widening (Figs. 16–17, 17–56) secondary to direct extension of tumor or, oc-

casionally, metastatic involvement of the spine is seen in about 20 per cent of abdominal neuroblastomas.[247]

Urography is positive in 75 to 100 per cent.[260] There is usually mass displacement of the kidney inferiorly and laterally (Figs. 17–50, 17–51, 17–55, 17–56) with some calyceal distortion from extrinsic pressure. Extensive extraperitoneal neuroblastoma may displace the kidney and ureter anteriorly (Fig. 17–52). Nonfunction of the kidney from invasion of the kidney or vascular pedicle is uncommon. When the site of origin is in the pelvis, striking displacement of the urinary bladder and lower ureters may be seen (Figs. 17–57, 17–58).[242]

Arteriography and venography are usually not performed in evaluation of neuroblastoma or ganglioneuroma. McDonald has shown that about 50 per cent of neuroblastomas exhibit pathologic circulation (Figs. 17–59), 17–60) and that many encase major branches of the abdominal aorta (Fig. 17–6).[248, 249] Arteriography may clearly document paraspinal intrathoracic extension of abdominal neuroblastoma. According to some, ganglioneuroma does not appear to have a pathologic circulation,[251] but others have demonstrated this.[229] Venography may discretely outline the mass of an adrenal neuroblastoma (Fig. 17–62).

Berger and associates found that a combination of ultrasonography and computed tomography yield diagnoses not possible with conventional urographic techniques in a series of children with neuroblastoma.[226]

Distant metastases to bone are generally bilateral and fairly symmetric.[241, 244, 247, 256] Most commonly involved are the skull, distal femurs, proximal humeri, pelvis, proximal tibias, vertebrae, and ribs. The lesions are primarily osteolytic, but patches of sclerosis are common. In the long bones, periosteal new bone formation is common and may be the only sign of skeletal involvement. In the skull, a typical finding is small lytic and sclerotic areas with vertical spicules of bone extending from the outer table into the soft tissue.

Thoracic neuroblastoma is evident as a posterior mediastinal mass originating in the paravertebral sulcus.[231, 241, 243, 261] It frequently contains calcifications (Figs. 17–63 to 17–65). Familial neuroblastoma may present as multiple tumors.[254]

ADRENAL CYST

Cysts of the adrenal gland are uncommon. Most are asymptomatic and discovered incidentally or at postmortem. Some of the larger ones may be palpable and associated with dull flank pain[262]; rarely, they may cause sciatica or a bruit from vascular compression.[266, 267] Adrenal cysts are generally classified into the following types[262, 265]:

1. *Pseudocysts.* These are the most common and are caused by hemorrhage with necrosis and cystic degeneration within a normal gland or a benign or malignant tumor. Hemorrhagic cystic degeneration of a tumor is usually evident clinically, radiologically, and histologically. Hemorrhage within the normal adrenal gland or a vascular neoplasm has been reported as a complication of anticoagulation.[267, 272] A history of preceding trauma is infrequent.[281] Pseudocysts have a thick hyaline fibrous capsule. Calcifications are present in about 15 per cent,[281] seen radiologically as typical curvilinear or spiculated densities around the periphery of the suprarenal mass (Figs. 16–15, 17–66.[268, 274, 275, 281, 282, 286] The pseudocysts are bilateral in about the same percentage of cases (Fig. 17–67). During the phase of total body opacification after urography or inferior venacavography (Fig. 17–68), the cyst appears radiolucent with a paper-thin cyst wall.[273] Arteriographic and venographic (Fig. 17–69) studies demonstrate vascular displacement about a nonopaque mass. Percutaneous puncture with fluid aspiration has been accomplished.[285] Ultrasonography and computed tomography have demonstrated adrenal pseudocyts clearly (Fig. 17–69a).[284, 287]

2. *Endothelial cysts.* These are divided into lymphangiectatic cysts, angiomatous cysts, and hamartomas. Lymphangiomatous cysts are the second most commonly encountered type. They are caused by ectasia of the lymphatic vessels of the adrenal capsule and medulla.[283] They may be single or multiple, usually small in size and project from one pole of the adrenal. Their presence is identified radiologically only rarely.[268, 274, 286]

3. *Parasitic cysts.* These are extremely rare and are generally caused by *Echinococcus.*[262]

4. *Epithelial cysts.* The fact that these are rarely encountered is explained by the lack of acini formation by either the cortex or medulla.[280]

MISCELLANEOUS STROMAL LESIONS

Simple connective tissue tumors, such as neurilemmoma, fibroma, neurofibroma, myoma, and lipoma are usually incidental postmortem findings. Particularly if calcified, they may be discovered incidental to radiographic study of other systems (Fig. 17–70). Hemangiomas and myelolipomas are rare but occasionally calcify or become large enough to displace the kidney.[290-294] Computed tomography may permit a specific diagnosis of myelolipoma by virtue of documenting its fatty content (Fig. 17–70a).[288]

ADRENAL METASTASES

The adrenal gland is the fourth most common site of metastasis by malignant tumors, following lung, liver, and bone. Adrenal metastases occur in 18 to 42 per cent of patients dying from lung cancer and 20 to 39 per cent of those dying from carcinoma of the breast.[295, 302, 303, 307] Other common primaries include carcinoma of the kidney and melanoma.[298, 300, 306] The metastatic deposits occur more frequently in the adrenal cortex and show a decided predilection for cortical "adenomas." Most are asymptomatic but rarely they cause adrenal insufficiency.[301]

If the metastasis achieves a large size, an adrenal mass may be seen on urography or nephrotomography. On arteriography, metastatic tumors most often show striking hypervascularity (Figs. 17–71 to 17–77). Secondary tumors rarely result in multiple avascular filling defects with vascular displacement.

Adrenal venography (Fig. 17–78) has been shown capable of detecting small metastatic deposits from 5 to 14 mm in diameter.[304] They are identifiable by displacement of adrenal veins that become slightly dilated and exhibit some stasis. The procedure may have a role in helping select the patients with breast carcinoma who should have palliative adrenalectomy.[295, 304]

Bernardino and co-workers have illustrated the ultrasonographic features of adrenal metastases,[297] and Dunnick and co-workers and Reynes and colleagues have clearly documented the condition by computed tomography (Fig. 17–78a).[299, 305]

NEONATAL ADRENAL HEMORRHAGE

Rapid involution of the large fetal adrenal glands normally occurs after birth. In a group of newborns, however, frank hemorrhage into the adrenals, either unilaterally or bilaterally, occurs. This condition is brought to clinical attention by the palpation of tumor masses or prolonged neonatal jaundice.[310, 315, 317, 318, 322, 324] The jaundice is secondary to hemoglobin breakdown within the hemorrhagic adrenal glands, and the high serum bilirubin is almost totally indirect. Although the bleeding may be massive, adrenal insufficiency is rarely found on follow-up even in bilateral cases.[321] It has been observed that, in many, the hemorrhage is localized to the fetal cortical zone and that the adult cortex is generally intact. Rarely, the glands rupture with exsanguinating hemorrhage into the peritoneal cavity.[315]

Most neonatal adrenal hemorrhages occur in large male babies.[308, 310, 314, 316, 322] The precipitating cause is unknown, but factors of involution of the large fetal gland, birth trauma, difficult extraction of large infants, and pre- or perinatal hypoxia may play a role. Predominant involvement of the right adrenal gland has been repeatedly noted. This has been attributed to its greater susceptibility both to compression between the liver and the spine and rapidly increasing venous pressure.[314]

Radiographic Findings. In the acute stage, urography shows depression of the kidney with perhaps lateral displacement of the upper pole on the affected side, with flattening of the upper calyces. The effect of total body opacification with the high-dose intravenous urogram may permit visualization of the avascular lucent adrenal mass, particularly on the right side.[318, 322] Ultrasonography is particularly useful in verifying a sonolucent suprarenal mass (Fig. 17–78b).[319, 320] The condition is to be differentiated from neonatal adrenal abscesses.[309, 310] Calcification develops rapidly, either as central flocculant areas or more commonly as calcific rims around the periphery of the mass (Figs. 17–79, 17–80).[312, 322, 324] It has been observed as early as 8 to 10 days after birth, but more commonly weeks to months may elapse before it is seen.[323] The calcifications then slowly contract to form triangular densities and the kidneys return to normal position and shape (Figs. 17–79, 17–80).

The asymptomatic adrenal calcifications occasionally encountered in the adult (Fig. 17–81) may represent the sequelae of unrecognized neonatal hemorrhage or perhaps traumatic focal adrenal hemorrhage.

WOLMAN'S DISEASE

Wolman's disease is a familial lipidosis characterized by the accumulation of large amounts of cholesterol and triglyceride in visceral foam cells.[325, 328, 332] Studies suggest that it may be caused by a deficiency of lysosomal esterolytic activity.[326] Xanthomatous infiltration, although involving particularly the adrenals, also involves the spleen, liver, lymph nodes, bone marrow, small bowel, lungs, and thymus. The course of the disease is short and lethal, owing to the severe adrenal insufficiency that dominates the clinical picture.

Radiologic examination of the abdomen is sufficient for a precise diagnosis, which may be confirmed by liver biopsy. Giant adrenal glands that reach three or four times the normal size and that show more or less intense calcification with preservation of their characteristic triangular shape are pathognomonic (Figs. 17–82, 17–83).[328, 330, 331] The calcifications are multiple, punctate, and symmetric. Although the superior pole of the adjacent kidney may be slightly flattened by the enlarged adrenal, it does not distort the pelvicalyceal system nor displace the kidney.[330] Hepatosplenomegaly is also evident.

In no other known abnormality resulting in enlargement and calcification of the adrenal glands is their normal shape retained. This distinguishes Wolman's disease from Niemann-Pick disease, neuroblastoma, adrenal hemorrhage, tuberculosis, and the Waterhouse-Friderichsen syndrome.

COMPUTED TOMOGRAPHY OF THE ADRENAL GLANDS

Albert A. Moss

Computed tomography (CT) is a noninvasive imaging technique that combines a high degree of spatial and density resolution and allows for an accurate display of both the normal adrenal glands and adrenal pathology.[333–342] Improvements in CT scanner technology permit precise delineation of normal-sized adrenal glands in 85 to 99 per cent of patients.[335] The CT findings in a variety of adrenal abnormalities have been described, and they indicate that CT is capable of accurately detecting the presence of adrenal tumors larger than 0.8 cm.[337–344] Computed tomography has rapidly become the imaging procedure of choice in the evaluation of patients with suspected adrenal abnormalities.

COMPUTED TOMOGRAPHIC TECHNIQUE

The patient is given 480 to 750 cc. of a 1 to 2 per cent solution of sodium diatrizoate approximately 30 minutes prior to CT scanning, with an additional 240 cc. of the same solution administered 5 minutes before scanning, so the intestine may be differentiated from other soft-tissue structures within the abdomen. Contiguous CT scans through the region of the adrenal glands are obtained with the patient supine and the CT gantry angled at 0°. In my experience, the 4- or 5-mm. thick slice appears superior to the slice 1 cm. or greater. CT scans should encompass at least 1 cm. above and below the adrenal gland to ensure that the entire gland has been imaged. Routine use of intravenous contrast material is not required to perform high-resolution adrenal CT scanning. However, in patients with a paucity of retroperitoneal fat, the CT scan must occasionally be repeated after intravenous contrast injection so that the adrenal gland may be distinguished from adjacent vessels, the upper pole of the kidneys, or the inferior vena cava. In the majority of patients, rapid infusion of 150 cc. of 30 per cent meglumine diatrizoate provides sufficient intravenous contrast to enable clear delineation of the adrenal glands from adjacent structures. Hypotonic agents such as intravenous glucagon should be administered if the CT scanner employed has a scanning cycle greater than 5 seconds.

NORMAL ADRENAL GLANDS

Right Adrenal. The body of the right adrenal gland is positioned just dorsal to the inferior vena cava at the level where the inferior vena cava becomes an intrahepatic structure. The body extends dorsally and slightly laterally for several millimeters along its long axis. The larger, more prominent medial limb of the gland arises from the body without a clear point of demarcation and extends dorsally in the retroperitoneal fat between the liver laterally and the diaphragm medially. The medial limb of the right adrenal gland is of variable length but has been noted to extend to the lateroposterior margin of the vertebral body.[333, 334]

The right adrenal gland has a variety of configurations on computed tomography (Fig. 17–84). Computed tomography depicts the right adrenal most frequently to be linear in shape with a course parallel to the diaphragmatic crura (Fig. 17–85a). With newer high-resolution CT scanners, the lateral limb of the right adrenal gland may be identified in the majority of cases and results in the adrenal gland having an inverted V shape (Fig. 17–85b). The lateral limb frequently is shorter than the medial limb and usually runs parallel to the medial limb, but, rarely, it is directed laterally at a right angle from the body of the adrenal gland. The right adrenal gland may also appear as a horizontal linear structure or have a K-shape configuration (Fig. 17–85c, d). The vast majority of right adrenal glands are positioned cephalad to the upper pole of the right kidney, and the lowermost portion of the right adrenal gland is always located cephalad to the right renal vasculature. The upper pole of the right adrenal gland, when compared to that of the left adrenal, is found by CT to be located higher in 34 per cent, at the same level in 51 per cent, and lower in 15 per cent of patients examined.[333, 334] The lower pole of the left adrenal gland is always located cephalad to the renal vessels, but more frequently it is in closer apposition to the left renal pedicle than to the right adrenal.

Left Adrenal. The shape of the left adrenal may vary considerably (Fig. 17–84). It most often has an inverted V or Y shape, but may appear triangular or linear in configuration (Fig. 17–85a to c). The body of the left adrenal most frequently splits into medial and lateral limbs at an acute angle (Fig. 17–85d). The lengths of each of the limbs of the left adrenal are usually equal, but not infrequently the lateral limb is seen to be several millimeters longer. The medial limb of the left adrenal gland is positioned lateral to the crus of the left hemidiaphragm but does not have a course as parallel to the diaphragm as does the medial limb of the right adrenal gland. The left adrenal is located anterior to the ventral vertebral body margin in over 90 per cent of instances,[334] but in all cases the left adrenal gland is positioned posterior to the anterior aortic tangent.[333, 334, 337] Most frequently, the upper pole of the left adrenal gland and the superior pole of the left kidney are seen on the same CT scan section.

The tail of the pancreas is located anterior or slightly lateral to the left adrenal gland. The tail of the pancreas is usually seen on at least one CT section with the left adrenal and serves as a good marker for identification of the left gland (Fig. 17–85d). The splenic vessels, when identified, are positioned just anteriorly to the lateral limb of the left adrenal. In most patients, the shape of the adrenal glands appears different depending on the particular CT section examined; thus it is difficult to ascribe only one shape to an adrenal gland in any one patient.[333–336]

Size of Normal Adrenal Glands. Montagne and co-workers described a method of measuring the length, width, and thickness of adrenal glands.[333] Adrenal gland length was defined as the cephalocaudal dimension as determined from the number of contiguous CT scans in which a gland was identified. Thickness of the adrenal gland was measured perpendicular to the long axis of the gland or one of its limbs and was defined as the greatest thickness measured at any site. This usually occurred at the junction of the adrenal gland body with its medial and lateral limbs. Gland width was measured by recording the greatest ventral–dorsal dimension of the gland.

Montagne found that 92 per cent of the right and 96 per cent of the left adrenal glands measured between 2 and 3 cm. in length.[333] However, these measurements are only approximations because the precise length of the adrenal glands is difficult to measure due to the associated partial volume averaging present in estimating the cephalad and caudal extent of each gland. Over 75 per cent of adrenal glands were found to have a maximum width ranging between 2 and 2.5 cm. However, great variations exist from patient to patient, and adrenal gland widths of more than 3 cm. have been described.[334]

Almost all adrenal glands are less than 1 cm. thick, except for triangular-shaped left adrenal glands (Fig. 17–85e).[333] The left adrenal gland is often slightly thicker than the right. Measurement of adrenal gland thickness is frequently difficult, and rather than attempt a measurement in each case, one may readily compare the thickness of the adrenal glands to the thickness of the diaphragmatic crus. In the majority of instances, adrenal gland thickness will be less than or equal to that of the crus of the diaphragm on the side of the gland that is being evaluated.

COMPUTED TOMOGRAPHY IN ADRENAL DISEASE

A number of authors have documented that CT is an accurate method for the detection of adrenal lesions that occur in a variety of diseases that affect the adrenal glands.[345-357] Computed tomography has rapidly become the imaging procedure of choice to evaluate the adrenals and has resulted in considerable reduction in invasive imaging procedures, such as adrenal arteriography and venography, and has emerged as the initial screening technique in suspected adrenal disease in many institutions.

Cushing's Syndrome. Cushing's syndrome is produced by continued exposure to elevated plasma corticosteroid levels. To institute appropriate therapy, it is necessary to differentiate patients with Cushing's syndrome due to an adrenal tumor from those with adrenocortical hyperplasia caused by excessive ACTH production. Although biochemical studies may allow this distinction to be made, the results are often equivocal and, even when an adrenal tumor is indicated, adrenal imaging is essential to localize the side with the tumor prior to surgery. Studies indicate that CT can accurately differentiate ACTH-dependent Cushing's syndrome from that due to an adrenal neoplasm in over 90 per cent of cases.[339, 341, 358]

Unilateral adrenal tumors responsible for Cushing's syndrome appear as solid mass lesions ranging in size from less than 2 cm. to 10 cm. in diameter (Fig. 17–86a, b). Adrenal adenomas and carcinomas may appear identical and may not be distinguishable by CT unless metastatic disease is present in the liver or retroperitoneum or unless intravenous extension of the neoplasm is demonstrated. Calcification has been identified in both adrenal adenomas (Fig. 17–86c) and carcinomas, and the administration of intravenous contrast medium does not appear to aid in distinguishing between these two neoplasms. The usual CT attenuation range of adrenal solid lesions is 30 to 50 Hounsfield units, but there are some adrenocortical neoplasms that have a low attenuation value, presumably due to the high lipid content of some adrenal tumors.[359, 360]

Normal adrenal glands have been reported as the most frequent CT finding in patients with Cushing's syndrome secondary to overproduction of ACTH.[339] Diffuse, bilateral adrenal gland enlargement with preservation of shape and configuration has been the second most frequent CT feature of ACTH-dependent Cushing's syndrome (Fig. 17–87a).[339] The nodular form of bilateral adrenal hyperplasia is unusual but may be detected by identification of a small nodule or nodules occurring in a diffusely enlarged adrenal gland (Fig. 17–87b).[339, 361] Associated findings in patients with Cushing's syndrome are an abnormally low attenuation value of the liver due to increased fat deposition within the liver (Fig. 17–87b) and an overall increase in retroperitoneal and subcutaneous fat. CT scans have not demonstrated contralateral adrenal atrophy in patients with a unilateral, functioning adrenal adenoma or carcinoma. However, after pituitary surgery, follow-up CT scans have demonstrated that the adrenal glands return to normal size. Because some patients with ACTH-dependent Cushing's syndrome will have normal adrenal glands both grossly and histologically, CT can never be used to exclude a diagnosis of ACTH-dependent Cushing's disease, but it can be used to diagnose accurately those patients with Cushing's syndrome due to adrenal neoplasm.

Pheochromocytoma. Pheochromocytoma is a tumor capable of secreting abnormal amounts of catecholamines, which produce paroxysmal attacks of hypertension, diaphoresis, tachycardia, and anxiety. The tumors are most frequently located in the adrenal medulla but may arise in the retroperitoneum, pelvis, or chest. Most tumors are solitary, but 10 per cent are multiple, 10 per cent ectopic in location, and many are associated with abnormalities of the thyroid and parathyroid glands. Computed tomography provides a rapid and accurate method of confirming or excluding the diagnosis of pheochromocytoma by virtue of its ability to scan the entire abdomen, pelvis, and chest.[339, 350, 351, 354-356] Most frequently, CT identifies a unilateral adrenal mass greater than 2 cm. in diameter and having a CT attenuation value of 16 to 70 Hounsfield units and a normal, contralateral gland (Fig. 17–88). Pheochromocytomas are frequently nonhomogeneous, with both cystic and solid components. Intravenous contrast media allow this nonhomogenicity to be better appreciated (Fig. 17–89) and also enable the tumor to be separated from nearby venous structures or allow a diagnosis of intravenous extension to be made. An ectopically positioned pheochromocytoma may be identified as a mass lesion in the retroperitoneum, chest, or pelvis (Fig. 17–90). Whenever a pheochromocytoma is found, additional CT scans through the liver should be performed to exclude hepatic metastasis.

The results of CT scanning in over 45 patients with pheochromocytomas have demonstrated CT to be almost 100 per cent accurate. CT has been recommended as the initial radiographic procedure in the evaluation of patients with clinical or biochemical suspicion of pheochromocytoma as well as for follow-up examination in patients with evidence of recurrent disease.[339, 350, 351, 354-356]

Primary Aldosteronism. Primary aldosteronism is a syndrome characterized by hypertension, hypokalemia, and reduced or absent plasma renin activity. Approximately 65 to 75 per cent of patients have a unilateral adrenal cortical adenoma, which rarely exceeds 3 cm. in size.[343, 344] The majority of the remaining patients have "idiopathic aldosteronism," usually termed bilateral adrenocortical hyperplasia, and adrenal glands in this group of patients are usually of normal size. Biochemical distinction between unilateral adrenal adenoma and bilateral hyperplasia is often unclear.[343] Adrenalectomy in a patient with a solitary adenoma is curative, but adrenal surgery is unlikely to be curative in patients with bilateral hyperplasia. Bilateral adrenal venography, venous sampling, and adrenal imaging with [131]I 19-iodocholesterol are currently employed to identify unilateral adenomas and bilateral adrenal hyperplasia. However, CT appears to be rapidly becoming the procedure of choice to evaluate patients with hyperaldosteronism.[343, 344, 358]

Computed tomography most frequently demonstrates a small, solid mass lesion frequently arising from one limb of the adrenal gland in patients with unilateral adenomas (Fig. 17–91).[343, 344] Adenomas ranging in size from 0.7 cm. in diameter may be identified by CT in greater than 85 per cent of instances.[343, 344] CT appears useful for the correct separation of patients with adenomas from those with bilateral adrenal hyperplasia (Fig. 17–92) and thus of use in directing the most appropriate method of therapy.[343]

Nonfunctioning Adrenal Tumors. Adrenal adenocarcinomas, which are nonfunctional, are detected by CT as solid mass lesions (Fig. 17–93a), which are either unilateral or bilateral. The CT findings alone cannot be used to distinguish between a benign or malignant solid adrenal lesion unless there is evidence of metastatic disease or direct tumor extension into adjacent organs (Fig. 17–93). Both adrenal carcinomas (Fig. 17–86c) and adrenal adenomas (Fig. 17–94) may become extremely large without producing any symptoms, and both may contain calcium. When a right adrenal gland tumor becomes large, it may be difficult by CT scanning to determine accurately on the axial scans alone whether the right upper quadrant mass is originating from the adrenal gland or from the liver. Re-formatting the axial CT image in the coronal or sagittal plane may allow such a distinction to be made more readily (Fig. 17–95). Following surgical removal of adrenal malignancy, CT scanning may be the preferred method to determine if there has been a recurrence of the adrenal carcinoma because no other imaging procedure allows complete evaluation of the surgical site.

Myelolipoma and Adenolipoma. Myelolipomas are rare tumors (present in 0.8 per cent of autopsies) of the adrenal cortex that contain varying proportions of bone marrow elements and fatty tissue; calcification is not an uncommon finding.[345, 346, 349] Adenolipomas are even rarer adrenal tumors that are composed predominantly of adipose tissue in which varying stages of degeneration, hemorrhage, fibrosis, and calcification are found.

Myelolipomas and adenolipomas are readily detected by CT as mass lesions within the adrenal gland that have low attenuation values and frequently contain areas of calcification (Fig. 17–96).

CT allows a specific diagnosis of a fatty adrenal tumor and permits distinction from adrenal carcinoma, adenoma, pheochromocytoma or metastasis.

Neuroblastoma. Infants with neuroblastoma usually have abdominal masses that have been diagnosed by palpation, plain abdominal radiography, or excretory urography. Computed tomography is useful to detect calcification not readily apparent by other imaging techniques and to provide precise anatomic information prior to surgery.[359] Neuroblastomas may contain calcium or appear as solid, noncalcified masses with or without cystic components (Fig. 17–97). Coronal and sagittal reconstruction allows demonstration of the relationship of the tumor to the diaphragm and determines the interthoracic extent of the lesion. CT can determine whether lesions are unilateral or bilateral and define the tumor's relationship to the liver, kidney, and surrounding vascular structures.

MISCELLANEOUS ADRENAL GLAND ABNORMALITIES

Adrenal Gland Metastasis. Adrenal gland metastases produce circumscribed mass lesions within the adrenal gland that alter the contour of the gland (Fig. 17–98). They may be unilateral but often are bilateral. Usually the attenuation coefficient of the metastasis is close to or identical to that of normal adrenal tissue, but if tumor necrosis has occurred, the lesion may be nonhomogeneous or even cystic. Metastasis to the liver, para-aortic lymph nodes, or lungs frequently is present when adrenal metastasis has occurred. Most patients with adrenal metastasis do not have a clinical picture of hypoadrenalism, and most adrenal metastases are detected when CT is performed to assess another clinical problem.

Hypoadrenalism. Hypoadrenalism has not been widely evaluated by CT. Normal adrenal glands have been reported in patients with hypoadrenalism secondary to pituitary irradiation or long-term steroid therapy.[339] However, CT may demonstate bilaterally enlarged adrenal glands in patients with acute hypoadrenalism secondary to adrenal hemorrhage (Fig. 17–99). This suggests that CT may be employed to identify patients with acute adrenal hemorrhage.

Adrenal Cysts. Adrenal cysts produce a rounded, low-density mass within the adrenal gland that may have a rim of calcification (Fig. 17–100).[353] The diagnosis of an adrenal cyst by CT, however, may be difficult because of the fact that adrenal tumors may have attenuation values near that of fluid, and both neoplastic and infectous processes are capable of resulting in adrenal calcification (Fig. 17–101).

CT has become the imaging procedure of choice in evaluation of the adrenal gland because of its capacity to image the normal adrenal gland in all its many variations in shape, to distinguish between adrenal tumors and adrenal hyperplasia, and to determine the extent and relationship of adrenal mass lesions to adjacent vascular and nonvascular structures. It has been valuable in the evaluation of the patient with suspected recurrent adrenal disease and in the location of ectopic adrenal abnormalities. Further refinements in CT technique and equipment should only serve to enhance further the capability of CT to image the adrenal glands.

CHAPTER 17, ILLUSTRATIONS

FIG. 17–1. Functional morphology of the adrenal gland.

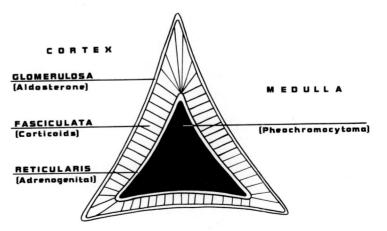

CORTEX

GLOMERULOSA
(Aldosterone)

FASCICULATA
(Corticoids)

RETICULARIS
(Adrenogenital)

MEDULLA

(Pheochromocytoma)

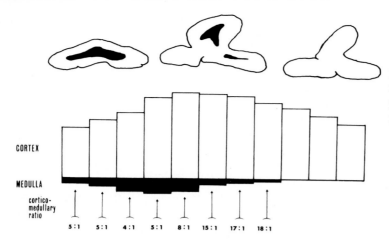

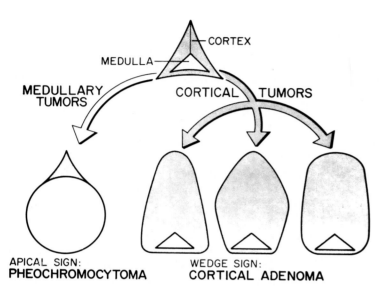

FIG. 17–2. The corticomedullary relationship in the different parts of the adrenal: base (*left*), body (*center*), and apex (*right*). (Modified from Symington, T., Functional Pathology of the Human Adrenal Gland, Baltimore, Williams & Wilkins, 1969)

FIG. 17–3. In pheochromocytomas, which arise from the medulla in the basal portion, the uninvolved apex containing most of the adrenal gland's cortical tissue may be clearly visualized. Cortical adenomas tend to produce proportionately greater enlargement in the upper third of the gland in the tissue of origin, yielding a wedge-shaped outline. (Meyers, M.A., Radiology, *87:*889, 1966)

FIG. 17–4. Apical sign on retroperitoneal pneumography. In two different cases, an intact apex (*small arrows*) of the adrenal gland involved with tumor is illustrated, a finding diagnostic of pheochromocytoma. (Meyers, M.A., Radiology, *87:*889, 1966)

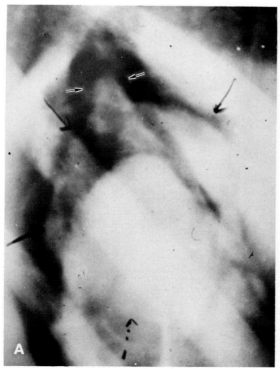

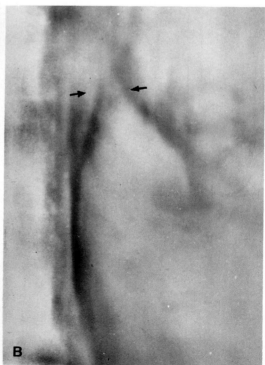

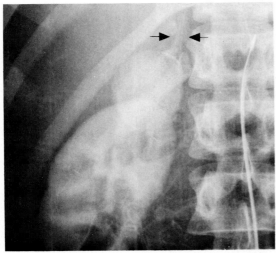

FIG. 17–5. Apical sign in capillary phase of abdominal aortography. The blush within a hypervascular adrenal tumor clearly shows an intact apex (*arrows*), indicating a pheochromocytoma. (Birnholz, J., Radiology, *109*:163, 1973)

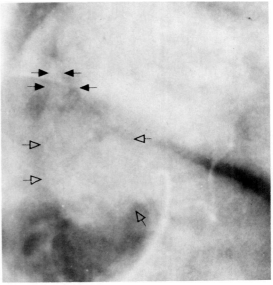

FIG. 17–6. Apical sign (*black arrows*) surmounting a tumor (*open arrows*) of the left adrenal gland indicates a pheochromocytoma in the late phase of this arteriogram.

FIG. 17–6a. Apical sign in left pheochromocytoma shown by computed tomography. **(A)** Section through upper portion of kidneys **(RK, LK)** shows intact apex of the left adrenal gland **(A)**. **(B)** Lower section transects bulk of the mass **(M)** of the adrenal pheochromocytoma compressing the upper renal pole.

FIG. 17–7. Plain tomogram outlines a large wedge-shaped mass of the adrenal gland **(A)** depressing the kidney **(K)**. The contour confirms the presence specifically of an adrenocortical adenoma.

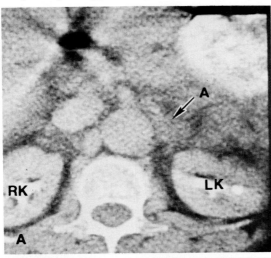

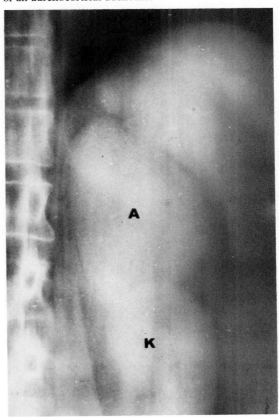

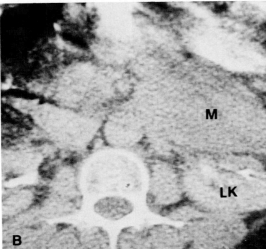

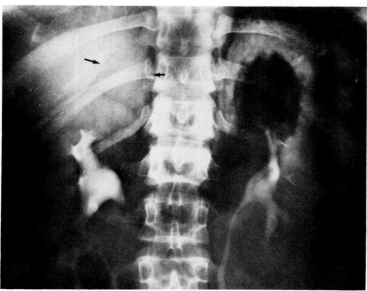

FIG. 17-8. Wedge sign of enlarged right adrenal (*arrows*), which causes mild flattening of upper renal pole. The shape is diagnostic of an adrenocortical adenoma.

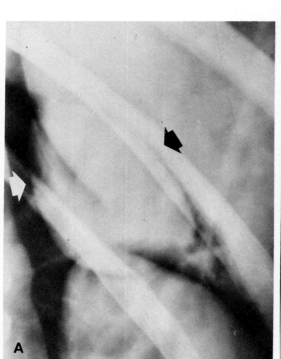

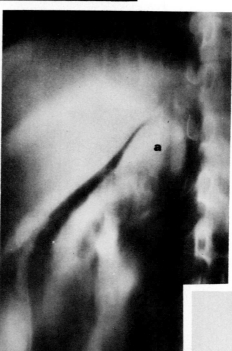

FIG. 17-9. Wedge sign on retroperitoneal pneumography. Two different cases **(A, B)** illustrating the wedge-shaped outline of the enlarged gland. This finding is specific for cortical adenoma. (Meyers, M.A., *Radiology*, *87*:889, 1966)

FIG. 17-10. Wedge sign in capillary phase of aortography. The case illustrates wedge-shaped contour of tumor enlargement of adrenal gland, which is diagnostic of cortical adenoma.

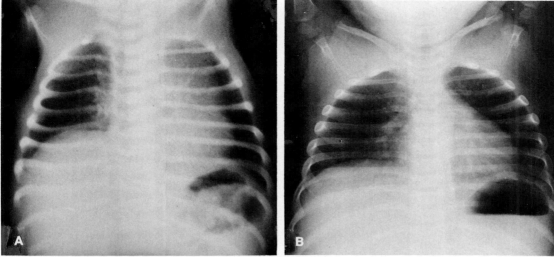

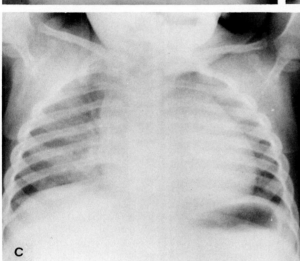

FIG. 17–11. Response of the thymus to Cushing's syndrome from adrenal carcinoma. (A) A routine chest film at 3 days of age shows a normal thymus. (B) At 11 months of age, and with clinical evidence of Cushing's syndrome, there is atrophy of the thymus. (C) Six months after adrenalectomy, there is a striking regrowth of the gland. (Darling, D.B., Loridan, L., and Senior, B.: Radiology, 96:503, 1970)

FIG. 17–12. Calcified left adrenal carcinoma (arrow) depresses the kidney in an infant with Cushing's syndrome and hemihypertrophy. Note the hypertrophy of the right kidney accompanying the increased size of the bony pelvis and ribs on the right. (Darling, D.B., Loridan, L., and Senior, B.: Radiology, 96:503, 1970)

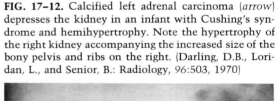

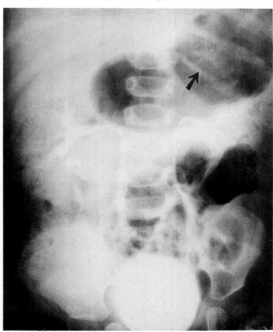

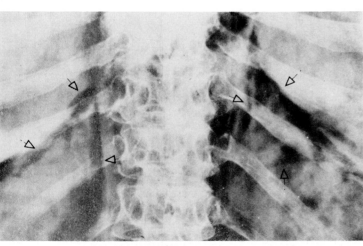

FIG. 17–13. Bilateral adrenal hyperplasia in Cushing's syndrome on retroperitoneal pneumography. The enlarged glands (arrows) are outlined. (Meyers, M.A.: Diseases of the Adrenal Glands: Radiologic Diagnosis. Springfield, Charles C Thomas, 1963)

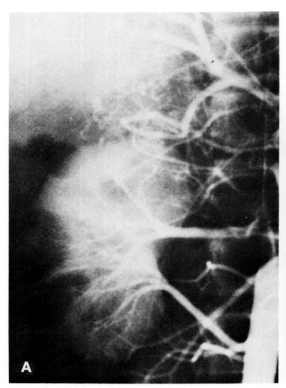

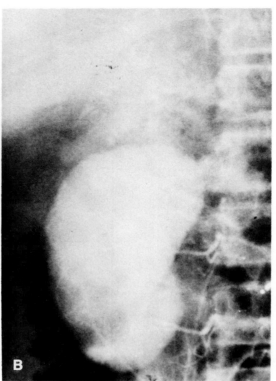

FIG. 17–14. Aortogram in a 10-year-old girl with mixed Cushing's and adrenogenital syndrome. A 4.5-cm. adenoma derives hypervascularity from enlarged, somewhat tortuous arteries (**A**) and shows areas of tumor blush in the capillary phase (**B**).

FIG. 17–15. Ten-year-old boy with features of Cushing's syndrome and sexual precocity. Hemihypertrophy of the right side of body clinically evident. (**A, B**) Selective renal arteriogram demonstrates enlarged inferior adrenal and renal capsular arteries supplying neovascularity with tumor stains within adrenal carcinoma. The mass contains scattered flecks of calcifications. (**C**) Selective celiac arteriogram demonstrates spreading of intrahepatic arteries, reflecting multiple liver metastases.

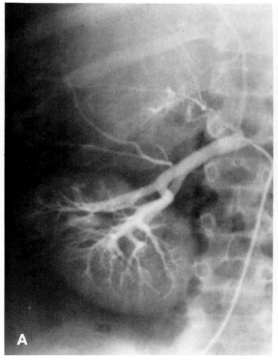

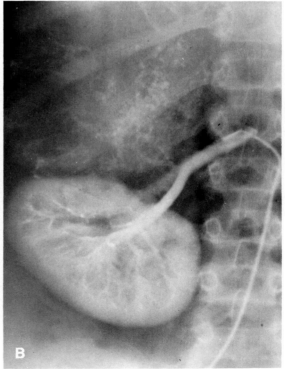

FIG. 17–16. Adrenal venography demonstrates circumferential displacement of veins around a 3-cm. tumor containing a reticular venous pattern. This represents an adenoma in a 23-year-old woman with a 3-year history of Cushing's syndrome.

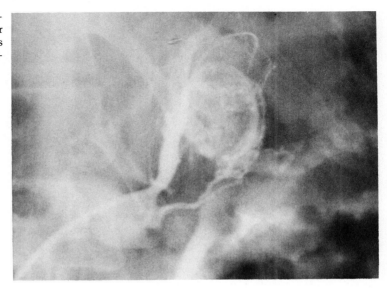

FIG. 17–17. Adrenal venogram in 72-year-old woman with Cushing's syndrome for 1 year. Wide convex displacement of veins outlines a 7-cm. adenoma.

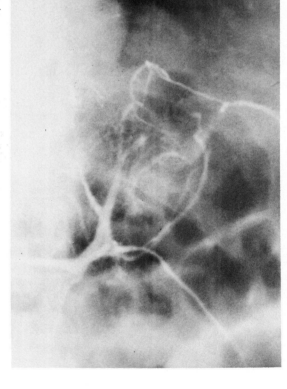

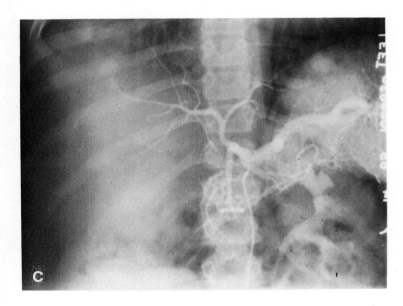

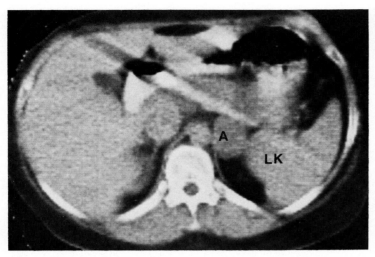

FIG. 17–17a. Computed tomography in 24-year-old woman with Cushing's syndrome demonstrates a 4.5 × 2 cm. adrenal cortical adenoma **(A)** anteromedial to upper pole of left kidney **(LK).**

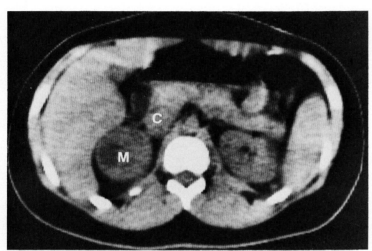

FIG. 17–17b. Adrenal carcinoma producing Cushing's syndrome in an 18-year-old woman. Computed tomography demonstrates a large inhomogeneous mass **(M)** arising within the right adrenal gland behind the inferior vena cava **(C).** (Courtesy of Carlos Reynes, M.D., Loyola University School of Medicine, Maywood, Illinois)

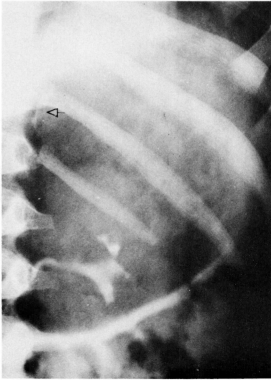

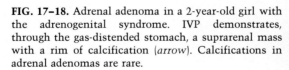

FIG. 17–18. Adrenal adenoma in a 2-year-old girl with the adrenogenital syndrome. IVP demonstrates, through the gas-distended stomach, a suprarenal mass with a rim of calcification (*arrow*). Calcifications in adrenal adenomas are rare.

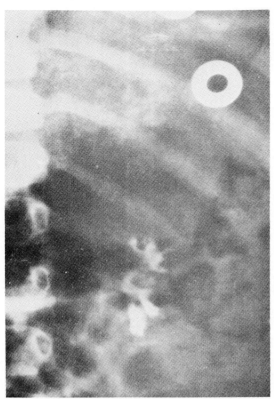

FIG. 17–19. Adrenal carcinoma in a 2-year-old boy with masculinization for 6 months. IVP shows flocculant calcifications in adrenal mass. (Meyers, M.A.: Diseases of the Adrenal Glands: Radiologic Diagnosis. Springfield, Charles C Thomas, 1963)

FIG. 17–20. A 23-year-old woman presented with hirsutism of 6 years' duration but no other signs of virilization. The 17-KS levels were elevated. Retroperitoneal pneumography outlines an unusually large left adrenocortical adenoma. (Meyers, M.A.: Diseases of the Adrenal Glands: Radiological Diagnosis. Springfield, Charles C Thomas, 1963)

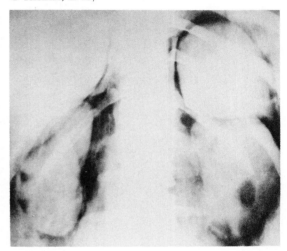

FIG. 17–21. Aortogram in a girl with the adrenogenital syndrome demonstrates hypervascularity to a round adrenal tumor (**A**), demonstrating a prominent diffuse blush in the parenchymal phase (**B**). Surgery confirmed a cortical adenoma.

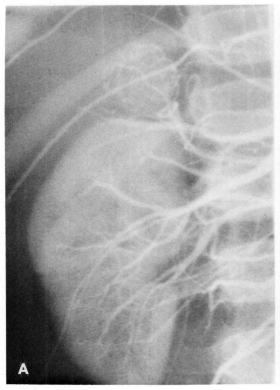

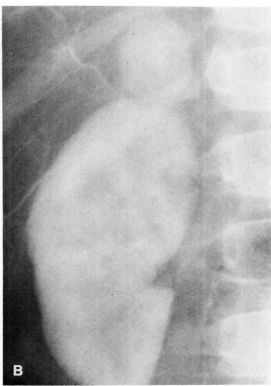

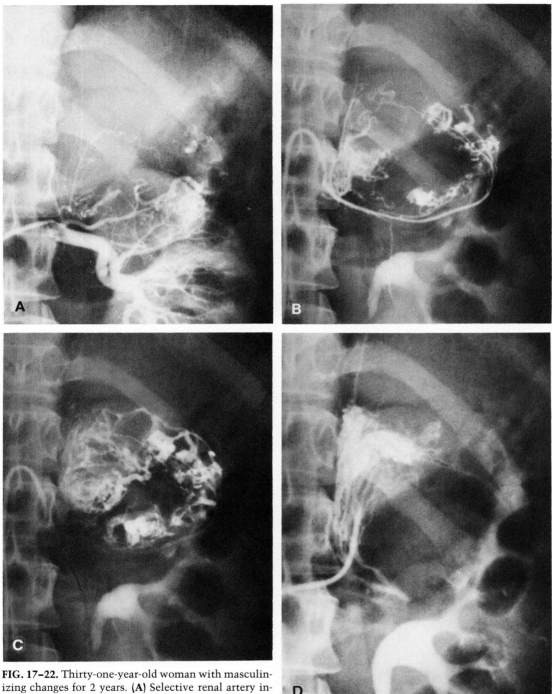

FIG. 17–22. Thirty-one-year-old woman with masculinizing changes for 2 years. **(A)** Selective renal artery injection shows some tumor vascularity from inferior adrenal artery to suprarenal mass. **(B** and **C)** Selective middle adrenal arteriogram demonstrates florid neovascularity, arteriovenous lakes, and early venous opacification. These changes document the presence of a carcinoma. **(D)** Adrenal venography shows mass compression and displacement of parenchymal veins. Bone and chest metastases developed after excision of the lesion.

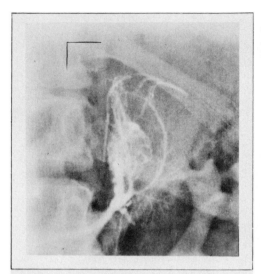

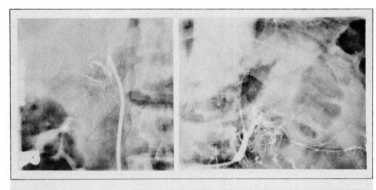

FIG. 17–23. Left adrenal venogram showing large adenoma in a patient with primary aldosteronism. Bilateral adrenal vein aldosterone levels are also shown. (Horton, R., and Finck, E.: Ann. Intern. Med., 76:885, 1972)

Adrenal Vein mµg/100ml		D.H.
Right 26		Left 1079

Adrenal Vein mµg/100mi		J.T.
Right 7670		Left 6466

FIG. 17–24. Bilateral adrenal venograms in primary aldosteronism. Wide displacement of numerous parenchymal veins indicates bilateral hyperplasia. The aldosterone level on both sides are seen to be high. (Horton, R., and Finck, E.: Ann. Intern. Med., 76:885, 1972)

FIG. 17–25. Left adrenal venograms (**A, B**) in two patients with aldosteronomas show characteristic circumferential displacement of veins with reticular channels through the lesion.

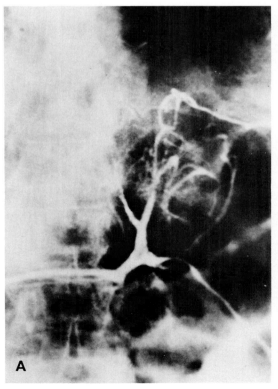

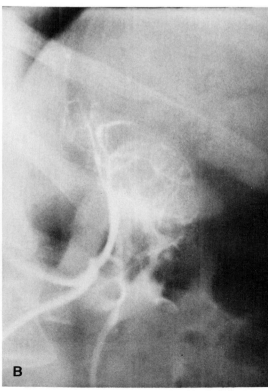

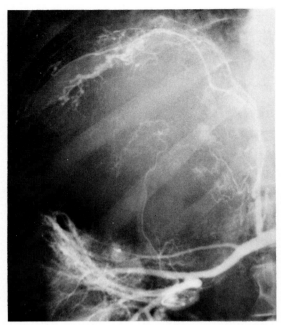

FIG. 17–26. Nonfunctioning adrenal carcinoma. Selective renal arteriogram demonstrates extreme hypervascularity to suprarenal mass, with grossly tortuous and irregular tumor vessels and areas of arteriovenous lakes.

FIG. 17–28. Nonhormonal adrenal carcinoma in 59-year-old man with right upper quadrant pain for 5 years. **(A)** Selective renal artery injection shows some blood supply from inferior adrenal and perforating renal capsular arteries. **(B)** Selective inferior phrenic arteriogram demonstrates extensive neovascularity and arteriovenous lakes. The lesion extended into the inferior surface of the liver, over the inferior vena cava, and across the aorta; it was inoperable.

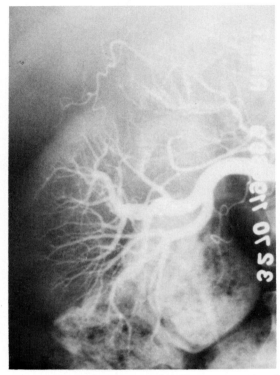

FIG. 17–27. Nonfunctioning adrenal carcinoma. Renal arteriogram demonstrates numerous irregular, tortuous tumor vessels arising from inferior adrenal artery.

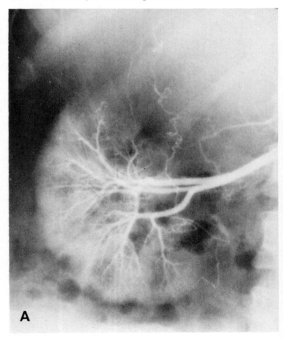

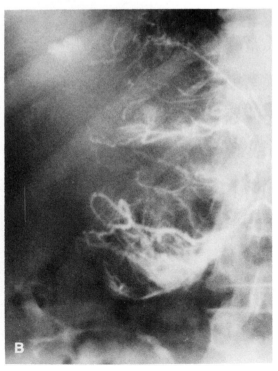

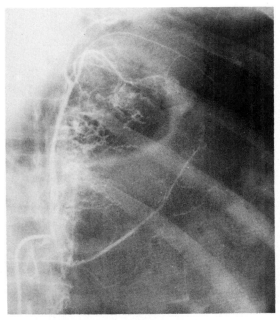

FIG. 17–29. Nonfunctioning adrenal carcinoma in a 43-year-old man. Inferior phrenic artery injection shows florid neovascularity from the superior adrenal branches and some blood supply from an enlarged middle adrenal artery.

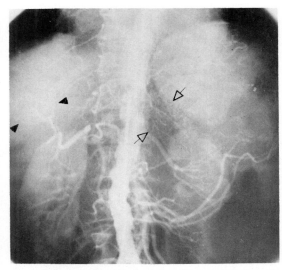

FIG. 17–30. Nonfunctioning adrenal carcinoma in a 68-year-old man. Aortogram reveals enlarged middle adrenal arteries (*arrows*) to left suprarenal mass and a metastasis in the liver displacing hepatic artery branches (*arrowheads*).

FIG. 17–30a. Nonfunctioning adrenal adenoma. Computed tomography demonstrates a low density mass (**M**) of the right adrenal gland, anterior to the upper pole of the right kidney (**K**). Fat-infiltrated adenoma identified at surgery. (Courtesy of Carlos Reynes, M.D., Loyola University School of Medicine, Maywood, Illinois)

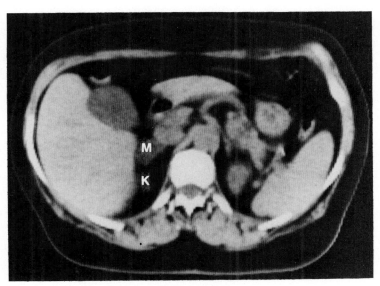

FIG. 17–31. Addison's disease. Dense multiple calcifications are present in both adrenals. Irregularity and partial atrophy of the gland substance are suggested.

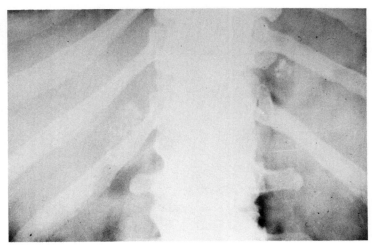

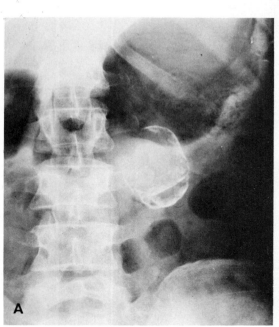

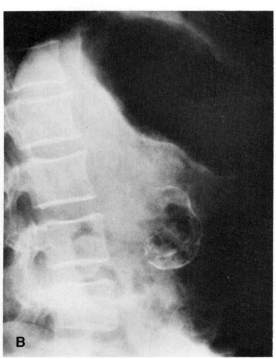

FIG. 17–32. "Egg-shell" calcification in a pheochromocytoma of the organ of Zuckerkandl. Note its characteristic position posteriorly and to the left of L-3. This occurred in a 55-year-old woman with long-standing hypertension. (Moir, W.M., and Crummy, A.B.: J. Urol., *107*:15, 1972)

FIG. 17–33. A 1.5-cm. calcified pheochromocytoma in a 28-year-old man with symptoms for 10 years. **(A)** IVP, AP view. **(B)** Presacral pneumogram. AP tomogram. Note also the convex lateral margin of the enlarged gland. (Meyers, M.A., and King, M.C.: Clin. Radiol., *20*:52, 1969)

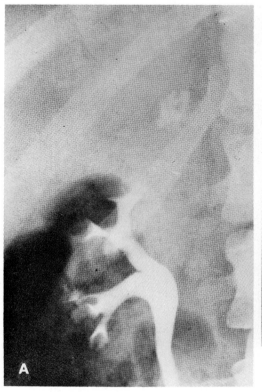

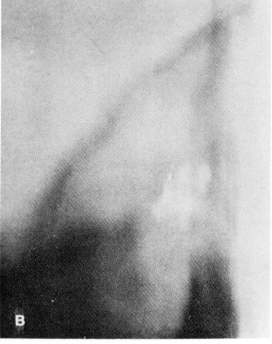

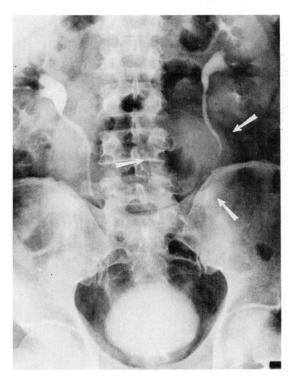

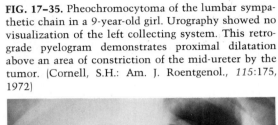

FIG. 17–34. Pheochromocytoma of the organ of Zuckerkandl in a 55-year-old man. IVP shows lateral deviation of the left ureter by a mass (*arrows*) at the level of L-4 and L-5. (Malter, I.J., and Koehler, P.R.: Radiology, *97*:57, 1970)

FIG. 17–35. Pheochromocytoma of the lumbar sympathetic chain in a 9-year-old girl. Urography showed no visualization of the left collecting system. This retrograde pyelogram demonstrates proximal dilatation above an area of constriction of the mid-ureter by the tumor. (Cornell, S.H.: Am. J. Roentgenol., *115*:175, 1972)

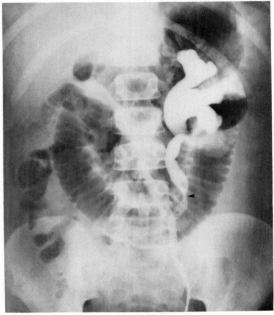

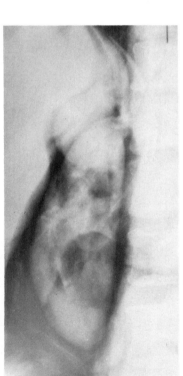

FIG. 17–36. Retroperitoneal pneumogram demonstrating a 4-cm. malignant pheochromocytoma. Microscopic pulmonary metastases were demonstrated at autopsy. Complete outlining of the tumor by the gas does not exclude the possibility of malignancy. (Meyers, M.A.: Diseases of the Adrenal Glands: Radiologic Diagnosis. Springfield, Charles C Thomas, 1963)

FIG. 17–37. Retroperitoneal pneumography outlines the mass density (*arrow*) of a pheochromocytoma of the organ of Zuckerkandl, overlying the left psoas muscle at the level of L-3. (Meyers, M.A., and King, M.C.: Clin. Radiol., *20*:52, 1969)

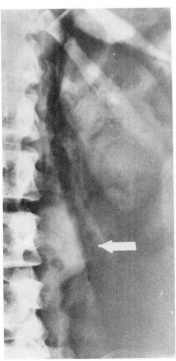

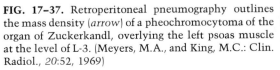

1091

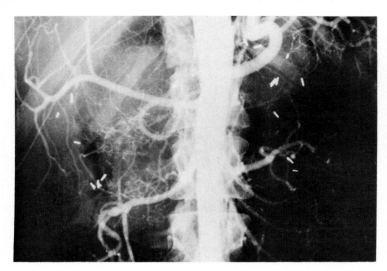

FIG. 17–38. Aortography demonstrates extreme hypervascularity to right adrenal mass. This represents a recurrent pheochromocytoma in a 23-year-old woman who had undergone resection of bilateral pheochromocytomas at the age of 4 years and then developed a medullary carcinoma of the thyroid at the age of 7 years.

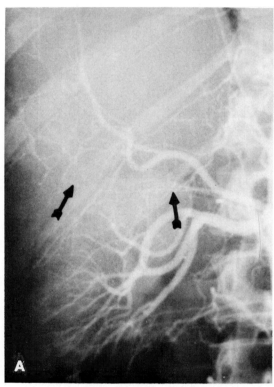

FIG. 17–39. Aortogram in a 35-year-old woman with neurofibromatosis and a 6-month history of headaches and hypertension. A right adrenal pheochromocytoma is supplied by an enlarged middle adrenal artery (A) and demonstrates several tortuous vascular channels (B).

FIG. 17–40. Malignant pheochromocytoma in a boy with metastases to the cervical spine. Aortography (A) demonstrates extreme hypervascularity from multiple enlarged arteries to right adrenal mass. Selective renal arteriography (B) shows these to advantage. In the late phase (C), there is persistent opacification of grossly irregular dilated tumor vessels in a bizarre "sunburst" or "fireworks" pattern.

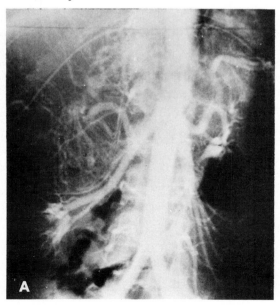

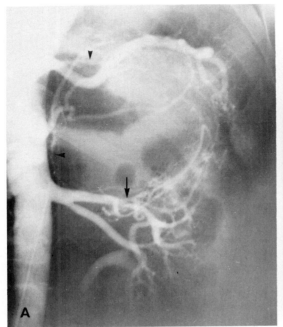

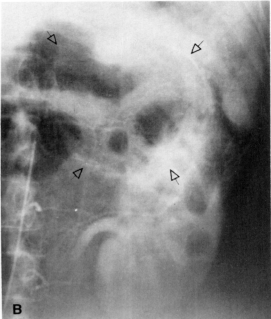

FIG. 17–41. Pheochromocytoma with central hemorrhage. **(A)** Aortogram shows depression of the renal artery (*arrow*), elevation of the splenic artery, and enlarged branches of the middle adrenal artery (*arrowheads*) displaced around a large adrenal mass. **(B)** Capillary phase demonstrates characteristic "lemon-peel" appearance of blush (*arrows*) surrounding central radiolucency of hemorrhage within the tumor.

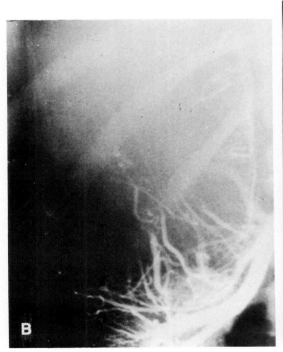

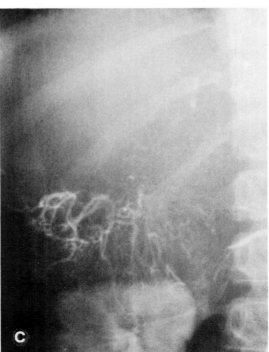

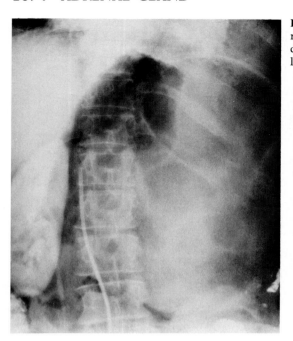

FIG. 17-42. Large pheochromocytoma with hemorrhagic pseudocyst formation. Aortogram in late phase demonstrates a thin halo of blush surrounding a central large, lucent, avascular mass.

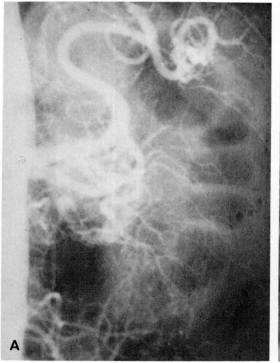
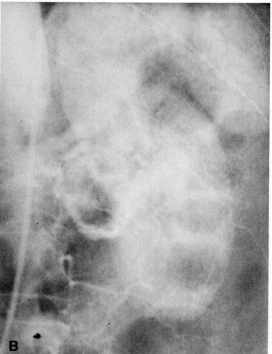

FIG. 17-43. Paraganglioma in left renal hilus. (A) Aortogram shows extreme hypervascularity to mass from branches of the renal and lumbar arteries. (B) Central radiolucency in capillary phase indicates hemorrhage and necrosis within the tumor.

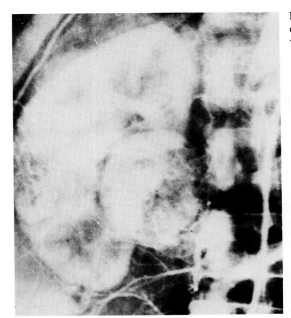

FIG. 17–44. Paraganglioma in right renal hilus. Parenchymal phase of aortogram shows a pronounced blush within the tumor.

FIG. 17–45. Malignant paragangliomas of the sympathetic chain. Arterial (**A**) and capillary (**B**) stages of aortography demonstrate a highly vascular bilateral pre- and paravertebral neoplasm (*arrows,* **B**), supplied primarily by the gonadal and the 2nd to 4th lumbar arteries (*arrows,* **A**), extending from the level of the renal arteries to the aortic bifurcation. (Baum, S., Stein, G., Roy, R., and Finkelstein, A.: Postgrad. Med., *38*:547–567, 1965)

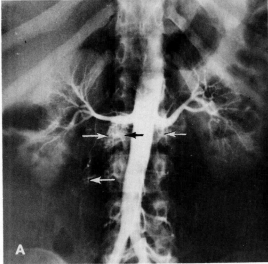

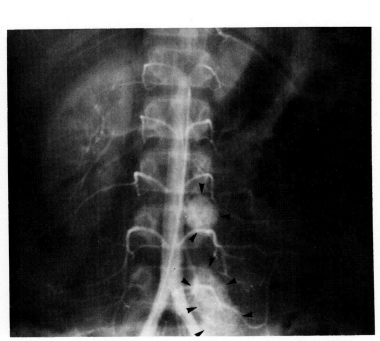

FIG. 17–46. Aortogram demonstrates two pheochromocytomas (*arrows*) of the lumbar sympathetic chain as discrete hypervascular tumor blushes. (Same case as Fig. 17–35.) (Cornell, S.H.: Am. J. Roentgenol., *115*:175, 1972)

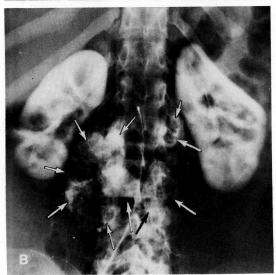

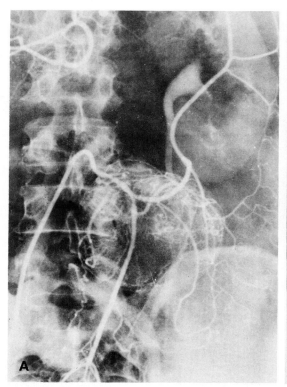

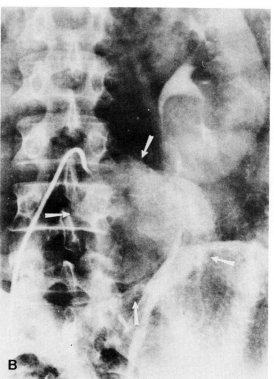

FIG. 17–47. Pheochromocytoma of the organ of Zuckerkandl. Inferior mesenteric arteriogram (**A**) identifies a vascular tumor just distal to its origin with encasement of some of the major arterial branches and considerable neovascularity. In the capillary phase (**B**), there is a pronounced homogeneous tumor blush (*arrows*). (Same case as Fig. 17–34.) (Malter, I.J., and Koehler, P.R.: Radiology, *97*:57, 1970)

FIG. 17–48. Pheochromocytoma of the organ of Zuckerkandl in a 54-year-old woman with hypertension. Selective inferior mesenteric arteriograms demonstrate displacement of the left colic arteries by a mass exhibiting neovascularity (**A**) and a distinct parenchymal blush (**B**). (Kinkhabwala, M.N., and Conradi, H.: J. Urol., *108*:666, 1972)

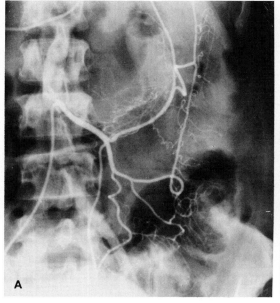

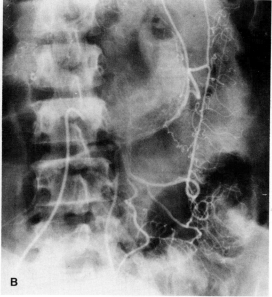

FIG. 17–49. Functioning nonchromaffin paraganglioma of the urinary bladder. Selective left hypogastric arteriogram demonstrates a highly vascular mass infiltrating the left bladder wall. Pathologic vessels extend along the base of the bladder. (Spitzer, R., Borrison, R., and Castellino, R.A.: Radiology, *98*:577, 1971)

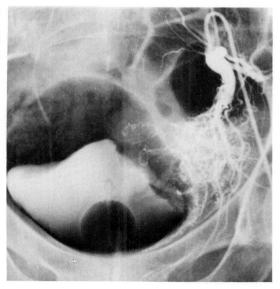

FIG. 17–49a. Cystic right pheochromocytoma in a 51-year-old man with paroxysmal hypertension. **(A)** Longitudinal ultrasonography demonstrates the mass with multiple compartmentalized echoes secondary to areas of necrosis and hemorrhage. **(B)** Computed tomography shows the 7.5 × 5 cm. partially cystic tumor mildly displacing the inferior vena cava anteriorly.

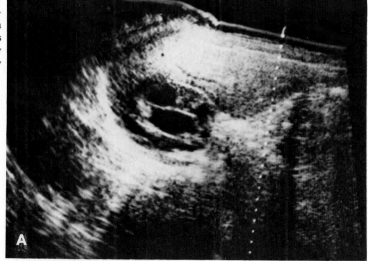

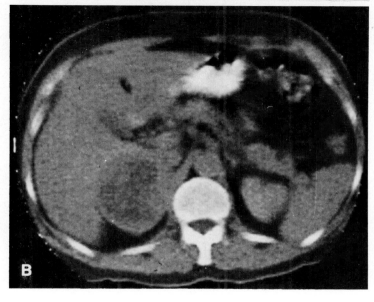

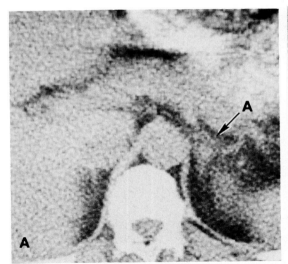

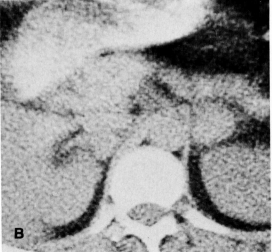

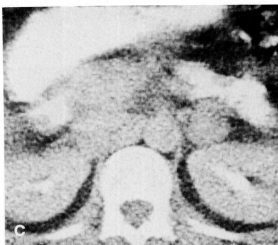

FIG. 17–49b. Bilateral adrenal pheochromocytomas in a 44-year-old female with Sipple's syndrome. Computed tomography. **(A)** Section demonstrates intact apex of left adrenal gland **(A)**. **(B)** Lower section illustrates 2-cm. tumor involving adrenal glands bilaterally. **(C)** After intravenous contrast, there is mild enhancement, reflecting hypervascularity.

FIG. 17–49c. Pheochromocytoma of organ of Zuckerkandl in a 71-year-old man with hypertension. Computed tomography. **(A)** Section through upper abdomen demonstrates normal suprarenal glands **(A)**. **(B, C)** Sections at and just below aortic bifurcation (aorta and common iliac arteries enhanced by IV contrast) reveal a $7 \times 5 \times 5$ cm. cystic, hemorrhagic mass with punctate calcifications.

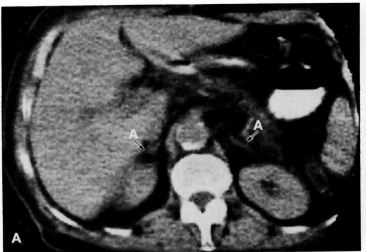

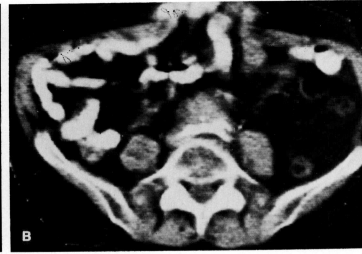

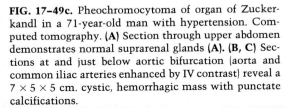

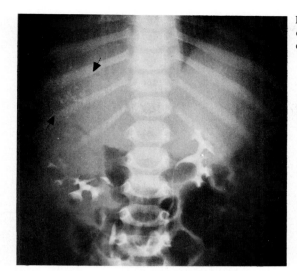

FIG. 17–50. Neuroblastoma. Right suprarenal mass containing a focus of stippled calcifications (*arrows*) displaces the kidney inferiorly and laterally.

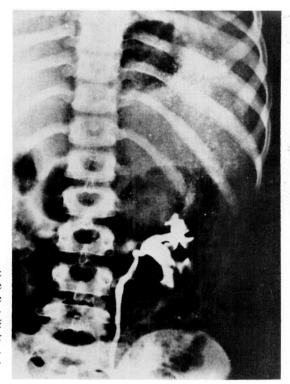

FIG. 17–51. Ganglioneuroblastoma. Lightly flocculant calcifications in adrenal mass with depression of the kidney. Eight-year-old girl with "enlarged spleen" since birth. Biopsy of mass at laparotomy showed an incompletely differentiated ganglioneuroma with foci of neuroblasts. Radiotherapy was given with no clinical or radiographic progression over 8-year follow-up. (Meyers, M.A.: Diseases of the Adrenal Glands: Radiologic Diagnosis. Springfield, Charles C Thomas, 1963)

FIG. 17–52. Neuroblastoma. Extensive extraperitoneal mass causing renal and ureteral displacement contains a cluster of fine calcifications (*arrow*).

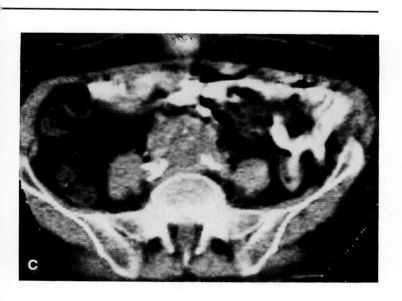

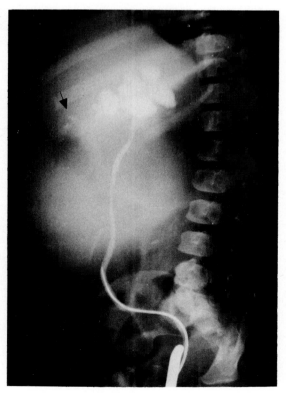

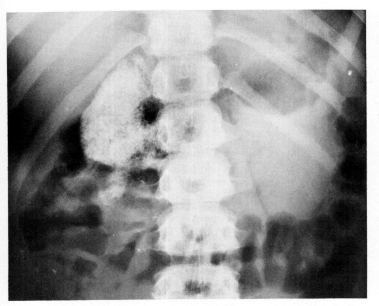

FIG. 17–53. Neuroblastoma. Dense adrenal calcifications extending beyond confines of gland.

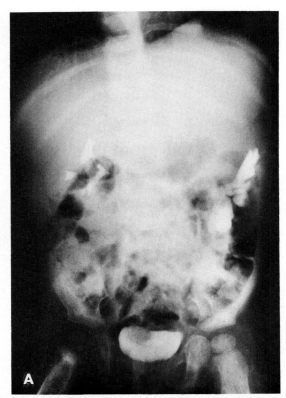

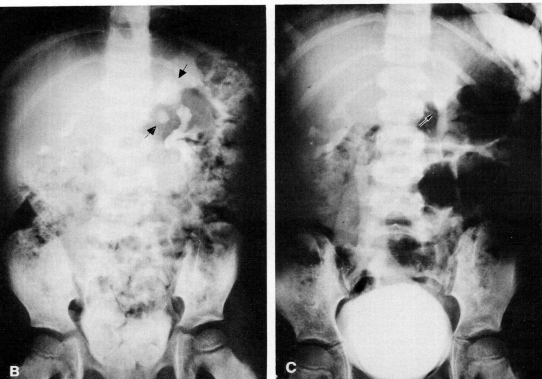

FIG. 17–54. Neuroblastoma. Fourteen-month-old child with unexplained fevers and left upper quadrant mass **(A)**. At admission, IVP demonstrated left adrenal mass with depression of kidney. Widespread osseous lytic metastases were evident. Biopsy of the tibia showed neuroblastoma. **(B)** After radiotherapy and chemotherapy to the abdominal mass, IVP 2 years later demonstrated calcifications in left suprarenal area (*arrows*) without evidence of mass. The bones now appear normal. **(C)** Four years after therapy, the calcifications have contracted even further.

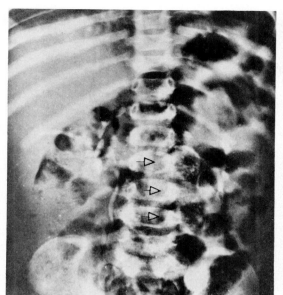

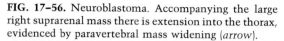

FIG. 17–55. Neuroblastoma. Left suprarenal mass with calcifications in metastatic paraortic lymph nodes to the left of the lumbar spine (*arrows*). (Meyers, M.A.: Diseases of the Adrenal Glands: Radiologic Diagnosis. Springfield, Charles C Thomas, 1963)

FIG. 17–56. Neuroblastoma. Accompanying the large right suprarenal mass there is extension into the thorax, evidenced by paravertebral mass widening (*arrow*).

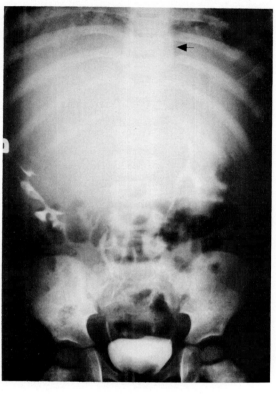

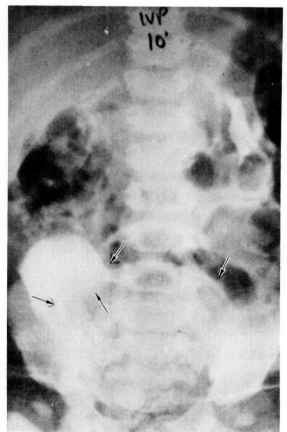

FIG. 17–57. Pelvic neuroblastoma in a child. IVP demonstrates gross distortion of the urinary bladder (*arrows*). (Meyers, M.A.: Diseases of the Adrenal Glands: Radiologic Diagnosis. Springfield, Charles C Thomas, 1963)

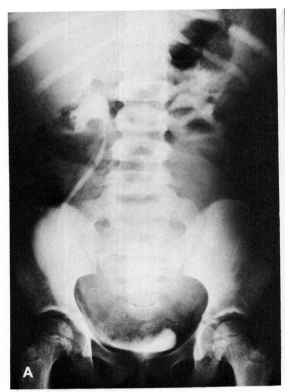

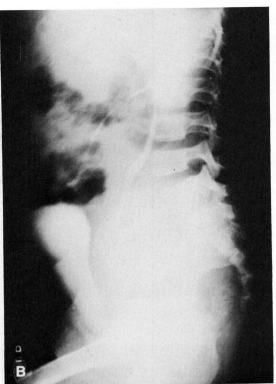

FIG. 17–58. Pelvic ganglioneuroma in a 4-and-one-half-year-old girl. The large mass displaces the ureters and urinary bladder laterally and anteriorly.

FIG. 17–59. Neuroblastoma in a 2-year-old boy with anemia and abdominal mass. **(A)** Aortogram shows downward stretching of right renal artery and rich tumor supply to mass. **(B)** Late film shows tumor blush and noninvaded nephrogram outline of right kidney. Operation revealed unresectable neuroblastoma.

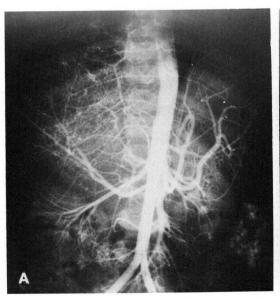

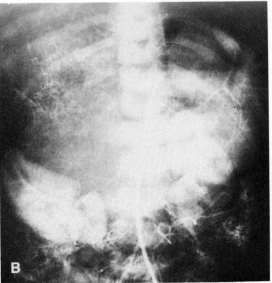

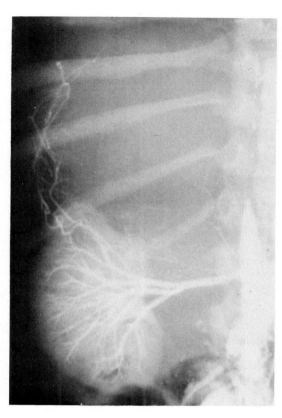

FIG. 17-60. Neuroblastoma. Selective renal arteriogram shows some neovascularity to the suprarenal tumor. (McDonald, P., and Harwood-Nash, D.C.F.: Am. J. Roentgenol., *112*:167, 1971)

FIG. 17-61. Neuroblastoma. Tumor encasement of the splenic artery on a selective celiac arteriogram is shown by smooth localized narrowing of the vessel close to its origin. (McDonald, P., and Harwood-Nash, D.C.F.: Am. J. Roentgenol., *112*:167, 1971)

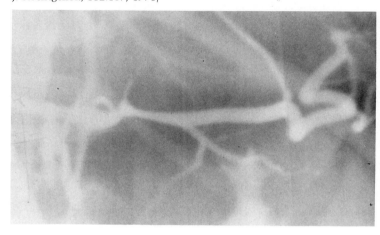

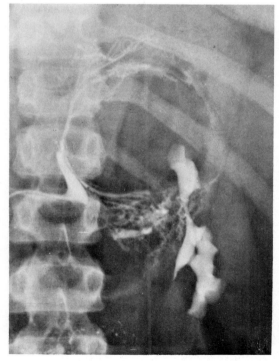

FIG. 17-62. Neuroblastoma. Adrenal venogram demonstrates circular displacement of veins by localized mass. (Cope, C., Isard, H.I., and Wesolowski, W.E.: Radiology, *90*:1105, 1968)

FIG. 17-63. Thoracic neuroblastoma. Posterior mediastinal extrapleural mass in a 4-year-old girl.

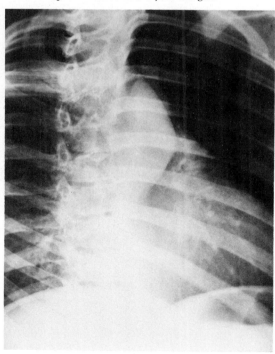

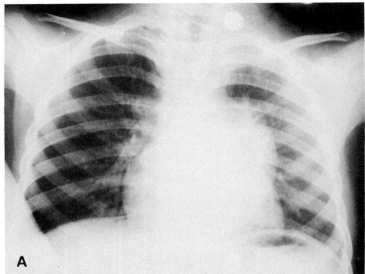

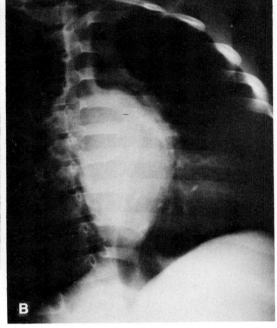

FIG. 17–64. (A,B) Thoracic neuroblastoma in a 4-year-old boy. Note the large paravertebral mass containing calcifications.

FIG. 17–65. Thoracic neuroblastoma in a 4-year-old girl. **(A)** Oblique Bucky chest film demonstrates speckled calcifications in large posterior mediastinal paravertebral mass (*arrows*). **(B)** Radiograph of resected specimen.

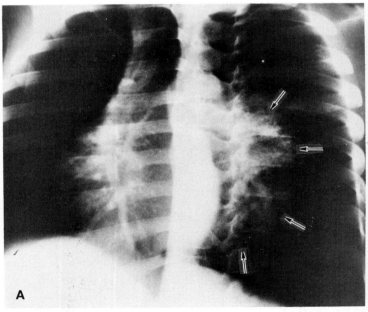

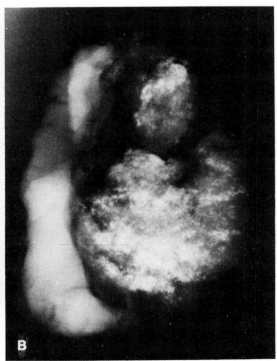

FIG. 17–66. Two cases of adrenal pseudocysts, demonstrating characteristic curvilinear and spiculated calcifications.

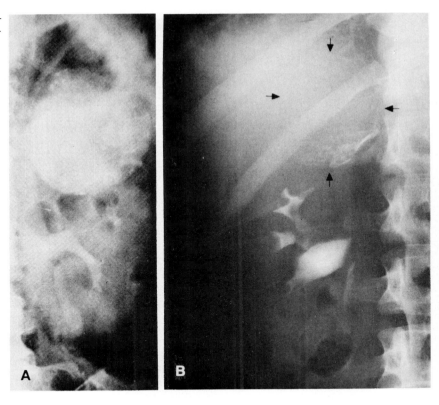

FIG. 17–67. Retroperitoneal pneumography demonstrating bilateral adrenal cysts in a woman who presented with a palpable left upper quadrant mass. The cyst on the left is dumbbell-shaped. (Courtesy of Harry Bergman, M.D.)

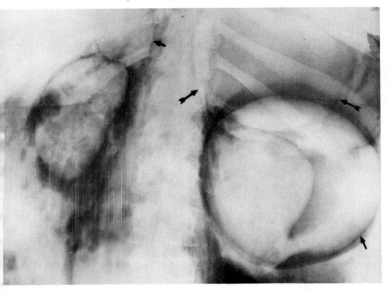

FIG. 17–68. Right adrenal pseudocyst outlined by virtue to total-body opacification during inferior venacavography. The mass is seen as a large lucent area surrounded by a thin rim of contrast material (*arrows*). The kidney is depressed and there is mild anterior displacement of the inferior vena cava.

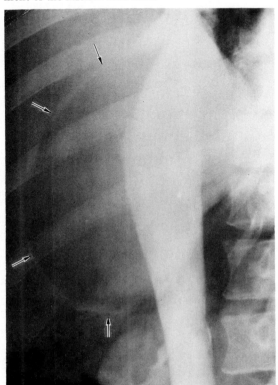

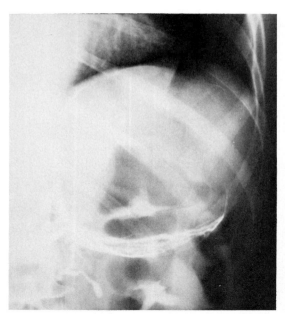

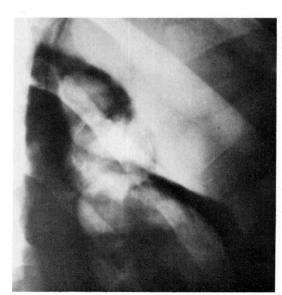

FIG. 17–69a. Right adrenal pseudocyst. Computed tomography after contrast enhancement demonstrates a smoothly contoured water-density mass with several flecks of calcium in its posterior border. (Courtesy of Carlos Reynes, M.D., Loyola University School of Medicine, Maywood, Illinois)

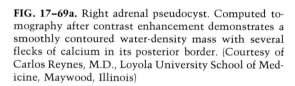

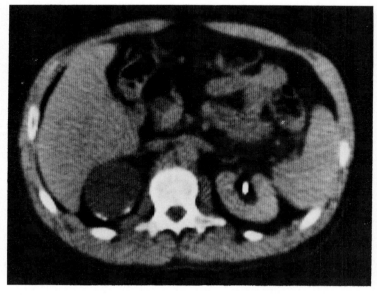

FIG. 17–70. Calcified neurofibroma of the left adrenal gland. In an 18-year-old woman, calcifications in suprarenal area were incidentally discovered on lumbosacral roentgenographic series. Retroperitoneal pneumogram outlines a lobulated mass of unusual contour, containing flakes of calcification. The tumor was actually composed of three discrete nodules, in total measuring 6 × 3.5 cm. (Meyers, M.A.: Diseases of the Adrenal Glands: Radiologic Diagnosis. Springfield, Charles C Thomas, 1963)

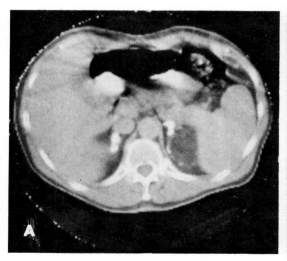

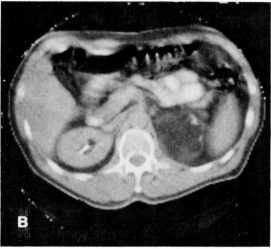

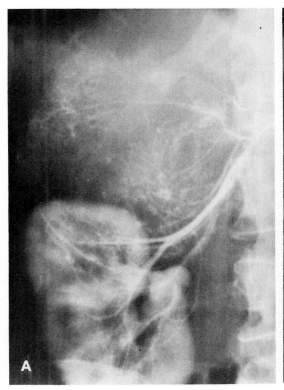

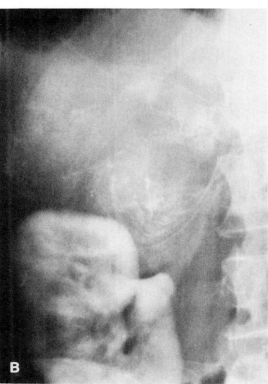

FIG. 17–71. Metastatic bronchogenic carcinoma to adrenal gland in a 65-year-old man. Renal arteriogram demonstrates tumor hypervascularity with areas of tumor staining and arteriovenous lakes.

FIG. 17–72. Bilateral adrenal metastases from bronchogenic carcinoma. Selective inferior phrenic artery injection outlines mass displacements of the superior adrenal artery branches. The metastasis within the left adrenal gland is hypervascular.

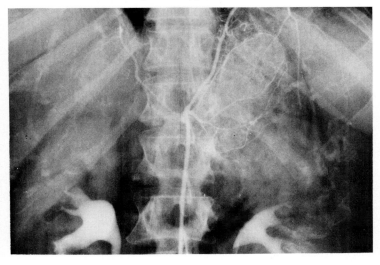

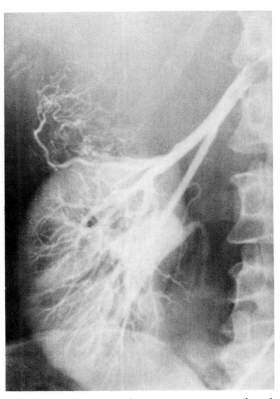

FIG. 17–70a. Myelolipoma of left adrenal gland. Computed tomography after IV contrast (**A** and **B**) demonstrates a 6.5 × 5 cm. hypovascular, predominantly fatty mass, with a calcified rim displacing the left kidney and pancreas. The findings are highly characteristic of myelolipoma.

FIG. 17–73. Metastatic breast carcinoma to adrenal. Selective renal arteriogram demonstrates plethora of irregular tumor vessels in right adrenal mass.

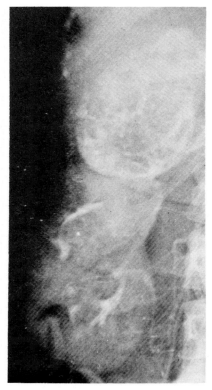

FIG. 17–74. Metastatic renal carcinoma to adrenal gland. Aortogram shows rich tumor circulation in a grossly enlarged gland. (Meyers, M.A.: Diseases of the Adrenal Glands: Radiologic Disorders. Springfield, Charles C Thomas, 1963)

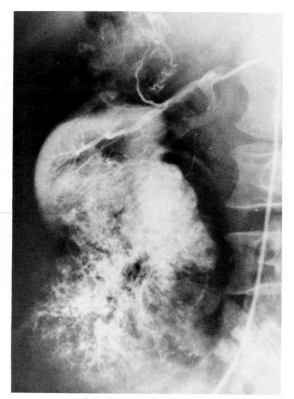

FIG. 17–75. Adrenal metastases from large, richly vascular hypernephroma of lower renal pole is shown on this selective renal arteriogram by tumor circulation from inferior adrenal artery.

FIG. 17–76. Melanoma metastatic to adrenal. In a 43-year-old woman 6 years after removal of a cutaneous malignant melanoma, selective renal arteriography demonstrates neovascularity from the inferior adrenal artery and tumor staining within a large suprarenal mass.

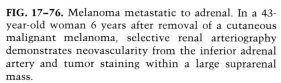

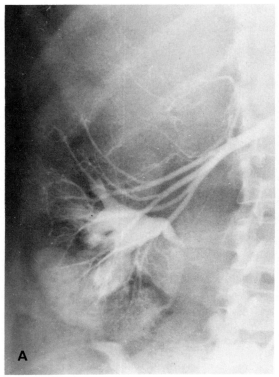

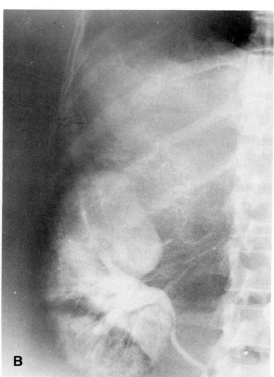

A

B

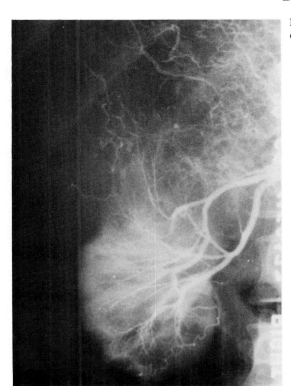

FIG. 17–77. Adrenal metastases from carcinoma of the ovary. Renal arteriogram reveals florid neovascularity.

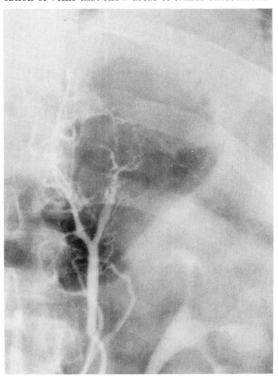

FIG. 17–78. Adrenal metastases from melanoma. Adrenal phlebography demonstrates diffuse mass with separation of veins that show areas of tumor encasement.

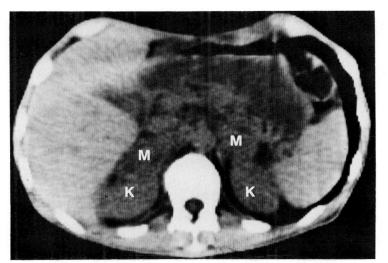

FIG. 17–78a. Bilateral adrenal metastases from bronchogenic carcinoma. Computed tomography demonstrates inhomogeneous masses (**M**) enlarging both adrenal glands. *K* = kidney. (Courtesy of Carlos Reynes, M.D., Loyola University School of Medicine, Maywood, Illinois)

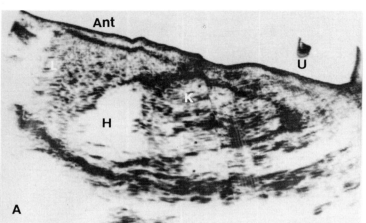

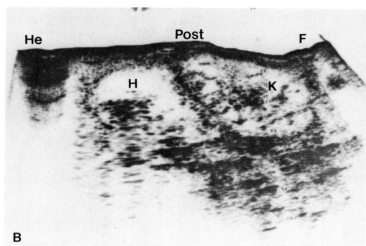

FIG. 17–78b. Neonatal adrenal hemorrhage. **(A)** Longitudinal sonogram of the right upper quadrant performed with the patient supine. The adrenal hemorrhage **(H)** is seen as an echo-free suprarenal mass. (*K* = kidney; *L* = liver; *U* = umbilicus; *Ant.* = anterior). **(B)** Longitudinal sonogram performed with the patient prone. The adrenal hemorrhage **(H)** now has an apparent echo-dense component, probably due to clot formation (*K* = kidney; *Post* = posterior; *He* = head; *F* = foot). (Mittelstaedt, C.A., Volberg, F.M., Mertenn, D.F., and Brill, P.W.: Radiology, *131*:453–457, 1979)

FIG. 17–79. Neonatal adrenal hemorrhage. Male infant presenting with prolonged jaundice. **(A)** IVP at 15 days of age demonstrates flattening of superior pole of right kidney and downward and lateral displacement of each kidney by lucent adrenal masses. Note rimlike calcification (*arrow*) in lateral aspect of right adrenal gland. **(B)** At 2 months of age, there is progressive calcification surrounding the adrenal masses. **(C)** At 3 months of age, plain film shows further regression of masses and assumption of triangular shape of calcifications. (Rose, J., Berdon, W.E., Sullivan, T., and Baker, D.H.: Radiology, *98*:263, 1971)

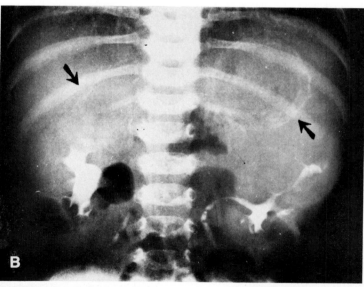

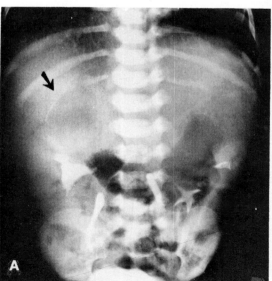

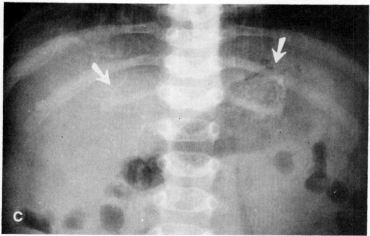

FIG. 17–80. Neonatal hemorrhage, asymptomatic. Bilateral adrenal calcifications in a two-and-one-half-month-old boy with a history of birth trauma and anoxia. Six years later, the areas of calcification had condensed.

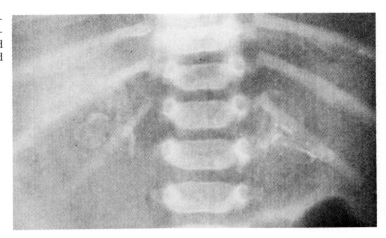

FIG. 17–81. Bilateral adrenal calcifications incidentally discovered on upper GI series in a 27-year-old man. There was no history of tuberculosis or definite trauma and no clinical evidence of adrenal disease. The calcifications are presumably the result of focal adrenal hemorrhages.

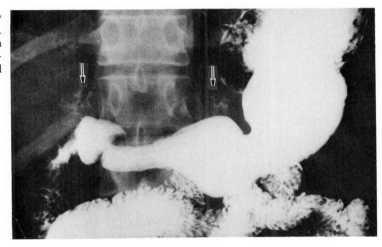

FIG. 17–82. Wolman's familial xanthomatosis. Characteristic bilateral calcifications within enlarged adrenal glands, which preserve their triangular shapes. The renal calyces are tipped down and laterally by the adrenal masses. (Rose, J., Berdon, W.E., Sullivan, T., and Baker, D.H.: Radiology, *98*:263, 1971)

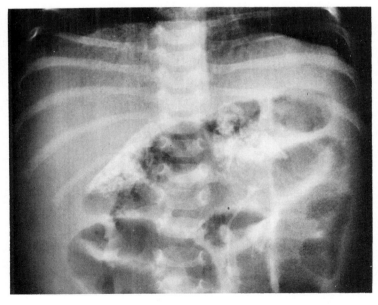

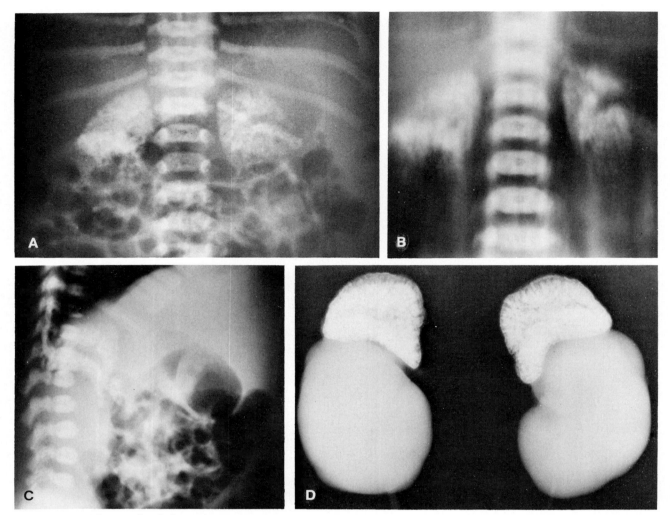

FIG. 17–83. Wolman's familial xanthomatosis in a seven-and-one-half-month-old boy. Plain film (**A**), tomogram (**B**), and lateral view (**C**) demonstrate typical, regularly distributed calcifications throughout enlarged adrenal glands that retain their triangular shapes. Postmortem radiograph (**D**) shows that these enlarged adrenals do not displace or distort the shape of the kidney. (Queloz, J.M., Captanio, M.A., and Kirkpatrick, J.A.: Radiology, *104*:357, 1972)

FIG. 17–84. The most frequent shapes of normal adrenal glands.

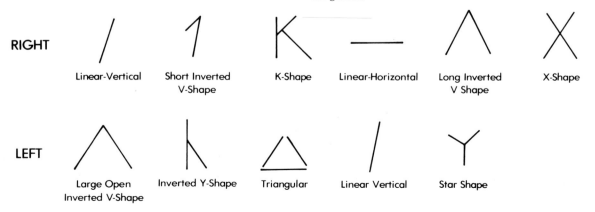

RIGHT

Linear-Vertical   Short Inverted V-Shape   K-Shape   Linear-Horizontal   Long Inverted V Shape   X-Shape

LEFT

Large Open Inverted V-Shape   Inverted Y-Shape   Triangular   Linear Vertical   Star Shape

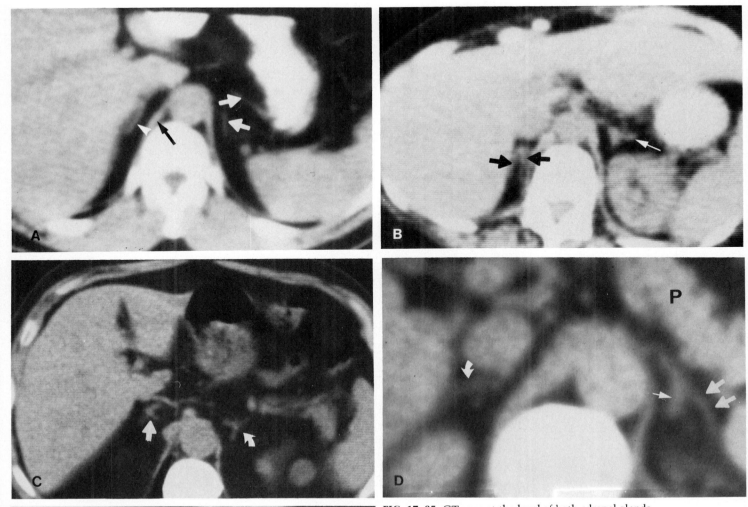

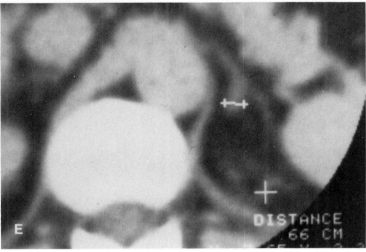

FIG. 17–85. CT scan at the level of both adrenal glands. **(A)** Right adrenal (*arrowhead*) is a linear structure coursing parallel to the diaphragmatic crura (*black arrow*) and liver. The left adrenal is shaped like an inverted V (*white arrows*). **(B)** The medial and lateral limbs of the right adrenal (*black arrows*) are clearly shown. The left adrenal (*white arrow*) is triangular in shape. **(C)** The right adrenal is K-shaped (*white arrow*) whereas the left adrenal has a Y shape (*curved arrow*). **(D)** Inverted Y-shaped left adrenal has medial limb (*arrow*) and lateral limbs (*arrows*) splitting at an acute angle. The right adrenal gland (*curved arrow*) is more horizontal in this patient. The pancreatic tail (*P*) is seen ventral to the left adrenal gland. **(E)** Thickness of the medial limb of the left adrenal is found to be 0.66 cm.

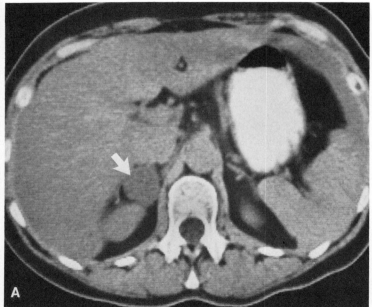

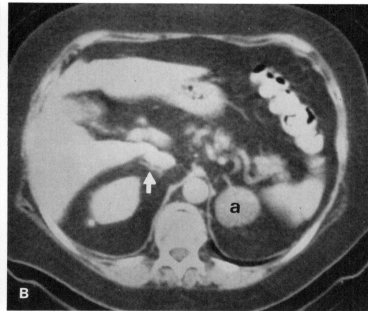

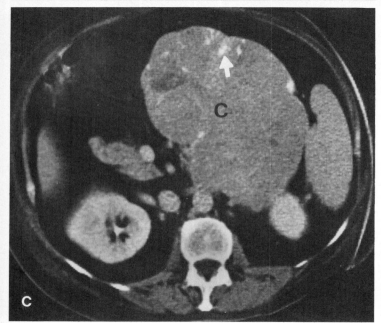

FIG. 17–86. CT scans of patients with adrenal neoplasms producing Cushing's disease. **(A)** Right adrenal adenoma (*arrow*). Note normal-sized left adrenal gland. **(B)** Rounded left adrenal adenoma (*a*) appearing as solid mass. A horizontal normal right adrenal gland (*arrow*) is present. **(C)** A very large left adrenal carcinoma (*C*) that contained calcium (*arrow*) and was hormonally active.

FIG. 17–87. CT scanning in patients with Cushing's syndrome. **(A)** CT scan in patient with pituitary tumor producing ACTH reveals diffusely thickened adrenal glands (*arrows*) that maintain a normal shape. **(B)** Bilateral nodular hyperplasia is demonstrated by CT. Both adrenal glands are thickened and contain areas of nodularity (*arrows*). The liver has a low CT attenuation due to excessive fat deposition secondary to the steroid excess.

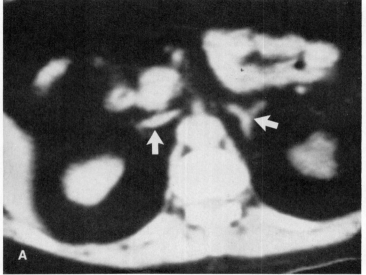

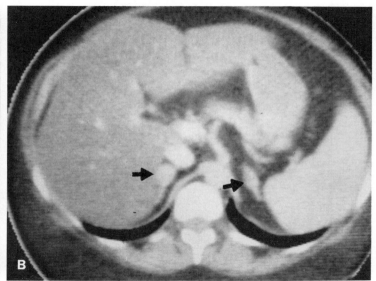

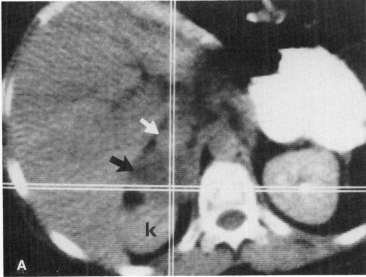

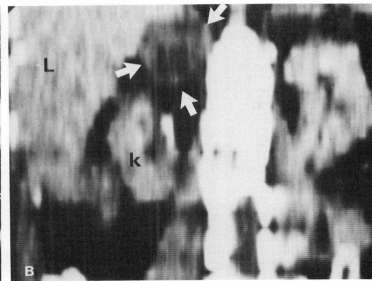

FIG. 17–88. Pheochromocytoma of right adrenal gland. **(A)** A solid mass (*black arrow*) is seen just above the right kidney (K) and posterior to the inferior vena cava (*white arrow*). The lines through the tumor are the planes of coronal and sagittal re-formation. **(B)** Axial CT image re-formatted into coronal plane demonstrates right kidney (*k*), liver (*L*), and round right pheochromocytoma (*arrows*).

FIG. 17–89. (A) CT scan demonstrating a right adrenal mass (*A*) in a patient with evidence of a pheochromocytoma. The mass appears solid on the noncontrast scan. **(B)** Following contrast administration, the mass is revealed to be nonhomogeneous with a peripheral solid component and a central lower density region (*arrow*) representing cystic degeneration of the tumor.

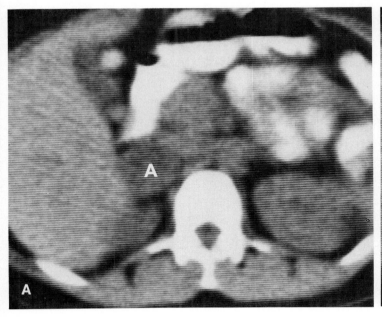

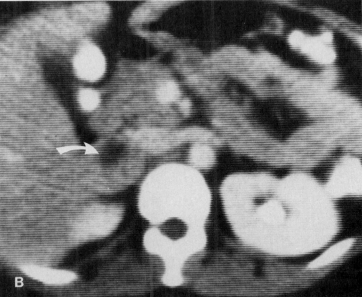

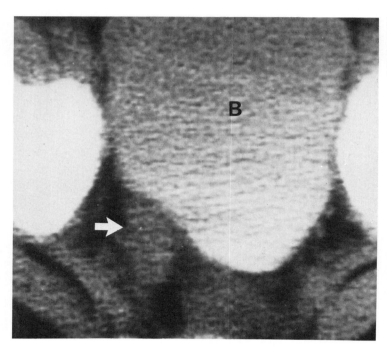

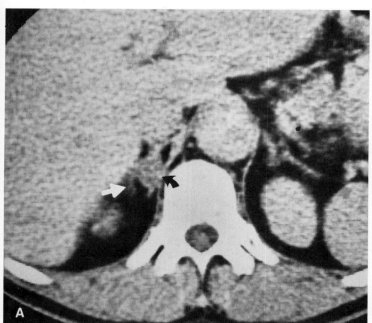

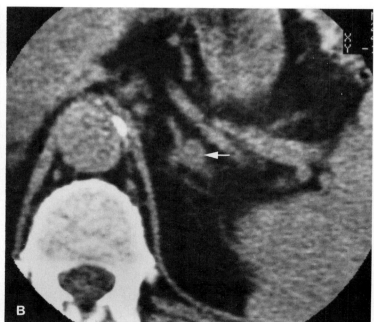

FIG. 17–90. A CT scan in a child with chemical evidence of a pheochromocytoma reveals a mass (*arrow*) in the right pelvis that distorts the bladder (*B*). An ectopic pheochromocytoma that had invaded the bladder wall was found at surgery.

FIG. 17–91. CT findings in patients with adrenal adenomas producing excess aldosterone. **(A)** Small adenoma (*black arrow*) arising in medial limb of right adrenal gland. The lateral limb (*white arrow*) of the right adrenal and the left adrenal gland are normal. **(B)** A small adenoma (*arrow*) originating from the lateral limb of the left adrenal. The tumor measured 0.7 × 1 cm. in size.

FIG. 17-92. CT scan in a patient with hyperaldosteronism produced by bilateral adrenal hyperplasia rather than by an adrenal adenoma. The outlines of the adrenal glands have been traced by the computer and demonstrate the adrenals to be bilaterally thickened but of normal shape.

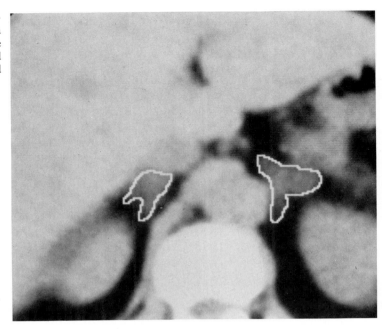

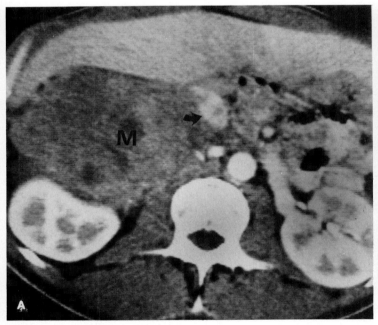

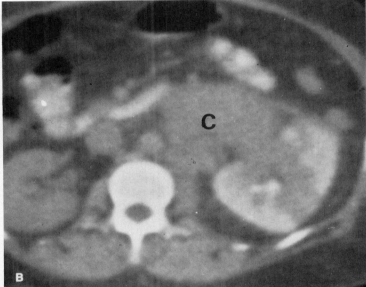

FIG. 17-93. CT findings in nonfunctioning adrenal carcinomas. **(A)** A large nonhomogeneous mass (*M*) arises in the right adrenal, depresses the right kidney, and elevates the inferior vena cava (*arrow*). **(B)** A large left adrenal carcinoma (*C*) invading the left kidney.

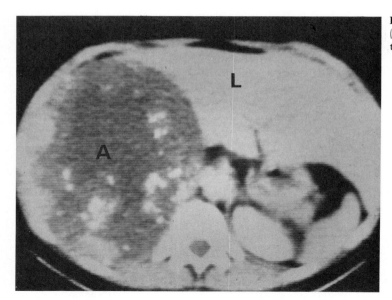

FIG. 17–94. An extremely large right adrenal adenoma (A) is demonstrated to contain calcium and to elevate the liver (L). The patient was asymptomatic.

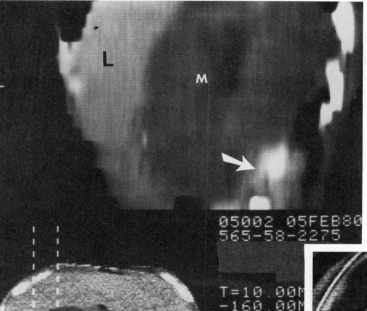

FIG. 17–95. A CT scan of a large right upper quadrant mass. In the axial display (*bottom figure*), it is difficult to determine whether the mass is adrenal or hepatic in origin. Re-formatting the axial image in the sagittal plane (*top figure*) allows the relationship of the liver (L), kidney (*arrow*), and mass (M) to be appreciated. The mass is seen to originate from the adrenal region posterior to the liver and superior to the kidney.

FIG. 17–96. A CT scan reveals a rounded mass in the left adrenal gland (*arrow*). The region-of-interest square measures the CT attenuation of the mass as −37 Old Hounsfield units. Note the normal right adrenal gland. A myelolipoma was found at surgery.

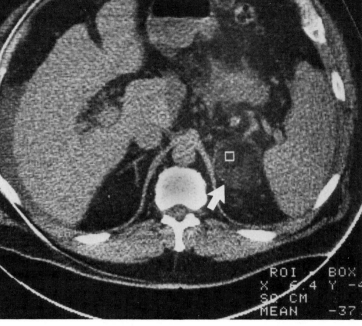

FIG. 17–97. A CT scan demonstrating a large left adrenal neuroblastoma (*N*) that contains some calcium (*arrow*).

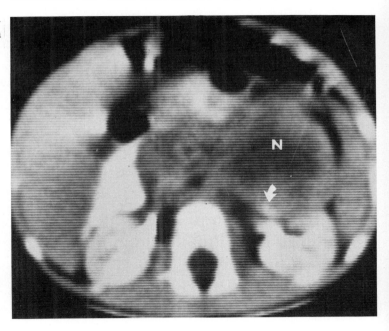

FIG. 17–98. Metastatic melanoma to both adrenal glands producing huge adrenal masses of varying CT attenuation values.

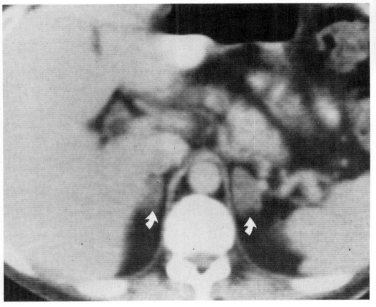

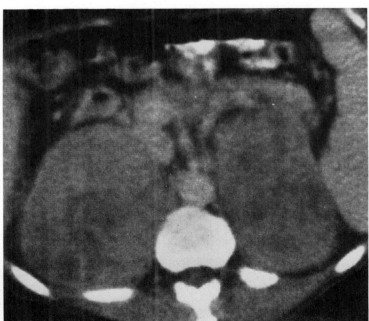

FIG. 17–99. Hypoadrenalism secondary to adrenal hemorrhage. Both adrenal glands (*arrows*) are seen to be diffusely enlarged.

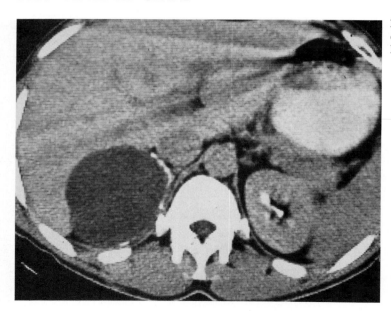

FIG. 17-100. A right adrenal cyst. CT clearly shows the cyst to have a rim of calcification and to be of uniform low density.

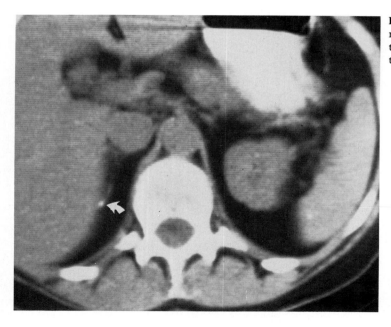

FIG. 17-101. A CT scan in a patient with histoplasmosis. There is a calcified granuloma in the spleen, and the right adrenal contains calcium (*arrow*). The patient's adrenal function was normal.

BIBLIOGRAPHY

Characteristic Shapes

1. Meyers, M.A.: Characteristic radiographic shapes of pheochromocytomas and adrenocortical adenomas. Radiology, *87*:889–892, 1966.

Cushing's Syndrome

2. Berardinelli, W., Paulione, F., Cordeiro, J.G., et al.: Sexual and somatic precocity with some features of Cushing's syndrome in a 2-year-old male. J. Clin. Endocr. Metab., *16*:674–679, 1956.

3. Bernardino, M.E., Goldstein, H.M., and Green, B.: Gray scale ultrasonography of adrenal neoplasms. A.J.R., *130*:741–744, 1978.

4. Cope, O., and Raker, J.W.: Cushing's disease. The surgical experience in the care of 46 cases. N. Engl. J. Med., *253*:119–127, 165–172, 1955.

5. Copple, P.J., and Duncan, W.Y., III: Congenital hemihypertrophy and adrenal carcinoma. Am. J. Dis. Child., *111*:419–420, 1966.

6. Cushing, H.: The basophil adenomas of the pituitary body and their clinical manifestations (pituitary basophilism). Bull. Johns Hopkins Hosp., *50*:137–195, 1932.

7. Darling, D.B., Loridan, L., and Senior, B.: The roentgenographic manifestations of Cushing's syndrome in infancy. Radiology, 96:503–508, 1970.

8. Dunnick, N.R., Schaner, E.G., Doppman, J.L., et al.: Computed tomography in adrenal tumors. A.J.R., *132*:43–46, 1979.

9. Farber, J.E., Gustina, F.J., and Postoloff, A.V.: Cushing's syndrome in children. Review of the literature and report of a case. A.M.A. Am. J. Dis. Child., 65:593–603, 1943.

10. Fraumeni, J.F., Jr., and Miller, R.W.: Adrenocortical neoplasms with hemihypertrophy, brain tumors, and other disorders. J. Pediatr., *70*:129–138, 1967.

11. Friedman, M., Marshall-Jones, P., and Ross, E.J.: Cushing's syndrome: adrenocortical hyperactivity secondary to neoplasms arising outside the pituitary–adrenal system. Q. J. Med., *35*:193–214, 1966.

12. Gilbert, M.G., and Cleveland, W.W.: Cushing's syndrome in infancy. Pediatrics, *46*:217–229, 1970.

13. Goldstein, H.M.: Cushing's syndrome due to tumor of adrenal cortex: report of a case of an eleven month old infant, with apparent operative cure. A.M.A. Am. J. Dis. Child., 78:260–278, 1949.

14. Guin, G.H., and Gilbert, E.F.: Cushing's syndrome in children associated with adrenal cortical carcinoma: a case report with review of the literature. A.M.A. Am. J. Dis. Child., 92:297–307, 1956.

15. Heinbecker, P., O'Neal, L.W., and Ackerman, L.V.: Functioning and nonfunctioning adrenal cortical tumors. Surg. Gynecol. Obstet., *105*:21–33, 1957.

16. Hinman, F., Jr., Steinbach, H.L., and Forsham, P.H.: Preoperative differentiation between hyperplasia and tumor in Cushing's syndrome. J. Urol., 77:329–338, 1957.

17. Hutter, A.M., and Kayhoe, D.E.: Adrenal cortical carcinoma. Clinical features of 138 patients. Am. J. Med., *41*:572–580, 1966.

18. Iannaccone, A., Gabrilove, J.L., Brahms, S.A., et al.: The roentgen diagnosis of adrenal tumor in Cushing's syndrome. A.M.A. Arch. Int. Med., *105*:257–263, 1960.

19. Jailer, J.W., Gold, J.J., and Wallace, E.Z.: Evaluation of the "cortisone test" as a diagnostic aid in differentiating adrenal hyperplasia from adrenal neoplasia. Am. J. Med., *16*:340–345, 1954.

20. Klevit, H.D., Campbell, R.A., Blair, H.R., et al.: Cushing's syndrome with nodular adrenal hyperplasia in infancy. J. Pediatr., *68*:912–920, 1966.

21. Knowlton, A.I.: Cushing's syndrome. Bull. N.Y. Acad. Med., *29*:441–465, 1953.

22. Koerner, H.J., and Sun, D.I-C.: Mediastinal lipomatosis secondary to steroid therapy. Amer. J. Roentgenol., 98:461–464, 1966.

23. Kovach, R.D., and Kyle, L.H.: Cushing's syndrome and bronchogenic carcinoma. Am. J. Med., 24:981–988, 1958.

24. Kyle, L.H., Meyer, R.J., and Canary, J.J.: Mechanism of adrenal atrophy in Cushing's syndrome due to adrenal tumor. N. Engl. J. Med., *257*:57–61, 1957.

25. Laidlaw, J.C., Reddy, W.J., Jenkins, D., et al.: Advances in diagnosis of altered states of adrenalcortical function. N. Engl. J. Med., *258*:747–753, 1955.

26. Liddle, G.W., Estep, H.L., Kendall, J.W., Jr., et al.: Clinical application of a new test of pituitary reserve. J. Clin. Endocrinol. Metab., *19*:875–894, 1960.

27. Liddle, G.W., and Givens, J.R., Nicholson, W.E., et al.: The ectopic ACTH syndrome. Cancer Res., *25*:1057–1061, 1965.

28. Liddle, G.W., Island, D.P., Ney, R.L., et al.: Nonpituitary neoplasms and Cushing's syndrome. Arch. Intern. Med., *111*:471–475, 1963.

29. Litt, R.E., and Altman, D.H.: Significance of the muscle cylinder ratio in infancy. Am. J. Roentgenol., *100*:80–87, 1967.

30. Loridan, L., and Senior, B.: Cushing's syndrome in infancy. J. Pediatr., *75*:349–359, 1969.

31. Madell, S.H., and Freeman, L.M.: Avascular necrosis of bone in Cushing's syndrome. Radiology, 83:1068–1070, 1964.

32. Marks, V., Samols, E., and Bolton, R.: Hyperinsulinism and Cushing's syndrome. Br. Med. J., *1*:1419–1420, 1965.

33. Meyers, M.A.: Diseases of the Adrenal Glands: Radiologic Diagnosis with Emphasis on the Use of Presacral Retroperitoneal Pneumography. Charles C Thomas, Springfield, Ill., 1963.

34. Miller, W.T., and Restifo, R.A.: Steroid arthropathy. Radiology, 86:652–657, 1966.

35. Mitty, H.A., Gabrilove, J.L., and Nicolis, G.L.: Nontumerous adrenal hyperfunction: Problems in angiographic-clinical correlation. Radiology, *122*:89–94, 1977.

36. Murray, R.O.: Steroids and the skeleton. Radiology, 77:729–743, 1961.

37. Neville, A.M., and Symington, T.: The pathology of the adrenal gland in Cushing's syndrome. J. Pathol. Bacteriol., *93*:19–35, 1967.

38. Plotz, C.M., Knowlton, A.I., and Ragan, C.: The natural history of Cushing's syndrome. Am. J. Med., *13*:597–614, 1952.

39. Powell, L.W., Jr., Newman, S., and Hooker, J.W.: Cushing's syndrome: report of a case in an infant twelve week's old. A.M.A. Am. J. Dis. Child., 90:417–420, 1955.

40. Reynes, C.J., Churchill, R., Moncada, R., et al.: Computed tomography of adrenal glands. Radiol. Clin. North Am., *17*:91–104, 1979.

41. Riggs, B.L., Jowsey, J., and Kelly, P.J.: Quantitative microradiographic study of bone remodeling in Cushing's syndrome. Metabolism, *15*:773–780, 1966.

42. Riggs, B.L., Jr., and Sprague, R.G.: Association of Cushing's syndrome and neoplastic disease. Arch. Int. Med., *108*:85–93, 1961.

43. Soffer, L.J., Iannaccone, A., and Gabrilove, J.L.: Cushing's syndrome—a study of fifty patients. Am. J. Med., *30*:129–146, 1961.

44. Steinbach, H.L., and Smith, D.L.: Extraperitoneal pneumography in diagnosis of retroperitoneal tumors. A.M.A. Arch. Surg., *70*:161–172, 1955.

45. Sussman, M.L., and Copleman, B.: The roentgenographic appearance of the bones in Cushing's syndrome. Radiology, *39*:288–292, 1942.

46. Tucci, J.R., Jagger, P.I., Lauler, D.P., et al.: Rapid dexamethasone suppression test for Cushing's syndrome. J.A.M.A., *199*:129–132, 1967.

47. Tyrrell, J.B., Brooks, R.M., Fitzgerald, P.A., et al.: Cushing's disease: Selective trans-sphenoidal resection of pituitary microadenomas. N. Engl. J. Med., *298*:753–758, 1978.

48. Wang, C.C., and Robbins, L.L.: Cushing's diseases: its roentgenographic findings. Radiology, *67*:17–25, 1956.

49. Weidner, M.G., Jr., and Towery, B.T.: Adrenocortical adenoma with Cushing's syndrome in infancy. Surgery, *39*:492–497, 1956.

50. Yeh, H.-C., Mitty, H.A., Rose, J., et al.: Ultrasonography of adrenal masses: Usual features. Radiology, *127*:467–474, 1978.

51. Yeh, H.-C., Mitty, H.A., Rose, J., et al.: Ultrasonography of adrenal masses: Unusual manifestations. Radiology, *127*:475–483, 1978.

Nelson's Syndrome

52. Moore, T.J., Dhuly, R.G., Williams, G.H., et al.: Nelson's syndrome: Frequency, prognosis, and effect of prior pituitary irradiation. Ann. Intern. Med., 85:731–734, 1976.
53. Nelson, D.H., Meakin, J.W., Dealy, J.B., Jr., et al.: ACTH-producing tumor of pituitary gland. N. Engl. J. Med., 259:161–164, 1958.
54. Hopwood, N., and Kenny, F.: Increased incidence of postadrenalectomy Nelson's syndrome in pediatric vs. adult Cushing's disease: Nationwide study. Pediatrics, 9:290, 1975.
55. Rovit, R.L., and Berry, R.: Cushing's syndrome and the hypophysis: Re-evaluation of pituitary tumors and hyperadrenalism. J. Neurosurg., 23:270–295, 1965.
56. Weinstein, M., Tyrell, B., and Newton, T.H.: The sella turcica in Nelson's syndrome. Radiology, 118:363–365, 1976.
57. Young, L.W., Lim, H.K., Forbes, G.B., et al.: Postadrenalectomy pituitary adenoma (Nelson's Syndrome) in childhood: Clinical and roentgenologic detection. Am. J. Roentgenol., 126:550–559, 1976.

Adrenogenital Syndrome

58. Bentinck, R.C., Hinman, F., Sr., Lisser, H., et al.: The familial congenital adrenal syndrome: Report of two cases and review of the literature. Postgrad. Med., 11:301–312, 1952.
59. Blair, A.J., and Reuter, S.R.: Adrenal venography in virilized women. J.A.M.A., 213:1623–1629, 1970.
60. Bongiovanni, A.M., and Root, A.W.: Adrenogenital syndrome. N. Engl. J. Med., 268:1283–1289, 1342–1351, 1391–1399, 1963.
61. Fischer, E., and Nowakowski, H.: Joint-like cleft formations in calcified cartilages of ribs in adrenogenital syndrome. Fortschr. a. d. Geb. d. Rontgenstrahlen, 84:57–61, 1956.
62. Gabrilove, J.L., Sharma, D.C., Wotiz, H.H., et al.: Feminizing adrenocortical tumors in the male. Medicine, 44:37–79, 1965.
63. Goldstein, A.E., Rubin, S.W., and Askin, J.A.: Carcinoma of adrenal cortex with adrenogenital syndrome in children. Complete review of the literature and report of a case with recovery in a child 8 months of age. A.M.A. Am. J. Dis. Child., 72:563–603, 1946.
64. Greenblatt, R.B., Chaney, R.H., and Clark, S.L.: Adrenal virilism in a three year old girl. Am. Surg., 17:760–769, 1951.
65. Gross, R.W., and Meeker, I.A., Jr.: Abnormalities of sexual development: Observations from 75 cases. Pediatrics, 16:303–324, 1955.
66. Heinbecker, P., O'Neal, L.W., and Ackerman, L.V.: Functioning and nonfunctioning adrenal cortical tumors. Surg. Gynecol. Obstet., 105:21–33, 1957.
67. Hiekkala, H., Sulamaa, M., and Takkanen, R.: Adrenogenital syndrome in children: Review of 22 cases. Ann. Paediatr. Fenn., 7:189–205, 1961.
68. Higgins, G.A., Brownlee, W.E., and Mantz, F.A.: Feminizing tumors of the adrenal cortex. Am. Surg., 22:56–79, 1956.
69. Hutter, A.M., and Kayhoe, D.E.: Adrenal cortical carcinoma. Clinical features of 138 patients. Am. J. Med., 41:572–580, 1966.
70. Huvos, A.G., Hajou, S.I., Brasfield, R.D., et al.: Adrenal cortical carcinoma: Clinicopathologic study of 34 cases. Cancer, 25:354–361, 1970.
71. Kurlander, G.J.: Roentgenology of the congenital adrenogenital syndrome. Am. J. Roentgenol., 95:189–199, 1965.

72. Levin, B., Rambar, A.C., and Shapiro, I.J.: Female pseudohermaphroditism. Report of a case proved roentgenologically. Am. J. Roentgenol., 69:948–952, 1953.
73. Maresh, M.: Changes in tissue widths during growth. Am. J. Dis. Child., 111:142–155, 1966.
74. Mellman, W.J., Bongiovanni, A.M., and Hope, J.W.: Diagnostic usefulness of skeletal maturation in endocrine clinic. Pediatrics, 23:530–544, 1959.
75. Paquin, A.J., Jr., Baker, D.H., Finby, N., et al.: Urogenital sinus: its demonstration and significance. J. Urol., 78:796–807, 1957.
76. Prader, V.A.: Der genitalbefund beim pseudohermaphroditismus femininus des kongenitalen adrenogenitalen syndroms. Acta Helv. Paediatr., 9:231–248, 1954.
77. Staubitz, W.J., Oberkircher, O.J., Lent, M.H., et al.: Feminization in an adult male with adrenal cortical carcinoma. N.Y. J. Med., 54:2565–2572, 1954.
78. Tristan, T.A., Eberlein, W.R., and Hope, J.W.: Roentgenologic investigation of patients with heterosexual development. Am. J. Roentgenol., 76:562–568, 1956.
79. Wagner, R., Cohen, M.M., and Hunt, E.E., Jr.: Dental development in idiopathic sexual precocity, congenital adrenocortical hyperplasia, and adrenogenic virilism. J. Pediatr., 63:566–576, 1963.
80. Weens, H.S., and Golden, A.: Adrenal cortical insufficiency in infants simulating high intestinal obstruction. Am. J. Roentgenol., 74:213–219, 1955.

Primary Aldosteronism

81. Brode, E., Grant, J.K., and Symington, T.: A biochemical and pathological investigation of adrenal tissues from patients with Conn's syndrome. Acta Endocrinol. Copenh., 41:411–431, 1962.
82. Cerny, J.C., Nesbit, R., and Conn, J.: Preoperative tumor localization by adrenal venography in patients with primary aldosteronism. J. Urol., 103:521–528, 1970.
83. Conn, J.W.: Primary aldosteronism: A new clinical syndrome. J. Lab. Clin. Med., 45:6–17, 1955.
84. Conn, J.W.: Aldosteronism in clinical medicine—past, present and future. A.M.A. Arch. Int. Med., 97:135–144, 1956.
85. Conn, J.W.: Aldosteronism and hypertension: primary aldosteronism versus hypertensive disease with secondary aldosteronism. Arch. Int. Med., 107:813–823, 1961.
86. Conn, J.W., Knopf, R.F., and Nesbit, R.M.: Clinical characteristics of primary aldosteronism from an analysis of 145 cases. Am. J. Surg., 107:159–172, 1964.
87. Conn, J.W., and Louis, L.W.: Primary aldosteronism, a new clinical entity. Ann. Int. Med., 44:1–15, 1956.
88. Dunnick, N.R., Schaner, E.G., Doppman, J.L., et al.: Computed tomography in adrenal tumors. A.J.R., 132:43–46, 1979.
89. Egdahl, R.H., Kahn, P.C., and Melby, J.C.: Unilateral adrenolectomy for aldosteronomas localized preoperatively by differential adrenal vein catheterization. Surgery, 64:117–125, 1968.
90. Foye, L.V., Jr., and Feichtmeir, T.V.: Adrenal cortical carcinoma producing solely mineralocorticoid effect. Am. J. Med., 19:966–975, 1955.
91. Horton, R., and Finck, E.: Diagnosis and localization in primary aldosteronism. Ann. Int. Med., 76:885–890, 1972.
92. Kahn, P.C., Kelleher, D., Egdahl, R.H., et al.: Adrenal arteriography and venography in primary aldosteronism. Radiology, 101:71–78, 1971.

93. Melby, J.C., Spark, R.F., Dale, S.L., et al.: Diagnosis and localization of aldosterone-producing adenomas by adrenal-vein catheterization. N. Engl. J. Med., 277:1050–1056, 1967.

94. Mitty, H., Nicolis, G.L., and Gabrilove, J.L.: Adrenal venography: Clinical–roentgenographic correlation in 80 patients. Am. J. Roentgenol., 119:564–575, 1973.

95. Reynes, C.J., Churchill, R., Moncada, R., et al.: Computed tomography of the adrenal glands. Radiol. Clin. North Am., 17:91–104, 1979.

96. Scoggins, B.A., Odie, C.J., Hare, W.S.C., et al.: Preoperative lateralisation of aldosterone-producing tumours in primary aldosteronism. Ann. Int. Med., 76:891–897, 1972.

97. Spark, R.F., Dale, S.L., Kahn, P.C., et al.: Activation of aldosterone secretion in primary aldosteronism. J. Clin. Invest., 48:96–104, 1969.

98. van Buchem, F.S.P., Doorenbos, H., and Elings, H.S.: Primary aldosteronism due to adrenocortical hyperplasia. Lancet, 2:335–337, 1956.

99. Yeh, H.-C., Mitty, H.A., Rose, J., et al.: Ultrasonography of adrenal masses: Usual features. Radiology, 127:467–474, 1978.

100. Yeh, H.-C., Mitty, H.A., Rose, J., et al.: Ultrasonography of adrenal masses: Unusual manifestations. Radiology, 127:475–483, 1978.

Nonfunctioning Cortical Tumors

101. Cleveland, M., and Knox, L.C.: Bilateral carcinoma of the adrenal cortex with metastasis to the iliac bone. A.M.A. Arch. Surg., 47:192–202, 1943.

102. Commons, R.R., and Callaway, C.D.: Adenomas of the adrenal cortex. Arch. Int. Med., 81:37–41, 1948.

103. Cottler, Z.R.: Nonhormonal adrenal cortical carcinoma: Report of a case with five year survival and relief of hypertension. J. Urol., 60:363–370, 1948.

104. Gordon, W.: Nonhormonal adrenal adenoma: A report of two cases. J. Urol., 75:579–585, 1956.

105. Heinbecker, P., O'Neal, L.W., and Ackerman, L.V.: Functioning and nonfunctioning adrenal cortical tumors. Surg. Gynecol. Obstet., 105:21–33, 1957.

106. Russi, S., Blumenthal, H.T., and Gray, S.H.: Small adenomas of the adrenal cortex in hypertension and diabetes. Arch. Int. Med., 76:284–291, 1945.

107. Sampliner, J., and Marks, C.: Non-functioning adrenocortical carcinoma. Am. Surg., 37:375–380, 1971.

Addison's Disease

108. Addison, T.: On the Constitutional and Local Effects of Disease of the Suprarenal Capsules. Highley, London, 1855.

109. Anderson, J.R., Buchanan, W.W., and Goudie, R.B.: Autoimmunity, Clinical and Experimental, p. 216. Charles C Thomas, Springfield, Ill., 1967.

110. Ball, R.G., Greene, C.H., Camp, J.D., et al.: Calcification in tuberculosis of the suprarenal glands: Roentgenographic study in Addison's disease. J.A.M.A., 48:954–961, 1932.

111. Barker, N.W.: The pathologic anatomy in twenty-eight cases of Addison's disease. Arch. Pathol., 8:432–450, 1929.

112. Baronchelli, A., and Rossi, L.: Retropneumoperitoneo e stratigrafia nella semeiologia delle ghiandole surrenali. Ann. Radiol. Diag., 27:261–297, 1954.

113. Blizzard, R.M., and Kyle, M.: Studies of the adrenal antigens and antibodies in Addison's disease. J. Clin. Invest., 42:1653–1660, 1963.

114. Camp, J.D., Ball, R.G., and Greene, C.H.: Calcification of the suprarenal glands in Addison's disease. Roentgenographic study. Am. J. Roentgenol., 28:594–597, 1932.

115. Cocchi, U.: Retropneumoperitoneum und Pneumomediastinum. Fortschr. Rontgenstrahl. ERG., 79:1–226, 1957.

116. Dunlop, D.: Eighty-six cases of Addison's Disease. Br. Med. J., 5362:887–891, 1963.

117. Guttman, P.H.: Addison's disease: A statistical analysis of five hundred and sixty-six cases and a study of the pathology. Arch. Pathol., 10:742–785, 1930.

118. Ingram, F.L.: Calcification of the suprarenals in Addison's disease. Br. J. Radiol., 23:232–233, 1950.

119. Jarvis, J.L., Jenkins, D., Sosman, M.C., et al.: Roentgenologic observations in Addison's disease. A review of 120 cases. Radiology, 62:16–28, 1954.

120. Jaudon, J.C.: Addison's disease in children. J. Pediatr., 28:737–755, 1946.

121. Morgan, H.E., Austin, J.H.M., and Follett, D.A.: Bilateral adrenal enlargement in Addison's disease caused by tuberculosis. Radiology, 115:357–358, 1975.

122. Rolleston, H.D., and Boyd, E.J.: Addison's disease in a boy with calcification of the adrenals, with remarks. Br. J. Child. Dis., 11:105–111, 1914.

123. Sanford, J.P., and Favour, C.B.: The interrelationships between Addison's disease and active tuberculosis: A review of 125 cases of Addison's disease. Ann. Int. Med., 45:56–72, 1956.

124. Sloper, J.C.: The pathology of the adrenals, thymus and certain other endocrine glands in Addison's disease: An analysis of 37 necropsies. Proc. Royal Soc. Med., 48:625–628, 1955.

125. Snelling, C.E., and Erb, I.H.: Suprarenal atrophy. J. Pediatr., 7:669–681, 1935.

126. Steinbach, H.L., and Smith, D.L.: Extraperitoneal pneumography in diagnosis of retroperitoneal tumors. A.M.A. Arch. Surg., 70:161–172, 1955.

127. Thorn, G.W.: Adrenal Insufficiency. Charles C Thomas, Springfield, Ill., 1951.

128. Weens, H.S., and Golden, A.: Adrenal cortical insufficiency in infants simulating high intestinal obstruction. Am. J. Roentgenol., 74:213–219, 1955.

Pheochromocytoma

129. Albers, D.D., Kalmon, E.H., and Back, K.: Pheochromocytoma: Report of five cases, one a spontaneous cure. J. Urol., 78:301–308, 1957.

130. Attia, A., Golden, R.L., and Ziffer, H.: Nonchromaffin-staining functional tumor of the organs of Zuckerkandl. N. Engl. J. Med., 264:1130–1133, 1961.

131. Bartels, E.C.: Malignant pheochromocytoma. S. Clin. N. Amer., 39:805–808, 1959.

132. Baum, S., Stein, G., Roy, R., and Finkelstein, A.: Arteriography in diagnosis of abdominal disease. Postgrad. Med., 38:547–567, 1965.

133. Besser, M.I.B., and Pfau, A.: Phaeochromocytoma of the urinary bladder. Br. J. Urol., 40:245–247, 1968.

134. Beer, E., King, F.H., and Prinzmetal, M.: Pheochromocytoma with demonstration of pressor (adrenalin) substance in the blood preoperatively during hypertensive crises. Ann. Surg., 106:85–91, 1937.

135. Bernardino, M.E., Goldstein, H.M., and Green, B.: Gray scale ultrasonography of adrenal neoplasms. A.J.R., 130:741–744, 1978.

136. Boijsen, E., Williams, C.M., and Judkins, M.P.: Angiography of Pheochromocytoma. Am. J. Roentgenol., *98*:225–232, 1966.

137. Bourne, R.B., and Beltaos, E.: Pheochromocytoma of the bladder: Case report and summary of literature. J. Urol., *98*:361–364, 1967.

138. Brines, O.A., and Jennings, E.R.: Paragangliomas: Review of subject and report of 5 original cases. Am. J. Pathol., *24*:1167–1197, 1948.

139. Cahill, G.F.: Pheochromocytoma: Diagnosis and treatment. J. Urol., *67*:779–795, 1952.

140. Carman, C.T., and Brashear, R.E.: Pheochromocytoma as an inherited abnormality. Report of the tenth affected kindred and review of the literature. N. Engl. J. Med., *263*:419–423, 1960.

141. Christenson, R., Smith, C.W., and Burko, H.: Arteriographic manifestations of pheochromocytoma. Am. J. Roentgenol., *126*:567–575, 1976.

142. Ciccantelli, M.J., Gallagher, W.B., Skemp, F.C., et al.: Fatal nephropathy and adrenal necrosis after translumbar aortography. N. Engl. J. Med., *258*:433–435, 1958.

143. Cohen, S.M., and Persky, L.: Malignant non-chromaffin paraganglioma with metastasis to the kidney. J. Urol., *96*:122–126, 1966.

144. Colapinto, R.F., and Steed, B.L.: Arteriography of adrenal tumors. Radiology, *100*:343–350, 1971.

145. Cornell, S.H.: Pheochromocytomas of the lumbar sympathetic chain demonstrated by angiography. Am. J. Roentgenol., *115*:175–178, 1972.

146. Cragg, R.W.: Concurrent tumors of the left carotid body and both Zuckerkandl Bodies. Arch. Pathol., *18*:635–645, 1934.

147. Davis, F.W., Hull, J.G., and Vardell, J.C.: Pheochromocytoma with neurofibromatosis. Am. J. Med., *8*:131–135, 1950.

148. DeCourcy, J.L.: Pheochromocytoma. Am. J. Surg., *86*:37–44, 1953.

149. Duffy, T.J., Erickson, E.E., Jordan, J.L., Jr., et al.: Megacolon and bilateral pheochromocytoma. Am. J. Gastroenterol., *38*:555–563, 1962.

150. Dunnick, N.R., Schaner, E.G., Doppman, J.L., et al.: Computed tomography in adrenal tumors. A.J.R., *132*:43–46, 1979.

151. Ellis, F.H., Jr., Dawe, C.J., and Claggett, O.T.: Cysts of the adrenal glands. Ann. Surg., *136*:217–227, 1952.

152. Engelman, K., and Sjoerdsma, A.: A new test for pheochromocytoma. Pressor responsiveness to tyramine. J.A.M.A., *189*:81–86, 1964.

153. English, J.T., Patel, S.K., and Flanagan, M.J.: Association of pheochromocytomas with brown fat tumors. Radiology, *107*:279–281, 1973.

154. Farley, S.E., and Smith, C.L.: Unusual location of pheochromocytoma in urinary bladder. J. Urol., *81*:130–132, 1959.

155. Feist, J., and Lasser, E.: Pheochromocytoma with large cytic calcification and associated sphenoid ridge malformation. Radiology, *76*:21–25, 1961.

156. Fries, J.G., and Chamberlin, J.A.: Extra-adrenal pheochromocytoma: literature review and report of a cervical pheochromocytoma. Surgery, *63*:268–279, 1968.

157. Fry, I.K., Kerr, I.H., Thomas, M.L., et al.: Value of aortography in diagnosis of pheochromocytoma. Clin. Radiol., *18*:276–281, 1967.

158. Ganem, E.J., and Cahill, G.F.: Pheochromocytomas coexisting in adrenal gland and retroperitoneal space with sustained hypertension. Report of a case with surgical cure. N. Engl. J. Med., *238*:692–697, 1948.

159. Gifford, R.W., Kvale, W.F., Maher, F.T., et al.: Clinical features, diagnosis and treatment of pheochromocytoma: A review of 76 cases. Mayo Clin. Proc., *39*:281–302, 1964.

160. Glushien, A.S., Mansuy, M.M., and Littman, D.S.: Pheochromocytoma: Its relationship to the neurocutaneous syndromes. Am. J. Med., *14*:318–327, 1953.

161. Graham, J.B.: Pheochromocytoma and hypertension. An analysis of 207 cases. Int. Surg. (Abstr.), *92*:105–121, 1951.

162. Grainger, R.G., Lloyd, G.A.S., and Williams, J.L.: Egg-shell calcification: A sign of phaeochromocytoma. Clin. Radiol., *18*:282–286, 1967.

163. Guttmann, G.E.: Pheochromocytoma: Case report of a pheochromocytoma in a 23-month-old child with survival. Wisconsin M.J., *56*:235–237, 1957.

164. Haberman, E.T., Millheiser, P.J., and Casten, D.F.: Pheochromocytoma in the organ of Zuckerkandl presenting with gastro-intestinal symptoms. J. Clin. Endocr., *24*:334–338, 1964.

165. Harrison, T.S., Bartlett, J.D., Jr., and Seaton, J.F.: Current evaluation and management of pheochromocytoma. Ann. Surg., *168*:701–712, 1968.

166. Harrison, T.S., Seaton, J.F., Cerny, J.C., et al.: Localization of pheochromocytoma by caval catheterization. Arch. Surg., *95*:339–343, 1967.

167. Haug, W.A., and Baker, H.W.: Malignant paraganglioma of the organ of Zuckerkandl. Arch. Path., *62*:335–339, 1956.

168. Hidalgo, F., and Williams, D.F.: Diagnóstico del feochromocitoma de la vesiga. Rev. Med. Chile, *97*:128–132, 1969.

169. Holsti, L.R.: Malignant extra-adrenal pheochromocytoma. Br. J. Radiol., *37*:944–947, 1964.

170. Hume, D.M.: Pheochromocytoma in the adult and in the child. Am. J. Surg., *99*:458–496, 1960.

171. James, R.E., Baker, H.L., Jr., and Scanlon, P.W.: The roentgenologic aspects of metastatic pheochromocytoma. Am. J. Roentgenol., *115*:783–793, 1972.

172. Joseph, L.: Malignant phaeochromocytoma of the organ of Zuckerkandl with functioning metastases. Br. J. Urol., *39*:221–225, 1967.

173. Kindler, H., and Kuemmerle, H.P.: Zur topischen Diagnostik des Phaochromozytoms. Fortschr. Rontgenstrahlen, *85*:330–333, 1956.

174. Kinkhabwala, M.N., and Conradi, H.: Angiography of extra-adrenal pheochromocytomas. J. Urol., *108*:666–668, 1972.

175. Kohler, R., and Holsti, L.R.: Angiographic localization of suprarenal tumors. Acta Radiol., *4*:21–32, 1966.

176. Koonce, D.H., Pollock, B.E., and Glassy, F.J.: Bilateral pheochromocytoma associated with neurofibromatosis. Am. Heart J., *44*:901–909, 1952.

177. Kvale, W.F., Roth, G.M., Manger, W.M., et al.: Pheochromocytoma. Circulation, *14*:622–630, 1956.

178. Kvale, W.F., Roth, G.M., Manger, W.M., et al.: Present-day diagnosis and treatment of pheochromocytoma: A review of 51 cases. J.A.M.A., *164*:854–861, 1957.

179. Lanner, L.O., and Rosencrantz, M.: Arteriographic appearances of pheochromocytomas. Acta Radiol., *10*:35–48, 1970.

180. Leestma, J.E., and Price, E.B., Jr.: Paraganglioma of the urinary bladder. Cancer, *25*:1063–1073, 1971.

181. Lepphart, C.J., and Nudelman, E.J.: Hibernoma masquerading as a pheochromocytoma. Radiology, *95*:659–660, 1970.

182. Lopez, J.F.: Pheochromocytoma of the adrenal gland with granulosa cell tumor and neurofibromatosis: Report of a case with fatal outcome following abdominal aortography. Ann. Int. Med., *8*:187–199, 1958.

183. Ludin, H., Fernex, M., and Waibel, W.: Aortographic demon-

stration of intra-thoracic para-aortic phaeochromocytoma. Acta Radiol., *3*:465–474, 1965.

184. Lulu, D.J.: Pheochromocytoma of the organs of Zuckerkandl. Arch. Surg., *99*:641–644, 1969.

185. Lund, R.R., Garcia, N.A., III, LeBlanc, G.A., et al.: Inferior vena cavography in preoperative localization of pheochromocytoma. J. Urol., *83*:768–773, 1960.

186. MacLaurin, J.C., and Arneil, G.C.: Phaeochromocytoma causing ureteric obstruction in a child. Lancet, *1*:426–429, 1961.

187. Maier, H.C.: Intrathoracic pheochromocytoma with hypertension. Ann. Surg., *130*:1059–1065, 1949.

188. Malter, I.J., and Koehler, P.R.: Angiographic findings in pheochromocytoma of the organs of Zuckerkandl. Radiology, *97*:57–58, 1970.

189. Mayo, C.H.: Paroxysmal hypertension with tumor of retroperitoneal nerve: report of a case. J.A.M.A., *89*:1047–1050, 1927.

190. McGuire, L.B., and Fox, L.M.: Recurrent pheochromocytoma with recognition of site of metastasis by means of venous catheterization. Ann. Int. Med., *60*:125–130, 1964.

191. Meany, T.F., and Buonocore, E.: Selective arteriography as a localizing and provocative test in the diagnosis of pheochromocytoma. Radiology, *87*:309–314, 1966.

192. Melicow, M.M.: Hibernating fat and pheochromocytoma. Arch. Pathol., *63*:367–372, 1957.

193. Melicow, M.: Tumors and hyperplasias of the adrenal gland, pp. 275–339. *In* Ariel, I.M., and Pack, G.T. (eds.): Cancer and Allied Diseases of Infancy and Childhood. Little, Brown, Boston, 1960.

194. Meyers, M.A.: Diseases of the Adrenal Glands: Radiologic Diagnosis with Emphasis on the Use of Presacral Retroperitoneal Pneumography. Charles C Thomas, Springfield, Illinois, 1963.

195. Meyers, M.A., and King, M.C.: Unusual radiologic features of pheochromocytoma. Clin. Radiol., *20*:52–56, 1969.

196. Moir, W.M., and Crummy, A.B.: Calcified pheochromocytoma of the para-aortic body. J. Urol., *107*:15–16, 1972.

197. Moser, M., Sheehan, G., and Schwinger, H.: Pheochromocytoma with calcification simulating cholelithiasis. Report of a case. Radiology, *55*:855–858, 1950.

198. Moloney, G.E., Cowdell, R.H., and Lewis, C.L.: Malignant phaeochromocytoma of the bladder. Br. J. Urol., *38*:461–470, 1966.

199. Mulholland, S.G., Atuk, N.O., and Walzak, M.P.: Familial pheochromocytoma associated with cerebellar hemangioblastoma: A case history and review of the literature. J.A.M.A., *207*:1709–1711, 1969.

200. Palmieri, G., Ikkos, D., and Luft, R.: Malignant Pheochromocytoma. Acta Endocrinol., *36*:549–560, 1961.

201. Pearson, K.D., Wells, S.A., and Keiser, H.R.: Familial medullary carcinoma of the thyroid, adrenal pheochromocytoma and parathyroid hyperplasia. Radiology, *107*:249–256, 1973.

202. Pincoffs, M.C.: A case of paroxysmal hypertension associated with suprarenal tumor. Trans. Assoc. Am. Physicians, *44*:295–299, 1929.

203. Reynes, C.J., Churchill, R., Moncada, R., et al.: Computed tomography of adrenal glands. Radiol. Clin. North Am., *17*:91–104, 1979.

204. Rosati, L.A., and Augur, N.A., Jr.: Ischemic enterocolitis in pheochromocytoma. Gastroenterology, *60*:581–585, 1971.

205. Rosenheim, M.L., Ross, E.J., Wrong, O.M., et al.: Unilateral renal ischemia due to compression of renal artery by pheochromocytoma. Am. J. Med., *34*:735–740, 1963.

206. Rossi, P.: Arteriography in adrenal tumours. Br. J. Radiol., *41*:81–98, 1968.

207. Rossi, P., Kaufman, L., Ruzicka, F., and Pauke, W.: Angiographic localization of pheochromocytoma. Radiology, *86*:266–275, 1966.

208. Rossi, J., Young, I.S., and Panke, W.F.: Techniques, usefulness, and hazards of arteriography of pheochromocytoma. Review of 99 cases. J.A.M.A., *205*:547–553, 19 August 1968.

209. Saltz, N.J., Luttwak, E.M., Schwartz, A., et al.: Danger of aortography in the localization of pheochromocytoma. Ann. Surg., *144*:118–123, 1956.

210. Schimke, R.N., Hartmann, W.H., Prout, T.E., et al.: Syndrome of bilateral pheochromocytoma, medullary thyroid carcinoma and multiple neuromas: A possible regulatory defect in the differentiation of chromaffin tissue. N. Engl. J. Med., *279*:1–7, 1968.

211. Schokett, E., and Teloh, H.A.: Aganglionic megacolon, pheochromocytoma, megaloureter and neurofibroma: Co-occurrence of several neural abnormalities. A.M.A. J. Dis. Child., *94*:185–191, 1957.

212. Sipple, J.H.: The association of pheochromocytoma with carcinoma of the thyroid gland. Am. J. Med., *31*:163–166, 1961.

213. Smithwick, R.H., Greer, W.E.R., Robertson, C.W., et al.: Pheochromocytoma. Discussion of signs, symptoms and procedures of diagnostic value. N. Engl. J. Med., *242*:252–257, 1950.

214. Snyder, C.H., and Rutledge, L.J.: Pheochromocytoma—localization by aortography. Pediatrics, *15*:312–316, 1955.

215. Snyder, C.H., and Vick, E.H.: Hypertension in children caused by pheochromocytoma: report of three cases and review of the literature. A.M.A. Am. J. Dis. Child., *73*:581–601, 1947.

216. Spitzer, R., Borrison, R., and Castellino, R.A.: Functioning nonchromaffin paraganglioma (chemodectoma) of the urinary bladder. Radiology, *98*:577–578, 1971.

217. Steinbach, H.L., and Smith, D.L.: Extraperitoneal pneumography in diagnosis of retroperitoneal tumors. A.M.A. Arch. Surg., *70*:161–172, 1955.

218. Straube, K.R., and Hodges, C.V.: Pheochromocytoma causing renal hypertension. Am. J. Roentgenol., *98*:222–224, 1966.

219. Weber, A.L., Janower, M.L., and Griscom, N.T.: Radiologic and clinical evaluation of pheochromocytoma in children: Report of 6 cases. Radiology, *88*:117–123, 1967.

220. West, G.B., Shepherd, D.M., Hunter, R.B., et al.: The function of the organs of Zuckerkandl. Clin. Sci., *12*:317–325, 1953.

221. Williams, E.D.: A review of 17 cases of carcinoma of the thyroid and phaeochromocytoma. J. Clin. Pathol., *18*:288–292, 1965.

222. Yeh, H.-C., Mitty, H.A., Rose, J., et al.: Ultrasonography of adrenal masses: Usual features. Radiology, *127*:467–474, 1978.

223. Yeh, H.-C., Mitty, H.A., Rose, J., et al.: Ultrasonography of adrenal masses: Unusual manifestations. Radiology, *127*:475–483, 1978.

224. Zuckerkandl, E.: Ueber Nebenorgane des Sympathicus im Retroperitonaelraum des Menschen. Anat. Anz., *19*:95–107, 1901.

Neuroblastoma and Ganglioneuroma

225. Beckwith, J.B., and Perrin, E.V.: In situ neuroblastomas: A contribution to the natural history of neural crest tumors. Am. J. Pathol., 43:1089–1104, 1963.
226. Berger, P.E., Kuhn, J.P., and Munschauer, R.W.: Computed tomography and ultrasound in the diagnosis and management of neuroblastoma. Radiology, 128:663–667, 1978.
227. Cushing, H., and Wolbach, S.B.: The transformation of a malignant paravertebral sympathicoblastoma into a benign ganglioneuroma. Am. J. Pathol., 3:203–216, 1927.
228. Doub, H.P.: The roentgen aspect of sympathetic neuroblastoma. J.A.M.A., 109:1188–1191, 1937.
229. Dunnick, N.R., and Castellino, R.A.: Arteriographic manifestations of ganglioneuromas. Radiology, 115:323–328, 1975.
230. Dyke, P.C., and Mulkey, D.A.: Maturation of ganglioneuroblastoma to ganglioneuroma. Cancer, 20:1343–1349, 1967.
231. Eklof, O., and Gooding, C.A.: Intrathoracic neuroblastoma. Amer. J. Roentgenol., 100:202–207, 1967.
232. Evans, A.R.: Congenital neuroblastoma. J. Clin. Pathol., 18:54–62, 1965.
233. Fortner, J.G., Nicastri, A., and Murphy, M.L.: Neuroblastoma: Natural history and results of treating 133 cases. Ann. Surg., 167:132–142, 1967.
234. Fulton, H., and Evans, W.A.: Roentgen evaluation in retroperitoneal tumors of children. A.M.A. Arch. Surg., 70:178–190, 1955.
235. Gellerstedt, N., and Hjelm, R.: Zur kasuistik der nebennierentumoren. Upsala läkaref. Förh., 34:271–288, 1928.
236. Goldman, R.L., Winterling, A.N., and Winterling, C.C.: Maturation of tumors of the sympathetic nervous system. Cancer, 18:1510–1516, 1965.
237. Goldring, D.: Neuroblastoma sympatheticum with metastases: Report of a case with apparent recovery. J. Pediatri., 38:231–234, 1951.
238. Green, M., Cook, R.E., and Lattanzi, W.: Occurrence of chronic diarrhea in three patients with ganglioneuromas. Pediatrics, 23:951–955, 1959.
239. Greenberg, R.E., and Gardner, L.I.: Catecholamine metabolism in a functioning neural tumor. J. Clin. Invest., 39:1729–1736, 1960.
240. Hansen, P.B.: Sympathicoblastoma of the adrenal medulla with osseous metastases. A report of three cases including one surviving eleven years after roentgen therapy. Acta Radiol., 40:500–510, 1953.
241. Hansman, C.F., and Girdany, B.R.: Roentgenographic findings associated with neuroblastoma. J. Pediatri., 51:621–633, 1957.
242. Harrison, F.G., Warres, H.L., and Fust, J.A.: Neuroblastoma involving the urinary tract. J. Urol., 63:598–612, 1950.
243. Jacobs, P.: Intrathoracic tumours of sympathetic nervous system, with report of two cases. J. Fac. Radiologists, 6:275–280, 1955.
244. Kincaid, O.W., Hodgson, J.R., and Dockerty, M.B.: Neuroblastoma: A roentgenologic and pathologic study. Am. J. Roentgenol., 78:420–436, 1957.
245. King, R.L., Storaasli, J.P., and Bolande, R.P.: Neuroblastoma: Review of twenty-eight cases and presentation of two cases with metastases and long survival. Am. J. Roentgenol., 85:733–747, 1961.
246. Koop, C.E., Kiesewetter, W.M., and Horn, R.C.: Neuroblastoma in childhood. Survival after major surgical insult to the tumor. Surgery, 38:272–278, 1955.
247. McAlister, W.H., and Koehler, P.R.: Diseases of the adrenal. Radiol. Clin. North Am., 5:205–220, 1967.
248. McDonald, P., and Harwood-Nash, D.C.F.: Arterial stenoses in neuroblastoma. Am. J. Roentgenol., 112:167–169, 1971.
249. McDonald, P., and Hiller, H.G.: Angiography in abdominal tumours in childhood with particular reference to neuroblastoma and Wilm's tumour. Clin. Radiol., 19:1–18, 1968.
250. Mandeville, F.B.: Sympathoblastoma (neuroblastoma), adrenal, abdominal and mediastinal. Urol. Cutan. Rev., 51:448–452, 1947.
251. Mindell, H.J., and Kupic, E.A.: Ganglioneuroblastoma: Angiographic-histologic correlation. Am. J. Roentgenol., 106:208–210, 1969.
252. Perez, C.A., Vietti, T.J., Ackerman, L.V., et al.: Treatment of malignant sympathetic tumors in children: Clinicopathological correlation. Pediatrics, 41:452–462, 1968.
253. Potter, E.L., and Parrish, J.M.: Neuroblastoma, ganglioneuroma and fibroneuroma in a stillborn fetus. Am. J. Pathol., 18 141–151, 1942.
254. Roberts, F.F., and Lee, K.R.: Familial neuroblastoma presenting as multiple tumors. Radiology, 116:133–136, 1975.
255. Ross, P.: Calcification in liver metastases from neuroblastoma. Radiology, 85:1074–1079, 1965.
256. Sherman, R.S., and Leaming, R.: The roentgen findings in neuroblastoma. Radiology, 60:837–849, 1953.
257. Stout, A.P.: Ganglioneuroma of the sympathetic nervous system. Surg. Gynecol. Obstet., 84:101–110, 1947.
258. Voorhess, M.L., and Gardner, L.I.: Value of serial catecholamine determinations in children with neuroblastoma: Report of a case. Pediatrics, 30:241–246, 1962.
259. Wittenborg, M.H.: Roentgen therapy in neuroblastoma: A review of seventy-three cases. Radiology, 54:679–687, 1950.
260. Wyatt, G.M., and Farber, S.: Neuroblastoma sympatheticum. Roentgenological appearances and radiation treatment. Am. J. Roentgenol., 46:485–495, 1941.
261. Young, L.W., Rubin, P., and Hanson, R.E.: The extra-adrenal neuroblastoma: High radiocurability and diagnostic accuracy. Amer. J. Roentgenol., 108:75–91, 1970.

Adrenal Cysts

262. Abeshouse, G.A., Goldstein, R.B., and Abeshouse, B.S.: Adrenal cyst: Review of the literature and report of three cases. J. Urol., 81:711–719, 1959.
263. Amador, E.: Adrenal hemorrhage during anticoagulant therapy: A clinical and pathological study of ten cases. Ann. Intern. Med., 63:559–571, 1965.
264. Anderson, M.X., Roberts, H.G., and Smith, E.T.: Calcified cyst of adrenal cortex without endocrine symptoms. Radiology, 54:236–241, 1950.
265. Barron, S.H., and Emanuel, B.: Adrenal cyst. A case report and a review of the pediatric literature. J. Pediatri., 59:592–599, 1961.
266. Dejardin, L.: Pseudo-kyste hémorragique surrénalien associe a une sciatique rebelle. Bull. Acad. Med. Belgique, 13:193–208, 1948.
267. Dorfman, J., and Kerr, B.G.: Adrenal Cyst. N.Y. J. Med., 62:260–262, 1962.
268. Ellis, F.H., Jr., Dawe, C.J., and Clagett, O.T.: Cysts of the adrenal glands. Ann. Surg., 136:217–227, 1952.
269. Falconer, C.D.: Adrenal apoplexy: A case of unilateral haemorrhage simulating a tumour of the kidney. Br. J. Urol., 25:183–186, 1953.
270. Feibelkorn, H.J.: Calcified adrenal cysts. Med. Klin., 47:186–187, 1952.

271. Hancock, R.A.: Adrenal cyst. J. Urol., 77:12–13, 1957.
272. Koehler, P.R., and McAlister, W.H.: Hemorrhage into a pheochromocytoma in a patient on anti-coagulants. J. Can. Assoc. Radiol., 18:404–405, 1967.
273. Kurti, D.J., and Patel, S.K.: Diagnosis of adrenal cysts utilizing the principle of total body opacification. Am. J. Roentgenol., 119:576–579, 1973.
274. Levison, P.: A case of bilateral adrenal cysts. Endocrinology, 17:372–376, 1933.
275. Lloyd, O.D., and Solomon, C.: Solitary cyst of the adrenal gland—report of a case. Calif. Med., 74:437–439, 1951.
276. Major, R.H., and Black, D.R.: A huge hemangioma of the liver associated with hemangiomata of the skull and bilateral cystic adrenals. Am. J. Med. Soc., 156:436–483, 1918.
277. Moore, F.P., and Cermak, E.G.: Adrenal cysts and adrenal insufficiency in an infant with fatal termination. J. Pediatri., 36:91–95, 1950.
280. Nowicki, W.: Zur Kenntnis der Nebennierenzystem. Virchow's Arch., 207:338–348, 1912.
281. Palubinskas, A.J., Christensen, W.R., Harrison, J.H., et al.: Calcified adrenal cysts. Am. J. Roentgenol., 82:853–861, 1959.
282. Parker, D.: Benign cysts of the adrenal gland: A case report. J. Urol., 68:1–5, 1952.
283. Rabson, S.M., and Zimmerman, E.F.: Cystic lymphangiectasia of the adrenal. Arch. Pathol., 26:869–872, 1938.
284. Reynes, C.J., Churchill, R., Moncada, R., et al.: Computed tomography of adrenal glands. Radiol. Clin. North Am., 17:91–104, 1979.
285. Scheible, W., Coel, M., Siemers, P.T., et al.: Percutaneous aspiration of adrenal cysts. Am. J. Roentgenol., 128:1013–1016, 1977.
286. Siceluff, J.G.: Benign adrenal cysts. J. Urol., 76 9–15, 1956.
287. Yeh, H.-C., Mitty, H.A., Rose, J., et al.: Ultrasonography of adrenal masses: Usual features. Radiology, 127:467–474, 1978.
288. Behan, M., Martin, E.C., Muecke, E.C., and Kazam, E.: Myelolipoma of the adrenal: Two cases with ultrasound and CT findings. Am. J. Roentgenol., 129:993–996, 1977.

Miscellaneous Stromal Lesions

289. Drucker, W.D., Longo, F.W., and Christy, N.P.: Calcification in a benign non-functioning tumor of the adrenal gland. J.A.M.A., 177:577–579, 1961.
290. Newman, P.H., and Silen, W.: Myelolipoma of the adrenal gland. Arch. Surg., 97:637–639, 1968.
291. Parsons, L., Jr., and Thompson, J.E.: Symptomatic myelolipoma of the adrenal gland. N. Engl. J. Med., 260:12–15, 1959.
292. Rothberg, M., Bastidas, J., Mattey, W.E., et al.: Adrenal hemangiomas: Angiographic appearance of a rare tumor. Radiology, 126 341–348, 1978.
293. Rubin, H.B., Hirose, F., and Benfield, J.R.: Myelolipoma of the adrenal gland: Angiographic findings and review of the literature. Am. J. Surg., 130:354–358, 1975.
294. Whittaker, L.D.: Myelolipoma of the adrenal gland. Arch. Surg., 97:628–631, 1968.
295. Aldrete, J.S., and Bohrod, M.G.: Adrenal metastases in cancer of breast: Their prognostic significance when found at adrenalectomy. Am. Surg., 33:174–178, 1967.
296. Alfidi, R.J., Gill, W.M., Jr., and Klein, H.J.: Arteriography of adrenal neoplasms. Am. J. Roentgenol., 106:635–641, 1969.
297. Bernardino, M.E., Goldstein, H.M., and Green, B.: Gray scale ultrasonography of adrenal neoplasms. A.J.R., 130:741–744, 1978.
298. Bullock, W.K., and Hirst, A.E., Jr.: Metastatic carcinoma of the adrenal. Am. J. Med. Sci., 226:521–536, 1953.
299. Dunnick, N.R., Schaner, E.G., Doppman, J.L., et al.: Computed tomography in adrenal tumors. A.J.R., 132:43–46, 1979.
300. Glomset, D.A.: The incidence of metastasis of malignant tumors to the adrenals. Am. J. Cancer, 32:57–61, 1938.
301. Hagvet, J.: Adrenocortical insufficiency due to metastatic infiltration of adrenal glands. Acta Med. Scandinav., 174:1–10, 1963.
302. Lumb, G., and Mackenzie, D.H.: The incidence of metastases in adrenal glands and ovaries removed for carcinoma of the breast. Cancer, 12:521–526, 1959.
303. Ochsner, A., and DeBakey, M.: Carcinoma of lung. Arch. Surg., 42:209–258, 1941.
304. Reuter, S.R.: Demonstration of adrenal metastases by adrenal venography. N. Engl. J. Med., 278:1423–1425, 1968.
305. Reynes, C.J., Churchill, R., Moncada, R., et al.: Computed tomography of adrenal glands. Radiol. Clin. North Am., 17:91–104, 1979.
306. Tenenbaum, J.: Hypernephroma associated with hyperplasia and metastatic carcinoma of the adrenals. Am. J. Surg., 52:120–128, 1941.
307. Willis, R.A.: Pathology of Tumours, pp. 242, 631. London, Butterworth, 1952.

Neonatal Adrenal Hemorrhage

308. Black, J., and Williams, D.I.: Natural history of adrenal hemorrhage in the newborn. Arch. Dis. Child., 48:183–190, 1973.
309. Blankenship, W.J., Bogren, H., Stadalnik, R.C., et al.: Suprarenal abscess in the neonate: A case report and review of diagnosis and management. Pediatrics, 55:239–243, 1975.
310. Carty, A., and Stanley, P.: Bilateral adrenal abscesses in a neonate. Pediatr. Radiol., 1:63–64, 1975.
311. Corcoran, W.J., and Strauss, A.A.: Suprarenal hemorrhage in newborn. J.A.M.A., 82:626–628, 1924.
312. Drucker, V., and Rodriguez, C.E.: Extensive bilateral calcification within adrenal hemorrhage. Radiology, 64:258–261, 1955.
313. Gabriele, O.F., and Sheehan, W.E.: Bilateral neonatal adrenal hemorrhage. Am. J. Roentgenol., 91:656–658, 1964.
314. Goldzieher, M.A., and Gordon, M.B.: The syndrome of adrenal hemorrhage in the new-born. Endocrinology, 16:165–181, 1932.
315. Gross, M., Kottmeier, P.K., and Waterhouse, K.: Diagnosis and treatment of neonatal adrenal hemorrhage. J. Pediatr. Surg., 2:308–312, 1967.
316. Jarvis, J.L., and Seaman, W.B.: Idiopathic adrenal calcification in infants and children. Am. J. Roentgenol., 82:510–520, 1959.
317. Kaplan, M., Straus, P., Grumbach, R., et al.: Hématomes surrénaliens unilaté raux chez le nouveauné à terme. A propos de deux observations. Ann. Pediatr., 11:405–417, 1964.
318. Kuhn, J., Jewett, T., and Munschauer, R.: The clinical and radiographic features of massive neonatal adrenal hemorrhage. Radiology, 99:647–652, 1971.
319. Mineau, D.E., and Koehler, P.R.: Ultrasound diagnosis of neonatal adrenal hemorrhage. A.J.R., 132:443–444, 1979.
320. Mittelstaedt, C.A., Volberg, F.M., Merten, D.F., et al.: The sonographic diagnosis of neonatal adrenal hemorrhage. Radiology, 131:453–457, 1979.
321. Moore, F.P., and Cermak, E.G.: Adrenal cysts and adrenal in-

sufficiency in an infant with fatal termination. J. Pediatr., 36:91–95, 1950.

322. Rose, J., Berdon, W.E., Sullivan, T., et al.: Prolonged jaundice as representing sign of massive adrenal hemorrhage in newborn. Radiographic diagnosis by IVP with total-body opacification. Radiology, 98:263–272, 1971.

323. Snelling, C.E., and Erb., I.H.: Hemorrhage and subsequent calcification of the suprarenal. J. Pediatr., 6:22–41, 1935.

324. Wagner, A.C.: Bilateral hemorrhagic pseudocysts of the adrenal glands in a newborn. Am. J. Roentgenol., 86:540–544, 1961.

Wolman's Disease

325. Abramov, A., Schorr, S., and Wolman, M.: Generalized xanthomatosis with calcified adrenals. A.M.A. J. Dis. Child., 91:282–286, 1956.

326. Lake, B.D., and Patrick, A.D.: Wolman's disease: Deficiency of E-600 resistant acid esterase activity with storage of lipids in lysosomes. J. Pediatr., 76:262–266, 1970.

327. Lough, J., Fawcett, J., and Wiegensberg, B.: Wolman's disease. An electron microscopic, histochemical, and biochemical study. Arch. Pathol., 89:103–110, 1970.

328. Marshall, W.C., Ockendon, B.G., Fosbrooke, A.S., et al.: Wolman's disease. A rare lipidosis with adrenal calcification. Arch. Dis. Child., 44:331–341, 1969.

329. Nelson, W.E., Vaughan, V.C., III, and McKay, R.J. ed: Textbook of Pediatrics, 9th ed., pp. 457, 1222. Saunders, Philadelphia, 1969.

330. Queloz, J.M., Capitanio, M.A., and Kirkpatrick, J.A.: Wolman's disease. Roentgen observations in 3 siblings. Radiology, 104:357–359, 1972.

331. Sandomenico, C., Tortora, M., and Gaetani, B.: Wolman's lipoidosis. Radiol. Med., 58:144–148, 1972.

332. Wolman, M., Sterk, V.V., Gatt, S., et al.: Primary familial xanthomatosis with involvement and calcification of the adrenals. Report of two more cases in siblings of a previously described infant. Pediatrics, 28:742–757, 1961.

Computed Tomography of the Adrenal Glands

333. Montagne, J.P., Kressel, H.Y., Korobkin, M., et al.: Computed tomography of the normal adrenal gland. Am. J. Roentgenol., 130:963–966, 1978.

334. Brownlie, K., and Kreel, L.: Computer assisted tomography of normal suprarenal glands. J. Comput. Assist. Tomogr., 2:1–10, 1978.

335. Wilms, G., Baert, A., Marchal, G., et al.: Computed tomography of the normal adrenal glands: Correlative study with autopsy specimens. J. Comput. Assist. Tomogr., 3:467–469, 1979.

336. Sample, F.W., and Sarti, D.A.: Computed tomography and gray scale ultrasonography of the adrenal gland: A comparative study. Radiology, 128:377–383, 1978.

337. Moss, A.A., and Goldberg, H.I.: Computed tomography of the adrenal glands. In Lohr, E. (ed.): Renal and Adrenal Tumors: Pathology, Radiology, Ultrasonography, Therapy, Immunology pp. 268–281, Berlin/Heidelberg/New York: Springer-Verlag, 1979.

338. Karstaedt, N., Sagel, S.S., Stanley, R.J., et al.: Computed tomography of the adrenal gland. Radiology, 129:723–730, 1978.

339. Korobkin, M., White, E.A., Kressel, H.Y., et al.: Computed tomography in the diagnosis of adrenal disease. Am. J. Roentgenol., 132:231–238, 1979.

340. Reyes, C.J., Churchill, R., Moncada, R., et al.: Computed tomography of adrenal glands. Radiol. Clin. North Am., 27:91–104, 1979.

341. Dunnick, N.R., Schaner, E.G., Doppman, J.L., et al.: Computed tomography in adrenal tumors. Am. J. Roentgenol., 132:43–46, 1979.

342. Curtis, J.A., Brennan, R.E., and Kurtz, A.B.: Evaluation of adrenal disease by computed tomography. Computerized Tomography, 4:165–168, 1980.

343. White, E.A., Schambelan, M., Rost, R.C., et al.: Use of computed tomography in diagnosing the cause of primary aldosteronism. N. Engl. J. Med., 303:1503–1507, 1980.

344. Linde, R., Coulam, C., Battino, R., et al.: Localization of aldosterone-producing adenomas by computed tomography. J. Clin. Endocrinol. Metab., 49:642–645, 1979.

345. Ganguly, A., Pratt, J.H., Kune, H.Y., et al.: Detection of adrenal tumors of computerized tomographic scan in endocrine hypertension. Arch. Intern. Med., 139:589–590, 1979.

346. Dunnick, N.R., Doppman, J.L., and Geelhoed, G.W.: Intravenous extension of endocrine tumors. Am. J. Roentgenol., 135:471–476, 1980.

347. Fink, D.W., Wurtzeback, L.R.: Symptomatic myelolipoma of the adrenal: Report of a case with computed tomographic evaluation. Radiology, 134:451–452, 1980.

348. Thomas, J.L., Bernardino, M.E., Samaan, N.A., et al.: CT of pheochromocytoma. Am. J. Roentgenol., 135:477–482, 1980.

349. Laursen, K., and Damgaard-Pedersen, K.: CT for pheochromocytoma diagnosis. Am. J. Roentgenol., 134:277–280, 1980.

350. Epstein, A.J., Patel, S.K., and Petasnick, J.P.: Computerized tomography of the adrenal gland. J.A.M.A., 242:2791–2794, 1979.

351. Daffner, R.H.: Evaluation of suprarenal mass. CT/T Clinical Symposium, Volume 1, Number 3.

352. Foley, W.D.: Ectopic pheochromocytoma. CT/T Clinical Symposium, Volume 3, Number 10.

353. Stewart, B.H., Bravo, E.L., Haaga, J., et al.: Localization of pheochromocytoma by computed tomography. N. Engl. J. Med., 299:460–461, 1978.

354. Hahn, L.C., Nadel, N.S., Bernstein, N.M., et al.: Localization of pheochromocytoma by computerized axial tomography. J. Urol., 120:349–351, 1970.

355. Costello, P., Clouse, M.E., Kane, R.A., et al.: Problems in the diagnosis of adrenal tumors. Radiology, 125:335–341, 1977.

356. Prosser, P.R., Sutherland, C.M., and Scullin, D.R.: Localization of adrenal aldosterone adenoma by computerized tomography. N. Engl. J. Med., 300:1278–1279, 1979.

357. Brasch, R.C., Korobkin, M., and Gooding, C.A.: Computed body tomography in children: Evaluation of 45 patients. Am. J. Roentgenol., 131:21–25, 1978.

358. Eghrari, M., McLoughlin, M.J., Rosen, I.E., et al.: The role of computed tomography in assessment of tumoral pathology of the adrenal glands. J. Comput. Assist. Tomogr., 4:71–77, 1980.

359. Behan, M., Martin, E.E., Muecke, E.C., et al.: Myelolipoma of the adrenal: Two cases with ultrasound and CT findings. Am. J. Roentgenol., 129:993–996, 1977.

360. Schaner, E.G., Dunnick, N.R., Doppman, J.L., et al.: Adrenal cortical tumors with low attenuation coefficients: a pitfall in computed tomography diagnosis. J. Comput. Assist. Tomogr., 2:11–15, 1978.

361. Federle, M.P., and Moss, A.A.: Adrenal abnormalities. CT/T Clinical Symposium, Volume 1, Number 4.

Part Four

URETER

The normal course and contour of the ureter have been discussed in Chapter 1, The Normal Kidney and Ureter. Variations in the course of the ureter often are associated with variations of renal structure or position. This is particularly true in ectopic kidney, malrotation of the kidney, segmentation of the renal pelvis, and horseshoe kidney.

The incidence of anomalies in the urinary tract is highest in the ureter. Ureteral anomalies produce clinical symptoms when the anomaly interferes with the transport of urine or when secondary infection or calculi are present. Anomalies must be excluded when persistent pyuria is present in young individuals. Campbell reported the incidence of reduplication to be 1:152 individuals, but in 1102 children with persistent pyuria it was present in 26 per cent.

The discussion of ureteral anomalies is based on a modification of Campbell's classification.

Anomalies of Number
    Agenesis and aplasia
    Duplication and triplication
    Blind-ending ureters
Anomalies of Structure and Caliber
    Congenital stricture
    Congenital valves and folds
    Congenital diverticula
    Aberrant vessels
    Megaloureter
    Megaureter
Anomalies of Origin and Termination
    Ectopia
    High insertion
    Ureterocele
    Retrocaval
    Herniation

The reader is referred to Chapter 2, Congenital Anomalies of the Kidney, for further discussion of some of these entities.

18

Congenital Lesions of the Ureter

ANOMALIES OF NUMBER

AGENESIS AND APLASIA

Bilateral ureteral agenesis is associated with bilateral renal agenesis. Unilateral agenesis, failure of the ureteral bud to develop, is associated with unilateral renal agenesis or aplasia. In aplasia the ureter may be a fibrous cord or have a small lumen in parts of its course. In agenesis cystoscopy usually reveals an absence of the ureteral orifice and corresponding half of the trigone. If the trigone is present there is usually an aplastic ureter and frequently an aplastic kidney (Fig. 18–1).

URETERAL DUPLICATION

Unilateral ureteral duplication is a common anomaly reported in over 0.5 per cent of autopsy material. In most cases the reduplication is incomplete, with the two ureters joining in the abdomen or more commonly in the pelvis just before entering the bladder. Over 10 per cent of the cases of complete duplication are bilateral. Obstruction and infection are more common in kidneys with duplication of the ureter, and duplications are more common in females. Partial or incomplete duplication may result in a blind-ending ureter (see next section) (Figs. 18–2 to 18–7).

As described in congenital anomalies of the kidney, complete ureteral duplication may be associated with ureteral ectopia, ureterocele, or reflux. With rare exceptions the ureter draining the upper renal segment enters the bladder below the ureter draining the lower renal segment, and this ureter may be ectopic (see Figs. 18–40, 18–41; Ectopic Ureteral Orifices, p. 1134). Reflux is more common in the ureter draining the lower renal segment (Fig. 18–8) when both orifices are on the trigone. As the ureter draining the upper segment becomes more ectopic (urethra, vagina), the reflux occurs to the upper segment. The two ureters frequently cross each other in the abdomen (Fig. 18–2) and may recross in the pelvis.

In incomplete duplications the ureters join in Y formation. A rare anomaly is the inverted Y (λ) duplication in which there are two orifices in the bladder but one ureter draining the kidney (Figs. 18–9, 18–10). In incomplete duplication ureteral dysperistalis may occur. (See Figure 22–39.)

Unusual variations of ureteral duplication include ureteral triplication (Figs. 18–11, 18–12). As many as six ureters have been reported in stillborns.

BLIND-ENDING URETERS

A blind-ending ureter may be 1 or 2 cm. in length, resembling a large diverticulum, or it may extend throughout most of the course of a reduplicated ureter without communicating with the renal structures. The remnants of an aplastic kidney are occasionally found at the termination of the ureter. Huge dilation of the blind-ending ureter may occur, forming a cystlike mass in the abdomen. Suggested causes include attempted reduplications or ureteral diverticula.

The most common type is the proximal blind end, which can be visualized radiographically by catheterization of the ureteral opening, but it is frequently not visualized during urography. Extremely rare variations are the distal blind end and both ends blind with the midportion patent (Fig. 18–13). The last two are usually visualized during urography (Figs. 18–13 to 18–17).

ANOMALIES OF STRUCTURE

CONGENITAL URETERAL STRICTURE

The majority of congenital ureteral strictures present in children at the ureterovesical or ureteropelvic junctions, with about 10 per cent occurring in the body of the ureter. The strictures are occasionally multiple and bilateral. The patient may be asymptomatic or may present with abdominal pain and infection.

The etiologic factors are unknown. Pathologically there may be an abnormal narrowing of the lumen, which may appear to be secondary to mucosal thickening or mucosal redundancies without inflammatory reaction or adventitial changes. The narrowed areas may be sharply localized or extended over 2 or 3 cm. In most individuals it is impossible to differentiate these lesions from inflammatory strictures (Figs. 18–18 to 18–21).

The true incidence of congenital stricture is unknown. Many of the ureteral dilatations may be associated with a normal ureterovesical orifice, and a retrograde catheter may pass with ease. In those cases in which no luminal change is noted the possibility of nonobstructive hydronephrosis from infection, reflux, or dysperistalsis (megaloureter) must be considered. Occasionally an area of deficient muscle occurs in the ureter; this interferes with peristalsis and may lead to severe proximal hydronephrosis.

The clinical finding is hydronephrosis, often massive. In the first year of life the most common cause of an abdominal mass is a hydronephrotic kidney.

Ureteral strictures must be differentiated from kinking of the ureter. Kinking seldom is congenital; more often it is secondary to a more distal obstruction, such as ureteral stone or stricture, to fixation of the ureter by fibrotic bands, or to excessive mobility of the kidney. Kinking without ureteral fixation rarely produces symptoms and can usually be differentiated from stricture by noting changes in the caliber and position of the ureter with changes in the position of the patient, for example, Trendelenberg. Apparent narrowing of the ureter without proximal distention should not be interpreted as stricture (Figs. 18-22, 18-23).

CONGENITAL URETERAL VALVES OR FOLDS

Pseudovalves consisting of transverse folds or redundant mucosa are common in the fetus and occur in about 10 per cent of newborns. They usually disappear in the first few months of life. A classification of valvelike lesions might include the following:

1. *True valves.* These lesions are rare and represent transverse folds of ureteral mucosa that contain some smooth muscle (Figs. 18-24, 18-25).

2. *Pseudovalves.* These represent transverse or redundant mucosa as already described, or mucosal hypertrophy simulating a valve secondary to chronic inflammation (Figs. 18-26, 18-27).

In all cases the findings are those of obstruction frequently with a sharp linear "cut-off" of the ureter. These lesions tend to occur in the body of the ureter, particularly the distal segment.

CONGENITAL DIVERTICULA

This is a rare congenital condition in which diverticula, presumably arising from accessory ureteral buds, present anywhere along the course of the ureter. There may be a single diverticulum or multiple diverticula. A single long diverticulum has the same appearance as a blind-ending ureter, and the distinction is frequently a semantic one. Occasionally a solitary diverticulum may become cystlike and present as a mass containing a good deal of fluid. A true ureteral diverticulum (or blind-ending ureter) should have the muscular walls of the ureter in the diverticulum. Unfortunately, after the muscular wall is destroyed by infection, it is frequently impossible to determine if the diverticulum is congenital or acquired (Figs. 18-28 to 18-30).

Multiple diverticula are less common and may arise from the ureteral anlage. Khonsari[170] hypothesized that they may also occur as pulsion diverticula with mucosal pouches protruding near sites of vessel penetration of the muscular wall, potential weak points. This is similar to the etiologic pattern of colonic diverticulosis (Figs. 18-31 to 18-32).

Solitary diverticula may be acquired from external trauma, perforation of a calculus, instrumentation, or surgery. This is particularly true of large diverticula that may represent pseudocysts of the ureter, fibrous tissue encapsulating a uriniferous collection that communicates with the ureter (Figs. 20-43 to 20-45).

CONGENITAL BANDS AND ABERRANT VESSELS

This subject has been discussed under Congenital Kidney and Obstructive Uropathy. Hydronephrosis secondary to congenital bands is rare. Imprints on ureters from aberrant vessels are common but rarely produce significant obstruction. As a ureter dilates, crossing vessels produce imprints on the ureter, which may suggest that these vessels are the primary cause of the obstruction. This is usually not the case; the imprints are secondary to the ureteral dilatation pressing upon the crossing vessel (Fig. 18-33).

MEGALOURETER AND MEGAURETER

Megaureter is a nonspecific term used to describe dilatations of the ureter, either secondary to mechanical obstruction (stone) or secondary to severe vesicoureteral reflux. Primary megaloureter (Figs. 22-36 to 22-38) is a term usually applied to congenital dilatation of the ureter in the absence of visible obstruction and in the presence of a relaxed, opened, nonrefluxing ureteral orifice.[202] The functional obstruction, a failure to transmit the peristaltic wave, occurs in the juxtavesical segment of the ureter. The clinical presentation is usually a young adult with vague lower quadrant pain. The urogram reveals a fusiform dilatation of the pelvic ureter, which may be minimal or as large as 4 or 5 cm. in diameter, just above the functionally obstructed juxtavesical segment. This latter narrowed area, which is easily visualized by pyelography, may be difficult to visualize in the urogram. Fluoroscopy reveals vigorous peristaltic churning in the dilated segment, but none will be seen in the narrowed juxtavesical segment. A retrograde catheter can be passed easily into the ureter. The lesion may be bilateral in 20 to 40 per cent. The proximal ureter may be normal or minimally dilated. Caulk suggests that the dilatation of the ureter is not accompanied by lengthening, angulation, tortuosity or kinking, such as is seen in the obstructive uropathies,[189] but this seems to depend upon the length of the dilated segment; the longer segments become more tortuous.

The dilatation of the pelvic ureter may remain unchanged for years unless infection or decompensation occurs; the latter represents inability to maintain normal urine flow by peristalsis. If this occurs there may be massive dilatation of the ureter and collecting system. Numerous possible causes have been suggested, such as persistence of the fetal ureter, neuromuscular dysfunction, achalasia, and muscular hypertrophy. McLaughlin and co-workers have stated in their review of the literature and assessment of the histopathology of 32 ureters that no single cause can be demonstrated. They divided their findings into four groups: (1) normal distal ureter; (2) abnormal orientation of smooth muscle; (3) mural fibrosis; and (4) muscle atrophy.[199]

Mild cases are usually discovered accidentally and require no therapy. Cases complicated by infection or calculi may require removal of the aperistaltic segment (Figs. 18–34 to 18–39).

Recently, cases of combined megaloureter and megacalyces have been observed (see Megacalyces).

Congenital absence of the abdominal musculature also can produce marked ureteral atony, together with marked dilatation of the bladder. In these cases the dysplastic ureters usually fall anteriorly against the lax abdominal wall and show marked redundancy. Marked ureteral dilatation can also be found in patients with neurogenic bladder, massive reflux, or infection and perhaps in congenital defective formation of the ureteral wall (Fig. 18–39).

ANOMALIES OF ORIGIN AND TERMINATION

ECTOPIC URETERAL ORIFICES (EXTRAVESICAL ORIFICES)

Ectopic ureteral orifices are four times as frequent in women as in men. In men the anomaly rarely is associated with incontinence, because it always lies within the control of the external sphincter. The ureter usually opens into the posterior urethra but occasionally into the vas deferens, the ejaculatory duct, or the seminal vesicle. In females 50 percent of the ectopic orifices lie beyond sphincteric control, and incontinence is frequently present. In the female the ectopic ureter frequently opens into the urethra but occasionally into the vagina or the uterus. Unusual sites, such as openings into urethral diverticula or the rectum, have been reported. There is a frequent association between ectopic ureteral orifices and reduplication of the ureter, the ectopia relating to the ureter draining the upper calyceal system, where the ureteral orifice is more caudal in the urinary tract. The majority of these cases are associated with stenosis of the ureteral opening and chronic urinary infection, which may produce hydroureter and hydronephrosis (Figs. 18–40 to 18–49).

Frequently, the renal segment associated with the ectopic orifice functions so poorly that it cannot be visualized in the urogram. The urogram may suggest a mass lesion, which actually represents the nonfunctioning hydronephrotic segment. Visualization of the ectopic ureteral orifice and retrograde injection permits confirmation of the diagnosis. Frequently the ectopic ureter may be seen through the contrast medium in the bladder, extending to the bladder neck. In such cases the ureter does not cross the midline (Figs. 18–40 to 18–41). The ureteral jet from peristalsis in a normally placed ureteral orifice always crosses obliquely to the opposite bladder wall (Fig. 1–115). Ultrasonography can be used in the diagnosis of ectopic ureter. The entire dilated ectopic duplicated system can be visualized.

HIGH INSERTION OF THE URETER

High insertion of the ureter may be congenital or acquired.

Congenital. Occasionally the proximal end of the ureter joins the renal pelvis cephalad to the most dependent portion of the pelvis. Embryologically this may occur if the ureteric bud enters the upper pole of the metanephros, with subsequent development of the renal pelvis and calyces in a caudal direction. This situation leads to poor drainage, producing hydronephrosis with a further increase in the ureteral angle and further obstruction (Figs. 18–50 to 18–52).

Acquired. When the renal pelvis dilates, the inferior portion below the ureteropelvic junction enlarges, elevating the ureteropelvic junction. This acquired relatively high position of the ureteropelvic junction secondary to pyelectasis is more common than the congenital variety (Fig. 18–52a).

URETEROCELE

Ureteroceles may be divided into two types — simple and ectopic. Simple ureteroceles usually occur with single renal systems; ectopic ureteroceles almost always occur in duplicated systems, usually involving the ureter draining the upper renal segment.

Simple Ureteroceles. These may be congenital or acquired. They usually occur in nonduplicated systems, and the ureter always enters the bladder in its normal position. A ureterocele is a prolapse of the dilated distal ureteral orifice into the bladder lumen (usually presents with distal ureteral dilatation). The cause is presumed to be a congenital or acquired narrowing or stenosis of the ureteral orifice, which produces a cystlike dilatation of the lower end of the ureter, which protrudes into the bladder lumen. The condition is common in children, women more than men, and may be bilateral. They may be seen in newborns. Most ureteroceles are small, but occasionally huge ureteroceles are seen that obstruct the vesical orifice. Hydronephrosis, infection, and calculi are commonly present.

The roentgenogram reveals a dilated distal segment of ureter within the bladder, separated from the contrast material in the bladder by a 2- or 3-mm. area of radiolucency representing the prolapsed walls of the ureter and the mucosa of the bladder. In the cystogram a radiolucent defect within the bladder near the ureteral orifice in children suggests a ureterocele even without visualization of the ureter. The combination of the bulbous dilatation of the protruding ureter and the surrounding radiolucent halo has been called the "cobra head appearance." Ureters with ureteroceles usually do not reflux. Following instrumental or surgical correction, reflux is common (Figs. 18–53 to 18–60).

Ectopic Ureteroceles. These are almost always associated with a duplicated system, the ureterocele arising from the ureter draining the upper segment. It is a congenital lesion usually found in children or young adults and is more symptomatic than the simple ureterocele (pyuria, dysuria, flank pain). The ectopic ureter enters the bladder wall near the normal site of insertion but does not communicate with the lumen. Instead it continues under the mucosa of the bladder for a variable distance before opening into the bladder neck or posterior urethra. If the orifice is stenotic, proximal distention of the ureter under the submucosa of the bladder produces the eccentric filling defect representing the ureterocele (Figs. 18–61 to 18–63).

It is more common in girls (7:1) and occurs bilaterally in 10 per cent. The upper pole of the kidney is usually severely damaged, whereas the lower pole may be pyelonephritic with reflux or hydronephrotic from obstruction. The contralateral side may be normal or may be duplicated with or without a ureterocele.

There are two types of ectopic ureteroceles: One is tense with a small or sealed-off orifice. Micturition does not affect the size of the mass as seen on the cystogram. The high pressure prevents reflux into the ipsilateral lower pole ureter. The other type is compressible with a wide orifice and low pressure in the ureterocele. On micturition the ureterocele may empty into the urethra or ureter, and reflux frequently occurs into the lower pole ureter.

The roentgenographic findings suggesting ectopic ureterocele are as follows:

1. A double kidney with hydronephrosis or non-visualization of the upper segment
2. The lower pole of the same side may be normal, but it is often pyelonephritic with reflux, or hydronephrotic from obstruction. It may be nonfunctioning.
3. The contralateral side may be duplicated without ureterocele, may present with an obstructed ureter without duplication, or may also present with a ureterocele.
4. Only one ureterovesical orifice visualized on cystoscopy on that side, the other ureter usually entering the posterior urethra.
5. In the lateral projection the defect is on the posterior bladder wall (Fig. 18–63).
6. On the cystogram, the tense type of ureterocele demonstrates an eccentric, frequently lobulated, radiolucent defect in the bladder adjacent to the vesical orifice. In tangential projection, contrast medium does not completely encircle the defect, which arises under the bladder mucosa.
7. In the compressible type, the distention of the bladder on the cystogram may compress the ureterocele, displacing the urine more proximally and decreasing or obliterating the defect in the bladder (Fig. 18–61).

A ureterocele rarely may prolapse through the bladder neck into the posterior urethra, producing some degree of urethral obstruction (Figs. 18–65, 18–66). Prolapsing ureteroceles usually occur during voiding, either intermittently or chronically. In girls they may present at the external meatus. In boys they do not pass the membranous urethra. Repeated prolapse may lead to necrosis and rupture.

The detrusor muscle posterior to the ureterocele occasionally is deficient or absent. The ureterocele may then protrude posteriorly or posterolaterally and appear to be outside of the bladder lumen (Fig. 18–64).

Other complications of ectopic ureteroceles include obstruction and rupture. Both are more common in prolapsing ureterocele, and obstruction is more common in men. Rupture may also occur following instrumentation. Following rupture, the ureterocele is seen as an irregular cavity outside the bladder outline or as an irregular filling defect within the bladder. Reflux occurs freely after rupture.

RETROCAVAL OR POSTCAVAL URETER

Normally the right ureter lies lateral to the inferior vena cava. The retrocaval ureter presents posteriorly and medially to the inferior vena cava in the region of L-2 or L-3. Embryologically the infrarenal segment of the inferior vena cava usually is formed from the supracardinal vein, which lies posterior to the ureter. If the subcardinal vein, which lies anterior to the ureter, forms the infrarenal segment of the inferior vena cava then the ureter passes behind the vena cava, lies medial to it, then crosses anteriorly usually over the common iliac vein to resume its normal course. This venous arrangement plus the medial displacement of the ureter as the vena cava migrates medially produces the typical hooklike deviation (Figs. 18–67 to 18–69). If an anomalous left inferior vena cava is present the left ureter may show the same roentgenographic changes (see Fig. 18–70). Although double inferior vena cava do occur rarely (Fig. 18–72), only one case of bilateral retrocaval ureter has been reported. The clinical importance of this entity arises from the frequent obstruction of the proximal ureter and collecting system secondary to compression of the ureter between the inferior vena cava and the posterior abdominal wall.

The radiographic appearance is usually characteristic. Near the junction of the mid- and the upper-third of the ureter, in the area of the third or fourth lumbar body, the ureter deviates medially as it passes behind the inferior vena cava from the lateral to the medial aspect. The medial deviation may be gradual or sharp but usually places the ureter over or medial to the pedicles. The ureter then gradually resumes its normal course. The kidney and proximal ureter may be normal, or varying grades of obstruction may be seen proximal to the anomalous crossing (Figs. 18–67 to 18–70).

The normal ureter as it crosses over the iliac artery and vein may show a vascular impression near L-5 to S-1. The ureter is occasionally retroiliac, and in such cases may show a marked vascular impression, slight medial displacement, and a varying degree of obstruction. Vascular studies in the steep oblique show the posterior position of the ureter (Figs. 18–73 to 18–73b).

HERNIATION OF THE URETER

There are three basic types of ureteral herniation: inguinal or femoral, sciatic, and internal.

Femoral or Inguinal (Scrotal) Hernia. This is a rare anomaly in which a redundant ureter follows an abnormal course into a femoral or inguinal hernia. The most common type is paraperitoneal, with the ureter lying alongside a peritoneal sac. The right ureter appears to be involved more commonly than the left. A clinical history of double voiding is common. In the urogram, if the hernia is small, the ureter may extend just to the inguinal ring and a *vertical redundancy* of the ureter may be seen just proximal to the ureterovesical orifice. If a major segment of ureter is involved, the portion of the ureter involved in the hernia may not fill, and the diagnosis may be missed. Following the passage of a retrograde catheter the diagnosis is established by the unusual appearance of the catheter entering the hernia. The primary complication is that of obstruction, frequently accompanied by infection (Figs. 18–74 to 18–76).

Sciatic Hernia. Although sciatic hernias were previously considered rare, with more attention to the diagnostic criteria, they have been found in increasing numbers. They are usually asymptomatic and occur as incidental findings in urograms, although rarely the ureter may be obstructed. They are usually unilateral. The hernia occurs through the suprapyriformis recess extending posteriorly into the sacrosciatic foramen. The urogram reveals a variable degree of *lateral angulation* of the pelvic ureter a few centimeters above the ureterovesical orifice. The diagnosis can be confirmed on the lateral film by visualizing the posterior deviation of the ureter into or through the sacrosciatic notch (Figs. 18–77, 18–78).

Internal Hernia. In these hernias the ureter becomes trapped under folds of peritoneum or iliac fascia or between the iliac vessels. This frequently results in some degree of obstruction. Internal hernias may occur following pelvic surgery (Fig. 18–79).

CHAPTER 18, ILLUSTRATIONS

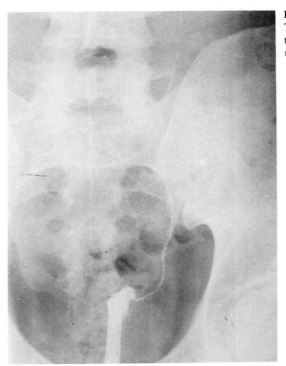

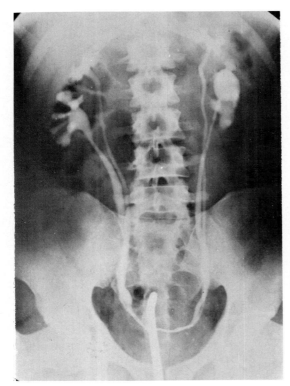

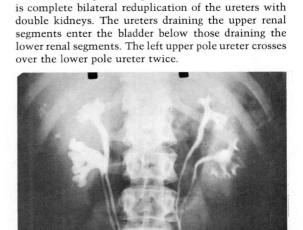

FIG. 18–1. Aplastic ureter. The left kidney was aplastic. The left trigone and ureteral orifice were present. Note the narrow lumen and corrugated appearance of the ureter, a frequent appearance in aplasia.

FIG. 18–2. Complete reduplication of the ureters. There is complete bilateral reduplication of the ureters with double kidneys. The ureters draining the upper renal segments enter the bladder below those draining the lower renal segments. The left upper pole ureter crosses over the lower pole ureter twice.

FIG. 18–3. Reduplication of the ureters. Bilateral double kidney and double ureters joining near the intramural portion of the bladder. Severe pyelonephritis and hydronephrosis are present in the lower half of the left kidney, possibly secondary to reflux, which occurs more commonly in the lower segment of double kidneys.

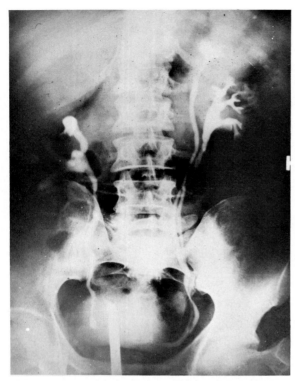

FIG. 18–4. Unilateral reduplication. The left kidney has a reduplicated ureter with two orifices in the bladder. The right kidney has a single ureter. The lower half of the double kidney contains numerous calyceal systems as compared with a single major calyceal system in the upper pole.

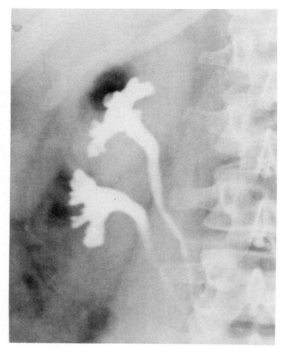

FIG. 18–5. Reduplication of the ureters. Less common appearance in which both the upper and lower renal segments have multiple major calyceal systems.

FIG. 18–6. Double right kidney with the two ureters joining at the level of L-3.

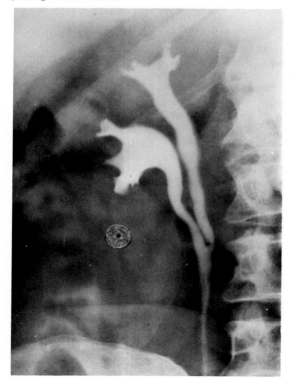

FIG. 18–7. Double right kidney and reduplicated ureter with both ureters joining at the level of S-1. Reduplicated ureters usually join prior to the ureterovesical junction.

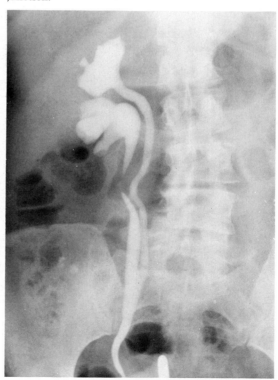

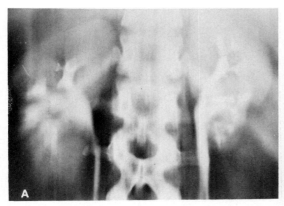

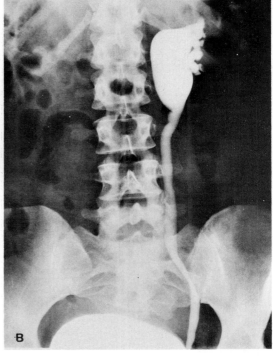

FIG. 18–8. Reflux tends to occur in the ureter supplying the lower renal segment, whereas the ureter from the upper renal segment may be ectopic. Tomogram of urogram (**A**) shows two renal segments; the lower segment is decreased in size (atrophy). The cystogram (**B**) shows marked reflux distending the lower renal segment.

FIG. 18–9. Inverted Y (⅄) ureter. Rare type of ureteral duplication. There are two ureteral orifices in the bladder and two ascending ureters, which join to form a single ureter over the ileum.

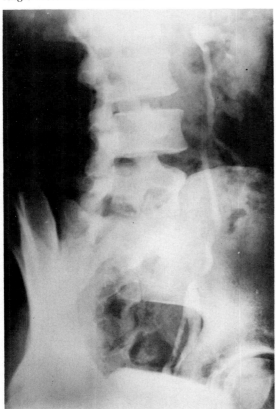

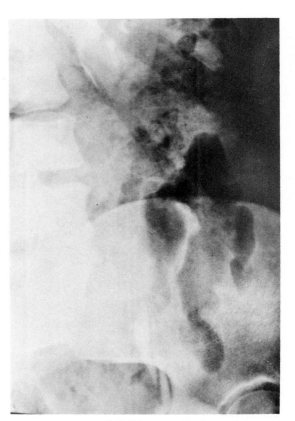

FIG. 18–10. Inverted Y (⅄) ureter. Single renal system, single proximal ureter and two pelvic ureters entering the bladder. (Courtesy of Leon Love, M.D.)

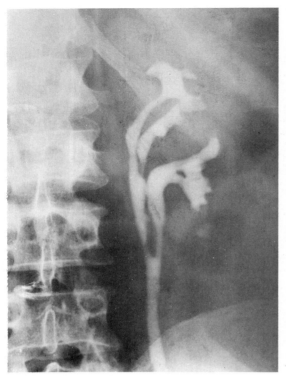

FIG. 18–11. Triplication of the ureter. There are three renal pelves, each leading to a major calyceal system. The three ureters join slightly below the ureteropelvic junctions. Triplication of the ureter is a rare anomaly.

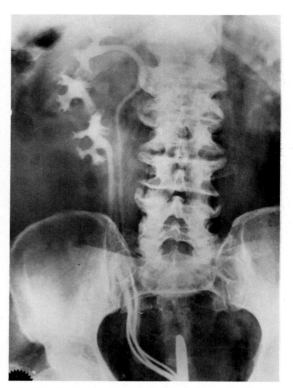

FIG. 18–12. Complete triplication of the ureter. During retrograde pyelography three ureteral orifices were catheterized on the right side of the bladder. The illustration shows the retrograde catheters in the lower thirds of the three ureters, with complete visualization of the trifid kidney and ureters. (Woodruff, S.R.: J. Urol., 46:376–379, 1941)

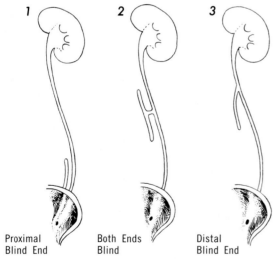

Proximal Blind End   Both Ends Blind   Distal Blind End

FIG. 18–13. Diagram of common types of blind-ending ureters. The blind segment may arise from any portion of the ureter. Short blind-ending ureters are identical to ureteral diverticula.

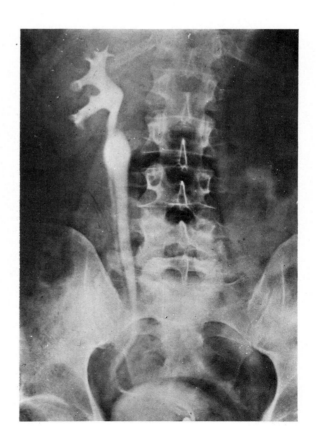

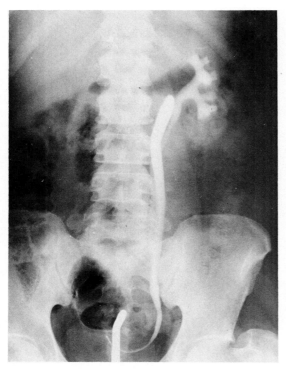

FIG. 18–15. Proximal blind-ending ureter. Similar to Figure 18–14 except that the blind ureter arose proximal to the ureterovesical orifice. There was only one ureteral opening in the bladder.

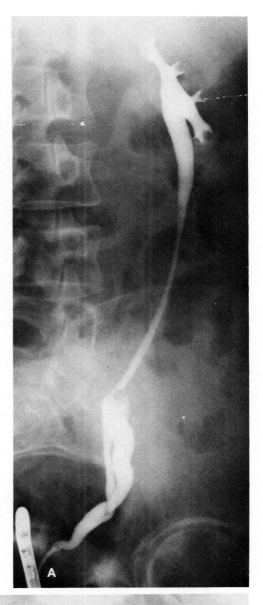

FIG. 18–16. Proximal blind-ending ureters. Two examples of short segments arising just proximal to the ureterovesical orifices. **(A)** Blind segment appears to be attached to ureter and impresses it. **(B)** Dilatation of the end of blind segment. This may lead to calculi or infection. (Fig. 18–16 **(A)** courtesy of Arthur Tessler, M.D.)

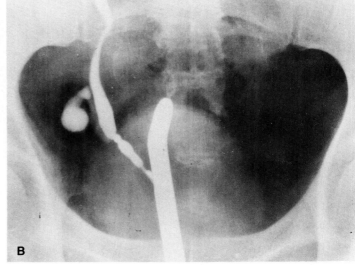

FIG. 18–14. Blind-ending ureter. Reduplication of the ureter with two ureteral orifices in the bladder. The ureter which normally would form the upper portion of the double kidney ends in a blind end. This is the commonest type of blind-ending ureter. Peristalsis may occur in blind-ending ureters. Infection and the formation of calculi are frequent.

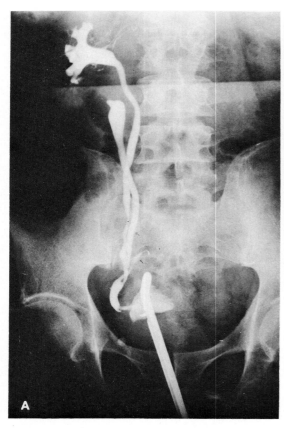

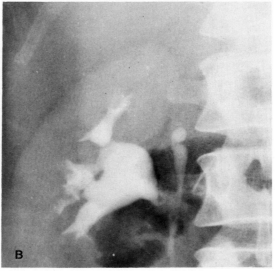

FIG. 18–17. (A) Multiple blind-ending ureters. A short (*lower arrow*) and long (*upper arrow*) blind-ending ureter, both originating from the same spot on the pelvic ureter. Attempt at triplication of the ureters. **(B)** Blind-ending ureter arising from the proximal ureter and ending blind cephalad to the renal pelvis.

FIG. 18–18. Ureteral stricture. A 12-year-old girl with pyuria and left flank pain. Urogram at 20 minutes **(A)** revealed severe left ureterectasis and moderate pelvicalyectasis. Delayed film **(B)** showed no contrast medium in the right kidney; the left ureter was completely filled with contrast material to the ureterovesical orifice. A catheter could not be passed through the orifice. Surgery revealed marked lumenal narrowing.

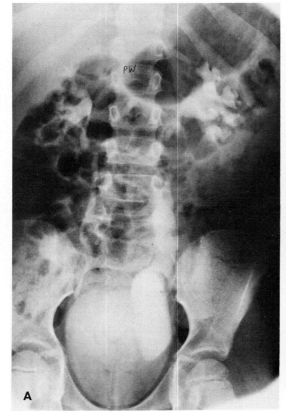

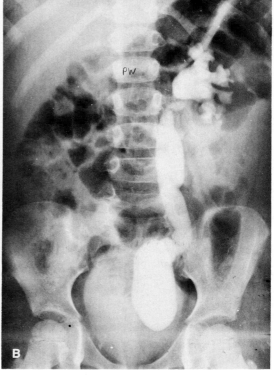

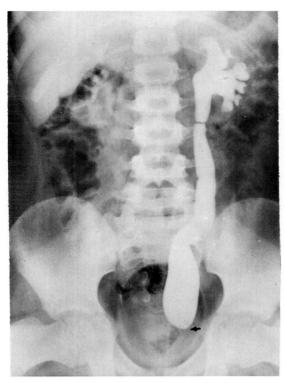

FIG. 18-19. Congenital ureteral stricture. Stricture at left ureterovesical junction (*arrow*). Marked hydroureter and hydronephrosis. The linear lucency crossing the proximal ureter was produced by a crossing vessel. Right kidney and ureter were normal. This child presented with pyuria and intermittent lower abdominal pain. Surgical correction was performed.

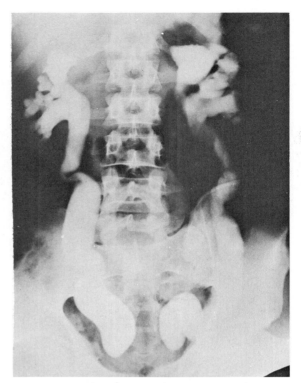

FIG. 18-20. Bilateral ureteral strictures at the ureterovesical junctions. Note marked tortuosity and redundancy of both ureters in the delayed film of the pyelogram, with severe hydroureter and hydronephrosis. Clinical signs of urinary tract infection were present. The contrast medium visible in the upper urinary tract remained within the ureters for several hours.

FIG. 18-21. Unilateral ureteral stricture. Right kidney is normal. This child presented with fever and pyuria secondary to a ureteral stricture at the left ureterovesical junction. The radiolucent defect crossing the upper ureter may represent a kink secondary to the ureterectasis or a crossing vessel.

FIG. 18-22. Ureteral kink. There is some question as to whether kinking of the ureter ever is congenital. In the illustration the kink in the proximal ureter was produced by adhesions secondary to previous surgery. Similar kinks have been reported in children that presumably were secondary to fixation of the ureter by congenital bands of connective tissue. Spiral twists, which may produce kinking of the ureter, are thought to be produced when the ureter fails to follow the normal rotation of the kidney.

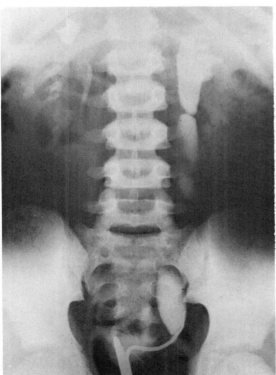

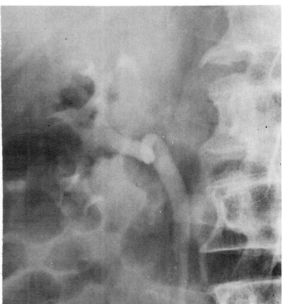

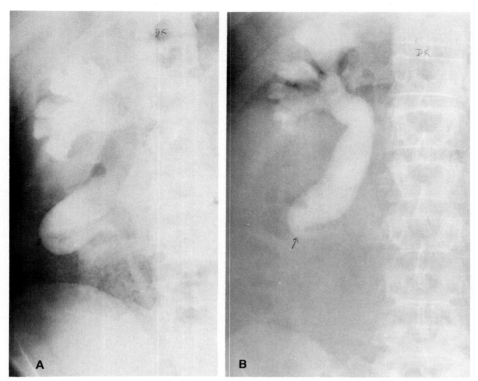

FIG. 18–23. Ureteral kink. Early (A) and late (B) films following retrograde injection of contrast medium. There is a sharp lateral angulation of the midureter (*arrow*). The kink is a residual from a previous ureterolithotomy.

FIG. 18–24. True ureteral valve. A 54-year-old man with ureteral colic. Scout film showed a calculus, which is obscured by contrast medium. Urogram (A) shows a defect in left ureter at site of valve (*arrowhead*). Pyelogram (B) shows area of narrowing, with Y-shaped lucent line (*arrows*) representing valve leaflets. Surgery revealed three leaflets with normal urothelium enclosing smooth muscle, a true ureteral valve. (Mering, J.H.: J. Urol., *107*:737–739, 1972. © 1972, The Williams & Wilkins Co., Baltimore)

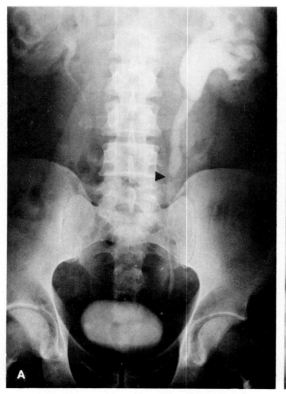

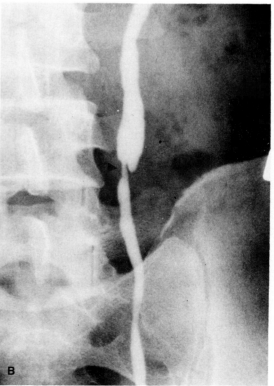

FIG. 18–25. True ureteral valves. Acute renal failure in a 3-year-old boy. BUN 144; creatinine 11. Following catheterization, marked diuresis occurred, and BUN dropped to 21 in 3 days. Urogram **(A)** revealed marked serpiginous tortuosity of both lumbar ureters. Ureterotomy **(B)** of right ureter revealed two flaplike ureter valves (*arrowheads*) that were covered with mucosa and contained smooth muscle. The ureter between the valves was redundant. Presumably a similar but nonobstructing valvular process is present in the left ureter. (Mering, J.H.: J. Urol., *107*:737–739, 1972. © 1972, The Williams & Wilkins Co., Baltimore.)

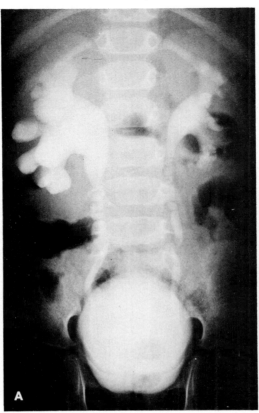

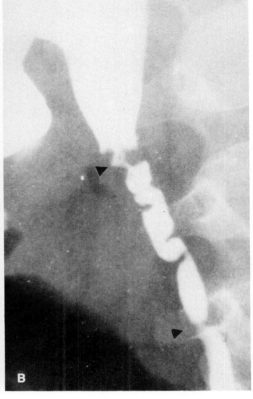

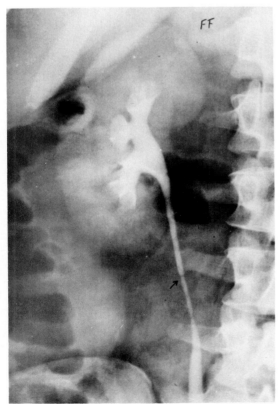

FIG. 18–25a. Valvelike lesion. Two separate urograms show the same nonobstructing defect in the proximal ureter (*arrow*). This may represent a nonobstructing mucosal flap or diaphragm.

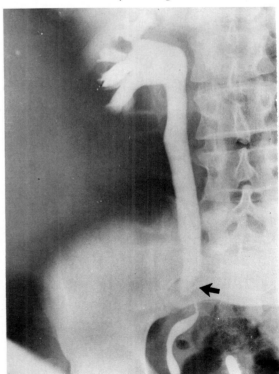

FIG. 18–26. Congenital ureteral valve. Young man who presented with pyuria. Urogram revealed marked hydronephrosis and dilatation of the proximal two-thirds of the right ureter. Pyelogram demonstrated a sharp oblique defect (*arrow*), which surgery showed to be a mucosal valve markedly reducing the ureteral lumen.

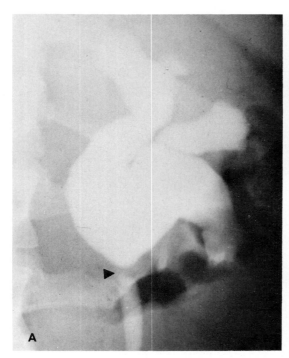

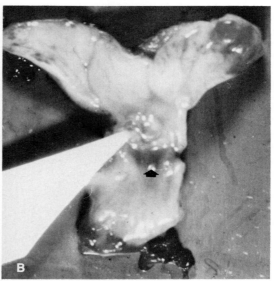

FIG. 18–27. Pseudovalve in a 29-year-old woman with repeated urinary tract infection. Urogram (**A**) showed left hydronephrosis with a sharp linear defect at the ureteropelvic junction (*arrowhead*). At surgery a chronic granuloma (**B**) (*pointer*) was present at the ureteropelvic junction. Just below the granuloma, mucosal hypertrophy produced a valvelike lesion (*arrow*), representing the defect in the urogram.

FIG. 18–28. Solitary ureteral diverticulum. Elongated solitary ureteral diverticulum arising from the midthird of right ureter (*arrow*). This illustrates the similarity between a ureteral diverticulum and a blind-ending ureter, previously illustrated. In this case the diverticulum has the appearance and the shape of an abortive ureter. No clinical symptomatology was present.

FIG. 18–29. Solitary ureteral diverticulum of proximal ureter with narrowing of the ureter at that point. This could be congenital or acquired (perforation) in origin, depending upon the clinical history.

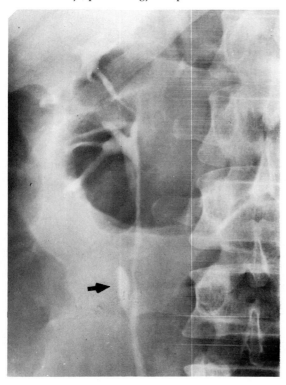

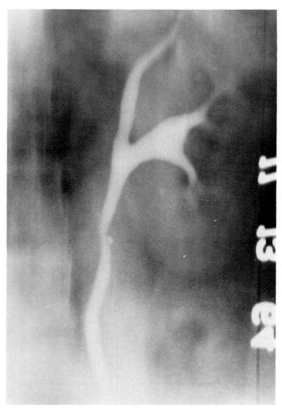

FIG. 18–30. Solitary diverticulum in the proximal third of the left ureter (*arrow*). A small calculus is present within the diverticulum and a moderate degree of ureteritis is present in the adjacent ureter. Calculi and infection are complications arising from stasis within diverticula.

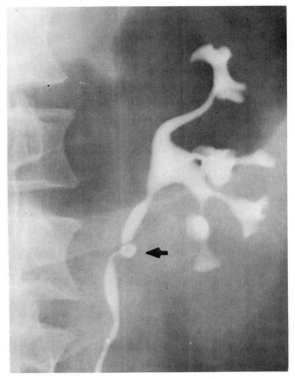

FIG. 18–31. Multiple diverticula. Illustrations reveal numerous small outpouchings from the midthirds of both ureters representing small ureteral diverticula. These are believed to arise from accessory ureteral buds along the course of the ureter. They are asymptomatic unless they become large in size, infected, or contain calculi. (Rank, W.B., Mellinger, G.T., and Spiro, E.: J. Urol., 83:566–569, 1960)

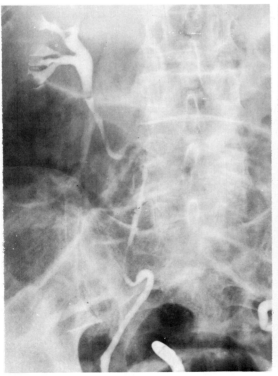

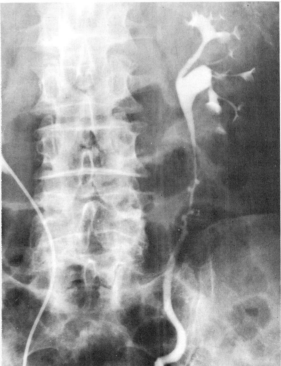

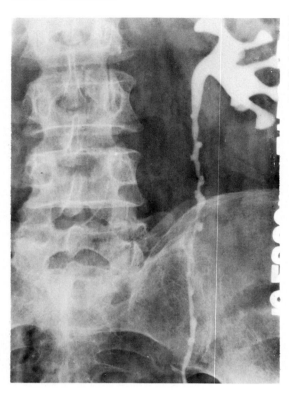

FIG. 18–32. Multiple congenital diverticula. Retrograde pyelography reveals numerous small diverticula along the entire course of the left ureter from the ureteropelvic junction to the ureterovesical junction. This was an incidental finding in a patient who had an intravenus urogram for right ureteral calculus. No clinical symptoms were present.

FIG. 18–33. Lower polar artery producing severe hydronephrosis. The ureter was fixed in position by fibrotic bands, allowing the extrinsic pressure of the vessel to produce obstruction. (See also Chapter 2, Congenital Anomalies of the Kidney.)

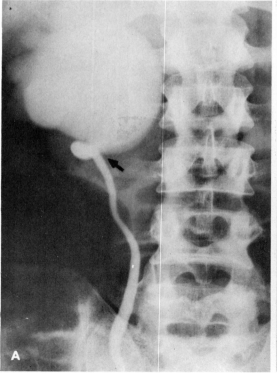

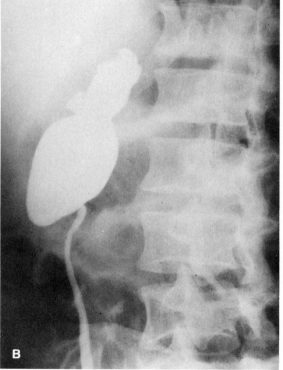

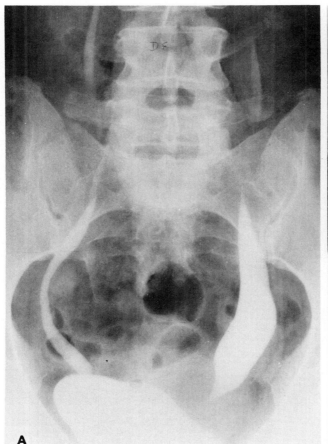

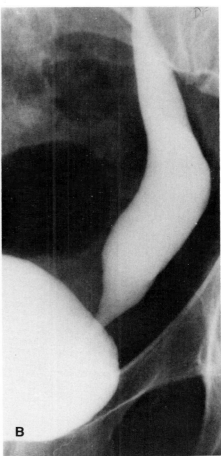

FIG. 18–34. Megaloureter. A 30-year-old woman with mild intermittent pelvic pain. The urogram (**A**) reveals fusiform dilatation of 3 or 4 cm. of the left pelvic ureter with a normal proximal ureter. The distal juxtavesical segment is not visualized. Spot film of the distal left ureter (**B**) shows the narrowed aperistaltic juxtavesical segment. As long as no significant complications or symptoms are present, conservative treatment will suffice. (Courtesy of Richard Pfister, M.D.)

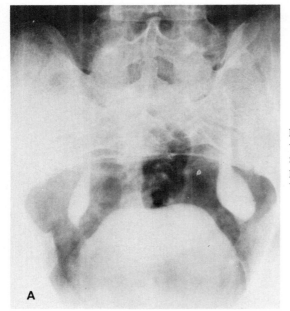

FIG. 18–35. Bilateral megaloureter. A 19-year-old man with mild pelvic pain. The urogram reveals bilateral fusiform dilatation of both pelvic ureters with normal proximal ureters. The narrowed aperistaltic segment is visualized on the right side.

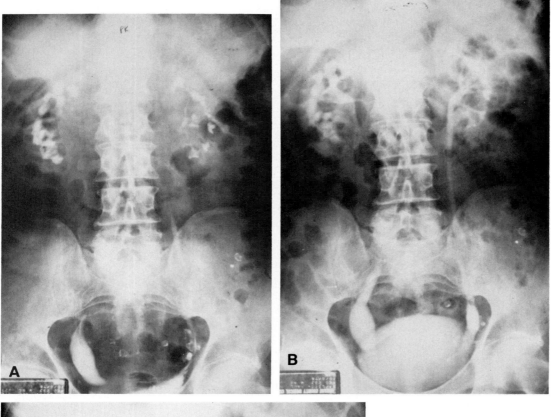

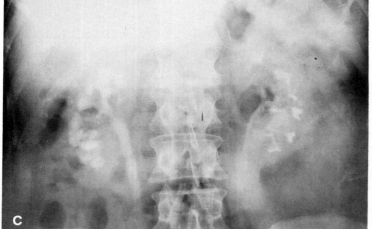

FIG. 18–35a. Megaloureter and megacalyces. Unusual association of two congenital lesions. (See Megacalyces.) The early **(A)** and later **(B)** roentgenograms of the urogram reveal the moderately dilated calyces with loss of normal cupping with normal cortex and renal pelvis **(C).** Bilateral megaloureter is present, more pronounced on the right side. (Courtesy of Alan Richman, M.D.)

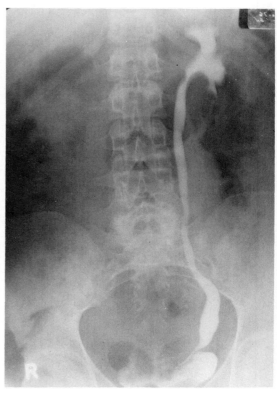

FIG. 18–36. Megaloureter. Withdrawal film showing mild dilatation of the pelvic ureter with contrast medium outlining the aperistaltic segment.

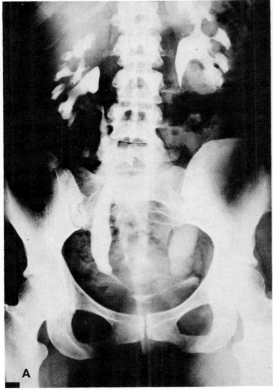

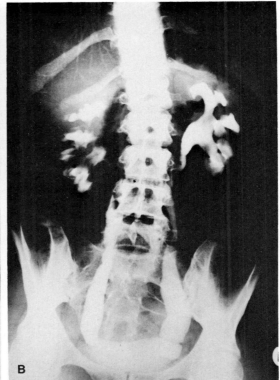

FIG. 18–37. Megaloureter and megacalyces in a 27-year-old man with occasional mild pelvic pain. Supine (A) and prone (B) films of the urogram show bilateral dilatation of the pelvic ureters that has progressed proximally. Note the narrowed aperistaltic segment delineated on the right (*arrow*). The renal pelves and most of the proximal ureters are normal. Bilateral megacalyces are present.

FIG. 18–37a. (A) Congenital megaloureter corrected surgically. Nephrostogram reveals dilatation of the entire ureter with the typical distal narrowed segment (*arrow*). (B) Urogram 10 years later after resection of the narrowed distal segment and 2 inches of excess ureteral length and reimplantation into the bladder. The collecting system shows minimal residual distention, and the ureter was essentially normal. (Courtesy of H. Hendren, M.D.)

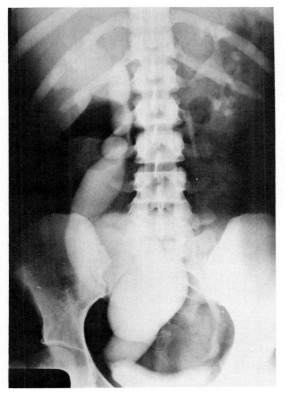

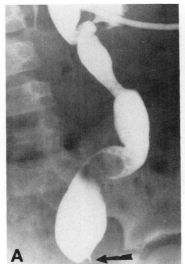
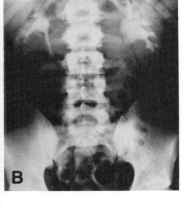

FIG. 18–38. Decompensated right megaloureter in a 35-year-old man with flank pain and pyuria. The entire ureter and collecting system are dilated. There is no mechanical obstruction. The dilatation probably results when peristalsis cannot maintain output equal to volume filtered and/or when infection occurs.

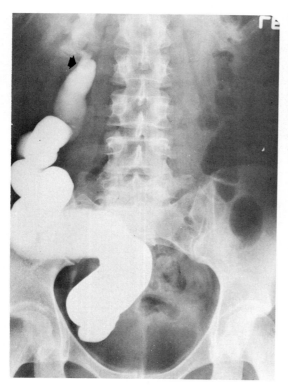

FIG. 18–39. Megaloureter. Retrograde study revealed a dilated, elongated, and tortuous right ureter. No peristalsis was observed. The proximal ureter (*arrow*) is not dilated, and there is no significant hydronephrosis. Following surgical resection, the proximal ureter had a normal muscular wall, whereas the dilated segment that extended to the ureterovesical junction did not reveal muscular fibers. This may represent faulty muscular development of the dilated segment of ureter or decompensated megaloureter with an extremely short aperistaltic segment that was not identified.

FIG. 18–40. Girl with persistent incontinence. Intravenous urogram (**A**) reveals the left kidney to be normal. A double kidney was present on the right with moderate hydronephrosis of the upper segment. The ureter draining the upper renal segment can be visualized through the contrast in the bladder (*arrow*) extending to the area of the posterior urethra. At cystoscopy only one orifice was visualized. An orifice was catheterized in the posterior urethra (*arrow*), and on pyelography (**B**) visualization of the upper renal segment was obtained. In girls, incontinence is common; in boys, it is uncommon.

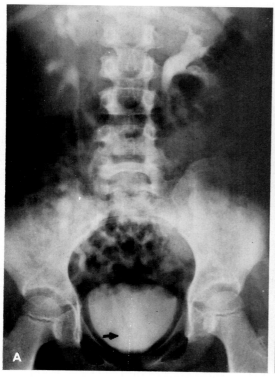

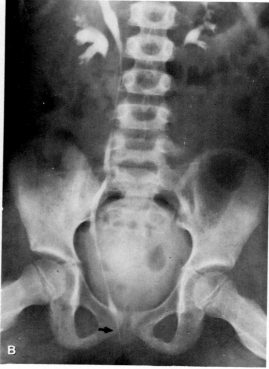

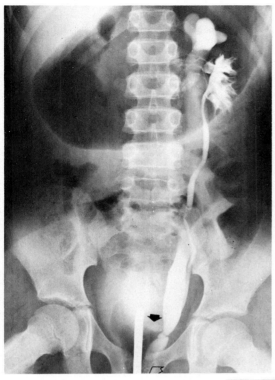

FIG. 18–41. A 10-year-old girl who presented with pyuria and incontinence. The illustration shows simultaneous catheterization of the ureteral orifice on the left side of the bladder (*dark arrow*) and an orifice in the posterior urethra (*light arrow*). Marked pyelorenal reflux has occurred in the lower renal segment, which is relatively normal. There is severe ureterectasis and pyelectasis of the upper renal segment draining through the ectopic orifice.

FIG. 18–42. Ectopic ureter. Urogram **(A)**, voiding cystourethrogram **(B)**, of a 3-year-old girl with incontinence. In the urogram the ureter is visualized to the bladder neck. Typical of ectopic ureters it does not cross the midline. In the voiding cystourethrogram the ureter fills from the posterior urethra (*arrowhead*) by reflux. (Courtesy of Keith Waterhouse, M.D.)

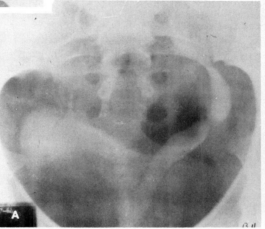
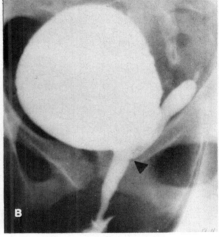

FIG. 18–43. Ectopic ureter in a 2-year-old girl with incontinence. The cystogram **(A)** demonstrated left ureteral reflux with contrast medium filling a distended collecting system. The voiding film **(B)** shows reflux into the ectopic left ureter filling from the junction of bladder and posterior urethra.

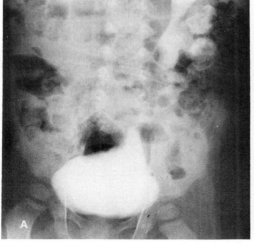
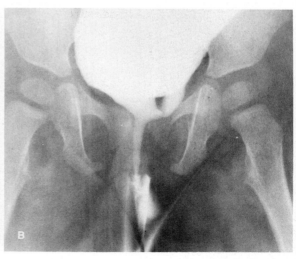

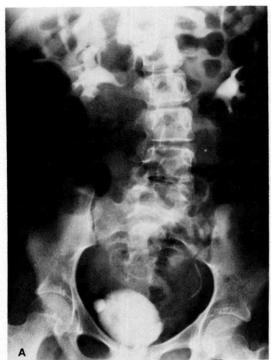

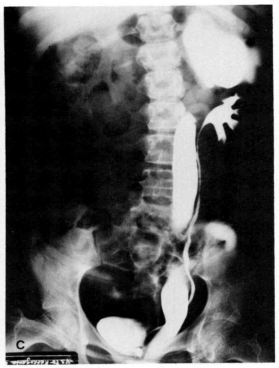

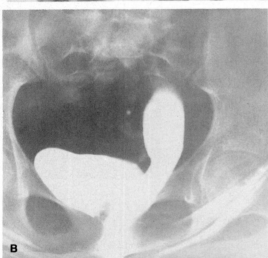

FIG. 18–44. Ectopic ureter in a woman. **(A)** Urogram shows abnormal tilt of left collecting system, suggesting a mass in the upper pole of the left kidney. Voiding cystourethrogram **(B)** reveals reflux into the dilated ectopic ureter. Retrograde catheterization of both left ureters was performed **(C)**. The dilated ectopic ureter to the upper pole opened into the posterior urethra.

FIG. 18–45. Ectopic ureter to seminal vesicle in young adult man. Seminal vesiculogram shows a dilated right seminal vesicle with reflux filling of right ureter (*arrowhead*). Contrast material is in the bladder. (Courtesy of Herbert Weber, M.D.)

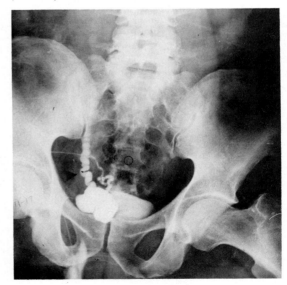

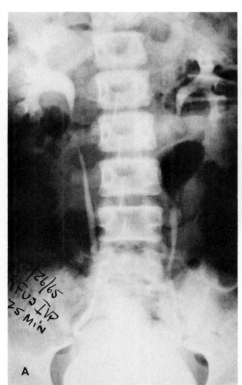 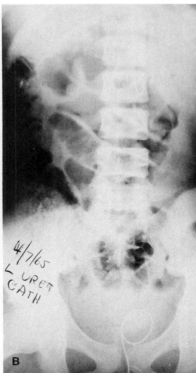 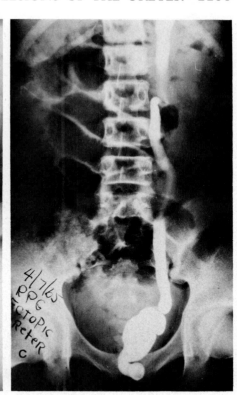

FIG. 18–46. Ectopic ureter to Gartner's duct cyst. Urogram **(A)** reveals faint visualization of a dilated double left upper collecting system. An ectopic ureteral orifice was found in the posterior urethra. The retrograde catheter coiled in the distal ectopic ureter **(B)**. Retrograde injection **(C)** revealed the ectopic ureter to enter a cystic mass that communicated with the urethra. This was confirmed by surgery. (Courtesy of Charles Rieser, M.D.)

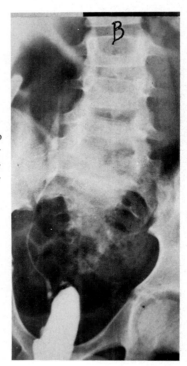

FIG. 18–47. Ectopic ureter into vagina. Young girl who presented with vaginal discharge. Vaginogram demonstrated filling of an ectopic ureter from the vagina, draining the upper pole of the right kidney. (Katzen, P., Trachtman, B.: J. Urol., 72:808, 1954)

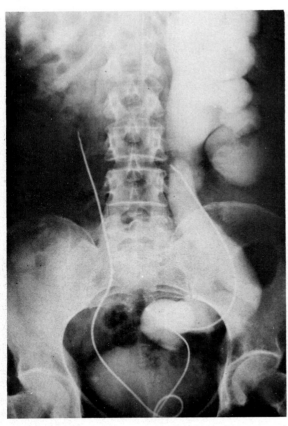

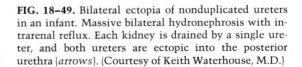

FIG. 18–48. Fifty-year-old woman who had incontinence since infancy and presented with renal tract infection and a palpable mass on the left side. Cystoscopy revealed a normal right ureteral orifice. No ureteral orifice could be seen on the left side. An orifice was found in the posterior urethra, and retrograde injection revealed ureterectasis and pyonephrosis (palpable mass). The ectopia occurred in a single system (no ureteral duplication), a rare occurrence.

FIG. 18–49. Bilateral ectopia of nonduplicated ureters in an infant. Massive bilateral hydronephrosis with intrarenal reflux. Each kidney is drained by a single ureter, and both ureters are ectopic into the posterior urethra (*arrows*). (Courtesy of Keith Waterhouse, M.D.)

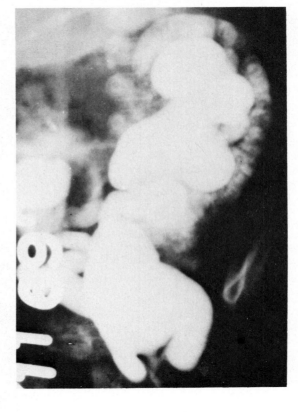

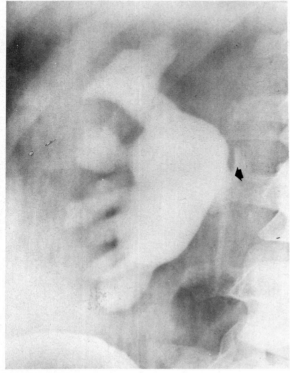

FIG. 18–50. intravenous urography revealed moderate calyectasis and pyelectasis. The right ureter (*arrow*) enters the superior aspect of the renal pelvis. Although most cases of high insertion occur secondary to pelvic dilatation, this amount of dilatation is insufficient to produce a secondary ureteral elevation of this degree. It is assumed that the congenital high position of the ureteropelvic junction did not allow adequate drainage, producing the moderate hydronephrosis seen.

FIG. 18–51. High insertion of the ureter. This insertion is similar to that in Figure 18–50, with less hydronephrosis. Normal drainage depends on the ureter being at the dependent part of the renal pelvis. High insertions tend to produce pyelectasis.

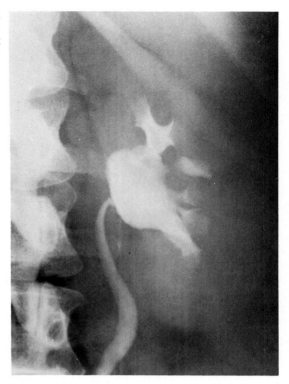

FIG. 18–52. High anterior insertion of the ureter. **(A)** In the frontal projection the ureter is noted to curve laterally prior to its insertion into the renal pelvis. **(B)** In the oblique projection the anterior position of the ureter is seen clearly without evidence of proximal obstruction. Although a minimal degree of malrotation cannot be excluded, this appears to represent a high anterior insertion of the ureter on a congenital basis.

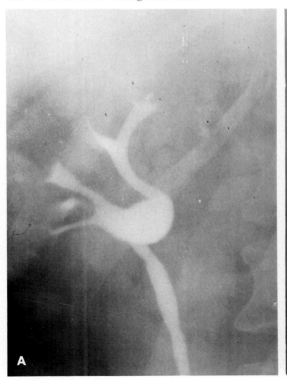

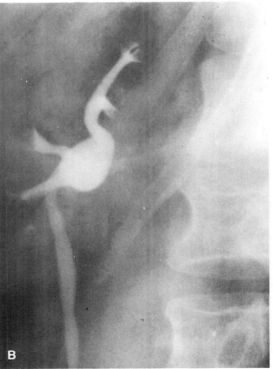

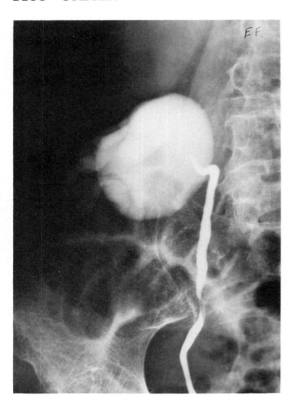

FIG. 18–52a. Acquired high insertion. Prior history of ureteral calculus and renal infection. The resulting marked pyeloectasis included dilatation of the inferior aspect of the renal pelvis with elevation of the ureteropelvic junction.

FIG. 18–53. Ureterocele. **(A)** Catheter is coiled within the lumen of the ureterocele. **(B)** Following injection, the ureterocele is visualized together with a normal ureter. **(C)** Following withdrawal of the catheter, contrast remains within the ureterocele. Contrast is also seen within the bladder.

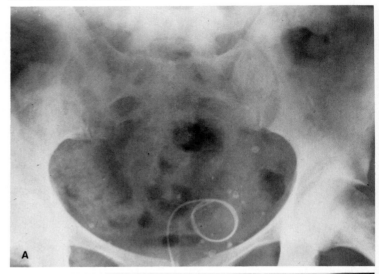

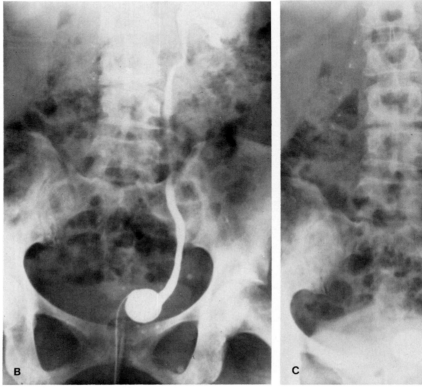

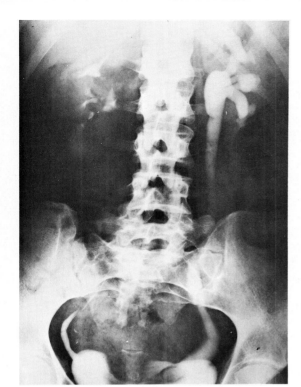

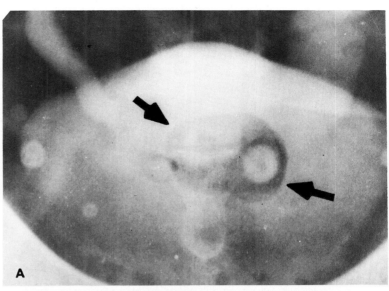

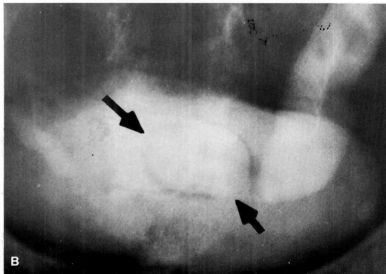

FIG. 18-53a. Ureterocele. There is moderate hydroureter and hydronephrosis on the left side. The distal end of the left ureter appears bulbous and protrudes into the bladder. The area of radiolucency around the bulbous tip represents the walls of the ureter and the mucosa of the bladder, separating the contrast material in the ureter from that in the bladder. This is a typical example of a moderate-sized ureterocele in a young adult, producing some proximal obstruction.

FIG. 18-54. Ureterocele seen by negative and positive contrast. **(A)** Supine position. A large radiolucent shadow is present near distal end of left ureter (*arrows*). This represents a ureterocele distended with nonopacified urine in the contrast-filled bladder. **(B)** Prone position a few minutes later. Contrast material now has filled ureterocele (*arrows*). Note radiolucent shadow around margins, representing ureteral and bladder walls.

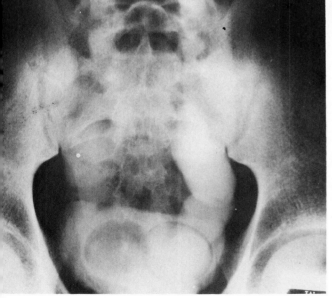

FIG. 18-55. Bilateral ureteroceles. Right ureterocele contains urine without contrast material; left ureterocele is contrast-filled with clear radiolucent halo. Bilateral partial ureteral obstruction is present.

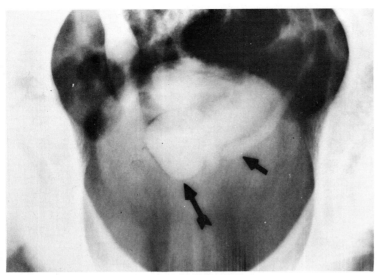

FIG. 18–56. Bilateral ureteroceles. Fifteen-minute urogram reveals a large ureterocele (*long arrow*) arising from the right ureter and a small ureterocele (*short arrow*) arising from the left ureter. Areas of radiolucency are present about both ureteroceles.

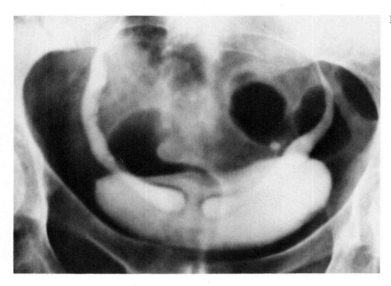

FIG. 18–57. Bilateral ureteroceles; nonobstructive.

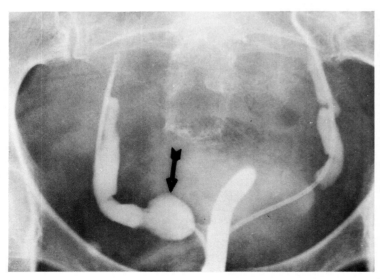

FIG. 18–58. Ureterocele. On the right side there is bulbous distention of the distal end of the right ureter. The ureter and the ureterocele (*arrow*) are filled with contrast material from retrograde injection, but the contrast material has not filled the bladder.

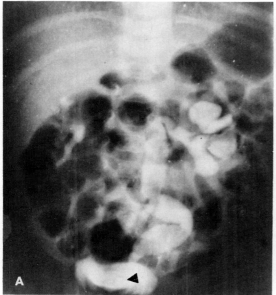

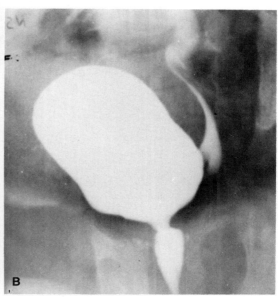

FIG. 18–59. Ureterocele in newborn. Urogram **(A)** shows left hydronephrosis from a left ureterocele (*arrowhead*) No reflux was present in the cystogram. Three weeks after surgery (unroofing) a cystogram **(B)** shows left ureterovesical reflux.

FIG. 18–59a. Obstructing ureterocele in infant. **(A)** Ten-minute urogram reveals the right collecting system to be faintly visualized and dilated. A large mass in the bladder is partially obstructing the left ureter. **(B)** Delayed roentgenogram reveals the mass to be a large ureterocele with right hydroureter. The ureterocele is so large that it partially obstructs the left ureterovesical orifice.

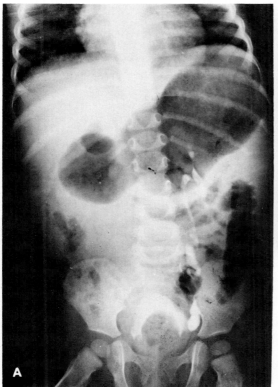

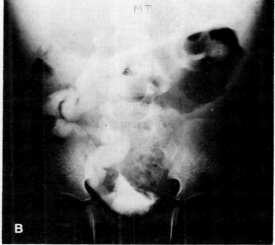

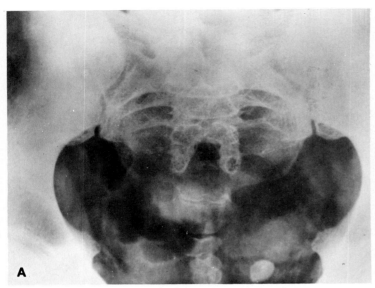

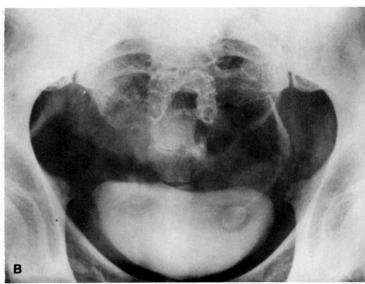

FIG. 18–60. Stone in ureterocele. (**A**) Scout film reveals large opaque calculus near left ureterovesical junction. (**B**) Urogram reveals no dilatation of left ureter. Persistent band of radiolucency around calculus shows it is within ureterocele.

FIG. 18–61. Ectopic ureterocele. Five-year-old girl with incontinence and pyuria. The urogram (**A**) showed a double right kidney, a hydronephrotic left kidney without visualization of the ureters, and a bilobed defect in the bladder. Pyelography (**B**) revealed two right and one left ureteral orifices in the bladder, with the eccentric lobulated bladder defect. A cystogram (**C**) revealed that the bladder defect could be obliterated by distention. The sequence suggested an ectopic ureterocele. The orifice was located in the posterior urethra. In (**D**) the ectopic ureter (*arrow*) and the normal orifice have been catheterized. Note the lobulation of the distal end of the ectopic ureter, which produced the bladder defect. A new orifice was created surgically. This series illustrates the typical findings of ectopic ureterocele, namely, (1) double kidney and ureter, (2) eccentric bladder defect, in which contrast in the bladder does not circle the defect completely, and (3) diminution or disappearance of the defect on increasing intracystic pressure by displacing the urine in the ureterocele proximally.

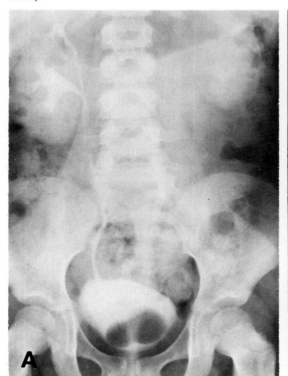

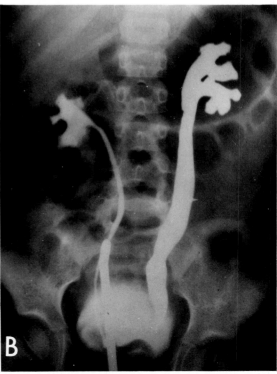

FIG. 18–62. Ectopic ureterocele in a 26-year-old woman with a long history of urinary tract infection and left flank pain. **(A)** Urogram reveals non-visualization of the upper left renal segments, with a large lucent defect in the bladder. **(B)** Retrograde catheterization revealed the ectopic orifice to be at the bladder neck. The distended ureter in the bladder submucosa produced the large bladder defect.

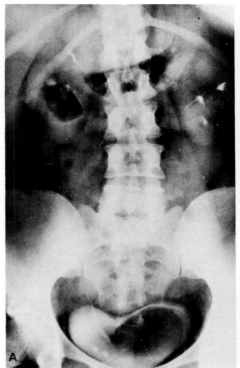
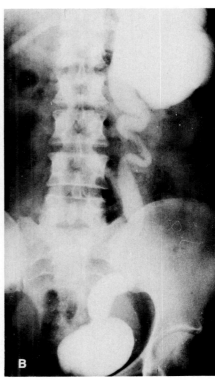
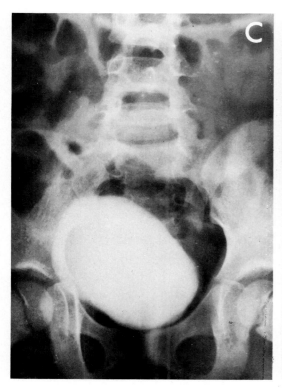
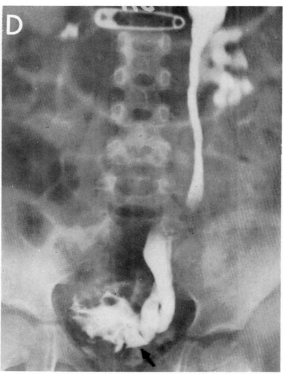

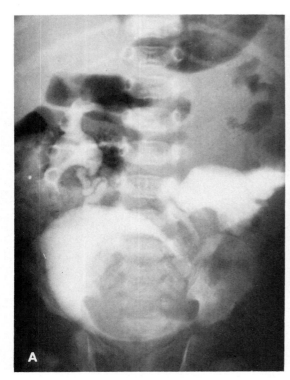

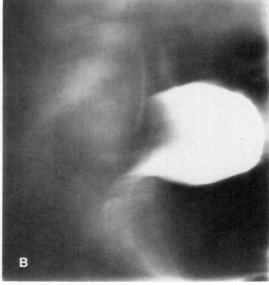

FIG. 18–63. Ectopic ureterocele. **(A)** Urogram showing a mass representing a dilated left upper pole compressing the lower renal segment. There is a large defect in the bladder, representing an ectopic ureterocele. **(B)** Lateral film showing posterior position of ureterocele. (Williams, D.I.: Br. J. Urol., *44*:417–433, 1971)

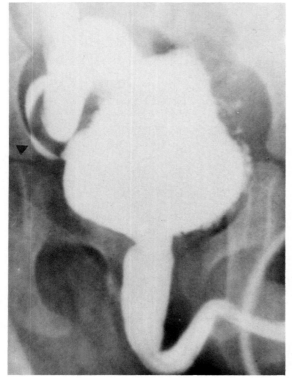

FIG. 18–64. Ectopic ureterocele projecting outside of bladder. Voiding cystogram with right ureteral reflux. The ureterocele (*arrowhead*) projects outside of the lumen. In such cases the detrusor muscle behind the ureterocele is poor or absent, and the ureterocele protrudes posteriorly. (Williams, D.I.: Br. J. Urol., *44*:417–433, 1971)

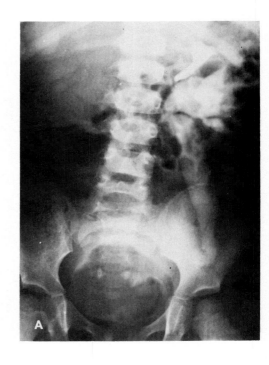

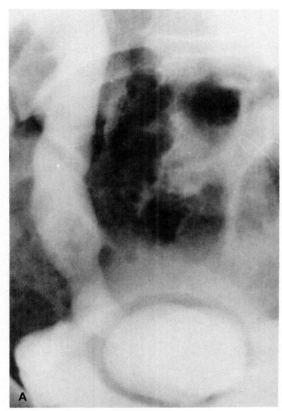

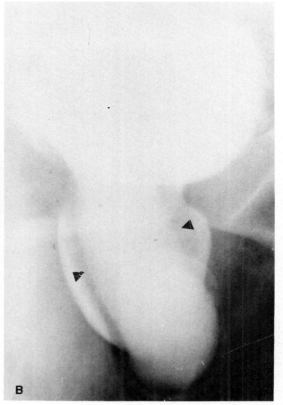

FIG. 18–66. Prolapsing ectopic ureterocele. Urogram (**A**) shows a large ureterocele in the bladder with proximal obstruction. Attempted voiding (**B**) shows prolapse of the ureterocele into the female urethra (*arrowheads*) and presenting at the urethral orifice. (Courtesy of Erich Lang, M.D.)

FIG. 18–67. Retrocaval ureter. Classic appearance of retrocaval ureter with localized medial deviation of proximal ureter as it passes behind inferior vena cava from lateral to medial side. Ureter posterior to inferior vena cava is pulled cephalad. Obstruction of proximal ureter with hydronephrosis of kidney has occurred secondary to compression of ureter between inferior vena cava and posterior abdominal wall. Ureter on the medial aspect of inferior vena cava overlies the pedicles.

FIG. 18–65. Prolapsing ectopic ureterocele in a young girl with bilateral duplex kidneys. The urogram (**A**) reveals nonvisualization of the right kidney and moderate left ureterectasis and pyelocalyectasis. The obstruction was secondary to a large right ectopic ureterocele. (**B**) Voiding cystourethrogram shows a filling defect at the base of the bladder projecting into the urethra (*arrowheads*), representing a prolapsing ectopic ureterocele. Rarely, ectopic ureteroceles chronically or intermittently prolapse into the urethra during voiding. In men, they are limited by the membranous urethra; in women, they may present at the external meatus. (Williams, D.I.: Br. J. Urol., *44*:417–433, 1971)

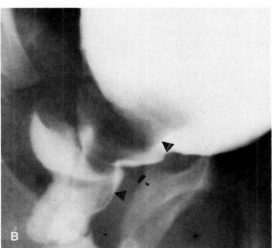

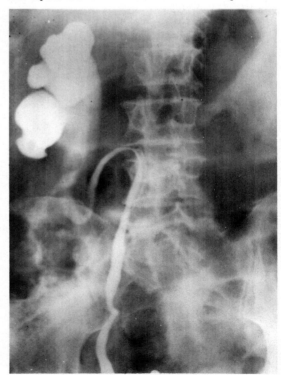

1165

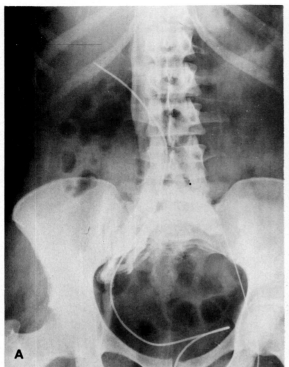 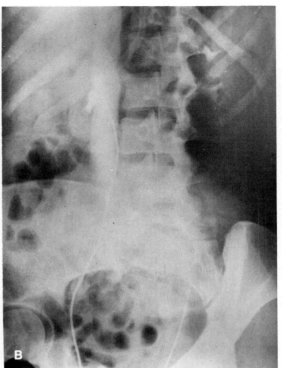

FIG. 18–68. Retrocaval ureter. Inferior venacavogram. (A) The retrograde catheter curves medially at L-3 behind inferior vena cava, which is outlined by contrast medium, to its medial aspect. The ureter then continues inferiorly, medial to the pedicles along medial aspect of vena cava to the pelvis. (B) Oblique projection. Inferior vena cava and collecting system of right kidney are outlined by contrast medium. Ureter is visualized behind inferior vena cava without elevation of this segment of ureter, as seen in Figure 18–67. The ureter crosses anterior to the vena cava near L-5 and resumes its normal course. There is no obstruction. (Courtesy of P. Ross, M.D.)

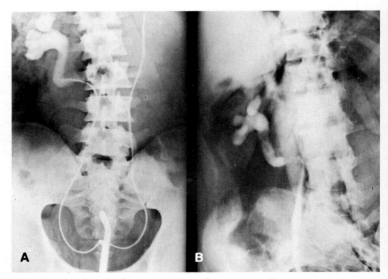

FIG. 18–69. Retrocaval ureter. Presacral oxygen study. (A) There is a sharp deviation of the ureter medial to the pedicles. A moderate degree of hydroureter and hydronephrosis is present. (B) Following presacral oxygen injection, the inferior vena cava is outlined by the oxygen. Demonstrated are the course of the ureter around the inferior vena cava and the site of compression of the ureter posterior to the inferior vena cava.

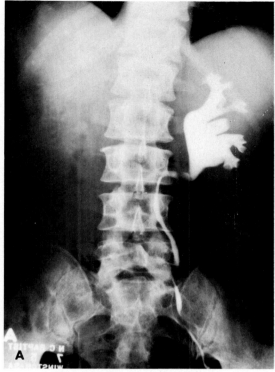

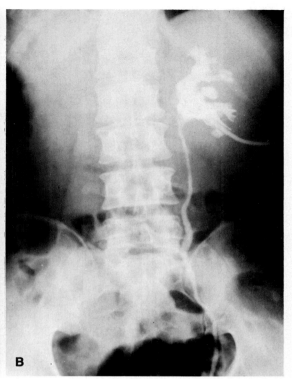

FIG. 18–70. Left retrocaval ureter. This 43-year-old man presented with left flank pain and a previous history of urinary infection. He had total situs inversus with cardiac anomalies. The urogram revealed a normal right kidney with a left hydronephrosis and marked delay in emptying. Left pyelogram (A) showed a smooth hook-like medial displacement of the proximal ureter medial to the pedicles, suggestive of a retrocaval ureter. Surgery revealed a left inferior vena cava associated with situs inversus. The ureter was divided and reanastomosis accomplished. The postoperative pyelogram (B) revealed satisfactory continuity. (Courtesy of Ralph E. Brooks, Jr., M.D.)

FIG. 18–71. Retrocaval ureter: Ureteral catheter outlining course of ureter. Between L-3–L-4 the ureter hooks sharply medial to the pedicles.

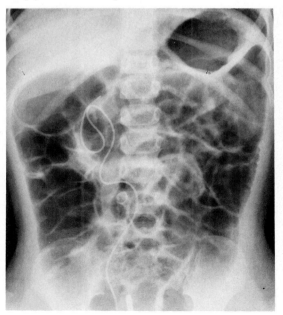

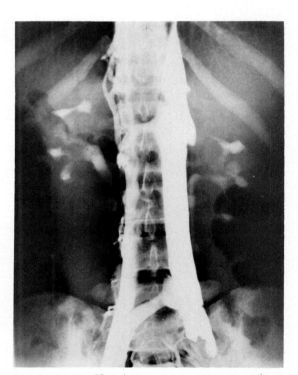

FIG. 18–72. Double inferior vena cava. Venogram showing bilateral inferior vena cava. (Courtesy of Lawrence Schechter, M.D.)

1167

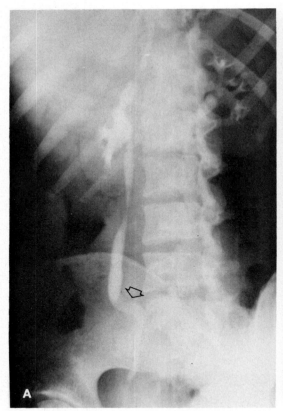
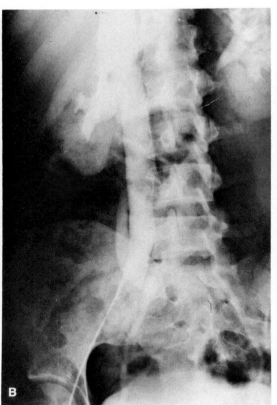

FIG. 18–73. Retroiliac ureter. **(A)** Oblique urogram reveals posterior angulation of the right ureter in front of L-5-S-1 (*arrow*). Note the impression of the iliac vein. **(B)** Venous study clearly outlines the right ureter posterior to the right iliac vein.

FIG. 18–73a. Retroiliac ureter in a 3-month-old boy with pyuria. The urogram shows sharp medial angulation of the left ureter (*arrow*) over S-1. This represented a left retroiliac ureter.

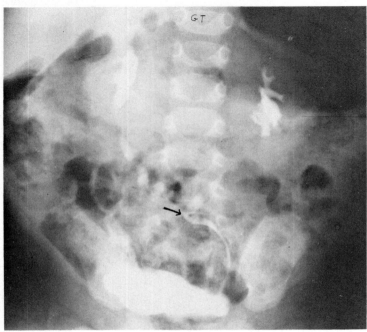

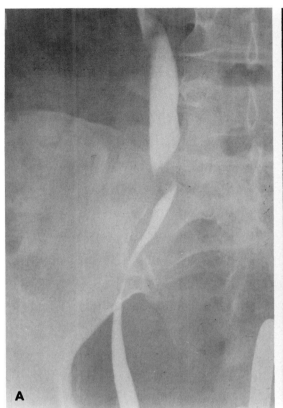 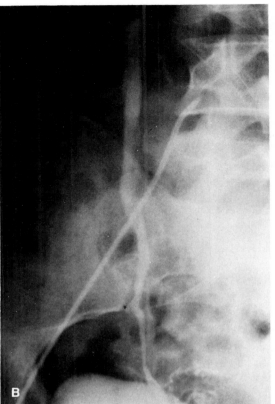

FIG. 18–73b. Retroiliac ureter. **(A)** Retrograde injection shows marked impression of iliac vein on the ureter. **(B)** Catheter in the right iliac vein shows the venous position to the right ureter in the oblique position. (Courtesy of Erich Lang, M.D.)

FIG. 18–74. Ureter in scrotal hernia. Nine-year-old boy investigated for hydronephrotic left kidney, pyuria, and left-sided pain. The intravenous urogram revealed severe hydronephrosis with poor visualization of the ureter. Retrograde catheterization showed the catheter to enter a left scrotal hernia with marked redundancy of the ureter within the hernial sac. Resection of the ureter within the hernial sac was performed. (Jewett, H.J., Harris, A.P.: J. Urol., *69*:184–187, 1953)

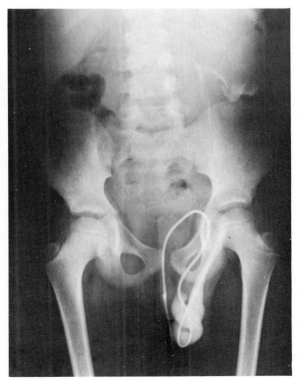

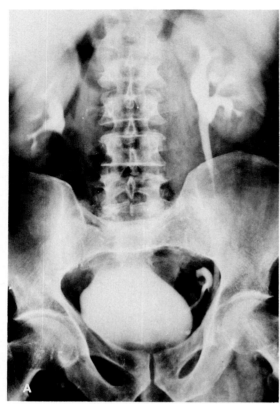

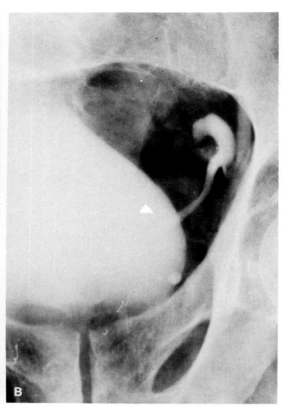

FIG. 18–75. Inguinal hernia in a 35-year-old man with mild left flank pain and pyuria. Urograms (**A, B**) show left hydronephrosis. There is a vertical redundancy of the distal left ureter frequently associated with inguinal hernias. The ureter was in the orifice of the left inguinal canal.

FIG. 18–76. Inguinal hernia. Frontal (**A**) and oblique (**B**) pyelogram shows vertical redundancy of pelvic ureter in (**A**) and angulation of ureter in (**B**). This patient had a femoral hernia with the ureter near the orifice of the hernia.

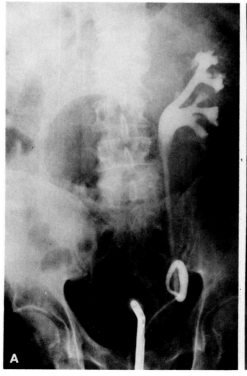

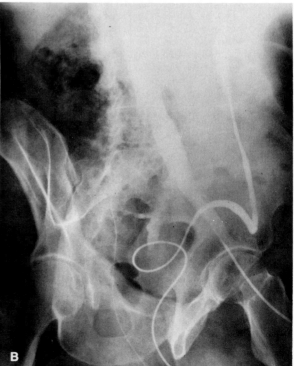

FIG. 18–76a. Ureter in inguinal hernias bilaterally. Both ureters show marked vertical redundancy as they extend into the orifices of the inguinal canal. The descending right ureter (*upper arrow*) and the distal ascending segment (*lower arrow*) are visualized. There was no obstruction.

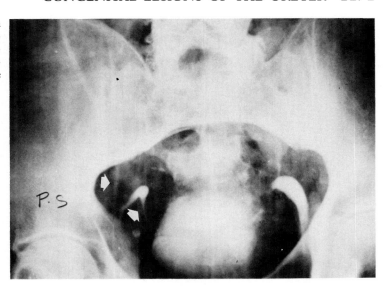

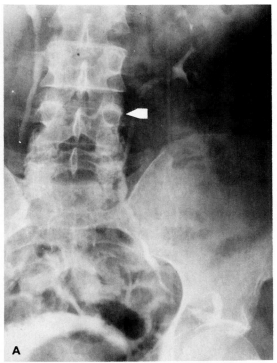

FIG. 18–77. Sciatic hernia in a 60-year-old man with prostatism. The urogram (**A**) shows sharp lateral angulation of the pelvic ureter (*arrow*) without obstruction. Lateral roentgenogram (**B**) shows the left ureter presenting posteriorly (*arrow*). This is a typical presentation of herniation through the sacrosciatic foramen. Obstruction rarely occurs.

FIG. 18–78. Sciatic hernia. Minor lateral redundancy of the right pelvic ureter (*arrow*) as it extends posteriorly into the sacrosciatic notch.

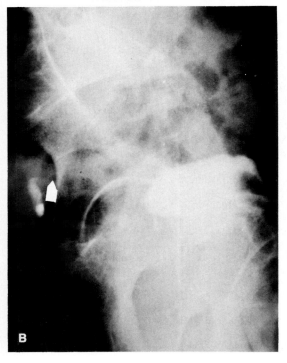

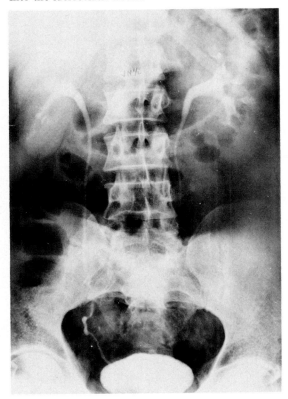

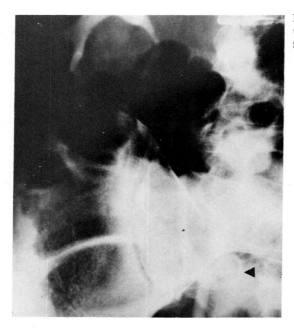

FIG. 18–79. Internal hernia. The right ureter loops in the pelvis (*arrow*), apparently caught in retroperitoneal folds around the right iliac vein.

BIBLIOGRAPHY

Congenital Ureter

General Ureteral Anomalies

1. Campbell, M.F. (ed.): Urology, 2nd ed. Vol. 1, p. 1618, Philadelphia, W.B. Saunders, 1963.
2. Currarino, G., and Allen, T.D.: Congenital anomalies of the upper urinary tract. Progr. Pediatr. Radiol., 3:211–217, 1970.
3. Meyer, R.R.: Normal and abnormal development of ureter in human embryo: Mechanistic considerations. Anat. Rec., 96:355–371, 1946.
4. Williams, D.: The ureter, the urologist, and the paediatrician. Proc. R. Soc. Med., 63:595–602, 1970.

Agenesis and Aplasia

See references at the end of Chapter 2.

Ureteral Aplasia and Hypoplasia

5. DeKlerk, D.P., Marshall, F.F., and Jeffs, R.D.: Multicystic dysplastic kidney. J. Urol., 118:306–308, 1977.
6. DeWolf, W.C., Fraley, E.E., and Markland, C.: Congenital hypoplasia of the proximal ureter. J. Urol., 113:236–237, 1975.
7. Gordon, M., and Reed, J.O.: Distal ureteral atresia. Am. J. Roentgenol., 88:579–584, 1962.
8. Griscom, N.T., Vawter, G.F., and Fellers, F.T.: Pelvo-infundibular atresia: The usual form of multicystic kidney; 44 unilateral and two bilateral cases. Seminar Roentgenol., 10:125–131, 1975.
9. Slater, G.S.: Ureteral atresia producing giant hydronephrosis. J. Urol., 78:130–137, 1951.

Ureteral Duplication

10. Amar, A.D., and Hutch, J.A.: Anomalies of the ureter. In Aiken, C.E., Dix, V.W., Goodwin, W.E., et al. (eds.): Encyclopedia of Urology, Vol. 7/1. New York, Springer-Verlag, 1968.
11. Ambrose, S.S., and Nicolson, W.P.: Ureteral reflex in duplicated ureter. J. Urol., 92:439–443, 1964.
12. Atwell, J.D., Coon, P.L., Howell, C.J., et al.: Familial incidence of bifid and double ureters. Arch. Dis. Child., 49:390–393, 1974.
13. Campbell, M.F.: Anomalies of the ureter. In Campbell, M.F., and Harrison, J.H. (eds.): Urology, 3rd ed., Chap. 37. Philadelphia, W.B. Saunders, 1970.
14. Christoffersen, J., and Iversen, H.G.: Partial hydronephrosis in a patient with horseshoe kidney and bilateral duplication of the pelvis and ureter. Scand. J. Urol. Nephrol., 10:91–93, 1976.
15. Colosimo, C.: Uretere doppio e uretre bifido (osservazioni 50 cases). Urologia, 5:239–267, 1938.
16. Dahl, D.S.: Bilateral complete renal duplication with total obstruction of both lower pole collecting systems. Urology, 6:727–729, 1975.
17. Dees, J.: Clinical importance of congenital anomalies of the upper urinary tract. J. Urol., 46:659–666, 1941.
18. Gutierrez, R.: Double kidney as a source of impaired dynamism: Its surgical treatment by heminephrectomy. Am. J. Surg., 65:256–267, 1944.
19. Hartman, G.W., and Hodson, C.J.: Duplex kidney and related anomalies. Clin. Radiol., 20:387–400, 1969.
20. Hawthorne, A.B.: Embryologic and clinical aspect of double ureter. J.A.M.A., 106:189–193, 1936.
21. Johnston, J.H.: Urinary tract duplication in childhood. Arch. Dis. Child., 36:180–189, 1961.

22. Kaplan, N., and Elkin, M.: Bifid renal pelves and ureters: Radiographic and cinefluorographic observations. Br. J. Urol., 40:235–244, 1968.

23. Kretschmer, H.L.: Hydronephrosis in infancy and childhood: Clinical data and a report of 101 cases. Surg. Gynecol. Obstet., 64:634–645, 1937.

24. Lenaghan, D.: Bifid ureters in children: An anatomical, physiological and clinical study. J. Urol., 87:808–817, 1962.

25. Mackie, C.G., and Stephens, F.D.: Duplex kidneys: A correlation of renal dysplasia with position of the ureteric orifice. Birth Defects, 13:313–321, 1977.

26. Meyer, R.: Normal and abnormal development of the ureter in the human embryo: A mechanistic consideration. Anat. Rec., 96:355–371, 1946.

27. Nation, E.F.: Duplication of the kidney and ureter: a statistical study of 230 cases. J. Urol., 51:456–465, 1944.

28. Nordmark, B.: Double formations of the pelves of the kidneys and the ureters. Embryology and clinical significance. Acta Radiol., 30:267–278, 1948.

29. Privett, J.T., Jeans, W.D., and Roylance, J.: The incidence and importance of renal duplication. Clin. Radiol., 27:521–530, 1976.

30. Ratner, I.A., Fisher, J.H., and Swenson, O.: Double ureters in infancy and childhood. Pediatrics, 28:810–815, 1961.

31. Stephens, F.D.: Double ureter in the child. Aust. N.Z. J. Surg., 26:81–94, 1956.

32. Stephens, F.D.: Anatomical vagaries of double ureters. Aust. N.Z. J. Surg., 28:27–33, 1958.

33. Swenson, O., and Ratner, I.A.: Pyeloureterostomy for treatment of symptomatic ureteral duplications in children. J. Urol., 88:184–190, 1962.

34. Thompson, I.M., and Amar, A.D.: Clinical importance of ureteral duplication and ectopia. J.A.M.A., 168:881–886, 1958.

35. Timothy, R.P., Dexter, A., and Perlmutter, A.D.: Ureteral duplication: Clinical findings and therapy in 46 children. J. Urol., 105:445–451, 1971.

36. Weigert, C.: Ureter einige Bildunsfehler der Ureteren. Virchow's Arch. (Pathol. Anat.), 70:490–501, 1877.

37. Wharton, L.R., Jr.: Double ureters and associated renal anomalies in early human embryos. Contrib. Embryol. Carnegie Inst., 33:103–112, 1949.

38. Whitaker, J., and Banks, D.M.: A study of the inheritance of duplication of the kidneys and ureters. J. Urol., 95:176–178, 1966.

39. Williams, D.I.: Bifid ureter: Complete duplication. *In* Williams, D.I. (ed.): Urology in Childhood, p. 128. New York, Springer-Verlag, 1972.

Inverted Y Ureter

40. Block, W.: Hydronephrosis from malformation of ureter. Z. Urol., 14:221–230, 1924.

41. Britt, D.B., Borden, T.A., and Woodhead, D.M.: Inverted Y ureteral duplication with a blind-ending branch. J. Urol., 108:387–388, 1972.

42. Hawthorne, A.B.: Embryologic and clinical aspect of double ureter. J.A.M.A., 106:189–193, 1936.

43. Klauber, G.T., and Reid, E.C.: Inverted Y reduplication of the ureter. J. Urol., 107:362–364, 1972.

44. Lenko, J., and Cieśliński, S.: Urete fibidus caudelis. Pol. Tyg. Lek., 14:915–919, 1959.

45. Rihmer, B.: Bifurcating ureter on left side, one branch emptying into vagina; urine passing from vagina for 17 years. Orv. Hetil, 73:1188–1189, 1929.

46. Saltykow, S.: Ureter bifidus caudalis. Centralbl. f. Allg. Path. u. Path. Anat., 52:177–179, 1931.

Dysperistalsis

47. Campbell, J.E.: Ureteral peristalsis in duplex collecting systems. Am. J. Roentgenol., 99:577–584, 1967.

48. Kaplan, N., and Elkin, M.: Bifid renal pelves and ureters: Radiographic and cinefluorographic observations. Br. J. Urol., 40:235–244, 1968.

49. Lenaghan, D.: Bifid ureters in children: An anatomical, physiological, and clinical study. J. Urol., 87:808–817, 1962.

Ureteral Triplication

50. Axilrod, H.D.: Triplicate ureter. J. Urol., 72:799–801, 1954.

51. Begg, R.C.: Sextuplicitas renum: a case of six functioning kidneys and ureters in an adult female. J. Urol., 70:686–693, 1953.

51a. Blumberg, N.: Ureteral triplication. J. Pediatr. Surg., 11:579–580, 1976.

51b. Burt, J.C., Lane, C.N., and Hamilton, J.C.: An unusual anomaly of the upper urinary tract. J. Urol., 46:235–240, 1941.

52. Demoullin, M., and Nickels, L.: Uberzahlige Nieren und Dystopien. Z. Urol., 48:183–185, 1955.

53. Gill, R.D.: Triplication of the ureter and renal pelvis. J. Urol., 68:140–147, 1952.

54. Gilmore, O.J.A.: Unilateral triplication of the ureter. Br. J. Urol., 46:585, 1974.

55. Ireland, E.F., Jr., and Chute, R.: A case of triplicate-duplicate ureters. J. Urol., 74:342–347, 1955.

56. Kohri, K., Magai, N., Kaneno, S., et al.: Bilateral trifid ureters associated with fused kidney, ureterovesical stenosis, left cryptorchidism and angioma of the bladder. J. Urol., 120:249–250, 1978.

57. Lau, F.T., and Henline, R.B.: Ureteral anomalies: report of a case manifesting three ureters on one side with one ending blindly in aplastic kidney and bifid pelvis with single ureter on other side. J.A.M.A., 96:587–591, 1931.

58. MacKelvie, A.A.: Triplicate ureter: case report. Br. J. Urol., 27:124, 1955.

59. McLean, J.T., and Harding, E.W.: Unilateral triplication of ureter and renal pelvis. J. Urol., 54:381–384, 1945.

60. Parker, R.M., Pohl, D.R., and Robison, J.R.: Ureteral triplication with ectopia. J. Urol., 103:727–731, 1970.

61. Parvinen, T.: Complete ureteral triplication. J. Pediatr. Surg., 11:1039–1041, 1976.

62. Patel, N.P., and Lavengood, R.M., Jr.: Triplicate ureter. Urology, 5:242–243, 1975.

63. Perkins, P.J., Kroovand, R.L., and Evans, A.T.: Triplication of ureter: A case report. Radiology, 108:533–538, 1973.

64. Redman, J.F.: Triplicate ureter with contralateral ureteral duplication. J. Urol., 116:805, 1976.

65. Ringer, M.G., Jr., and MacFarlan, S.M.: Complete triplication of the ureter: A case report. J. Urol., 92:429–430, 1964.

66. Smith, I.: Triplicate ureter. Br. J. Surg., 34:182–185, 1946.

67. Soperdahl, D.W., Shirani, I.W., and Schamber, D.T.: Bilateral ureteral quadruplication. J. Urol., 116:255–256, 1976.

68. Spangler, E.B.: Complete triplication of the ureter. Radiology, 80:795–797, 1963.

69. Withycombe, J.F.R.: A case of trifid ureter and segmental hydroureter. Br. J. Surg., 38:113–116, 1950.

70. Wolpowitz, A., Evan, P., and Botha, R.A.G.: Triplication of ureter on one side and duplication on the other. Br. J. Urol., 47:622, 1975.

71. Woodruff, S.R.: Complete unilateral triplication of the ureter and renal pelvis. J. Urol., 46:376–379, 1941.

72. Wright, H.B., and McFarlane, D.J.: Unilateral triplication of the ureter; report of patient with three renal pelves the three ureteral orifices. J.A.M.A., 158:1166–1168, 1955.

Blind-Ending Ureter

73. Albers, D.D., Geyer, J.R., and Barnes, S.D.: Blind-ending branch of bifid ureter. Report of 3 cases. J. Urol., 99:160–164, 1968.

74. Albers, D.D., Geyer, J.R., and Barnes, S.D.: Clinical significance of the blind-ending branch of a bifid ureter: report of 3 additional cases. J. Urol., 105:634–637, 1971.

75. Bacher, E.: Ureter bifidus with blind end forked branch. Z. Urol., 51:326–328, 1958.

76. Barbalias, G.A., and Digioacchino, R.: Rudimentary branched ureter. A report of four cases. Del. Med. J., 46:511–516, 1974.

77. Baurys, W., and Wentzell, R.A.: Bifid blind ending ureter. Am. J. Surg., 94:499–501, 1957.

78. Campbell, M.F.: Diverticulum of the ureter. Am. J. Surg., 34:385–390, 1936.

79. Culp, O.S.: Ureteral diverticulum: Classification of the literature and report of an authentic case. J. Urol., 58:309–321, 1947.

80. Dublin, A.B., Stadalnik, R.C., DeNardo, G.L., et al.: Scintigraphic imaging of a blind-ending ureteral duplication. J. Nucl. Med., 16:208–209, 1975.

81. Engel, W.J.: Aberrant ureters ending blindly: Report of two cases, one of which simulated acute surgical abdomen. J. Urol., 42:674–683, 1939.

82. Hamilton, J.L.: Hypoplasia of ureter with renal agenesis. J. Urol., 56:530–534, 1946.

83. Hanley, H.G.: Blind ending duplication of the ureter. Br. J. Urol., 17:50–54, 1945.

84. Harlin, J.C., Atkinson, H.D., Fort, C.A., et al.: Blind ending branch of a bifid ureter. Urol. Cut. Rev., 55:83–85, 1951.

85. Harris, A.: Ureteral anomalies with special reference to partial duplication with one branch ending blindly: A report of two cases with renal obstruction cured by surgical resection. J. Urol., 38:442–454, 1937.

86. Haschek, H., and Kaiser, E.: Uber einen Fall von Ureter bifidus mit einem blinden Ast. Z. Urol., 46:745–748, 1953.

87. Hillenbrand, H.J.: Ureter bifidus mit bindem Ast. Z. Urol., 48:488–492, 1955.

88. Kontturi, M., and Kaski, P.: Blind-ending bifid ureter with uretero-ureteral reflux. Scand. J. Urol. Nephrol., 6:91–93, 1972.

89. Kretschmer, H.L.: Duplication of the ureters at their distal ending, one pair ending blindly: So-called diverticula of the ureters. J. Urol., 30:61–73, 1933.

90. Lenaghan, D.: Bifid ureters in children: An anatomical and physiological clinical study. J. Urol., 87:808–817, 1962.

91. McGraw, A.B., and Culp, O.S.: Diverticulum of the ureter: Report of another authentic case. J. Urol., 67:262–265, 1952.

92. Miller, E.V., and Tremblay, R.E.: Symptomatic blindly ending bifid ureter. J. Urol., 92:109–112, 1964.

93. Peterson, L.J., Grimes, J.H., Weinerth, J.L., et al.: Blind-ending branches of bifid ureters. Urology, 5:191–195, 1975.

94. Rao, K.G.: Blind-ending bifid ureter. Urology, 6:81–83, 1975.

95. Rubinstein, A.B., Jablokow, V.R., and Lloyd, F.A.: Differentiation of a bifid ureter from ureteral diverticulum. I. M. J., 134:33–35, 1968.

96. Szokoly, V., Veradi, E., and Szporny, G.: Blind ending bifid and double ureters. Int. Urol. Nephrol., 6:174–176, 1974.

Congenital Ureteral Stricture

97. Allen, T.O.: Congenital ureteral stricture. J. Urol., 104:196–204, 1970.

98. Campbell, M.F.: Ureteral obstruction in children. J. Urol., 4:660–678, 1939.

99. Kosto, B.: Congenital mid-ureteral stricture in a solitary kidney. J. Urol., 106:529–531, 1971.

100. Mehta, H.J.: Development of the ureter. *In* Bergman, H. (ed.): The Ureter, p. 19. New York, Harper & Row, 1967.

Ureteropelvic Obstruction

101. Allen, R.P., Condon, V.R., and Collins, R.E.: Multilocular cystic hydronephrosis secondary to congenital (ureteropelvic junction) obstruction: An adjunct to diagnosis with intravenous urography. Radiology, 80:203–207, 1963.

102. Allen, T.D.: Congenital ureteral stricture. J. Urol., 104:196–204, 1970.

103. Amar, A.D.: Congenital hydronephrosis of lower segment in duplex kidney. Urology, 7:480–485, 1976.

104. Campbell, M.: Hydronephrosis in infants and children. J. Urol., 65:743–747, 1951.

105. Cannon, J.F.: Hereditary unilateral hydronephrosis. Ann. Intern. Med., 41:1054–1060, 1954.

106. Creevy, C.D.: Unusual types of obstruction of the ureteropelvic junction. Trans. Am. Assoc. Genitourin. Surg., 34:115–122, 1941.

107. Dunbar, J.S., Nogrady, N.B., and MacEwan, D.W.: The crescent sign: A pyelographic sign of severe hydronephrosis. Presented at the Sixty-third Annual Meeting of the American Roentgen Ray Society, Washington, D.C. Oct. 2–5, 1962.

108. Ericsson, N.O., Rudhe, U.G., Livaditis, A.: Hydronephrosis associated with aberrant vessels in infants and children. Surgery, 50:687–690, 1961.

109. Feyder, S., and Deming, C.L.: Congenital hydronephrosis in lower half of a kidney: Report of a case. N. Engl. J. Med., 225:220–223, 1942.

110. Foley, F.E.B., McMartin, W.J., Culp, O.S., et al.: Panel discussion on hydronephrosis. Urol. Surv., 7:91–114, 1957.

111. Foote, J.W., Blennerhassett, J.B., Wiglesworth, F.W., et al.: Observations on the ureteropelvic junction. J. Urol., 104:252–257, 1970.

112. Freed, A., Ney, C., and Miller, H.L.: Unilateral hydronephrosis affecting the contralateral kidney and ureter. Radiology, 104:33–37, 1972.

113. Hanley, H.G.: The pelviureteric junction: A cine-pyelography study. Br. J. Urol., 31:277–354, 1959.

114. Hanna, M.K., Jeffs, R.D., Sturgess, J.M., et al.: Ureteral stricture and ultrastructure, Part II: Congenital ureteropelvic junction obstruction and primary obstructive megaureter. J. Urol., 117:725–730, 1976.

115. Hellstrom, J.: A contribution to the knowledge of the relation of abnormally running renal vessels to hydronephrosis and an investigation of the arterial condition of 50 kidneys. Acta Chir. Scand., 61:289–330, 1927.

116. Henline, R.B., and Hawes, C.J.: Ureteropelvic obstruction: Symptoms and treatment: Report of 70 cases, 62 operations. J.A.M.A., *137*:777–782, 1948.

117. Hinman, F.: Obstructive hydro-ureteral angularity with hydronephrosis in children. Arch. Surg., *18*:21–62, 1929.

118. Hoffman, H.A.: Massive hydronephrosis. J. Urol., *59*:784–794, 1948.

119. Jewell, J.H., and Buchert, W.I.: Unilateral hereditary hydronephrosis: A report of four cases in three consecutive generations. J. Urol., *88*:129–136, 1962.

120. Jewett, H.J.: Stenosis of the ureteropelvic junction: Congenital and acquired. J. Urol., *44*:247–258, 1940.

121. Jewett, H.J.: Symposium on pediatric urology: Upper urinary tract obstruction in infants and children: diagnosis and treatment. Pediatr. Clin. North Am., *2*:720–754, 1955.

122. Johnston, J.H.: The pathogenesis of hydronephrosis in children. Br. J. Urol., *41*:724–734, 1969.

123. Johnston, J.H., Evans, J.P., Glassberg, J.I., et al.: Pelvic hydronephrosis in children: A review of 219 personal cases. J. Urol., *117*:97–101, 1977.

124. Kelalis, P.P., Culp, D.S., Stickler, G.B., et al.: Ureteropelvic obstruction in children: Experience with 109 cases. J. Urol., *106*:418–422, 1971.

125. Lebowitz, R.L., and Griscom, N.T.: Neonatal hydronephrosis: 146 cases. Radiol. Clin. North Am., *15*:49–59, 1977.

126. LeVine, M., Allen, A., Stein, J.L., et al.: The crescent sign. Radiology, *81*:971–973, 1963.

127. Lich, R., Jr.: The obstructed ureteral pelvic junction. Radiology, *58*:337–344, 1957.

128. Lich, R., Jr., and Barnes, M.L.: A clinical pathologic study of ureteropelvic obstruction. J. Urol., *77*:382–387, 1957.

129. Lich, R., Jr., and Maurer, J.E.: Congenital hydronephrosis. J.A.M.A., *157*:577–579, 1955.

130. Lowry, E.C., Hayward, J.C., and Beard, D.E.: Hydronephrosis caused by accessory renal vessels. J. Urol., *52*:492–496, 1944.

131. Mayo, W.J., Braasch, W.F., and MacCarty, W.C.: Relation of anomalous renal blood vessels to hydronephrosis. J.A.M.A., *52*:1383–1388, 1909.

132. McLoughlin, W.L., and Bowler, J.P.: Excretory urography in the diagnosis of ureteropelvic obstruction. J. Urol., *57*:1012–1018, 1952.

133. Murnaghan, G.F.: The dynamics of the renal pelvis and ureter with reference to congenital hydronephrosis. Br. J. Urol., *30*:321–329, 1958.

134. Murnaghan, G.F.: The mechanism of congenital hydronephrosis with reference to the factors influencing surgical treatment. Ann. R. Coll. Surg. Engl., *23*:25–46, 1958.

135. Murnaghan, G.F.: Experimental aspects of hydronephrosis. Br. J. Urol., *31*:370–376, 1959.

136. Nesbit, R.M.: Diagnosis of intermittent hydronephrosis: Importance of pyelography during episodes of pain. J. Urol., *75*:767–771, 1956.

137. Nixon, H.H.: Hydronephrosis in children: a clinical study of seventy-eight cases with special reference to the role of aberrant vessels and the results of conservative operation. Br. J. Surg., *40*:601–609, 1953.

138. Ostling, K.: The genesis of hydronephrosis. Acta Chir. Scand. (Suppl. 72), *85*:1–122, 1942.

139. Robson, W.J., Rudy, S.M., and Johnston, J.H.: Pelviureteric obstruction in infancy. J. Pediatr. Surg., *11*:57–61, 1976.

140. Rolleston, G.L., and Reay, E.R.: The pelvi-ureteric junction. Br. J. Radiol., *30*:617–625, 1957.

141. Shopfner, C.E.: Ureteropelvic junction obstruction. Am. J. Roentgenol., *98*:148–159, 1966.

142. Squitieri, A.A., Ceccarelli, F.E., and Wurster, J.C.: Hypertension with elevated renal vein renins secondary to ureteropelvic junction obstruction. J. Urol., *111*:284–287, 1974.

143. Swenson, O., and Marchant, D.: Uretero-pelvic obstruction in infants and children: Clinical, radiological and experimental studies on eleven patients. J. Urol., *73*:945–950, 1955.

144. Tolson, H.L.: Massive congenital hydronephrosis: Ruptured hydronephrosis. Urol. Cut. Rev., *39*:768–774, 1935.

145. Whitaker, R.H.: Reflex induced pelviureteric obstruction. Br. J. Urol., *48*:555–560, 1976.

146. Wilder, W.O., and Doolittle, L.H.: "Gigantic" hydronephrosis. J. Urol., *34*:356–358, 1935.

147. Williams, D.I., and Karlaftis, C.M.: Hydronephrosis due to pelviureteric obstruction in the newborn. Br. J. Urol., *38*:128–144, 1966.

148. Williams, D.I., and Kenawi, M.M.: The prognosis of pelviureteric obstruction in childhood: A review of 190 cases. Eur. Urol., *2*:57–63, 1976.

149. Zimet, R.R., and Kappel, L.: Giant hydronephrosis as a cause of pyelonephrosis in the opposite kidney. J. Urol., *56*:515–519, 1946.

Valves of the Ureter

150. Cabot, R.C.: Case records of the Massachusetts General Hospital, case 13072: Two diagnoses are better than one. Boston Med. Surg. J., *196*:276–279, 1927.

151. Cussen, L.J.: The morphology of congenital dilatation of the ureter: Intrinsic ureteral lesions. Aust. N.Z. J. Surg., *41*:185–194, 1970.

152. Cussen, L.J.: Valve of the ureter. *In* Bergsma, D., and Duckett, J.W., Jr. (eds.): Urinary System Malformation in Children: Birth Defects: Original Article Series, Vol. 13, No. 5, pp. 19–20. New York, Alan R. Liss, 1977.

153. Foroughi, E., and Turner, J.A.: Congenital ureteral valve. J. Urol., *81*:272–284, 1959.

154. Hunner, G.L., and Wharton, L.R.: The pathological findings in cases clinically diagnosed as ureteral stricture. J. Urol., *15*:57–91, 1926.

155. MacLean, J.T.: Congenital valve in the upper ureter. J. Urol., *54*:374–380, 1945.

156. Mering, J.H., Steel, J.F., and Gittes, R.F.: Congenital ureteral valves. J. Urol., *107*:737–739, 1972.

157. Passaro, E., Jr., and Smith, J.P.: Congenital ureteral valves in children: A case report. J. Urol., *84*:290–292, 1960.

158. Roberts, R.R.: Complete valve of the ureter: Congenital ureteral valves. J. Urol., *76*:62–65, 1956.

159. Samellas, W.: Congenital ureteral valve. J. Urol., *88*:363–364, 1962.

160. Seitzman, D.M., Montoro, G.G., and Miele, A.J.: Congenital ureteral valves. J. Urol., *101*:152–156, 1969.

161. Simon, H.B., Culp, O.S., and Parkhill, E.M.: Congenital ureteral valves: Report of two cases. J. Urol., *74*:336–341, 1955.

162. Wall, B., and Wachter, H.E.: Congenital ureteral valve; its role as a primary obstructive lesion: Classification of the literature and report of an authentic case. J. Urol., *68*:684–690, 1952.

163. Williams, D.I.: Discussion. *In* Bergsma, D., and Duckett, J.W., Jr. (eds.): Urinary System Malformations in Children. Birth Defects: Original Article Series, Vol. 13, No. 5, p. 39. New York, Alan R. Liss, 1977.

Single Diverticulum of the Ureter

164. Campbell, M.F.: Diverticulum of the ureter. Am. J. Surg., 34:385–390, 1936.
165. Culp, O.S.: Ureteral diverticulum: Classification and report of an authentic case. J. Urol., 58:309–321, 1947.
166. Mayers, M.M.: Diverticulum of the ureter. J. Urol., 61:344–350, 1949.
167. McGraw, A.B., and Culp, O.S.: Diverticulum of the ureter: Report of another authentic case. J. Urol., 67:262–265, 1952.

Multiple Ureteral Diverticula

168. Dolan, P.A., and Kirkpatrick, W.E.: Multiple ureteral diverticula. J. Urol., 83:570–571, 1960.
169. Holly, L.E., and Sumead, B.: Diverticular ureteral changes: A report of four cases. Am. J. Roentgenol., 78:1053–1060, 1957.
170. Khonsari, H., and Oliver, J.A.: Multiple ureteral diverticula. J. Urol., 105:183–185, 1971.
171. Norman, C.H., Jr., and Dubowy, J.: Multiple ureteral diverticula. J. Urol., 96:152–154, 1966.
172. Pratt, J.G., Gahagan, H.Q., and Fischman, J.L.: Ureteral diverticula: Review of the literature and report of two additional cases. J. Urol., 58:322–326, 1947.
173. Rank, W.B., Mellinger, G.T., and Spiro, E.: Ureteral diverticula: Etiologic considerations. J. Urol., 83:566–569, 1960.
174. Rathbun, N.P.: Bilateral diverticula of ureter. J. Urol., 18:347–362, 1927.
175. Scarello, N.S., and Humar, S.: Multiple ureteral diverticula. J. Urol., 106:36–71, 1971.
176. Tynes, W.V., II, Devine, C.J., Jr., Buttarazzi, P.J., et al.: Ureteral embryology and resultant anomalies. Va. Med., 95:395–403, 1968.
177. Webber, M.M., and Kaufman, J.J.: Multiple ureteral diverticula. Am. J. Roentgenol., 90:26–27, 1963.

Aberrant Vessels

178. Campbell, M.F.: Vascular obstruction of the ureter in juveniles. Am. J. Surg., 22:527–541, 1933.
179. Campbell, M.F.: Vascular obstruction of the ureter in children. J. Urol., 36:366–387, 1936.
180. Greene, L.F., Priestley, J.T., Simon, H.B., et al.: Obstruction of the lower third of the ureter by anomalous blood vessels. J. Urol., 71:544–548, 1954.
181. Hyams, J.A.: Aberrant blood vessels as a factor in lower ureteral obstruction: Preliminary report. Surg. Gynecol. Obstet., 48:474–479, 1929.
182. Javadhpour, N., Solomon, T., and Bush, I.M.: Obstruction of the lower ureter by aberrant vessels in children. J. Urol., 108:340–342, 1972.
183. Young, J.D., Jr., and Kiser, W.S.: Obstruction of the lower ureter by aberrant blood vessels. J. Urol., 94:101–106, 1965.

Megaloureter

184. Budin, E., and Eichwald, M.: Achalasia of the ureter. Radiology, 75:757–765, 1960.
185. Campbell, E.W.: Megalo-ureter. J. Urol., 60:31–45, 1948.
186. Campbell, M.F.: Primary megalo-ureter. J. Urol., 68:584–590, 1952.
187. Carlson, H.E.: The intrapsoas transplant of megaloureter. J. Urol., 72:172–177, 1954.

188. Carver, J.H.: Megaloureter: Report of 2 cases. Br. J. Surg., 36:168–172, 1948.
189. Caulk, J.R.: Megaloureter: The importance of the ureterovesical valve. J. Urol., 9:315–330, 1923.
190. Creevy, C.D.: The atonic distal ureteral segment (ureteral achalasia). J. Urol., 97:457–463, 1967.
191. Fortescue-Brickdale, J.M.: A note of congenital dilatation of the ureters. Bristol Med. Chir. J., 23:231–233, 1905.
192. Gloor, H.U.: Causes of megaloureter. Schweiz. Med. Wochenschr., 69:1080–1084, 1939.
193. Grana, L., Donnellan, W.L., and Swenson, O.: Effects of gram-negative bacteria on ureteral structure and function. J. Urol., 99:539–550, 1968.
194. Hurst, A.F., and Jones, J.G.: Case of megaloureter due to achalasia of the ureterovesical sphincter. Br. J. Urol., 3:43–52, 1931.
195. Lewis, E.L., and Cletsoway, R.W.: Megaloureter. J. Urol., 75:643–649, 1956.
196. Lewis, E.L., and Kimbrough, J.C.: Megaloureter: New concept of treatment. South. Med. J., 45:171–177, 1952.
197. Mackinnon, K.J., Foote, J.W., Wiglesworth, F.W., et al.: The pathology of the adynamic distal ureteral segment. J. Urol., 103:124–137, 1970.
198. Mark, L.K., and Moel, M.: Primary megaloureter. Radiology, 93:345–349, 1969.
199. McLaughlin, A.P., III, Pfister, R.L., Leadbetter, W.F., et al.: The pathophysiology of primary megaloureter. J. Urol., 109:805–811, 1973.
200. Nesbit, R.M., and Withycombe, J.: The problem of primary megaloureter. J. Urol., 72:167–171, 1954.
201. Ockerblad, N.F.: Congenital dilatation of the ureter. J. Urol., 13:325–328, 1925.
202. Pfister, R.C., McLaughlin, A.P., III, and Leadbetter, W.F.: Radiological evaluation of primary megaloureter: The aperistaltic distal ureteral segment. Radiology, 99:503–510, 1971.
203. Swenson, O., MacMahon, H.E., Jaques, W.E., et al.: A new concept of the etiology of megaloureters. N. Engl. J. Med., 246:41–46, 1952.
204. Wayman, T.B.: Surgical treatment of megalo-ureter. J. Urol., 61:883–903, 1949.

Megaureter

205. Hendren, W.H.: Operative repair of megaureter in children. J. Urol., 101:491–507, 1969.
206. Hendren, W.H.: Functional restoration of decompensated ureter in children. Am. J. Surg., 119:477–482, 1970.
207. Hendren, W.H.: Restoration of function in the severely decompensated ureter. In Johnston, J.H., and Scholtmeyer, R.S. (eds.): Problems in Paediatric Urology, pp. 1–56. Amsterdam, Excerpta Medica, 1972.
208. Johnston, J.H., and Farkas, A.: The congenital refluxing megaureter: Experience with surgical reconstruction. Br. J. Urol., 47:153–159, 1975.
209. Weber, A.L., Pfister, R.C., James, A.E., Jr., et al.: Megaureter in infants and children: Roentgenologic, clinical, and surgical aspects. Am. J. Roentgenol., 112:170–177, 1971.

Ectopia of the Ureter

210. Abeshouse, B.S.: Ureteral ectopia: Report of a rare case of ectopic ureter opening in uterus and review of literature. Urol. Cut. Rev., 47:447–465, 1943.

211. Abeshouse, B.S., Goldstein, A.E., and Tankin, L.H.: Ectopic ureteral orifice: Report of 4 cases. Urol. Cut. Rev., 54:7-17, 1950.

212. Abeshouse, B.S., Heller, E., and Salik, J.O.: Vasoepididymography and vasoseminal vesiculography. J. Urol., 72:983-991, 1954.

213. Alfert, H.J., and Gillenwater, J.Y.: Ectopic vas deferens communicating with lower ureter. Embryological considerations. J. Urol., 108:172-173, 1972.

214. Allansmith, R.: Ectopic ureter terminating in seminal vessels; unilateral polycystic kidney: Report of a case and review of the literature. J. Urol., 80:524-534, 1958.

215. Bard, R.H., and Welles, H.: Nonduplication of upper urinary tract associated with horseshoe kidney and bilateral ureteral ectopia. Urology, 5:784-786, 1975.

216. Borger, J.A., and Belman, A.B.: Uretero-vas deferens anastomosis associated with imperforate anus: Embryologically predictable occurrence. J. Pediatr. Surg., 10:255-257, 1975.

217. Brannon, W., and Henry, H.H., II: Ureteral ectopia: Report of 39 cases. J. Urol., 109:192-195, 1973.

218. Burford, C.E., Glenn, J.E., and Burford, E.H.: Ureteral ectopia: A review of the literature and two case reports. J. Urol., 62:211-218, 1949.

219. Campbell, J.H., Pasquier, C.M., Jr., and St. Martin, E.C.: Ureteral ectopia in adult male patients. J. Urol., 81:99-104, 1959.

220. Campbell, M.F.: Ectopic ureteral orifice: Report of 17 cases in children. Surg. Gynecol. Obstet., 64:21-29, 1937.

221. Cendron, J., and Bonhomme, C.: Urétère a terminaison ectopique extravesical chez des sujers due sexe masculin (à propos de 10 cas). J. Urol. Nephrol., 74:31-35, 1968.

222. Chidlow, J.H., and Utz, D.C.: Ureteral ectopia in vestibule of vagina with urinary continence. South. Med. J., 63:423-425, 1970.

223. Clarke, B.G., Mitchell, G.W., and Feeley, J.R.: Ureteral ectopia in the female. N. Engl. J. Med., 251:135-136, 1954.

224. Cohen B.: The ectopic ureter. Med. J. Aust., 2:856-860, 1964.

225. Constantian, H.M.: Ureteral ectopia, hydrocolpos, and uterus didelphys. J.A.M.A., 197:54-57, 1968.

226. Cox, C.E., and Hutch, J.A.: Bilateral single ectopic ureter: A report of 2 cases and review of the literature. J. Urol., 95:493-497, 1966.

227. Crenshaw, J.L., and Buchtel, H.A.: Ectopic ureter with extravesical orifice. J. Urol., 35:190-205, 1936.

228. Davis, D.M.: Urethral ectopic ureter in the female without incontinence. J. Urol., 23:463-476, 1930.

229. DeWeerd, J.H., and Feeney, D.P.: Bilateral ureteral ectopia with urinary incontinence in a mother and daughter. J. Urol., 98:335-337, 1967.

230. DeWeerd, J.H., and Litin, R.B.: Ectopia of ureteral orifice (vestibular) without incontinence: Report of case. Mayo Clin. Proc., 33:81-86, 1958.

231. Dickinson, K.M.: Ectopic ureter entering a seminal vesicle. Br. J. Surg., 50:858-860, 1963.

232. Eckerbom, H., and Liliequist, B.: Ectopic ureter: Report of case. Acta Radiol., 38:420-427, 1952.

233. Eisendrath, D.N.: Ectopic opening of ureter. Urol. Cut. Rev., 42:404-411, 1938.

234. Ellerker, H.G.: The extravesical ectopic ureter. Br. J. Surg., 45:344-353, 1958.

235. Engel, W.J.: Ureteral ectopic opening into seminal vesicle. J. Urol., 60:46-49, 1948.

236. Farr, J.L.: Ectopic ureteral opening into seminal vesicle. J. Urol., 83:108-112, 1960.

237. Freeman, I.: Urethral ectopic ureter in the female without incontinence: a case report. J. Urol., 39:398-402, 1938.

238. Fuselier, H.A., and Peters, D.H.: Cyst of seminal vesicle with ipsilateral renal agenesis and ectopic ureter: Case report. J. Urol., 116:833-835, 1976.

239. Goldstein, A.E., and Heller, E.: Ectopic ureter opening into a seminal vesicle. J. Urol., 75:57-62, 1956.

240. Gordon, H.L., and Kessler, R.: Ectopic ureter entering the seminal vesicle associated with renal dysplasia. J. Urol., 108:389-391, 1972.

241. Goyanna, R., and Greene, L.F.: The pathologic and anomalous condition associated with duplication of the renal pelvis and ureter. J. Urol., 54:1-9, 1945.

242. Grossman, H., Winchester, P.H., and Muecke, E.C.: Solitary ectopic ureter. Radiology, 89:1069-1072, 1967.

243. Hepler, A.B.: Bilateral pelvic and ureteral duplication with uterine ectopic ureter. J. Urol., 57:94-105, 1947.

244. Honke, E.M.: Ectopic ureter. J. Urol., 55:460-463, 1946.

245. Idbohrn, H., and Sjostedt, S.: Ectopic ureter not causing incontinence until adult life. Acta Obstet. Gynecol. Scand., 33:457-464, 1954.

246. Johnston, J.H., and Davenport, T.J.: The single ectopic ureter. Br. J. Urol., 41:428-433, 1969.

247. Katzen, P., and Trachtman, B.: Diagnosis of vaginal ectopic ureter by vaginogram. J. Urol., 72:808, 1954.

248. Kesavan, P., Ramakrishnan, M.S., and Fowler, R.: Ectopia in unduplicated ureters in children. Br. J. Urol., 49:481-493, 1977.

249. Kittredge, R.D., and Levin, D.C.: Unusual aspect of renal angiography in ureteric duplication. Am. J. Roentgenol., 119:805-811, 1973.

250. Kjellberg, S.R., Ericsson, N.O., and Rudhe, U.: The Lower Urinary Tract in Childhood: Some Correlated Clinical and Roentgenologic Observations, p. 248. Chicago, Year Book Medical Publishers, 1957.

251. Koyanagi, T., Tsuji, I., Orika, S., et al.: Bilateral single ectopic ureter: Report of a case. Int. Urol. Nephrol., 9:123-127, 1977.

252. Landes, R.R.: Ureteral ectopia associated with renal dystopia. J. Urol., 66:115-118, 1951.

253. Leef, G.S., and Leader, S.A.: Ectopic ureter opening into the rectum: A case report. J. Urol., 87:338-342, 1962.

254. Levisay, G.L., Holder, J., and Weigel, J.W.: Ureteral ectopia associated with seminal vesicle cyst and ipsilateral renal agenesis. Radiology, 114:575-576, 1975.

255. Lucius, G.F.: Klinik und therapie der dystopen: Harnleitermundungen in die Samenuege. Urologe, 2:360-363, 1963.

256. Malek, R.S., Kelalis, P.P., Stickler, G.B., et al.: Observations on ureteral ectopy in children. J. Urol., 107:308-313, 1972.

257. McKay, R.W., and Baird, H.H.: Bilateral single ureteral ectopia terminating in urethra. J. Urol., 63:1013-1018, 1950.

258. Mellin, H.L., Kjaer, T.B., and Madsen, P.O.: Crossed ectopia of seminal vesicles, renal aplasia and ectopic ureter. J. Urol., 115:765-766, 1976.

259. Mogg, R.A.: The single ectopic ureter. Br. J. Urol., 46:3-10, 1974.

260. Moore, T.: Ectopic openings of the ureter. Br. J. Urol., 24:3-18, 1952.

261. Moore, T.D.: The diagnosis and management of ureteral ectopia. J. Urol., 60:50-62, 1948.

262. Mulholland, S.G., Edson, M., and O'Connell, K.J.: Congenital uretero-seminal vesicle fistula. J. Urol., 106:649-651, 1971.

263. O'Brien, H.A., and Mitchell, J.D.: Ectopic ureteral orifices: A

report of five cases. New Orleans Med. Surg. J., *104*:585–589, 1952.

264. Ogawa, A., Kakizawa, Y., and Akaza, H.: Ectopic ureter passing through the external urethral sphincter: Report of a case. J. Urol., *116*:109–110, 1976.

265. Orquisa, C.S., Ghayani, B.N., Berry, J.L., et al.: Ectopic opening of the ureter into the seminal vesicle; report of case. J. Urol., *104*:532–535, 1970.

266. Palmer, J.M., and Russ, M.F.: Persistent urogenital sinus with absence of the bladder and urethra. J. Urol., *102*:590–594, 1970.

267. Pasquier, C.M., Jr., and Womack, R.K.: Ectopic opening of ureter into seminal vesicle. J. Urol., *70*:164–167, 1953.

268. Prewitt, L.H., Jr., and Lebowitz, R.L.: The single ectopic ureter. Am. J. Roentgenol., *127*:941–948, 1976.

269. Redman, J.F., and Sulieman, J.S.: Bilateral vasal-ureteral communication. J. Urol., *116*:808–809, 1976.

270. Riba, L.W., Schmidlapp, C.J., and Bosworth, N.L.: Ectopic ureter draining into the seminal vesicle. J. Urol., *56*:332–338, 1946.

271. Rusche, C.F., and Morrow, F.R.: Ureteral ectopia in infancy and children: Report of case. South. Med. J., *49*:1328–1337, 1956.

272. Schnitzer, B.: Ectopic ureteral opening into seminal vesicle. J. Urol., *93*:576–581, 1965.

273. Schulman, C.C.: The single ectopic ureter. Eur. Urol., *2*:64–69, 1976.

274. Seitzman, D.M., and Patton, J.F.: Combined ureteral and vas deferens anomaly. J. Urol., *84*:604–608, 1960.

275. Stephens, F.D.: Correlation of ureteral orifice position with renal morphology. Trans. Am. Assoc. Genitourin. Surg., *58*:53–55, 1978.

276. Sullivan, M., Halpert, L., and Hodge, C.F.: Extravesical ureteral ectopia. Urology, *11*:577–580, 1978.

277. Uson, A.C., and Donovan, J.T.: Ectopic ureteral orifice. Am. J. Dis. Child., *98*:152–161, 1959.

278. Uson, A.C., and Schulman, C.C.: Ectopic ureter emptying into the rectum: Report of a case. J. Urol., *108*:156–158, 1972.

279. Uson, A.C., Womack, C.D., and Berdon, W.E.: Giant ectopic ureter presenting as an abdominal mass in a newborn infant. J. Pediatr., *80*:473–476, 1972.

280. Vanhoutte, J.J.: Ureteral ectopia with a Wolffian duct remnant (Gartner duct or cyst) presenting as a urethral diverticulum in two girls. Am. J. Roentgenol., *110*:540–545, 1970.

281. Varney, D.C., and Ford, M.D.: Ectopic ureteral remnant persisting as cystic diverticulum of the ejaculatory duct: Case report. J. Urol., *72*:802–807, 1954.

282. Weiss, J.M., and Dykhuizen, R.F.: An anomalous vaginal insertion into the bladder: A case report. J. Urol., *98*:610–612, 1967.

283. Wiggishoff, C.C., and Kiefer, J.H.: Ureteral ectopia: Diagnostic difficulties. J. Urol., *96*:671–673, 1966.

284. Williams, D.I.: The ectopic ureter: Diagnostic problems. Br. J. Urol., *26*253–260, 1954.

285. Williams, D.I., and Lightwood, R.G.: Bilateral single ectopic ureter. Br. J. Urol., *44*:267–273, 1972.

286. Williams, D.I., and Royle, M.: Ectopic ureter in the male child. Br. J. Urol., *41*:421–427, 1969.

287. Willmarth, C.L.: Ectopic ureteral orifice within a urethral diverticulum: Report of a case. J. Urol., *59*:47–49, 1948.

288. Zielinski, J., Sosnierz, M., and Marquardt, M.: Abouchement de l'uretere dans la vesicule seminale avec syndrome clinique extraordinaire. J. Urol. Nephrol., *68*:381–390, 1962.

Simple Ureterocele

289. Amar, A.D.: Simple ureterocele at the distal end of a blinding-ending ureter. J. Urol., *106*:423–424, 1971.

290. Emmett, J.L., and Logan, G.B.: Ureterocele with prolapse through the urethra. J. Urol., *51*:19–23, 1944.

291. Gross, R.F.: The Surgery of Infancy and Childhood. Philadelphia, W.B. Saunders, 1953.

292. Merricks, J.W., and Herbst, P.H.: Treatment of ureterocele in adults. J. Urol., *64*:643–645, 1950.

293. Orr, L.M., and Glanton, J.B.: Prolapsing ureterocele. J. Urol., *70*:180–186, 1953.

294. Thompson, G.S., and Greene, L.F.: Ureterocele: A clinical study and a report of thirty-seven cases. J. Urol., *47*:806–809, 1942.

Ectopic Ureterocele

295. Aas, T.N.: Ureterocele: a clinical study of sixty-eight cases in fifty-two adults. Br. J. Urol., *32*:133–144, 1960.

296. Aas, T.N., and Nilson, A.E.: Ureterocele in adults: Clinical and roentgenographic follow-up. Acta Chir. Scand., *116*:263–267, 1959.

297. Bauer, S.B., and Retik, A.B.: The non-obstructed ectopic ureterocele. J. Urol., *119*:804–807, 1978.

298. Berdon, W.E., Baker, D.H., Becker, J.A., et al.: Ectopic ureterocele. Radiol. Clin. North Am., *6*:205–214, 1968.

299. Brock, W.A., and Kaplan, G.W.: Ectopic ureterocele in children. J. Urol., *119*:800–803, 1978.

300. Cremin, B.J., Funston, M.R., and Aaronson, I.A.: The intraureteric diverticulum, a manifestation of ureterocele intussusception. Pediatr. Radiol., *6*:92–96, 1977.

301. Dorst, J.P., Cussen, G.H., and Silverman, F.N.: Ureteroceles in children with emphasis on the frequency of ectopic ureterocele. Radiology, *74*:88–89, 1960.

302. Eklöv, O., Lohr, G., Ringertz, H., et al.: Ectopic ureterocele in the male infant. Acta Radiol., *19*:145–153, 1978.

303. Eklöv, O., and Mäkinen, E.: Ectopic ureterocele. A radiological appraisal of 66 consecutive cases. Pediatr. Radiol., *2*:111–120, 1974.

304. Ericsson, N.O.: Ectopic ureterocele in infants and children: Clinical study. Acta Chir. Scand. (Suppl.), *197*:1–192, 1954.

305. Fendel, H.: The radiology of the vesico-ureteric junction. In Eklöv, O. (ed.): Current Concepts of Pediatric Radiology. Springer-Verlag, New York, 1977.

306. Friedland, G.W., and Cunningham, J.: The elusive ectopic ureterocele. Am. J. Roentgenol., *116*:792–811, 1972.

307. Johnson, J.H., and Johnson, L.M.: Experience with ectopic ureteroceles. Br. J. Urol., *41*:61–70, 1969.

308. Malek, R.S., Kelalis, P.P., Burke, J.C., et al.: Simple and ectopic ureterocele in infancy and childhood. Surg. Gynecol. Obstet., *134*:611–616, 1972.

309. Mertz, H.O., Hendricks, J., and Garrett, R.A.: Cystic ureterovesical protrusion: Report of four cases in children and two in adults. J. Urol., *61*:506–516, 1949.

310. Mogg, R.A.: Some observations on the ectopic ureter and ureterocele. J. Urol., *97*:1003–1012, 1967.

311. Sidaway, N.F.: Ureterocele in infancy and childhood. Clin. Radiol., *13*:297–303, 1962.

312. Stephens, D.F.: Ureterocele in infants and children. Aust. N.Z. Surg., *27*:288–295, 1958.

313. Stephens, D.: Congenital Malformations of the Rectum, Anus, and Genito-Urinary Tracts. Edinburgh, E. & S. Livingstone, 1963.

314. Stephens, D.: Caecoureterocele and concepts of the embryology and etiology of ureteroceles. Aust. N.Z. J. Surg., 40:239–246, 1971.

315. Subbiah, N., and Stephens, D.: Stenotic ureterocele. Aust. N.Z. J. Surg., 41:257–263, 1972.

316. Thornbury, J.R.: The roentgen diagnosis of ureterocele in children. Am. J. Roentgenol., 90:15–25, 1963.

317. Williams, D.I.: Ureteroceles. In Encyclopedia of Urology, Suppl. XV, Urology in Childhood. New York, Springer-Verlag, 1974.

318. Williams, D.I., Ray, R., and Lillie, J.G.: The functional radiology of ectopic ureterocele. Br. J. Urol., 44:417–433, 1972.

319. Williams, D.I., and Royle, M.: Ectopic ureter in the male child. Br. J. Urol., 41:421–427, 1969.

320. Williams, D.I., and Woodard, J.R.: Problems in management of ectopic ureteroceles. J. Urol., 92:635–652, 1964.

Retrocaval Ureter

321. Abeshouse, B.S., and Tankin, L.H.: Retrocaval ureters: Report of a case and review of the literature. Am. J. Surg., 84:383–393, 1952.

322. Bateson, E.M., and Atkinson, D.: Circumcaval ureter: A new classification. Clin. Radiol., 20:173–177, 1969.

323. Blundon, K.E.: The treatment of retrocaval ureter in the solitary kidney. J. Urol., 8829–32, 1962.

324. Brooks, R.E., Jr.: Left retrocaval ureter associated with situs inversus. J. Urol., 88484–487, 1962.

325. Cathro, A.J.M.: Section of inferior vena cava for retrocaval ureter: new method of treatment. J. Urol., 67:464–475, 1952.

325a. Cenoron, J., and Reis, C.F.: L'uretèrê rétrocave chez l'enfant. A propos de 4 cas. J. Urol. Nephrol. (Paris), 59:254–255, 1972.

325b. Considine, J.: Retrocaval ureter. Brit. J. Urol., 38:412–423, 1966.

326. Corbus, B.C., Estrem, R.D., and Hunt, W.: Retroiliac ureter. J. Urol., 84:67–68, 1960.

327. Creevy, C.D.: Recognition and surgical correction of retrocaval ureter. J. Urol., 60:26–30, 1948.

328. Crosse, J.E., Soderdahl, D.W., Teplick, S.K., et al.: Nonobstructive circumcaval (retrocaval) ureter: A report of 2 cases. Radiology, 116:69–71, 1975.

329. Dupp, P.A.: Retrocaval ureter: Case report. J. Urol., 63:496–499, 1950.

330. Ekstrom, T., and Nilson, A.E.: Retrocaval ureter. Acta Clin. Scand., 118:53–59, 1959.

331. Fletcher, E.W.L., and Lecky, J.W.: Retrocaval ureter obstructed by an aberrant renal artery. J. Urol., 106:184–185, 1971.

332. Gladstone, R.J.: An acardiac foetus. J. Anat. Physiol., 40:71–80, 1905.

333. Goodwin, W.E., Burke, D.E., and Muller, W.H.: Retrocaval ureter. Surg. Gynecol. Obstet., 104:337–345, 1957.

334. Goyanna, R., Cook, E.N., and Counseller, V.S.: Circumcaval ureter. Mayo Clin. Proc., 21:356–360, 1946.

335. Greene, L.F., and Kearns, W.M.: Circumcaval ureter with consideration of the preoperative diagnosis and successful plastic repair. J. Urol., 5552–59, 1946.

336. Grossman, S.L., and Fehr, J.U.: Retrocaval ureter. Am. J. Surg., 84:679–682, 1953.

337. Gruenwald, P., and Surks, S.N.: Pre-ureteric vena cava and its embryological explanation. J. Urol., 49:195–201, 1943.

338. Harrill, H.C.: Retrocaval ureter: Report of a case with operative correction of the defect. J. Urol., 44:450–457, 1940.

339. Heslin, J.E., and Mamonas, C.: Retrocaval ureter: Report of four cases and review of literature. J. Urol., 65:212–222, 1951.

340. Hida, H.: Retrocaval ureter in children: Report of two cases. Eur. Urol., 4:127–131, 1978.

341. Hradcova, L., and Kalka, V.: Retrocaval ureter in childhood. Urol. Int., 16:103–116, 1963.

342. Kenawi, M.M., and Williams, D.I.: Circumcaval ureter: A report of four cases in children with a review of the literature and a new classification. Br. J. Urol., 48:183–192, 1976.

343. Laughlin, V.C.: Retrocaval (circumcaval) ureter associated with solitary kidney. J. Urol., 71:195–199, 1954.

344. Mayer, R.F., and Mathes, G.F.: Retrocaval ureter. South. Med. J., 51:945–950, 1958.

345. McClure, C.F.W., and Butler, E.G.: The development of the vena cava inferior in man. Am. J. Anat., 35:331–384, 1925.

346. McElhinney, P.P.B., and Dorsey, J.W.: Retrocaval ureter: Case report. J. Urol., 59:497–500, 1948.

347. Olson, R.O., and Austen, G., Jr.: Postcaval ureter: Report and discussion of case with successful surgical repair. N. Engl. J. Med., 242:963–968, 1950.

348. Parks, R.E., and Chase, W.E.: Retrocaval ureter: Report of two cases diagnosed preoperatively in childhood. Am. J. Dis. Child., 82:442–445, 1951.

349. Pick, J.W., and Anson, B.J.: Retrocaval ureter: Report of a case with a discussion of its clinical significance. J. Urol., 43:672–685, 1940.

350. Pitt, D.C.: Retrocaval ureter: Report of a case diagnosed preoperatively by intravenous and retrograde pyelography. Radiology, 84:699–702, 1965.

351. Presman, D., and Raymond, F.: A diagnostic method for retrocaval ureter. Am. J. Surg., 92:628–631, 1956.

352. Randall, A., and Campbell, E.W.: Anomalous relationship of right ureter to the vena cava. J. Urol., 34:564–583, 1935.

353. Rowland, H.S., Jr., Bunts, R.C., and Iwano, J.H.: Operative correction of retrocaval ureter: A report of four cases and review of the literature. J. Urol., 83:820–833, 1960.

354. Salem, R.J., and Luck, R.J.: Midline ensheathed ureters. Br. J. Urol., 48:18, 1976.

355. Sesboue, P.: L'uretere retro-cave. These No. 824, Paris, Universite Faculte de Medecine, 1952.

356. Shown, T.E., and Moore, C.A.: Retrocaval ureter: 4 cases. J. Urol., 105:497–501, 1971.

Postiliac Artery Ureter

357. Corbus, B.C., Estren, R.D., and Hunt, W.: Retro-iliac ureter. J. Urol., 84:67–68, 1960.

358. Dees, J.E.: Anomalous relationship between ureter and external iliac artery. J. Urol., 44:207–215, 1940.

359. Hanna, M.K.: Bilateral retro-iliac artery ureters. Br. J. Urol., 44:339–344, 1972.

360. Seitzman, D.M., and Patton, J.F.: Ureteral ectopia: Combined ureteral and vas deferens anomaly. J. Urol., 84:604–608, 1960.

Hernia of the Ureter

361. Barquin, O.P., Madsen, P.O.: Scrotal herniation of the lower urinary tract. J. Urol., 98:508–511, 1967.

362. Beck, W.C., Baurys, W., Brochu, J., et al.: Herniation of the ureter into the sciatic foramen ("curlique ureter"). J.A.M.A., *149*:441–442, 1952.

363. Bohnert, W.W.: Ureteral sciatic hernias: Case report of an infant with bilateral ureteral herniation into the sciatic foramen. J. Urol., *106*:142–143.

364. Carli, C.: L'ernia dell'uretere. Ann. Ital. Chir., *11*:2078–2104, 1932.

365. Dourmashkin, R.L.: Scrotal hernia of the ureter associated with unilateral fused kidney: Case report. J. Urol., *38*:455–467, 1937.

366. Fotopoulos, J.P., Burkhead, H.C.: Herniation of the ureter: A review and report of a case. Arch. Surg., *82*:290–292, 1961.

367. Franken, E.A., Jr., and Smith, E.E.: Sciatic hernia: Report of three cases including two with bilateral ureteral involvement. Am. J. Roentgenol., *107*:791–795, 1969.

368. Jewett, H.J., and Harris, A.P.: Scrotal ureter: Report of a case. J. Urol., *69*:184–187, 1953.

369. Lebowitz, R.: Ureteral sciatic hernia. Pediatr. Radiol., *1*:178–182, 1973.

370. Lindbom, A.: Unusual ureteral obstruction by herniation of ureter into sciatic foramen: Report of case. Acta Radiol., *28*:225–226, 1947.

371. Mallough, C., and Pellman, C.M.: Scrotal herniation of ureter. J. Urol., *106*:38–41, 1971.

372. Ney, C., Miller, H.L., and Gardimer, H.: Preinguinal canal herniation of the ureter: Value of the curlicue sign direction. Arch. Surg., *105*:633–634, 1972.

373. Page, B.H.: Obstruction of ureter in internal hernia. Br. J. Urol., *27*:254–255, 1955.

374. Pollack, H.M., Popky, G.L., and Blumberg, M.L.: Hernia of the ureter: An anatomic roentgenographic study. Radiology, *117*:275–281, 1975.

375. Rothchild, T.P.: Ureteral hernia. Report of a case of herniation of the ureter into the sciatic foramen. Arch. Surg., *98*:96–98, 1969.

376. Swithinbank, A.H.: Intrathoracic deviation of a ureteric loop. Br. J. Surg., *45*:379–381, 1958.

377. Tripathi, V.N., and Flint, L.D.: Ureteral herniation. Ann. Surg., *169*:417–419, 1969.

Inflammatory diseases of the ureter are associated intimately with inflammatory lesions of the kidney, and they have in general been covered under that section. Particular emphasis is placed in this chapter on relatively specific conditions or diseases in which the ureteral changes are of paramount importance.

URETERITIS

Ureteritis may be primary or secondary. Primary ureteritis is associated most commonly with pyelonephritis or cystitis, with the ureter becoming involved in the inflammatory process. Ureteritis may be associated with ureteral anomalies, such as ureterocele or stricture, which produce stasis and infection proximal to the lesion. It is associated commonly with ureteral calculi and is seen occasionally following instrumental trauma, surgery, or radiation therapy. Secondary ureteritis consists of involvement of the ureter from inflammations in areas outside the urinary system, usually salpingitis, seminal vesiculitis, appendicitis, or regional ileitis.

In acute ureteritis the segment of involved ureter may become aperistaltic and remain moderately dilated throughout the examination. If moderate dilatation is the only finding, reflux must be excluded before this is attributed to a ureteral abnormality. In chronic ureteritis the ureter may become thickened and fibrotic with narrowing or stricture. Multiple or long areas of narrowing or stricture is most common in ureteral tuberculosis (Figs. 19–19 to 19–23). In chronic ureteritis the ureter becomes thickened and fibrotic, with the roentgenographic appearance of irregular narrowing and stricture (Figs. 19–1 to 19–9).

19

Diseases
of the
Ureter

STRIATIONS IN THE UPPER URINARY TRACT

A fine parallel linear striated pattern of relative lucency may be seen, primarily in the renal pelvis and proximal ureter in urograms of infants, children, and less commonly in adults. It resembles the fine mucosal pattern of the esophagus. Originally it was thought to represent a reaction to infection and was described as "pyelitis." More recently it appears that the most common denominator is reflux. In children the pattern may be caused by stretching and deepening of folds in a redundant system that has been overstretched by reflux.[14, 16]

Although most of the children with mucosal striations had refluxing ureters, many of them also had urinary tract infection. The rare case of striations in the adult is almost always associated with infection. Striations also occur with leukoplakia in the adult (see below), but in leukoplakia the striations appear more coarse and irregular and are frequently associated with filling defects.

Although the clinical significance of this finding is still not certain, the finding of mucosal striations should suggest reflux, reflux and/or infection, and, if reflux is not demonstrated, infection (Figs. 19–10 to 19–14).

STRICTURE

Ureteral strictures may be congenital or acquired. Congenital strictures are most common at the ureteropelvic or the ureterovesical junction.

The presence of ureteral dilatation by itself is not sufficient to diagnose stricture; dilatation may be secondary to infection or megaloureter. There must be compromise of the lumen and proximal dilatation. (Narrowing of the lumen in retrograde studies does not necessarily represent stricture, since irritation from catheter manipulation may produce ureteral spasm). If stricture is present, in most instances it is impossible to determine if it is congenital or acquired. In the acquired form it may be the end result of inflammatory disease (ureteritis) or secondary to instrumental or surgical trauma, neoplasm, extrinsic inflammations or, occasionally, radiotherapy. The clinical importance of stricture relates to the degree of dilatation of the proximal urinary tract, the effect on function and the presence of infection (Figs. 19–8, 19–9, 19–15 to 19–17).

TUBERCULOSIS

Tuberculosis of the ureter is almost always associated with tuberculosis of the kidney and frequently the bladder. (See Tuberculosis of the Kidney.) Although involvement of the ureter from distant tuberculous foci has been reported, the ureter usually is affected through the ureteral lumen from the kidney. Roentgenograms in the early stages reveal dilatation of the ureter, possibly secondary to atonicity of the ureter or from edema secondary to involvement of the ureterovesical orifice.

The following is an outline of the roentgenographic findings in ureteral tuberculosis (Figs. 19–18 to 19–24).

1. Early
   a. Mild to moderate ureteral dilation (see above). There may be no renal findings (Fig. 19–18).
   b. Ulcerative ureteritis. Long segments of ragged irregular ureteral mucosa having a "motheaten" appearance. This is associated with tuberculous abscesses or calyceal destruction in the kidney (Figs. 19–19, 19–20).
2. Late
   a. Strictures. The strictures occur in the areas of ulcerative ureteritis. If the infection is limited to the mucosa, following treatment a normal pattern may return. If the infection destroys muscle, the fibrosis may lead to a stricture. Multiple strictures are common because of the long areas of ulcerative ureteritis (Fig. 19–20). If the strictures occur close together, a "beaded" appearance may result (Figs. 19–21 to 19–23).
   b. Calcifications. Ureteral calcifications are rare and may be mottled or linear and are usually associated with renal calcification. Calcifications in the proximal ureter are usually secondary to tuberculosis (Fig. 19–23b). Calcifications in the distal ureter associated with calcifications of the bladder are usually from schistosomiasis (Figs. 19–45 to 19–48).
   c. Total ureteral involvement may lead to a thin "pipe-stem" ureter encased in a chronically infected thick ureteral wall. Varying patterns of narrowing and dilatation may occur (see Figs. 19–23a, 19–24). (For other illustrations, see Chapter 6, Tuberculosis of the Kidney.)

URETERITIS CYSTICA

In this entity multiple inflammatory cysts, varying in size from 1 or 2 mm to large cysts that may partially obstruct the lumen, project from the urothelial lining of the ureter. Ureteritis cystica is more frequently unilateral and is frequently associated with pyelitis cystica and less often with cystitis cystica. The etiology is not known, but there is a definite association with chronic urinary infection. Whether infection leads to metaplasia of the surface urothelium or leads to degeneration of the submucosal cell nests of von Brunn is not known. The cysts contain a watery or viscid fluid. The suburothelial cysts are more common in the renal pelvis and proximal ureter. The urogram and pyelogram define the cystic lesions as smooth, round, or oval filling defects of diverse size that protrude into the lumen. They may vary from a few scattered cysts to complete involvement of the ureteral mucosa. In pyelograms they occasionally mimic air bubbles (Fig. 19-25), but if care is taken to obtain multiple projections the cysts are seen tangentially arising from the wall of the ureter, whereas air bubbles always remain centered in the ureteral lumen. In addition, air bubbles, in contradistinction to cysts, usually change position in multiple films. The ureter also may show irregular areas of dilatation and constriction (Figs. 19-25 to 19-31a).

Cystic blebs similar to ureteritis cystica may rarely occur secondary to an allergic response of the ureteral mucosa in which the blebs protrude into the lumen. This has been seen in Stevens–Johnson syndrome where the ureteral mucosa may respond in a similar manner to other mucosal surfaces (Lopez, F., personal communication). In the latter situation, the kidney does not reveal changes of chronic urinary infection, and the process is reversible (Fig. 19-32).

FISTULA

Fistula of the ureter may occur from a variety of causes. Most commonly they occur following surgery (ureterolithotomy and gynecologic procedures) or trauma (rupture of the ureter); in the latter instance the fistulous tract usually extends cutaneously. Following pelvic surgery, fistulization may occur to the vagina, the seminal vesicles, rectum, and so forth. The most common site in the female is to the vagina. Rarely fistulization is seen to intraperitoneal organs, such as the small or the large intestine, or even to the bronchi, usually secondary to severe inflammation or tumor (Figs. 19-33, 19-34). (Additional illustrations are found in Chapter 20, Trauma to the Ureter.)

RETROPERITONEAL FIBROSIS

Retroperitoneal fibrosis is an entity of unknown etiology (see discussion below) in which there is a fibrous mass or plaque in the retroperitoneal area, usually in the region of the sacral promontory, which envelops the retroperitoneal structures, including the ureters, but usually does not invade them. Although it may present unilaterally it is usually bilateral (60–70%). The age of incidence varies from 8 to 80 years but is most common from 40 to 60 years (Figs. 19-35 to 19-42).

There is an overall male predominance of 2 or 3:1, although this appears to be less marked in younger patients. The disease appears to have two stages: (1) *Early* – a fibrotic productive disease, with variable symptoms, primarily back or flank pain frequently with associated weight loss, urinary frequency, and an elevated sedimentation rate. (2) *Late* – the disease itself is quiescent. The symptoms relate to the secondary changes of ureteral or vascular obstruction or to random involvement of other organs by the pannus of fibrotic granulation tissue.

The lesion may involve any portion of the urinary tract from the kidney to the bladder, but it occurs most commonly around the fourth and fifth lumbar vertebrae.

The typical presentation is a man, around 50 years of age, with a history of several months of back pain frequently associated with dysuria. The radiologic findings consist of dilatation of the proximal urinary tract, with narrowing and frequently medial deviation of both ureters in the area between L-5 and S-2. The ureteral narrowing is smooth and conical and may involve a long segment. Vascular structures in the pelvis, particularly veins, may become obstructed by the fibrotic reaction. Arger and coworkers reported that medial deviation alone is not a reliable sign to suggest retroperitoneal fibrosis.[108] Although functional obstruction is frequently present, retrograde catheters usually are passed through the involved area without difficulty (Fig. 19-36). CT (Fig. 19-40c) and ultrasound (Fig. 19-40d) are excellent methods of demonstrating the localized mass.

Pathologically the plaquelike mass of fibroblasts and inflammatory cells may randomly involve the ureters, inferior vena cava, iliac vessels, or rectum and rectosigmoid. Skeel and co-workers reported two cases of retroperitoneal fibrosis in which intrinsic involvement of the ureteral muscular wall occurred in contradistinction to the usually reported extrinsic compression or encasement.[167]

The etiology is not known. The lesion was previously labeled idiopathic, but many cases fall into subgroups that are associated with this disease. It has been suggested that this entity may represent a form of collagen disease secondary to an unknown antigen, the disease representing an allergic or autoimmune reaction. Deposits of IgG, IgM, and IgA have been found in the fibrotic tissue. Many feel that this lesion is basically a vasculitis related to polyarteritis. A frequent association with drug ingestion has been shown, including methysergide, ergot derivatives, phenacetin, and others. The disease has also been related to numerous malignancies (particularly the lymphoma group), arteritides, and pyelosinus extravasation. It is probable that there are numerous etiologic causes affecting different patients under variable situations. The usual treatment consists of steroids and/or surgery to free the involved areas (Figs. 19–38, 19–39). The ureters when freed may be placed intraperitoneally. It appears that in some cases in the late phase of the disease spontaneous regression may occur.

Numerous variants of this entity have been reported (i.e., Gerota fasciitis), some involving the proximal ureters and others involving single segments of a ureter. For the present we have considered idiopathic retroperitoneal fibrosis as that entity which involves any segment of the ureters in association with other retroperitoneal tissues and is usually bilateral. Bilateral metastatic lesions occasionally may encase the ureters mimicking retroperitoneal fibrosis (Fig. 19–42).

A similar process occurs in the mediastinum (fibrosing mediastinitis), the common bile duct (sclerosing cholangitis), retro-orbital pseudotumor, retractile mesenteritis, Riedel's thyroiditis, and around the urinary bladder (sclerosing fibrolipomatosis). Whether these are of similar etiology is still speculative.

PERIURETERAL FIBROSIS

Periureteral fibrosis is a variant of retroperitoneal fibrosis, which involves one ureter, often a fairly long segment, with progressive narrowing of the ureter, producing proximal dilatation. It is not associated pathologically with the massive retroperitoneal involvement seen in idiopathic retroperitoneal fibrosis, but the inflammatory tissue is limited to the ureteral walls (Fig. 19–41).

PELVIC FIBROLIPOMATOSIS (LIPOMATOSIS)

This may be a variant of retroperitoneal fibrosis (see Bladder, p. 1525). It differs in that it is located within the bony pelvis, has a more marked male predominance, and is more common in blacks. Histology shows a fibrofatty tissue with fat much more predominant than the usual retroperitoneal fibrosis. Clinically the disease is milder, but the character of the involvement is similar to retroperitoneal fibrosis. The new tissue compresses and elevates the bladder, frequently producing a teardrop appearance;

the ureters are compressed and medially deviated in the pelvis (Fig. 19–42a), and the rectum is compressed and elongated (Fig. 19–42c). The patients may present with ureterectasis, hydronephrosis, or bowel symptoms. The presence of excess fat in the pelvis is frequently visible in a scout abdomen. A large number of cases, perhaps half of the total, are noted incidentally in patients without symptoms. Individuals under the age of 50 presenting with this lesion appear more likely to have progressive lesions and symptomatology. In patients over the age of 60 presenting with this entity, the disease appears to be more stable without progression. It is important not to confuse pelvic fibrolipomatosis with renal sinus lipomatosis, which refers to excess fat in the renal sinus.

SCHISTOSOMIASIS

Schistosomiasis is endemic in Egypt, much of Africa, western Asia, India, Pakistan, and Japan. It is several times more common in men than in women. With the increased mobility of people, the disease is present all over the world and increasing in the United States. The life cycle of the *Schistosoma haematobium* has been described by Vermooten (see Reference 173 in Chapter 26, Inflammation of the Bladder.) Infestation is acquired from bathing in infested water. The ureteral lesions are secondary to the presence of *S. haematobium* in the venules beneath the mucosa of the ureter. The ova are deposited in the subepithelial layer and lead to hyperplasia of the urothelium, with the formation of nodules that may protrude into the lumen. This is followed by fibrosis, mucosal atrophy, and ulceration, which lead to scarring, stricture, calcification (areas of necrosis and dead ova), loss of peristalsis, and secondary calculi. The predominant findings occur in the urinary bladder. The ureter is involved in about half of the bladder cases. Primary changes are in the pelvic ureter with the proximal ureter and kidney affected by the secondary changes of calculi and hydronephrosis.

Radiographic findings usually are limited to the bladder and the distal thirds of the ureters. In the early stages there is dilatation of the lower ends of the ureters secondary to infestation of the ureteral walls and the urinary bladder. Nodular lesions (hyperplasia) may protrude into the lumen of the bladder and ureter associated with acute interstitial cystitis and ureteritis (Figs. 19–43, 19–44). This progresses to intermittent areas of dilatation and stenosis of the ureter with proximal hydronephrosis.

The end stage may show strictures, aperistalsis, linear calcification, and occasionally punctate calcification within the distal ureters. Ureteral calcification is almost always associated with calcification of the wall of the bladder. Large bladder and ureteral calculi may be present. Papillomas may develop and occasionally calcify, leading to the term "hanging calculus" (Figs. 19–45 to 19–48).

ENDOMETRIOSIS

Endometriosis involves the urinary tract in about 1 per cent of the total cases. Involvement of the bladder is more common than involvement of the ureter, usually the distal pelvic ureter. Renal involvement is extremely rare. Symptoms are variable and include dysuria, hematuria, and obstruction. The diagnosis of endometriosis is suspect when women of late childbearing age (35–40 years) present with pelvic pain, menorrhagia, dysmenorrhea, and hematuria in association with their menstrual periods. However only about 50 per cent of patients present with this classic syndrome. Sixty-seven cases of ureteral endometriosis were reported as of 1972. Involvement of the ureter may be divided into an intrinsic or extrinsic type, but the division is arbitrary and both types may present in the same patient.

In intrinsic or primary ureteral endometriosis, endometrial tissue is present within the muscular wall or lumen of the pelvic ureter. Occasionally an intraluminal mass, an endometrioma, is present, indistinguishable from a ureteral tumor. Strictures may occur leading to severe ureteral obstruction (Figs. 19–49, 19–50).

In the extrinsic type (four times more common) ureteral deviation or obstruction is secondary to external pressure from masses associated with pelvic endometriosis without ureteral invasion. The sigmoid colon is frequently involved in the same process (Figs. 19–51 to 19–53).

In both types the obstruction is usually below the level of the pelvic brim. Suggested causes include extruded uterine tissue into the peritoneal cavity, vascular or lymphatic transport of endometrial tissue, metaplasia, and implantation of endometrial cells during pelvic surgery.

LEUKOPLAKIA

The definition of leukoplakia varies among different authors. It is probably best defined as an end stage of squamous metaplasia of the transitional epithelium with white membranous patches on the epithelium that contain areas of stratification and keratinization. Squamous metaplasia may occur without leukoplakia. Leukoplakia is an uncommon disease that usually follows long-standing chronic infection. About half of the patients have renal calculi. The areas usually involved are the bladder and renal pelvis and less often the proximal ureter. Leukoplakia is considered a precancerous lesion, with probably under 50 per cent of the patients developing squamous carcinoma. The lesion is usually unilateral.

Unilateral ureteral involvement usually is associated with leukoplakia of the renal pelvis. The radiographic findings consist of irregularity of the pelvic and ureteral walls with multiple small filling defects and, in the more severe cases, strictures or stenoses. Linear striations are frequently visualized in the renal pelvis and proximal ureter, produced by thickening of the mucosa involved in the squamous metaplasia. Calculi may be present (Figs. 19–54 to 19–56).

In the renal pelvis irregular striations and filling defects, occasionally concentric, resembling "onion skin," may occur depending on the amount of keratin. If leukoplakia obstructs the renal pelvis with masses of keratin, a cholesteatoma (inflammatory tumor) results. If a cholesteatoma forms, the chance of malignancy appears to decrease.

MALACOPLAKIA

Malacoplakia is far more common in the bladder than in the ureter (25 per cent of cases involve kidney and ureter). It is also found in the gastrointestinal tract (stomach and colon), prostate, testes, and retroperitoneum. The cause is unknown, but it appears to represent a response to long-standing chronic inflammatory disease. The lesion consists of soft yellowish, frequently umbilicated, plaques in the submucosa, which may be discrete or confluent. Histologic examination reveals large histiocytic cells containing Michaelis–Gutmann bodies, which are specific for this entity. Terner and Lattes have shown that the Michaelis–Gutmann bodies are products of phagocytized bacteria, suggesting the inflammatory nature of this disease.[283]

The roentgenogram may show single or multiple irregular plaquelike areas projecting into the lumen, which may produce a scalloped appearance, with areas of narrowing or dilatation. Single lesions may produce obstruction and suggest a tumor (Figs. 19–57, 19–58). (See Chapter 5, Infections of the Kidney, for illustrations of renal malacoplakia.)

AMYLOIDOSIS

Amyloidosis may present as a primary lesion (Figs. 19–58a to 19–60), may occur secondary to chronic inflammatory lesions such as tuberculosis, regional enteritis or rheumatoid arthritis, or secondary to malignant lesions such as myeloma. Rarely, amyloidosis occurs as a primary focal lesion in one systemic area, frequently the urinary tract.[294]

When amyloidosis involves the urinary tract it is most common in the renal parenchyma, with the amyloid deposits in the glomeruli and vessels (see Chap. 11, Medical Diseases of the Kidney and Chap. 5, Infections of the Kidney). Over 50 per cent of these patients develop the nephrotic syndrome, and renal vein thrombosis is not uncommon. When amyloid involves the renal pelvis the appearance may mimic leukoplakia. Calcifications may be seen in the walls of the infundibula, pelvis, or ureter (Figs. 19–61 to 19–63). Linear calcifications of the walls of the collecting system should suggest amyloidosis. Occasionally, amyloid deposits may obstruct the lumen.

Primary, secondary, or focal (localized) amyloidosis may involve a segment of the ureters. The radiographic findings are not characteristic. The ureters appear to be somewhat rigid and narrowed and occasionally are constricted. Proximal hydronephrosis is frequently present (Figs. 19–58a, 19–60).

Nagata in 1971 reviewed 50 cases of localized amyloid.[296] Most occurred in the bladder, but 15 involved the ureter or renal pelvis. The clinical features were similar to those of stricture or neoplasm. Of the ten occurring in the ureter seven were in the lower half.

POLYARTERITIS NODOSA

Polyarteritis is a systemic disease of small and medium-sized arteries that involves the kidney in approximately 80 per cent of cases (see Chap. 11, Medical Diseases of the Kidney). The small perforating arteries of the ureter may often be involved in a similar process. The pathologic feature is a fibrinoid necrosis of the media of the arterial wall, which frequently produces visible aneurysms in the kidney but in the ureter presents as irregular notching, usually larger and more rigid than that produced by vascular collaterals. Steroid therapy has been used with varying results. We have seen notching in a young person with polyarteritis that disappeared with steroid therapy (Figs. 19–64 to 19–65).

VASCULAR NOTCHING OF THE URETER

Vascular notching from dilatation of the periureteral or gonadal vessels may be arterial or venous, congenital or acquired (Figs. 19–64 to 19–70). Notching usually occurs in the proximal ureters. The findings must be persistent on multiple films, since peristalsis may mimic notching on a single film.

Some causes of vascular notching are outlined below.

1. Arterial
   a. Renal artery stenosis or occlusion: frequently seen in renal hypertension with collateral flow to the kidney through periureteral arteries (Fig. 19–66)
   b. Renal tumor: hypervascular tumor receiving additional supply from periureteral arteries
   c. Arteriovenous aneurysm: shunting decreases blood supply to kidney and additional supply may come through collaterals.
   d. Polyarteritis (see above): (Figs. 19–64, 19–65).
2. Venous
   a. Congenital varicosities (Fig. 19–68)
   b. Occlusion of the renal vein: Periureteral veins dilate as they assist in venous drainage of kidney (Fig. 19–67a).
   c. Renal tumor with occlusion of the renal vein (Fig. 19–67): Venous drainage by way of the collateral network
   d. Systemic venous hypertension, cardiac failure: Increased venous pressure may dilate periureteral veins.
   e. Occlusion of the inferior vena cava at or above the renal veins: The effect is more pronounced on the right kidney where periureteral and other collaterals may be prominent. Venous drainage of the left kidney continues by the ascending lumbar vein arising from the left renal vein and joining the azygous system and by reverse flow through the gonadal vein (Fig. 19–68a).
   f. Occlusion of the inferior vena cava below the renal veins: This may produce notching of the distal ureters. The ureteral veins may be used to by-pass the site of occlusion (Fig. 19–69).
   g. Portal hypertension: This may produce notching of the left renal pelvis and proximal ureters as retroperitoneal splenorenal veins are used to shunt blood from the portal to the systemic circulation (Fig. 19–70).

OVARIAN VEIN SYNDROME

The significance of this syndrome as a clinical entity is not certain. The ovarian veins tend to dilate during pregnancy, and after several pregnancies, the veins may not involute and may remain enlarged, occasionally becoming as large as the inferior vena cava. Because the right ovarian vein crosses over the ureter at about the level of S-1 to enter the inferior vena cava, it may compress the ureter at that point. Many clinicians do not feel that the enlarged vein by itself is the primary cause of the ureteral obstruction. It has been suggested that when obstruction is present it may relate to periureteral fibrosis. There has also been recent speculation that this syndrome may occur primarily in those individuals with variations of the right ovarian vein, such as multiple veins occurring around the ureter or the ureter and vein in a common sheath. Although the ovarian vein syndrome has been described on the left side, the left ovarian vein usually drains directly into the left renal vein and does not cross the ureter.

The roentgenograms reveal mild to moderate dilatation of the upper half of the right ureter, with mild proximal hydronephrosis. An impression may occur at the level of the iliac vessels (Fig. 19–72a) or at the point where the ovarian vein crosses the right ureter, usually around the first sacral segment (Figs. 19–71 to 19–74). Smaller scalloped pressure deformities may occur in the proximal ureter, representing ureteral varicosities.

It has been suggested that this entity, which affects the right ureter and kidney, may explain several abnormalities in women that statistically are more common on the right side:

1. Pyelonephritis of pregnancy is predominantly right sided.
2. The hydronephrosis and hydroureter of pregnancy occur primarily on the right side.
3. Unilateral ptosis is more common in women and more common on the right side.

The presence of a dilated ovarian vein within 8 or 10 weeks of pregnancy should not be considered significant. Dilatation must persist and produce significant obstruction or renal infection before surgery is contemplated. Resection of an enlarged vein does not always produce a beneficial effect.

FUNGAL INFECTION

Fungal infection has been considered in Chapter 5. Rarely the ureter may have roentgenographic findings in association with renal lesions (Figs. 19–75, 19–76, 19–77).

CHAPTER 19, ILLUSTRATIONS

FIG. 19–1. Long segment of ureteritis. Long-standing right pelvic pain. On excretory urography the right kidney was moderately hydronephrotic. The lower portion of the right ureter was not seen. The retrograde study revealed a long narrowed segment of terminal ureter with marked irregularity and considerable narrowing of the ureteral lumen. Some dilatation of the proximal ureter is present. This probably represents an area of ureteritis, but the possibility of spasm secondary to the retrograde study must be considered.

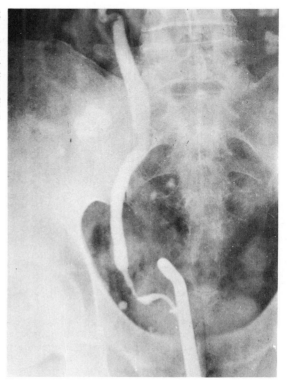

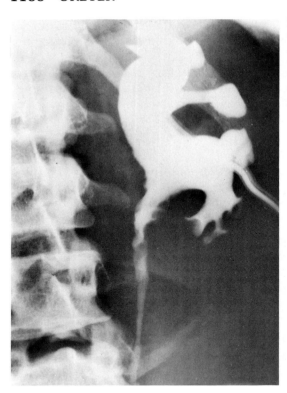

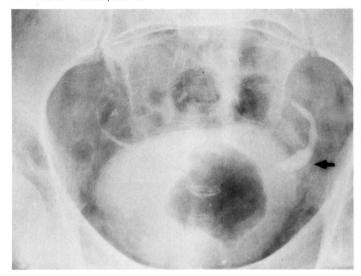

FIG. 19–2. Ureteritis. Following surgery for a ureteropelvic obstruction, a nephrostomy was performed. A tube pyelogram five days later revealed an acute ureteritis of the proximal ureter secondary to the surgery, with irregular contours and marginal defects. Following removal of the nephrostomy tube, the ureteritis disappeared.

FIG. 19–3. Secondary ureteritis. Elderly man with left seminal vesiculitis. This patient had a catarrhal seminal vesiculitis that involved the distal end of the left ureter. Dilatation and atony were persistent in this segment of the ureter (*arrow*).

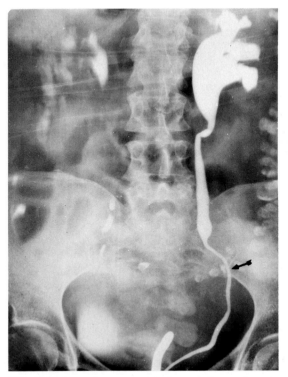

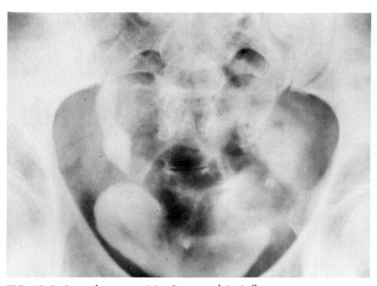

FIG. 19–4. Secondary ureteritis. Large tubo-ovarian abscess involving the ureteral wall (*arrow*). The abscess adhered to the ureter with marked local inflammation of the ureteral wall, producing narrowing and adhesions of the ureter.

FIG. 19–5. Secondary ureteritis. Severe pelvic inflammatory disease had involved the distal end of the right ureter. There was a constriction slightly above the ureterovesical orifice with dilatation and atony proximal.

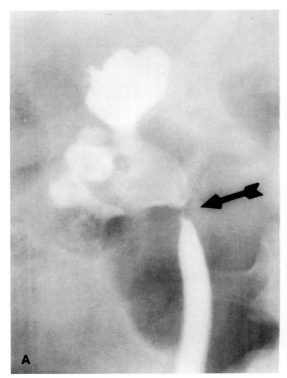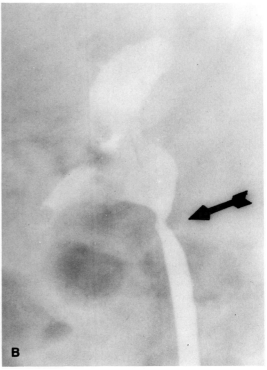

FIG. 19–6. Ureteritis from calculus. Large calculus in the right renal pelvis. **(A)** The retrograde pyelogram revealed a persistent narrowed area at the ureteropelvic junction (*arrow*). **(B)** Following removal of the pelvic calculus, a repeat retrograde study three months later revealed dilatation of this previously narrowed segment (*arrow*). This area had not been touched at the time of surgery. This finding demonstrates a severe ureteritis or spasm that improved following removal of calculus and restoration of adequate drainage.

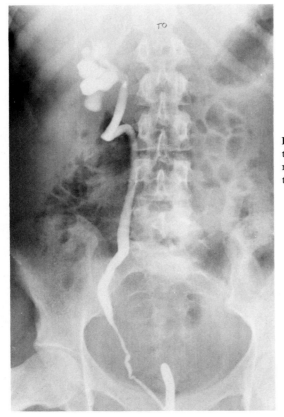

FIG. 19–7. Secondary ureteritis. Long area of distal ureteral narrowing and proximal hydronephrosis. The narrowed ureter represented secondary ureteritis from a tubo-ovarian abscess.

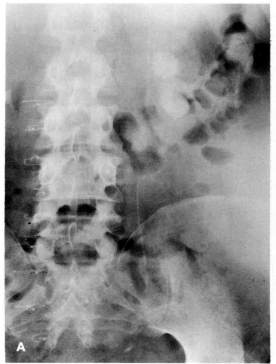

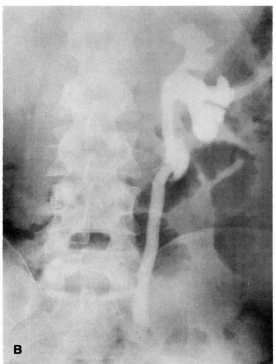

FIG. 19–8. Secondary ureteritis. Regional ileitis had directly involved the left ureter, producing ureteritis and stricture. (A) The urogram revealed severe proximal hydronephrosis with poor definition of the ureter. (B) The withdrawal film of the pyelogram visualized the proximal ureter to the stricture over the sacrum. Extravasation occurred proximally.

FIG. 19–9. Regional enteritis obstructing ureter. Urogram (A) shows a lateral deviation and partial obstruction of the left ureter near the pelvic brim. There is mild proximal hydronephrosis. Film of the small bowel (B) shows typical pattern of regional enteritis affecting multiple loops of ileum. Although the right ureter is usually involved, in this instance it is the left.

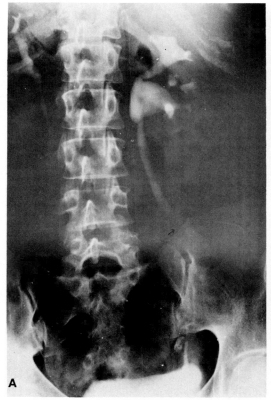

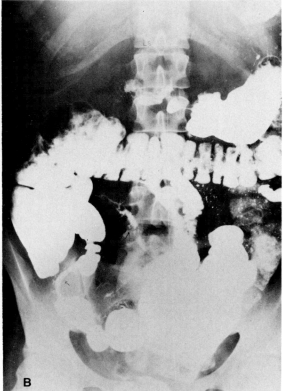

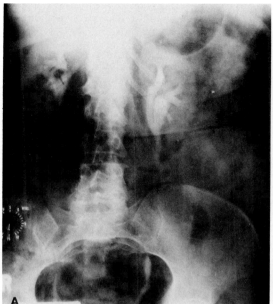

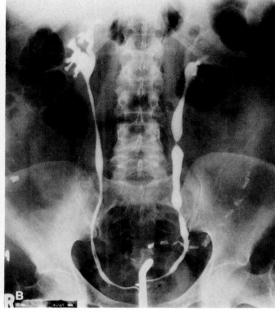

FIG. 19–9a. Nonspecific granulomatous ureteritis. **(A)** Urogram shows moderate left pelvicalyceal dilatation with poor ureteral visualization. **(B)** Retrograde injection shows two areas of narrowing in the mid left ureter. At surgery, nonspecific granulomatous reaction produced the ureteral narrowing. Etiology was not known. (Storm, P.: J. Urol., *117*:323, 1977)

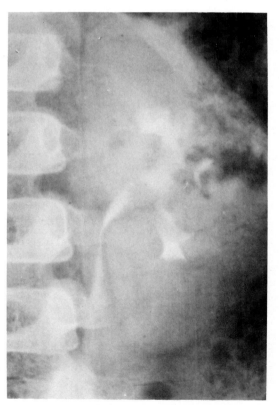

FIG. 19–10. Mucosal striations. A 4-year-old girl presented with urinary tract infection. Reflux could not be demonstrated at this time. There is a linear pattern of mucosal striations in the renal pelvis, infundibula, and proximal ureter.

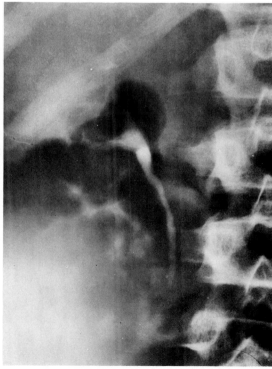

FIG. 19–11. Mucosal striations. Young boy with pyelonephritis. The illustration demonstrates a coarse mucosal pattern of the renal pelvis and the proximal ureter, presumably secondary to mucosal thickening.

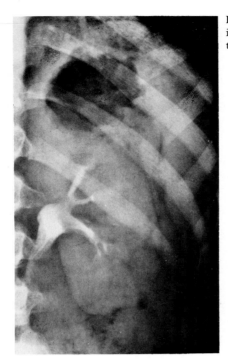

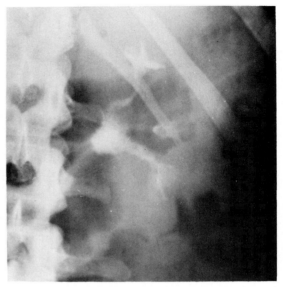

FIG. 19–12. Mucosal striations. Coarse pelvic and proximal ureteral striations in a young girl with urinary tract infection and reflux.

FIG. 19–13. Coarse striations. Young woman with fever and pyuria. Marked irregularity of the mucosa of the renal pelvis secondary to infection.

FIG. 19–15. Stricture of the proximal ureter. Ureteral calculus at the level of L-4 with chronic pyelonephritis of the left kidney. A stricture has developed (*arrow*) secondary to the pyelonephritis and ureteritis. Note that the dilatation occurs primarily above the stricture rather than proximal to the calculus.

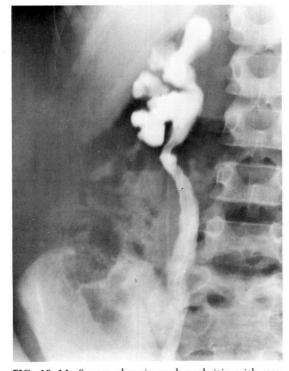

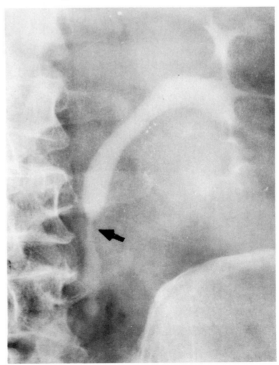

FIG. 19–14. Severe chronic pyelonephritis with ureteritis. Diffuse ureteritis with marked thickening and edema of the ureteral mucosa, producing within the ureter a linear, coarse mucosal pattern. At autopsy, the mucosa was cicatrized and thickened with irregular, coarse folds.

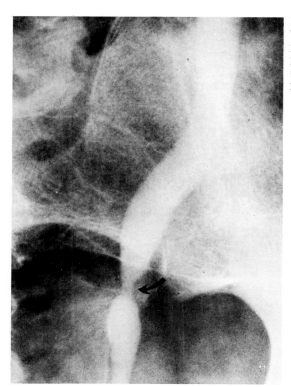

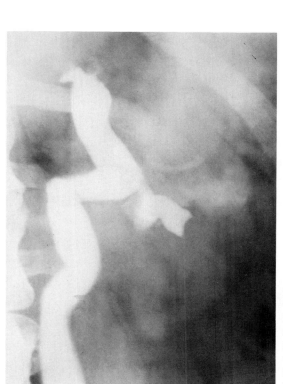

FIG. 19–16. Stricture of the lower third of the ureter. This patient had a previously impacted calculus that passed spontaneously. Pyuria and left flank pain were persistent. The retrograde study reveals a short stricture (*arrow*) in the lower third of the ureter with moderate proximal ureterectasis.

FIG. 19–17. Stricture at the ureterovesical junction. An elderly man with chronic right flank pain and pyuria. Excretory urography failed to visualize the right kidney. Delayed film of the pyelogram revealed massive right hydronephrosis with ureterectasis, tortuosity, and redundancy of the ureter. It is impossible to differentiate radiographically the congenital from the acquired stricture, although this site is a common one for congenital stricture.

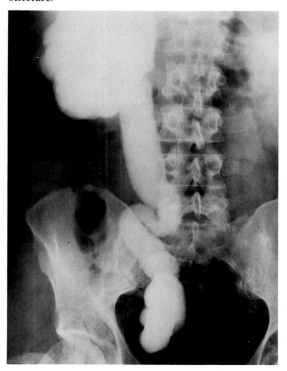

FIG. 19–18. Early changes of tuberculosis of the ureter. There is a tuberculoma present in the midportion of the left kidney. Strictures of many infundibula have occurred, with obliteration of peripheral calyces. There is diffuse dilatation of the ureter without evidence of stricture. Dilatation of the ureter is usually the initial finding in tuberculous ureteritis and may progress to ulceration.

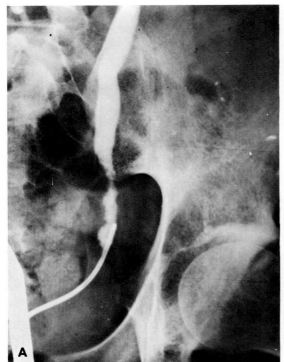
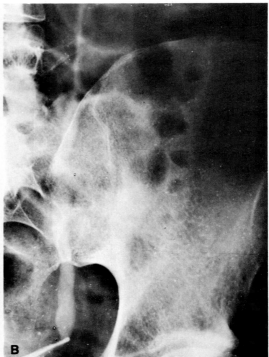

FIG. 19–19. Localized tuberculous ureteritis. (A) Severe ulcerative ureteritis affecting the distal end of the left ureter with marked irregularity and narrowing of the ureteral lumen. The proximal ureter was dilated. Renal tuberculosis was present. (B) Six months after the institution of therapy a repeat pyelogram reveals marked improvement of the ureteritis, with the ureteral lumen appearing smooth and minimally dilated. (Sol Unger, M.D.)

FIG. 19–20. Advanced tuberculous ureteritis. Right renal tuberculosis with a tuberculous abscess in the right kidney and severe ulcerative ureteritis. The very ragged appearance of the entire ureter mimics the findings seen in ureteritis cystica (see below). There is marked destruction of the mucosa of the ureter with long ulcerated segments in the proximal and distal ureter and a segmental area of dilatation in the midureter. (Bernard Loitman, M.D.)

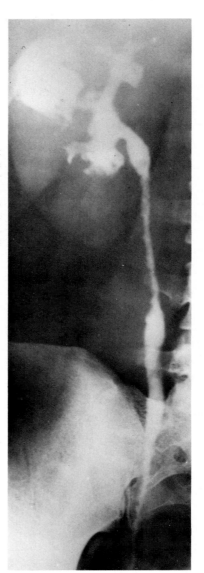

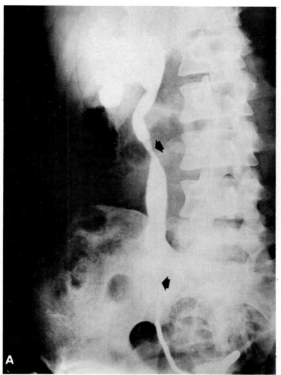

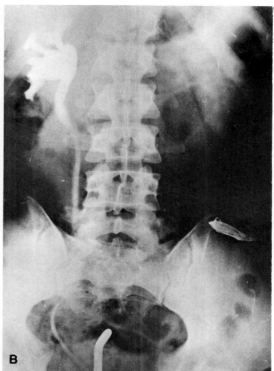

FIG. 19–21. Tuberculous ureteritis. Tuberculosis of the right kidney and ureter. (A) Delayed pyelogram following withdrawal of the catheter. Multiple strictures of the ureter are visualized (*arrows*) in areas of tuberculous ureteritis, with moderate dilatation of the proximal ureter and right hydronephrosis. (B) In a repeat retrograde study 10 months after initiation of therapy, the calyectasis and the ureterectasis have disappeared. The strictures have regressed, and there is no evidence of significant ureteritis.

FIG. 19–22. Tuberculous ureteritis. (A) Right renal tuberculosis and tuberculosis of the right ureter. Segmental areas of dilatation and contraction of the right ureter with multiple strictures, producing a corkscrew appearance of the proximal ureter. (B) Another example of tuberculous ureteritis with multiple constrictions, producing a corkscrew appearance. Although multiple strictures of the ureter are suggestive of tuberculosis, similar findings may occur in pyelonephritis.

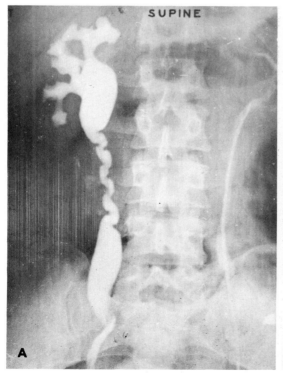

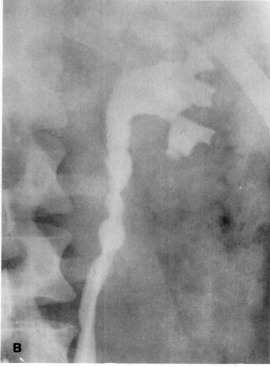

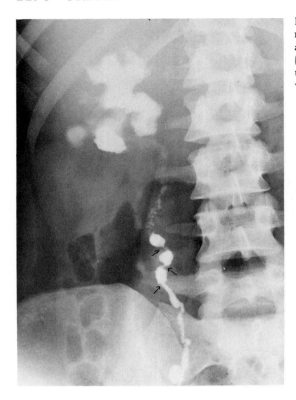

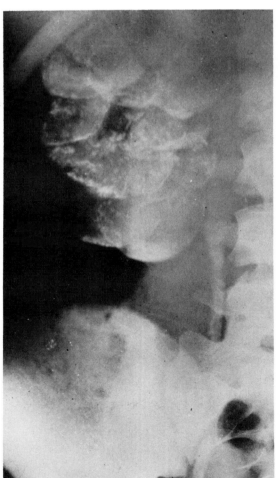

FIG. 19–23. Advanced tuberculosis. Diffuse involvement of the entire ureter with mucosal ulcerations and areas of attempted healing by stricture formation (*arrows*). There are areas of segmental dilatation between strictures; the entire kidney and ureter are involved.

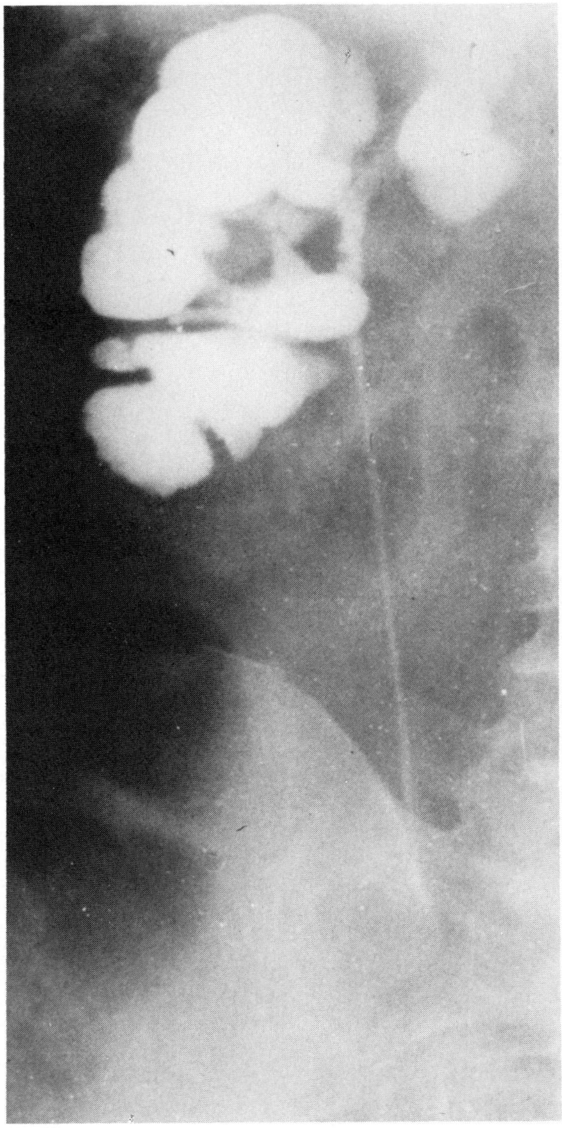

FIG. 19–23a. End-stage tuberculous ureteritis. Narrow ureteral lumen that is encased by granulomatous tissue. This variant of end-stage ureteritis has been termed a pipe-stem ureter.

FIG. 19–23b. Calcification of kidney and ureter. Scout film shows massive renal and ureteral calcification in end-stage tuberculosis.

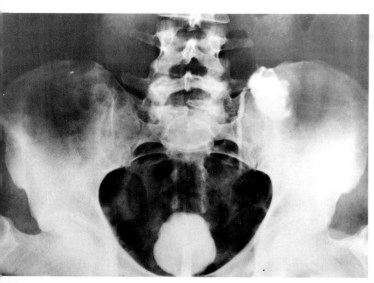

FIG. 19–24. Tuberculous empyema. The patient had a previous left nephrectomy for renal tuberculosis. In such cases the ureter usually is resected, as areas of involvement in the ureter are common even though the radiograph may appear normal. The pyelogram reveals marked irregularity and narrowing (pipe stem) of the ureteral stump, with a tuberculous abscess at the proximal end of the stump. (Courtesy of Sol Unger, M.D.)

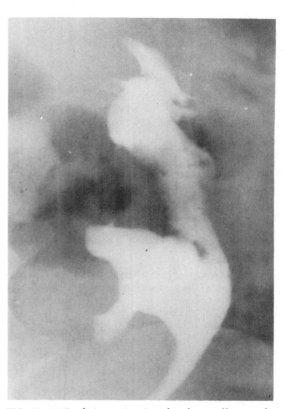

FIG. 19–26. Pyelitis cystica. Localized area affecting the upper infundibulum. Clinical diagnosis was neoplasm, and nephrectomy was performed. Pathology was pyelitis cystica. (Courtesy of A.J. Palubinskas: Syllabus: Genitourinary Tract Radiol., 1978. Radiological Society of North America)

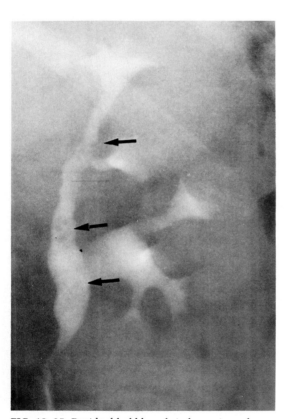

FIG. 19–25. Residual bubbles of air from air pyelogram simulating pyelitis cystica. (Courtesy of A.J. Palubinskas: Syllabus: Genitourinary Tract Radiol., 1978. Radiological Society of North America)

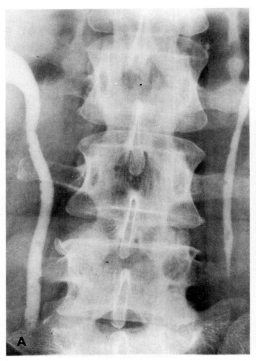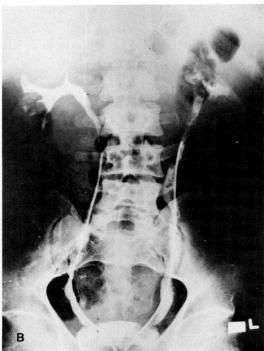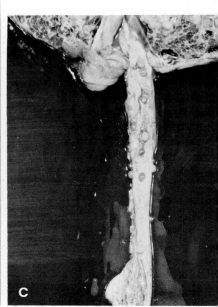

FIG. 19–27. Early case of ureteritis cystica. **(A)** Discrete, widely separated marginal cysts are present in both ureters. When seen tangentially, the cysts arising from the ureteral wall form a half circle projecting into the ureteral lumen. **(B)** Retrograde injection showing numerous cysts within the left ureter. The left kidney did not function. **(C)** Specimen showing the cysts projecting above the opened ureter. (Courtesy of Jack Lapides, M.D.)

FIG. 19–28. Bilateral ureteritis cystica. Chronic pyelonephritis associated with pyelitis cystica and ureteritis cystica. The cystic areas are seen to best advantage in the left proximal ureter. Note that when they are seen tangentially, the base of the cyst arises from the ureteral wall and projects into the ureteral lumen. This helps to differentiate cysts from air bubbles, which would be within the lumen and surrounded by contrast medium on all sides. (Courtesy of Bernard Loitman, M.D.)

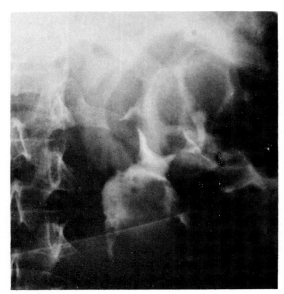

FIG. 19–29. Pyelitis and ureteritis cystica. This is a good example of cysts in renal pelvis, both enface and tangential views.

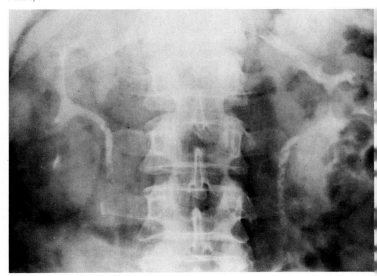

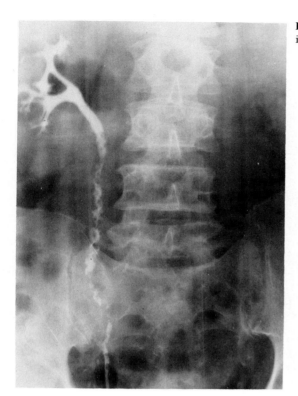

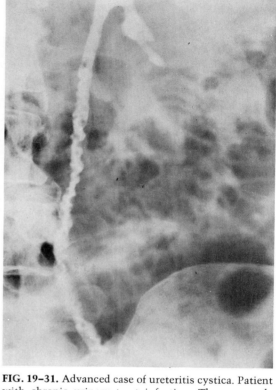

FIG. 19–30. Ureteritis cystica. Large number of coalescing cysts that mimic tuberculous ureteritis.

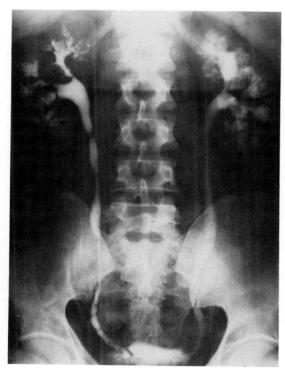

FIG. 19–31. Advanced case of ureteritis cystica. Patient with chronic urinary tract infection. The retrograde study reveals marked scalloping and irregularity of the entire ureter. Innumerable cysts are present, producing marked mucosal distortion. Cysts arising from the anterior or the posterior wall of the ureter are seen as complete circular lesions surrounded by contrast material.

FIG. 19–31a. Ureteritis and pyelitis cystica. Advanced case showing an unusual number of cysts in the calyces.

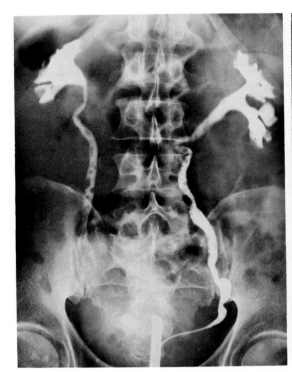 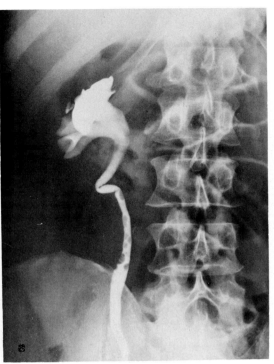

FIG. 19–32. Stevens–Johnson syndrome in a 23-year-old woman. Numerous allergic cysts or blebs are present mimicking ureteritis cystica. The blebs are larger and more irregular in shape than the usual cystica. There was no history of urinary tract infection. The patient had severe mucosal desquamation of all mucosa surfaces of the body. The lesion eventually resolved. (Courtesy of F. Lopez, M.D.)

FIG. 19–33. Ureterocutaneous fistula. Following ureterolithotomy there was a persistent cutaneous fistula communicating with the distal third of the ureter. A retrograde pyelogram revealed satisfactory visualization of the kidney and the proximal ureter. Contrast material extended laterally (*arrow*) from the distal third of the ureter through a fistula to the skin. Corrective surgery was performed.

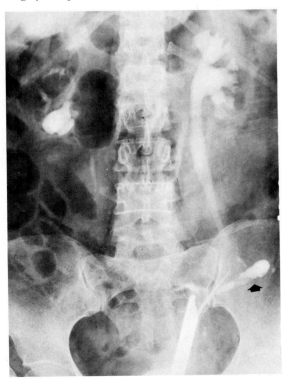

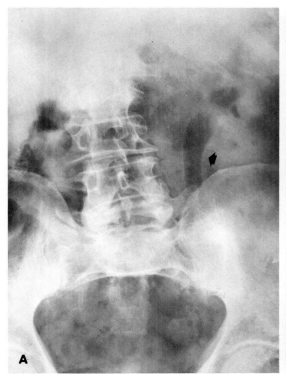

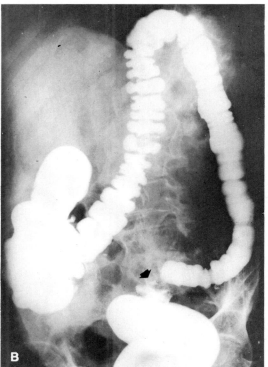

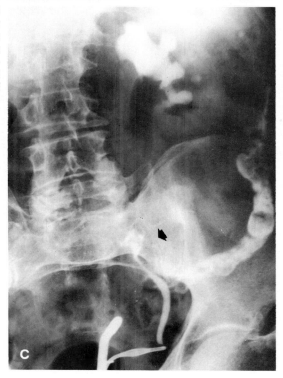

FIG. 19–34. Ureterocolonic fistula. Patient admitted with left flank pain and fever. **(A)** Scout film revealed air within the left ureteral lumen (*arrow*). **(B)** A barium enema revealed severe localized diverticulitis affecting the distal sigmoid (*arrow*). **(C)** Following retrograde injection of the left ureter, the contrast material flowed freely through a fistulous tract from the distal third of the ureter (*arrow*) to the sigmoid colon. A large pericolonic abscess was present.

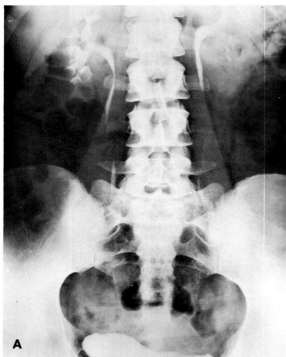

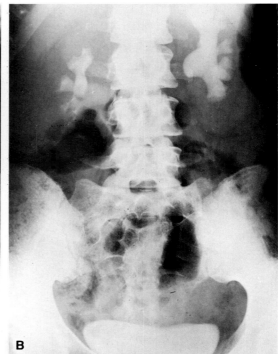

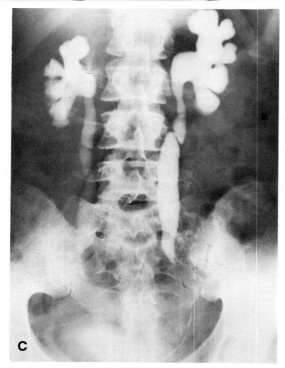

FIG. 19–35. Retroperitoneal fibrosis. These films illustrate the typical radiographic progression of idiopathic retroperitoneal fibrosis. **(A)** An excretory urogram obtained for unrelated pathology reveals the urinary tract to be within normal limits. Six months later the patient presented with backache and flank pain, and a repeat excretory urogram **(B)** revealed moderately severe hydronephrosis with poor visualization of the ureters. Five months later the patient again was reexamined and at this time marked hydronephrosis **(C)** was present bilaterally, together with bilateral ureterectasis above the sacral promontory. Below this point both ureters, where visualized, appeared to be normal in caliber. There was no evidence of ureteral deviation. This is a classic example of progressive idiopathic retroperitoneal fibrosis, with obstruction in the region of the sacral promontory and with gradual tapering of the ureters without evidence of a mass lesion. (J. A. Hejtmancik, M.D.)

FIG. 19–36. Unilateral retroperitoneal fibrosis. The presenting symptom was right-sided colic. Urography revealed a normal left kidney without visualization of the right kidney. Right retrograde examination revealed the classic medial deviation of the ureter (*arrow*) over the sacral promontory, with marked dilatation of the proximal ureter and severe hydronephrosis. At surgery the lesion presented unilaterally. (Courtesy of H. Bergman, M.D.)

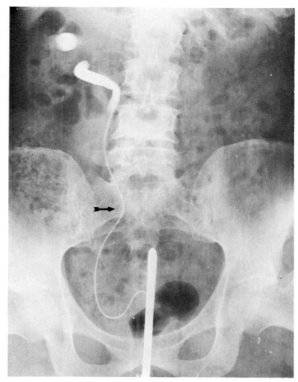

FIG. 19–37. Retroperitoneal fibrosis. A 52-year-old man presented with back pain. Urogram (**A**) shows moderate right hydronephrosis. The left kidney is normal. Withdrawal film (**B**) of the pyelogram shows a long tapered area of narrowing of the distal ureter. The lesion presented unilaterally.

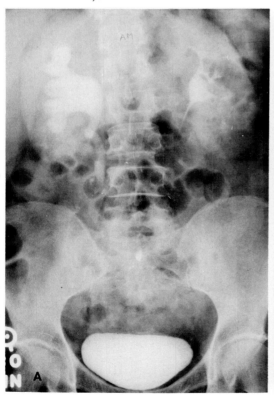

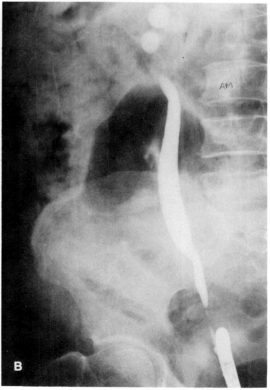

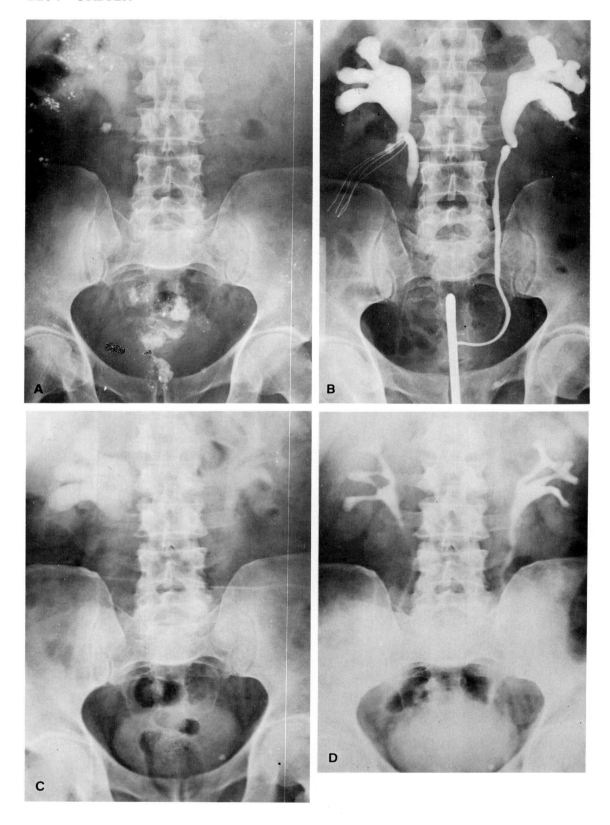

FIG. 19–38. Retroperitoneal fibrosis. Bilateral flank pain, weight loss and anorexia of 2 months' duration. The urogram **(A)** shows hydronephrosis on the right without visualization of the left kidney. Pyelography **(B)** revealed bilateral hydronephrosis with proximal ureterectasis. Seven weeks after left ureterolysis **(C)** the urogram reveals marked improvement in the left kidney. **(D)** Four months after left ureterolysis and ten weeks after right ureterolysis there is marked improvement in both kidneys. (Shaheen, D.J., Johnston, A.: J. Urol., *82*:51–57, 1959)

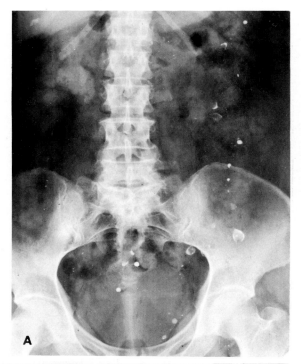

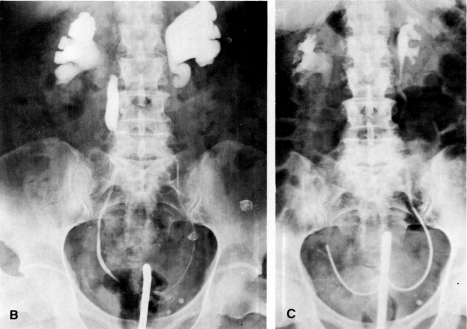

FIG. 19–39. Retroperitoneal fibrosis. Nausea, anorexia, and weight loss of 4 weeks' duration. The urogram **(A)** and the retrograde pyelogram **(B)** show bilateral calyectasis, pyelectasis, and proximal ureterectasis. There is minimal medial deviation of the ureters at L-5 to S-1. **(C)** Pyelogram 15 months after right ureterolysis reveals marked bilateral improvement. (Shaheen, D.J., Johnston, A.: J. Urol., *82*:51–57, 1959)

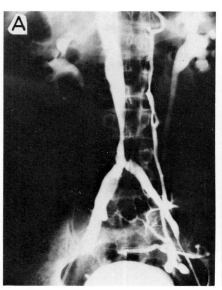
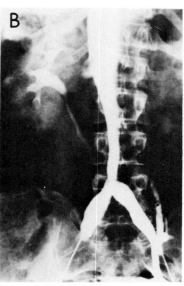
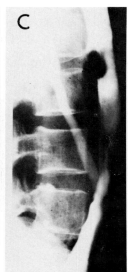
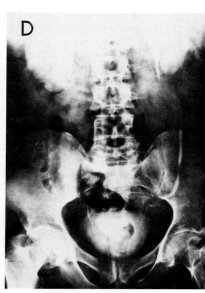

FIG. 19–40. Retroperitoneal fibrosis. A 32-year-old man presented with left flank pain. Preoperative cavogram (**A** and **C**) demonstrates compression with collateral filling and left hydroureteronephrosis. In the lateral films (**C**), anterior displacement and narrowing are present. Following left ureterolysis with lateral placement of ureter and steroid therapy, a repeat cavogram (**B**) and urogram (**D**) one year later show improved caval filling with no collateral filling and lateral placement of a normal ureter without hydronephrosis. (Kearney, G.P., Mahoney, E.M., Sciammas, F.D. et al.: J. Urol., *115*:32–35, 1976)

FIG. 19–40a. Retroperitoneal fibrosis (Gerota's fascitis). Woman, age 25, presented with back pain. The urogram (**A**) reveals bilateral pelvicalyectasis that is more pronounced on the left. The ureters appeared normal. Angiogram (**B**) showed numerous small retroperitoneal vessels retaining contrast medium for a prolonged time. Surgery revealed retroperitoneal fibrosis around the kidney partially enveloping the ureteropelvic areas. The fibrosis may have been secondary to pyelosinus urinary extravasation secondary to the ureteropelvic obstruction.

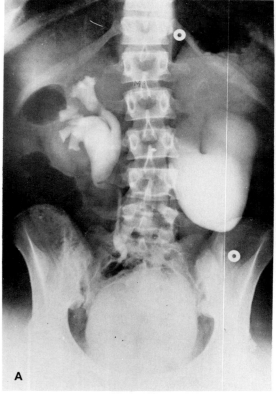
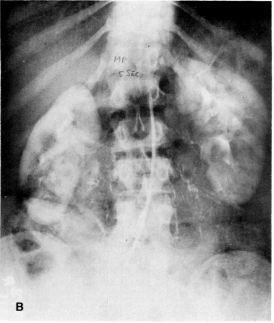

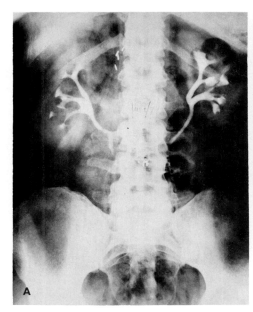

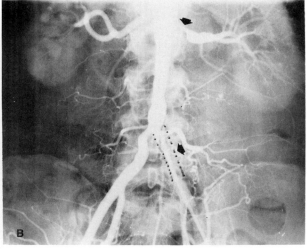

FIG. 19–40b. Retroperitoneal fibrosis. **(A)** Minimal narrowing of the distal two-thirds of both ureters from retroperitoneal fibrosis in this patient with primarily vascular involvement. **(B)** Aortogram shows unusual vascular involvement with diffuse tapering of the left iliac artery (*lower arrow*) and narrowing of the proximal renal artery (*upper arrow*). This patient presented with renovascular hypertension. (Courtesy of Murray Mazer, M.D.)

FIG. 19–40c. Retroperitoneal fibrosis in a 50-year-old man with increasing back pain. **(A)** Urogram shows moderate bilateral calyectasis with slight proximal ureteral dilatation and medial deviation. **(B)** CT at L-4 shows calcified aorta displaced anteriorly and surrounded by a diffuse mass that extends to the psoas. This was confirmed surgically.

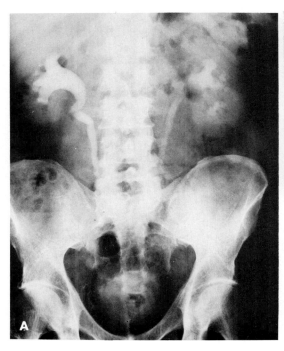

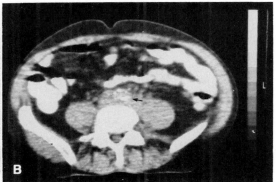

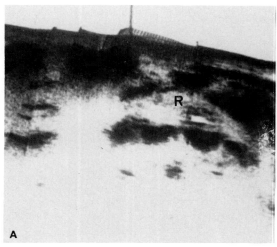

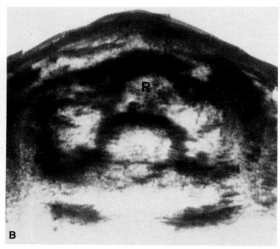

FIG. 19–40d. Ultrasonograms of retroperitoneal fibrosis. **(A)** Longitudinal sonographic section shows smooth-bordered, moderately echo-filled mass **(R)** anterior to the sacral promontory. **(B)** Transverse section shows a slightly irregular mass **(R)** just anterior to the sacral promontory. This is an excellent method of detecting the mass of retroperitoneal fibrosis. (Courtesy of Roger C. Sanders, M.D.)

FIG. 19–41. Periureteral fibrosis. Excretory urography revealed a normal left kidney with poor visualization of the right kidney. Right retrograde study revealed moderate hydronephrosis with renal reflux. There is a long narrowed segment of proximal ureter (*arrow, both films*) that is tapered at both ends without a sharp cutoff. Air bubbles are present in the proximal ureter. There is no evidence of ureteral deviation. At surgery a localized periureteritis was found without specific etiology. This is a variant of retroperitoneal fibrosis, where retroperitoneal tissues other than the ureter are not involved. Satisfactory function was restored following surgery.

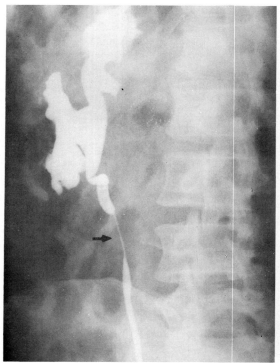

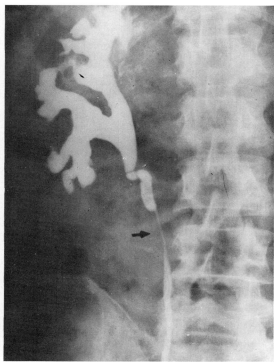

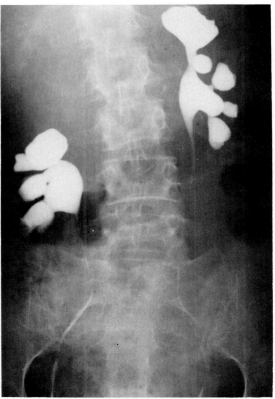

FIG. 19–42. Metastatic lesions mimicking retroperitoneal fibrosis. Patient presented with back pain and known history of breast carcinoma. Urogram shows bilateral hydronephrosis with finely tapered ureters produced by diffuse retroperitoneal metastases. (Skeel, D.A., Shols, D.W., Sullivan, M.J. et al.: J. Urol., *113*:166–169, 1975)

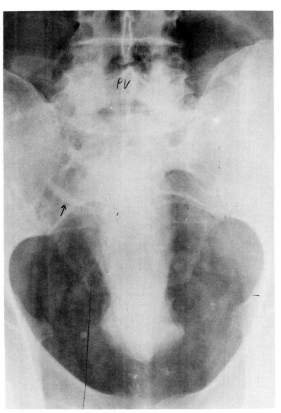

FIG. 19–42a. Pelvic lipomatosis. Marked compression and elevation of the bladder by fibrofatty tissue. Note the elevation and medial position of the right ureter (*arrow*), which is not obstructed.

FIG. 19–42b. Pelvic lipomatosis. Compression and elevation of the bladder and ureters. The left ureter is partially obstructed.

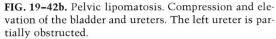

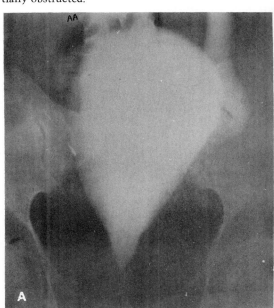

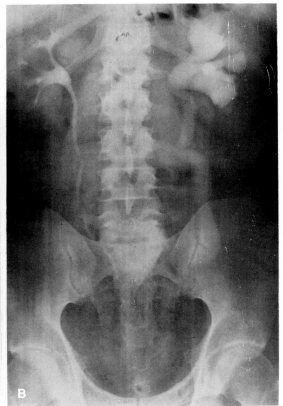

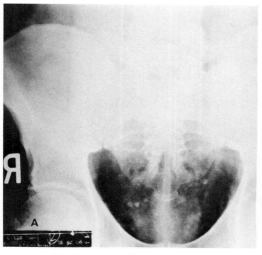

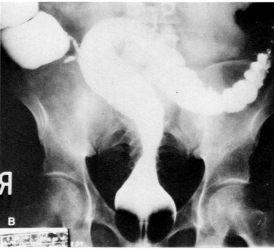

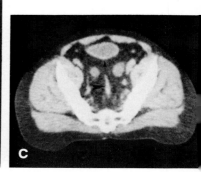

FIG. 19–42c. Pelvic lipomatosis. **(A)** Scout film of the pelvis reveals marked increase in fatty tissue around the bladder. **(B)** Barium enema shows narrowing of the rectosigmoid from compression by the fibrofatty proliferative tissue. **(C)** CT scan shows diffuse fibrofatty tissue throughout the pelvis compressing the bladder (*arrows*), arteries, and the rectosigmoid (*arrow*) posteriorly.

FIG. 19–43. Acute schistosomiasis. Young man presented with dysuria and intermittent gross hematuria. The urogram **(A)** shows hyperplastic nodules protruding into both distal ureters, with a large defect in the left proximal ureter (*arrow*). The bladder **(B)** shows numerous nodules protruding into the lumen. Peristalsis is still adequate. No calcifications or calculi are present.

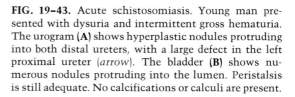

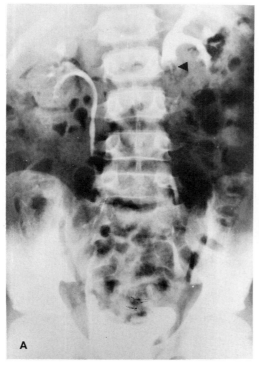

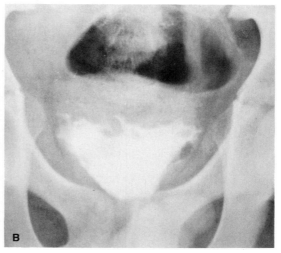

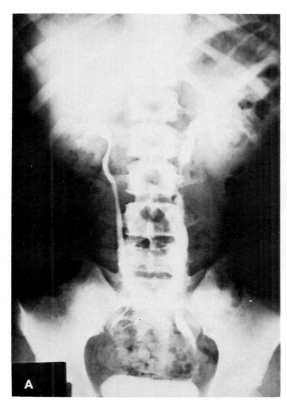

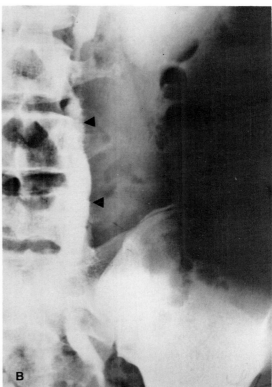

FIG. 19–44. Acute schistosomiasis in a 25-year-old Egyptian man. Urogram (**A**) and area of left ureter (**B**). Note the fine hyperplastic nodular pattern along the entire two-thirds of the left ureter (*arrows*) associated with areas of ureteritis, edema, and spasm. Similar but less marked changes are present in the distal right ureter.

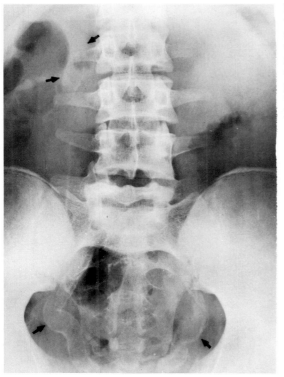

FIG. 19–45. Schistosomiasis. Scout film of a young man with poor renal function revealed linear calcifications of the ureteral walls and marked dilatation of the ureters. The calcifications are most prominent in the distal ureters (*lower arrows*), but in this case calcification extends up the entire right ureter to the renal pelvis (*upper arrows*). Calcification of the proximal ureters and the renal pelves is unusual. (Courtesy of P. Jamison, M.D., Tanta, Egypt)

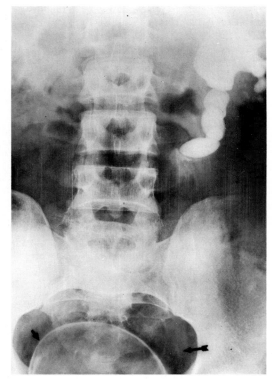

FIG. 19–46. Schistosomiasis. Young man with a large staghorn calculus in the left kidney and numerous calculi in the proximal ureter. There is calcification of the entire bladder wall (*short arrow*). No contrast medium is present. There is faint linear calcification of the distal ureters, most marked on the left side (*long arrow*). (Courtesy of P. Jamison, M.D., Tanta, Egypt)

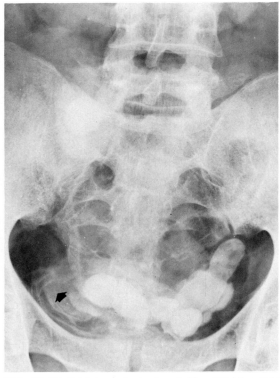

FIG. 19–47. Schistosomiasis. Scout film. Middle-aged man with numerous calculi in the bladder, a solid linear calcification in distal end of the left ureter and a large laminated calculus in right midureter. Marked calcification of the bladder is seen as numerous folds of calcification in the bladder wall (*arrow*). This illustrates the association of vesical wall calcification, ureteral wall calcification and calculi formation. (Courtesy of P. Jamison, M.D., Tanta, Egypt)

FIG. 19–48. Schistosomiasis. Enormous dilatation of the distal ureters with calcification of the walls of the ureters (*long arrows*). In this scout film there is a large solitary calculus within the bladder, together with marked calcification of the bladder wall (*short arrow*). (Courtesy of P. Jamison, M.D., Tanta, Egypt)

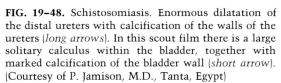

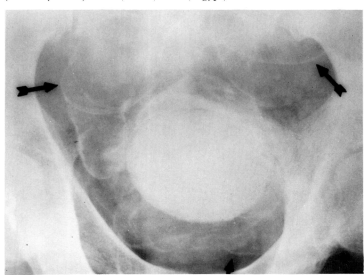

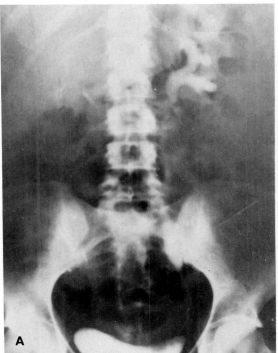

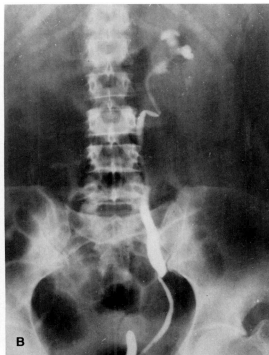

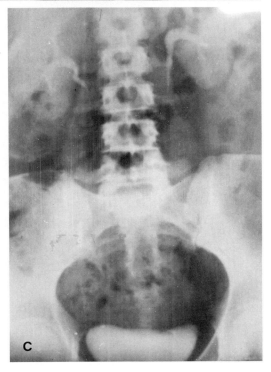

FIG. 19–49. Endometriosis. Young woman with pain and hematuria associated with her menstrual cycle. (**A**) The urogram revealed partial obstruction of the pelvic portion of the left ureter. (**B**) The pyelogram shows a transition from normal to dilated ureter without an intraluminal defect. This was produced by endometrial implants in the ureteral wall at this site. (**C**) Following surgery the urogram was normal. (Courtesy of R.S. Hotchkiss, M.D.)

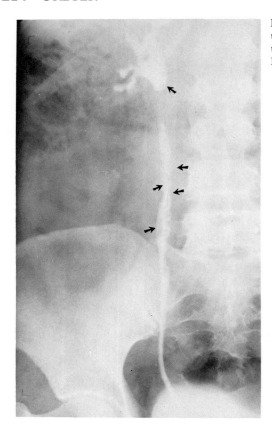

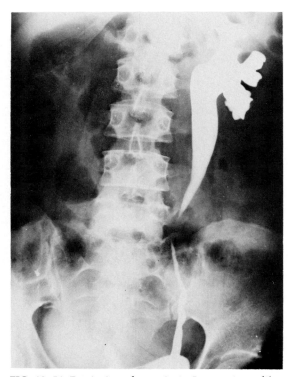

FIG) 19–50. Diffuse intraluminal defects (*arrows*) throughout the right ureter representing endometrial tissue projecting into the lumen. (Courtesy of Erich Lang, M.D.)

FIG. 19–51. Extrinsic endometriosis. Long stricturelike lesion from endometriosis compressing the midureter with considerable proximal distention. The lesion is at the pelvic brim higher than the usual lesion from endometriosis.

FIG. 19–52. Extrinsic ureteral endometriosis in a 38-year-old woman with dysuria. Multiple pelvic masses are present. There is marked compression of the distal right ureter with moderate obstruction leading to hydronephrosis. The endometrial mass did not invade the ureter.

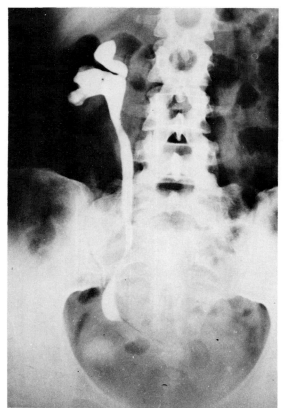

FIG. 19–53. Bilateral endometriosis. There are mass imprints on both pelvic ureters, with proximal obstruction. In some cases bilateral endometriosis may show intrinsic involvement on one side and extrinsic on the other side.

FIG. 19–54. Leukoplakia. Severe involvement of the renal pelvis with extension into the proximal ureter. Numerous filling defects are present with marginal irregularity of the ureteral wall (*arrow*) (keratin-displacing contrast medium). (Radiology Department, Mt. Sinai Hospital, New York, N.Y.)

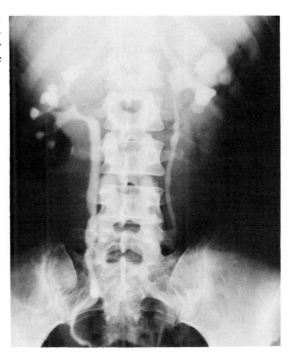

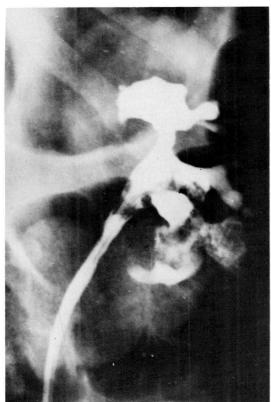

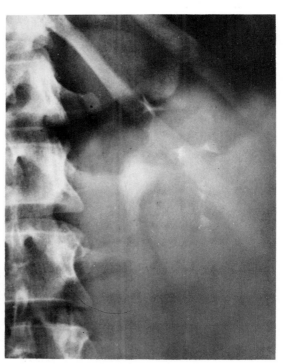

FIG. 19–55. Leukoplakia. Note the coarse, striated appearance of renal pelvis and proximal ureter. This appearance is produced by displacement of contrast medium by irregular deposits of stratified epithelium or keratin. (Courtesy of Howard Pollack, M.D.)

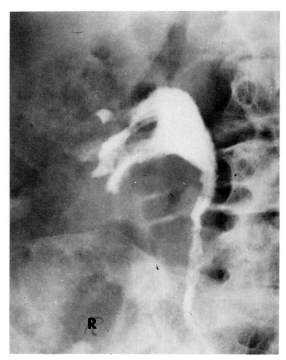

FIG. 19–56. Leukoplakia. Irregular striations in calyces, pelvis, and proximal ureter. (Courtesy of Howard Pollack, M.D.)

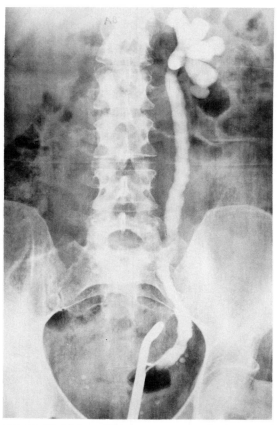

FIG. 19–57. Malacoplakia in a woman with a history of chronic urinary tract infection. Diffuse marginal scalloping of the entire ureter with proximal hydronephrosis. At surgery this represented diffuse malacoplakia. (Courtesy of Richard Pfister, M.D.)

FIG. 19–58. Malacoplakia. Left ureteral obstruction. Antegrade pyelography demonstrated the involvement of the distal ureter, with obstruction at the ureterovesicle junction. The ureteral lesion was secondary to bladder malacoplakia. (Courtesy of E. Lang, M.D.)

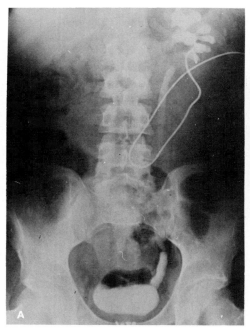

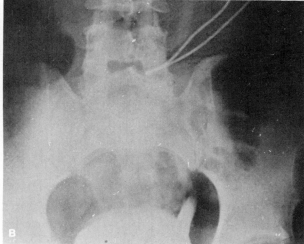

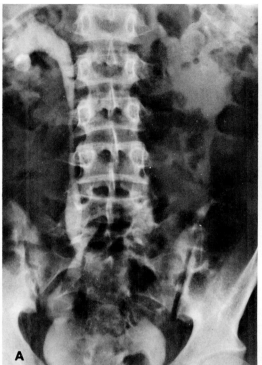

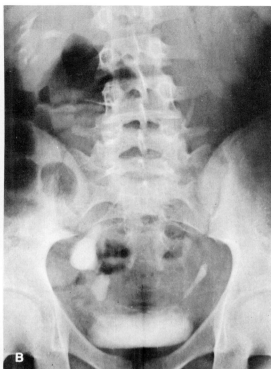

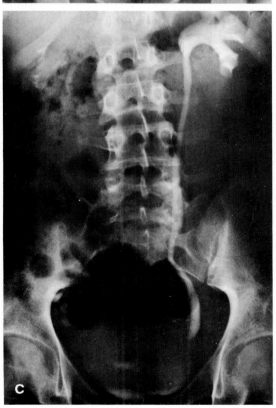

FIG. 19–58a. Primary ureteral amyloidosis. Seventeen-year-old man admitted with dull, aching right flank pain and gross painless hematuria. (**A** and **B**) The urogram revealed right hydronephrosis and hydroureter, presumably secondary to a stricture of the pelvic portion of the ureter. Retrograde catheterization of the right ureter beyond 3 mm was not possible. The left kidney and ureter appeared to be normal. Lower ureter and a cuff of the bladder were resected, and a ureterocystostomy was performed. There was amyloid infiltration throughout all layers of the ureteral wall, which measured up to 1 cm in thickness.

The patient was readmitted one year later, again with gross hematuria and left flank pain. (**C**) Excretory urography at this time revealed left hydronephrosis and hydroureter. A catheter could not be passed through the left ureteral orifice. Exploration revealed an edematous thick wall of the distal ureter similar to the gross appearance previously encountered on the right side. The histologic diagnosis again was amyloidosis, and complete investigation revealed no evidence of systemic disease. (Johnson, H.W., Ankenman, G.J.: J. Urol., *92:*275–277, 1964)

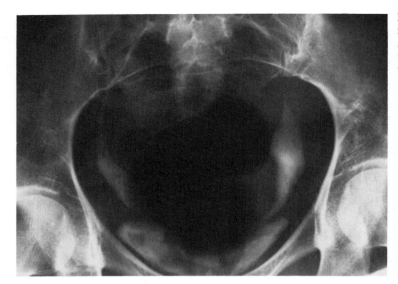

FIG. 19–59. Pelvic amyloid. Dilatation of the segments of both ureters suggesting primary megaloureter. At surgery primary amyloidoses of the ureters produced the distal narrowing most marked on the left, leading to the proximal dilatation.

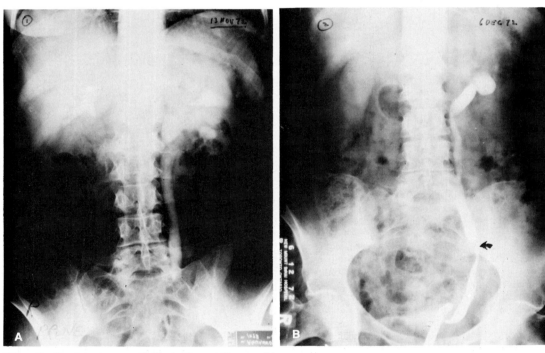

FIG. 19–60. Primary amyloidosis in a 65-year-old woman with hematuria. Urogram (**A**) shows a partially obstructing lesion of the distal ureter with proximal hydronephrosis. Retrograde injection (**B**) shows a narrow segment in the distal ureter (*arrow*) suggesting a stricture. At surgery, a long lesion several centimeters in length was present, involving the distal ureter, which represented primary amyloidosis. (Klotz, P.G.: Brit. J. Urol., 47:518, 1975)

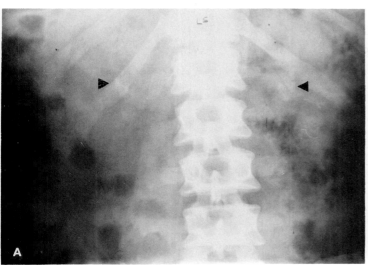

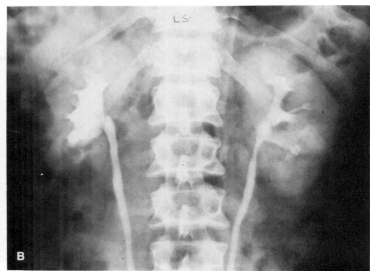

FIG. 19–61. Amyloid. Scout film (**A**) shows linear calcifications bilaterally in the walls of the renal pelves (*arrows*). Urogram (**B**) shows multiple filling defects in the pelves and proximal ureters.

FIG. 19–62. Amyloid. Scout tomogram (**A**) shows marked calcifications outlining the walls of the pelves and infundibula. Urogram (**B**) shows mottled defects from amyloid deposits with calyectasis in left. (Courtesy of Howard Pollack, M.D.)

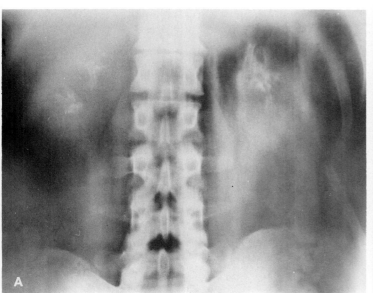

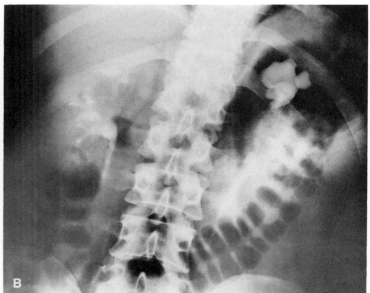

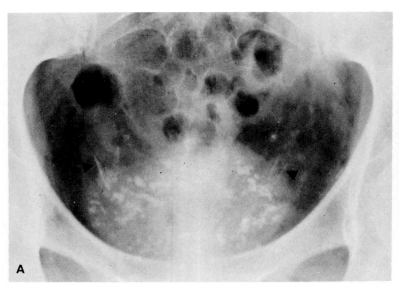

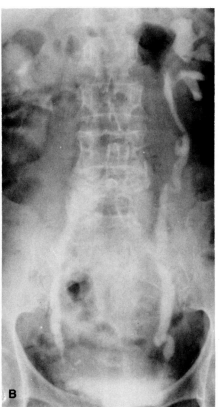

FIG. 19–63. Amyloid. An 80-year-old woman presented with a history of chronic urinary infection. Scout film **(A)** shows mottled calcification of the bladder wall and linear calcifications of the walls of the distal ureters (*arrows*). Urogram **(B)** shows narrowing of the distal ureters secondary to amyloid deposits, with moderate proximal ureterectasis and hydronephrosis. (Courtesy of Howard Pollack, M.D.)

FIG. 19–64. Polyarteritis nodosa. Middle-aged man with known polyarteritis nodosa. **(A)** The retrograde pyelogram revealed large marginal irregularities in the proximal third and the midthird of the left ureter simulating vascular notching. **(B)** An enlarged view demonstrates similar changes in the renal pelvis. At postmortem the ureteral walls were found to be thickened with diffuse necrotizing arteritis of the medium and the smaller arteries. (Radiology Department, Montefiore Hospital, Bronx, N.Y.)

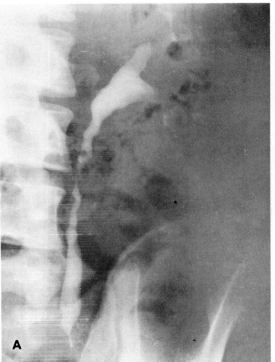

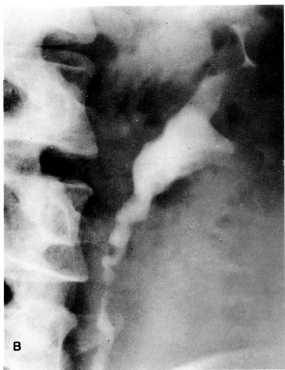

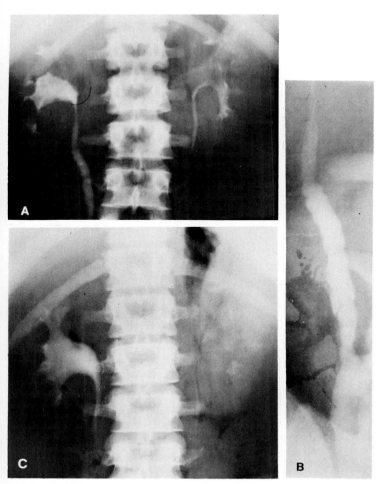

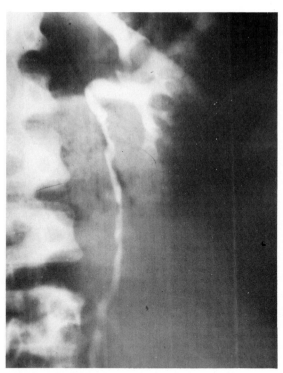

FIG. 19–66. Vascular notching of ureter. Numerous marginal defects similar to those in the preceding illustration, produced by enlarged ureteral arteries following partial occlusion of the renal artery. (Radiology Department, Mt. Sinai Hospital, New York, N.Y.)

FIG. 19–65. Polyarteritis. Young girl with symptomatic polyarteritis. (A and B) Urogram and closeup of right ureter show irregular marginal notching of the right renal pelvis and ureter, presumably from the associated small vessel arteritis. (C) Urogram 3 weeks after cortisone therapy shows a normal marginal outline. (Courtesy of Sam Schorr, M.D.)

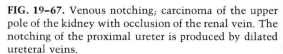

FIG. 19–67. Venous notching; carcinoma of the upper pole of the kidney with occlusion of the renal vein. The notching of the proximal ureter is produced by dilated ureteral veins.

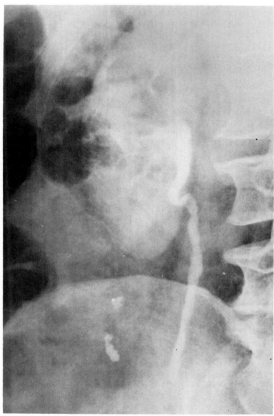

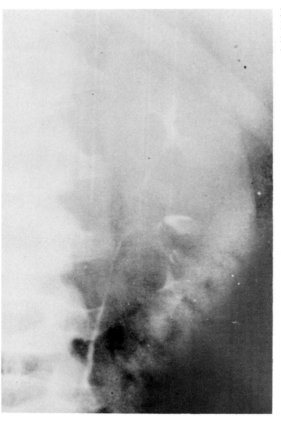

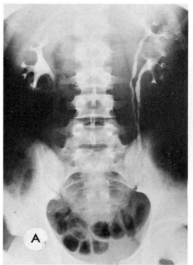 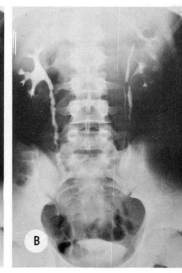

FIG. 19–67a. Left renal vein thrombosis from trauma. Fine scalloped notching defects are present along the margin of the proximal ureter from dilated ureteral veins.

FIG. 19–68. (A and **B)** Varices of ureter. The urogram revealed scalloping of the single right and the bifid left ureters, produced by periureteral varices. (Kaufman, J.J., Maxwell, M.H.: Am. J. Roentgen., *92*:346–350, 1964)

FIG. 19–68a. Obstruction of the inferior vena cava secondary to carcinoma of the pancreas. **(A)** Urogram shows marked marginal notching from ureteral collaterals draining the renal venous blood flow. **(B)** Late film of the arteriogram shows markedly dilated ureteral and gonadal veins. The left kidney showed no abnormality (see text).

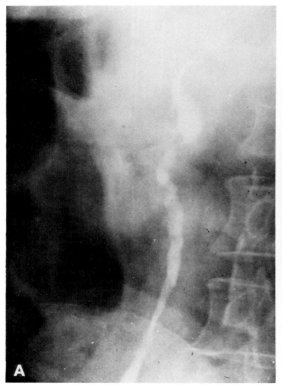 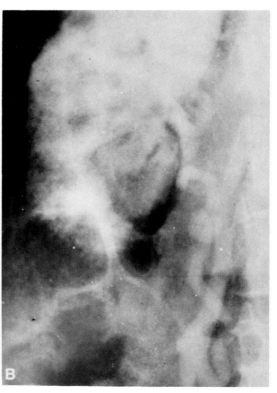

FIG. 19–69. Obstruction of the inferior vena cava below renal veins by tumor. Pyelogram shows vascular notching of the lower third of the right ureter.

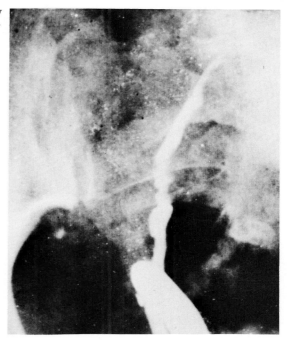

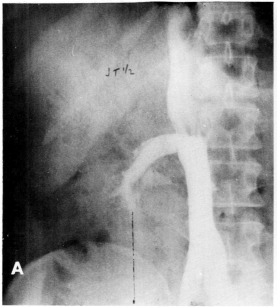

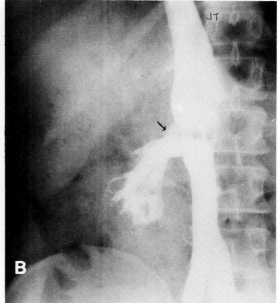

FIG. 19–69a. Unusual complication of caval plication for pulmonary emboli. The surgeon did not realize that two renal veins were present on the right. The umbrella was placed between the two veins, creating a venous shunt. **(A)** Early film of the cavogram shows considerable obstruction at the umbrella with contrast material flowing into the lower right renal vein and returning to the cava **(B)** (*arrow*) through the second renal vein.

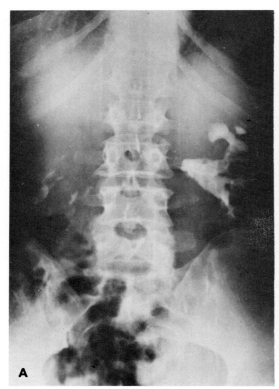

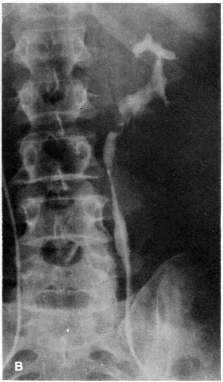

FIG. 19–70. Varices. Thirty-nine-year-old woman, alcoholic, admitted with severe left flank pain and hematuria. The urogram (**A**) and the pyelogram (**B**) revealed multiple small filling defects involving the proximal ureter, the renal pelvis, and the superior infundibulum. (**C**) At surgery large dilated veins encompassed the left renal pelvis and ureter, producing the marginal defects seen in the urogram. The dilated ureteral, pelvic, and renal veins were secondary to the enlarged collateral shunt between the portal and the caval systems (*arrow*), which had developed secondary to partial occlusion of the portal system from cirrhosis. This produces only left-sided notching.

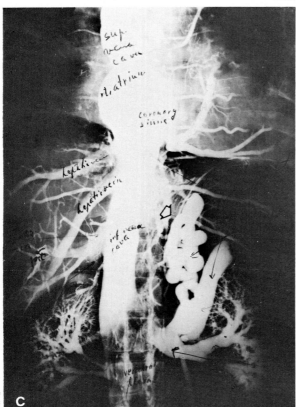

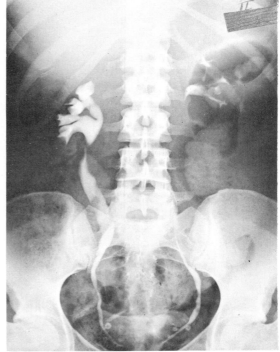

FIG. 19–71. Ovarian vein syndrome. Flattening of the right midureter around the first sacral segment, with proximal dilatation secondary to pressure where the right varicosed ovarian vein crosses the ureter. (Courtesy of R.F. Dykhuizen, M.D.)

1224

FIG. 19–72. Ovarian vein syndrome. Multiparous woman with typical impression on the right ureter at S-1, with proximal ureterectasis and hydronephrosis.

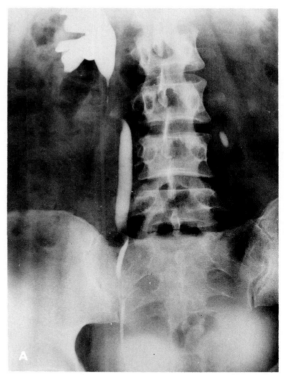

FIG. 19–72a. Iliac artery impression on ureter. **(A)** Young woman with mild calyectasis. Pyelogram shows impression on right ureter near S-3 (*arrow*). Note difference in position of impression from Figure 19–72. **(B)** Pelvic arteriogram shows iliac artery crossing ureter at that point (*arrow*).

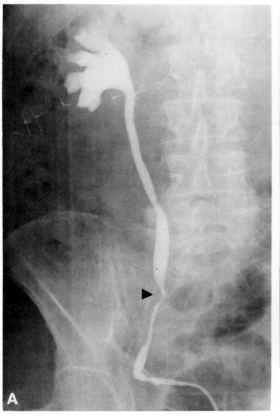

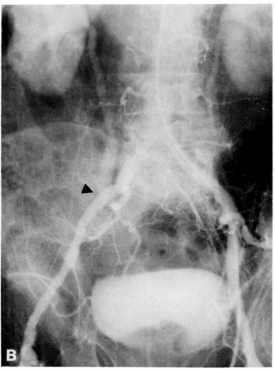

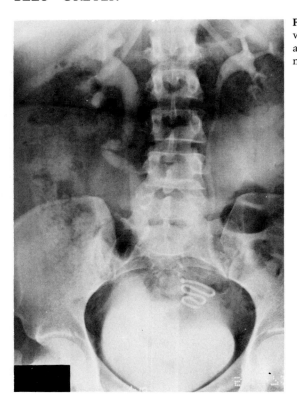

FIG. 19–73. Ovarian vein syndrome in a multiparous woman. There was dilatation of the right lumbar ureter and pelvicalyceal system from pressure on the ureter near S-1 by the ovarian vein.

FIG. 19–74. Ovarian vein syndrome. Young woman with right flank pain. **(A)** Pyelogram confirms the extrinsic impression on the right ureter (*arrow*) previously noted on urogram. **(B)** Injection of contrast medium into the uterine myometrium fills the venous plexus around the uterus and ovary and drains into the ovarian vein (*arrow*). The dilated vein crosses the ureter at the site of the defect.

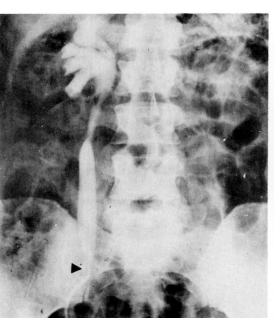

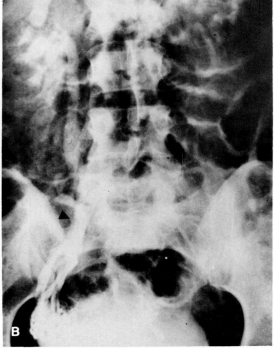

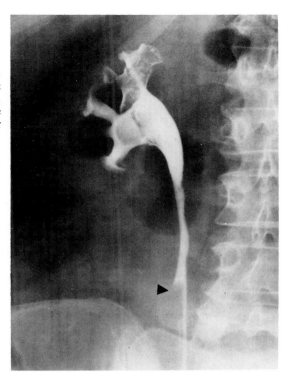

FIG. 19-75. Candidiasis. Candidiasis is the most common fungal infection of the kidney. Occasionally, part of a fungus ball may break off and impact in the ureter, producing renal colic and/or obstruction. Note large fungus ball in renal pelvis with fragment in midureter (*arrow*). (Courtesy of Montreal General Hospital.)

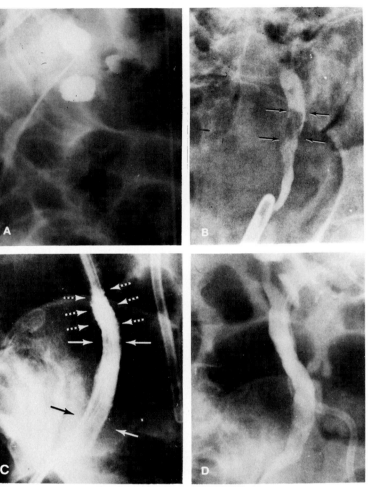

FIG. 19-76. Ureteral candidiasis. **(A)** Retrograde pyelogram shows proximal ureterectasis and calyectasis. **(B)** Large irregular filling defect (*arrows*) in the distal left ureter representing a fungus ball. **(C)** Following surgery and extrusion of the debris from the distal left ureter, the postoperative pyelogram revealed shaggy areas of intraluminal scalloping, presumably representing candida infection and mucosal edema. **(D)** Following anphotericin B, marked improvement in contour of left ureter is observed.

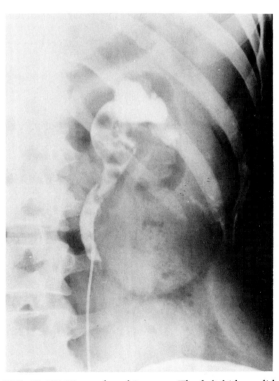

FIG. 19-77. Ureteral ecchinoccus. The left kidney did not function on urography. Pyelogram reveals a large mass in the lower pole, which was a hydatid cyst. The cyst had ruptured into the collecting system, and numerous daughter cysts were growing in the renal pelvis and ureter (radiolucencies in pyelogram). (Courtesy of Montreal General Hospital)

1227

BIBLIOGRAPHY

Ureteritis

1. Bissada, N.K., and Finkbeiner, A.E.: Idiopathic segmental ureteritis. Urology, 12:64–66, 1978.
2. Braasch, W.F., and Hurley, M.V.: Granulomas in urinary tract. J. Urol., 18:595–605, 1927.
3. Dreyfuss, W., and Goodsitt, E.: Acute regional ureteritis. J. Urol., 79:202–208, 1958.
4. Henke, R., and Lubarsch, O.: Handbuch der speciellen pathologischen. Anat. Histol. B.V. 1/2, 1934.
5. Israel, J., and Israel, W.: Chirurgie der Niere und des Harnleiters, pp. 524. Leipzig, 1925.
6. Kaufman, E.: Lehrbuch der speciellen pathologischen Anatomie, pp. 876. Berlin, 1911.
7. Litzky, G.M., and Seidel, R.F.: Obstructing intrinsic granuloma of the ureter. J. Urol., 103:426–428, 1970.
8. Mininberg, D.T., Andronaco, J., Nagamatsu, G.R., et al.: Nonspecific regional ureteritis. J. Urol., 98:664–668, 1967.
9. Mougenot, B., Mitrofanoff, P., Bouisson, F., et al.: Stenosing ureteritis during Henoch-Schonlein purpura in children. Ann. Radiol., 21:215–222, 1978.
10. Noring, O.: Nonspecific ureteritis elucidated by a case of primary ureteritis. J. Urol., 79:701–706, 1958.
11. O'Flynn, W.R., and Sandrey, J.G.: Nonspecific granulomata of the ureter and bladder. Br. J. Urol., 35:267–276, 1963.
12. Storm, P.B., and Fallon, E.: Nonspecific granulomatous ureteritis. J. Urol., 117:794–795, 1977.
13. Thackston, L.P., Price, N.C., and Richardson, A.G.: Use of antispasmodics in treatment of spastic ureteritis. J. Urol., 73:487–493, 1955.

Striations

14. Friedland, G.W., and Forsberg, L.: Striations of the renal pelvis in children. Clin. Radiol., 23:58–60, 1972.
15. Gwinn, J.L., and Barnes, G.R., Jr.: Striated ureters and renal pelvis. Am. J. Roentgenol., 91:666–668, 1964.
16. Kirks, D.R., Currarino, G., and Weinberg, A.G.: Transverse folds in the proximal ureter: A normal variant in infants. Am. J. Roentgenol., 130:463–464, 1978.
17. Poole, C.A., Ferris, A.J., Jr., and Haukohl, R.S.: Radiolucent folds in the upper urinary tract. Am. J. Roentgenol., 110:529–539, 1970.
18. Vezina, J.A., Leger, L.P., Raymond, O., et al.: Mucosal folds of upper urinary tract. J. Can, Assoc. Radiol., 14:10–19, 1963.

Strictures

19. Allen, T.D.: Congenital ureteral strictures. Birth Defects, 13:17–18, 1977.
20. Campbell, M.: The dilated ureter in children: Brief consideration of its cause, diagnosis and treatment. Am. J. Surg., 39438–451, 1938.
21. Campbell, M.F.: Urology, 2nd ed., pp. 895–1862, pp. 1681–1712. Philadelphia, W.B. Saunders, 1963.
22. Church, C.K.: Urinary stasis, with emphasis on stasis due to stricture of the ureter. J. Int. Coll. Surg., 30:46–54, 1958.
23. Coyle, J.K., and McDonald, D.F.: The relationship between repeated instrumentation and urinary tract infections. J. Urol., 98:260–262, 1967.

24. Hunner, G.L.: Ureteral stricture: Report of 100 cases. Bull. Hopkins Hosp., 29:1–15, 1918.
25. Hunner, G.L.: Ureteral stricture, an important etiologic factor in so-called essential hematurias. J.A.M.A., 79:1731–1739, 1922.
26. Hunner, G.L.: Ureteral strictures and chronic pyelitis in children. Am. J. Dis. Child., 34:603–623, 1927.
27. Hunner, G.L.: Ureteral stricture; its frequency and diagnosis. South. Med. J., 34:885–890, 1941.
28. Sargent, J.W.: Primary stricture of the ureter. J. Urol., 88:181–183, 1962.

Tuberculosis of Ureter

29. Barrie, H.J., Kerr, W.K., and Gale, G.L.: The incidence and pathogenesis of tuberculous strictures of the renal pyelus. J. Urol., 98:584–589, 1967.
30. Claridge, M.: Ureteric obstruction in tuberculosis. Br. J. Urol., 42:688–692, 1970.
31. Feldstein, M.S., Sullivan, M.J., and Banowsky, L.H.: Ureteral involvement in genitourinary tuberculosis: Review of 20 cases encountered over three years. Urology, 6:175–181, 1975.
32. Friedenberg, R.M., Ney, C., and Stachenfeld, R.A.: Roentgenographic manifestations of tuberculosis of ureter. J. Urol., 99:25–29, 1968.
33. Puigvert, A.: The ureter in renal tuberculosis. Br. J. Urol., 27:258–266, 1955.
34. Rees, R.W.M., and Hollands, F.G.: The ureter in renal tuberculosis. Br. J. Urol., 42:693–696, 1970.
35. Viollet, G.: The ureter of the urogenital tuberculotic. Vie. Med., 44:895–960, 1963.

Ureteritis Cystica

36. Hinman, F., Johnson, M., and McCorkle, J.: Pyelitis and ureteritis cystica. J. Urol., 35:173–189, 1936.
37. Joelson, J.J.: Pyelitis, ureteritis, and cystitic cystica: Report of a case showing urographic evidence of the lesion in the ureter and pelvis. Arch. Surg., 18:1570–1583, 1929.
38. Kamens, L.: Ureteritis cystica: Diagnosis by antegrade pyelography. Urology, 6:209–211, 1975.
39. Kindall, L.: Pyelitis cystica and ureteritis cystica. J. Urol., 24:645–659, 1933.
40. Knutsson, F.: The roentgen appearance in ureteritis cystica. Acta Radiol., 16:43–47, 1935.
41. Mahboubi, S., Duckett, J.N., and Spackman, T.J.: Ureteritis cystica after treatment of cyclophosphamide-induced hemorrhagic cystitis. Urology, 7:521–523, 1976.
42. Patch, F.S.: Pyelitis, ureteritis and cystitis cystica. N. Engl. J. Med., 220:980–987, 1939.
43. Wershub, L.P., Kirwin, T.J., and Biel, L.: Bilateral pyelitis cystica and ureteritis cystica. J. Int. Coll. Surg., 18:443–455, 1952.

Fistulas

Ureterocutaneous Fistula

44. Aubert, J., Roland, D., and Casamayou, J.: Uretero-cutaneous fistula following resection of the rectum. J. Urol. Nephrol., 82:100–106, 1976.

45. Fraser, R.A., and Leary, F.J.: Ureterocutaneous fistula following percutaneous renal biopsy. J. Urol., *109*:931–933, 1973.
46. Rohner, T.J.: Delayed ureteral fistula from high velocity missiles: Report of 3 cases. J. Urol., *105*:63–64, 1971.

Ureterolymphatic Fistula

47. Ehrlich, R.M., Hecht, H.G., and Veenema, R.J.: Chyluria following aorto-iliac bypass graft: A unique method of radiologic diagnosis and review of the literature. J. Urol., *107*:302–303, 1972.

Ureteroarterial Fistula

48. Cowen, R.: Uretero-arterial fistula. J. Urol., *73*:801–803, 1955.
49. Davidson, O.W., and Smith, R.P.: Uretero-arterial fistula. J. Urol., *42*:257–262, 1939.
50. Reiner, R.J., Conway, G.F., and Threlkeld, R.: Ureteroarterial fistula. J. Urol., *113*:24–25, 1975.
51. Rennick, J.M., Link, O.P., and Palmer, J.M.: Spontaneous rupture of an iliac artery aneurysm into a ureter: A case report and review of the literature. J. Urol., *116*:111–113, 1976.
52. Shultz, M.L., Ewing, D.D., and Lovett, V.F.: Fistula between iliac aneurysm and distal stump of ureter with hematuria: A case report. J. Urol., *112*:585–586, 1974.
53. Taylor, W.N., and Reinhart, H.L.: Mycotic aneurysm of common iliac artery with rupture into right ureter. J. Urol., *42*:21–26, 1939.
54. Whitmore, W.F., Jr.: Uretero-arterial fistula and ureterovaginal fistula: report of case. Urologia, *21*:184–188, 1954.

Ureterouterine Fistula

55. Galka, M., and Dlugopolski, S.: Uretero-uterine fistulas. Ginekol. Pol., *46*:989–994, 1975.
56. Barton, J.J., Grier, E.A., and Mutchnik, D.L.: Uretero-uterine fistula as a complication of elective abortion. Obstet. Gynecol., *52*:815–845, 1978.
57. Hardt, W., and Borgmann, V.: Uretero-uterine fistula after abortion. Z. Urol. Nephrol., *68*:761–764, 1975.

Ureteroperitoneal Fistula

58. Alleman, R., Cauduro, J.B., and Ramos, L.D.: Acute abdomen caused by spontaneous ureteroperitoneal fistula. Rev. Paul. Med., *61*:270–272, 1962.
59. Arduino, G.J.: Ureteroperitoneal fistula: Case report of a late bullet wound complication. J. Urol., *73*:890–994, 1955.
60. Bourdeau, G.V.: Urinary ascites secondary to ureteroperitoneal fistula. Urology, *4*:209–211, 1974.
61. Everett, H.S.: Ureteroperitoneal fistula with urinary ascites. J. Urol., *78*:585–591, 1957.
62. Hunner, G.L., and Everett, H.S.: Ureteroperitoneal fistula with urinary ascites and chronic peritonitis. J.A.M.A., *95*:327–333, 1930.
63. Hunner, G.L., and Everett, H.S.: Ureteroperitoneal fistula with urinary ascites: A second case. J. Urol., *28*:333–341, 1932.

Ureterovaginal Fistula

64. Brunschwig, A., and Frick, H.C.: Urinary tract fistulas following radical surgical treatment of carcinoma of the cervix. Am. J. Obstet. Gynecol., *72*:479–488, 1956.
65. Burch, J.C., Chalfont, R.L., and Johnson, J.W.: Technique for prevention of uretero-vaginal fistula following abdominal hysterectomy: Preservation of uterine blood supply. Ann. Surg., *161*:832–837, 1965.
66. Calame, R.J., and Nelson, J.H., Jr.: Ureterovaginal fistula as a complication of radical pelvic surgery. Arch. Surg., *94*:876–880, 1967.
67. Carter, R.G.: Ureterovaginal fistula. J. Urol., *71*:200–207, 1954.
68. Cid, L.: Ureterovaginal fistula: Report of a case with a fused kidney and double ureter cured by heminephrectomy. J. Urol., *86*:54–56, 1961.
69. Gitsch, E.: Prophylaxis of urologic and surgical complications resulting from radical operations for cervical carcinoma. Wien Klin. Wochenschr., *82*:579–582, 1970.
70. Green, T.H., Jr.: Ureteral suspension for prevention of ureteral complications following radical Wertheim hysterectomy. Obstet. Gynecol., *28*:1–11, 1966.
71. Gurevich, M.N.: On a case report contribution to the pathogenesis of ureteral vaginal fistula. Urologia. Moskva, *26*:60–61, 1961.
72. Higgins, C.C.: Ureteral injuries during surgery: A review of 87 cases. J.A.M.A., *199*:82–88, 1967.
73. Koyangi, T., Takamatsu, T., Kaneta, T., et al.: A spontaneous vesico-ectopic uretero-vaginal fistula in a girl. J. Urol., *118*:871–872, 1977.
74. Lee, R.A., and Symmonds, R.E.: Ureterovaginal fistula. Am. J. Obstet. Gynecol., *109*:1032–1035, 1971.
75. Macasaet, M.A., Lu, T., and Nelson, J.H., Jr.: Ureterovaginal fistula as a complication of radical pelvic surgery. Am. J. Obstet. Gynecol., *124*:757–760, 1976.
76. Meigs, J.V.: Surgical Treatment of Cancer of the Cervix, p. 149. New York, Grune & Stratton, 1954.
77. Nelson, J.H., Jr.: Atlas of Radical Pelvic Surgery. New York, Appleton-Century-Crofts, 1969.
78. Prosser, I., and Velati, G.: Acquired uretero-vaginal fistulas. Rass. Int. Clin. Ter., *42*:1159–1177, 1962.
79. Symmonds, R.E.: Morbidity and complications of radical hysterectomy and pelvic lymph node dissection. Am. J. Obstet. Gynecol., *91*:663–678, 1966.
80. Talbert, L.M., Palumbo, L., Shingleton, H., et al.: Urologic complication of radical hysterectomy for carcinoma of the cervix. South. Med. J., *58*:11–17, 1965.
81. Ten Cate, H.W., Emmett, J.L., and Pratt, J.H.: Unusual ureterovaginal fistula: Report of a case. J. Urol., *88*:477–479, 1962.
82. Tueter, K.J., and Mathison, W.: Uretero-vaginal fistula. Ann. Chir. Gynaecol., *65*:408–411, 1976.
83. Vianna, J.B.: Ureteral complications following Wertheim-Meigs operation for cancer of the cervix. Urol. Int., *19*:271–279, 1965.
84. Wallace, D.M.: Uretero-vaginal fistula. Br. J. Urol., *44*:617–622, 1972.

Ureteroileal Fistula

85. Appleyard, I., and Lloyd-Jones, W.: A case of complete uretero-ileal fistula. Br. J. Urol., *49*:494, 1977.

86. Blumgart, L.H., and Thakur, K.: Uretero-ileal fistula due to Crohn's disease. Brit. J. Surg., *58*:469–470, 1971.

87. Critchley, C.F.: A case of uretero-ileal fistula. Br. J. Surg., *54*:812–813, 1967.

88. Flaster, S.L., and Bush, I.M.: Ureteroileal fistula: Report of a case complicated by increased chloride reabsorption from the ildeal segment. J. Urol., *109*:589–591, 1973.

89. Goodwin, W.E., Winter, C.C., and Turner, R.D.: Fistula between bowel and urinary tract. J. Urol., *84*:95–105, 1960.

90. Haysom, A.H.: Case of spontaneous left ureterocolonic fistula associated with abscess in left loin and fecal fistula. Br. J. Surg., *43*:646–649, 1956.

91. Scott, W.P.: Uretero-ileal fistula. Br. J. Radiol., *38*:957–958, 1963.

92. Shiozaki, H., Takai, S., and Iwamota, T.: Idiopathic ureteroduodenal fistula. J. Urol., *113*:714–715, 1975.

93. Wilson, J.D., Emmett, J.L., and Pratt, J.H.: Uretero-ileal fistula: Report of a case. Mayo Clin. Proc., *42*:155–160, 1967.

Ureterocolic Fistula

94. Earlam, M.S.: Migration of a ureteric calculus to the bladder via a ureterocolic and a vesicocolic fistula. Aust. N.Z. J. Surg., *47*:519–520, 1977.

95. Haysom, A.H.: Case of spontaneous left ureterocolonic fistula associated with abscess in left loin and fecal fistula. Br. J. Surg., *43*:646–649, 1956.

96. Krishna, A.U., Dhar, N., Pletman, R.J., et al.: Spontaneous closure of ureterocolic fistula secondary to diverticulitis. J. Urol., *118*:476–477, 1977.

97. Sankaran, R., Chesley, A.E., and Khadilkar, M.C.: Ureterocolic fistula associated with Hodgkin's disease. Urology, *4*:450–453, 1974.

98. Simon, O., Yuval, E.: Chronic cecoureteral fistula following cystectomy and cutaneous ureterostomy: A case report. Eur. Urol., *3*:243–244, 1977.

99. Winter C.C.: Ureterocolic fistula. J. Urol., *108*:396–398, 1972.

100. Winter, C.C., Linderholm, B.E., and Shiraki, I.W.: Ureterocolic fistula. Am. J. Surg., *125*:338–342, 1973.

Ureteral Fistulas After Renal Transplantation

101. Malek, G.H., Mehling, D.T., Daduk, A.A., et al.: Urological complication of renal transplantation. J. Urol., *109*:173–176, 1973.

102. Schiff, M., Jr., McGuire, E.J., Weiss, R.M., et al.: Management of urinary fistulas after renal transplantation. J. Urol., *115*:251–256, 1976.

103. Starzl, T.E., Groth, C.G., Putnam, C.W., et al.: Urological complications in 216 human recipients of renal transplants. Ann. Surg., *172*:1-22, 1970.

Retroperitoneal Fibrosis

104. Abbott, D.L., Skinner, D.G., Yalowitz, P.A., et al.: Retroperitoneal fibrosis associated with abdominal aortic aneurysms: an approach to management. J. Urol., *109*:987–989, 1973.

105. Abrams, M.: Idiopathic retroperitoneal fibrosis. J. Urol., *90*:163–166, 1963.

106. Albarran, J.: Medecine operatoire des voies urinaires, 991 pp. Paris, Masson et Cie, 1909.

107. Aptekar, R.G., Mitchinson, M.J.: Retroperitoneal fibrosis in two patients previously exposed to LSD. Calif. Med., *113*:77–79, 1970.

108. Arger, P.H., Stolz, J.L., and Miller, W.T.: Retroperitoneal fibrosis: An analysis of the clinical spectrum and roentgenographic signs. Am. J. Roent. Rad. Ther. Nucl. Med., *119*:812–821, 1973.

109. Bartholomew, L.G., Cain, J.C., Woolner, L.B., et al.: Sclerosing cholangitis: its possible association with Riedel's struma and fibrous retroperitonitis: Report of two cases. N. Engl. J. Med., *296*:8–12, 1963.

110. Bianchine, J.R., and Friedman, A.P.: Metaolism of methysergide and retroperitoneal fibrosis. Arch. Intern. Med., *126*:252–254, 1970.

111. Brown, K.A., Staubitz, W.J., Oberkircher, O.J., et al.: A review of retroperitoneal fibrosis. J. Urol., *92*:323–330, 1964.

112. Buckberg, G.D., Dilley, R.B., and Longmire, W.P.: The protean manifestations of sclerosing fibrosis. Surg. Gynecol. Obstet., *123*:729–736, 1966.

113. Cerny, J.L., and Scott, T.: Non-idiopathic retroperitoneal hemorrhage. J. Urol., *105*:49–55, 1972.

114. Clouse, M.D., Fraley, E.E., and Litwin, S.: Lymphangiographic criteria for diagnosis of retroperitoneal fibrosis. Radiology, *83*:1–5, 1964.

115. Corriere, J.N., Jr., Mackie, J.A., and Murphy, J.J.: Retroperitoneal fibrosis presenting with large bowel symptoms: Report of two cases. J. Urol., *96*:161–166, 1966.

116. Friedel, W.E., Smith, T.R., and Herman, J.R.: Anuria caused by perianeurysmal retroperitoneal fibrosis. J. Urol., *110*:516–518, 1973.

117. Furlong, J.H., Jr., and Connerty, H.V.: Compression of the aorta and the ureters by a retroperitoneal inflammatory mass: Case report. Del. Med. J., *30*:63–67, 1958.

118. Gleeson, M.H., Taylor, S., and Dowling, R.H.: Multifocal fibrosclerosis. Proc. R. Soc. Med., *63*:1309–1311, 1970.

119. Goddard, J.W.: Granuloma, a characteristic "qualitative" change in focal anaphylactic inflammation. Am. J. Pathol., *23*:943–965, 1947.

120. Grabstald, H., and Kaufman, R.: Hydronephrosis secondary to ureteral obstruction by metastatic heart cancer. J. Urol., *102*:569–576, 1969.

121. Graham, J.R.: Cardiac and pulmonary fibrosis during methysergide therapy for headache. Am. J. Med. Sci., *254*:1–12, 1967.

122. Graham, J.R., Suby, H.I., Lecompte, P.R., et al.: Fibrotic disorders associated with methysergide therapy for headache. N. Engl. J. Med., *274*:359–368, 1966.

123. Guistra, P.E., Killoran, P.J., Opper, L., et al.: Abnormal excretory urogram and lymphangiogram in retroperitoneal panniculitis. Radiology, *106*:545–546, 1973.

124. Hache, L., Utz, D.C., and Woolner, L.B.: Idiopathic fibrous retroperitonitis. Surg. Gynecol. Obstet., *115*:737–744, 1962.

125. Hache, L., Woolner, L.B., and Bernatz, P.E.: Idiopathic fibrous mediastinitis. Am. J. Dis. Chest, *41*:9–25, 1962.

126. Hackett, E.: Idiopathic retroperitoneal fibrosis: A condition involving the ureters, the aorta, and the inferior vena cava. Br. J. Surg., *46*:3–9, 1958.

127. Hahn, R.D.: The use of lymphangiography for the diagnosis of idiopathic retroperitoneal fibrosis. Am. J. Obstet. Gynecol., *94*:539–542, 1966.

128. Halverstadt, D.B.: Problems in the use of urography and lymphangiography in the diagnosis of idiopathic retroperitoneal fibrosis. J. Urol., *99*:423–426, 1968.

129. Harlin, H.C., and Hamm, F.C.: Urologic disease resulting from nonspecific inflammatory conditions of the bowel. J. Urol., *68*:383–392, 1952.

130. Hewett, A.L., and Headstream, J.W.: Pericystitis plastica. J. Urol., *83*:103–107, 1960.

131. Hoffman, W.W., and Trippel, O.N.: Retroperitoneal fibrosis: Etiologic considerations. J. Urol., 86:222–231, 1961.

132. Jones, E.A., and Alexander, M.K.: Idiopathic retroperitoneal fibrosis associated with an arteritis. Am. Rheum. Dis., 25:356–360, 1966.

133. Kay, R.G.: Retroperitoneal vasculitis with perivascular fibrosis. Br. J. Urol., 35:284–291, 1963.

134. Kearney, G.P., Mahoney, E.M., Scrammas, F.D., et al.: Venacavography, corticosteroids and surgery in the management of idiopathic retroperitoneal fibrosis. J. Urol., 115:32–35, 1976.

135. Kerr, W.S., Jr., Suby, H.I., Vickery, A., et al.: Idiopathic retroperitoneal fibrosis: Clinical experience with 15 cases 1956–1967. J. Urol., 99:575–584, 1968.

136. Kittredge, R.D., and Nash, A.D.: The many facets of sclerosing fibrosis. Am. J. Roent., Rad. Ther., Nucl. Med., 122:288–298, 1974.

137. Koep, L., and Zuidema, G.D.: The clinical significance of retroperitoneal fibrosis. Surgery, 81:250–257, 1977.

138. Lalli, A.F.: Retroperitoneal fibrosis and unapparent obstructive uropathy. Radiology, 122:339–342, 1977.

139. Leffall, L.D., Jr., White, J.E., and Mann, M.: Retroperitoneal fibrosis: Two unusual cases. Arch. Surg., 89:1070–1076, 1964.

140. Lemmon, W.T., Jr., and Kiser, W.S.: Idiopathic retroperitoneal fibrosis: Diagnostic enigma: Report of a case simulating diabetes insipidus and a review of the literature. J. Urol., 96:658–667, 1966.

141. Lepor, H., and Walsh, P.C.: Idiopathic retroperitoneal fibrosis. J. Urol., 122:1–6, 1979.

142. Longley, J.R., Bush, J., and Brunsting, C.D.: Occult neoplasm causing syndrome of retroperitoneal fibrosis. Calif. Med., 103:279–282, 1965.

143. Margoles, J.S., and McQueeney, A.J.: Ormond's syndrome. Arch. Surg., 81:660–667, 1960.

144. Miller, J.M., Lapin, R.J., Meisel, H.J., et al.: Bilateral ureteral obstruction due to compression by chronic retroperitoneal inflammation. J. Urol., 68:447–451, 1952.

145. Mitchinson, M.J.: Systemic idiopathic fibrosis and systemic Weber-Christian disease. J. Clin. Pathol., 18:645–649, 1965.

146. Mitchinson, M.J.: The pathology of idiopathic retroperitoneal fibrosis. J. Clin. Pathol., 23:681–689, 1970.

147. Mitchinson, M.J., Bird, D.R.: Urinary leakage and retroperitoneal fibrosis. J. Urol., 105:56–58, 1971.

148. Morin, L.J., and Zuerner, R.T.: Retroperitoneal fibrosis and carcinoid tumor. J.A.M.A., 216:1647–1648, 1971.

149. Mulvaney, W.P.: Periureteritis obliterans: A retroperitoneal inflammatory disease. J. Urol., 79:410–417, 1958.

150. Nitz, G.L., Hewitt, C.B., Straffon, R.A., et al.: Retroperitoneal malignancy masquerading as benign retroperitoneal fibrosis. J. Urol., 103:46–49, 1970.

151. Ormond, J.K.: Bilateral ureteral obstruction due to envelopment and compression by an inflammatory retroperitoneal process. J. Urol., 59:1072–1079, 1948.

152. Ormond, J.K.: Idiopathic retroperitoneal fibrosis: An established clinical entity. J.A.M.A., 174:1561–1568, 1960.

153. Ormond, J.K.: Idiopathic retroperitoneal fibrosis: A discussion of the etiology. J. Urol., 94:385–390, 1965.

154. Pallette, E.M., Pallette, E.C., and Harrington, R.W.: Sclerosing lipogranulomatosis the reversal abdomen. Arch. Surg., 94:803–810, 1967.

155. Paull, D.P., Causey, J.C., and Hodges, C.V.: Perinephritis plastica. J. Urol., 73:212–216, 1955.

156. Pophan, B.I., and Stevenson, T.D.: Idiopathic retroperitoneal fibrosis associated with a coagulation defect (factor VII deficiency): Report of a case and review of the literature. Ann. Intern. Med., 52:894–906, 1960.

157. Raper, F.P.: Idiopathic retroperitoneal fibrosis involving the ureters. Br. J. Urol., 28:436–446, 1956.

158. Raper, F.P.: Bilateral symmetrical periureteric fibrosis. Proc. R. Soc. Med., 48:736–740, 1955.

159. Reidbord, H.E., and Hawk, W.A.: Idiopathic retroperitoneal fibrosis and necrotizing vasculitis: Report of a case, with autopsy findings and etiologic consideration. Cleve. Clin. Q., 32:19–27, 1965.

160. Robertson, J.A.: Retroperitoneal fibrosis. Urol., 3:741–746, 1974.

161. Ross, J.C., and Goldsmith, H.J.: The combined surgical and medical treatment of retroperitoneal fibrosis. Br. J. Surg., 58:422–427, 1971.

162. Salmon, H.W.: Combined mediastinal and retroperitoneal fibrosis. Thorax, 23:158–164, 1968.

163. Sanders, R.C., Duffy, T., McLoughlin, M.G., et al.: Sonography in the diagnosis of retroperitoneal fibrosis. J. Urol., 118:944–946, 1977.

164. Saxton, H.M., Kilpatrick, F.R., Kinder, C.H., et al.: Retroperitoneal fibrosis: A radiological and follow-up study of fourteen cases. Q. J. Med., 38:59–81, 1969.

165. Schneider, C.F.: Idiopathic retroperitoneal fibrosis producing vena caval, biliary, ureteral and duodenal obstructions. Ann. Surg., 159:316–320, 1964.

166. Scully, R.E., Galdabini, J.J., and McNeely, B.U.: Case records of the Massachusetts General Hospital. N. Engl. J. Med., 293:1034–1039, 1975.

167. Skeel, D.A., Shols, D.W., Sullivan, M.J., et al.: Retroperitoneal fibrosis with intrinsic ureteral involvement. J. Urol., 113:166–169, 1975.

168. Stecker, J.F., Jr., Rawls, H.P., Devine, C.J., Jr., et al.: Retroperitoneal fibrosis and ergot derivatives. J. Urol., 112:30–32, 1974.

169. Suby, H.I., Kerr, W.S., Jr., Graham, J.R., et al.: Retroperitoneal fibrosis: A missing link in the chain. J. Urol., 93:144–152, 1965.

170. Thomas, M.H., Chisholm, G.D.: Retroperitoneal fibrosis associated with malignant disease. Br. J. Cancer, 28:453–458, 1973.

171. Trevor, R.N.: Reticulum-cell sarcoma producing retroperitoneal and periureteric fibrosis: Report of a case. N. Engl. J. Med., 258:268–270, 1958.

172. Usher, S.M., Brendler, H., and Ciavarra, V.A.: Retroperitoneal fibrosis secondary to metastatic neoplasm. Urology, 9:191–194, 1977.

173. Utz, D.C., and Henry, J.D.: Retroperitoneal fibrosis. Med. Clin. North Am., 50:1091–1099, 1966.

174. Utz, D.C., Rooke, E.D., Spittell, J.A., Jr., et al.: Retroperitoneal fibrosis in patients taking methysergide. J.A.M.A., 191:983–985, 1965.

175. Virtama, P., and Helela, T.: Lymphography and cavography in retroperitoneal fibrosis. Br. J. Radiol., 40:231–232, 1967.

176. Wagenknecht, L.V., and Auvert, J.: Symptoms and diagnosis of retroperitoneal fibrosis. Analysis of 31 cases. Urol. Int., 26:185–195, 1971.

177. Wagenknecht, L.V., and Madsen, P.O.: Bilateral ureteral obstruction secondary to aortic aneurysm. J. Urol., 103:732–736, 1970.

178. Webb, A.J.: Cytological studies in retroperitoneal fibrosis. Br. J. Surg., 54:375–378, 1967.

179. Webb, A.J., and Dawson-Edwards, P.: Non-malignant retroperitoneal fibrosis. Br. J. Surg., 54:508–518, 1967.

180. Weigel, J.W.: Unusual aspects of retroperitoneal fibrosis.

Abstr. Proc. Kimbrough Urological Seminar, Vol. *X, 23rd Meeting, Tacoma, 5–9 October 1975.

Periureteral Fibrosis

181. Hejtmancik, J.H., and Magid, M.A.: Bilateral periureteritis plastica. J. Urol., 76:57–61, 1956.
182. Houston, W.: Periureteritis plastica: Report of case with indication of probable pathology. Br. J. Urol., 29:38–41, 1957.
183. MacDonald, S.A., and deDomenico, I.J.: Periureteral fibrosis. Can. J. Surg., 1:162–166, 1958.
184. Millard, D.G., and Wyman, S.M.: Periureteric fibrosis: Radiographic diagnosis. Radiology, 72:191–196, 1959.
185. Mulvaney, W.P.: Periureteritis obliterans: A retroperitoneal inflammatory disease. J. Urol., 79:410–417, 1958.
186. Oppenheimer, G.D., and Goldman, H.: Periureteral fibrosis: An unusual complication of renal biopsy. J. Urol., 88:611–615, 1962.
187. Park, H., and Jones, I.: Periureteric fibrosis. Lancet, 1:195–196, 1958.
188. Passaro, E.P., Rose, R.S., and Taylor, J.N.: Periureteritis fibrosis: Review of literature and presentation of two cases. J. Urol., 85:506–511, 1961.
189. Ross, J.: Periureteral fibrosa, with note on 3 cases. J. Fac. Radiologist, 9:142–146, 1958.
190. Trabucco, A., and Marquez, F.J.: Ureteritis plastica as a sequel of periappendicular abscess. Rev. Argent. Urol., 19:214–216, 1950.
191. Twigg, H.L., Jr.: Periureteral fibrosis. Am. J. Roentgenol., 84:876–885, 1960.
192. Vest, S.A., and Barelare, B., Jr.: Periureteritis plastica: Report of 4 cases. J. Urol., 70:38–50, 1953.

Pelvic Lipomatosis

193. Abbott, D.A., and Skinner, D.G.: Congenital venous anomalies associated with pelvic lipomatosis (a case report). J. Urol., 112:739–742, 1974.
194. Ambos, M.A., Bosniak, M.A., Lafleur, R.S., et al.: The pear-shaped bladder. Radiology, 122:85–88, 1977.
195. Amoe, H.E., Jr., and Lewis, R.E.: Urographic and barium enema appearance in inferior vena cava obstruction. Radiology, 108:307–308, 1973.
196. Barry, J.M., Bilbao, M.K., and Hodges, C.V.: Pelvic lipomatosis: A rare cause of suprapublic mass. J. Urol., 109:592–594, 1973.
197. Becker, J.A., Weiss, R.M., Schiff, M., Jr., and Lytton, B.: Pelvic lipomatosis: A consideration in the diagnosis of intrapelvic neoplasms. Arch. Surg., 100:94–96, 1970.
198. Bender, L., and Kass, M.: Periureteral lipomatosis: Case report. J. Urol., 103:293–295, 1970.
199. Blau, J.S., and Janson, K.L.: Pelvic lipomatosis: Consideration of the urinary tract complications. Arch. Surg., 105:498–500, 1972.
200. Carpenter, A.A.: Pelvic lipomatosis: successful surgical treatment. J. Urol., 110:397–399, 1973.
201. Engels, E.P.: Sigmoid colon and urinary bladder in high fixation: roentgen changes simulating pelvic tumor. Radiology, 72:419–422, 1959.
202. Flaherty, J.J., Kelley, R., Burnett, B., et al.: Relativity of pelvic bone fracture patterns to injury of the urethra and bladder. J. Urol., 99:297–300, 1965.
203. Fogg, L.B., and Smyth, J.W.: Pelvic lipomatosis: A condition simulating pelvic neoplasm. Radiology, 90:558–564, 1968.

204. Gellhorn, A., and Marks, P.A.: The composition and biosynthesis of lipid in human adipose tissue. J. Clin. Invest., 40:925–932, 1961.
205. Golding, P.L., Singh, M., and Worthington, B.: Bilateral ureteral obstruction caused by benign pelvic lipomatosis. Br. J. Surg., 59:69–72, 1972.
206. Goldstein, H.M., and Vargas, C.A.: Pelvic lipomatosis in females. J. Can. Assoc. Radiol., 25:65–68, 1974.
207. Grimmett, G.M., Hall, M.G., Jr., Aird, C.C., and Kurtz, L.H.: Pelvic lipomatosis. Am. J. Surg., 125:347–349, 1973.
208. Hall, R., and Jenkins, J.D.: Intravenous pyelography in acute idiopathic vena cava thrombosis. Br. J. Radiol., 43:781–786, 1970.
209. Harrow, B.R.: Retroperitoneal fibrosis following sclerosing injection for inguinal hernia and hemorrhoids. Am. J. Roentgenol., 99:90–95, 1967.
210. Hewett, A.L., and Headstream, J.W.: Pericystitis plastica. J. Urol., 83:103–107, 1960.
211. Leuzinger, D.E., Bahr, R.D., Miller, C.D., and Shipman, G.A.: Case report of high fixation of bladder and sigmoid colon. J. Urol., 85:163–165, 1961.
212. Long, W.W., Jr., Kellett, J.W., Gardner, W.A., and Lynch, K.M., Jr.: Perivesical lipomatosis. J. Urol., 109:238–241, 1973.
213. Lucey, D.T., and Smith, M.J.V.: Pelvic lipomatosis. J. Urol., 105:341–345, 1971.
219. Mahlin, M.S., and Dovitz, B.W.: Perivesical lipomatosis. J. Urol., 100:720–722, 1968.
215. Malter, I.J., and Omell, G.H.: Pelvic lipomatosis in a woman: A case report. Obstet. Gynecol., 37:63–66, 1971.
216. Missal, M.E., Robinson, J.H., and Tatum, R.W.: Inferior vena cava obstruction: clinical manifestations, diagnostic methods, and related problems. Ann. Intern. Med., 62:133–161, 1965.
217. Morretin, L.B., and Wilson, M.: Pelvic lipomatosis. Am. J. Roentgenol., 113:181–184, 1971.
218. Moss, A.A., Clark, R.E., Goldberg, H.I., and Pepper, H.W.: Pelvic lipomatosis: A roentgenographic diagnosis. Am. J. Roentgenol., 115:411–419, 1972.
219. Nussbaum, P.S.: Carcinoma of the prostate presenting as pelvic lipomatosis. Surg. Clin. North Am., 52:405–414, 1972.
220. O'Dea, M.J., and Malek, R.S.: Foreign body in bladder and perivesicular inflammation masquerading as pelvic lipomatosis. J. Urol., 116:669–670, 1976.
221. Pepper, H.W., Clement, A.R., and Drew, J.E.: Pelvic lipomatosis causing urinary obstruction. Br. J. Radiol., 44:313–315, 1971.
222. Puckette, S.E., Jr.: X-ray films of the month. J. Can. Med. Assoc., 66:248, 1970.
223. Radinsky, S., Cabal, E., and Shields, J.: Pelvic lipomatosis. Urol., 7:108–111, 1976.
224. Rosenberg, B., Hurwitz, A., and Hermann, H.: Dercum's disease with unusual retroperitoneal and paravesical fatty infiltration. Surgery, 54:451–455, 1963.
225. Sacks, S.A., and Drenick, E.J.: Pelvic lipomatosis: Effect of diet. Urology 5:609–615, 1975.
226. Schechter, L.S.: Venous obstruction in pelvic lipomatosis. J. Urol., 111:757–759, 1974.
227. Steinberg, A., Madayag, M., Bosniak, M.A., et al.: Demonstration of two unusually large pelvic lymphcysts by lymphography. J. Urol., 109:477–478, 1973.
228. Yalla, S.V., Ivker, M., Burros, H.M., and Dorey, F.: Cystitis glandularis with perivesical lipomatosis: frequent association of two unusual proliferative conditions. Urology, 5:383–386, 1975.

Schistosomiasis of the Ureter

229. Fagerstrom, D.P.: 1958, quoted in Herbut, P.A.: Urological Pathology, Vol. 1, p. 394. London, Kimpton, 1952.
230. Fairley, N.H.: Egyptian bilharziosis: Its recent pathological symptomatology and treatment. Proc. Roy. Soc. Med., 13:1–18, 1919.
231. Fam, A.: The problem of the bilharzial ureter. Br. J. Urol., 36:211–219, 1964.
232. Gelfand, M.: Bilharzial affection of ureter, study of 110 consecutive necropsies showing vesical bilharziosis. Br. Med. J., 1:1228–1230, 1948.
233. Ghorab, M.M.A.: Ureteritis calcinosa, a complication of bilharzial ureteritis and its relation to primary ureteric stone formation. Br. J. Urol., 34:33–43, 1962.
234. Honey, R.M., and Gelford, M.: The urological aspects of bilharziasis in Rhodesia. Cent. Afr. J. Med., 6:1–51, 58–61, 109–111, 153–155, 199–212, 248–259, 1960.
235. Ibrahim, A.B.: Bilharziasis of ureter. Lancet, 2:1184–1186, 1923.
236. James, W.B.: Urological manifestations in Schistosoma haematobium infestation. Br. J. Radiol., 36:40–45, 1963.
237. Maden, F.C.: The Surgery of Egypt. Cairo, Nile Misc., 1919.
238. Makar, N.: The bilharzial ureter: Some observations on the surgical pathology and surgical treatment. Br. J. Surg., 36:148–155, 1948.
239. Payer, J., and Skutil, V.: Urological schistosomiasis. Cas. Lek. Cesk., 102:403–404, 1963.
240. Saad, S.A., and Hanafy, H.M.: Bilharzial (schistosomal) urethritis cystica. Urol., 6:261–266, 1974.
241. Tarabulcy, E.Z.: The radiographic aspect of urogenital schistosomiasis. J. Urol., 90:470–475, 1963.
242. Tardos, R.: Radiologic study of the ureteral and renal lesions of urinary bilharziosis. J. Radiol. Electr. Med. Nucl., 44:187–190, 1963.
243. Young, S.W., Khalid, K.H., Farid, Z., et al.: Urinary tract lesions of Schistosoma haematobium. Radiology, 111:81–84, 1974.

Endometriosis of the Ureter

244. Abdel-Shahid, R.B., Beresford, J.M., and Curry, R.H.: Endometriosis of the ureter with vascular involvement. Obst. Gynecol., 43:113–117, 1974.
245. Bates, J.S., and Beecham, C.T.: Retroperitoneal endometriosis with ureteral obstruction. Obstet. Gynecol., 34:242–248, 1963.
246. Beahrs, O.H., Hunter, J.S., Jr., and Sloss, P.T.: Intramural obstructing endometriosis of the ureter. Mayo Clin. Proc., 67:73–77, 1957.
247. Beecham, C.T., and McCrea, L.E.: Endometriosis of the urinary tract. Urol. Surv., 7:2–24, 1957.
248. Berlin, L., Waldman, I., White, F.H., et al.: Endometriosis of the ureter. Am. J. Roentgenol., 92, No. 2:351–353, 1964.
249. Brock, D.R.: Ureteral obstruction from endometriosis. J. Urol., 83:100–102, 1960.
250. Bulkley, G.J., Carrow, L.A., and Estensen, R.D.: Endometriosis of the ureter. J. Urol., 93:139–143, 1965.
251. Chinn, J., Horton, R.K., and Rusche, C.: Unilateral ureteral obstruction as sole manifestation of endometriosis. J. Urol., 77:144–150, 1957.
252. Colby, F.H.: Massachusetts General Hospital case records, Case 46322. N. Engl. J. Med., 263:303–306, 1960.
253. deLorimier, A.A., Moehring, H.G., and Hannan, J.R.: Clinical Roentgenology, p. 355. Springfield, Ill., Thomas, 1956.

254. Fujita, K.: Endometriosis of the ureter. J. Urol., 116:664, 1976.
255. Grayburn, R.W.: Ureteric obstruction due to endometriosis. J. Obstet. Gynaec. Br. Emp., 67:74–75, 1960.
256. Lichtenheld, F.R., McCauley, R.T., and Staples, P.P.: Endometriosis involving urinary tract; a collective review. Obstet. Gynecol. Ann., 17:762–768, 1961.
257. Mazzola, V.P., Mazzola, N.J., Mitchell, F.V., et al.: Extraperitoneal pelvic tumors following total hysterectomy. J. Int. Coll. Surg., 24:689–696, 1955.
258. Meyer, E.G.: Unilateral ureteral obstruction due to endometriosis. Can. J. Surg., 3:171–175, 1960.
259. Navratil, E.: Ureteral obstruction due to extensive pelvic endometriosis. Wien. Klin. Wchnschr., 58:661–666, 1946.
260. O'Conor, V.J., and Greenhill, J.P.: Endometriosis of bladder and ureter. Surg. Gynecol. Obstet., 80:113–119, 1945.
261. Ostenfeld, J.: Endometriosis of the ureter. Nord. Med., 41:227, 1949.
262. Randall, A.: Endometrioma of the bladder and ureter. J. Urol., 46:419–422, 1941.
263. Ratliff, R.K., and Crenshaw, W.B.: Ureteral obstruction from endometriosis. Surg. Gynecol. Obstet., 100:414–418, 1955.
264. Reddy, A., and Evans, A.T.: Endometriosis of the ureter. J. Urol., 111:474–480, 1974.
265. Simon, H.B., Zimet, R.R., Schneider, E., et al.: Bilateral ureteral obstruction due to endometriosis. J.A.M.A., 183:487–489, 1963.
266. Stanley, K.E., Jr., Utz, D.C., and Dockerty, M.B.: Clinically significant endometriosis of the urinary tract. Surg. Gynecol. Obstet., 120:491–498, 1965.
267. Stiehm, W.D., Becker, J.A., and Weiss, R.M.: Ureteral endometriosis. Radiology, 102:563–564, 1972.
268. Yates-Bell, A.J., Molland, E.A., and Pryor, J.P.: Endometriosis of the ureter. Br. J. Urol., 44:58–67, 1972.

Leukoplakia of the Ureter

269. Falk, C.C.: Leukoplakia of renal pelvis and ureter. J. Urol., 72:310–315, 1954.
270. Kretschmer, H.L.: Leukoplakia of bladder and ureter. Surg. Gynecol. Obstet., 31:325–327, 1920.
271. Laughlin, V.C., and Bilotta, J.F.L.: Leukoplakia of urinary tract: Report of unusual case of leukoplakia of ureter. J. Urol., 44:358–366, 1940.
272. Patch, F.S.: The association between leukoplakia and squamous cell carcinoma in the upper urinary tract. N. Engl. J. Med., 200:423–436, 1929.
273. Politano, V.A.: Leukoplakia of renal pelvis and ureter. J. Urol., 75:633–642, 1956.
274. Taylor, W.N.: Leukoplakia of the kidney pelvis and ureter. Am. J. Surg., 32:335–342, 1936.
275. Torres, L.F., Jr., and Recio, P.M.: Ureteral leukoplakia: Review of literature with case report (successful resection of ureter with reimplantation into urinary bladder). J. Philipp. Med. Assoc., 23:153, 1947.
276. Wilson, C.L., and Wilson, M.C.: Leukoplakia of the ureter. Trans. Southeast. Sect. Am. Urol. Assoc., pp. 23–27, Oct. 1955.

Malacoplakia of Ureter

277. Gibson, T.E., Bareta, J., and Lake, G.C.: Malakoplakia: Report of a case involving the bladder and one kidney and ureter. Urol. Int., 1:5–14, 1955.
278. Lewis, J.E., Vieralves, G., Landes, R.R., et al.: Malakoplakia

of the renal pelvis, calyces and upper ureter: Case report. J. Urol., 85:243–245, 1961.

279. Schneiderman, C., and Simon, M.A.: Malacoplakia of the urinary tract. J. Urol., 100:694–698, 1968.

280. Scott, E., Van, Z., and Scott, W.F., Jr.: A fatal case of malakoplakia of the urinary tract. J. Urol., 79:52–56, 1958.

281. Scullin, D.R., and Hardy, R.: Malacoplakia of the urinary tract with spread to the abdominal wall. J. Urol., 107:908–910, 1972.

282. Sunshine, B.: Malacoplakia of the upper urinary tract. J. Urol., 112:362–363, 1974.

283. Terner, J.Y., and Lattes, R.: Malakoplakia of colon and retroperitoneum: Report of a case with a histochemical study of the Michaelis-Gutmann inclusion bodies. Am. J. Clin. Pathol., 44:20–31, 1965.

Amyloidosis of the Ureter

284. Andreas, B.F., and Oosting, M.: Primary amyloidosis of the ureter. J. Urol., 79:929–931, 1958.

285. DeRosena, R., Koss, M.N., and Pirani, C.: Demonstration of amyloid fibril in urinary sediment. N. Engl. J. Med., 293:1131–1133, 1975.

286. Forssell, A., and Isaksson, B.: Nephroangiography in amyloidosis. Acta Radiol. (Diagn.) (Stockh.), 17:797–804, 1976.

287. Gilbert, L.W., and McDonald, J.R.: Primary amyloidosis of renal pelvis and ureter: Report of a case. J. Urol., 58:137–139, 1952.

288. Higbee, D.R., and Millett, W.D.: Localized amyloidosis of the ureter: Report of a case. J. Urol., 75:424–427, 1956.

289. Johnson, H.W., and Ankenman, G.J.: Bilateral ureteral primary amyloidosis. J. Urol., 92:275–277, 1964.

290. Klotz, P.G.: Primary amyloidosis of ureter: Case report. Br. J. Urol., 47:518, 1975.

291. Kyle, R.A., and Bayrd, E.D.: Amyloidosis: Review of 236 cases. Medicine, 54:271–299, 1975.

292. Lee, K.T., and Deeths, T.M.: Localized amyloidosis of ureter. Radiology, 120:60, 1976.

293. Linke, R.P.: Urinary amyloid fibrils in the absence of amyloidosis (letter). Br. Med. J., 2:1259, 1976.

294. Magri, J., and Atkinson, E.A.: Primary amyloidosis of the ureter. Br. J. Urol., 42:37–42, 1970.

295. Neale, T.J.: Amyloid fibrils in urinary sediment (letter). N. Engl. J. Med., 294:444–445, 1976.

296. Takaha, M., Nagata, H., and Sonoda, T.: Localized amyloid tumor of the ureter: Report of a case. J. Urol., 105:502–503, 1971.

297. Yalowitz, P.A., and Kelalis, P.P.: Primary amyloidosis of ureter: Report of case. J. Urol., 96:668–670, 1966.

Polyarteritis Nodosa

298. Fisher, R.S., and Howard, H.H.: Unusual ureterograms in a case of periarteritis nodosa. J. Urol., 60:308–404, 1948.

299. Samellas, W., Bellonias, E., and Papacharalampous, N.: Polyarteritis nodosa: Ureteral involvement. J. Urol., 105:186–187, 1971.

Notching of the Ureter

300. Chait, A., Matagar, K.W., Fabian, C.B., et al.: Vascular impression on the ureters. Am. J. Roentgenol., 111:729–749, 1971.

301. Cleveland, R.H., Fellows, K.E., and Lebowitz, R.L.: Notching of the ureter and pelves in children. Am. J. Roentgenol., 129:837–844, 1977.

302. Eisen, S., Friedenberg, M.J., and Klahr, S.: Bilateral ureteral notching and selective renal phlebography in the nephrotic syndrome due to renal vein thrombosis. J. Urol., 93:343–346, 1965.

303. Friedenberg, R.M., and Bergman, H.: Vascular notching of the ureter. N.Y. State J. Med., 70:1211–1212, 1976.

304. Gray, S.R., Carrington, C.B., and Cornog, J.L.: Lymphangiomyomatosis: Report of a case with ureteral involvement and chyluria. Cancer, 35:490–498, 1975.

305. Halpern, M., and Evans, J.A.: Coarctation of the renal artery with "notching" of the ureter: A roentgenologic sign of unilateral renal disease as a cause of hypertension. Am. J. Roentgenol., 88:159–164, 1962.

306. Love, L., and Bush, I.M.: Early demonstration of renal collateral arterial supply. Am. J. Roentgenol., 104:296–301, 1962.

307. Norfray, J.F., and Nudelman, E.J.: Visceral collateral arterial circulation: Another cause of ureteral notching. J. Urol., 112:172–173, 1974.

308. Taylor, D.A., and Boyes, T.D.: Filling of a varicose left ovarian vein following retrograde pyelography: A new cause of notching of the ureter. Br. J. Radiol., 37:625–627, 1964.

309. Thomas, R.G., and Levin, N.W.: Ureteric irregularity with renal artery obstruction: A new radiological sign. Br. J. Radiol., 34:438–440, 1961.

310. Woodward, J.R.: Vascular imprints of the upper ureter. J. Urol., 87:666–668, 1962.

Ovarian Vein

311. Bellina, J.H.: Ovarian vein syndrome. J. Abdom. Surg., 15:21–25, 1973.

312. Bucker, J., and Sildiroglu, A.I.: Ureterobstrucktion durch die Vena ovarian im Gefolgen einer Schivwangerschaft. Fortschr. Roentgenstr., 116:357–363, 1972.

313. Clark, J.C.: The right ovarian vein syndrome. In Witten, D.M., Myers, C.H., Jr., and Utz, D.C. (eds.): Emmett's Clinical Urography, 4th ed., pp. 2149–2155. Philadelphia, W.B. Saunders, 1977.

314. DeBruin, T.R., and Udding, H.: Linea innominata syndroom. Ned. Tijdschr Geneeskol., 111:2011–2020, 1967.

315. Derrick, F.C., Jr., Rosenblum, R., and Frensilli, F.J.: Right ovarian vein syndrome: Six-year critique. Urology, 1:383–385, 1973.

316. Derrick, F.C., Jr., Rosenblum, R.R., and Lynch, R.M., Jr.: Pathological association of the right ureter and right ovarian vein. J. Urol., 97:633–640, 1967.

317. Dykhuizen, R.F.: Right ureteral obstruction related to ovarian vein varicosities. J. Am. Operating Room Nurses, 51–54, 1967.

318. Dykhuizen, R.F., and Roberts, J.A.: The ovarian vein syndrome. Surg. Gynec. Obstet., 130:443–452, 1970.

319. Hubmer, G.: The ovarian vein syndrome. Eur. Urol., 4:263–268, 1978.

320. Mackler, M.A., and Royster, H.P.: Right ovarian vein thrombophlebitis and ovarian arteritis. J. Urol., 100:683–686, 1968.

321. Melnick, G.S., and Bramwit, D.N.: Bilateral ovarian vein syndrome. Am. J. Roentgenol., 113:509–519, 1971.

322. Pereira, R.M., Ferreira, A.A., and Lane, E.: Diagnosis of the right ovarian vein syndrome. Am. J. Obstet. Gynecol., 103:888–890, 1969.

Ureteral injury relates mainly to instrumental and surgical procedures, primarily pelvic surgery performed for carcinoma of the gynecologic organs.

Injury of the upper ureter is usually secondary to instrumentation or penetration injuries. Traumatic closed rupture of the ureter from external trauma is rare, since the ureters are well protected throughout their entire course. Acute hyperextension of the spine or acute lateral flexion of the trunk (compressing the contralateral kidney against the twelfth rib or upper lumbar transverse process) may produce tearing or avulsion of the ureter near the ureteropelvic junction.

Trauma to the lower ureter is usually secondary to instrumentation or surgical intervention, and it most commonly occurs where the ureter crosses the common iliac vessels or where it enters the bladder.

COMPLICATIONS

The major complications of ureteral trauma include (1) complete ureteral obstruction leading to loss of renal function unilaterally or bilaterally; (2) ureteral stricture leading to hydronephrosis; (3) abscess formation, frequently with a sinus tract to the skin; (4) pseudocyst from extravasation of urine; and (5) fistula formation, primarily ureterovaginal and ureterocutaneous.

CLASSIFICATION

The following classification outlines the major causes of ureteral trauma:

I. Surgical
   A. Direct injury: cutting, tying, kinking, or clamping of the ureter. This may occur in any type of gynecologic, abdominal, or genitourinary surgery (Figs. 20–1 to 20–3, 20–6, 20–8 to 20–14).

20

Trauma to the Ureter

B. Indirect injury: This refers to postsurgical adhesions or inflammatory lesions that involve the ureter, producing obstructive phenomena. Loss of blood supply causes stricture and necrosis. Indirect injury may occur secondary to delivery or use of a pessary (Figs. 20-4, 20-5).

II. Instrumentation
    A. Perforation by catheter (Figs. 20-15 to 20-18, 20-20 to 20-26)
    B. Rupture from pressure of injection distal to an obstruction, usually occurring in a diseased ureter (Fig. 20-19)

III. External trauma
    A. Penetrating wounds, such as stab wounds or bullet wounds (Figs. 20-7, 20-28 to 20-32)
    B. Major external trauma to the abdomen without penetration (acute hyperextension or lateral flexion (Figs. 20-33, 20-34)

IV. Radium or radiotherapy
    A. Usually later stricture following radiotherapy for carcinoma of the cervix (Fig. 20-40)

V. Foreign body
    A. Broken pieces of catheter, such as basket or loop catheters, are the most common foreign bodies (Figs. 20-35 to 20-39).
    B. Wires, bullet, and so forth, also have been reported within the ureteral lumen.

SURGICAL TRAUMA

In any surgical procedure in which there is a reasonably high potential for ureteral damage (extensive pelvic surgery), a urogram should be performed prior to surgery to evaluate the function of the kidneys and ureters and to exclude significant congenital variations in the course or caliber of the ureters.

It is difficult to assess the amount of ureteral injury, since routine pre- and postoperative urograms are not obtained, and unilateral injury without fistula formation is frequently asymptomatic and unrecognized. Higgins in 1967 reported on 87 patients with ureteral injury secondary to surgery.[20] Women accounted for 80 per cent of the injuries, relating to the high incidence of injury in gynecologic procedures. Approximately 10 per cent were bilateral. It has been estimated that ureteral injuries occur in as many as 2 per cent of patients undergoing hysterectomy for benign conditions and three or four times this number in patients with malignant disease.[36] During surgery one or both ureters may be sectioned, causing the formation of a local abscess and/or nonfunction of the involved kidney. If anuria is present for 8 to 10 hours after major pelvic surgery, the possibility of bilateral ureteral injury must be suspected. Cutting or ligating the ureters usually produces prompt symptoms. Kinking, crushing, or clamping of the vascular supply to the ureters may not produce evidence of injury until several weeks after surgery, when necrosis of the ureteral wall may occur (Figs. 20-4, 20-5). The most common complication in such cases is ureterovaginal or ureterocutaneous fistula. Ureteroenteric fistulas are rare. In such cases the sooner the fistula is corrected, the better are the functional results (Figs. 20-1 to 20-14).

Bilateral ureteral injury producing anuria is extremely serious but is usually recognized shortly after surgery. Unilateral injury that does not produce anuria may not be recognized. In any instance in which injury is suspected, a urogram should be performed. If ureteral injury has occurred, prompt drainage must be instituted. Repair of the injured ureter can be delayed until the patient's clinical condition permits.

INSTRUMENTAL TRAUMA

Retrograde pyelography is the single most common cause of traumatic perforation of the ureter. Fortunately, with the decreased use of retrograde catheterization, instrumental injuries are now less common. It occurs most often in diseased ureters or distal to a stricture or stone. In a normal ureter perforation is most common at the ureterovesical junction. The use of specialized catheters such as stone extractors, bulb catheters, and the like leads to perforation more commonly than the use of routine ureteral catheters (Figs. 20-15 to 20-25).

In most instances of catheter rupture spontaneous healing occurs within 1 or 2 weeks without surgical intervention and without ureteral splinting. This is similar to the extravasation seen at the site of anastomosis following ureteral lithotomy. The ureter heals spontaneously in 1 or 2 weeks, provided that there is no obstruction to the passage of urine down the ureter (Fig. 20-15).

Occasionally, kinking or pseudodiverticula may occur at the site of perforation (see Figs. 22-1 to 22-3, Chap. 22). Ureteral perforation may not heal when a distal ureteral obstruction is present, because of the increased proximal luminal pressure. Continuous extravasation may lead to the formation of a ureteral pseudocyst communicating with the ureter and often containing large volumes of urine (Figs. 20-42 to 20-45).

At the ureterovesical junction three types of perforation with extravasation are observed. The first type is perforation of the ureter proximal to its entrance into the bladder, with retroperitoneal and occasionally subserosal extravasation. The remaining two types occur in the short intravesical segment of ureter, and they consist of intramural and submucosal extravasation. Examples illustrating the typical roentgenographic appearance of the usual retroperitoneal extravasation as compared with the intramural and the submucosal extravasations are included (Figs. 20–21 to 20–25).

In dilated ureters or hydronephrotic kidneys, kinking or knotting of the ureteral catheters occasionally occurs, which makes it difficult or even impossible to withdraw the retrograde catheters (Fig. 20–26).

EXTERNAL TRAUMA

As previously stated, the ureters are well protected throughout their course. Lying deep in the retroperitoneal area adjacent to the lumbar spine, they rarely rupture from external blows or even crushing injuries. So-called spontaneous rupture representing pyelosinus backflow from increased intrapelvic pressure has been discussed previously. True spontaneous rupture, if it occurs, would be very uncommon and would occur in patients with severe pelviureteral disease (Fig. 20–27).

Ureteral injury occurring in association with fractures of the transverse processes is more common than with other spinal fractures.

The usual type of external trauma affecting the ureter consists of gunshot or stab wounds. There are less than 60 cases of missile injury reported in the literature (see Figs. 20–28 to 20–32).

AVULSION AT THE URETEROPELVIC JUNCTION

This unusual type of traumatic closed rupture, which occurs more often in children, is secondary to torsion and stretching of the ureter against the upper lumbar transverse processes by hyperextension or severe lateral flexion of the trunk. The latter type has been referred to as a "car bumper" type of injury, in which the patient is struck on the lateral aspect of the knee with acute lateral flexion of the trunk. The urogram reveals the contrast medium extending from the renal pelvis directly into the retroperitoneal space. The ureter does not fill but may be seen as a negative shadow outlined by the contrast medium. Prompt surgical repair is required (Figs. 20–33, 20–34).

FOREIGN BODY

Foreign bodies within the ureteral lumen are almost always the result of instrumental manipulation. Most foreign bodies are produced by a catheter breaking within the ureter or separation of the tip of an instrumental catheter. Rare instances of foreign bodies migrating from the bladder to the ureter by reflux or secondary to ureterointestinal or nephrointestinal fistula have been reported. If the foreign body is large, surgical removal may be necessary (Figs. 20–35 to 20–39).

RADIUM AND RADIOTHERAPY

The ureter is extremely resistant to radiation damage in doses of up to 8000 rads. Radiotherapy treatment to the pelvis, usually administered for carcinoma of the body of the uterus or cervix, may result in gradual fibrosis around the pelvic portion of the ureter, leading to eventual stricture and obstruction. The stricture usually occurs 1 or 2 cm. above the ureterovesical orifice. The obstruction usually presents several months to years after treatment, and it may be bilateral. In most cases the ureter was originally involved with carcinoma, and following radiotherapy, necrosis of the carcinoma and secondary fibrosis lead to stricture. Obstruction occurring years after radiation therapy is more likely from recurrent carcinoma than fibrosis (Fig. 20–40).

LATE SEQUELAE FROM URETERAL TRAUMA

The findings vary according to the site and severity of trauma. (Also see Chapter 8, Trauma to the Kidney.) The roentgenograms may reveal stricture, extravasation, pseudocyst, hydroureter and hydronephrosis, fistula, and, in late stages, renal atrophy (Fig. 20–41).

The formation of a ureteral pseudocyst is similar to that described for traumatic renal pseudocysts. There is usually injury with ureteral extravasation. The ureteral tear may not heal, either because of disease of the ureter or because of increased intralumenal pressure secondary to a distal obstruction (Figs. 20–42 to 20–45).

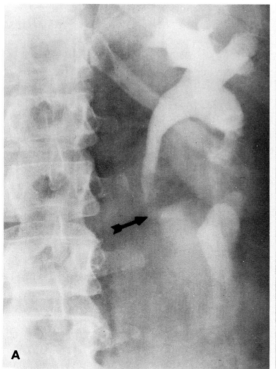 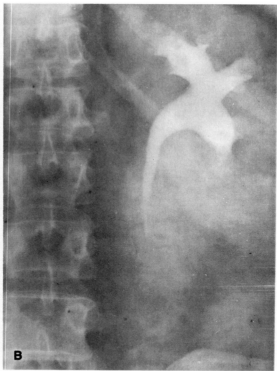

FIG. 20–1. Surgical trauma. **(A)** Excretory urography 6 days postureterolithotomy revealed extravasation (*arrow*) at the operative site with minimal proximal hydronephrosis. **(B)** A repeat excretory urogram 10 days later fails to reveal any extravasation outside the ureteral lumen. The proximal hydronephrosis has decreased, and faint visualization of the distal ureter is observed. Extravasation for several days following ureterolithotomy is common and rarely of significance.

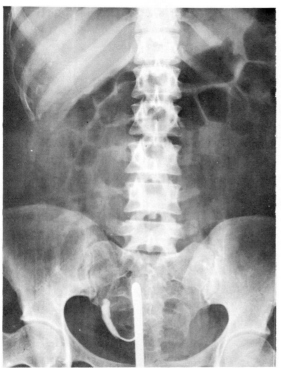

FIG. 20–2. Surgical trauma. Accidental ligation of the right ureter during hysterectomy. Two weeks later the patient developed right flank pain. Excretory urography revealed no function on the right side. Retrograde pyelography (illustration) revealed filling of the distal stump of the right ureter to the point of ligation. Following a temporary nephrostomy, an unsuccessful attempt was made to establish continuity of the ureter. Nephrectomy finally was performed. (Friedenberg, R.M., Ney, C., and Elkin, M.: Am. J. Roentgenol., *90*:28–36, 1963)

FIG. 20-3. Surgical trauma by suture. Three days after hysterectomy for fibroid uterus the patient developed persistent left flank pain. Pyelogram (illustration) revealed marked kinking slightly above the ureterovesical junction, with moderate proximal ureterectasis and calyectasis. Presumably, the periureteral tissues had been caught in a suture at the time of the previous surgery. Since the obstruction was incomplete, and satisfactory function was present, conservative treatment was instituted with catheter dilatation. The ureterectasis and the calyectasis decreased, and the patient retained satisfactory function. (Friedenberg, R.M., Ney, C., and Elkin, M.: Am. J. Roentgenol., *90*:28–36, 1963)

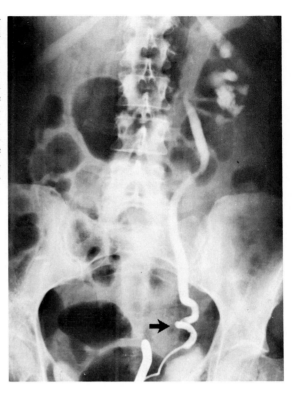

FIG. 20-4. Ureteral stricture following surgery. Increasing right flank pain developed 6 months postureterolithotomy. Retrograde revealed narrowing (*arrow*) of a short segment of the proximal ureter with severe proximal hydronephrosis. Serial examinations revealed the hydronephrosis to be progressive. Surgical correction with resection of the stricture and end-to-end anastomosis was performed. (Friedenberg, R.M., Ney, C., and Elkin, M.: Am. J. Roentgenol., *90*:28–36, 1963)

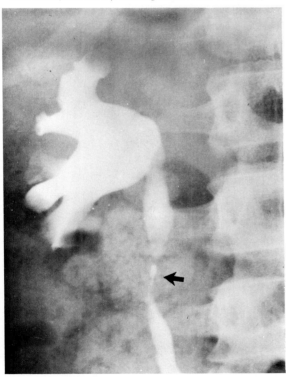

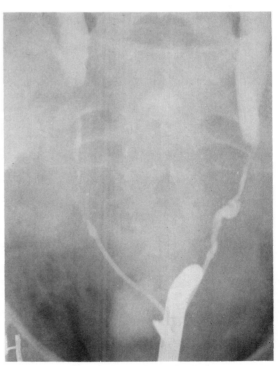

FIG. 20-5. Avascular necrosis. Following hysterectomy, bilateral hydronephrosis developed secondary to lower ureteral obstruction. Pyelogram shows long, irregular, narrowed areas of both ureters. The strictures were secondary to avascular necrosis from loss of blood supply. (Courtesy of Erich Lang, M.D.)

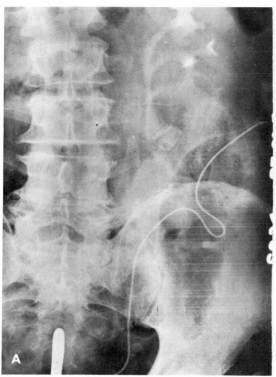
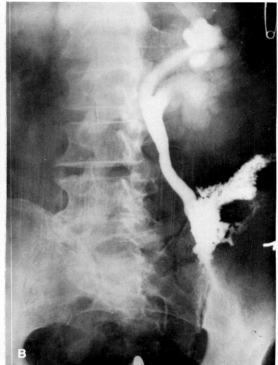

FIG. 20–6. Surgical trauma with secondary cutaneous fistula. Following ureterolithotomy the patient developed a draining fistula in the left flank. Urography visualized the calyces and the proximal ureter. Immediately following urography retrograde catheterization was performed. **(A)** The retrograde catheter deviates laterally, extending to the cutaneous fistula in the left flank. Following withdrawal of the catheter into the lower third of the ureter, retrograde injection **(B)** revealed filling of an abscess cavity in the left retroperitoneal area draining to the left flank, with surprisingly good visualization of the proximal ureter. (Friedenberg, R.M., Ney, C., and Elkin, M.: Am. J. Roentgenol., *90*:28–36, 1963)

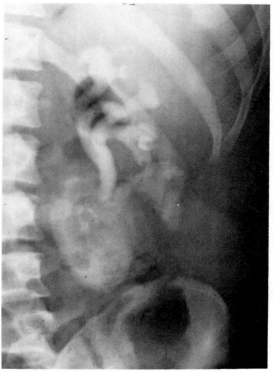

FIG. 20–7. Ureterocutaneous fistula. Gunshot injury transecting proximal ureter. Urogram reveals pooling of contrast medium in retroperitoneal area and then draining to flank. Presence of fistula preserves renal function.

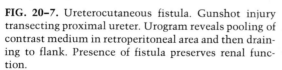

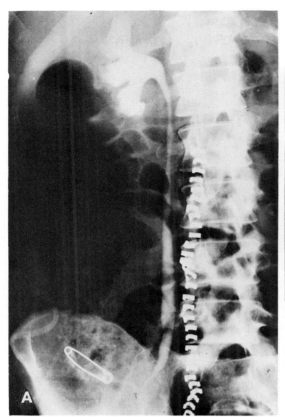

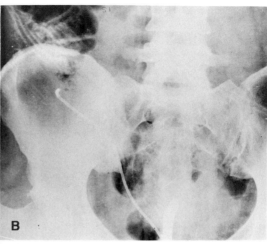

FIG. 20–8. Ureterocutaneous fistula following hysterectomy. **(A)** Urogram shows moderate hydronephrosis with ureter continuously filled to pelvis. Cutaneous fistula (*arrow*) is present in the flank. **(B)** Catheter passed from ureter into fistula tract.

FIG. 20–9. Surgical trauma with secondary fistula. Following an extensive surgical procedure for invasive rectal carcinoma the patient developed fever and left pelvic pain. A cutaneous fistula was present over the pelvic area. Excretory urography revealed poor function on the left side with severe hydronephrosis. Injection of the left vas deferens (illustration) revealed filling of the left ureter from the vas deferens (*arrow*). This represented a fistula extending from the left ureter to the left vas and the skin. (Friedenberg, R.M., Ney, C., and Elkin, M.: Am. J. Roentgenol., *90*:28–36, 1963)

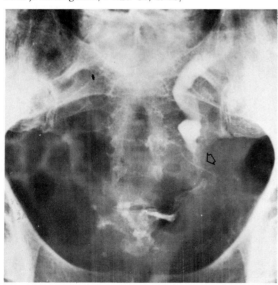

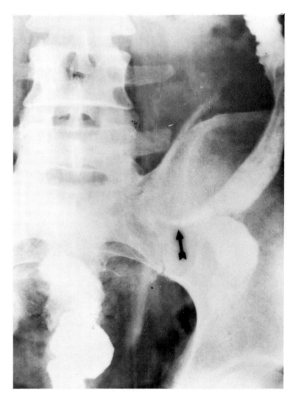

FIG. 20–10. Ureterocolonic fistula. Following surgery for sigmoid diverticulitis the patient developed left flank pain, fever and diarrhea. Urography failed to visualize the left ureter. A repeat barium enema several days later faintly outlined the left ureter through a fistulous tract to the colon (*arrow*). Nephrectomy was performed.

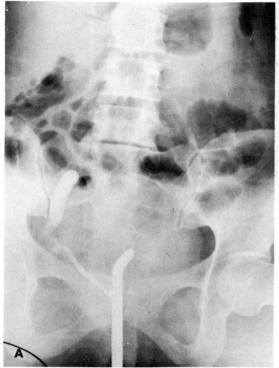

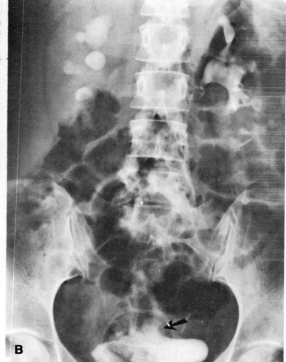

FIG. 20–11. Surgical trauma resulting in ureterovaginal fistula. The right ureter accidentally was tied during a hysterectomy. Ten days later the patient reported urine leaking from the vagina. **(A)** Retrograde study revealed filling of the distal stump of the ureter to the point of the ligation. **(B)** Excretory urography revealed moderate hydronephrosis of the right kidney. The ureter proximal to the ligation communicated with the vagina (*arrow*). The persistence of renal function following ureteral ligation usually indicates the presence of a fistulous tract. At a later date reimplantation of the proximal ureter to the bladder was performed. (Friedenberg, R.M., Ney, C., and Elkin, M.: Am. J. Roentgenol., *90*:28–36, 1963)

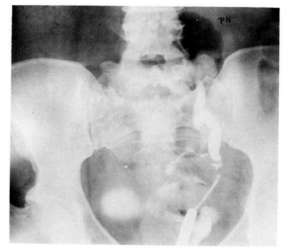

FIG. 20–12. Ureterovaginal fistula following hysterectomy. The patient noted vaginal draining 8 days postsurgery. Urogram showed poor visualization of left kidney. Pyelogram shows a fistulous tract to the vagina from the pelvic ureter. The distal ureter was partially ligated.

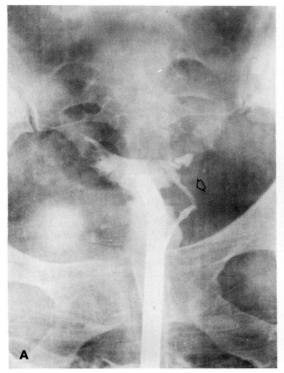

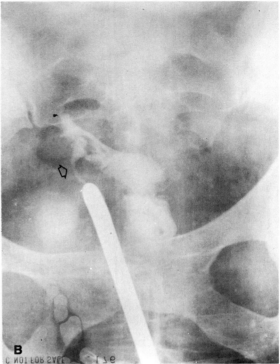

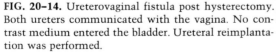

FIG. 20–13. Surgical trauma resulting in bilateral ureterovaginal fistulas. Three days after hysterectomy for fibroids the patient noted copious amounts of urine being discharged from the vagina. She was not voiding urine spontaneously, and catheterization of the bladder revealed no residual urine. (**A**) Following insertion of a bulb catheter into the distal end of the left ureter, retrograde injection revealed a direct communication with the vagina (*arrow*), with excellent visualization of the vaginal outline. (**B**) A similar injection into the distal end of the right ureter revealed a similar fistulous tract, again outlining the vagina. Reimplantation of both ureters into the bladder was performed. (Friedenberg, R.M., Ney, C., and Elkin, M.: Am. J. Roentgenol., 90:28–36, 1963)

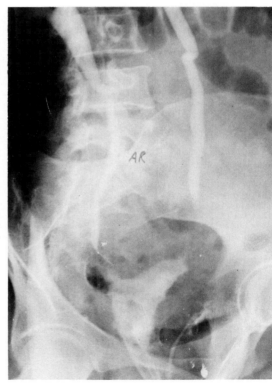

FIG. 20–14. Ureterovaginal fistula post hysterectomy. Both ureters communicated with the vagina. No contrast medium entered the bladder. Ureteral reimplantation was performed.

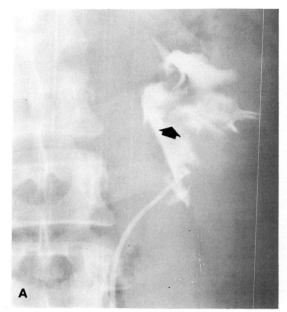

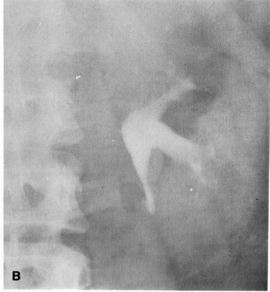

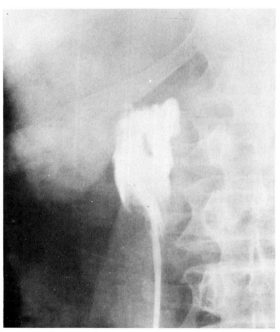

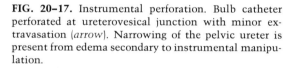

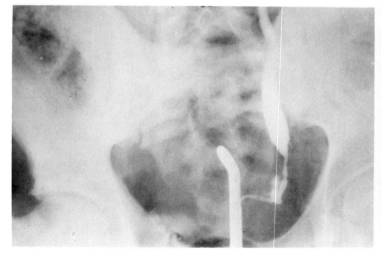

FIG. 20–15. Instrumental perforation. The retrograde catheter perforated the proximal left ureter at the site of a ureteral kink. **(A)** Following contrast injection extravasation is observed outside the ureteral lumen retroperitoneally along the psoas margin and around the renal pelvis. Contrast material has entered the peripelvic area, with the renal pelvis outlined as a radiolucent shadow (*arrow*). **(B)** Excretory urography 8 days later reveals normal calyceal and pelvic outlines without evidence of extravasation.

FIG. 20–17. Instrumental perforation. Bulb catheter perforated at ureterovesical junction with minor extravasation (*arrow*). Narrowing of the pelvic ureter is present from edema secondary to instrumental manipulation.

FIG. 20–16. Instrumental perforation. During pyelography the catheter perforated the proximal ureter just below the ureteropelvic junction. The illustration reveals extravasation of the contrast medium in the retroperitoneal area around the ureter. In perforations of the proximal ureter the contrast material usually extends proximal to the site of perforation, whereas in perforations of the distal ureter the contrast material extends distal to the site of perforation. In each instance this is explained simply by the slope of the ureter. Spontaneous closure of instrumental perforation occurs if the distal ureter is patent. Excretory urography 1 week later revealed no evidence of extravasation in this patient. (Friedenberg, R.M., Ney, C., and Elkin, M.: Am. J. Roentgenol., *90*:28–36, 1963)

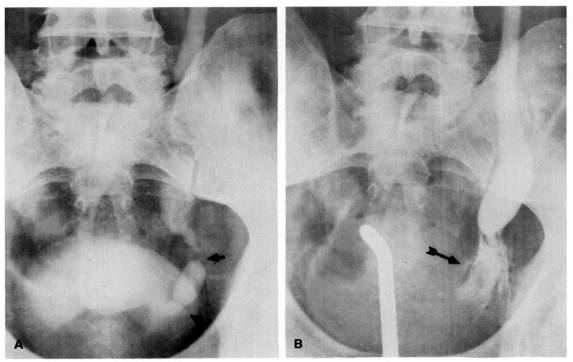

FIG. 20–18. Instrumental perforation. Excretory urography was performed for evaluation of colicky left pelvic pain. **(A)** The urogram revealed multiple strictures in the distal end of the left ureter (*arrows*) with localized ureteritis and segmental areas of dilatation and contraction. The cause of the ureteral stricture is not known. **(B)** Retrograde pyelography was attempted. The catheter perforated the terminal ureter with contrast medium in the fascial planes of the pelvic retroperitoneal region (*arrow*). Perforation of the ureter in the presence of ureteral abnormalities is common. In this case surgical correction was performed with reanastomosis of the ureter to the bladder.

FIG. 20–19. Perforation of the ureter secondary to the force of injection. **(A)** A calculus was present (*arrow*), completely obstructing the right ureter, with no function visible on excretory urography. Retrograde injection was performed below the calculus. The proximal ureter was dilated markedly with pyonephrosis of the right kidney. **(B)** The diseased proximal ureter perforated, with contrast material extending retroperitoneally around the ureteropelvic junction (*arrow*). Spontaneous perforation following retrograde injection usually occurs when a ureter is severely diseased, or when injection is performed into a closed system, such as that produced by an obstructing calculus proximal and a Braasch bulb catheter distal.

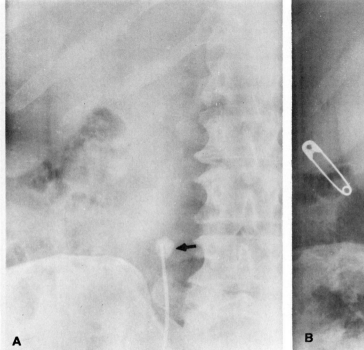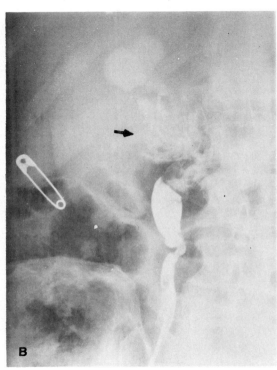

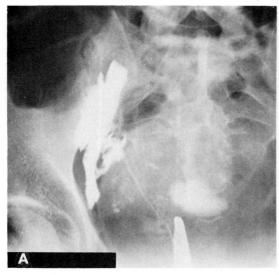

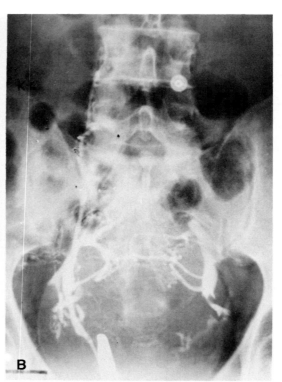

FIG. 20–20. Instrumental perforation. **(A)** Contrast material has extravasated around the pelvic ureter. Perforation evidently occurred into pelvic venous pelxus. **(B)** Immediate filling of pelvic veins occurred.

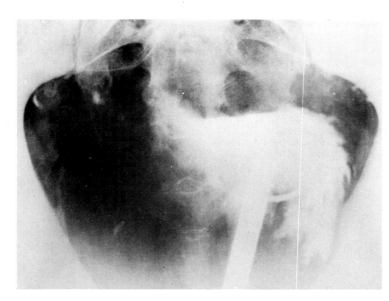

FIG. 20–21. Retroperitoneal rupture at the ureterovesical orifice. Considerable difficulty was encountered in catheterizing the left ureteral orifice. After several unsuccessful attempts to pass the ureteral catheter into the proximal ureter, an injection was performed with the catheter in the distal segment of ureter. Contrast material extended inferiorly around the base of the bladder into the retroperitoneal area limited by fascial planes. This is the usual type of extravesical retroperitoneal rupture. Spontaneous healing occurred. (Friedenberg, R.M., and Ney, C.: Am. J. Roentgenol., *90*:72–74, 1963)

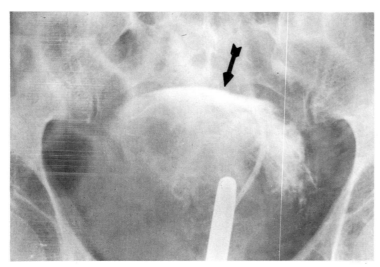

FIG. 20–22. Subserosal extravasation at the uterovesical junction. Ureteral catheter had perforated the intravesical ureter. Following injection, contrast has extended subserosally over the dome of the bladder (*arrow*) and retroperitoneally around the left lateral aspect of the bladder. The adventitia of the bladder in its retroperitoneal portion is thin and easily ruptured, while the dome of the bladder is covered by peritoneum, which prevents rupture in that area. (Friedenberg, R.M., and Ney, C.: Am. J. Roentgenol., *90*:72–74, 1963)

FIG. 20–23. Intramural extravasation. Nonopaque calculus in the distal third of the right ureter. Retrograde examination was performed following the insertion of a Braasch bulb catheter into the right ureteral orifice. This consisted of an injection into a short closed segment of ureter where the intraureteral pressure will increase rapidly. The illustration reveals intramural extravasation in the ureteral segment which is within the wall of the bladder surrounded by circular muscle. Note the sharp localization of contrast on each side of the ureter, with the ureter appearing to be relatively radiolucent. Usually free retroperitoneal extravasation follows rapidly. (Friedenberg, R.M., and Ney, C.: Am. J. Roentgenol., *90:*72–74, 1963)

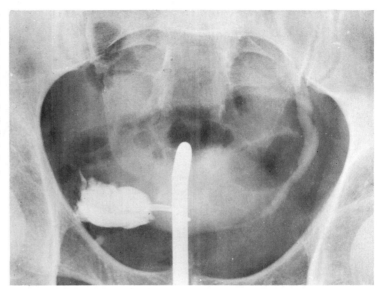

FIG. 20–24. Submucosal extravasation following multiple attempts to catheterize the right ureteral orifice. Injection was performed with the ureteral catheter just at the margin of the orifice. This resulted in a submucosal extravasation (illustration) of the contrast around the ureteral orifice. Note the feathery, fanlike appearance of the margins of the extravasation without evidence of retroperitoneal extension. (Friedenberg, R.M., and Ney, C.: Am. J. Roentgenol., *90:*72–74, 1963)

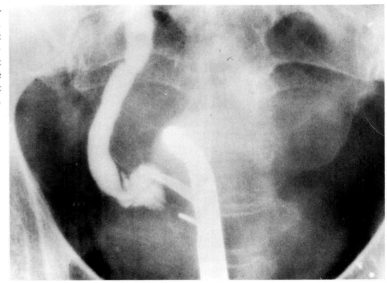

FIG. 20–25. Large submucosal extravasation, again following difficulty in catheterization of a ureteral orifice, this time the left. Some contrast material appears to be free within the bladder. Again note the localized collection of contrast medium with irregular, feathery margins under the mucosa.

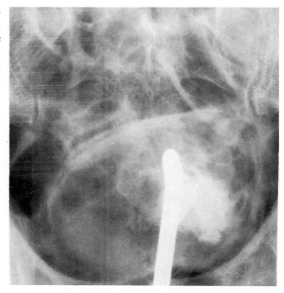

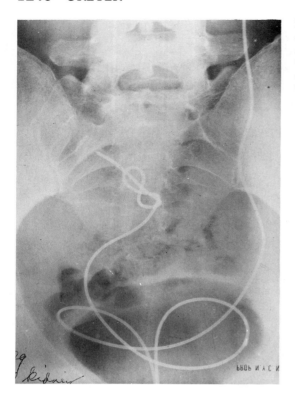

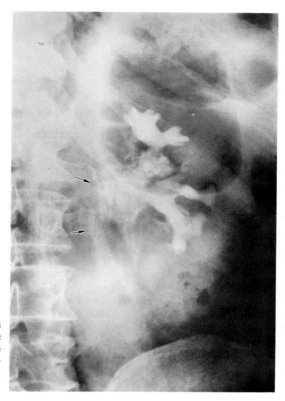

FIG. 20–26. Catheter knot. Following catheterization of a moderately hydronephrotic right sacral kidney, a knot occurred in the ureteral catheter within the pelvis of the kidney. It was impossible to withdraw the catheter, and pyelotomy was performed. (Friedenberg, R.M., Ney, C., and Elkin, M.: Am. J. Roentgenol., *90*:28–36, 1963)

FIG. 20–27. "Spontaneous rupture." Renal infection and calculi. Urogram reveals extravasation around the renal pelvis and proximal ureter (*arrows*). In spite of the severe disease present, the extravasation is probably caused by pyelosinus backflow.

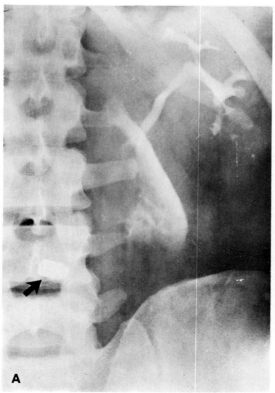

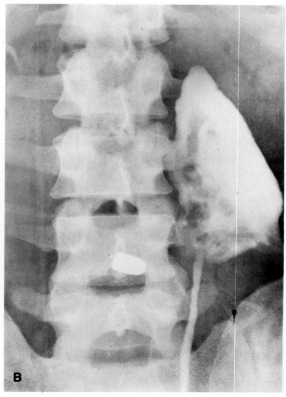

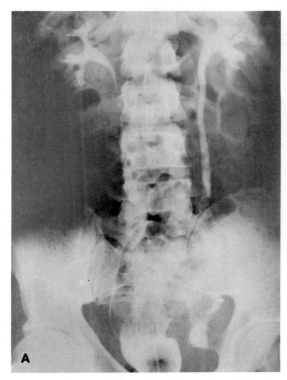

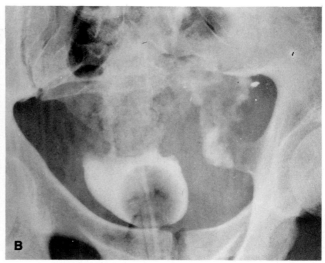

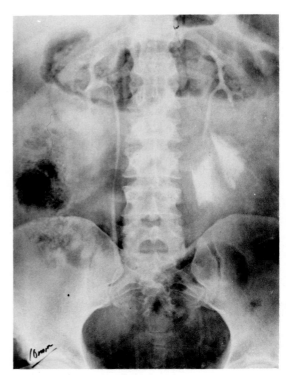

FIG. 20–29. External trauma. Bullet perforated the distal third of the left ureter and the bladder. The bladder rent was repaired immediately. **(A)** Twelve days later urography revealed residual deformity of the bladder with an extravesical hematoma. Contrast medium is pooling around the distal third of the left ureter draining through a cutaneous fistula. **(B)** Small fragments of the bullet surround the contrast medium extravasating from the left ureter. Reanastomosis of the ureter into the bladder was performed.

FIG. 20–28. External trauma. Bullet wound that severed proximal ureter. Urine was draining through the cutaneous opening. **(A)** Excretory urography revealed satisfactory function of the kidney with extravasation from the proximal ureter extending retroperitoneally along the psoas margin. The distal ureter was not visualized. **(B)** Pyelography revealed complete extravasation of the contrast medium at L-4 without filling of the proximal ureter. Drainage occurred through the cutaneous fistula. Satisfactory anastomosis could not be performed, and the kidney was removed. (Friedenberg, R.M., Ney, C., and Elkin, M.: Am. J. Roentgenol., *90*:28–36, 1963)

FIG. 20–30. Stab wound in left ureter. Urogram shows contrast medium extravasating from transected ureter. There is no proximal hydronephrosis, since there was free drainage through the cutaneous opening.

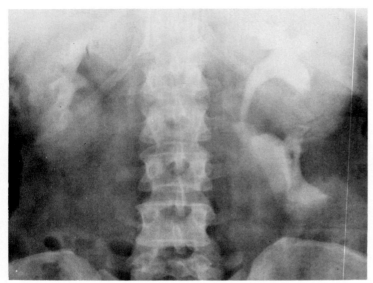

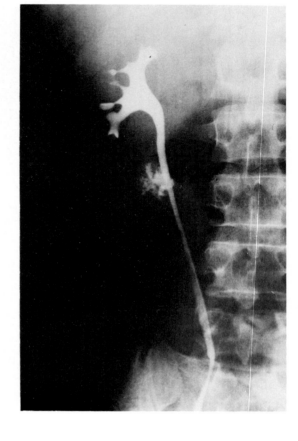

FIG. 20–31. Stab wound of the left ureter. Extravasation from proximal ureter at site of laceration.

FIG. 20–31a. Stab wound of the right ureter. Pyelogram shows minor extravasation from a small nick in the proximal ureter.

FIG. 20–32. External trauma with ureteroperitoneal fistula. Two weeks prior to admission the patient had repair of an intestinal perforation from a bullet wound. There was no history of hematuria or urinary fistula at that time. On admission, paracentesis yielded 5700 ml. of slightly hemorrhagic fluid. Excretory urography showed satisfactory function bilaterally, and right retrograde pyelography was normal. Following retrograde injection into the left ureter **(A)**, contrast material pooled in two areas: along the psoas margin in the region of the metallic bullet and more proximally in the left flank. The retrograde catheter, when passed proximally **(B)**, extended laterally and anteriorly into the left flank, where it was intraperitoneal. The upper area of extravasation (*large arrow*) is intraperitoneal, whereas the lower area (*small arrow*) is retroperitoneal. It is not known whether the complicated fistulous tracts arose from the time of injury or following the previous intestinal surgery. Nephroureterectomy was performed. (Arduino, L.J.: J. Urol., *73*:990–994, 1955)

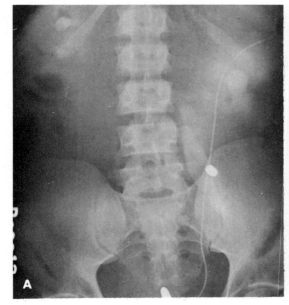

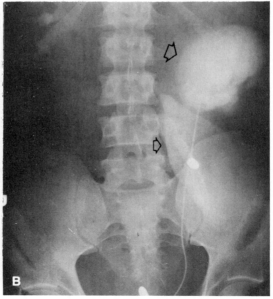

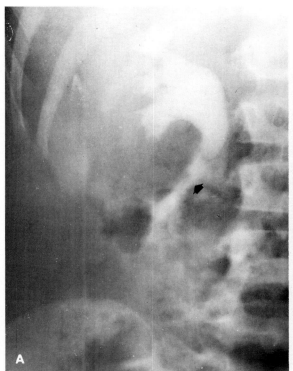

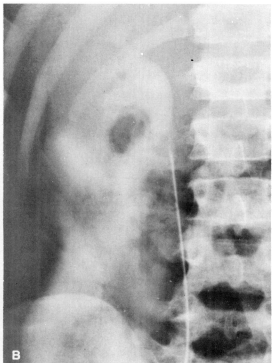

FIG. 20–33. Blunt trauma. Closed rupture of the ureter. Following blunt trauma with lateral flexion of the trunk, the patient presented with right flank pain and hematuria. **(A)** An immediate urogram revealed mild right hydronephrosis with contrast medium extending retroperitoneally (*arrow*). The ureter was not visualized. **(B)** Immediate retrograde pyelography with the catheter in the proximal ureter revealed massive retroperitoneal extravasation without further contrast material entering the renal pelvis. At surgery there was a complete avulsion of the ureter at the ureteropelvic junction. Continuity was restored. Avulsion of the ureter secondary to severe lateral flexion of the trunk always occurs at the ureteropelvic junction.

FIG. 20–34. Avulsion of the ureter from blunt trauma in a 4-year-old boy with avulsion of the right ureter at the ureteropelvic junction. **(A)** Massive extravasation of contrast medium is present in the retroperitoneum. **(B)** Slight lateral position of the proximal ureter following surgical repair.

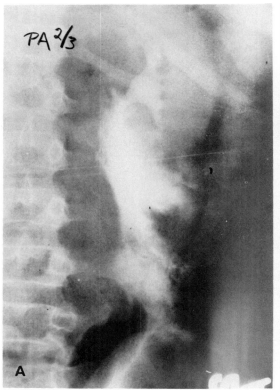

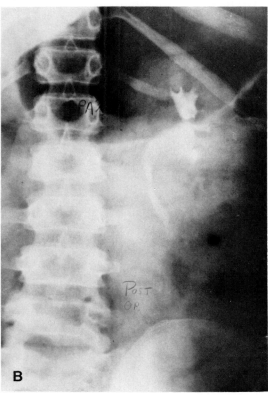

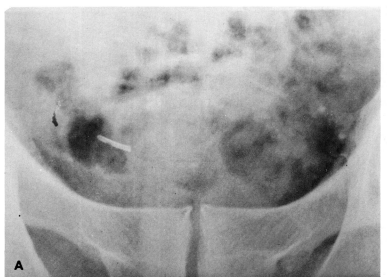

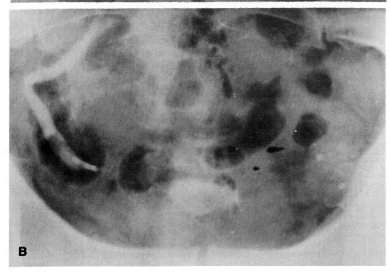

FIG. 20–35. Foreign body in ureter. During pyelography the distal portion of the ureteral catheter broke off and remained within the right ureter. **(A)** The scout film reveals a small segment of catheter lying in the lower third of the ureter. **(B)** In the excretory urogram the catheter partially obstructs the ureter slightly above the ureterovesical junction. Spontaneous passage into the bladder occurred in 3 days. (Friedenberg, R.M., Ney, C., and Elkin, M.: Am. J. Roentgenol., *90*:28–36, 1963)

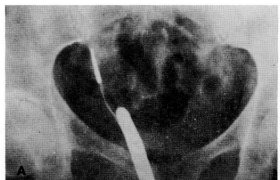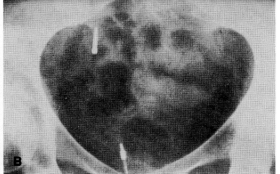

FIG. 20–36. Foreign body in ureter. **(A)** A Johnson basket stone extractor was introduced into the right ureter in an attempt to remove an impacted ureteral calculus. **(B)** The tip of the catheter separated and remained within the ureteral lumen. (Beneventi, F.A., Creighton, F.S.: Am. J. Surg., *89*:1086–1087, 1955)

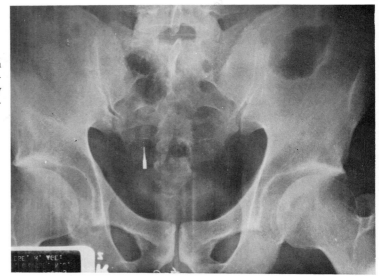

FIG. 20–37. Foreign body in ureter. The scout film reveals the metallic tip of a ureteral catheter (stone extractor) within the right ureter. It passed spontaneously into the bladder and was removed. (Courtesy of Maxwell Malament, M.D.)

FIG. 20–38. Foreign body in ureter. Thirty-five-year-old woman admitted with left colicky pain. The scout film reveals a large ureteral calculus slightly above the left ureterovesical junction. Within the calculus is a short dense linear opacity representing a segment of ureteral catheter, which presumably broke off during a previous retrograde pyelography 3 years earlier. Segments of catheter within the ureter usually are passed spontaneously. It is unusual for one to remain within the lumen for this length of time. It became the nidus for a calculus.

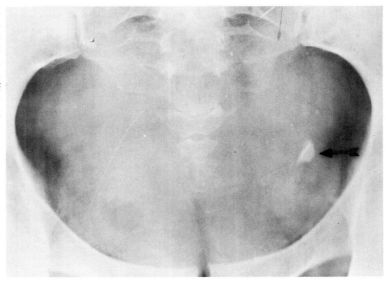

FIG. 20–39. Foreign body. Scout film (**A**) shows wooden toothpick in the right ureter (*arrows*). In the urogram (**B**) the toothpick is faintly visible in the distal ureter through the bladder contrast medium. Proximal ureterectasis and calyectasis are present.

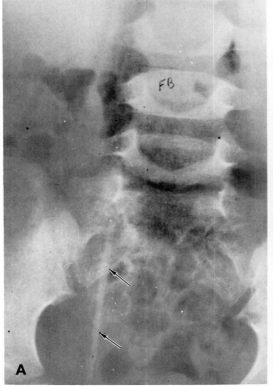

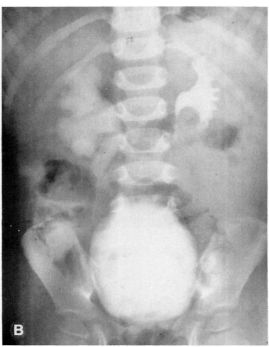

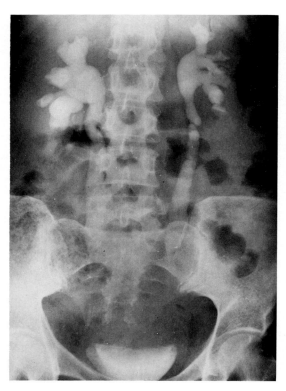

FIG. 20-40. Radiotherapy stricture. Three years after the administration of radium and x-ray therapy for carcinoma of the uterine cervix the patient developed a gradual progressive hydroureter and hydronephrosis. The illustration is a 30-minute pyelogram revealing marked bilateral dilatation extending from the pelvic portion of both ureters proximally. The lower thirds of the ureters are not visualized. There was no clinical or radiologic evidence of recurrence of the carcinoma or of metastases. (Friedenberg, R.M., Ney, C., and Elkin, M.: Am. J. Roentgenol., *90:*28–36, 1963)

FIG. 20-41. Scout film (**A**) shows multiple areas of calcification in the right flank with deformity of the second lumbar transverse process from an old gunshot wound. The urogram failed to visualize the right kidney. Retrograde study (**B**) reveals a severe stricture of the proximal ureter with poor visualization of the calyces secondary to renal atrophy. Nephrectomy revealed the ureteral stricture to be secondary to an organized periureteral hematoma and fibrosis. (Department of Radiology, Montefiore Hospital, Bronx, N.Y.)

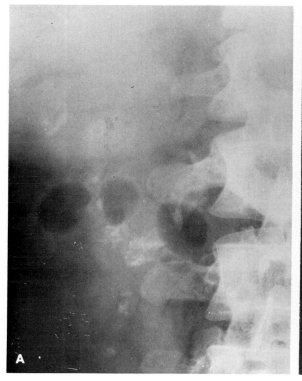

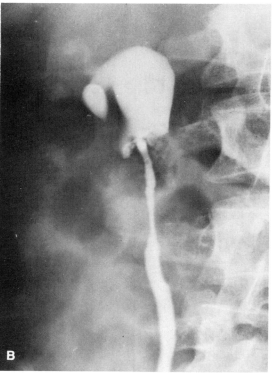

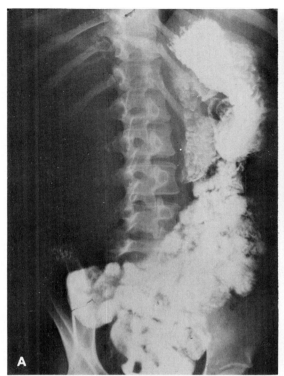

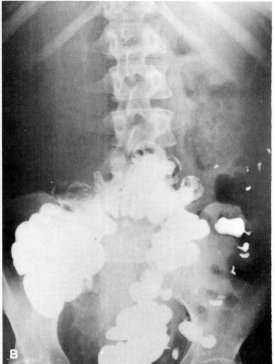

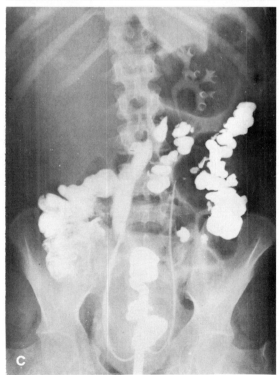

FIG. 20–42. Traumatic pseudocyst of ureter. The patient presented with a large right upper quadrant mass 2 months after an automobile accident. Previous urogram 4 years prior to admission was normal. (**A**) The upper gastrointestinal series revealed the stomach and the small bowel to be displaced anteriorly and to the left. (**B**) The barium enema showed the hepatic flexure to be displaced inferiorly. (**C**) Retrograde pyelography revealed the left kidney and the ureter to be normal. The right ureter was displaced medially, with an apparent obstruction in the proximal third of the ureter. A large mass which could not be separated from the right kidney was producing the displacement of the ureter and the bowel. Surgery revealed a large cyst, containing 4000 ml. of sterile urine, adherent to the peritoneum, the perirenal fascia and the lower pole of the kidney. The proximal ureter entered the cyst, and the distal ureter was necrotic. Nephroureterectomy was performed. Traumatic rupture of the proximal ureter allows urine drainage into the perirenal tissues. If the rupture does not close promptly, a pseudocyst is formed. Symptoms may be minimal for months. (Davis, J.E., Cortijo, R., and Beneventi, F.A.: Urol. Int., *16*:91–102, 1963)

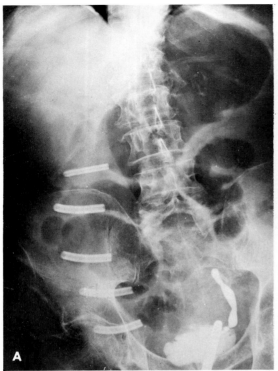

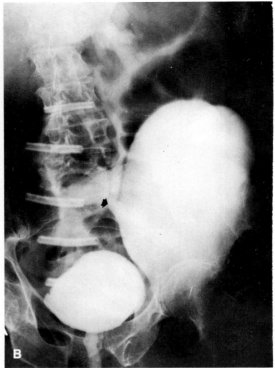

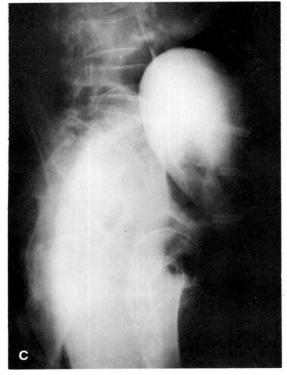

FIG. 20–43. Paraureteral pseudocyst. Elderly man who presented with a large cystic mass about 10 × 15 cm. in the left lower quadrant 4 months after an abdominoperineal resection for carcinoma of the rectum. Excretory urography did not visualize the left kidney. Left pyelogram (**A**) outlined the distal segment of ureter, which was obstructed at the pelvic brim. The mass was visualized by percutaneous injection (**B, C**). The communication with the proximal ureter (*arrow*) is well defined. The combination of a ureteral rent and distal ureteral obstruction leading to the paraureteral pseudocyst occurred at the time of the abdominoperineal resection. (Samellas, E.B., Le-Veen, H.H.: J. Urol., *89*:578–580, 1963)

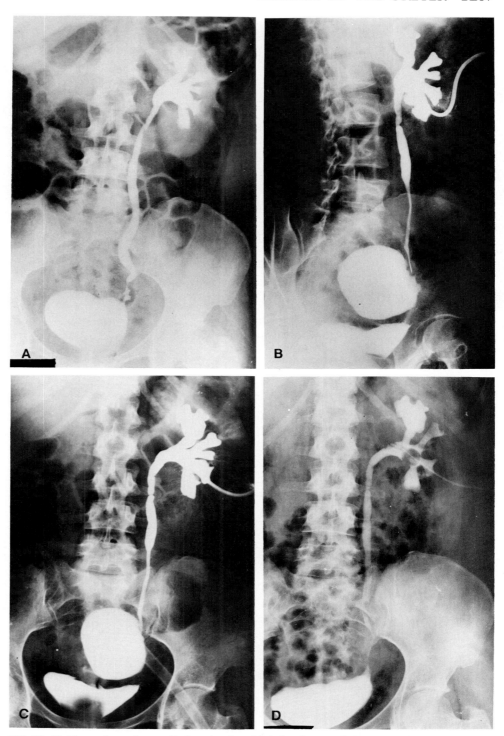

FIG. 20–44. Ureteral pseudocyst. Patient developed left distal ureteral obstruction (**A**) after hysterectomy and radiotherapy for cervical carcinoma. Nephrostomy was performed, followed by ureteral reimplantation into bladder. Six weeks later contrast medium injected through the nephrostomy (**B** and **C**) revealed a large pseudocyst at the surgical site. There was a stricture at the ureterovesical junction. Drainage of the cyst and surgical correction of the ureterovesical junction led to a satisfactory result (**D**).

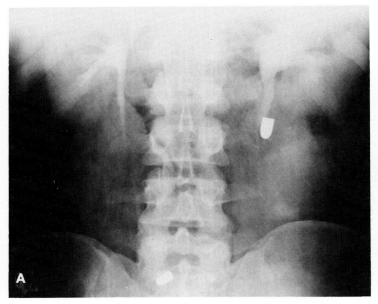

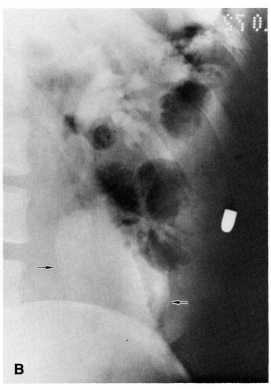

FIG. 20–45. Pseudocyst ureter. Bullet wound with proximal ureteral injury led to formation of pseudocyst (urinoma). The urogram (**A** and **B**) shows contrast medium in the cyst (*arrows*). (Courtesy of F. Lopez, M.D.)

BIBLIOGRAPHY

Trauma to the Ureter: General

1. Aschner, P.: Accidental injury to ureters and bladder in pelvic surgery. J. Urol., *69*:774–786, 1953.
2. Baird, H.H., and Justis, H.R.: Surgical injuries of ureter and bladder. J.A.M.A., *162*:1357–1361, 1956.
3. Barbaric, Z.L., Wolfe, D.E., and Segal, A.J.: Intraoperative ureteral trauma: A radiologic approach. J. Can. Assoc. Radiol., *29*:40–43, 1978.
4. Benson, R.C., and Hinman, F., Jr.: Urinary tract injuries in obstetrics and gynecology. Am. J. Obstet. Gynecol., *70*:467–485, 1955.
5. Brown, R.B.: Surgical and external ureteric trauma. Aust. N.Z. J. Surg., *47*:471–476, 1977.
6. Carlton, C.E., Jr., Guthrie, A.G., and Scott, R., Jr.: Surgical correction of ureteral injury. J. Trauma, *9*:457–464, 1969.
7. Carlton, C.E., Jr., Scott, R., Jr., and Guthrie, A.G.: The initial management of ureteral injuries. J. Urol., *108*335–340, 1971.
8. Conger, K., Beecham, C.T., and Horrax, T.M.: Ureteral injury in pelvic surgery: Current thought on incidence, pathogenesis, prophylaxis and treatment. Obstet. Gynecol., *3*:343–357, 1954.
9. Derrick, F.C., Jr., and Kretkowski, R.C.: Trauma to kidney, ureter, bladder, and urethra: Diagnosis and management. Postgrad. Med., *55*:183–192, 1974.
10. Evans, R.A., and Smith, M.J.: Violent injuries to the upper ureter. J. Trauma, *16*:558–561, 1976.
11. Everett, H.S., and Mattingly, R.F.: Urinary tract injuries resulting from pelvic surgery. Am. J. Obstet. Gynecol., *71*:502–514, 1956.
12. Falk, H.C.: Urologic Injuries in Gynecology, 2nd ed., Philadelphia, Davis, 1964.
13. Feiner, D.: Operative injuries of the ureter. Surg. Gynecol. Obstet., *66*:790–796, 1938.
14. Forsythe, W.E., and Persky, L.: Operative ureteral injuries. A.M.A. Arch. Surg., *79*:861–863, 1959.
15. Freda, V.C., and Tacchi, D.: Ureteral injury discovered after pelvic surgery. Am. J. Obstet. Gynecol., *83*:406–409, 1962.
16. Friedenberg, R.M., Ney, C., and Elkin, M.: Trauma to the ureter. Am. J. Roentgenol., *90*:28–36, 1963.
17. Halverstadt, D.B., and Fraley, E.E.: Avulsion of the upper ureter secondary to blunt trauma. Br. J. Urol., *39*:588–593, 1967.
18. Heckel, N.J., and McDonald, J.H.: Injuries to the ureter. I. M. J., *109*:227–230, 1956.
19. Herman, L.: Accidental bilateral occlusion of the ureters. J. Urol., *9*:151–179, 1923.
20. Higgins, C.C.: Ureteral injury during surgery: A review of 87 cases. J.A.M.A., *199*:82–88, 1967.
21. Holloway, H.J.: Injury to urinary tract as a complication of gynecological surgery. Am. J. Obstet. Gynecol., *60*:30–40, 1950.
22. Ihse, I., Arnesjö, B., and Jonsson, G.: Surgical injuries of the ureter: A review of 42 cases. Scand. J. Urol., Nephrol., *9*:39–44, 1975.
23. Jackson, J.T.: Report on a series of hysterectomies, with particular reference to complications in the urinary tract. J. Tenn. Med. Assoc., *54*:81–83, 1961.

24. Mannes, H., Zimskind, P.D., Subbarao, Y., et al.: Crush injury of the lower ureter: An experimental study. J. Urol., *108*:548–552, 1972.

25. Meigs, J.V.: Radical hysterectomy with bilateral pelvic lymph node dissections: Report of 100 patients operated on five or more years ago. Am. J. Obstet. Gynecol., *62*:854–870, 1951.

26. Moore, T.D.: Management of the surgically traumatized ureter. J. Urol., *59*:712–725, 1948.

27. Newman, H.R., Hotchkiss, R., and Gordon, S.: Ureteral injuries in pelvic surgery. Am. J. Surg., *94*:421–430, 1957.

28. Pfister, R.C., and Newhouse, J.H.: Radiology of ureter. Urology, *12*:15–39, 1978.

29. Raney, A.M.: Ureteral trauma: Effects of ureteral ligation with and without deligation—experimental studies and case reports. J. Urol., *119*:326–329, 1978.

30. Rusche, C.F.: Injury of the ureter. Nebraska Med. J., *41*:271–279, 1956.

31. St. Martin, E.C., et al.: Ureteral injuries in gynecological surgery. J. Urol., *70*:51–57, 1953.

32. Schneiderman, C., and Strean, G.J.: Ureteral and urethral injuries associated with gynecologic and obstetric practice. J. Int. Coll. Surg., *35*:484–494, 1961.

33. Senger, F.L., and Johnson, S.: Severe surgical injuries to both ureters with subsequent restoration of function. J. Urol., *44*:35–39, 1940.

34. Slutsky, N.: Ligation of both ureters, unilateral nephrostomy, recovery. Am. J. Obstet. Gynecol., *36*:1045–1047, 1936.

35. Smith, M.J.V., Nanson, E.M., and Campbell, J.M.: An unusual case of closed rupture of the kidney. J. Urol., *83*:277–278, 1960.

36. Solomons, E., Levin, E.J., Bauman, J., et al.: Pyelographic study of ureteric injuries sustained during hysterectomy for benign conditions. Surg. Gynec. Obstet., *111*:41–48, 1960.

37. Spence, H.M., and Boone, T.B.: Injuries to the ureter due to external violence. Am. Surg., *24*:423–430, 1958.

38. Stone, H.H., and Jones, H.Q.: Penetrating and nonpenetrating injuries to the ureter. Surg. Gynecol. Obstet., *114*:52–56, 1962.

39. Symmonds, R.E.: Ureteral injuries associated with gynecologic surgery: Prevention and management. Clin. Obstet. Gynecol., *19*:623–644, 1976.

40. TeLinde, R.W., Meigs, J.V., Ulfelder, H., et al.: Forum on the ureter. Am. J. Obstet. Gynecol., *68*:1272–1278, 1954.

41. Waterhouse, K., and Gross, M.: Trauma to the genitourinary tract: A 5-year experience with 251 cases. J. Urol., *101*:241–246, 1969.

42. Wishard, W.N., Jr.: Surgical injuries of the ureter and bladder. J. Urol., *72*:1009–1014, 1955.

Surgical Trauma

Injuries Secondary to General Surgery

43. Aboulker, P., Lance, P., and Giovanola, P.: Les fistules de l'uretere apres appendicectomie. J. Urol. Nephrol. Paris, *62*:94–95, 1956.

44. Andersson, A., and Bergdahl, L.: Urologic complications following abdominoperineal resection of the rectum. Arch. Surg., *111*:969–971, 1976.

45. Bandler, C.G., and Roen, P.R.: Urologic complications of left colon surgery. Ann. Surg., *128*:80–88, 1948.

46. Reference deleted.

47. Brown, J.Y., Engelbach, W., and Carman, R.D.: Anatomic, pathologic and clinical studies of lesions involving the appendix and right ureter. J.A.M.A., *54*:1491–1497, 1910.

48. Carli: Injuries to a ureter in a hernia. Ann. Ital. Chir., *11*:2078–2104, 1932.

49. Coplan, M.M., Woods, F.M., and Melvin, P.D.: The recognition and management of injuries to the lower ureters and bladder resulting from pelvic and recto-sigmoid colon surgery. Proc. North Cent. Sec. Am. Urol. Assoc., *pp. 64–74, 1955.*

50. Eickenberg, H.O., Amin, M., Klompus, W., et al.: Urologic complications following abdominoperineal resection. J. Urol., *115*:180–182, 1976.

51. Ewert, E.E.: Comparative analysis of the urological complications following large bowel surgery. J. Urol., *46*:764–776, 1941.

52. Ewert, E.E.: Urologic complications following large bowel surgery and their management. Surg. Clin. N. Am., *26*:695–702, 1946.

53. Graham, J.W., and Goligher, J.C.: The management of accidental injuries and deliberate resection of the ureter during excision of the rectum. Br. J. Surg., *42*:151–160, 1954–1955.

54. Gyory, G.: Accidental injuries of the ureters and bladder in surgery and late sequelae. Zentralbl Gynaekol., *80*:1318–1327, 1958.

55. Harrington, S.W.: The effect on the kidney of various surgical procedures on the blood supply, capsule, and on ureters. Arch. Surg., *2*:547, 1921.

56. Jones, T.E.: Complications of one-stage abdominoperineal resection of rectum. J.A.M.A., *120*:104–107, 1942.

57. Marino, H., and Veppo, A.A.: Appendicitis: fistula ureteral post-operatoria. Arch. Argent. Enferm. d'ap digest y de la nutricion, *11*:107–114, 1935–1936.

58. Samellas, E.B., and LeVeen, H.H.: Traumatic paraureteral pseudocyst. J. Urol., *89*:578–580, 1963.

59. Zol'nikov, S.M.: Ureteral injury during appendectomy. Urologia, *23*, No. 4:56–57, 1958.

Complications Secondary to Aortofemoral Bypass Operation

60. Dorfman, L.E., and Thomford, N.R.: Unusual ureteral injury following aorto-iliac bypass graft. J. Urol., *101*:25–27, 1969.

61. Lytton, B.: Ureteral obstruction following aortofemoral bypass graft. Surgery, *59*:918–922, 1966.

62. Petrone, A.F., Dudzinski, J., and Mamatis, W.: Ureteral obstruction secondary to aortic femoral bypass. Ann. Surg., *179*:192–196, 1974.

63. Wallijn, E., Renders, G., and Vereecken, L.: Urological complications following aortofemoral bypass graft. Br. J. Urol., *47*:617–621, 1975.

Injuries Secondary to Laminectomies and Other Orthopaedic Procedures

64. Billig, R., and Baker, R.: Ureteral injury during a hip nailing procedure. J.A.M.A., *235*:1724, 1976.

65. Borski, A.A., and Smith, R.A.: Ureteral injury in lumbar disc operation. J. Neurosurg., *17*:925–928, 1960.

66. Kern, H.B., Barnes, W., and Malament, M.: Lumbar laminectomy and associated ureteral injury. J. Urol., *102*:675–677, 1969.

67. Sandoz, I., and Hodges, C.V.: Ureteral injury incident to lumbar disk operation. J. Urol., *93*:687–689, 1965.

Obstetric, Uterine, Total Manipulations

68. Beneventi, F.A., and Twinem, F.P.: Transection of the ureter following uterine instrumentation. J. Urol., *62*:224–227, 1950.
69. Howkins, J.: Unusual ureteric catastrophe. J. Obstet. Gynaec. Brit. Emp., *59*:850–852, 1952.
70. Irvin, T.T., Goligher, J.C., and Scott, J.S.: Injury to the ureter during laparascopic tubal sterilization. Arch. Surg., *110*:1501–1503, 1975.
71. Kramer, K.W.: Letale Urinphlegmone infolge Harnleiterverletzung durch Zertrummerung eines Harnleitersteines bei Zangeneutbindung. Zentralbl. Gynaekol, *62*:526–528, 1938.
72. Popoff, P.M.: Re:Avulsion of the ureter from both ends as a complication of interruption of pregnancy with a vacuum aspirator (letter). J. Urol., *118:1073–1074, 1977.*

Spontaneous Rupture of the Ureter

73. Albarran, M.: Calculs, fistules et retrecissements de la portion lomboiliaque de l'uretere. Ann. Mal. Organ Genitourin., *13*:193–216, 1895.
74. Amin, M., and Howerton, L.W.: Spontaneous rupture of the ureter. South. Med. J., *67*:1398–1501, 1974.
75. Berry, J.: Perforation of the ureter by calculus: Extravasation of urine: death from uremia and sepsis. Br. J. Surg., *8*:372–374, 1921.
76. Bhargava, B.N.: Spontaneous rupture of the ureter. J. R. Coll. Surg. Edinb., *22*:293–295, 1977.
77. Brillembourg, B.J.: Flegmon lumbar periureteral por ruptura no traumatica del ureter, Rev. Policlin. Caracas, *15*:94–101, 1946.
78. Collins, A.N., and Clement, G.: Ureteral stone with periureteral extravasation. Minn. Med., *13*:910–911, 1930.
79. Curtis, H.L.: Three cases of partial rupture of the ureter due to ureteral calculi with extravasation of urine into abscess pocket. Maine Med. J., *29*:69–72, 1938.
80. Foulds, G.S., and Varey, D.H.: Extravasation of urine from the ureter secondary to ureteral calculus, Br. J. Urol., *6*:27–36, 1934.
81. Freshman, E.: Extravasation of urine following spontaneous rupture of the ureteropelvic junction, Brit. J. Urol., *7*:267–270, 1935.
82. Orkin, L.A.: Spontaneous or nontraumatic extravasation from the ureter. J. Urol., *67*:272–283, 1952.
83. Ramsey, E.W., Jarzylo, S.V., and Bruce, E.W.: Spontaneous extravasation of urine from the renal pelvis and ureter. J. Urol., *110*:507–512, 1973.
84. Rathbun, N.P.: Necrosis of the ureter, perforation, periurethral abscess. J. Urol., *17*:329–335, 1927.
85. Smith, S.: Spontaneous ureteral rupture with periureteral abscess formation. Am. J. Surg., *45*:139–141, 1939.
86. Surraco, L.A.: Spontaneous pyeloureteral rupture, J. Urol., Paris, *43*:34–51, 1937.

Cystoscopic Injuries

86a. Ellik, M.: Stones in the ureter: their extraction by looped catheter. J. Urol., *57*:473–478, 1947.
87. Goldstein, A.G., and Conger, K.B.: Perforation of the ureter during retrograde pyelography. J. Urol., *94*:658–664, 1965.
87a. Levant, B.: A new stone basket. J. Urol., *72*:992–994, 1954.
87b. Martin, L.A., Estes, E.E., Jr., and Headstream, J.W.: Ureteral

calculi: evaluation of management. J. Arkansas Med. Soc., *59*:442–445, 1963.

Bilateral Injuries and Avulsions of Upper Ureter

88. Ainsworth, T., Weems, W.L., and Merrell, W.H., Jr.: Bilateral ureteral injury due to nonpenetrating external trauma. J. Urol., *96*:439–442, 1966.
89. Boston, U.E., and Smyth, B.T.: Bilateral pelvi-ureteric avulsion following closed trauma. Br. J. Urol., *47*:149–151, 1975.
90. Ford, W.D., and Kirkland, I.S.: Avulsion of the pelvi-ureteric junction after minor trauma complicated by anaphylactoid purpura. J. Roy. Coll. Surg. Edinb., *23*:44–46, 1978.
91. Heath, A.D., and May, A.: Bilateral avulsion of the upper ureters. Br. J. Urol., *47*:387, 1975.

Foreign Bodies in the Ureter

92. Klika, M.: Kompakt Ainsel oder ein Neirstein und eine spontane Knotung des ureter-katheters im ureter. Z. Urol., *25*:590–593, 1931.
93. Konuralp, H.Z., Barcas, G.S., and Altung, K.Y.: An unusual foreign body in the ureter. Br. J. Urol., *40*:233–234, 1968.
94. Oldfield, J.: Fracture of ureteric catheter, Br. J. Urol., *31*:166–167, 1959.
95. Rusche, C.F., and Bacon, S.K.: Injury of ureter due to surgery, intra-ureteral instrumentation, external violence and foreign bodies: Report of 50 cases. J.A.M.A., *114*:201–207, 1940.
96. Valenta, J.C., and Chenoweth, C.V.: Foreign bodies in ureter: A complication from use of electrodes for ureteral meatotomy. J. Urol., *69*:492–495, 1953.
97. Wishard, W.N., Jr.: Stone in lower third of ureter with report of instance incarcerated basket. J. Urol., *50*:775–783, 1943.

Radiation Effects

98. Albers, D.D., Dee, A.L., Kalmon, E.H., et al.: Irradiation injury to the ureter and surgical tolerance; an experimental study. Invest. Urol., *14*:229–232, 1976.
99. Buchler, D.A., Kline, J.C., Peckham, D.M., et al.: Radiation reaction in cervical cancer therapy. Am. J. Obstet. Gynecol., *111*:745–750, 1971.
100. Graham, J., and Abad, R.S.: Ureteral obstruction due to radiation. Am. J. Obstet. Gynecol., *99*:405–415, 1967.
101. Kirchhoff, H.: Complications: Abundant changes in the urinary tract after radiotherapy of cervical carcinoma. Geburtsh Frauenheilk, *20*:34–39, 1960.
102. Kottmeier, H.L.: Complications following radiation therapy in carcinoma of the cervix and their treatment. Am. J. Obstet. Gynecol., *88*:854–866, 1964.
103. Lang, E.K., Wood, M., Brown, R., et al.: Complications in the urinary tract related to treatment of carcinoma of the cervix. South. Med. J., *66*:228–236, 1973.
104. Shingleton, H.M., Fowler, W.C., and Pepper, F.D.: Ureteral strictures following therapy for carcinoma of the cervix. Cancer, *24*:77–83, 1969.
105. Slater, J.M., and Fletcher, G.H.: Ureteral strictures after radiation therapy for carcinoma of the uterine cervix. Am. J. Roentgenol., *111*:269–272, 1971.
106. Taylor, J.S.: The behaviour of the ureters following radiotherapy and Wertheim hysterectomy. Br. J. Urol., *49*:203–206, 1977.

107. Underwood, P.B., Lutz, M.H., and Smoak, D.L.: Ureteral injury following irradiation therapy for carcinoma of the cervix. Obstet. Gynecol., 49:663–669, 1977.

Gunshot Wounds and Knife Injuries of the Ureter

108. Busch, F.M., Chenault, O.W., Jr., Zinner, N.R., et al.: Urological aspects of veterans' war injuries. J. Urol., 97:763–765, 1967.
109. Byers, W.L.: Pertinent data in 27 wounds to ureter among 3154 abdominal cases. In Forward Surgery of the Severely Wounded, Vol. 1, pp. 373–377. Headquarters, 2nd Auxiliary Surgical Group, U.S. Army, 1945.
110. Clarke, G.B., and Leadbetter, W.F.: Management of wounds and injuries of genito-urinary tract: A review of reported experience in World War II. J. Urol., 67:719–739, 1952.
111. Culp, O.S.: War wounds of the genito-urinary tract. J. Urol., 57:1117–1128, 1947.
112. Eickenberg, H.U., and Amin, M.: Gunshot wounds to the ureter. J. Trauma, 16:562–565, 1976.
113. Elkin, D.C., and Ward, W.C.: Gunshot wounds of the abdomen. Ann. Surg., 118:780–787, 1943.
114. Everidge, J., and Barnes, D.R.: Gunshot wounds of the ureter: Three cases with preservation of ureter in two. Br. J. Urol., 18:166–175, 1946.
115. Fisher, S., Young, D.A., Malin, J., et al.: Ureteral gunshot wounds. J. Urol., 108:238–239, 1972.
116. Fronstein, R.M., and Epstein, I.M.: On injuries of kidney and ureter, abstract. Bull. War Med., 5:19–20, 1944.
117. Fullerton, A.: Gunshot wounds of the kidney and ureter as seen at the base. Br. J. Surg., 5:248–285, 1917.
118. Gordon-Taylor, B.: Complicated injuries of the urinary tract. Br. J. Urol., 12:1–28, 1940.
119. Graham, W.H.: Management of injuries to the genitourinary system during war. J. Urol., 57:73–78, 1947.
120. Hawes, L.E.: Late effects of battle wounds in the genitourinary tract. J. Urol., 56:561–583, 1946.
121. Heller, E.: War wounds of the upper urinary tract. J. Urol., 72:149–161, 1954.
122. Holder, S., Hicks, C.C., O'Brien, D.P., et al.: Gunshot wounds of the ureter: A 15-year review of 63 consecutive cases. J. Urol., 116:562–564, 1976.
123. Howley, C.P., and Howley, T.F.: Gunshot wounds of the ureter. Am. J. Surg., 27:513–517, 1939.
124. Kimbrough, J.C.: War wounds of the urogenital tract. J. Urol., 55:179–189, 1946.
125. Kimbrough, J.C.: Urology in the European theater of operations. J. Urol., 57:1105–1116, 1947.
126. Lankford, R., Block, N.L., and Politano, V.A.: Gunshot wounds of the ureter: A review of 10 cases. J. Trauma, 14:848–852, 1974.
127. Liroff, S.A., Pouter, J.E., Pierce, J.N., Jr.: Gunshot wounds of the ureter: 5-year experience. J. Urol., 118:552–553, 1977.
128. Lloyd, F.A.: Historical notes on Twelfth General Hospital (U.S.): War injuries of the ureter. Quart. Bull. Northwest. Univ. Med. Sch., 30:74–79, 1956.
129. O'Heeron, M.K.: The management of trauma of the genitourinary tract in battle casualties at an evacuation hospital during the Northern and Central Burma Campaigns 1944 and 1945. J. Urol., 57:1184–1193, 1947.
130. Pugh, W.S.: Cases of ureteral injury. Am. Med., 41:227–230, 1935.
131. Pumphrey, J.D., Joslin, A.H., and Lich, R., Jr.: Missile wounds of the ureter. J. Trauma, 2:89–95, 1962.
132. Rajo Rao, A.K., and Walter, J.F.: Arteriographic diagnosis of a gunshot injury to the ureter. Radiology, 121:322, 1976.
133. Robinson, J.N., Culp, O.S., Suby, H.I., et al.: Injuries to the genito-urinary tract in the European theatre of operations. J. Urol., 56:498–507, 1946.
134. Rohner, T.J., Jr.: Delayed ureteral fistula from high velocity missiles: Report of 3 cases. J. Urol., 105:63–64, 1971.
135. Rouffilange, F., Neveux, J.Y., and Guilmet, D.: Nine cases of war wounds of the ureter. J. Urol. Med. Chir., 65:478–486, 1959.
136. Rusche, C.F.: Injury of the ureter due to gunshot wounds. J. Urol., 60:63–75, 1948.
137. Salvatierra, O., Rigdon, W.O., Norris, D.M., et al.: Vietnam experience with 252 urological war injuries. J. Urol., 101:613–620, 1969.
138. Swersie, A.K.: Experiences and lessons of emergency urological surgery in war. J. Urol., 57:938–944, 1947.
139. Van Buskirk, K.E., and Kimbrough, J.C.: Urological surgery in combat. J. Urol., 71:639–646, 1954.
140. Walker, J.A.: Injuries of the ureter due to external violence. J. Urol., 102:410–413, 1969.
141. Whitby, T.E.: Injury of the ureter. Br. J. Urol., 13:165–168, 1941.
142. Young, H.H.: Wounds of the urogenital tract in modern warfare. J. Urol., 47:59–108, 1942.

Late Results of Ureteral Injury

143. Auvigne, J.: Les résultats élongés de l'urétérotomie pour calcul. J. Urol. Paris, 60:884–898, 1954.
144. Auvray, P.: Late results of reparative surgery of the ureter. Acta. Urol. Belg., 29:91–93, 1961.
145. Davis, J.E., Cortijo, R., and Beneventi, F.A.: Traumatic pseudocyst of ureter. Urol. Int., 16:91–102, 1963.
146. De Laet, M.: Les Sequelles Traumatiques. Paris, Masson, 1952.
147. Dossogne, M.: Late results of reparative surgery of the ureter. Acta. Urol. Belg., 29:95, 1961.
148. Eddy, R.W., and Miller, F.H.: Postoperative urinary tract sequelae in total hysterectomy. Am. J. Obstet. Gynec., 33:85–90, 1937.
149. Judd, E.S.: The results of operations for the removal of stones from the ureter. Ann. Surg., 71:128–138, 1920.
150. Rhamy, R.K., and Stander, R.W.: Postradiation ureteral stricture. Surg. Gynecol. Obstet., 113:615–622, 1961.
151. Ribeiro, B.F., and Quartey, J.K.M.: Traumatic avulsion of the ureter with obstruction, pseudocyst formation and hypertension. Br. J. Urol., 48:107–110, 1976.
152. Silagy, J.M., and Leichtling, J.J.: Ureteral fistula following surgery for inflammatory retrocecal mass. J. Mount Sinai Hosp. N.Y., 28:444–450, 1961.
153. Vanwelkenhuyzen, P.: Résultats eloinges de la chirurgie de l'uretère. Acta. Urol. Belg., 29:93–94, 1961.
154. Wincqz, P.J.: Résultats eloinges de la chirurgie reparatrice de l'uretère. Acta. Urol. Belg., 29:89–91, 1961.

Trauma-Induced Fistulas

Ureterolymphatic Fistulas

155. Ehrlich, R.M., Hecht, H.G., and Veenema, R.J.: Chyluria following aorto-iliac bypass graft: A unique method of radiologic diagnosis and review of the literature. J. Urol., 107:302–303, 1972.

Ureterocutaneous Fistulas

156. Aubert, J., Roland, D., and Casamayou, J.: Uretero-cutaneous fistula following resection of the rectum. J. Urol. Nephrol., (Paris) 82:100–106, 1976.
157. Fraser, R.A., and Leary, F.J.: Ureterocutaneous fistula following percutaneous renal biopsy. J. Urol., 109:931–933, 1973.
158. Rohner, T.J.: Delayed ureteral fistula from high velocity missiles: Report of 3 cases. J. Urol., 105:63–64, 1971.

Ureteroarterial Fistulas

159. Cowen, R.: Uretero-arterial fistula. J. Urol., 73:801–803, 1955.
160. Davidson, O.W., and Smith, R.P.: Uretero-arterial fistula. J. Urol., 42257–262, 1939.
161. Reiner, R.J., Conway, G.F., and Threlkeld, R.: Ureteroarterial fistula. J. Urol., 113:24–25, 1975.
162. Rennick, J.M., Link, O.P., and Palmer, J.M.: Spontaneous rupture of an iliac artery aneurysm into a ureter. A case report and review of the literature. J. Urol., 116:111–113, 1976.
163. Shultz, M.L., Ewing, D.D., and Lovett, V.F.: Fistula between iliac aneurysm and distal stump of ureter with hematuria: A case report. J. Urol., 112:585–586, 1974.
164. Taylor, W.N., and Reinhart, H.L.: Mycotic aneurysm of common iliac artery with supture into right ureter. J. Urol., 42:21–26, 1939.
165. Whitmore, W.F., Jr.: Uretero-arterial fistula and uretero-vaginal fistula: Report of case. Urologia, 21:184–188, 1954.

Ureterouterine Fistulas

166. Barton, J.J., Grier, E.A., and Mutchnik, D.L.: Uretero-uterine fistula as a complication of elective abortion. Obstet. Gynecol., 52:815–845, 1978.
167. Galka, M., and Dlugopolski, S.: Uretero-uterine fistulas. Ginekol. Pol., 46:989–994, 1975.
168. Hardt, W., and Borgmann, V.: Uretero-uterine fistula after abortion. Z. Urol. Nephrol., 68:761–764, 1975.

Ureteroperitoneal Fistulas

169. Alleman, R., Cauduro, J.B., and Ramos, L.D.: Acute abdomen caused by spontaneous ureteroperitoneal fistula. Rev. Paul. Med., 61:270–272, 1962.
170. Arduino, G.J.: Ureteroperitoneal fistula: Case report of a late bullet wound complication. J. Urol., 73:990–994, 1955.
171. Bourdeau, G.V.: Urinary ascites secondary to ureteroperitoneal fistula. Urology, 4:209–211, 1974.
172. Everett, H.S.: Ureteroperitoneal fistula with urinary ascites. J. Urol., 78:585–591, 1957.
173. Hunner, G.L., and Everett, H.S.: Ureteroperitoneal fistula with urinary ascites and chronic peritonitis. J.A.M.A., 95:327–333, 1930.
174. Hunner, G.L., and Everett, H.S.: Ureteroperitoneal fistula with urinary ascites, a second case. J. Urol., 28:333–341, 1932.

Ureterovaginal Fistulas

175. Brunschwig, A., and Frick, H.C.: Urinary tract fistulas following radical surgical treatment of carcinoma of the cervix. Am. J. Obstet. Gynecol., 72:479–488, 1956.

176. Burch, J.C., Chalfont, R.L., and Johnson, J.W.: Technic for prevention of uretero-vaginal fistula following abdominal hysterectomy: Preservation of uterine blood supply. Ann. Surg., 161:832–837, 1965.
177. Calame, R.J., and Nelson, J.H., Jr.: Ureterovaginal fistula as a complication of radical pelvic surgery. Arch. Surg., 94:876–880, 1967.
178. Carter, R.G.: Ureterovaginal fistula. J. Urol., 71:200–207, 1954.
179. Cid, L.: Ureterovaginal fistula: Report of a case with a fused kidney and double ureter cured by heminephrectomy. J. Urol., 86:54–56, 1961.
180. Gitsch, E.: Prophylaxis of urologic and surgical complications resulting from radical operations for cervical carcinoma. Wien Klin. Wochenschr., 82:579–582, 1970.
181. Green, T.H., Jr.: Ureteral suspension for prevention of ureteral complications following radical Wertheim hysterectomy. Obstet. Gynecol., 28:1–11, 1966.
182. Gurevich, M.N.: On a case report contribution to the pathogenesis of ureteral vaginal fistula. Urol. Nephrol. Mosk., 26:60–61, 1961.
183. Higgins, C.C.: Ureteral injuries during surgery: A review of 87 cases. J.A.M.A., 199:82–88, 1967.
184. Koyangi, T., Takamatsu, T., Kaneta, T., et al.: A spontaneous vesico-ectopic ureterovaginal fistula in a girl. J. Urol., 118:871–872, 1977.
185. Lee, R.A., and Symmonds, R.E.: Ureterovaginal fistula. Am. J. Obstet. Gynecol., 109:1032–1035, 1971.
186. Macasaet, M.A., Lu, T., and Nelson, J.H., Jr.: Ureterovaginal fistula as a complication of radical pelvic surgery. Am. J. Obstet. Gynecol., 124:757–760, 1976.
187. Meigs, J.V.: Surgical Treatment of Cancer of the Cervix, p. 149. New York, Grune & Stratton, 1954.
188. Nelson, J.H., Jr.: Atlas of Radical Pelvic Surgery. New York, Appleton-Century-Crofts, 1969.
189. Prosser, I., and Velati, G.: Acquired uretero-vaginal fistulas. Rass. Int. Clin. Ter., 42:1159–1177, 1962.
190. Symmonds, R.E.: Morbidity and complications of radical hysterectomy and pelvic lymph node dissection. Am. J. Obstet. Gynecol., 91:663–678, 1966.
191. Talbert, L.M., Palumbo, L., Shingleton, H., et al.: Urologic complication of radical hysterectomy for carcinoma of the cervix. South. Med. J., 58:11–17, 1965.
192. Ten Cate, H.W., Emmett, J.L., and Pratt, J.H.: Unusual ureterovaginal fistula: Report of a case. J. Urol., 88:477–479, 1962.
193. Tueter, K.J., and Mathison, W.: Uretero-vaginal fistula. Ann. Chir. Gynaecol., 65:408–411, 1976.
194. Vianna, J.B.: Ureteral complications following Wertheim-Meigs operation for cancer of the cervix. Urol. Int., 19:271–279, 1965.
195. Wallace, D.M.: Uretero-vaginal fistula. Br. J. Urol., 44:617–622, 1972.

Ureterocolic Fistulas

196. Earlam, M.S.: Migration of a ureteric calculus to the bladder via a ureterocolic and a vesicocolic fistula. Aust. N.Z. J. Surg., 47:519–520, 1977.
197. Haysom, A.H.: Case of spontaneous left ureterocolonic fistula associated with abscess in left loan and fecal fistula. Br. J. Surg., 43:646–649, 1956.
198. Krishna, A.U., Dhar, N., Pletman, R.J., et al.: Spontaneous closure of ureterocolic fistula secondary to diverticulitis. J. Urol., 118:476–477, 1977.

199. Sankaran, R., Chesley, A.E., and Khadilkar, M.C.: Ureterocolic fistula associated with Hodgkin's disease. Urology, *4*:450–453, 1974.

200. Simon, O., Yuval, E.: Chronic cecoureteral fistula following cystectomy and cutaneous ureterostomy: A case report. Eur. Urol., *3*:243–244, 1977.

201. Winter, C.C.: Ureterocolic fistula. J. Urol., *108*:396–398, 1972.

202. Winter, C.C., Linderholm, B.E., and Shiraki, I.W.: Ureterocolic fistula. Am. J. Surg., *125*:338–342, 1973.

Ureteroileal Fistulas

203. Appleyard, I., and Lloyd-Jones, W.: A case of complete uretero-ileal fistula. Br. J. Urol., *49*:494, 1977.

204. Blumgart, L.H., and Thakur, K.: Uretero-ileal fistula due to Crohn's disease. Br. J. Surg., *58*469–470, 1971.

205. Critchley, C.F.: A case of uretero-ileal fistula. Br. J. Surg., *54*:812–813, 1967.

206. Flaster, S.L., and Bush, I.M.: Ureteroileal fistula: Report of a case complicated by increased chloride reabsorption from the ileal segment. J. Urol., *109*:589–591, 1973.

207. Goodwin, W.E., Winter, C.C., and Turner, R.D.: Fistula between bowel and urinary tract. J. Urol., *84*:95–105, 1960.

208. Scott, W.P.: Uretero-ileal fistula. Br. J. Radiol., *38*:957–958, 1963.

209. Shiozaki, H., Takai, S., Iwamoto, T., et al.: Idiopathic ureteroduodenal fistula. J. Urol., *113*:714–715, 1975.

210. Wilson, J.D., Emmett, J.L., and Pratt, J.H.: Uretero-ileal fistula: Report of a case. Mayo Clin. Proc., *42*:155–160, 1967.

When considering tumors of the urothelium of the upper urinary tract, the calyces, renal pelvis and ureter must be considered as a continuum. Therefore there is some overlap with Chapter 10, Tumors of the Kidney. Renal carcinomas constitute about 85 to 87 per cent of all upper urinary tract tumors with about 10 to 12 per cent representing carcinomas of the renal pelvis and 1 to 2 per cent, sarcomas. Approximately 1 per cent of all malignant tumors of the upper urinary tract occur in the ureter.

CLASSIFICATION OF PELVIC AND URETERAL TUMORS

I. Primary Tumors
    A. Epithelial (malignant)
        1. Transitional cell carcinoma (papillomas)
        2. Squamous cell carcinoma
        3. Adenocarcinoma: rare
    B. Mesodermal (malignant)
        Sarcomas: rare
    C. Mesodermal (benign): polypoid or sessile
        Fibromas, fibromyomas, hemangioma, lymphangioma
II. Secondary Tumors
    A. By way of urinary tract: implants from bladder or kidney
    B. By direct extension: from cervix and body of uterus, rectosigmoid, and rarely, from other retroperitoneal tumors
    C. Metastases through the blood or the lymphatics: from primary tumor in prostate, stomach, cervix, bladder, breast, bowel, lung, or ovary

21

Tumors of the Ureter

All epithelial tumors are considered malignant. The term papilloma implies a low-grade papillary transitional cell carcinoma. The polyp (see below) represents a mesenchymal benign tumor covered by epithelium that projects into the lumen. The term papillary refers to the histologic appearance of the lesion and is not synonymous with polypoid. Papillary tumors may be polypoid or sessile. The following graph illustrates the types of lesions, their incidence, and the tendency toward multiplicity. The figures given are approximate.

TUMORS OF THE UROTHELIUM OF THE PELVIS AND URETER

—Benign tumors 10%
—Sarcoma (rare)
—Adenocarcinoma (rare)
—Squamous carcinoma (rare) 5% to 6%
—Transitional cell carcinoma 80% to 85%
    Transitional cell carcinoma can be subdivided as follows:

Transitional Cell Carcinoma

Nonpapillary 20%   Papillary 80%
All infiltrating,
Single lesions   Infiltrating   Noninfiltrating
                        50%   50%
                Approximately 40%
                to 50% are multiple.

The incidence of infiltrating papillary tumors is less in the ureter (35–40%) than in the renal pelvis (50%).

Multiplicity is ipsilateral in 85 per cent. Whether this represents multicentric growth, direct extension (seeding or mucosal) or extension by way of lymphatics or blood vessels, or combinations of the above is not known.

Multiplicity is more common in the ureter (50%) than in the renal pelvis (40%).

The cure rate by histologic criteria is best for papillary noninfiltrating, next for papillary infiltrating (see Fig. 21–15) and least for nonpapillary infiltrating (see Figs. 21–16, 21–17).

Renal pelvic carcinomas are three times more frequent in men and tend to occur in the older population over the age of 60. As noted previously, approximately 40 to 50 per cent of papillary lesions tend to be multiple, primarily on the ipsilateral side affecting the ureter or bladder. It is not known whether these are independent multiple foci, lymphatic or hematogenous extensions, or luminal seeding of tumor cells, but the first consideration is the most probable and most generally accepted. *If a papillary tumor is present, careful investigation of the ipsilateral ureter and bladder must be made for possible multiple lesions* (see Figs. 21–10 to 21–13).

The nonpapillary transitional cell carcinomas (see Figs. 21–16, 21–17) (20%) are usually single, are infiltrating tumors, and have a worse prognosis. Squamous cell carcinoma (see Figs. 21–14, 21–20) is rare, is usually associated with chronic infection, calculi, or leukoplakia, whereas adenocarcinoma (mucus producing) is even rarer and is almost always associated with calculi and infection.

PRIMARY URETERAL TUMORS

Primary malignant tumors of epithelial origin usually are found in elderly patients (5th to 7th decade), predominantly male, with the primary symptoms of painless hematuria. The usual ureteral tumor is papillary transitional cell carcinoma with a lower incidence of infiltration than in the renal pelvis. Approximately 50 per cent of these lesions are multiple, either initially or with a second lesion occurring at a later date in the distal ureter or bladder (see Figs. 21–10 to 21–13). Nonpapillary transitional cell carcinomas are less common than in the renal pelvis but are difficult to diagnose because they may present as a stricturelike lesion (see Figs. 21–16, 21–17).

The diagnostic triad consists of pain, hematuria, and a palpable mass in the renal area. Pain is present in over 50 per cent of the cases and is secondary to distention of the ureter. Hematuria is present in over 75 per cent of the cases. A palpable mass representing a hydronephrotic kidney is present in approximately 40 per cent of cases. Although pain is a frequent finding, it is far less frequent than in ureteral calculi, and therefore *painless hematuria always must be regarded as a possible indication of a ureteral tumor.*

Owing to an awareness of the clinical symptomatology and the development of more adequate diagnostic techniques, earlier diagnoses are now being made. It is not uncommon in the early lesions that are not obstructing to obtain excellent visualization of the upper urinary tract without evidence of hydronephrosis or ureterectasis.

The majority of ureteral carcinomas occur in the

lower third of the ureter (50%), a segment of the ureter that is frequently poorly visualized in urography. There are several important maxims to be stressed in the diagnostic work-up of patients suspected of having carcinoma of the ureter:

1. In all patients past middle age with recurrent or persistent gross hematuria, when a lesion is not visualized in the kidney, the entire ureter must be clearly visualized. If this cannot be obtained in the urogram, a bulb tip retrograde study is indicated.

2. In young patients (under 35 years) with unexplained hematuria with a normal urogram, the possibility of a small hemangioma or arteriovenous malformation must be considered.

3. Hydronephrosis of unknown etiology in middle-aged or elderly patients should always be suggestive of pelvic or ureteral carcinoma.

4. A stricture of unknown etiology in the lower third of the ureter may represent ureteral carcinoma (Figs. 21–16, 21–17).

The major roentgenographic features of primary papillary transitional cell carcinoma (Figs. 21–1 to 21–15) of the ureter are as follows:

1. *Intraluminal filling defect with local dilatation of the ureter.* The defect frequently appears "pock-marked" owing to the irregular papillary surface (Fig. 21–2). The dilatation due to mucosal infiltration may be more striking than the filling defect in some nonobstructive lesions.

2. *Cupping of the contrast medium around the superior or inferior margin of the growth* (Fig. 21–6). This is produced by the leading edge of the tumor protruding into the lumen.

3. *Fixation of the lesion to the ureteral wall.*

4. *Varying degrees of proximal obstruction* (Figs. 21–3, 21–9).

5. *Coiling of the retrograde catheter below the lesion* (Figs. 21–7, 21–8). The growing intraluminal mass produces dilatation of the ureter below the tumor, allowing the catheter to coil upon itself when striking the obstructing lesion. The dilatation may also be observed with contrast medium (Figs. 21–6, 21–10). With obstructing calculi, the ureter immediately below the lesion is collapsed, and the lumen usually is not of sufficient size to allow coiling of the catheter (Fig. 21–1).

Infiltrating lesions, either papillary or nonpapillary, but particularly the latter, may present as short or long strictures of the ureter. Squamous cell carcinoma is rare, less common than in the renal pelvis. These malignant lesions resemble inflammatory strictures and metastatic lesions (Figs. 21–14 to 21–17).

Angiography is rarely required for diagnosis of ureteral carcinoma. The angiogram usually suggests a hypovascular lesion. There is usually some increase in vascularity, and if the tumor is large enough, a faint stain may be seen. Vessel encasement is common and proximal hydronephrosis may be present. These changes are similar to those seen in renal pelvic carcinoma and frequently mimic an inflammatory lesion or abscess (Figs. 21–18 to 21–21).

In functioning kidneys, a ureteral tumor can be visualized by urography or pyelography. In nonfunctioning kidneys, pyelography may visualize the lesion. If pyelography is contraindicated or unsuccessful and if ultrasound demonstrates a dilated collecting system, a skinny needle puncture can be performed followed by an antegrade pyelogram (Fig. 21–9). Following the method described in Chapter

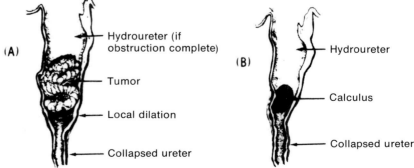

FIG. 21–1. Carcinoma of the ureter. **(A)** Localized dilatation of the ureter below the tumor, allowing space for catheter coiling. Such dilatation is common with expanding intraluminal lesions. **(B)** Calculus producing proximal hydroureter but with collapse of the distal ureter. (Bergman, H., Friedenberg, R.M., Sayegh, V.: Am. J. Roentgen., 86:707–717, 1961)

20 for percutaneous nephrostomy, a brush biopsy can be performed.

Primary malignant tumors of mesodermal origin are extremely rare. They consist of varying types of sarcomas, with the same symptom complex as that produced by papillary carcinomas of the ureter. The radiographic appearance is identical with that of the primary infiltrating carcinomas, but the prognosis is poor.

Benign Tumors of the Ureter. The symptomatology and the radiographic findings are similar to those of their malignant counterparts. The true polyps may be defined more clearly; a pedicle may be demonstrated, and because they do not invade the ureteral wall they rarely obstruct the ureter. The papilloma (carcinoma) is more common in the lower third of the ureter, whereas the polyp occurs most frequently in the proximal third. Although polyps are common in young adults, transitional cell carcinoma is uncommon prior to 40 years of age in the United States. As mentioned previously the polyp represents a mesenchymal tumor consisting of a thick core of fibrous connective tissue covered by normal epithelium. The polyp may grow to several centimeters in length, with most of its mass lying free in the lumen. Therefore, in different films it may move in position and, on the retrograde study, reverse its direction from that in the urogram. The epithelial carcinoma (papilloma) is usually villous or sessile, whereas the ureteral polyp frequently arises on a pedicle (Table 21-1). The radiographic diagnosis of polyp is usually not difficult, because it is frequently outlined by a rim of contrast material that surrounds the intralumenal mass (Figs. 21-28 to 21-31).

Nonpolypoid, benign lesions of the ureter are rare and are frequently missed on urography. Similar to tumors of the renal pelvis, they may represent any form of mesenchymal tumor. They occur submucosally and are fixed in position. One type of benign tumor reported in children is fibrous polyps, which may cause obstruction and pain. They usually occur in the proximal ureter and are frequently multiple (Figs. 21-29 to 21-31).

SECONDARY TUMORS OF THE URETER

Extension Within the Urinary System. The most common secondary ureteral tumor is from a similar lesion in the calyx (usually transitional cell carcinoma), renal pelvis, or proximal ureter (Figs. 21-32 to 21-35). The tendency for multiplicity of lesions has been discussed previously. The lesions in the ureter may arise synchronously or at widely spaced intervals. If multiple lesions present simultaneously, the usual approach is to consider the proximal lesion primary and the distal secondary. Obviously both may be primary, that is, multifocal lesions. This is why surgery usually requires removal of the kidney, ureter, and bladder cuff to avoid missing multiple lesions or lesions which will appear in future months or years. Some surgical attempts at local resection have been performed in an effort to preserve renal function. This is particularly true in some endemic areas (Yugoslavia) where bilateral lesions and endemic nephropathy, producing renal failure, are relatively common or in cases in which preservation of renal function is important, that is, damaged contralateral kidney. The clinical diagnosis and the radiographic findings in secondary tumors are no different from those seen in primary tumors of the ureter, except that the picture may be complicated by metastatic involvement elsewhere in the body. Occasionally, adenocarcinomas of the kidney metastasize to the ureter (Figs. 21-35 to 21-36).

TABLE 21-1

A Comparison of the Stromal Ureteral Polyp and the Epithelial Papilloma*

Polyp
1. Usually young adults, 20 to 40 years of age
2. Intermittent pain, usually without bleeding
3. Mainly upper third of ureter
4. Roentgenogram
A. Long, narrow filling defect
B. Pedicle frequently seen
C. Margins of lesion smooth
D. Obstruction not common

Papilloma
1. Usually older patients, 50 to 70 years of age
2. Usually asymptomatic until it bleeds
3. Often lower third of ureter
4. Roentgenogram
A. Shorter defect, similar to that of carcinoma
B. No pedicle
C. Margins shaggy and irregular
D. Frequent obstruction

* Adapted from E.J. Collier.

Extension From Distant Sources. Metastases to the ureter from distant sources are rare. They may occur from almost any organ in the body but have been reported with slightly greater frequency from the prostate, stomach, breast, lung, and colon (Figs. 21–36 to 21–43). It is difficult to state whether a lymphomatous process such as Hodgkin's disease metastasizes to a ureter or whether the ureter is involved in a multicentric origin of the lymphoma. These metastatic lesions may occur at any site along the ureter and frequently are seen in both ureters. The lesion tends to involve the ureteral wall, frequently presenting as a "stricture-like" or encasing tumor. The ureter is usually not an early site of metastasis, and in most cases other evidence of distant metastasis is present. Metastatic lesions are brought to the ureter through the blood vessels or the lymphatics.

Direct Extension From Neighboring Lesions. A third method of metastatic involvement of the ureters is by direct extension from neighboring malignant lesions, which invade the ureter from the serosal side to the lumen. This is seen most commonly from carcinoma of the cervix but may occur from other retroperitoneal tumors and occasionally from extensive carcinoma involving the rectum or the sigmoid (Figs. 21–44 to 21–46).

Many malignant lesions, particularly the lymphomas, may displace the ureters without actual invasion. This occurs when marked retroperitoneal nodal involvement is present with deviation of the ureters laterally by the massive nodes (Figs. 21–47, 21–48). Other lesions, such as tumors or cysts of the kidneys, retroperitoneal tumors, abscesses, and ovarian cysts also cause displacement of the ureters. Deviations of the ureter are considered separately in Chapter 22, Miscellaneous Conditions of the Ureter.

CHAPTER 21, ILLUSTRATIONS

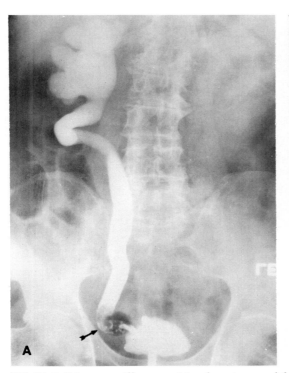
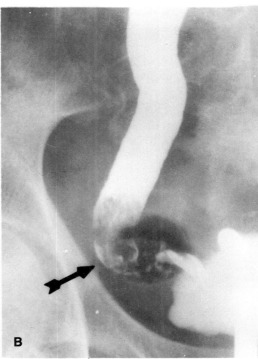

FIG. 21–2. Primary papillary transitional carcinoma of the ureter. Elderly man with renal colic and hematuria. The urogram revealed poor function with severe hydronephrosis. **(A)** The pyelogram demonstrated a sausage-shaped filling defect near the ureterovesical junction. **(B)** In the enlarged view of this area, note the irregular areas of contrast in marginal crevices of the tumor. The lesion was prolapsing through the ureteral orifice. The tumor was removed by nephroureterectomy, including a large bladder cuff.

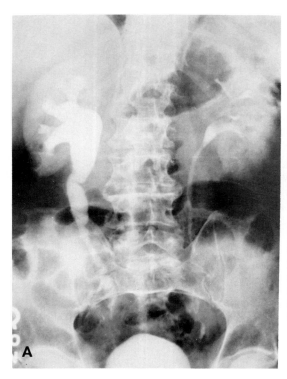

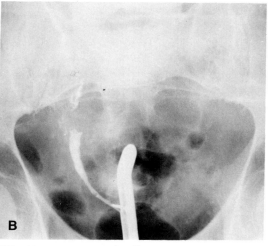

FIG. 21–3. Transitional cell carcinoma. Urogram (**A**) shows right pyelocalyectasis and proximal ureterectasis from distal ureteral obstruction. The lesion is not well defined. Pyelogram (**B**) shows typical cupped obstructive lesion.

FIG. 21–4. Primary carcinoma of the ureter in a 55-year-old man with painless hematuria. (**A**) The urogram revealed poor visualization of the proximal ureter. Small crescentic cupping (*arrow*) slightly above the 5th lumbar transverse process seen in one film of the urogram was ignored in the original report. (**B**) Pyelographic study revealed a large filling defect within the ureteral lumen at the junction of the lower and the middle thirds of the ureter. This finding is typical of the mass lesion seen in primary tumors of the ureter, with segmental dilatation of the ureter as the mass enlarges within the lumen. There is no ureterectasis, because obstruction has not occurred. A primary papillary carcinoma of the ureter was removed by nephroureterectomy. (Bergman, H., Friedenberg, R.M., Sayegh, V.: Am. J. Roentgen., 86:707–717, 1961)

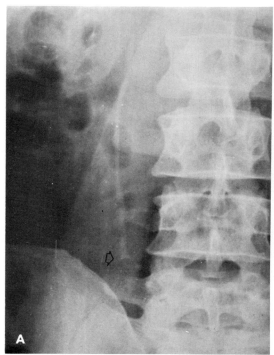

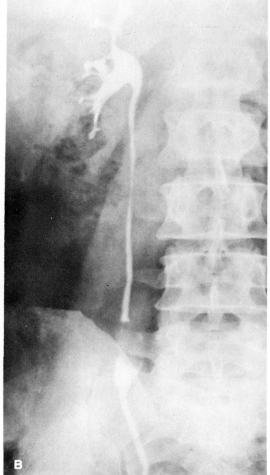

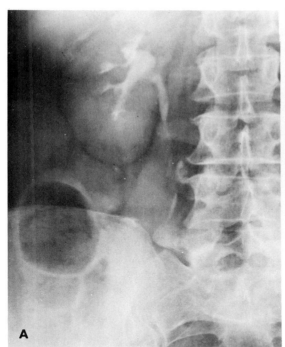

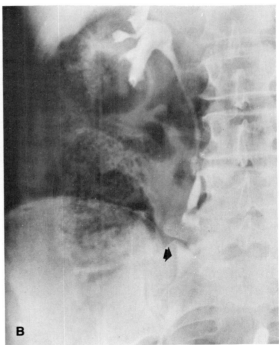

FIG. 21–5. Primary ureteral carcinoma. Elderly man presenting with renal colic and hematuria. **(A)** Excretory urography was interpreted as normal. Because of the persistent hematuria, a pyelogram was performed. **(B)** A mass lesion was observed at the level of L-5, producing a filling defect within the ureter with segmental dilatation. Note the increased width of the ureteral lumen below the tumor *(arrow)*. This case again emphasizes the necessity of obtaining a complete ureterogram in cases of hematuria. Surgery confirmed the presence of a papillary carcinoma of the ureter. (Bergman, H., Friedenberg, R.M., Sayegh, V.: Am. J. Roentgen., *86:707–717, 1961)*

FIG. 21–6. Primary carcinoma of the ureter. Elderly man with painless hematuria. Urography revealed pyelonephritis of the left kidney with poor visualization of the ureter. **(A)** Retrograde demonstrated an irregular filling defect in the distal end of the ureter, representing a primary carcinoma *(arrow)*. **(B)** A withdrawal film of the retrograde study reveals in better detail the expanding mass lesion completely within the ureteral lumen, with secondary dilatation of the ureter proximal and distal.

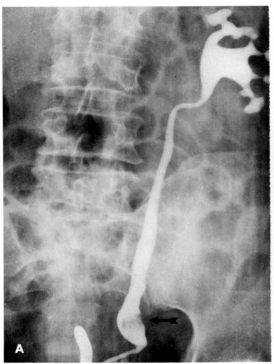

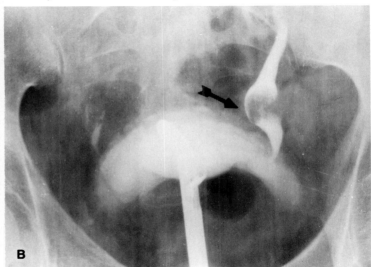

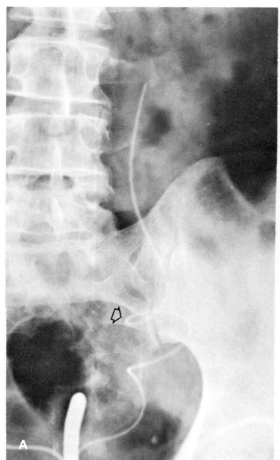

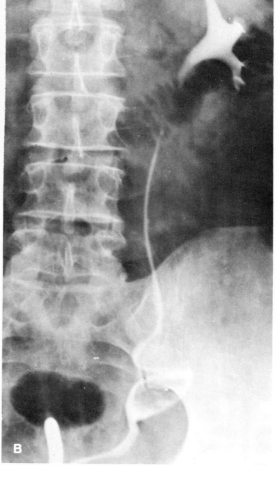

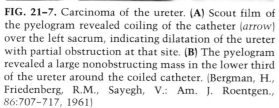

FIG. 21–7. Carcinoma of the ureter. **(A)** Scout film of the pyelogram revealed coiling of the catheter (*arrow*) over the left sacrum, indicating dilatation of the ureter with partial obstruction at that site. **(B)** The pyelogram revealed a large nonobstructing mass in the lower third of the ureter around the coiled catheter. (Bergman, H., Friedenberg, R.M., Sayegh, V.: Am. J. Roentgen., 86:707–717, 1961)

FIG. 21–8. Primary carcinoma of the ureter, causing obstruction. Elderly man with persistent gross hematuria of several weeks' duration. There was nonfunction of the right kidney in the urogram. Retrograde (illustration) revealed a complete obstruction in the lower third of the ureter with coiling of the tip of the catheter just below the obstructing lesion, indicating dilatation of the ureter distal to the obstruction. Surgery confirmed the presence of a primary carcinoma, completely obstructing the ureter. (Bergman, H., Friedenberg, R.M., Sayegh, V.: Am. J. Roentgen., 86:707–717, 1961)

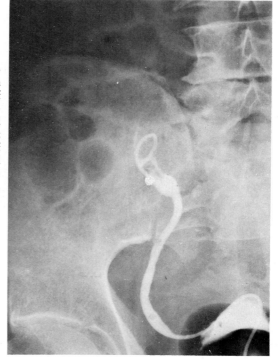

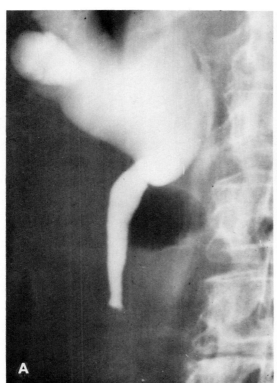

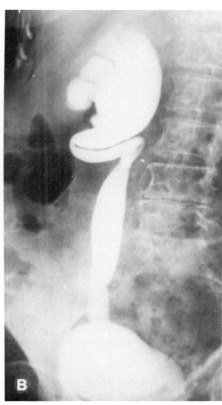

FIG. 21-9. Antegrade pyelogram. Two cases of transitional cell carcinoma of the ureter with proximal hydronephrosis confirmed by ultrasound. Percutaneous puncture of the renal pelvis was performed followed by injection of contrast medium. (**A**) Total obstruction in the right midureter. (**B**) Severe obstruction at the ureterovesical orifice.

FIG. 21-10. Bilateral ureteral carcinomas. Elderly man presented with back pain, flank pain, and hematuria. Bilateral pyelograms reveal intraluminal lesions in the distal thirds of both ureters. The lesion in the right ureter (**A**) was not obstructing, whereas the lesion in the left ureter (**B**) was obstructing. Whereas polyps rarely obstruct despite their large size, carcinomas frequently obstruct the ureter.

FIG. 21-11. Multiple papillary transitional cell carcinomas. Two separate lesions were present in the distal ureter (*arrows*). The proximal lesion was infiltrating (grade 4), the distal, noninfiltrating (grade 1). (Courtesy of Erich Lang, M.D.)

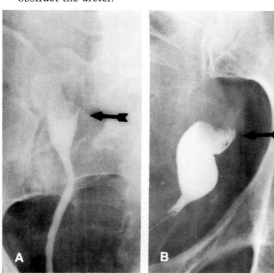

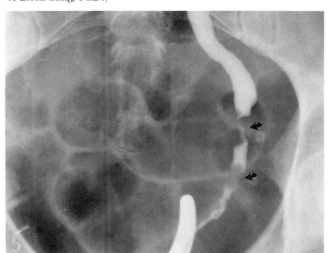

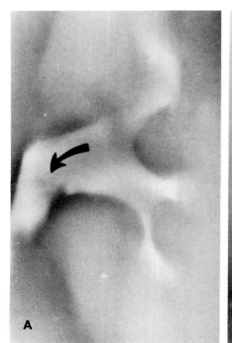

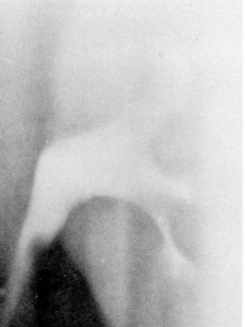

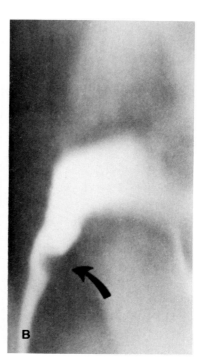

FIG. 21–12. Multiple papillary transitional cell carcinomas. Series of tomographic sections. **(A)** Lesion (*arrow*) at junction of pelvis and ureter. **(B)** Second separate lesion (*arrow*) in proximal ureter. (Courtesy of E.J. Palubinskas, M.D.)

FIG. 21–12a. Multiple ureteral carcinomas. **(A)** Pyelogram demonstrates a transitional cell carcinoma of the midureter. Segmental resection was performed with preservation of ureteral continuity. **(B)** Two months after surgery, a urogram showed good bilateral renal function. Note some irregularity of the left distal ureter (*arrow*), which was not well visualized and not noted at that time. Two and a half years later, the patient had several episodes of gross hematuria. **(C)** Left pyelogram shows a second carcinoma (*arrow*) of the distal ureter. Multiple carcinomas occur in 40 to 50% of patients with papillary transitional cell carcinoma of the renal pelvis or ureter.

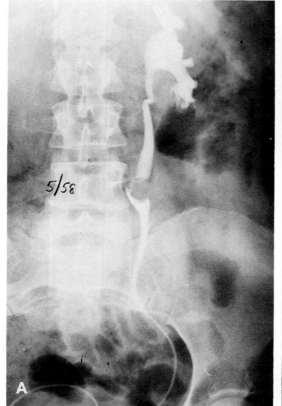

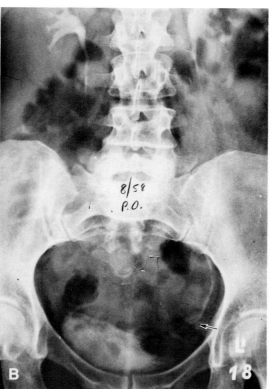

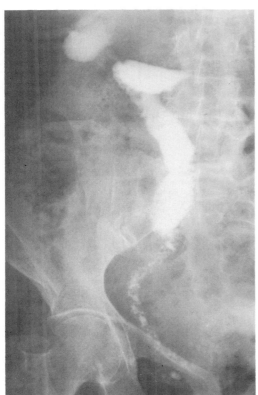

FIG. 21–13. Papillomatosis of ureter. The entire ureteral mucosa is covered with small grade 1 papillomas. The appearance mimics ureteritis cystica. The lesions varied in size from 1 to 2 mm to 7 or 8 mm in size. Nephrectomy and ureterectomy were performed. (Courtesy of Erich Lang, M.D.)

FIG. 21–14. Squamous cell carcinoma in a 74-year-old woman with a long history of chronic infection. Previous urograms suggested pyelitis and ureteritis. Current admission for gross hematuria. Pyelogram shows stricture of proximal ureter with mucosal infiltration throughout the renal pelvis. The entire lesion consisted of infiltrating squamous cell carcinoma.

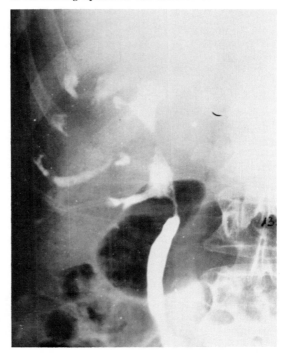

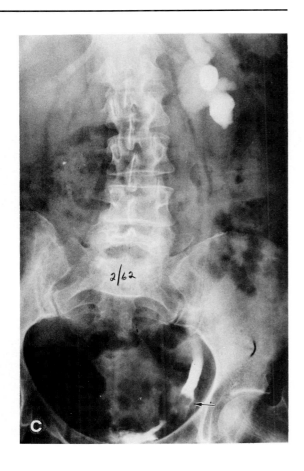

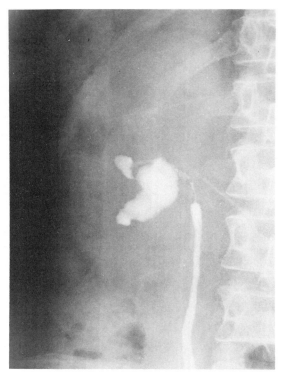

FIG. 21–15. Infiltrating papillary transitional cell carcinoma. Pyelogram reveals diffuse infiltrating lesion of proximal ureter and renal pelvis. Note the resemblance to the case shown in Fig. 21–14.

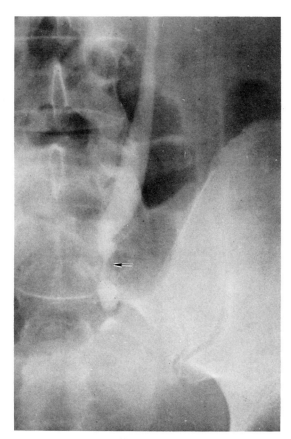

FIG. 21–16. Nonpapillary infiltrating transitional carcinoma. The lesion presented as a stricture (*arrow*) of the distal ureter in a 55-year-old man. Any unexplained stricture in the cancer age group must be suspect of carcinoma.

FIG. 21–17. (A, B) Nonpapillary infiltrating transitional cell carcinoma. Unusually long stricture of the pelvic ureter with proximal obstruction. Note the irregularity of the walls of the stricture suggesting irregular tumor growth. (Courtesy of Erich Lang, M.D.)

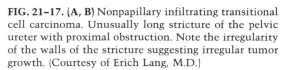

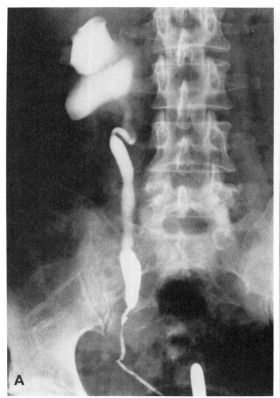

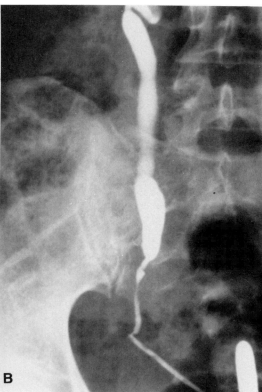

FIG. 21–17a. Infiltrating carcinoma of the ureter. A nephrostomy was performed because of severe hydronephrosis. Injection through the nephrostomy tube revealed a long, irregular, compressed proximal ureter with intraluminal defects. Surgery revealed a papillary infiltrating transitional cell carcinoma.

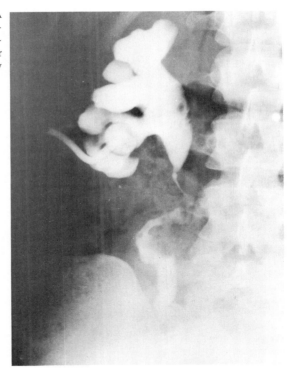

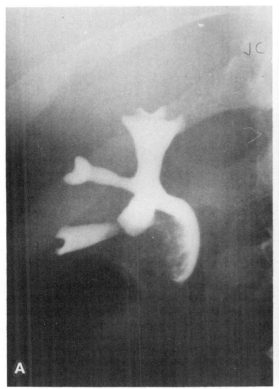

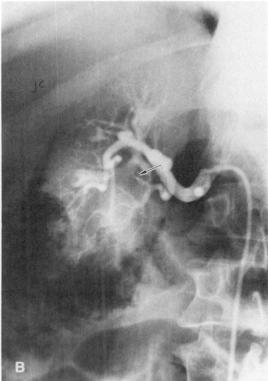

FIG. 21–18. Transitional carcinoma. **(A)** Pyelogram reveals irregular filling defect in renal pelvis. **(B)** Angiogram shows encasement (*arrow*) of a segmental vessel without significant increased vascularity.

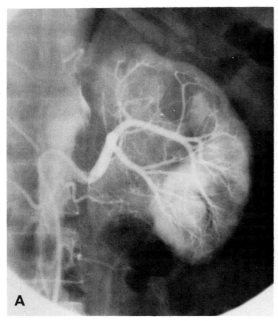

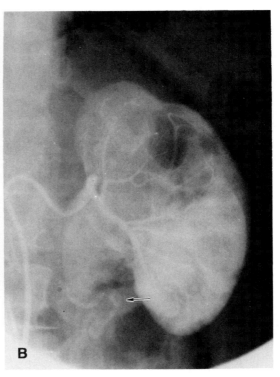

FIG. 21–19. Transitional carcinoma of the renal pelvis. Early film of the arteriogram **(A)** reveals increased vascularity in the renal pelvis. Late film **(B)** shows a tumor stain in the renal pelvis with large draining pelvic veins (*arrow*). The parenchymal changes were secondary to hydronephrosis.

FIG. 21–20. Squamous carcinoma of renal pelvis and proximal ureter. Scout film revealed calculi in renal pelvis and calcifications in renal parenchyma. There was no visualization in the urogram. Pyelogram **(A)** shows an obstructing, irregular, stricturelike lesion of proximal ureter (*arrow*) that was squamous carcinoma. Early **(B)** and late **(C)** angiograms showed complete replacement of renal parenchyma by a vascular tumor. ▶

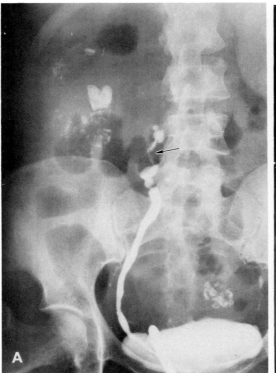

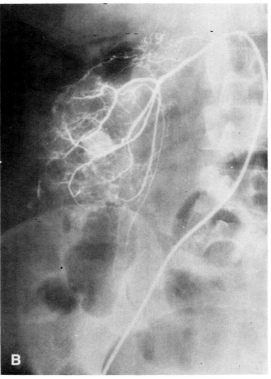

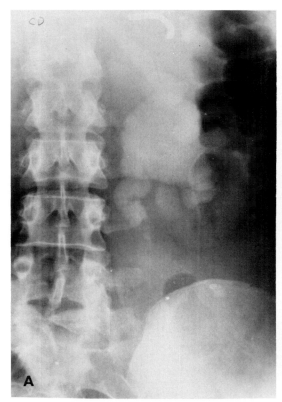

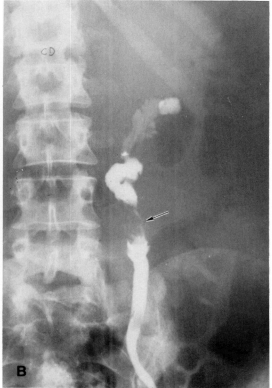

FIG. 21-21. Transitional carcinoma of ureter. Urogram (A) shows an obstructing lesion of the proximal ureter. Pyelogram (B) shows a long irregular filling defect (*arrow*) with distal cupping. This was an intraluminal tumor. The arteriogram (C) demonstrates renal hydronephrosis with a large pelvis outlined by a pelvic artery (*upper arrow*). Increased vasculature is present (*arrows*) in and around the ureteral tumor from ureteral and capsular arteries. (Courtesy of Morton Bosniak, M.D.)

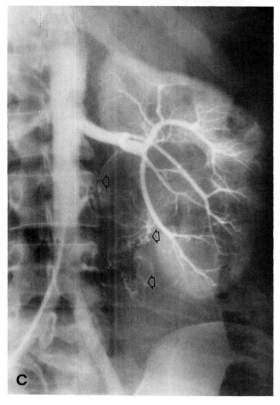

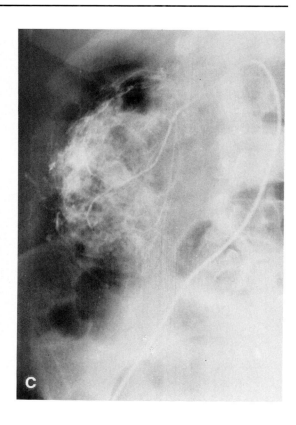

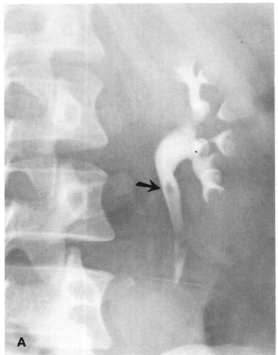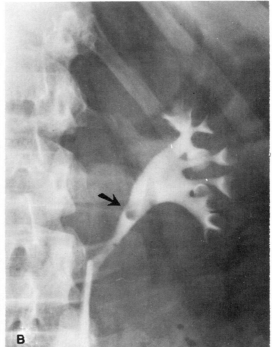

FIG. 21–22. Ureteral polyp. Middled-aged man admitted with intermittent colic and occasional hematuria. (A) The excretory urogram reveals an elongated filling defect in the proximal ureter, representing a ureteral polyp on a long stalk attached to the ureteral mucosa at the proximal end of the filling defect. The polyp conforms to the shape of the lumen of the ureter. (B) Pyelogram reveals the free end of the polyp to extend proximally into the renal pelvis. The *arrows* in the two films indicate the point of attachment to the ureteral wall. The change in direction of the polyp was produced by the retrograde injection. This demonstrates the free movement of a polyp, the lack of invasion or irregularity of the ureteral wall, the smooth, regular contour of the lesion, and the lack of obstruction despite the large size of the polyp. (Courtesy of Heino Provet, M.D.)

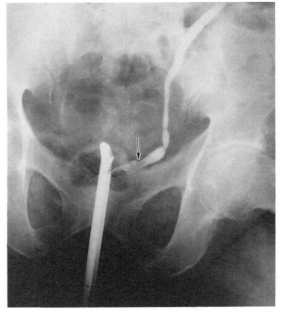

FIG. 21–23. Ureteral polyp. Small polyp (*arrow*) that, because of its location at the ureterovesical junction, was symptomatic.

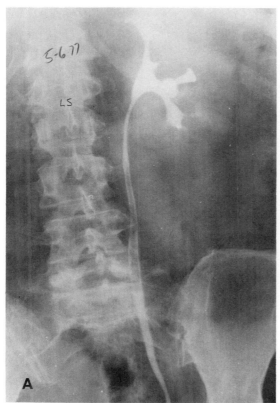

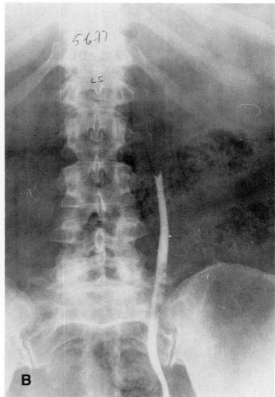

FIG. 21–24. Ureteral polyp. Urogram (**A**) shows typical defect of polyp outlined by contrast medium coating the ureteral wall. There is no obstruction. The polyp conforms to the size of the ureteral lumen. Pyelogram (**B**) produced temporary obstruction by displacing the polyp superiorly.

FIG. 21–25. Ureteral polyp. Fibroma in one of the duplicated ureters on the right side. Note pedicle just above *arrow*. (Courtesy of Jack Lapides, M.D.)

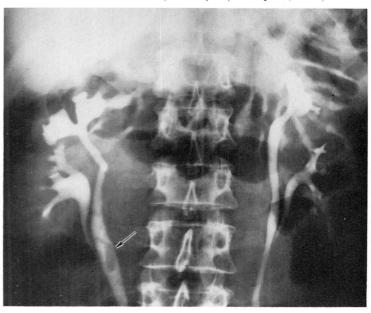

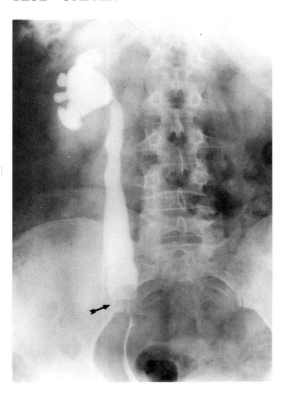

FIG. 21–26. Ureteral polyp. Intraluminal mass in lower third of the left ureter, partially obstructing. The border of the mass has smooth margins. Differentiation from carcinoma is not possible. (Courtesy of Keith Waterhouse, M.D.)

FIG. 21–27. Ureteral polyp. Right retrograde pyelogram revealed a large intraluminal filling defect in the distal third of the right ureter. Marked ureteral dilatation is present, but there was no significant obstruction in the urogram. At surgery this giant polyp, measuring 10 cm × 3 cm, was found to be attached to the ureter just below the ureteropelvic junction by a narrow pedicle (not visible in the illustrations). Two small 5-mm calculi also were present. (Howard, T.L.: J. Urol., 79:397–402, 1958)

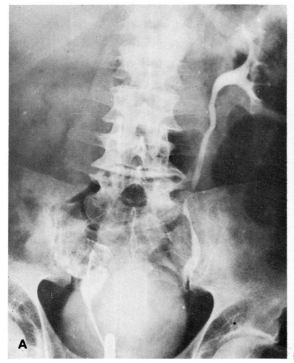 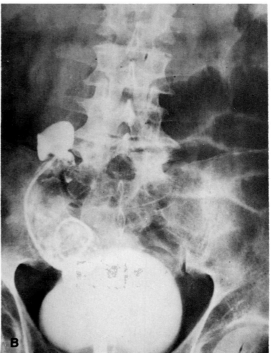

FIG. 21–28. Calyceal polyp. Child 6 years old with microscopic hematuria. Urogram failed to visualize a right mid calyx. Pyelogram shows large right mid calyx with a lucent intraluminal filling defect (*arrow*). Intrarenal reflux is present. Surgery revealed a submucosal benign polyp in the calyx.

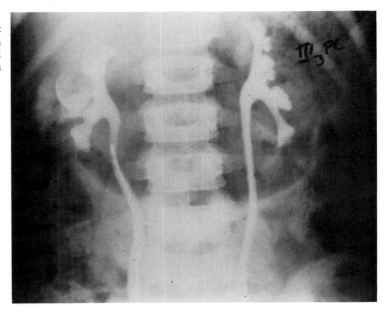

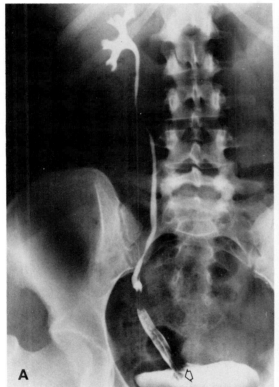

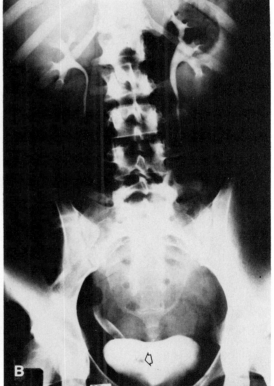

FIG. 21–28a. Ureteral polyp in a young man with intermittent pain and hematuria. (**A, B**) The radiolucent defect of the long polyp can be seen in the distal ureter of both films of the urogram. Part of the polyp has prolapsed into the bladder producing a radiolucent defect (*arrows*) and the clinical symptom of pain.

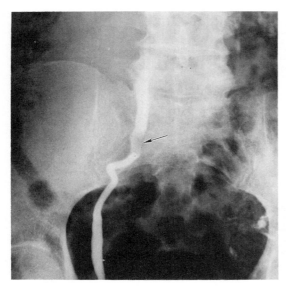

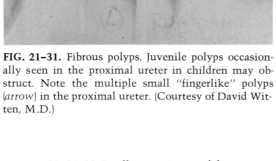

FIG. 21–31. Fibrous polyps. Juvenile polyps occasionally seen in the proximal ureter in children may obstruct. Note the multiple small "fingerlike" polyps (*arrow*) in the proximal ureter. (Courtesy of David Witten, M.D.)

FIG. 21–29. Fibroma of ureter. Sessile submucosal fibroma protruding into the lumen. Sessile mesenchymal tumors are less common than the polypoid lesion. Although they rarely obstruct, it is impossible to differentiate them from malignant papillomas. (Courtesy of Erich Lang, M.D.)

FIG. 21–30. Fibroma of ureter (*arrow*). This sessile mesenchymal lesion is similar to that seen in Fig. 21–29.

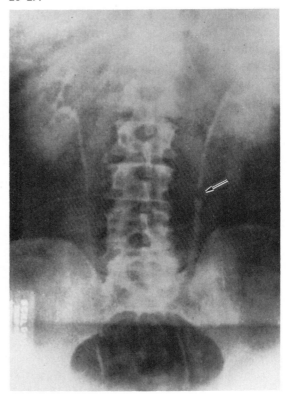

FIG. 21–32. Papillary carcinoma of the ureter associated with papillary carcinoma of the renal pelvis. Pyelogram reveals numerous intraluminal filling defects throughout the right ureter, with complete obstruction of the proximal ureter. Presumably, these are multifocal lesions of transitional epithelia.

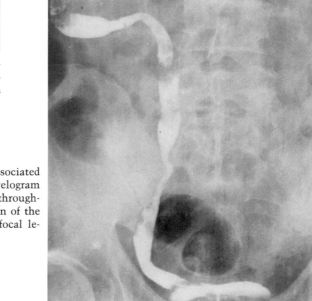

FIG. 21–33. Secondary papillary carcinoma of the ureter. This patient had known papillary carcinoma of the bladder for three years. Readmission for recurrent hematuria and left flank pain. Pyelogram demonstrates an intraluminal filling defect at the distal end of the ureter. Biopsy of this lesion showed that it was identical histologically with the papillary carcinoma of the bladder.

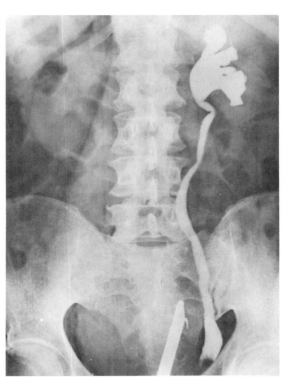

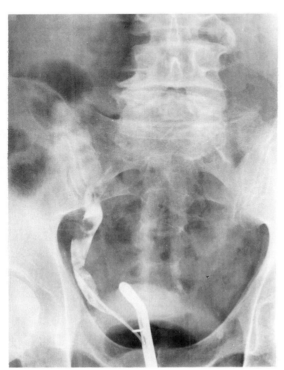

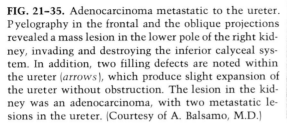

FIG. 21–34. Papillary transitional cell carcinoma of the ureteral stump. This patient had a previous nephrectomy for papillary carcinoma of the renal pelvis. At the time of surgery, because of the patient's poor condition, a nephrectomy and a partial ureterectomy were performed. The present ureterogram reveals multiple large filling defects within the ureteral stump, which represent multifocal lesions of transitional epithelia.

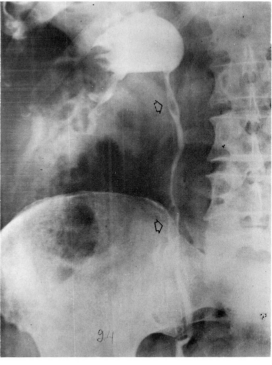

FIG. 21–35. Adenocarcinoma metastatic to the ureter. Pyelography in the frontal and the oblique projections revealed a mass lesion in the lower pole of the right kidney, invading and destroying the inferior calyceal system. In addition, two filling defects are noted within the ureter (*arrows*), which produce slight expansion of the ureter without obstruction. The lesion in the kidney was an adenocarcinoma, with two metastatic lesions in the ureter. (Courtesy of A. Balsamo, M.D.)

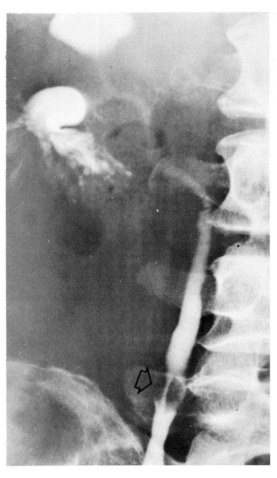

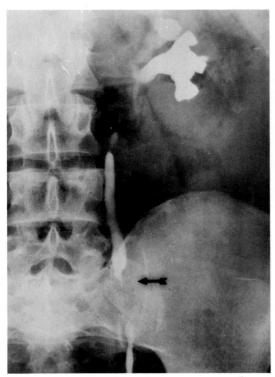

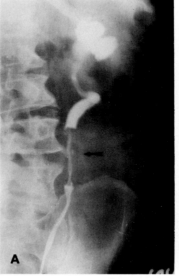 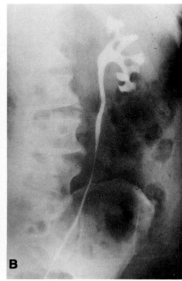

FIG. 21–36. Metastic carcinoma of the ureter from clear cell carcinoma of the opposite kidney, removed 14 months prior to the present study. Pyelogram reveals a localized narrowing of the midureter (*arrow*), representing metastatic intramural carcinoma. Severe renal infection is present secondary to the obstruction. (Courtesy of Herman Wechsler, M.D.)

FIG. 21–37. Metastatic seminoma to left ureter. **(A)** Long lesion of the midthird of the ureter, producing considerable obstruction. Although a cupping type of defect is present proximally similar to that seen with intraluminal lesions, the length of the lesion and the narrowing of the ureter suggest that the intramural and serosal portions of the ureter are involved. **(B)** Following radiation therapy, the ureter has returned to a normal appearance.

FIG. 21–38. Metastatic carcinoma of the distal ureter from carcinoma of the pancreas (*arrow*). A metastatic lesion from a primary outside the urinary tract usually involves the serosa of the ureter and presents as an extrinsic lesion resembling a stricture. Occasionally, these lesions may extend into the lumen of the ureter, presenting as an intraluminal mass. In this illustration the lesion is primarily serosal, with marked narrowing of the ureteral lumen and proximal hydronephrosis.

FIG. 21–39. Metastatic melanoma. Melanoma is one of the more common metastatic lesions that mimics a primary intraluminal tumor. It is most common in the bladder. Urogram reveals an intraluminal filling defect (*arrow*) in the left pelvis that was melanoma. (Courtesy of Howard Pollack, M.D.)

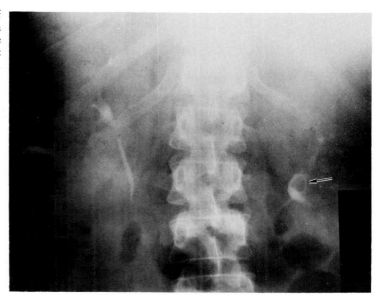

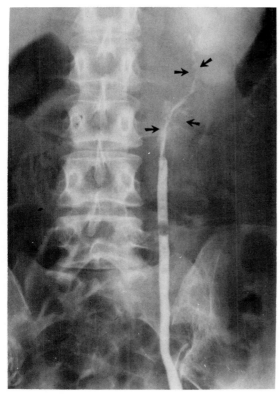

FIG. 21–40. Ovarian metastases. Pyelogram shows diffuse narrowing of the proximal ureter with marked irregularity of the lumen. The metastases had encased the ureter and extended into the lumen destroying the mucosa. Note the spiculated contrast medium (*arrows*) extravasating through ulcerations. (Courtesy of Erich Lang, M.D.)

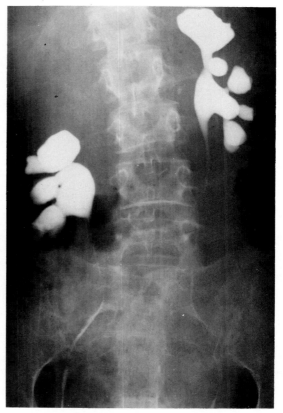

FIG. 21–41. Metastases from breast carcinoma. Diffuse encasement of both ureters by retroperitoneal metastases from carcinoma of the breast.

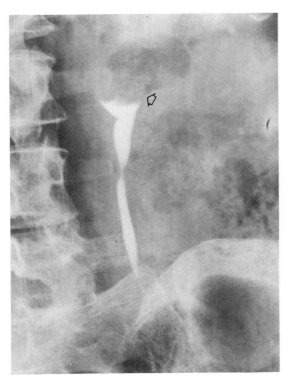

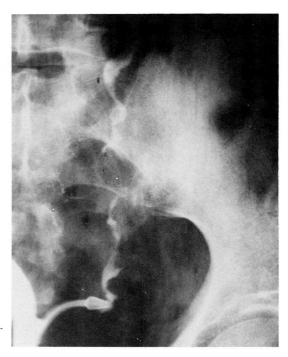

FIG. 21–42. Metastatic lesion of the ureter. Metastatic tumor from the colon, involving the proximal end of the left ureter (*arrow*). The lesion is indistinguishable from a primary carcinoma of the ureter. The authors have seen three cases of colonic metastases to the ureter presenting as intraluminal lesions.

FIG. 21–43. Prostatic metastases. Diffuse nodular implants along the entire ureter, producing a curlicue appearance. (Courtesy of Erich Lang, M.D.)

FIG. 21–44. Direct invasion from carcinoma of the cervix. Encasement of the distal ureter (*arrow*) from direct extension from cervix. The typical area involved is usually about 1 cm. above the ureterovesical junction.

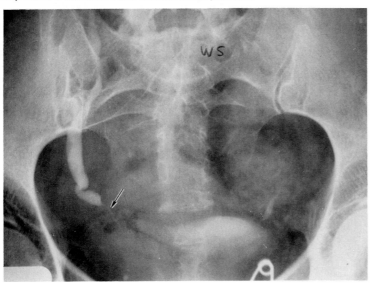

FIG. 21–45. Carcinoma of the sigmoid involving the ureter by direct extension. There is considerable obstruction of both ureters at the level of the second sacral body more caudal than the obstruction seen in retroperitoneal fibrosis. In addition, there is marked medial deviation of both ureters, a common finding when pelvic carcinoma involves the ureters secondarily.

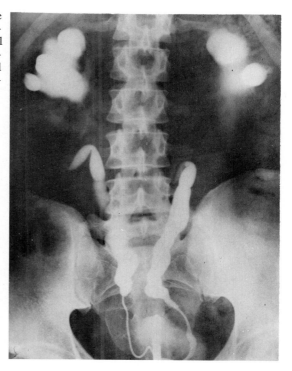

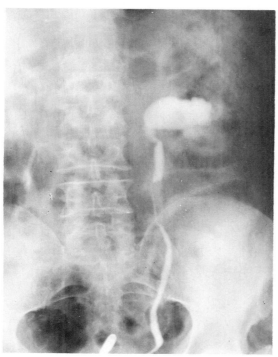

FIG. 21–46. Retroperitoneal sarcoma involving the midportion of the left ureter by direct extension. Moderate proximal hydronephrosis is present. (Courtesy of J.A. Evans, M.D.)

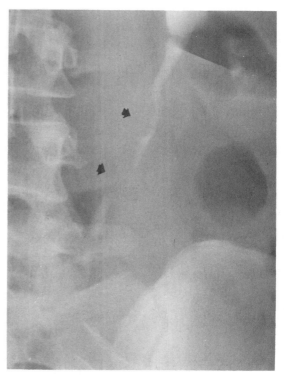

FIG. 21–47. Retroperitoneal nodes. Lymphoma producing discrete scalloped impressions (*arrows*) on the left ureter from enlarged retroperitoneal nodes. (Courtesy of Erich Lang, M.D.)

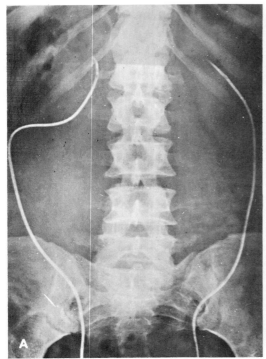
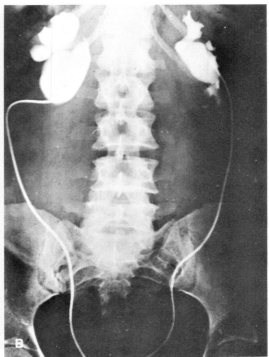
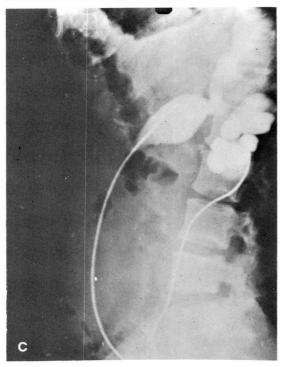

FIG. 21–48. Massive enlargement of the retroperitoneal lymph nodes, producing lateral deviations of the mid thirds of the ureters. **(A)** Lymphosarcomatous nodes have produced marked lateral deviation of both ureters, more pronounced on the right side. When marked lateral deviation occurs **(B)**, anterior deviation of the ureter usually is present **(C)**. Enlarged retroperitoneal nodes are the most common cause of lateral deviation of either the proximal or the midthirds of the ureters. (Courtesy of Herbert Kenyon, M.D.)

BIBLIOGRAPHY

Primary Malignant Tumors of the Ureter—Epithelial in Origin

Transitional Cell Tumors

1. Abeshouse, B.S.: Primary benign and malignant tumors of ureter: Review of literature and report of one benign and 12 malignant tumors. Am. J. Surg., 91:237-271, 1956.
2. Arger, P.H., and Stolz, J.L.: Ureteral tumors: The radiologic evaluation of a differential diagnosis "thrown-in." Am. J. Roentgenol., 116:812-821, 1972.
3. Beck, A.D., Heslin, J.E., Milner, W.A., et al.: Primary tumors of ureter: Diagnosis and management. J. Urol., 102:683-688, 1969.
4. Bergman, H., Friedenberg, R.M., and Sayegh, V.: New roentgenologic signs of carcinoma of the ureter. Am. J. Roentgenol., 86:707-717, 1961.
5. Bergman, H., and Hotchkiss, R.S.: Ureteral tumors. In Bergman, H. (ed.): The Ureter, pp. 439-464. New York, Hoeber, 1967.
6. Bloom, N.A., Vidune, R.A., and Lytton, B.: Primary carcinoma of ureter: Report of 102 new cases. J. Urol., 103:590-598, 1970.
7. Witten, D.M., Myers, G.H., Jr., and Utz, D.C. (eds.): Emmett's Clinical Urography, 4th ed. Philadelphia, W.B. Saunders, 1977.
8. Fisher, H.E., Jr.: Exfoliative cytology of primary tumors of the ureter: A report of 3 cases. J. Urol., 102:180-183, 1969.
9. Hanchi-Olsen, A., and Seland, P.: Primary tumors of the ureter: Report of 2 cases. Scand. J. Urol. Nephrol., 2:143-144, 1968.
10. Holtz, F.: Papillomas and primary carcinoma of ureter: Report of 20 cases. J. Urol., 88:380-385, 1962.
11. Jönsson, G.: Primary tumours of ureter: Report of 17 cases. Acta. Chir. Scand., 126:368-378, 1963.
12. Newsam, J.E.: Diagnosis of ureteric tumors. Br. J. Urol., 38:268-273, 1966.
12a. Petkovic, S.B.: Epidemiology and treatment of renal, pelvic and ureteral tumors. J. Urol., 114:858-865, 1975.
13. Whitlock, G.F., McDonald, J.R., and Cook, E.N.: Primary carcinoma of ureter: Pathologic and prognostic study. J. Urol., 73:245-253, 1955.
14. Wood, L.G., and Howe, G.E.: Primary tumors of the ureter: Case reports. J. Urol., 79:418-430, 1958.

Bilateral Tumors of the Ureter

15. Antonio, P., Jr.: Primary bilateral cancer of the ureters. J. Philippine Med. Assoc., 33:165-170, 1957.
16. Barber, J.W.: Bilateral simultaneous primary carcinomas of the ureters. Radiology, 90:318-319, 1968.
17. Barroso, C.H., Jr., Florence, T.J., and Scott, C., Jr.: Bilateral papillary carcinoma of the ureters: Presentation of a case and 2-year follow-up report. J. Urol., 96:451-454, 1966.
18. Crassweller, P.O.: Bilateral primary carcinoma of the ureter with the use of ileal graft for ureteral replacement: A case report. Br. J. Urol., 30:152-160, 1958.
19. Felber, E.: Asynchronous bilateral benign papilloma of the ureter with subsequent carcinoma of the ureteral stump, bladder and vagina. J. Med. Assoc. Ga., 42:198-200, 1953.

20. Gaca, A.: Das doppelseitige papillare Harnleiterkorzinom. Z. Urol., 53:925-928, 1958.
21. Gillenwater, J.Y., Howard, R.S., and Paquin, A.J., Jr.: Bilateral primary carcinoma of the ureters. J.A.M.A., 197:1040-1041, 1966.
22. Gracia, V., and Bradfield, E.O.: Simultaneous bilateral transitional cell carcinoma of the ureter: A case report. J. Urol., 79:925-928, 1958.
23. Hauge, A.: Bilaterale Harnleiterpapillome. Z. Urol., 57:807-811, 1964.
24. Levine, R.L., and Airhart, R.A.: Bilateral synchronous transitional ureteral carcinoma: Two additional cases. South. Med. J., 70:1418-1420, 1977.
25. Perlmutter, A.D., Retik, A.B., and Harrison, J.H.: Simultaneous bilateral carcinoma of ureter present for 5 years before surgery. J. Urol., 93:582-587, 1965.
26. Ratliff, R.K., Baum, W.C., and Butler, W.J.: Bilateral primary carcinoma of the ureter: A case report. Cancer, 2:815-818, 1949.
27. Scarzella, G.I., and MacDonald, G.R.: Asynchronous bilateral primary epithelial tumors of the ureter: Report of a case. J. Urol., 97:464-468, 1967.
28. Sozer, I.T.: Simultaneous bilateral carcinoma of ureters. Urology, 16:217-219, 1974.
29. Talavera, J.M., Carney, J.A., and Kelalis, P.P.: Bilateral synchronous primary transitional cell carcinoma of the ureter: Report of 2 cases and review of literature. J. Urol., 104:679-683, 1970.
30. Utz, D.C., Brunsting, C.D., and Harrison, E.G., Jr.: Bilateral ureteral and vesical carcinomas occurring asynchronously: A case report. J. Urol., 88:488-493, 1962.
31. Vanwelkenhuyzen, N.P.: Tumeru double de l'uretere. Acta Urol. Belg., 29:368-371, 1961.
32. Viek, N.F., Uhlman, R.C., and Verrilli, R.: Simultaneous bilateral transitional cell carcinoma of kidney. J. Urol., 89:49-52, 1963.

Adenocarcinoma of the Ureter

33. Jacob, N.H., Jr., and Mau, W.: Metaplasia of ureteral epithelium resulting in intestinal mucosa and adenocarcinomatous transformation: Report of two cases. J. Urol., 65:20-24, 1951.
34. Ray, P., and Lingard, W.F.: Primary adenocarcinoma of ureter: A case report. J. Urol., 106:655-657, 1971.
35. Stahl, D.M.: Unusual primary hypernephroma (renal cell carcinoma) of the ureter in a child. J. Urol., 80:176-179, 1958.

Carcinoma in Situ of Ureter

36. Khan, A.U., Farrow, G.M., and Zinche, H., et al.: Primary carcinoma in situ of the ureter and pelvis. J. Urol., 121:681-683, 1979.
37. Linker, O., and Whitmore, W.F., Jr.: Ureteral carcinoma in situ. J. Urol., 113:777-780, 1975.
38. Schade, R.O.K., Serck-Hanssen, A., and Swinney, J.: Morphological changes in the ureter in cases of bladder carcinoma. Cancer, 27:1267-1272, 1971.
39. Sharma, T.C., Melamed, M.R., and Whitmore, W.F., Jr.: Car-

cinoma in situ of the ureter in patients with bladder carcinoma treated by cystectomy. Cancer, 26:583–587, 1970.

Angiography of Ureteral Tumors

40. Boijsen, E.: Angiographic diagnosis of ureteric carcinoma. Acta Radiol. (Stockh), 38172–176, 1962.
41. Lang, E.K.: The arteriographic diagnosis of primary and secondary tumors of the ureter and renal pelvis. Radiology, 93:799–805, 1969.
42. Lambeth, J.T., and Ranniger, K.: Arteriographic diagnosis of primary and secondary tumors of ureter or ureter and renal pelvis. Radiology, 93:799–805, 1969.
43. Siegelman, S.S., Hoyt, D.B., Annes, G.P., et al.: Angiography in carcinoma of the proximal ureter. Radiology, 91:925–928, 1968.

Malignant Nonepithelial Tumors of the Ureter

44. D'Aunoy, R., and Zoeller, A.: Primary carcinoma of the ureter: Report of a case and review of the literature. Arch. Pathol., 9:17–30, 1936.
45. Alznauer, R.L.: Leiomyosarcoma of right ureter: Report of a case. Arch. Pathol., 59:94–99, 1955.
46. Fein, R.L., and Hamm, F.C.: Hemangiosarcoma of the ureter: A case report. J. Urol., 93:684–686, 1965.
47. Kraus, J.E.: Primary sarcoma of the ureter. Urol. Cutan. Rev., 48:522–525, 1944.
48. Rademaker, L.: Primary sarcoma of the ureter: Case report and review of the literature. Am. J. Surg., 62:402–406, 1943.
49. Renner, M.J.: Primary malignant tumor of the ureter. Surg. Gynecol. Obstet., 52:793–803, 1931.
50. Rossien, A.Y., and Russell, T.H.: Leiomyosarcoma involving the right ureter. Arch. Pathol., 41:655–660, 1946.
51. Senger, F.L., and Furey, C.A., Jr.: Primary ureteral tumors with a reivew of the literature since 1943. J. Urol., 69:243–258, 1953.
52. Smith, G.G.: Neoplasms of the kidney and ureter: A report of 40 cases. Am. J. Surg., 30:130–140, 1935.
53. Werner, J.R.K., Ligensmith, W., and Denko, J.V.: Leiomyosarcoma of the ureter: Case report and review of literature. J. Urol., 82:68–71, 1959.

Nonpolypoid, Nonepithelial Benign Tumors of Ureter

54. Auerbach, S., Lewis, H.Y., and McDonald, J.R.: Recurrent polypoid hamartoma and epithelial cell nests in the ureter and renal pelvis of an adolescent. J. Urol., 95:691–696, 1966.
55. Brodny, M.L., and Hershman, H.: Pedunculated hemangioma of the ureter. J. Urol., 71:539–543, 1954.
56. Cooney, C.J.: Fibroma of the ureter. J. Urol., 47:651–657, 1942.
57. Elson, E.C., and McLaughlin, A.P., II: Xanthomatous ureteral polyp. Urology, IV:214–216, 1976.
58. Galbraith, W.N.: Pedunculated vascular tumor of the ureter. Br. J. Urol., 22:195–200, 1950.
59. Hamer, H.G., Mertz, H.O., and Wishard, W.N., Jr.: Ureteral granulomata. J. Urol., 29:43–49, 1933.
60. Hudson, H.C., and Howland, R.L., Jr.: Primary benign ureteral tumor of mesodermal origin. J. Urol., 105:794–796, 1971.

61. Jeppeson, F.B.: Lymphangioma of the ureter. J. Urol., 70:410–414, 1953.
62. Leighton, K.M.: Leiomyoma of the ureter. Br. J. Urol., 27:256–257, 1953.
63. Patch, F.S.: Granuloma of the ureter. J. Urol., 25:193–201, 1931.
64. Ravich, A.: Neurofibroma of the ureter: Report of a case with operation and recovery. Arch. Surg., 30:442–445, 1935.
65. Roen, P.R., and Kandalaft, S.: Primary benign mesodermal ureteral tumor. J. Urol., 96:890–891, 1961.
66. Uhlir, K.: Hemangioma of the ureter. J. Urol., 110:647–649, 1973.
67. Wöller, A.: Hemangioma des Ureters. Z. Urol., 46:668–670, 1953.

Polyps of the Ureter

68. Bose, B., and Williams, J.P.: Benign polypoidal tumor of ureter. Br. J. Surg., 58:144–151, 1971.
69. Cavallo, T., and Crocker, D.W.: Benign tumor of ureter: Case report. J. Natl. Med. Assoc., 64:421–423, 1972.
70. Chauvine, E., and Romieu, M.: Bilateral polyps and capillary adenomata of ureter. Urol. Cut. Rev., 35:415–418, 1931.
71. Colgon, J.R., Skaist, L.E., and Morrow, J.W.: Benign ureteral tumors in childhood: Case report and plea for conservative management. J. Urol., 109:308–310, 1973.
72. Compere, D.E., Begley, G.F., Isaacks, H.E., et al.: Ureteral polyps. J. Urol., 79:209–214, 1958.
73. Crum, D.M., Sayegh, E.S., Sacher, E.C., et al.: Benign ureteral polyps. J. Urol., 102:678–682, 1969.
74. Davides, K.L., and King, I.M.: Fibrous polyps of the ureter. J. Urol., 115:651–653, 1976.
75. Gerdes, G., and Nordquist, L.: Intussusception of ureter caused by primary benign tumor. Acta Chir Scand., 132:397–402, 1966.
76. Howard, T.L.: Giant polyp of ureter. J. Urol., 79:397–402, 1958.
77. Hudson, H.C., and Howland, R.L., Jr.: Primary benign ureteral tumor of mesodermal origin. J. Urol., 105:794–796, 1971.
78. Hughes, F.A., III, and Davis, C.S., Jr.: Multiple benign ureteral polyps. Am. J. Roentgenol., 126:723–727, 1975.
79. Hussaini, M.A., Marden, H.E., Jr., and Woodruff, M.W.: Multiple fibrous polyps of ureter. Urology, 2:563–565, 1973.
80. Knackstredt, J., Pirozynski, W., and Oliver, J.A.: Benign fibroepithelial polyps of ureter. Br. J. Urol., 43:284–288, 1971.
81. Lambeth, J.T., and Ranniger, K.: Arteriographic diagnosis of primary and secondary tumors of ureter or ureter and renal pelvis. Radiology, 93:799–805, 1960.
82. Neal, J.M., and Arbuckle, L.D.: Benign fibrous polyp of ureter: Case report. J. Urol., 108:230–232, 1972.
83. Palmer, J.K., and Greene, L.F.: Benign fibromucous polyp of the ureter: Report of a case. Surgery, 22:562–565, 1947.
84. Pinto, R.S., Fauver, E., and Anderson, J.R.: Benign fibroepithelioma of the ureter. Urology, 3:747–749, 1974.
85. Schneiderman, C., Simon, M., and Sedlezky, I.: Benign polyp of the ureter. Br. J. Urol., 31:168–175, 1959.
86. Soderdahl, D.W., and Schuster, S.R.: Benign ureteral polyp in newborn. J.A.M.A., 207:1714–1715, 1966.
87. Stuppler, S.A., and Kanozari, S.J.: Fibroepithelial polyps of the ureter: A benign ureteral tumor. Urology, 5:553–558, 1975.

88. Yong, S.L., and Rajamani, R.: A case of giant ureteric polyp. Aust. N.Z. J. Surg., *42*:266–271, 1973.

Ureteral Stump

89. Amar, A.D.: Squamous cell carcinoma of ureteral stump 40 years after nephrectomy. J. Urol., *91*:337–339, 1964.
90. Loef, J.A., and Casella, P.A.: Squamous cell carcinoma occurring in the stump of a chronically infected ureter many years after nephrectomy. J. Urol., *67*:159–163, 1962.
91. Malek, R.S.: Primary tumours of the ureteric stump. Br. J. Urol., *45*:391–394, 1973.
92. Malek, R.S., Moghaddam, A., Furlow, W.L., et al.: Symptomatic ureteral stump. J. Urol., *106*:522–528, 1971.
93. Sozer, I.T.: Squamous cell carcinoma and calculi in ureteral stump: 12 years post nephrectomy. J. Urol., *99*:264–265, 1968.
94. Strong, D.W., Pearse, H.D., Tank, E.S., Jr., et al.: The ureteral stump after nephroureterectomy. J. Urol., *115*:654–655, 1976.
95. Wisheart, J.D.: Primary tumour of the ureteric stump following nephrectomy: Presentation of a case and a review of the literature. Br. J. Urol., *40*:344–349, 1968.

Transitional Cell Carcinoma of Renal Pelvis and Similar Lesions in Ureter

96. Kaplan, J.H., McDonald, J.R., and Thompson, G.J.: Multicentric origin of papillary tumors of urinary tract. J. Urol., *66*:792–804, 1951.
97. Kimball, F.N., and Ferrer, H.W.: Papillomatous tumors of renal pelvis associated with similar tumors in ureter and bladder. J. Urol., *31*:257–304, 1934.
98. Lang, E.H.: The arteriographic diagnosis of primary and secondary tumors of the ureter and renal pelvis. Radiology, *93*:799–805, 1969.
99. McDonald, J.R., and Priestley, J.T.: Carcinoma of the renal pelvis. J. Urol., *51*:245–258, 1944.
100. O'Connor, V.J.: The diagnosis of tumors of the renal pelvis and ureter. J. Urol., *75*:416–423, 1956.

Metastases to Ureter from Adenocarcinoma of Kidney

101. Chordia, M.L., Ockuly, E.A., Ockuly, J.J., et al.: Ureteral and vesical metastases from parenchymal renal carcinoma: case report and review of the literature. J. Urol., *102*:298–301, 1969.
102. Gross, M., and Minkowitz, S.: Ureteral metastasis from renal adenocarcinoma. J. Urol., *106*:23–26, 1971.
103. Heslin, J.E., Wilner, W.A., and Garlick, W.B.: Lower urinary tract implants or metastases from clear cell carcinoma of the kidney. J. Urol., *73*:39–46, 1955.
104. Hook, G., and Scheiman, L.S.: Ureteral stump metastasis from renal adenocarcinoma. Urol., *3*:352–353, 1974.
105. Hovenanian, M.S.: Implantation of renal parenchymal carcinoma. J. Urol., *64*:188–192, 1950.
106. Hudson, H.C., and Windsor, J.L.: Ureteral metastasis from hypernephroma of the contralateral kidney. South. Med. J., *64*:618–620, 1971.
107. Kato, T., and Okado, K.: Renal cell carcinoma with metastases to the ureter: Report of a case. Acta Urol., Japan, *17*:528–531, 1971.
108. LeBlanc, G.A.: Contralateral ureteral metastasis from renal adenocarcinoma. J. Urol., *86*:316–318, 1961.
109. MacAlpine, J.B.: Implantation of secondaries from a renal carcinoma (hypernephroma) within the ureteric lumen. Br. J. Surg., *36*:164–168, 1948.
110. Mitchell, J.E.: Ureteric secondaries from a hypernephroma. Br. J. Surg., *45*:392–394, 1958.
111. Sargent, J.W.: Ureteral metastasis from renal adenocarcinoma presenting a bizarre urogram. J. Urol., *83*:97–99, 1960.
112. Sinner, W.: Carcinoma inoculation metastasis to the ureteral stump after nephrectomy for a solid kidney carcinoma. J. Urol., *52*:673–679, 1959.
113. Wechsler, H., and Spivak, L.: Metastasis in ureter from adenocarcinoma of the contralateral kidney. N.Y. State J. Med., *57*:1942–1944, 1957.
114. Young, I.S.: Ureteral implant from renal adenocarcinoma: Report of a case and review of the literature. J. Urol., *95*:661–663, 1967.

Metastases to Ureter from Sources Outside Kidney

115. Bartels, E.C.: Carcinoma of stomach with bilateral ureteral metastases. Minn. Med., *16*:578–579, 1933.
116. Brotherus, J.V., and Westerlund, R.M.: Metastatic carcinoma of the ureter: A report of three cases. Scand. J. Urol. Nephrol., *5*:86–90, 1971.
117. Carson, W.J.: Metastatic carcinoma in the ureter: Report of additional cases. Ann. Surg., *86*:549–555, 1927.
118. Cohen, W.M., Freed, S.Z., and Hasson, J.: Metastatic cancer to the ureter: A review of the literature and case presentation. J. Urol., *112*:188–189, 1974.
119. Grabstald, H., and Kaufman, R.: Hydronephrosis secondary to ureteral obstruction by metastatic heart cancer. J. Urol., *102*:569–574, 1969.
120. Judd, R.L.: Melanoma of the ureter: A case report. J. Urol., *87*:805–807, 1962.
121. Kirschbaum, J.D.: Metastatic tumors of ureter. J. Urol., *30*:665–677, 1933.
122. Kleiman, A.H.: Carcinoma of the ureter secondary to neoplasm of the descending colon. J. Urol., *57*:120–125, 1947.
123. Klinger, M.E.: Secondary tumors of the genitourinary tract. J. Urol., *65*:144–153, 1951.
124. Kost, L.V., and Leberman, P.R.: Metastatic carcinoma to the ureter: A case report. J. Urol., *93*:367–369, 1965.
125. MacKenzie, D.W., and Ratner, M.: Metastatic growth in the ureter: A report of 3 cases and a brief review of the literature. Can. Med. Assoc. J., *25*:265–270, 1931.
126. McCrea, L.E., and Peale, A.R.: Metastatic carcinoma to the ureter. Urol. Cut. Rev., *55*:11–22, 1951.
127. Presman, D., and Ehrlich, L.: Metastatic tumors of the ureter. J. Urol., *59*:312–325, 1948.
128. Richie, J.P., Withers, G., and Ehrlich, R.M.: Ureteral obstruction secondary to metastatic tumors. Surg. Gynecol. Obstet., *148*:355–357, 1979.
129. Robbins, J.J., and Lich, R., Jr.: Metastatic carcinoma of the ureter. J. Urol., *75*:242–243, 1956.
130. Samellas, W., and Marks, A.R.: Metastatic melanoma of the urinary tract. J. Urol., *85*:21–23, 1961.
131. Stearns, D.B., Farmer, D.A., and Gordon, S.K.: Ureteral me-

tastases secondary to gastric carcinoma: Case report. J. Urol., *80*:214–217, 1958.

132. Tock, E.P.C., and Wee, A.S.T.: Bilateral ureteric metastases causing complete anuria. Br. J. Urol., *40*:421–424, 1968.

133. Woodruff, S.R.: Secondary tumors of the ureter. J.A.M.A., *105*:925–931, 1935.

Direct Invasion of Ureter

134. Graves, R.C., Kickham, C.J.E., and Nathanson, I.T.: The ureteral and renal complication of carcinoma of the cervix. J. Urol., *36*:618–642, 1936.

135. Kaufman, J.J.: Unusual causes of extrinsic ureteral obstruction, part 1. J. Urol., *87*:319–327, 1962.

136. Kaufman, J.J.: Unusual causes of extrinsic ureteral obstruction. J. Urol., *87*:328–337, 1962.

137. Kickham, C.J.E.: Urologic pitfalls in the management of carcinoma of the cervix. J. Urol., *80*:229–236, 1958.

138. Miller, W.A., and Speark, J.L.: Periureteral and ureteral metastases from carcinoma of cervix. Radiology, *107*:533–535, 1973.

139. Perch, C.A.: Carcinoma of cervix involving the upper urinary tract. J. Urol., *106*:562–564, 1971.

The following unrelated topics are included in this chapter:

1. Postoperative ureteral complications and illustrations of the ureter following ureteral diversion; interventional approach to the ureter
2. Vesicoureteral and intrarenal reflux (see also Part V, Bladder and Part IX, Pediatric Urology)
3. Abdominal masses, inflammatory conditions, and urinary anomalies that produce relatively characteristic deviations of the ureter

POSTOPERATIVE URETER

Following surgery on the ureter or surgery on neighboring organs in which the ureter is inadvertently injured, strictures, fistulas, diverticula, abscesses, urinomas, and other less severe ureteral deformities (deviations) may result during the postoperative period. Complications following direct ligations and injury secondary to periureteral trauma (necrosis, kinking) have been illustrated in Chapter 20, Trauma to the Ureter. Different minor deformities may occur following instrumentation and surgery that usually do not affect ureteral function, namely, the transport of urine. In most cases instrumental perforations heal rapidly without sequelae unless more than 50 per cent of the circumference of the ureter is involved or unless distal obstruction is present (Figs. 22–1 to 22–3).

Following ureteral reimplantation or diversion, different types of roentgenograms are obtained, depending on the procedure performed. Each procedure has its advantages and disadvantages, its advocates and critics. We will just list some of the more common procedures under major subgroups.

22

Miscellaneous Conditions of the Ureter

ISOLATED LOOP

The isolated intestinal loop removed from the fecal stream and draining cutaneously has in most hands proved to be the most desirable form of diversion with the best chance of maintaining renal function for a prolonged period (Figs. 22–5 to 22–10). All intestinal loops have the advantage of being isoperistaltic segments that aid in the transport of urine to the exterior. The *ureteroileocutaneous* anastomosis has been used successfully for 25 years. The *ureterosigmoidcutaneous* and *ureterotransversecutaneous* anastomoses have gained in popularity because it is easier to obtain a good antireflux procedure with colic loops. In addition, the transverse colon provides a reservoir distinct from pelvic pathology.

URETEROSTOMY

With improved surgical procedures and improved appliances that are watertight and prevent skin wetting, a ureterostomy has become more acceptable (Figs. 22–11 to 22–13). However, the incidence of complications is much higher than in isolated loops, and maintenance of normal renal function for a prolonged time is less likely. They are utilized more commonly with a dilated ureter. The *ureterocutaneous diversion* may be unilateral or bilateral. It is frequently utilized as an interim procedure pending final surgical correction. A variation of this is *transureteroureterostomy* (TUU) in which one ureter is anastomosed to the other (Figs. 22–14 to 22–17). There are many variations: The single ureter may be brought to the skin or reimplanted to the bladder or into the bowel. This procedure is usually done when one ureter is either damaged distally or has lost its functional ability distally. The normal ureter is, of course, placed at risk by joining it with the abnormal or diseased ureter. In long-standing cases, carcinoma of the colon can occur.[5a]

TO INTACT COLON

The use of *ureterosigmoidostomy* or the placement of the ureter into any area of functioning bowel where ascending infection may occur is usually reserved for terminally ill patients in whom long-term renal function will not be required (Figs. 22-18 to 22-21). With the better surgical technique providing antireflux anastomosis, some surgeons are using these procedures more frequently, but long-term renal infection, abscesses, and loss of function are common.

INTERPOSITION OF BOWEL (URETERAL REPLACEMENT)

Loss of one or both ureters with normal bladder function requires ureteral replacement usually with an isolated segment of ileum (Figs. 22–22 to 22–26). The ileum may replace the lower half or more of one ureter, both ureters, or replace the ureters completely if both upper ureters are damaged. In the latter instance a Roux-in-Y anastomosis may be performed with two segments of ileum, one from each renal pelvis joining into one segment that enters the bladder. Antireflux procedures have been introduced for the ileum–bladder anastomosis. Ureteral replacement by ileum, although it frequently functions satisfactorily, is only performed when no other direct anastomosis is possible.

There are many variations to the few procedures just described, many dictated by particular patient problems (Figs. 22–24 to 22–26).

INTERVENTIONAL APPROACH TO THE URETER

Along with the new interventional therapy in the kidney for arteriovenous aneurysms, aneurysms, massive hematuria, and inoperable carcinomas, new approaches have developed for ureteral diseases:

1. *Antegrade pyelography* (percutaneous)
   The indicators for antegrade pyelography are as follows (Figs. 21–9, 22–4):
   a. If pyelography is contraindicated or if it is impossible to pass a catheter from below
   b. If nephrostomy is indicated for severe urosepsis, anuria, or for other conditions requiring immediate drainage
   c. In children in whom retrograde pyelography is difficult or impossible
   d. To avoid administering general anesthesia
   e. To obtain urodynamics
      This procedure is utilized in cases of supravesical urinary obstruction. It is also the first step toward passing catheters through obstructing ureteral lesions or for manipulating calculi from above. A skinny needle puncture can be performed utilizing ultrasound or, if the kidneys excrete contrast, fluoroscopy after urography.
2. *Needle aspiration of renal masses*
   Percutaneous needle aspiration can be employed to drain abscesses, urinomas, hematomas, and lymphoceles and to perform a biopsy of masses producing ureteral obstruction.
3. *Stent catheters* (Gibbons, Fig. 22-4a; pigtail, Fig. 22-4, 22-26a, 22-26b)
   The renal pelvis is opacified by urography or by skinny needle puncture. An 18-gauge needle is inserted through the renal parenchyma (to prevent leakage) into the renal pelvis. Under fluoroscopic control, a guide

wire and then a stenting catheter are passed into the renal pelvis (*i.e.*, pigtail, 8.3 or 10F). The catheter can usually be passed through obstructing lesions into the bladder, permitting continuous urinary drainage for months or years. If necessary, the catheter can be replaced. (See diagram, Fig. 22–26b).

REFLUX

There are two major types of urinary reflux that may be associated with renal pathology: vesicoureteral reflux and intrarenal reflux. Although reflux is considered an abnormal and potentially dangerous radiologic finding, it is not always associated with significant pathology.

VESICOURETERAL REFLUX

Vesicoureteral reflux, the backward flow of urine from the bladder to the ureter, is considered an abnormal variant in the human (Fig. 22–27). The intravesical ureter is constructed to perform the functions of a valve, to allow urine to flow freely into the bladder, but to prevent backward flow into the ureter. The intravesical ureter is open during ureteral peristalsis, but at other times it is closed. The ability of the intravesical segment to withstand reflux depends on the length of the segment (usually over 1 cm.), its structural integrity, and probably an innate ability to remain closed until peristalsis is initiated.[87, 88] A poorly developed trigone may predispose to reflux. In addition to the status of the intravesical ureter, changes in structure of the bladder near the ureterovesical orifice and/or inflammation of the bladder tend to produce reflux. In the former instance, sacculations or diverticula that involve the intravesical ureter reduce its effective length and structural integrity (see Fig. 22–33). Inflammation of the bladder involving the intravesical ureter may (1) convert it into a rigid tube that cannot be compressed and closed and (2) produce edema in the surrounding mucosa that would straighten out the intraveiscal ureter and restrict its movement.[88, 89]

The usual causes of vesicoureteral reflux can be divided into primary and secondary categories. (See also the illustrations in Part V, Bladder, and Part IX, Pediatric Urology.)

PRIMARY CONGENITAL CAUSES

Primary congenital causes include the following:
1. *Structural abnormalities of the ureterovesical junction.* These are frequently associated with lateral placement of the ureteral orifices. This condition is usually referred to as primary reflux (Figs. 22–28, 22–29).

2. *Complete double ureters entering the bladder.* Reflux usually occurs into the ureter draining the lower renal segment (see Fig. 22–38).

3. *Ureteral ectopia,* usually in a complete double system with one ureter ectopic to the bladder neck or urethra. Reflux may occur into the ectopic ureter that drains the upper renal segment (Fig. 22–30).

4. *Congenital syndromes* such as loss of the abdominal musculature (prune belly) and exstrophy (Fig. 22–31).

Primary reflux is the most common type, occurring especially in Caucasian girls. The intravesical ureter is usually short and the orifice more lateral and gaping. It may be bilateral, unilateral, or alternately unilateral. The left side appears to be affected more frequently. Primary reflux is present in infancy but frequently ceases spontaneously before puberty.

There have been reports suggesting that reflux may be transmitted as a familial sex-linked genetic abnormality with variable penetrance.[115, 116, 147]

In primary reflux the urine is frequently sterile because the reflux depends on an anatomic defect; secondary reflux is frequently associated with infection and infected urine.

SECONDARY (ACQUIRED) CAUSES

Secondary (acquired) causes include the following:

1. Bladder inflammation either bacterial or chemical (cyclophosphamide) (Fig. 22–32)
2. Obstruction of the urethra (valves) (Fig. 22–33)
3. Neurogenic bladder (see Fig. 22–27)
4. Secondary to previous ureterovesical surgery
5. Secondary to loss of efflux (Figs. 22–34, 22–35)

Reflux is a radiologic finding, not a disease. The grading of reflux is arbitrary. Many different schemes have been proposed including the degree of ureteral and calyceal filling and dilatation and grading based on reflux at different pressure gradients (high and low pressure gradients). Probably the simplest method consists of grading according to the volume of reflux. This may be divided into 4 grades with grades 3 and 4 considered severe reflux.

Grade 1—Lower ureteral filling
Grade 2—Filling of the ureteral and pelvicalyceal system without clubbing or significant dilatation of the calyces and without ureteral tortuosity
Grade 3—Ureteral and pelvicalyceal filling with dilatation, calyceal clubbing, and ureteral tortuosity
Grade 4—Severe hydronephrosis and hydroureter

Reflux is an evanescent finding, present on one examination, absent on the next. Whether reflux can be demonstrated in any single examination may depend upon many variables including the position of the patient, the degree of intracystic pressure, and the state of hydration. Reflux may occur in the decubitus position, but not in the supine position. It may occur only with low intracystic pressure or only with high pressure, or it may occur throughout the examination. Reflux may occur during low renal output and disappear during diuresis. Therefore the classification has limited value because it may vary in different examinations on the same patient. The significance of reflux is still under investigation, and there are wide differences of opinion on how to handle the patient with reflux. In the infant or young child with reflux, without urinary tract infection or radiologic evidence of renal injury, most urologists will observe the patient because the reflux may cease as the child grows. Persistent reflux associated with repeated urinary tract infection or pyelonephritis is usually corrected surgically. The presence of intrarenal reflux (see below) in association with vesicoureteral reflux may lead to progressive renal changes. Whether surgical correction should be performed in such cases even in the absence of renal changes is under review. In patients without severe congenital abnormalities or marked ureterectasis, the condition can be corrected surgically in about 95% of cases.

The occurrence of reflux into the stumps of unused ureters after proximal diversion even though reflux had not occurred prior to diversion has been reported.[98] The reflux persisted after antireflux surgery on the ureteral stump but disappeared after reestablishment of ureteral continuity and flow down the distal ureter (Figs. 22–34, 22–35).

Because reflux is common in children and relatively rare in adults, the spontaneous cessation of reflux has been generally accepted. Hutch promulgated the theory of maturation—that changes take place around puberty that result in the cessation of reflux.[40] Many authors feel that reflux is less likely to stop in cases with ureteral dilatation or in those where it has been present for more than 2 or 3 years.

ROENTGENOGRAPHIC FINDINGS IN VESICOURETERAL REFLUX

The urogram is usually normal although, during reflux, reflux hydronephrosis may occur (see Figs. 22–29, 22–38). Occasionally there may be moderate to marked dilatation of one or both ureters with increased redundancy and dilatation of the renal pelvis and calyces. Mucosal striations may be present in the renal pelvis and proximal ureters. If atrophic pyelonephritis is present, the typical focal calyceal and cortical changes will be present. *Atrophic pyelonephritis (reflux nephropathy) is so frequently associated with reflux that a voiding cystourethrogram should be performed in all such instances.* One of the major problems associated with reflux is the perpetuation of urinary tract infection by constant reinfection of the kidney from bladder urine.

In children, reflux is much more common in girls. In older adults reflux is frequently associated with chronic lower tract obstruction (prostatic hypertrophy) and is more common in men. Many adults with reflux show renal changes such as pyelonephritis or back-pressure atrophy.

REFLUX AND BACK PRESSURE ATROPHY

The relationship between small kidneys and severe reflux is still under investigation. The possibility that massive reflux in the adult may lead to diffuse renal atrophy has also been suggested. Whether this might relate directly to intermittent increases in intrarenal pressure, is secondary to ischemia, or involves other, different mechanisms is not known. Hodson and others have suggested that generalized blunting or recession of the renal papillae, fairly uniform in degree, may occur together with fairly uniform narrowing of the renal substance and decreased renal size.[83-85] It has been suggested that, in children, massive reflux may interfere with normal renal growth even in the absence of infection. There have been scattered reports that sterile reflux may retard normal growth and that correction of reflux may lead to accelerated growth. End-stage kidneys of interstitial nephritis may be the result of sterile reflux. Although in some patients reflux and atrophy are seen, many patients have significant reflux without atrophy (Figs. 22–36 to 22–38).

URETERAL DYSPERISTALSIS

This condition was discussed earlier. Occasionally, a double ureter in which the two segments join prior to entering the bladder may have reflux up one ureter with proximal hydronephrosis of that segment. This situation has been referred to as "seesawing" of ureteral peristalsis. In a duplex system, peristalsis can be initiated in either segment, although in the author's experience it appears to initiate more commonly in the upper segment. Upon reaching the point of junction of duplex ureters, the peristaltic wave may proceed retrogradely up the other ureter as well as toward the bladder. This in effect is a nonmechanical obstruction that may lead to proximal hydronephrosis. The retrograde peristalsis and proximal hydronephrosis appear to occur more commonly in the lower segment (Fig. 22–39).

INTRARENAL REFLUX

Vesicoureteral reflux occasionally may be associated with intrarenal pyelotubular or pyelointerstitial reflux (Figs. 22–40, 22–41). It is presumed that intrarenal reflux relates to incompetency of the openings of the collecting ducts that penetrate the cribiform membrane into the calyx. Incompetence may be secondary to congenital variations (compound calyces) or secondary to destruction of portions of the renal papillae. The role of intrarenal reflux in producing renal damage is not clear. The incidence of intrarenal reflux in children with vesicoureteral reflux has been reported to be 5% to 27%.[159, 171, 172] These children usually had a history of infection, and intrarenal reflux would be an excellent method for bacteria to gain access to the renal parenchyma. It has been suggested that intrarenal reflux in the absence of infection may lead to focal renal atrophy similar to that seen in atrophic pyelonephritis.[161, 162] Hodson experimentally demonstrated renal scarring similar to that seen in pyelonephritis following intrarenal reflux in the presence of sterile urine in young pigs. Other observers state that sterile reflux generally does not produce renal deterioration.[173] Rollestan, Maling and Hodson found intrarenal reflux in 16 out of 386 children with vesicoureteral reflux and history of infection.[171] Of the 20 kidneys that showed intrarenal reflux, scarring developed in 13, usually conforming exactly to the site of intrarenal reflux. There were 45 additional kidneys that developed scarring in which intrarenal reflux had not been demonstrated.

Intrarenal reflux appears to be more common at the poles of the kidney conforming to the usual sites of focal pyelonephritic scarring. It has been suggested that intrarenal reflux is more common in compound calyces that usually occur in the upper pole. (See discussions under Chronic Pyelonephritis, Etiology, Chapter 5. See Figures 5–7 to 5–15.)

DEVIATIONS OF THE URETER

A survey of numerous lesions of the genitourinary tract reveals a number of relatively consistent ureteral deviations in specific abnormalities. Although exceptions have been found to all types of deviations that are presented, it is felt that a selected differential diagnosis may be offered by the roentgenologist or the urologist through careful consideration of the type of ureteral deviation present.

There are no absolute definitions for ureteral course. Generally, a ureter that crosses over a pedicle is suspect of abnormal medial placement whereas a ureter that lies entirely medial to a pedicle is considered abnormally placed. Contours and mass impressions obviously add information. Lateral deviation is more difficult to define. Most ureters lie within a centimeter of the transverse process. The larger or more muscular the individual, the more likely the ureter is to be laterally placed (Fig. 22–42).

In many instances the type of deviation from a mass lesion is not specific, simply depending on the character of growth of the mass and its chance impingement on the ureter (Figs. 22–43 to 22–49).

Benign retroperitoneal tumors may produce severe deviation of the ureter without significant obstruction. Malignant retroperitoneal tumors are more likely to obstruct the ureter and usually fix the ureter in position before marked deviation occurs. Certain slow-growing, well-encapsulated malignancies behave like benign lesions. It is uncommon for benign intraperitoneal lesions to produce complete obstruction of the ureters. Therefore, complete obstruction from an intraperitoneal lesion usually indicates that the lesion is malignant.

The most common proximal ureteral deviation is secondary to enlarged retroperitoneal lymph nodes, which deviates the ureters laterally (see Figs. 22–60, 22–61). Most retroperitoneal tumors such as lipomas occur laterally to the ureter and tend to displace the ureter medially. Any significant lateral or medial ureteral displacement usually deviates the ureter anteriorly (see Figs. 22–44 and 22–61).

In the pelvis the most common mass is uterine fibroids, which tend to deviate the ureters laterally. Interligamentous fibroids may displace the ureter medially (Fig. 22–49). Ovarian cysts may displace the ureter in either direction.

The following deviations, which occur less commonly, are characteristic enough to suggest the diagnosis.

UPPER THIRD OF THE URETER (RENAL AREA)

Lesions affecting the upper third of the ureter often affect the kidney, and therefore no proper separation of renal and upper ureteral deviations can be offered. In this region lateral displacement (retroperitoneal nodes) is far more common than medial displacement.

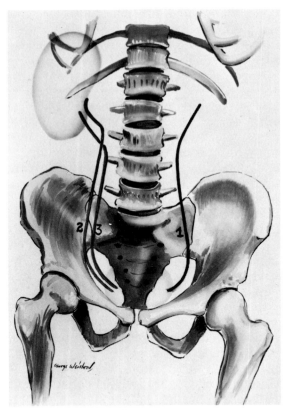

FIG. 22–50. Diagram of specific deviations of the proximal ureter. 1 = Malrotation; 2 = pyelectasis; 3 = peripelvic cyst.

The diagram in Figure 22–50 illustrates three fairly specific lesions producing lateral deviation of the proximal ureter. They are as follows:

1. Malrotation of the kidney. Because of the anterior or posterior position of the renal pelvis, the ureter arises more laterally than normal. There is no mass impression (Fig. 22–51).
2 & 3. Peripelvic cyst or pyelectasis. Both lesions may produce a mass impression "sitting" on the proximal ureter. In peripelvic cyst, function is usually good. In obstructive hydronephrosis the dilated pelvis may be seen as a soft tissue mass displacing the ureter inferiorly and laterally even when contrast visualization of the renal pelvis does not occur (Figs. 22–52, 22–53).

Medial deviation of the ureter is uncommon and nonspecific and occurs in cysts or tumors of the lower pole of the kidney (Fig. 22–54) and retroperitoneal tumors located lateral to the ureter. In the former, the renal architecture usually is distorted, whereas in the latter the renal architecture usually is normal. Obviously displacement of the kidney by an enlarged spleen, tumors or cysts of the adrenal, pancreas or retroperitoneal tumors may displace the ureter as well as the kidney (see Chap. 3, Rotation and Displacement of the Kidney).

MIDDLE THIRD OF THE URETER

The diagram in Figure 22–55 illustrates three of the more informative deviations seen along the course of the middle third of the ureters. These represent the following:

1. Medial deviation of the ureter opposite the body of L-3, associated with a retrocaval ureter (see Chap. 18, Congential Lesions of the Ureter, Figs. 18–67 to 18–69). The ureter gradually returns to its normal position near L-5. The deviation in this case is sharp and almost plateaulike, because the ureter hooks posteriorly to the inferior vena cava (Figs. 22–56, 22–57).
2. Medial deviation produced by retroperitoneal fibrosis, which usually is bilateral and may be associated with moderately severe ureteral ob-

FIG. 22–55. Diagram of specific deviations of the middle third of the ureter. 1 = Retrocaval; 2 = retroperitoneal fibrosis; 3 = aortic or iliac aneurysm.

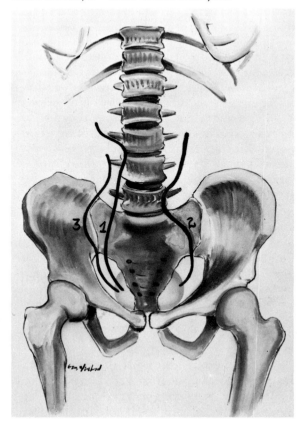

struction opposite the body of L-5 and S-1. The deviation may be associated with a mass imprint. Retroperitoneal fibrosis may occur without ureteral deviation (see Fig. 19–35).

3. Lateral deviation of the ureter in the region of the lower lumbar spine associated with aneurysm of the aorta or iliac arteries (Fig. 22–58, 22–59).

Lateral deviation in the middle third of the ureter is far more common than medial deviation, and again the most common cause is enlarged retroperitoneal nodes, either metastatic or from lymphomatous involvement (Figs. 22–60, 22–61).

Medial deviation of the midthird of the ureter, similarly to that of the proximal third, is usually nonspecific, aside from retrocaval ureter and retroperitoneal fibrosis.

THE PELVIC URETER

Deviations of the pelvic ureter are far more important than those of the proximal two-thirds and appear to be more constant and specific. The diagram in Figure 22–62 illustrates five types of ureteral deviations:

1. The usual lateral deviation of the ureter associated with a large central pelvic mass, such as an ovarian cyst or uterine fibroids (Fig. 22–63)

2. Sharp medial angulation slightly above the ureterovesical orifice, often associated with diverticulum of the bladder arising near the orifice. Characteristically, the deviation extends to the ureterovesical orifice (Fig. 22–66).

3. Gradual medial deviation of both ureters over the middle sacral segments similar to the deviation frequently seen in retroperitoneal fibrosis at a higher level. This bilateral medial deviation over S-1 to S-3 is seen in two associated conditions.

   a. Following abdominoperineal surgery during which the posterior peritoneum is divided, the ureters tend to deviate medially, probably following the pelvic curvature. In such cases there is no evidence of obstruction unless recurrent carcinoma is present (Fig. 22–64).

   b. Pelvic carcinomatosis, most commonly from carcinoma of the rectosigmoid, may trap the ureters and deviate them medially over the sacrum. This deviation is similar to the one in (a), but is associated with some degree of uretreal obstruction (Figs. 22–65, 22–67).

4. Incomplete distal ureteral obstruction that has

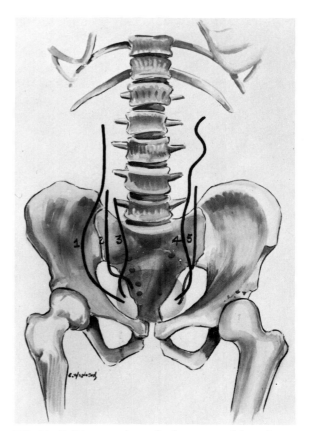

FIG. 22–62. Diagram of specific deviations of the pelvic ureter. 1 = Uterine fibroid; 2 = bladder diverticulum; 3 = post abdominoperineal surgery; 4 = distal obstruction; 5 = pelvic nodes.

been present for some time tends to produce characteristic deviations secondary to ureteral redundancy. There is a proximal lateral deviation just below the ureteropelvic junction and a distal medial sacral deviation. The proximal lateral deviation is often an acute angle, a buckling or redundancy of the proximal ureter, whereas the medial sacral deviation is more gradual over a longer segment following the medial slope over the sacrum (Figs. 22–68, 22–69).

5. The most valuable of the pelvic deviations is the medial deviation of the pelvic ureter just below the pelvic brim. Normally the ureter in this area is convex laterally following the contour of the inner margin of the iliac bone. Straightening of the ureter in this region is suspect, but convexity medially is abnormal. This deviation may be secondary to two lesions.

   a. Enlarged retroperitoneal nodes, usually secondary to prostatic, bladder, or uterine carcinoma or to lymphoma (Fig. 22–70). Rarely, an inflammatory mass may produce the deviation (Fig. 22–71).

    b. Aneurysm or aneurysmal widening of the internal iliac (hypogastric) artery. Vascular calcifications are frequently seen in the area (Figs. 22–72, 22–73). This deviation differs from that of bladder diverticulum in that the ureter returns to its normal contour prior to entering the bladder.

Although none of the ureteral deviations is specific, an awareness of the usual deviations seen in different entities will aid the examiner in making a more selective differential diagnosis. We have found the pelvic deviations, especially those associated with bladder diverticulum, enlarged retroperitoneal nodes, and pelvic carcinoma, to be of diagnostic assistance.

CHAPTER 22, ILLUSTRATIONS

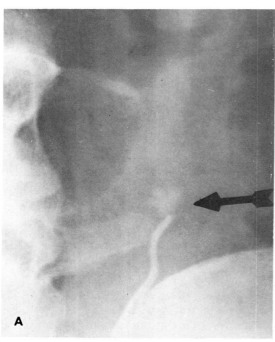

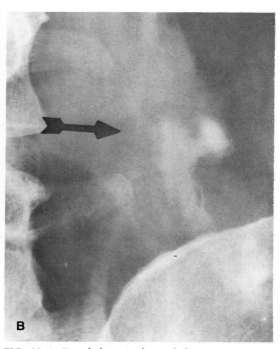

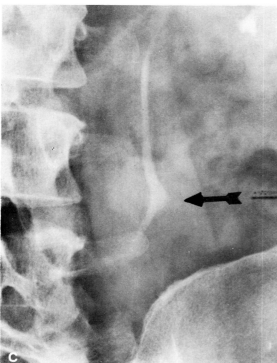

FIG. 22–1. Pseudodiverticulum of the ureter. Patient admitted with left renal colic. **(A)** A ureteral calculus is present opposite the tip of the 4th lumbar transverse process, with the retrograde catheter just below the calculus (*arrow*). Following manipulation the calculus passed spontaneously. A urogram the following day **(B)** revealed extensive extravasation just above the site of the previously impacted calculus (*arrow*). The extravasation follows the contour of the psoas margin. No surgery was performed. The patient was readmitted 4 years later for unrelated pathology. At this time a repeat excretory urogram **(C)** revealed a small pseudodiverticulum (*arrow*) at the site of the previous rupture. It is surprising that such deformities are not encountered more often following ureteral rupture.

FIG. 22–2. Postoperative ureteral deformity. Following surgery for unilateral idiopathic retroperitoneal fibrosis, a drain was inserted in the vicinity of the right ureter near S-1. When the drain was removed, it pulled the ureter laterally, producing the sharp angulation seen in the illustration. A repeat pyelogram several months later revealed the same deformity without evidence of obstruction. (Other examples of minor deformities following surgery are included in Chapter 20, Trauma to the Ureter.)

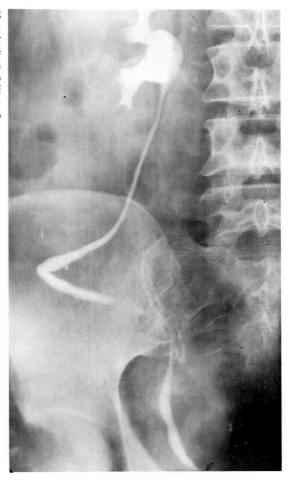

FIG. 22–3. (A) Nephrostomy following ligation of the distal right ureter (*arrow*) during hysterectomy. **(B)** Injection through nephrostomy tube following reimplantation of ureter into bladder.

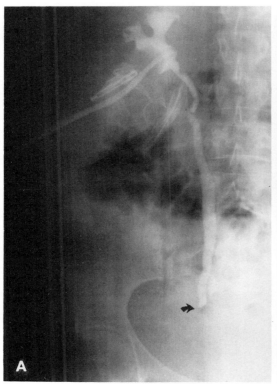

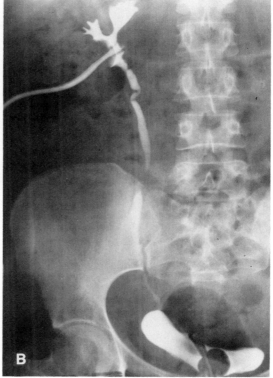

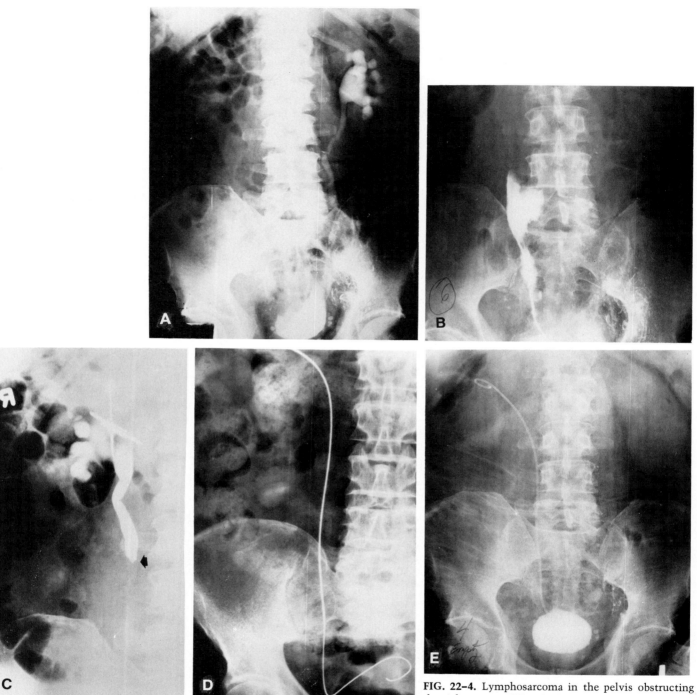

FIG. 22–4. Lymphosarcoma in the pelvis obstructing the right ureter. BUN 30. Creatinine 1.8. **(A)** Urogram showing nonfunction of the right kidney with mild left hydronephrosis, and mass impressing right superior aspect of bladder. **(B)** Attempted pyelogram was unsuccessful with extravasation of contrast medium. **(C)** Percutaneous pyelogram with contrast medium defining the level of obstruction (*arrow*). **(D)** Catheter was passed through obstruction allowing for urine drainage. **(E)** Pigtail stent replaced catheter and was left in place during radiotherapy; proximal curled end in renal pelvis, distal end in bladder. (Courtesy of Murray Mazer, M.D.)

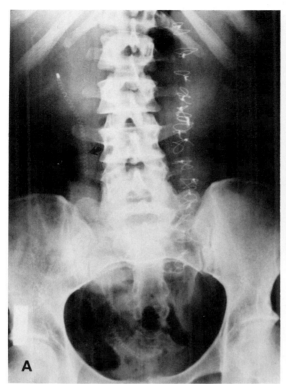

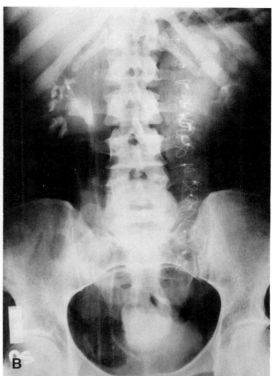

FIG. 22–4a. Ureteral splint by catheter. **(A)** Scout film shows coiled spring of catheter (*arrow*) splinting right ureter. **(B)** Maintenance of ureteral lumen by catheter allows for normal renal function.

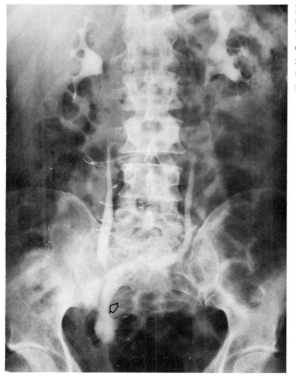

FIG. 22–5. Ileal loop (ureteroilealcutaneous). Both ureters were transplanted into an isolated loop of ileum because of advanced inoperable carcinoma of the bladder. The left ureter courses across the sacrum to the terminal ileum. Note that there is no significant proximal ureterectasis or pyelectasis. Contrast filling of the ileum (*arrow*) is seen readily.

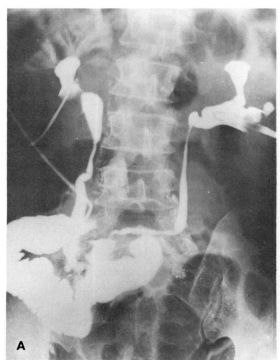

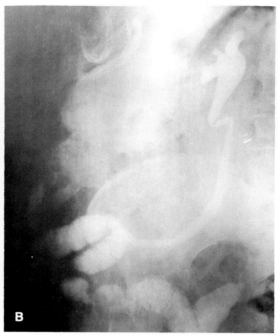

FIG. 22–6. Ileal loop. Illustrations of good functioning ureteroileostomies performed for inoperable carcinoma of the bladder (**A**) and for severe interstitial cystitis (**B**).

FIG. 22–7. Ileal loop. Urogram 7 years after ureteroileocutaneous anastomosis showing excellent function of both kidneys.

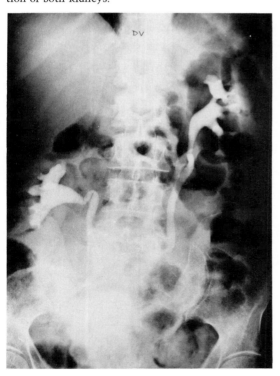

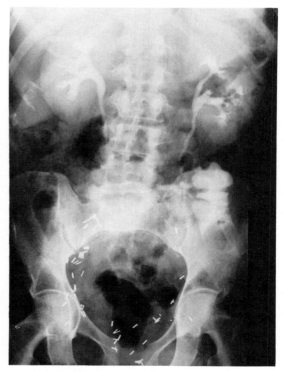

FIG. 22–8. Ureterosigmoidcutaneous anastomosis. Both ureters drain into an isolated sigmoid loop that is out of the pelvic area where the primary pathologic function was located. Renal function is excellent. (Courtesy of A. Tessler, M.D.)

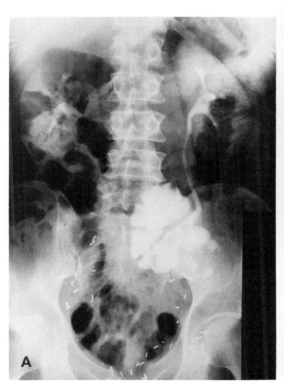

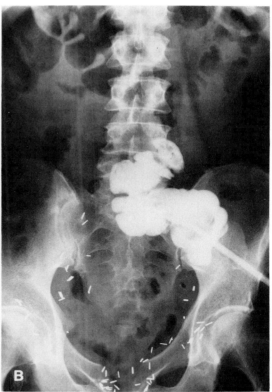

FIG. 22–9. Ureterosigmoidcutaneous anastomosis. Urogram (**A**) shows excellent renal function with prompt drainage into the isolated sigmoid loop. (**B**) Retrograde injection of the sigmoid loop shows no ureteral reflux. Using colic loops, there is less chance of ureteral reflux. (Courtesy of A. Tessler, M.D.)

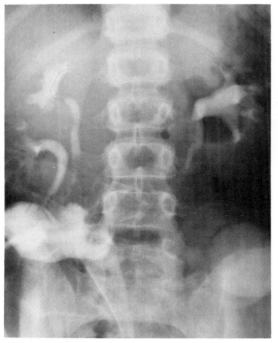

FIG. 22–10. Nonrefluxing transverse colon conduit. Two right ureters and left ureter diverted into an isolated segment of transverse colon. Prior pelvic exenteration operation with colostomy and ileal loop, the latter now replaced by colon loop. (Courtesy of W. Hardy Hendren)

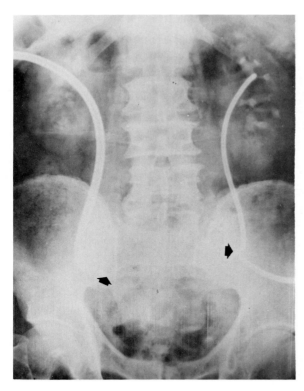

FIG. 22–11. Ureterostomies. Both ureters were transplanted cutaneously following total cystectomy for carcinoma of the bladder. The illustration, a 30-minute urogram, reveals minimal bilateral hydronephrosis. On the right side the tip of the catheter is inserted in the cutaneous opening of the ureter (*arrow*), with the remainder of the catheter lying externally on the skin. On the left side the catheter enters the cutaneous opening of the ureter (*arrow*) and then is passed up the ureter into the renal pelvis.

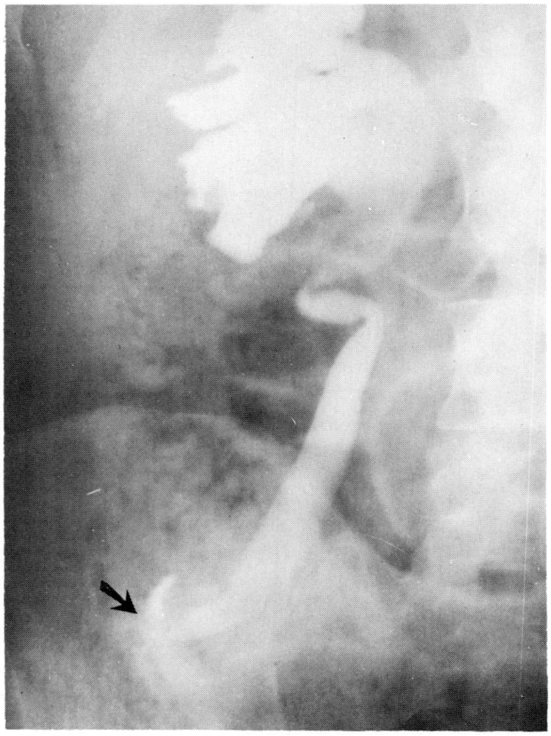

FIG. 22–12. Ureterostomy. The excretory urogram reveals severe hydronephrosis of the right kidney. The ureter is well visualized to the point of the ureterostomy. At this point contrast medium is noted to be spilling on the skin (*arrow*).

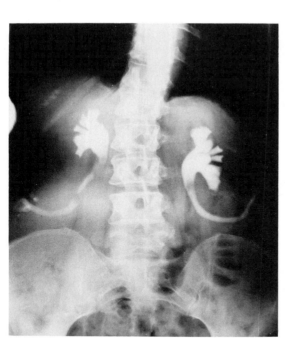

FIG. 22–13. Bilateral cutaneous ureterostomies following extensive pelvic surgery.

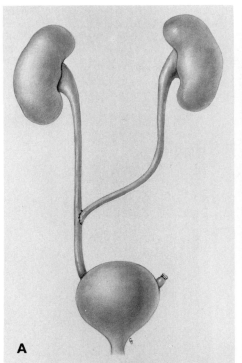 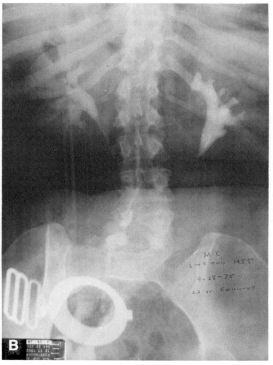

FIG. 22–14. Transureteroureterostomy. **(A)** Diagram of procedure. **(B)** Urogram of patient 23 years after TUU. (Courtesy of Clarence V. Hodges, M.D.)

FIG. 22–15. Functioning right-to-left transureteroureterostomy performed after resection of right ureteral stricture. Moderate hydronephrosis from partial left ureteral obstruction distal to anastomosis. (Courtesy of Moneer K. Hanna, M.D.)

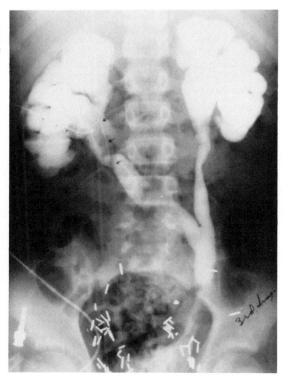

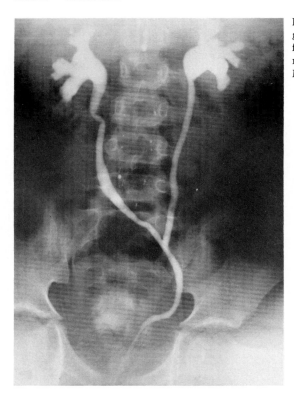

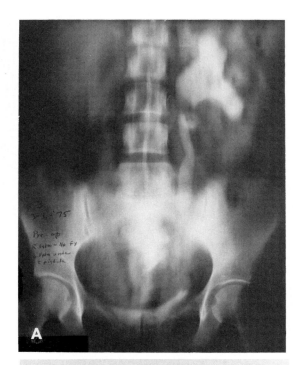

FIG. 22–16. Transureteroureterostomy. Ten-year-old girl who had bilateral ureteral vesical implants with failure on the right side. Retrograde 6 months after right-to-left TUU. (Courtesy of W. Hardy Henaren, M.D.)

FIG. 22–17. Transureteroureterostomy. **(A)** Right kidney nonfunctioning. Left hydronephrosis secondary to distal ureteral obstruction. **(B)** Excellent function of left kidney 8 months after left-to-right TUU. **(C)** Diagram of procedure. (Courtesy of Clarence V. Hodges, M.D.)

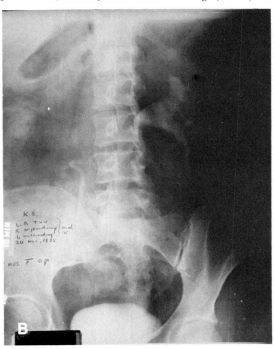

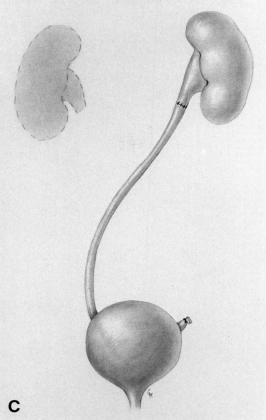

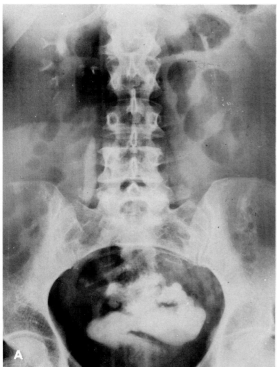

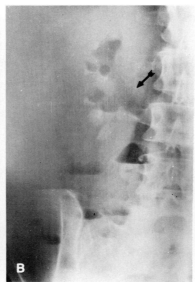

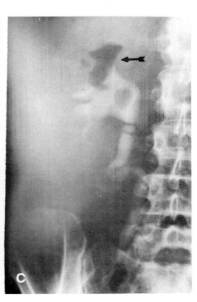

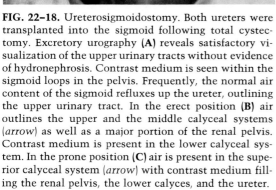

FIG. 22–18. Ureterosigmoidostomy. Both ureters were transplanted into the sigmoid following total cystectomy. Excretory urography (**A**) reveals satisfactory visualization of the upper urinary tracts without evidence of hydronephrosis. Contrast medium is seen within the sigmoid loops in the pelvis. Frequently, the normal air content of the sigmoid refluxes up the ureter, outlining the upper urinary tract. In the erect position (**B**) air outlines the upper and the middle calyceal systems (*arrow*) as well as a major portion of the renal pelvis. Contrast medium is present in the lower calyceal system. In the prone position (**C**) air is present in the superior calyceal system (*arrow*) with contrast medium filling the renal pelvis, the lower calyces, and the ureter.

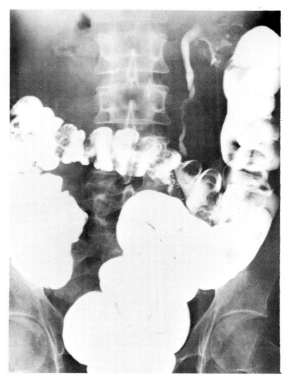

FIG. 22–19. Ureterosigmoidostomy. Both ureters were implanted into the sigmoid because of inoperable obstructing carcinoma of the bladder. Barium enema reveals filling of the left ureter and kidney with barium. There is no reflux into the right ureter. Such reflux filling of the urinary system following colonic implant tends to produce severe pyelonephritic changes and ureteritis. Better surgical techniques now provide antireflux anastomoses.

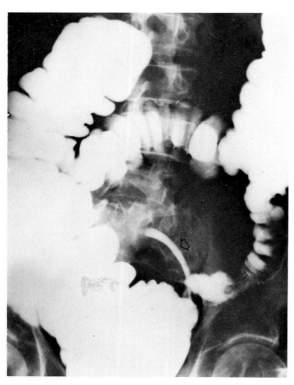

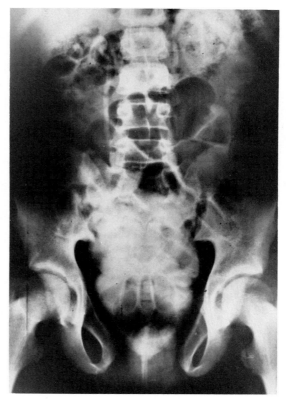

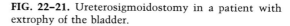

FIG. 22–20. Ureterosigmoidostomy. Following total cystectomy for carcinoma of the bladder, both ureters were transplanted into the sigmoid. The barium enema reveals reflux up the right ureter, which crossed the midline (*arrow*). There is no reflux up the left ureter. Excretory urography revealed satisfactory visualization of both upper urinary tracts with slight hydronephrosis on the right side.

FIG. 22–21. Ureterosigmoidostomy in a patient with extrophy of the bladder.

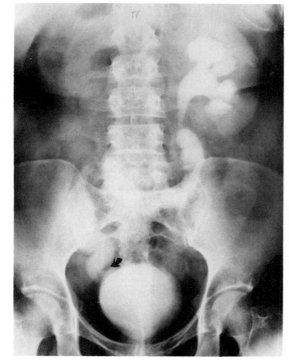

FIG. 22–22. Ureteral replacement. Urogram 1 year after anastomosis of both proximal ureters to an isolated loop of ileum that is implanted into the right side of the bladder (*arrow*). A stricture at the site of anastomosis of the right ureter to the ileum resulted in atrophy of the right kidney.

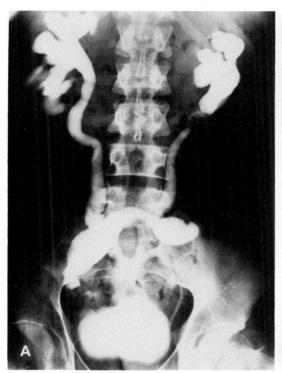

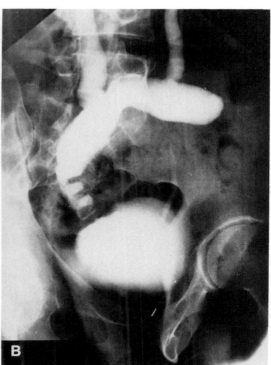

FIG. 22–23. Interposition of bowel. **(A)** Both ureters were connected to a loop of ileum that was then connected to the bladder. Function was satisfactory but bilateral reflux was present. In **(B)**, note reflux from bladder up distal segment of unused left ureter.

FIG. 22–24. Ileocystopathy. Small bladder secondary to chronic interstitial cystitis. A closed loop of ileum has been anastomosed to the bladder to increase the capacity of the bladder. The ureters still enter the bladder in their normal position.

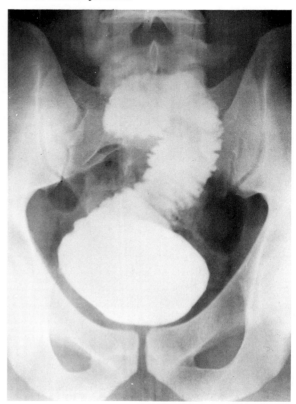

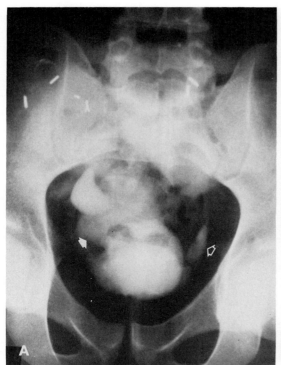
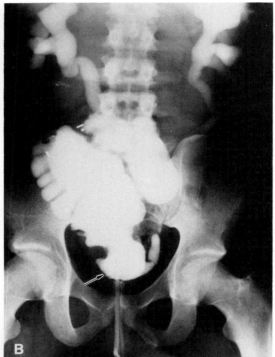

FIG. 22–25. Interposition of bowel following partial cystectomy. **(A)** Urogram filling the cecum (*white arrow*), which is connected to the residual bladder. Both ureters enter the isolated cecum. Note reflux up unused distal left ureter (*open arrow*). **(B)** Cystogram shows bilateral reflux up both ureters and unused segment of left ureter. The cecum is connected to the small residual bladder (*arrow*).

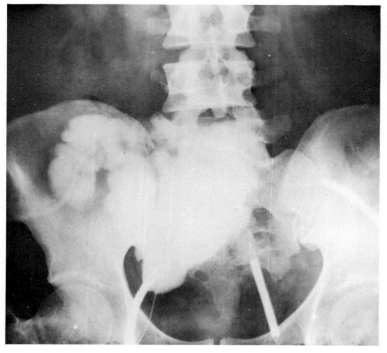

FIG. 22–26. Cecal bladder. Both ureters were transplanted into the cecum, with the cecum and the terminal ileum isolated from the remainder of the bowel. A catheter is present in the terminal ileum, draining cutaneously. Retrograde injection of contrast medium has filled the entire cecum and the terminal ileum. There is no reflux up either ureter.

FIG. 22–26a. Pig-tail catheter extending from renal pelvis to bladder providing drainage through a metastatic lesion that had occluded the right ureter.

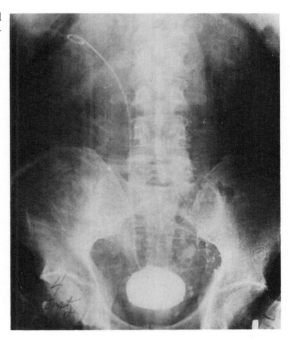

FIG. 22–26b. Pig-tail catheter used as stent. Diagram shows introduction of needle (**A**), guide wire (**B**), catheter over guide wire (**C**), placement of catheter into renal pelvis and withdrawal of guide wire (**D** & **E**), and finally catheter in position for drainage (**F**). Curled tails in renal pelvis and bladder prevent slipping of catheter. (Courtesy of B. Mazer)

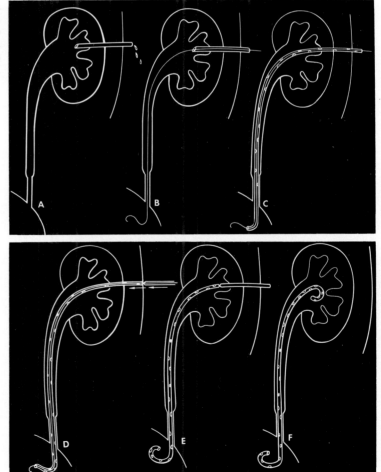

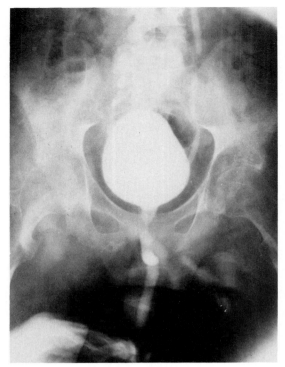

FIG. 22–27. Voiding cystourethrography in a man with neurogenic bladder. Bilateral ureteral reflux is more pronounced on left side.

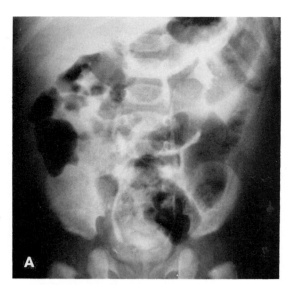

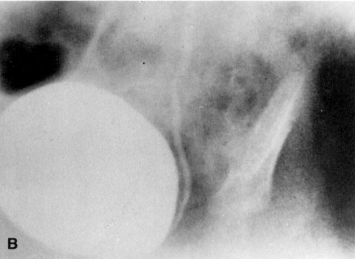

FIG. 22–28. Primary left ureteral reflux. **(A)** Girl, 1 month old, with normal urogram. The distal right ureter appears slightly dilated, suggesting the possibility of right ureteral reflux, but this is often misleading. **(B)** Cystourethrogram reveals left ureteral reflux. The left ureteral orifice was laterally placed and gaping.

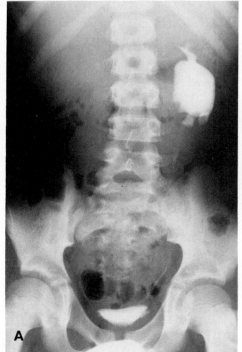

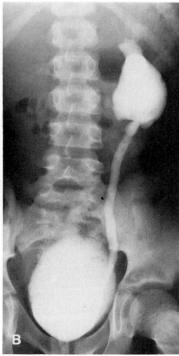

FIG. 22–29. Solitary left kidney with ureteropelvic junction obstruction and reflux. Young boy with intermittent left flank pain. **(A)** Urogram shows moderate ureteropelvic junction obstruction of left renal pelvis and no visualization of the right kidney. The left ureter appears normal. **(B)** Cystourethrogram reveals grade 3 reflux with further distention of the renal pelvis and calyces.

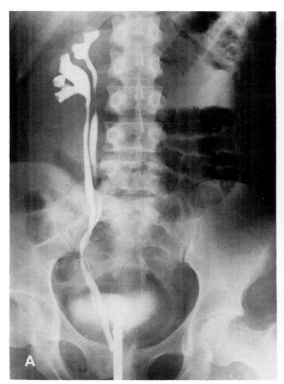

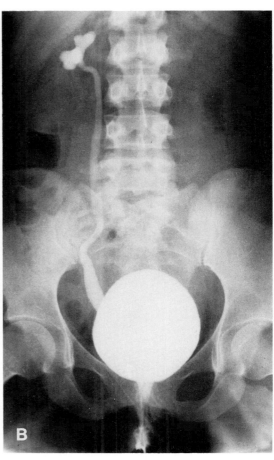

FIG. 22–30. Double right kidney with reflux into the ectopic ureter draining the upper pole. **(A)** Pyelogram with ureter draining the upper pole entering the posterior urethra. **(B)** Voiding cystourethrogram with grade 3 reflux into ectopic ureter.

FIG. 22–31. Cystogram in a child with loss of abdominal musculature. Note the massive bilateral ureteral reflux associated with renal hypoplasia and ureteral redundancy.

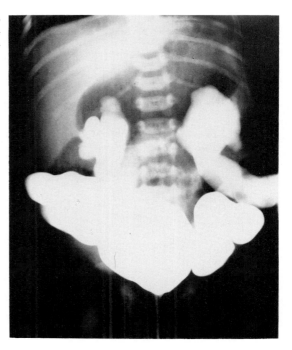

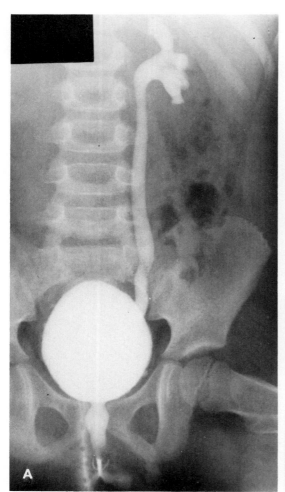

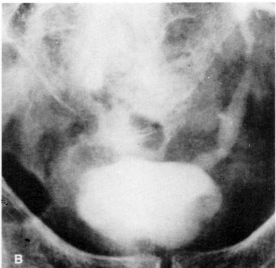

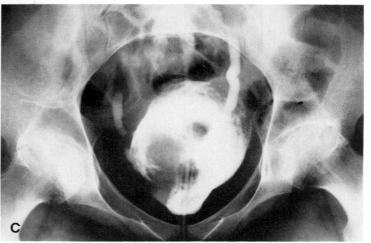

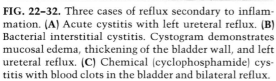

FIG. 22–32. Three cases of reflux secondary to inflammation. **(A)** Acute cystitis with left ureteral reflux. **(B)** Bacterial interstitial cystitis. Cystogram demonstrates mucosal edema, thickening of the bladder wall, and left ureteral reflux. **(C)** Chemical (cyclophosphamide) cystitis with blood clots in the bladder and bilateral reflux.

FIG. 22–33. Posterior urethral valve. Lateral film of a young boy showing the dilated posterior urethra (*arrow*) secondary to a posterior urethral valve. Note the trabeculated bladder and the massive bilateral ureteral reflux.

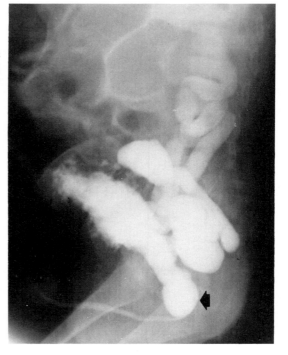

FIG. 22–34. Reflux after loss of efflux. Girl, age 6 years, with clinical diagnosis of neurogenic bladder. **(A)** Prediversion urogram showing bilateral hydronephrosis. **(B)** Cystogram shows markedly deformed bladder without reflux. **(C)** Following diversions, bilateral reflux occurred into the nonused ureteral stump *(arrows)*. **(D)** After diagnosis of chronic cystitis and good response to therapy, de-diversion was performed. Cystogram revealed no reflux. (Teele, R.: J. Urol., *115*:310–313, 1976)

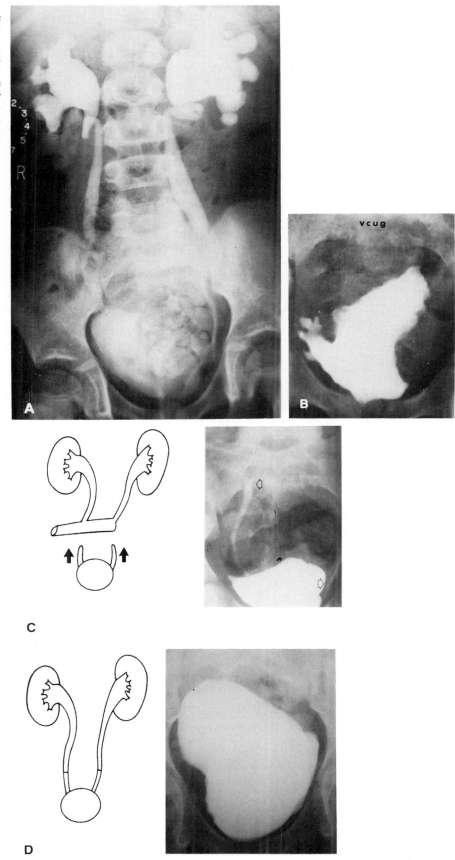

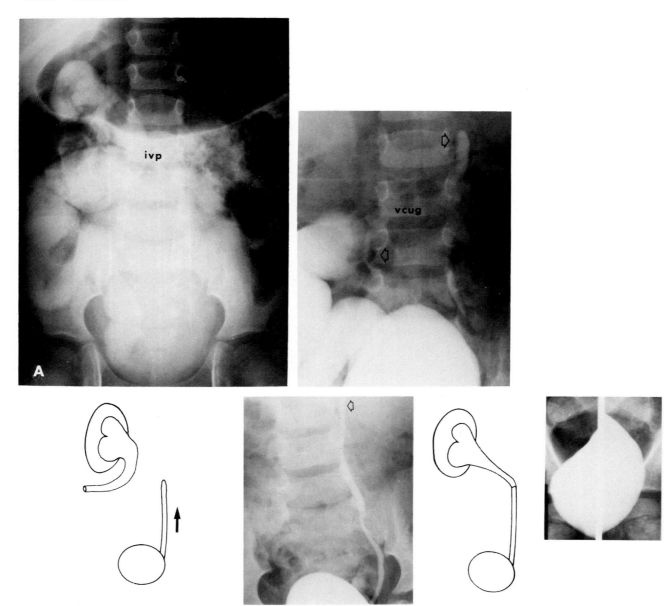

B

FIG. 22–35. Young boy with congenital right hydroureteronephrosis and dysplastic left kidney. **(A)** *Left:* Urogram showing dilatation of the right ureter and collecting system. *Right:* Cystogram showing bilateral reflux *(arrows).* **(B)** *Left:* A right ureterostomy was performed and the left kidney removed. The left unused ureter was reimplanted. Cystogram shows persistent reflux. *Right:* The right kidney was connected to the left ureter (transureteroureterostomy). As soon as flow commenced through the left ureter, reflux ceased (cystogram). ivp = intravenous urogram; vcug = vesicoureterogram. (Teele, R.: J. Urol., *115*:310–313, 1976)

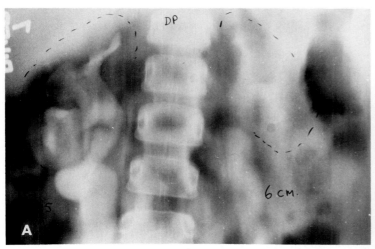

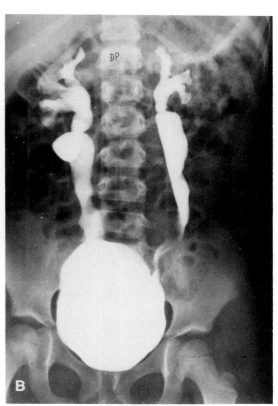

FIG. 22–36. Renal atrophy, infection, and reflux. Five-year-old girl with multiple episodes of renal infection. Tomogram of the urogram (**A**) reveals poor function bilaterally. There is calyectasis, ureterectasis, and renal atrophy. Cystogram (**B**) shows massive reflux bilaterally, grade 4.

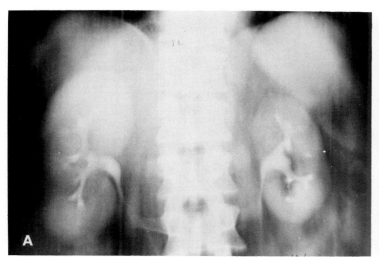

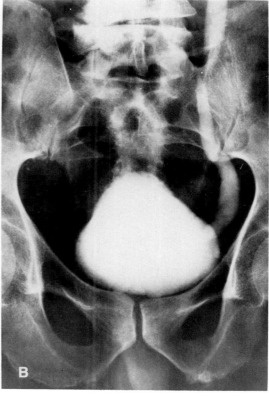

FIG. 22-37. Reflux and a small kidney in a 63-year-old woman with no previous history of urinary tract disease. (**A**) Tomogram of the urogram performed prior to a hysterectomy reveals the left kidney to be small, measuring 10.6 cm., whereas the right kidney measures 14.3 cm. There are no abnormalities of the calyces or parenchyma. A cystogram (**B**) revealed grade 3 left ureteral reflux. The relationship between the reflux and the small kidney is controversial (see text).

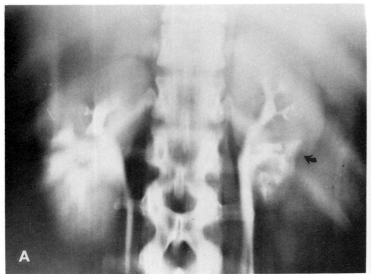

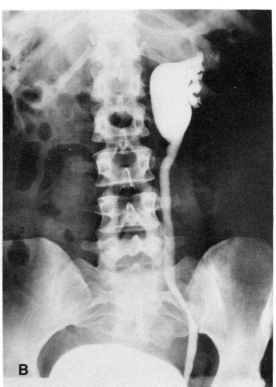

FIG. 22–38. Reflux and renal atrophy in a 26-year-old woman with no history of urinary tract pathology. Tomogram of urogram (**A**) reveals a double collecting system on the left. The upper system is normal, the lower atrophic with a thin cortical rim. Note the sharp demarcation (*arrow*) between the upper and lower systems. Cystogram (**B**) reveals grade 4 reflux into the lower system with reflux hydronephrosis. Urine culture was sterile. As in Fig. 22–37, one may conjecture on the relation of the segmental atrophy to the reflux.

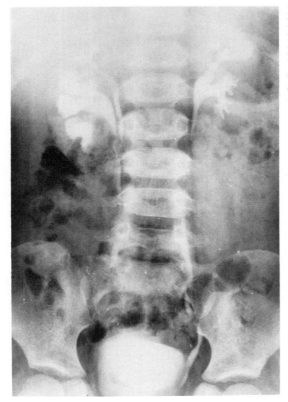

FIG. 22–39. Dysperistalsis. Pelvicalyectasis of the lower half of the double right collecting system with the two ureters joining at L-3. Fluoroscopy revealed dominant peristalsis from the upper segment continuing down the ureter to the junction of the two ureters. The peristaltic wave split, continuing down the lumbar ureter and also up retrogradely in the ureter to the lower renal segment producing calyectasis.

FIG. 22–40. Cystogram with bilateral ureterovesical reflux. Note the intrarenal reflux in the left kidney (*arrow*). This may introduce bacteria into the renal parenchyma or in noninfected urine produce focal renal destruction.

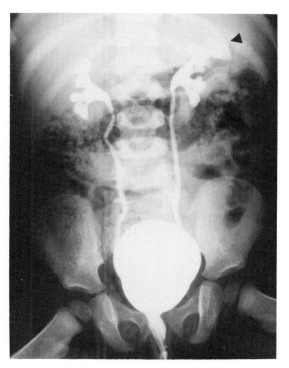

FIG. 22–41. Vesicoureteral reflux with intrarenal reflux primarily in the upper pole. Intrarenal reflux appears to be more common in the polar areas and provides bacteria access to the renal parenchyma. Sterile intrarenal reflux may produce destruction of parenchyma and a focal scar similar to that caused by bacterial infection.

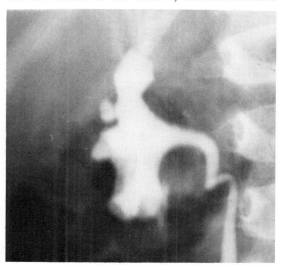

FIG. 22–42. Normal lateral course of ureter in a muscular 28-year-old man. Urogram (**A**) shows lateral bowing of the left ureter opposite L-4 (*arrow*). CT scan at the renal level (**B**) shows both ureters (*arrows*) in normal position. (**C**) CT scan at L-4–L-5 shows the left ureter (*arrow*) to be displaced anteriorly and laterally by thick psoas muscle. (Courtesy of G. Hartman, M.D.)

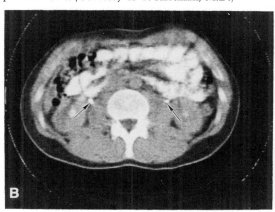

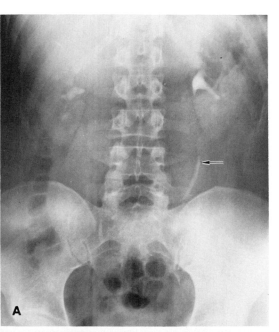

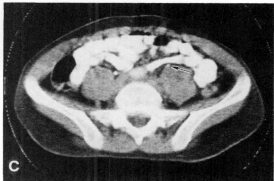

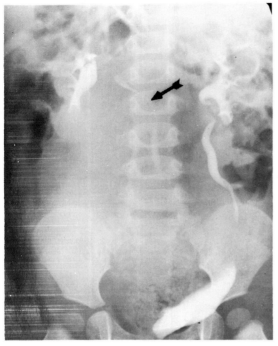

FIG. 22–43. Retroperitoneal sarcoma. Young child with a massive abdominal tumor extending down into the pelvis and laterally on both sides of the spine. Excretory urography reveals marked medial displacement of the right ureter over the midline of the spine (*arrow*). Slight lateral deviation of the mid left ureter is present. The urinary bladder is displaced to the left. In most cases, the type of displacement is nonspecific, depending on the location of the lesion with respect to the varying portions of the urinary system.

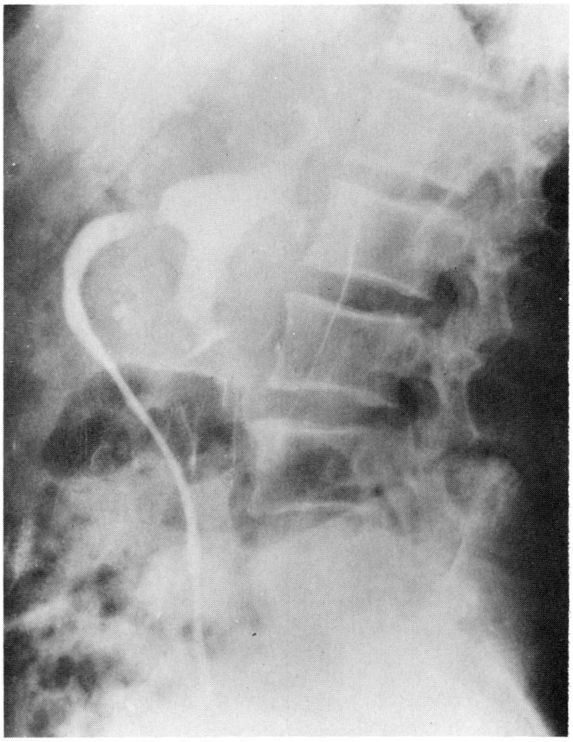

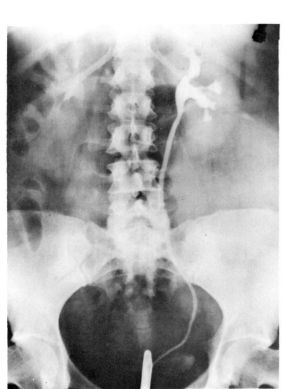

FIG. 22–44. Retroperitoneal sarcoma. In the frontal projection the left ureter was deviated laterally. Lateral deviation of the ureter is usually associated with anterior deviation of the ureter in the lateral projection.

FIG. 22–45. Benign retroperitoneal cyst. Large well-defined mass lesion in the left flank. The ureter is slightly deviated medially.

FIG. 22–46. Retroperitoneal myoliposarcoma. Marked lateral deviation of the right ureter associated with a large right retroperitoneal mass that is poorly defined. The right ureter lies on top of the mass and is pulled laterally with it. In the lateral projection, anterior deviation was present. (Courtesy of R. Hyman, M.D.)

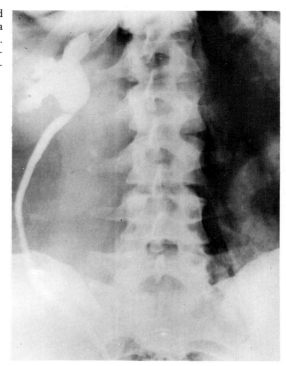

FIG. 22–47. Carcinoma of the ascending colon and the cecum, deviating the right ureter. This patient presented with a large right flank mass. In the barium enema, a large carcinoma of the ascending colon and the cecum was demonstrated (**A**, *arrow*), which had extended outside the cecum into the surrounding tissues. Excretory urography (**B**) revealed marked medial deviation of the ureter (*arrow*) without evidence of obstruction. We have seen cases of carcinoma of cecum that have produced obstruction of the right ureter.

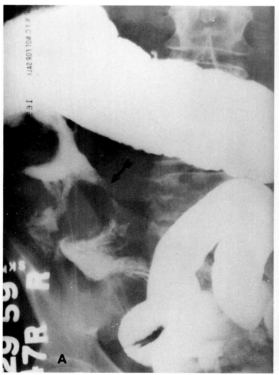

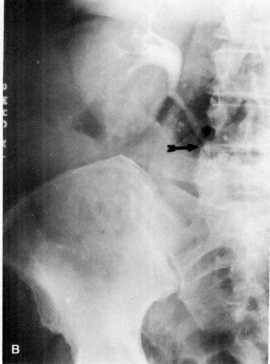

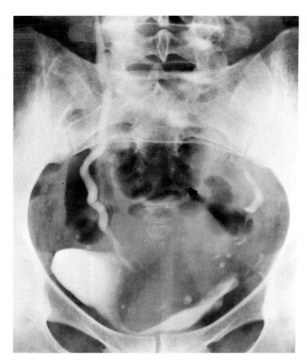

FIG. 22–48. Fibroid uterus indenting, distorting, and almost bisecting the bladder. The pelvic mass is well outlined by the intestinal gas content (*arrow*). It is difficult to distinguish the noncalcified fibroid uterus from an ovarian cyst. Marked deviation and distortion of bladder architecture are more common with a fibroid, since the uterus is in intimate association with the superior surface of the bladder.

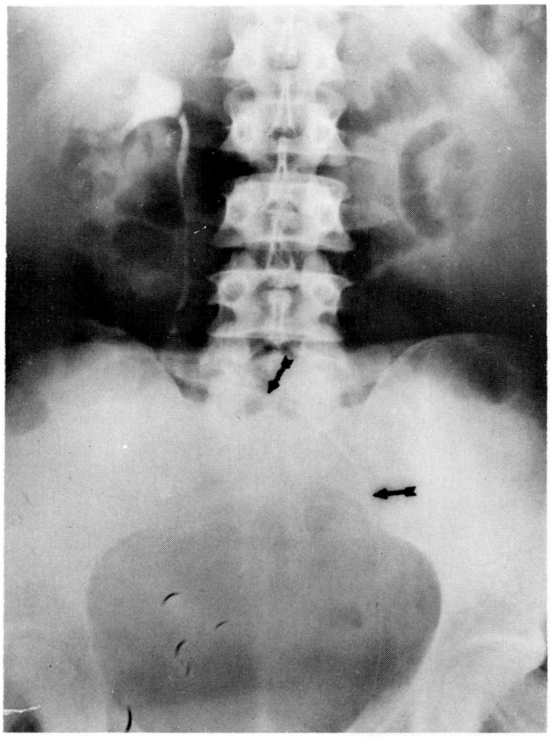

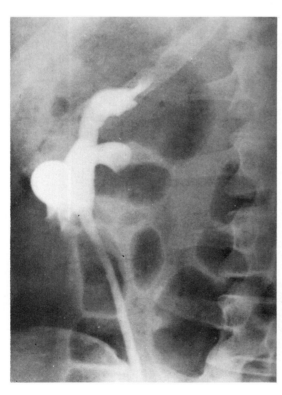

FIG. 22–49. Interligamentous fibroid. Most fibroids deviate the uterus laterally. Interligamentous fibroids may produce bizarre deviations of the ureter. This large right interligamentous fibroid has caught the right ureter and deviated it markedly to the left (*arrows*). Fibroids in this area are associated intimately with the pelvic ureter and may displace it medially or laterally.

FIG. 22–51. Malrotation of the kidney. The proximal ureter is deviated laterally secondary to nonrotation of the kidney with lateral placement of the renal pelvis. This type of deviation is smooth without evidence of a mass lesion impinging on the ureter.

FIG. 22–52. Peripelvic cyst. A peripelvic cyst (*upper arrow*) that presents medially to the renal pelvis displaces the pelvis laterally in a manner similar to that seen with malrotation. However, in this case a mass lesion is present, and mass impingement on the ureter is demonstrated (*lower arrow*). The lateral deviation of the ureter usually is more marked than that seen in simple malrotation, and the lower pole of the kidney is placed more laterally from the spine than the upper pole.

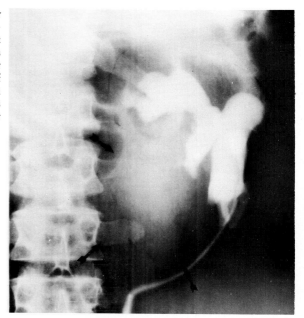

FIG. 22–53. Pyelectasia producing lateral deviation of the proximal ureter. Marked dilatation of the renal pelvis, usually secondary to an obstruction near the ureteropelvic junction, produces sharp lateral angulation of the proximal ureter (**A,** *arrow*). The greater the pelvic dilatation, the more prominent is the ureteral impression. (**B**) Another example of massive dilatation of the pelvis and calyces. The dilated renal pelvis has deviated the proximal ureter inferiorly and laterally (*arrow*) and displaced the midthird of the ureter medially.

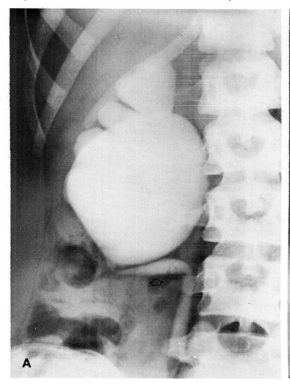

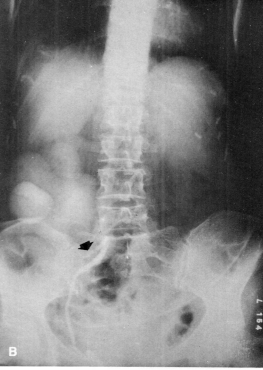

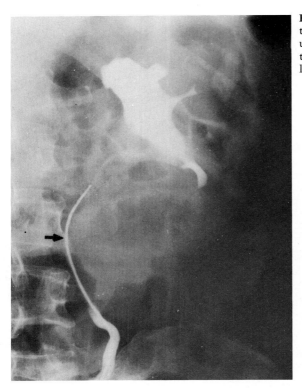

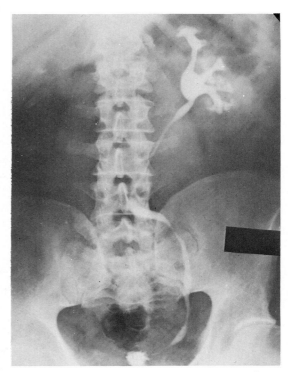

FIG. 22–54. Large hypernephroma of the inferior pole of the left kidney impinging on and deviating the left ureter medially. Cysts or tumors of the lower pole of the kidney frequently produce medial deviation of the left ureter.

FIG. 22–56. Medial deviation of the left ureter. This is an unusual, sharply localized medial deviation of the ureter, with the apex of the deviation at L-4. It is similar to the deviation seen with retrocaval ureter on the right side. We have seen two such cases, both unproved, which suggest the possibility of a retro-aortic ureter, the ureter possibly being hooked behind the abdominal aorta in a manner similar to that seen with the ureter on the right side passing behind the inferior vena cava. The possibility of a left-sided or double inferior vena cava must be excluded. No surgery was performed on this case. (Courtesy of P. Ross, M.D.)

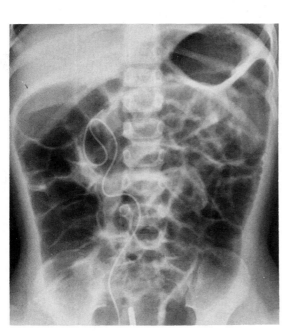

FIG. 22–57. The catheter shows the typical sharp medial deviation near L-3–L-4 by a retrocaval ureter.

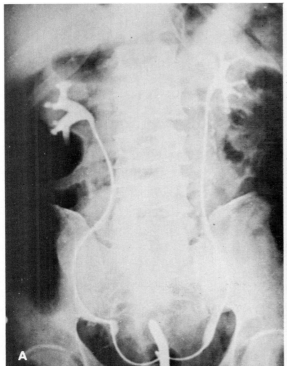
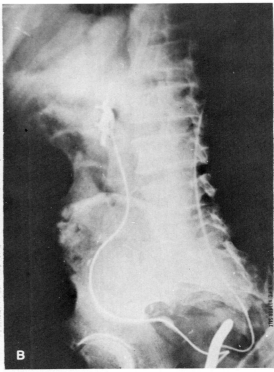

FIG' 22–58. Aneurysm of the aorta, producing lateral deviation of the ureter. **(A)** There is a well-circumscribed, partially calcified aneurysm of the aorta arising at the bifurcation, producing marked lateral deviation of the right ureter and anterior displacement **(B)** in the oblique projection. This type of deviation is not uncommon with large aortic aneurysms in this region.

FIG. 22–59. Large abdominal aortic aneurysm deviating both ureters laterally in the midabdomen.

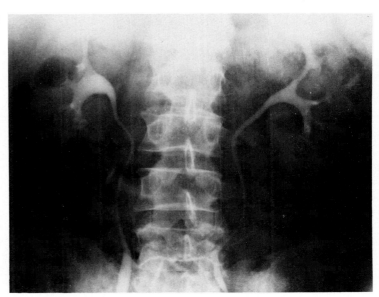

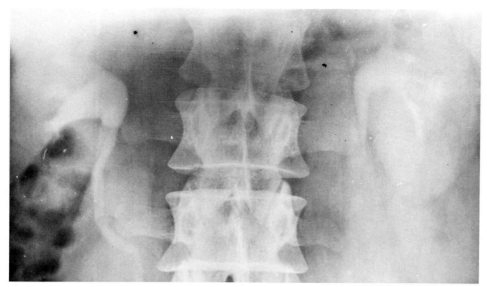

FIG. 22–60. Enlarged retroperitoneal nodes metastatic from carcinoma of the testes deviating the proximal ureter. This is by far the most common cause of lateral deviation of the proximal ureter and usually indicates lymphoma or metastatic malignant disease.

FIG. 22–61. Massive enlargement of the retroperitoneal lymph nodes, producing lateral deviations of the mid-thirds of the ureters (**A**). When marked lateral deviation occurs (**B**), anterior deviation of the ureter usually is present (**C**). Enlarged retroperitoneal nodes are the most common cause of lateral deviation of either the proximal or the midthirds of the ureters. (Courtesy of Herbert Kenyon, M.D.)

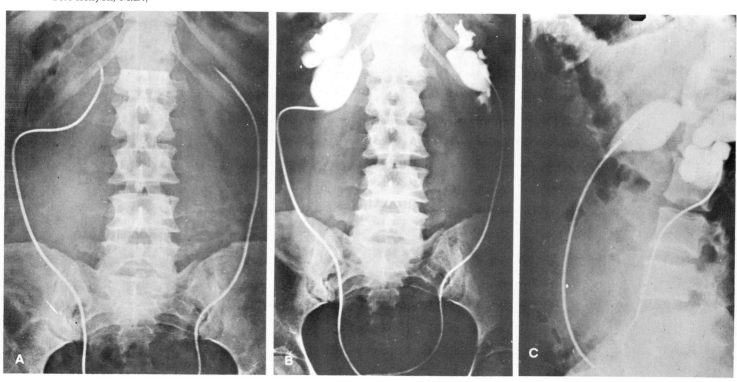

FIG. 22–63. Fecal impaction deviating ureters. In early infancy this patient had been operated on for anal stricture. Following surgery, a slowly progressive anal stenosis had developed. The illustration, an excretory urogram at age 14, reveals a markedly dilated sigmoid containing a large quantity of fecal material, producing marked lateral deviation of both ureters (*arrows*) similar to that seen with any centrally located pelvic mass, such as uterine fibroid or ovarian cyst.

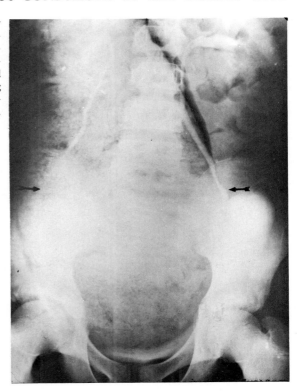

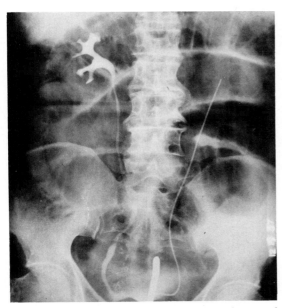

FIG. 22–64. Medial deviation after abdominal perineal surgery. Pyelogram reveals medial deviation of both ureters over S-1 and S-2 without obstruction, secondary to loss of peritonealization of the pelvic floor. Unless recurrent carcinoma is present, there is no evidence of proximal obstruction.

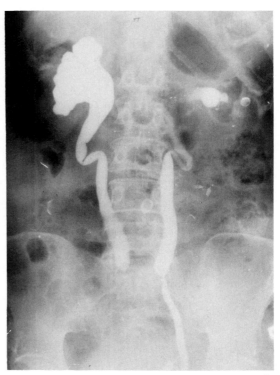

FIG. 22–65. Medial deviation of both ureters over the sacrum secondary to diffuse pelvic carcinomatosis from carcinoma of the rectosigmoid. Some degree of obstruction with proximal hydronephrosis is usually present.

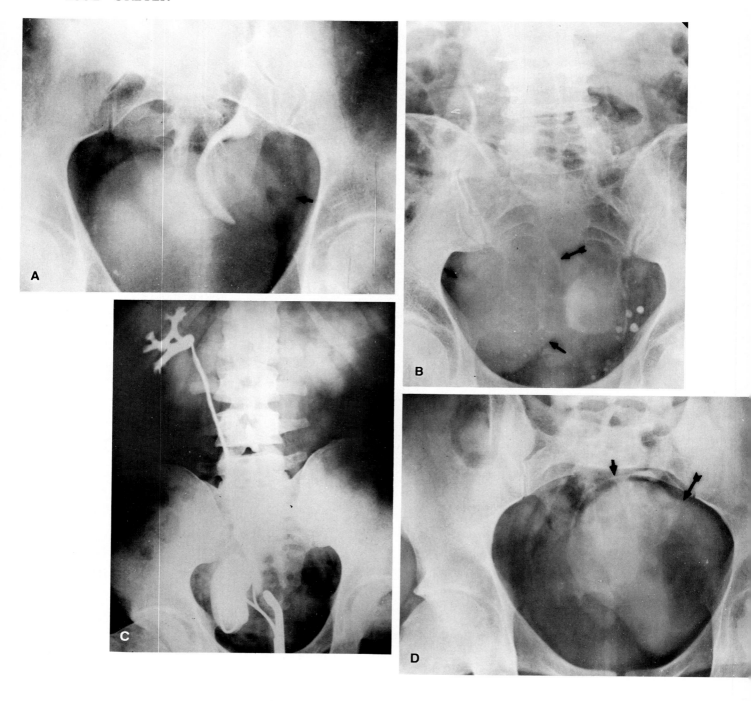

FIG. 22–73. Aneurysmal dilatation of the internal iliac artery producing medial deviation of the right ureter. The *arrows* point to faint arterial wall calcifications.

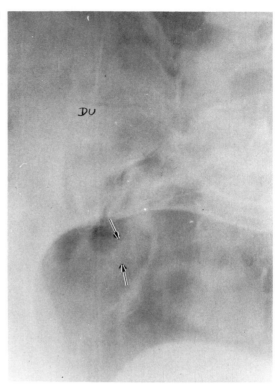

FIG. 22–74. Prolapse of the bladder. **(A)** Both ureters (*arrows*) descend below the symphysis in the urogram. **(B)** Cystogram demonstrates bladder prolapse.

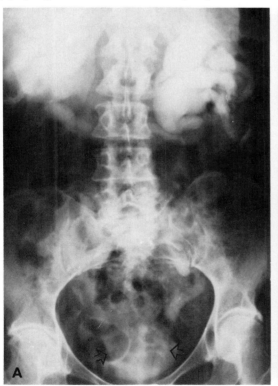

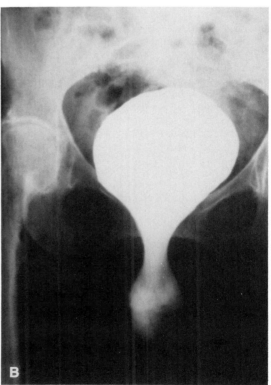

BIBLIOGRAPHY

Ureterosigmoidostomy

1. Bennett, A.H.: Exstrophy of bladder treated by ureterosigmoidostomies: Long term evaluation. Urol., 2:165–168, 1973.
2. Cardonnier, J.J.: Ureterosigmoid anastomosis. J. Urol., 63:276–283, 1950.
3. Carswell, J.J., III, Skeel, D.A., Witherington, R., et al.: Neoplasms at site of ureter sigmoidostomy. J. Urol., 115:750–752, 1976.
4. Leadbetter, W.F.: Consideration of problems incident to performance of ureteroenterostomy: Report of a technique. J. Urol., 65:818–830, 1931.
5. Leadbetter, W.F., and Clarke, B.G.: Five years' experience with ureterosigmoidostomy by the "combined" technique. J. Urol., 73:67–82, 1955.
5a. Leadbetter, G.W., Jr., Zickerman, P., Pierce E.: Ureterosigmoidoscopy and carcinoma of the colon. J. Urol. 121:732–735, 1979.
6. Megalli, M., and Lattimer, J.K.: Review of the management of 140 cases of extrophy of the bladder. J. Urol., 109:246–248, 1973.
7. Spence, H.M.: Ureterosigmoidostomy for exstrophy of the bladder: Results in a personal series of thirty-one cases. Br. J. Urol., 38:36–43, 1966.

Transureteroureterostomy

8. Anderson, H.V., Hodges, C.V., Behman, A.M., et al.: Transureteroureterostomy (contralateral uretero-ureterostomy): Experimental and clinical experience. J. Urol., 84:543–601, 1960.
9. Derrick, F.C., Jr., Lynch, K.M., Jr., Price, R., Jr., et al.: Transureteroureterostomy. J.A.M.A., 200:987–990, 1967.
10. Halpern, G.N., King, L.R., and Belman, A.B.: Transureteroureterostomy in children. J. Urol., 109:504–509, 1973.
11. Harbach, L.B., Kaufman, J.J., and Goodwin, W.E.: Experiment in ureterosigmoidostomy: Transureteroureterostomy combined with ureterosigmoidostomy to allow a single ureterocolic anastomosis. J. Urol., 104:395–401, 1970.
12. Hecker, G.N., and Ocker, J.M., Jr.: Why transureteroureterostomy? J. Urol., 108:710–711, 1972.
13. Higgins, C.C.: Transuretero-ureteral anastomosis: Report of a clinical case. J. Urol., 34:349–355, 1935.
14. Hodges, C.V., Moore, R.J., Lehman, T.H., et al.: Clinical experience with transureteroureterostomy. J. Urol., 90:552–562, 1963.
15. Jacobs, D., Politano, V.A., and Harper, J.M.: Experience with transureteroureterostomy. J. Urol., 97:1013–1016, 1967.
16. Schmidt, J.D., Flocks, R.H., and Arduino, L.: Transureteroureterostomy in the management of distal ureteral disease. J. Urol., 108:240–245, 1972.
17. Smith, I.: Trans-uretero-ureterostomy. Br. J. Urol., 41:14–22, 1969.
18. Smith, R.B., Harbach, L.B., Kaufman, J.J., et al.: Crossed ureteroureterostomy: Variation of uses. J. Urol., 106:204–208, 1971.
19. Udall, D.A., Hodges, C.V., Pearse, H.M., et al.: Transureteroureterostomy: A neglected procedure. J. Urol., 109:817–820, 1973.

Dysperistalsis (Uncoordinated Peristalsis)

20. Boyarsky, S., Labay, P., and Lenaghan, D.: Transureteroureterostomy, bifid ureters and ureteral dyskinesia. J. Urol., 99:156–159, 1968.
21. Dudzinski, P.J., Painter, M.R., and Lewin, E.L.: Urodynamics in transureteroureterostomy. J. Urol., 103:738–739, 1970.
22. Kaplan, N., and Elkin, M.: Bifid renal pelvis and ureter. Br. J. Urol., 40:235–244, 1968.
23. Tressider, G.C., Blandy, J.P., and Murray, R.S.: Pyelopelvic and ureteropelvic reflux. Br. J. Urol., 42:728–735, 1970.

Aneurysms of Abdominal Aorta

24. Albers, D.D., and Bettaglio, A.: Ureteral obstruction from an unsuspected aortic aneurysm: Case report. J. Urol., 55:249–250, 1961.
25. Culp, O.S., and Bernatz, P.E.: Urologic aspects of lesions in the abdominal aorta. J. Urol., 86:189–195, 1961.
26. Crane, J.F.: Ureteral involvement by aortic aneurysm. J. Urol., 79403–409, 1958.
27. DeWeerd, J.H., Ringo, M.G., Jr., Pool, T.L., et al.: Aortic aneurysm causing bilateral ureteral obstruction. J. Urol., 57:78–81, 1955.
28. Goodwin, W.E., and Shumacher, H.B., Jr.: Aneurysm of the hypogastric artery producing urinary tract obstruction. J. Urol., 57:839–844, 1947.
29. Labardini, M.M., and Ratliff, R.K.: The abdominal aortic aneurysm and the ureter. J. Urol., 98:590–596, 1967.
30. Pearlman, C.K., and Mackey, J.F., Sr.: Anuria resulting from abdominal aneurysm. J. Urol., 83:184–187, 1960.
31. Pinck, B.D.: Aneurysms of the aorta simulating urologic disease. J. Urol., 86:798–818, 1961.
32. Schloss, W.A., and Kaplan, B.J.: Spontaneous extravasation from ureter secondary to aneurysm of the abdominal aorta. N. Engl. J. Med., 249:802–804, 1953.
33. Shumacker, H.B., Jr., and Garrett, R.A.: Obstructive uropathy from abdominal aortic aneurysm. Surg. Gynecol. Obstet., 100:758–761, 1955.
34. Wagenknecht, L.V., and Madsen, P.O.: Bilateral ureteral obstruction secondary to aortic aneurysm. J. Urol., 103:732–736, 1970.

Colon Conduit

35. Hendren, W.H.: Nonrefluxing colon conduit for temporary or permanent urinary diversion in children. J. Pediatr. Surg., 10:381–398, 1975.
36. Hendren, W.H.: Exstrophy of the bladder: An alternative method of management. J. Urol., 115:195–202, 1976.
37. Richie, J.P., and Skinner, D.G.: Urinary diversion: The physiological rationale for nonrefluxing colonic conduit. Br. J. Urol., 47:269–273, 1975.
38. Skinner, D.G., Gottesman, J.E., and Richie, J.P.: The isolated sigmoid segment: its value in temporary urinary diversion and reconstruction. J. Urol., 118:614–618, 1975.

Ileal Loop

39. Arnarson, D., and Straffon, R.A.: Clinical experience with the ileal conduit in children. J. Urol., 102:768–771, 1969.
40. Bricker, E.M.: Substitution for the urinary bladder by the use of isolated ileal segments. Surg. Clin. North Am., 36:1117–1130, 1956.
41. Ellis, L.R., Udall, D.A., and Hodges, C.V.: Further clinical

experience with intestinal segments for urinary diversion. J. Urol., 105:354–357, 1971.

42. Engel, R.M.: Complications of bilateral uretero-ileo cutaneous urinary diversions: a review of 208 cases. J. Urol., 101:508–512, 1969.

43. Gregory, J.G., Gursahani, M., and Schoenberg, H.W.: Five-year radiographic review of ileal conduits. J. Urol., 112:327–331, 1974.

44. Malek, R.S., Burke, E.C., and DeWeerd, J.H.: Ileal conduit diversions in children. J. Urol., 105:892–906, 1971.

45. Mueller, C.S., and Thornbury, J.R.: Adenocarcinoma of the colon complicating ureterosigmoidostomy: A case report and review of the literature. J. Urol., 109:225–227, 1973.

46. Murphy, J.J., and Schoenberg, H.M.: Survey of long-term results of total urinary diversion. Br. J. Urol., 39:700–703, 1967.

47. Schmidt, S.D., Hawtrey, C.E., Flocks, A.H., et al.: Complications, results and problems of ileal conduit diversion. J. Urol., 109:210–216, 1973.

Ureteroileosigmoidostomy

48. Houtappel, H.C.: Experience with uretero-ileosigmoidostomy. Br. J. Urol., 35:277–283, 1963.

Vesicoureteral Reflux

49. Amar, A.D.: Familial vesicoureteral reflux. J. Urol., 108:969–971, 1972.

50. Ambrose, S.S., and Nicolson, N.P.: Ureteral reflux in duplicated ureters. J. Urol., 92:439–444, 1964.

51. Apperson, J.W., Atkins, H., and Fleming, R.: The value of the isotope cystogram in determining pressure and volume at which ureteral reflux occurs. J. Urol., 89:405–413, 1963.

52. Auer, J., and Seager, L.D.: Experimental local bladder oedema causing urine reflux into ureter and kidney. J. Exp. Med., 66:741–754, 1937.

53. Bailey, R.: The relationship of vesicoureteric reflux to urinary tract infection and chronic pyelonephritis-reflux nephropathy. In Pepper, S. (ed.): Clinical Nephrology, pp. 132–141. Boston, Little, Brown, 1971.

54. Baker, R., Maxted, W., Mayloth, J., et al.: Relation of age, sex and infection to reflux: Data indicating high spontaneous cure rate in pediatric patients. J. Urol., 95:27–32, 1966.

55. Bakshandeh, K., Lynne, C., and Carrion, H.: Vesicoureteric reflux and end stage renal disease. J. Urol., 116:557–558, 1976.

56. Bialestock, D.: Renal malformation and pyelonephritis: The role of vesico-ureteral reflux. Aust. N.Z. J. Surg., 33:114–127, 1963.

57. Blight, E.M., and O'Shaughnessy, P.: Vesico-ureteral reflux in children. J. Urol., 102:44–46, 1969.

58. Bruce, A.W., and Awad, S.A.: Reflux in the residual ureter. J. Urol., 92:278–281, 1964.

59. Bunge, R.G.: Delayed cystograms in children. J. Urol., 70:729–732, 1953.

60. Burger, R.H.: Familial and hereditary vesicoureteral reflux. J.A.M.A., 216:680–681, 1971.

61. Burger, R.H.: A theory on the nature of transmission of congenital vesicoureteral reflux. J. Urol., 108:249–254, 1972.

62. Castro, J.E., and Fine, H.: Passive antireflux mechanism in the human cadaver. Br. J. Urol., 41:554–563, 1969.

63. Cooper, D.E.W.: Bladder studies in children with neurogenic incontinence. Br. J. Urol., 40:157–174, 1968.

64. Culp, O.S., Rusche, C.F., Johnson, S.H. III, et al.: Hydronephrosis and hydroureter in infancy and childhood. J. Urol., 88:443–450, 1962.

65. Cussen, L.J.: Cystic kidneys in children with congenital urethral obstruction. J. Urol., 106:939–941, 1971.

66. Dwoskin, J.Y., and Perlmutter, A.D.: Vesicoureteral reflux in children: A computerized review. J. Urol., 109:888–890, 1972.

67. Edwards, D.: In Symposium on Urinary Infections. London, Oxford University, 1969.

68. Ekman, H., Jacobson, B., Kock, N.G., et al.: High diuresis, a factor in presenting vesicoureteral reflux. J. Urol., 95:511–515, 1961.

69. Ericsson, N.O., and Ivemark, B.I.: Renal dysplasia and pyelonephritis in infants and children. Arch. Pathol., 66:255–263, 1958.

70. Ericsson, N.O., and Ivemark, B.I.: Renal dysplasia and urinary tract infections. Acta Chir. Scand., 115:58–65, 1958.

71. Fisher, J.H., and Darling, D.B.: The course of vesico-ureteric reflux associated with urinary infection in children. J. Pediatr. Surg., 2:221–224, 1967.

72. Foote, J.W., Blennerhassett, J.B., Siglesowrth, R.W., et al.: Observations on the ureteropelvic juncture. J. Urol., 104:252–257, 1970.

73. Forsythe, W.I., and Wallace, I.R.: The investigation and significance of persistent and recurrent urinary infections in children. Br. J. Urol., 30:297–302, 1958.

74. Forsythe, W.I., and Whelan, R.F.: The occurrence and significance of vesico-ureteral reflux in chidlren. Br. J. Urol., 30:189–197, 1958.

75. Fridjofsson, A., and Sundinn, T.: Studies of renal function in vesicoureteric reflux. Br. J. Urol., 38:445–452, 1966.

76. Fryjordet, A.: Sympathectomy and ureteral reflux. Scand. J. Urol. Nephrol., 2:196–198, 1968.

77. Garrett, R.A., Rhamy, R.K., and Carr, J.R.: Nonobstructive vesico-ureteral regurgitation. J. Urol., 87:350–354, 1962.

78. Gibson, H.M.: Ureteral reflux in the normal child. J. Urol., 62:40–43, 1949.

79. Hackler, R.H., Dalton, J.J., Jr., and Bunts, R.C.: Changing concepts in the preservation of renal function in the paraplegic. J. Urol., 94:107–111, 1965.

80. Harrow, B.B.: Ureteral reflux in children: concepts for conservative versus surgical treatment. Clin. Pediatr., 6:83–93, 1967.

81. Hinman, F., Jr., Miller, E.R., Hutch, J.A., et al.: Low pressure reflux: Relation of vesicoureteral reflux to intravesical pressure. J. Urol., 88:758–765, 1962.

82. Hinman, F., Jr., and Hutch, J.A.: Atrophic pyelonephritis from ureteral reflux without obstructive signs. ("Reflux pyelonephritis"). J. Urol., 87:230–242, 1962.

83. Hodson, C.J.: Obstructive atrophy of the kidney in children. Ann. Radiol., 10:273–276, 1967.

84. Hodson, C.J.: Chronic atrophic pyelonephritis: A review of present concepts. Presented at New York Roentgen Society Spring Meeting, New York, N.Y., Apr. 26–28, 1973.

85. Hodson, C.J., and Edwards, D.: Chronic pyelonephritis and vesicoureteric reflux. Clin. Radiol., 11:219–234, 1960.

86. Hutch, J.A.: Vesicoureteral reflux in the paraplegic: Causes and correction. J. Urol., 68:457–467, 1952.

87. Hutch, J.A.: The Ureterovesical Junction. Los Angeles, University of California, 1958.

88. Hutch, J.A.: Theory of maturation of the intravesical ureter. J. Urol., 86:534–538, 1961.

89. Hutch, J.A.: The role of the ureterovesical junction in the natural history of pyelonephritis. J. Urol., 88:354–362, 1962.

90. Hutch, J.A., Hinman, F., Jr., and Miller, E.R.: Reflux as a

cause of hydronephrosis and chronic pyelonephritis. J. Urol., 88:169–175, 1962.

91. Iannacone, G., and Panzironi, P.E.: Ureteral reflux in normal infants. Acta Radiol., 46:451–456, 1955.

92. Jeffs, R.D., and Allen, M.S.: The relationship between ureterovesical reflux and infection. J. Urol., 58:694–695, 1962.

93. Jones, B.W., and Headstream, J.W.: Vesicoureteral reflux in children. J. Urol., 80:114–115, 1958.

94. Kaveggia, C., King, L.R., Ghana, L., et al.: Pyelonephritis: A cause of vesicoureteral reflux. J. Urol., 95:158–163, 1966.

95. Kerr, W.S., Jr., Leadbetter, B.W., Jr., and Donohue, J.: An evaluation of internal urethrotomy in female patients with urethral or bladder neck obstruction. J. Urol., 95:218–221, 1966.

96. King, L.R., and Idriss, F.S.: Effect of vesico-ureteral reflux on renal function in dogs. Invest. Urol., 4:419–427, 1967.

97. King, L.R., Surian, M.A., Wendel, R.M., et al.: Vesico-ureteric reflux. J.A.M.A., 203:169–174, 1968.

98. Kirkland, I.S., Ross, J.A., Edmond, P., et al.: Ureteral function in vesico-ureteral reflux. Br. J. Urol., 43:289–296, 1971.

99. Kjellberg, S.R., Ericsson, N.D., and Rudhe, V.: The Lower Urinary Tract in Childhood. Chicago, Year Book Publishers, 1957.

100. Krepler, P.: The incidence of radiologically detectable changes in children with urinary infections. Z. Kinderheilk, 104:103–114, 1968.

101. Lattimer, J.K., Apperson, J.W., Gleason, D.M., et al.: The pressure at which reflux occurs: An important indication of prognosis and treatment. J. Urol., 89:395–404, 1963.

102. Lattimer, J.K., Leuzinger, D., Justice, M., et al.: When should the child with reflux be operated upon? J. Urol., 85:275–279, 1961.

103. Leadbetter, G.W., Jr., Duxbury, J.H., and Dreyfuss, J.P.: Absence of vesicoureteral reflux in normal adult males. J. Urol., 84:69–70, 1960.

104. Lenaghan, D.: Experimental neurogenic vesico-ureteral reflux. Br. J. Urol., 41:606–607, 1969.

105. Lenaghan, D., Cass, A.S., Cussen, L.J., et al.: Long term effect of vesico-ureteral reflux on upper urinary tract of dogs, I. Without urinary infection. J. Urol., 107:755–757, 1972.

106. Lenaghan, D., Cass, A.S., Cussen, L.J., et al.: Long term effect of vesico-ureteral reflux on upper urinary tract of dogs, II. With urethral obstruction. J. Urol., 107:758–761, 1972.

107. Lich, R., Homerton, L.W., Goode, L.S., et al.: The ureterovesical junction of the newborn. J. Urol., 92:436–438, 1964.

108. MacGregor, M., and Freeman, P.: Subclassification of childhood urinary tract infections as an aid to diagnosis. *In* Grady, F.D., and Brumfitt, W. (eds.): Urinary Tract Infections, pp. 95–102. London, Oxford University Press, 1968.

109. Marchetti, L.J., and Gonick, P.: A comparison of renal function in spinal cord injury patients with and without reflux. J. Urol., 104:365–367, 1970.

110. McGovern, J.H., and Marshall, V.F.: Reimplantation of ureters into the bladders of children. J. Urol., 99:572–574, 1968.

111. McGovern, J.H., Marshall, V.F., and Paquin, A.J., Jr.: Vesicoureteral regurgitation in children. J. Urol., 83:122–149, 1960.

112. Mebust, W.K., and Foret, J.D.: Vesicoureteral reflux in identical twins. J. Urol., 108:630–636, 1972.

113. Melick, W.F., Brodeur, A.E., and Naryke, J.J.: The results of treatment of ureteral reflux by revision of bladder neck. J. Urol., 96:36–38, 1966.

114. Melick, W.F., and Naryke, J.J.: Pressure studies of the normal and abnormal ureters in children by means of the strain gauge. J. Urol., 83:267–276, 1960.

115. Middleton, G.W., Howard, S.S., and Gillenwater, J.Y.: Sex-linked familial reflux. J. Urol., 114:36–39, 1975.

116. Miller, H.C., and Caspari, E.W.: Ureteral reflux as genetic trait. J.A.M.A., 220:842–843, 1972.

117. Mobley, D.F.: Familial vesicoureteral reflux. Urology, 2:514–518, 1973.

118. Mulcahy, J.J., Kelalis, P.P., Stickler, G.B., et al.: Familial vesicoureteral reflux. J. Urol., 104:762–764, 1970.

119. O'Donnell, B., Moloney, M.A., and Lynch, V.: Vesico-ureteric reflux in infants and children. Br. J. Urol., 41:6–13, 1969.

120. Paquin, A., Marshall, V.F., and McGovern, J.H.: The megacystic syndrome. J. Urol., 83:634–646, 1960.

121. Pellman, C.: The neurogenic bladder in children with congenital malformation of the spine: A study of 61 patients. J. Urol., 89:696–701, 1963.

122. Ransley, P.G., and Risdon, R.A.: Renal papillae and intrarenal reflux in the pig. Lancet, 2:1114, 1974.

123. Ross, J.C., Damanski, M., and Gibbon, N.: Ureteric reflux in the paraplegic. Br. J. Surg., 47:636–642, 1960.

124. Ross, G., and Thompson, I.M.: Relationship of non-obstructive reflux and chronic pyelonephritis. J. Urol., 70:391–394, 1963.

125. Rudhe, V., and Ericsson, N.O.: Congenital bladder neck obstruction in infancy and childhood. Ann. Radiol., 9:3–15, 1966.

126. St. Martin, E.C., Campbell, J.H., and Pesquier, C.M.: Cystography in children. J. Urol., 75:151–159, 1956.

127. Schmidt, J.D., Hawtrey, C.E., Flocks, R.H., et al.: Vesicoureteral reflux: An inherited lesion. J.A.M.A., 220:821–824, 1972.

128. Scott, J.E.: Results of anti-reflux surgery. Lancet, II:68–71, 1969.

129. Scott, J.E., and Stansfeld, J.M.: Ureteric reflux and kidney scanning in children. Arch. Dis. Child., 43:468–470, 1968.

130. Sherwood, T.: Ureteric reflux 1973: Chronic pyelonephritis v. reflux nephropathy. Br. J. Radiol., 46:653–654, 1973.

131. Shopfner, C.: Vesico-ureteral reflux five year re-evaluation. Radiology, 95:637–648, 1970.

132. Silber, I., and McAlister, W.H.: Longitudinal folds as an indirect sign of vesicoureteral reflux. J. Urol., 103:89–91, 1970.

133. Simpson, J.L., and German, J.: Familial urinary tract anomalies. J.A.M.A., 212:2264–2265, 1970.

134. Smith, D.R.: Critique of the concept of vesical neck obstruction in children. J.A.M.A., 207:1686–1692, 1969.

135. Spence, H.M., Murphy, J.J., McGovern, J.H., et al.: Urinary tract infection in infants and children. J. Urol., 91:623–628, 1964.

136. Stecker, J.F., Jr., Rose, J.G., and Gillenwater, J.Y.: Dysplastic kidneys associated with vesicoureteral reflux. J. Urol., 110:341–343, 1973.

137. Stephens, F.D., Joska, R.A., and Simmons, R.T.: Megaureter with vesicoureteric reflux in twins. Aust. N.Z. J. Surg., 24:192–194, 1955.

138. Stephens, F.D., and Lenaghan, D.: The anatomical basis and dynamics of vesicoureteral reflux. J. Urol., 87:669–680, 1962.

139. Stewart, C.M.: Delayed cystogram. J. Urol., 70:588–593, 1953.

140. Stewart, C.M.: Delayed cystography and voiding cystourethrography. J. Urol., 74:749–759, 1955.

141. Tanagho, E.A., Guthrie, T.H., and Lyon, R.F.: The intravesical ureter in primary reflux. J. Urol., 101:824, 832, 1964.

142. Tanagho, E.A., and Hutch, J.A.: Primary reflux. J. Urol., 93:158–164, 1965.
143. Tanagho, E.A., Hutch, J.A., Meyers, F.H., et al.: Primary vesicoureteral reflux experimental studies of the etiology. J. Urol., 93:165–176, 1965.
144. Tanagho, E.A., Meyers, F.H., and Smith, D.P.: The trigone: Anatomical and physiological configuration, I. In relation to the ureterovesical junction. J. Urol., 100:623–632, 1968.
145. Tanagho, E.A., Meyers, F.H., and Smith, D.P.: The trigone: Anatomical and physiological configuration, II. In relation to the bladder neck. J. Urol., 100:632–639, 1968.
146. Teele, R.L., Lebowitz, R.L., and Colodny, A.H.: Reflux and the unused ureter. J. Urol., 115:310–313, 1976.
147. Tobenkin, M.: Hereditary vesicoureteral reflux. South. Med. J., 57:139–147, 1964.
148. Waterhouse, K.: Discussion. In Glenn, J.F. (ed.): Ureteral Reflux in Children, p. 200. Washington, D.C., Nat. Acad. of Science, Nat. Research Council, 1963.
149. Weiss, R.M., Schiff, M., Jr., and Lytton, R.: Reflux and trapping. Radiology, 118:129–131, 1976.
150. Williams, D.I.: Urology in Childhood. Springer-Verlag, New York, 1974.
151. Williams, D.I., and Eckstein, H.B.: Surgical treatment of reflux in children. Br. J. Urol., 37:13–24, 1965.
152. Williams, D.I., Ray, R., and Lillie, J.G.: The functional radiology of ectopic ureterocele. Br. J. Urol., 44:417–437, 1972.
153. Williams, D.I., and Taylor, J.S.: A rare congenital uropathy: Vesico-urethral dysfunction with upper tract anomalies. Br. J. Urol., 41:307–313, 1969.

Intrarenal Reflux

154. Amar, A.D.: Calicotubular backflow with vesicoureteral reflux: Relation to pyelonephritis. J.A.M.A., 213:293–294, 1970.
155. Angel, J.R., Smith, T.W., Jr., and Roberts, J.A.: The hydrodynamics of pyelorenal reflux. J. Urol., 122:20–26, 1979.
156. Aperia, A., Broberger, O., Ekengren, K., et al.: Correlation between kidney parenchymal area and renal function in vesicoureteral reflux of different degrees. Ann. Radiol. (Paris), 20:141–144, 1977.
157. Bauer, D.: Pyelorenal backflow. Am. J. Roentgenol., 78:296–316, 1957.
158. Bourne, H.H., Condon, V.R., Hoyt, T.S., et al.: Intrarenal reflux and renal damage. J. Urol., 115:304–306, 1976.
159. Brodeur, A.E., Goyer, R.A., and Melick, W.: A potential hazard of barium cystography. Radiology, 85:1080–1084, 1965.
160. Hodson, C.J., Maling, T.M.J., McNamamon, P.J.: The pathogenesis of reflux nephropathy (chronic atrophic pyelonephritis). Br. J. Radiol. (Suppl.), 13:1–26, 1975.
161. Hodson, C.J.: The effect of disturbance of flow in the kidney. J. Infect. Dis., 120:56–60, 1969.
162. Kill, F.: The Function of the Ureter and Renal Pelvis. Philadelphia, W.B. Saunders, 1957.
163. Kohler, R.: Investigations on backflow in retrograde pyelography: Roentgenologic and clinical study. Acta Radiol. (Suppl.), 99:1–92, 1953.
164. Maling, T.M.J., and Rolleston, G.L.: Intra-renal reflux in children demonstrated by micturating cystography. Clin. Radiol., 25:81–85, 1974.
165. Mellins, H.Z.: Chronic pyelonephritis and renal medullary necrosis. Sem. Roentgenol., 6:292–308, 1971.
166. Ransley, P.G.: The renal papilla and intrarenal reflux. In Williams, D.I., and Chisholm, G.D. (eds.): Scientific Foundations in Urology, Vol. 1, pp. 79–87. Chicago, Year Book Medical Publishers, 1976.
167. Ransley, P.G.: Intrarenal reflux: Anatomical, dynamic, and radiological studies, Part I. Urol. Res., 5:61–69, 1977.
168. Ransley, P.G., and Risdon, R.A.: Renal papillary morphology and intrarenal reflux in the young pig. Urol. Res., 3:105–109, 1975a.
169. Ransley, P.G., and Risdon, R.A.: Renal papillary morphology in infants and children. Urol. Res., 3:111–113, 1975b.
170. Roberts, J.A.: The urinary system. In Fiennes, R.N.T.W. (ed.): Pathology of Simian Primates, pp. 821–840. Basel, S. Karger, 1972.
171. Rolleston, G.C., Maling, T.M.J., and Hodson, C.J.: Intrarenal reflux and the scarred kidney. Arch. Dis. Child., 49:531–539, 1974.
172. Rose, J.S., Glassberg, K.I., and Waterhouse, K.: Intrarenal reflux and its relativity to renal scarring. J. Urol., 113:400–403, 1975.
173. Ross, J.A.: One thousand retrograde pyelograms and manometric pressure records. Br. J. Radiol., 31:133–140, 1959.
174. Smellie, J.M., and Normond, I.C.S.: Bacteriuria, reflux and renal scarring. Arch. Dis Child., 50:581–585, 1975.
175. Tamminen, T.E., and Kaprio, E.A.: The relation of the shape of renal papillae and of collecting duct openings to intrarenal reflux. Br. J. Urol., 49:345–354, 1972.

Deviations of the Ureter

176. Drouillard, J., Bruneton, J.N., Resca, J.R., et al.: Lumbar ureteral deviation and hypertrophy of the psoas: A radiological lesion (author's translation). Ann. Radiol. (Paris), 20:557–562, 1977.
177. Friedenberg, R.M., Ney, C., Lopez, F.A., et al.: Clinical significance of deviation of the pelvic ureter. J. Urol., 96:146–151, 1966.
178. Gerlock, A.J.: Left testicular vein varices simulating retroperitoneal lymph-node enlargement. Radiology, 93:873–874, 1969.
179. Haines, J.O., and Kyaw, M.M.: Anterolateral deviation of ureter by psoas muscle hypertrophy. J. Urol., 106:831–832, 1971.
180. Haller, J.O., Berdon, W.E., Slovis, T.L., et al.: Excretory urographic demonstration of ureteral displacement by sigmoid fecal impaction simulating retroperitoneal tumor. J. Urol., 115:302–303, 1976.
181. Levine, R.B., Forrester, D., and Halpern, M.: Ureteral deviation due to iliopsoas hypertrophy. Am. J. Roentgenol., 107:756–759, 1969.
182. Saldino, R.M., and Palubinskas, A.J.: Medical placement of the ureter: A normal variant which may simulate retroperitoneal fibrosis. J. Urol., 107:582–585, 1972.
183. Ziter, F.M.: Unilateral ureteral deviation due to unilateral iliopsoas muscle hypertrophy. J. Can. Assoc. Radiol., 25:327–328, 1974.

Part Five

BLADDER

SHAPE OF THE BLADDER

The shape of the normal bladder is influenced by the degree of filling and the pressure of adjacent organs. The outline of the normal bladder is smooth, and its shape varies. It may be round (Fig. 23-1), oval (Fig. 23-2), oblong, or square (Fig. 23-3). Its greater diameter can be either transverse or vertical. The transverse diameter is more likely to be greater in females. In the intravenous urogram, the urinary bladder at various stages of filling reveals the indentations of adjacent organs. In the female the normal uterus produces an indentation (Figs. 23-11, 23-12) on the upper surface of the bladder, which usually is located centrally but may be slightly eccentric. The sigmoid colon may indent the upper surface of the bladder (Figs. 23-10, 23-20) on the left side. Complete filling usually erases these impressions. The base of the bladder may be indented slightly in the male by a prostate of even normal size. The levator ani (Fig. 23-5) may produce a slight elevation of the floor of the bladder in either sex. The penis can give a false impression on the cystogram (Figs. 23-16, 23-17). Other masses, such as bone lesions, can produce actual defects or false impressions on the bladder (Fig. 23-18). Recesses (Fig. 23-19) seen in females are pockets of normal bladder wall situated at the posterior lateral area of the bladder at the floor. These appear to be the result of the uterus pushing up the central part of the floor and allowing the lateral edges to balloon out.

POSITION OF THE BLADDER

In the newborn infant, both male and female, the bladder lies higher than it does in adult life. In many instances the internal sphincter lies well above the symphysis pubis. Gradually, as the child grows and

23

Normal
Bladder

becomes upright, the bladder descends until the vesical neck lies either at the upper border of the symphysis or just below. Disse considered that the internal sphincter did not reach the adult position until after puberty.[3] However, it would appear that by the first or second year of life the bladder in a child should be at the adult level. Hansen believes that the fundus (the portion around the vesical orifice) is higher in children and adult males than in females, but he added that there is no difference in the level in children and men.[6] The bladder is located centrally, and significant deviations are abnormal.

SIZE OF THE BLADDER

The size of the bladder varies, depending on such factors as exposure to cold, psychic phenomena, and inflammations. The anatomic capacity of the bladder is greater than its physiologic capacity. To determine the size of the bladder by x-ray study, the bladder is filled with an opaque material until discomfort occurs or until the pressure has reached at least 26 cm. of water.

In the child the upper border of the bladder should not rise above the level of the lumbosacral joint. Certainly, if the bladder reaches the level of the junction of the fourth and the fifth lumbar vertebrae, it is definitely enlarged. In the adult the bladder should not reach above the second or the third sacral segment. As to breadth, we believe that the sacroiliac joints represent the upper margin of the normal bladder in the adult. In the child we have found no definite anatomic limit that is useful in determining the normal breadth.

It should be emphasized that, because of the wide variations in the shape and size of pelves, these are not hard and fast rules. Attempts to correlate the appearance on the cystogram with the actual measurement of bladder volume have not been entirely satisfactory.

The trigone (Fig. 23–20) and the interureteric ridge (Figs. 23–8, 23–9) occasionally are visualized on an excretory cystogram. Visualization of the area is better in males than in females. It is most often seen when the bladder is partially distended with diluted contrast medium in the supine position. The interureteric ridge gives a crescentric appearance, with the concavity facing cranially (Figs. 23–8, 23–9). The increased density above the concave margin represents pooling of contrast material in the supine position. The ureters enter caudal to the crescent.[4] Defects in the area due to edema or inflammation can be seen in low ureteral stones and postcatheterizations of the ureter.[2]

On performing intravenous urography, a prone view is taken at 25 minutes for better evaluation of lesions of the anterior bladder wall, since it has been established that dependent areas of the urinary bladder are visualized better, owing to two factors: (1) Greater opacification results from the layering effect (the heavier opacified urine becomes dependent to the nonopacified urine); and (2) stretching results from the weight of the contained fluid.[5] In general, in the prone view the normal bladder appears to be elongated cephalically (Figs. 23–13, 23–14), owing to the anterior prolongation, and in the abnormal bladder lesions of the anterior wall (Fig. 23-15) can be visualized more satisfactorily.

CHAPTER 23, ILLUSTRATIONS

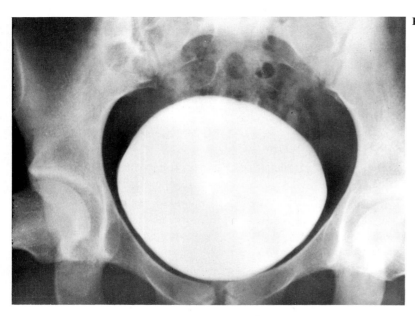

FIG. 23–1. Round bladder.

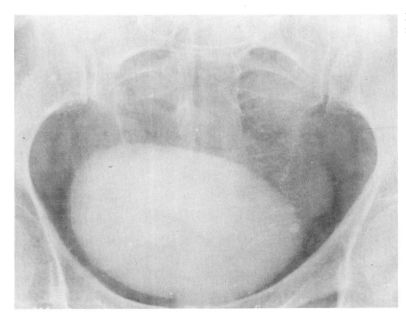

FIG. 23–2. Oval bladder. Bladder is elongated in horizontal axis.

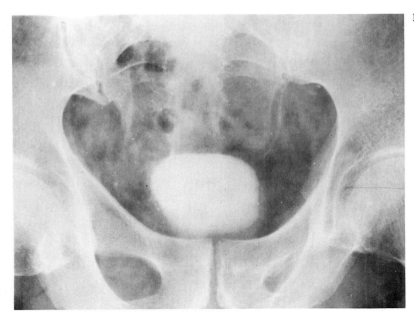

FIG. 23–3. Square bladder.

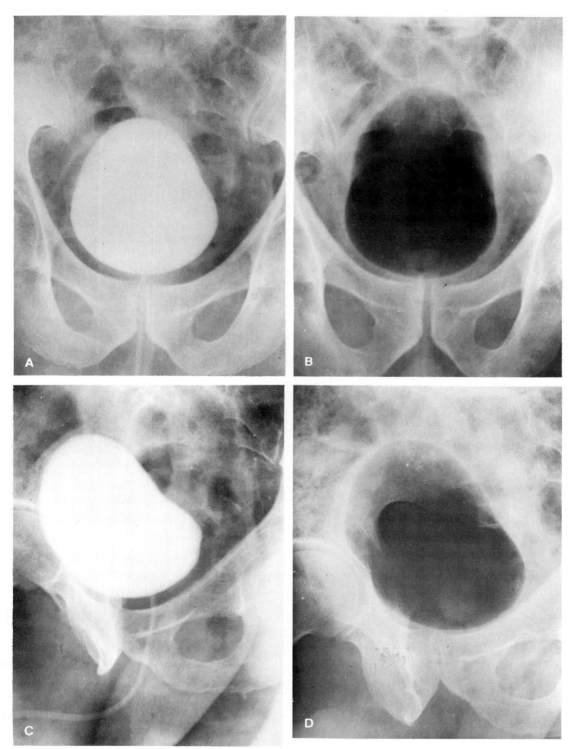

FIG. 23–4. Normal cystogram and pneumocystogram in AP and oblique views on the same patient. Bladder is elongated in vertical axis. **(A)** AP contrast cystogram. **(B)** AP pneumocystogram. **(C)** Right oblique contrast cystogram. **(D)** Right oblique pneumocystogram.

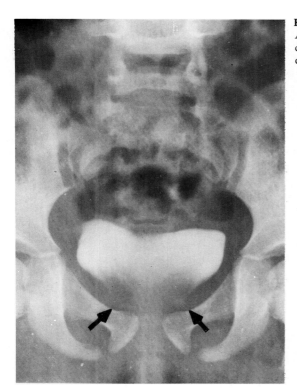

FIG. 23–5. Intravenous pyelogram in a 2½-year-old girl. *Arrows* point to indentations on either side of the bladder, probably owing to activity of the levator ani muscles.

FIG. 23–6. (A) *Arrows* point to double contrast that appears to be a diverticulum. (B) On oblique view one sees an elongated bladder, apparently folded on itself. No diverticulum was seen on cystoscopy.

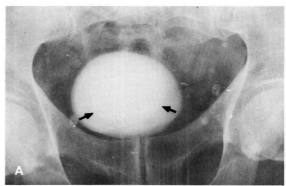

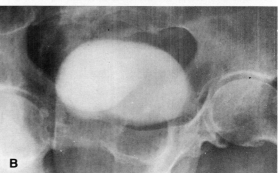

FIG. 23–7. (A) Supine view. Apparent diverticular formation. (B) Prone view. Complete filling of bladder. No diverticulum is seen. The appearance in the left film was due to cephalic elongation of the anterior wall of the bladder.

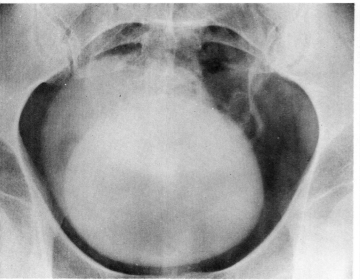

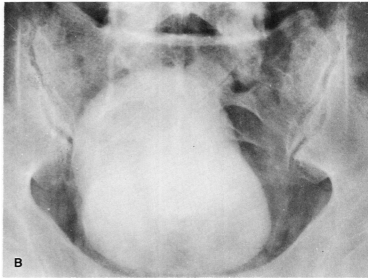

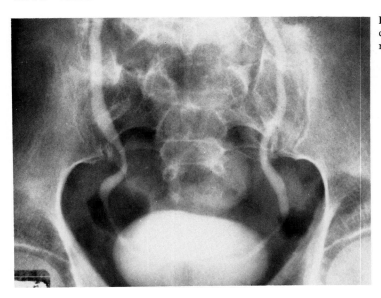

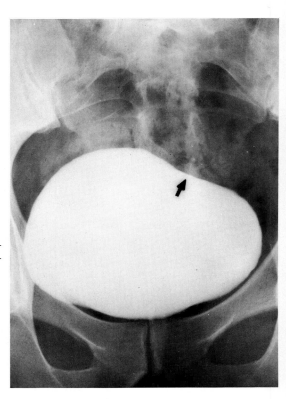

FIG. 23-8. Course of ureters in bladder. Note dense collection of contrast medium behind the interureteric ridge.

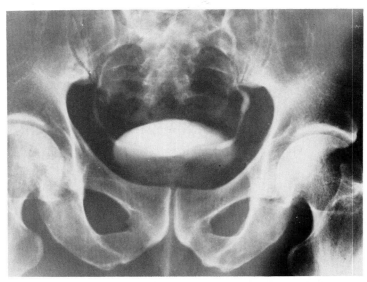

FIG. 23-9. Cystogram on intravenous urogram. Note the dense area cephalad to the course of the ureters within the bladder. This represents pooling of contrast material behind interureteric ridge.

FIG. 23-10. Retrograde cystogram showing the impression of the sigmoid on the bladder (*arrow*) in a 24-year-old man.

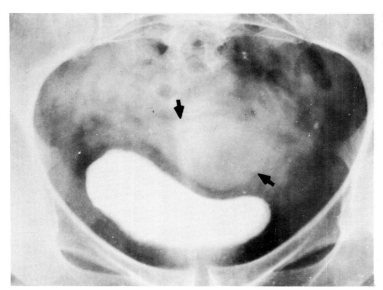

FIG. 23–11. Intravenous urogram. The indentation on the upper surface, which is somewhat asymmetric, is caused by a normal uterus (*arrows*).

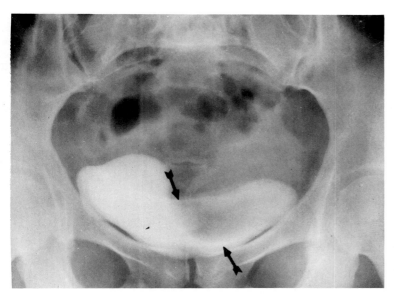

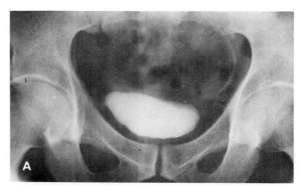

FIG. 23–12. Excretory cystogram. Fibroid and normal uterine impression on the bladder. Normal indentation of uterus (*upper arrow*); fibroid pressure (*lower arrow*).

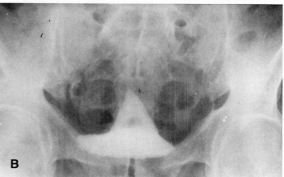

FIG. 23–13. Excretory cystogram in a man. (**A**) Supine view. (**B**) Prone view. Note cephalic prolongation of the anterior wall of the bladder with peaking from attachment of fibrous remnant of urachus. The anterior segment of the bladder is visualized best in the prone position.

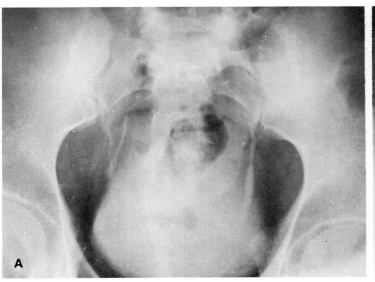

FIG. 23–14. Excretory cystogram in a man. **(A)** Supine view. **(B)** Prone view. Note the cephalic prolongation on the prone film with better visualization of the anterior wall of the bladder.

FIG. 23–15. To show the value of prone film in lesions of the anterior wall of the bladder. **(A)** Supine film. Normal cystogram. The defect of the Foley bag can be seen. **(B)** Prone film. Irregular outline of upper right side of bladder represents a carcinoma of the bladder. (Elkin M.: Radiology, 78:904, 1962)

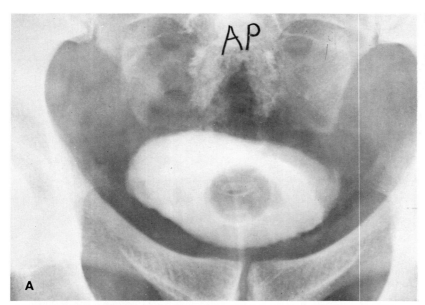

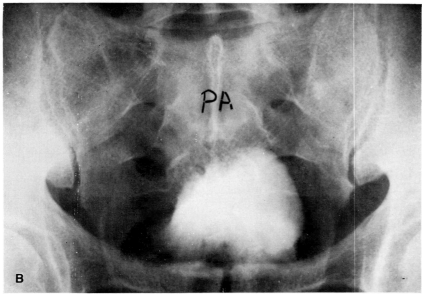

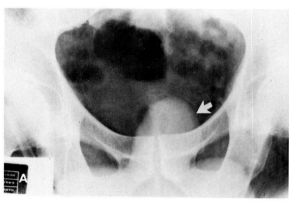

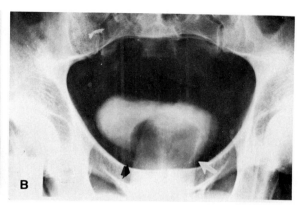

FIG. 23–16. Normal bladder to show imprint of penis (*arrow*). (**A**) Scout film. (**B**) Excretory cystogram. *Black arrow* points to penis superimposed on bladder. *White arrow* indicates air in rectum overlying bladder.

FIG. 23–17. (**A**) Elongated bladder; could be confused with neurogenic bladder. (**B**) Penis; overlying bladder was the cause of the upper projection in the bladder contour.

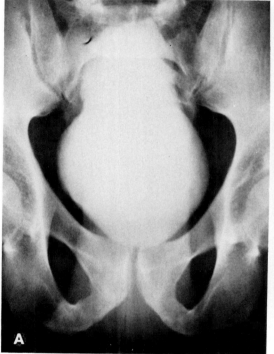

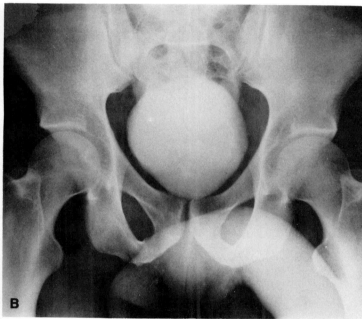

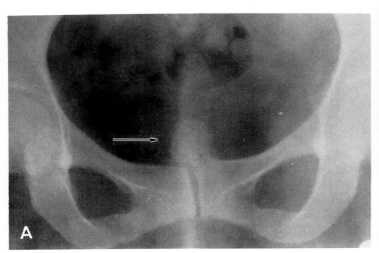

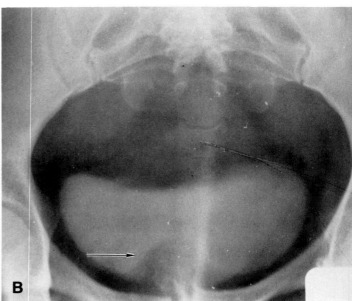

FIG. 23–18. (A) Osteochondroma pubis (*arrow*). **(B)** Cystogram; apparent defect in the bladder (*arrow*).

FIG. 23–19. Recesses (*arrows*) on either side of bladder. These are normal variations.

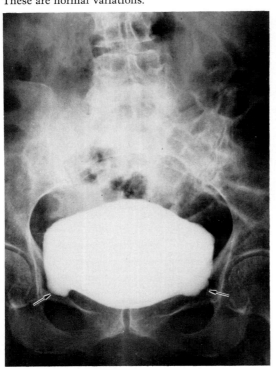

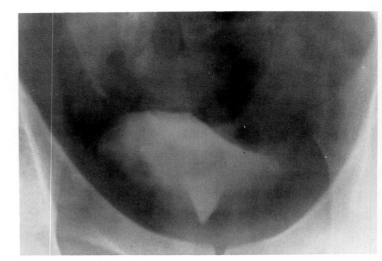

FIG. 23–20. Man; visualization of trigone on intravenous urogram cystogram. Note sigmoid indentation on the upper left side of bladder.

BIBLIOGRAPHY

1. Campbell, M.F.: Clinical Pediatric Urology. Philadelphia, Saunders, 1951.
2. Cunningham, J.J.: Radiologic features of the interureteric ridge. Am. J. Roentgenol., *125*:688–691, 1975.
3. Disse, J.: Harnorgane. In Handb. d. Anat. d. Menschen, Bd. 7, T. 1, Jena, Fischer, 1902.
4. Edling, N.P.G.: Further studies of the interureteric ridge of the bladder. Acta Radiol., *30*:67–75, 1948.
5. Elkin, M.: Supine and prone positions in intravenous urography for diagnosis of bladder lesions. Radiology, *78*:904–912, 1962.
6. Hansen, L.K.: Micturition cystourethrography with automatic serial exposures. Acta. Radiol. (Stockholm) (Suppl.), *207*:11–138, 1961.
7. Kjellberg, S.R., Ericsson, N., and Rudhe, U.: The Lower Urinary Tract in Childhood: Some Correlated Clinical and Roentgenological Observations. Chicago, Year Book Publishers, 1957.

CLASSIFICATION AND DESCRIPTION OF BLADDER ANOMALIES

The major vesical anomalies are as follows:

Agenesis
Hypoplasia
Diverticula
Reduplication
Abnormalies of the urachus
Exstrophy
Cloacal formation

VESICAL AGENESIS

Agenesis of the urinary bladder (Figs. 24–1, 24–2) is a rare anomaly usually associated with absence of the urethra and with other congenital abnormalities incompatible with life. These abnormalities include anencephalia, absence of kidneys and ureters, imperforate anus, penile absence, polycystic kidneys, meningocele, and polydactylism. Most reported cases have been at autopsy or in stillborn infants. Only seven cases have survived.[3] Only one proved case has been in a male.[2] Graham's case was unusual in that the urethra was present.[3] Occasionally the dilated ureters entering the urethra can act as bladders.[4]

HYPOPLASIA

Dwarf bladder, as hypoplasia is sometimes called, is extremely rare and is usually associated with other anomalies of the urinary tract (Figs. 24-3, 24-4). Campbell reported a case in a stillborn boy with hypospadias and horseshoe kidney.[8] Currarino published two cases associated with agenesis of the kidneys.[9]

24

Congenital Anomalies of the Bladder

DIVERTICULA

Diverticula (Figs. 24–6, 24–7) are considered in Chapter 27, Herniation and Diverticula of the Bladder.

REDUPLICATION

The various malformations included in this category have been classified in many ways and with marked variations in terminology. Probably the best term would be "bladder division." Diverticula have been considered by Cacciarelli and co-workers to fall in this group, but for practical purposes we have considered them in the chapter on diverticula in general (Chap. 27).

CONGENITAL BLADDER DIVISIONS

The following is a classification (Fig. 24–8) of congenital bladder divisions as presented by Senger and Santare.[28] These are similar to those described by Burns and co-workers except in the case of multi-locular bladders.[14] Senger and Santare separate these from other septal bladders,[28] whereas Burns considers them as sagittal septums or frontal septums.

1. Sagittal or longitudinal divisions
   Complete reduplication of the bladder
   Incomplete reduplication of the bladder
   Complete sagittal septum
   Incomplete sagittal septum
2. Frontal or transverse divisions
   Complete frontal septum
   Incomplete frontal septum
   Hourglass bladder
3. Multilocular and multiseptated bladders

Sagittal Divisions

Complete reduplication (Figs. 24–9, 24–11, 24–12) of the bladder occurs when there are two bladders lying side by side, each draining through a separate urethra. Each bladder receives a ureter from the ipsilateral side. The walls of the bladder are separated by a peritoneal fold of varying depth and consist of mucosal and muscular layers. This anomaly is frequently associated with duplications of the genital and distal gastrointestinal tracts and external genitalia.[10, 27, 29, 30]

Incomplete duplication is less common than complete reduplication (Fig. 24–10).[10, 22] The bladders lie side by side, separated by a peritoneal fold of varying depth, and each side receives the ipsilateral ureter. There is free communication between the two halves, and they empty through a common urethra. There is much lower incidence of accompanying anomalies.

Complete sagittal septum of the bladder occurs when a sagittal septum, which may be muscular, mucosal, or both, separates the bladder into right and left chambers, which may be equal or unequal. The external contour of the bladder is essentially normal. There is only one urethra, usually draining only one cavity. One or more ureters enter into each cavity. If the ureter to the cavity not joining the urethra is functioning, the kidney becomes hydronephrotic, aplastic, or dysplastic. The distended blind chamber may obstruct the opposite one. Senger and Santare would call these multilocular,[28] whereas Burns and co-workers would classify them as complete sagittal septums.[14]

The incomplete sagittal septum is somewhat similar to the complete sagittal septum except that the septum does not completely separate the two chambers.

Frontal or Transverse Divisions

In complete frontal septum the bladder is divided into two chambers by a frontal septum. The anterior cavity is usually connected with the urethra, whereas the posterior cavity is closed off. Usually one ureter enters each cavity. Singh and co-workers in 1973 reported a case of complete frontal septation of the bladder with two separate urethras in a 6-month-old boy.[29] The ureters opened to the posterior bladder structure. The urethra draining the blind anterior bladder was located in front of the functioning urethra and opened to the dorsum of the penis in its midportion.

Incomplete frontal septum (Fig. 24–13) is similar to complete frontal septum except that the frontal septum is not complete, and the two chambers that are anterior and posterior communicate with each other. The ureters may open into the posterior inferior chamber or into each one.

Hourglass divisions represent an incomplete transverse indentation dividing the bladder into upper and lower chambers (Fig. 24–14). Caulk[17] and Young[33] reported such cases. The transverse bands or septums were felt only in the posterior portions of the bladder. It was generally thought that the hourglass appearance was caused by a contraction of the muscle in the line of the transverse septum. The portions of the bladder above and below the constriction must be normal. These must be differentiated from urachal diverticula and possibly posterior urethral valves.

Cases of multilocular bladder have been classified separately by Senger and Santare.[28] The loculus always contains a ureter, and usually the ureter has failed to perforate the mucosa of the bladder wall. The ureter is obstructed, and the loculus is a cystic dilatation of the lower end of the ureter, occurring in the bladder cavity. Occasionally, the cystlike dilatation may perforate, providing a communication between the two cavities. Actually, there can be as many loculations as there are ureters. Senger and Santare believe that ureteroceles are probably a minor form of this type of bladder.

Multiseptated bladders may be another variety of this type of bladder. Externally the bladder appears normal, but internally it is divided by septa into multiple communicating chambers. The anomaly is rare. Kohler reported this condition in a 10-day-old infant.[20]

URACHAL ANOMALIES

CLASSIFICATION

Urachal anomalies are related closely to the development of the bladder (Figs. 24–15 to 24–21). The various types of anomalies that exist depend directly on what portions of the urachus persist or become obliterated. There have been various classifications, especially by Trimingham and McDonald,[83] Nix and co-workers,[76] and Long.[67] A modification of these classifications follows:

1. Patent
   a. Persistence of fetal bladder without descent. The bladder opens at the level of the umbilicus through a widely patent urachus (Fig. 24–15).
   b. Persistence of fetal bladder with descent. The bladder has descended but is formed abnormally, and the urachus is a double funnel, narrowed in its middle segment.
   c. Arrested closure of urachus. The bladder is normal in position and shape. The urachus is a narrow tube of fairly uniform diameter. This is the type one usually sees in the so-called acquired type of umbilical urinary fistula (Fig. 24–16).
2. Partially patent
   a. Open at the umbilical end and not connected with the bladder (umbilical urachal sinus) (Fig. 24–17)
   b. Open in the bladder but closed at the umbilical end (Figs. 24–18, 24–19)

3. Urachal cyst
   The urachus is closed at both ends with cyst formation between (Fig. 24–21).

DEVELOPMENT

Although these anomalies have been well documented, there still exists a great deal of controversy concerning the development of the urachus. Originally it was thought that the allantois formed the apex of the bladder and that a remnant of the allantois formed the urachus, which connected the apex of the bladder with the umbilicus. Arey,[35] Begg,[39] and Felix[52] thought that the allantois contributed nothing to the formation of the bladder or the urachus and should be considered a true vestigial structure.

Kjellberg, Ericsson, and Rudhe considered that the bladder floor, chiefly the trigone, originates from the urogenital sinus, whereas the cephalic part of the bladder is given off by the allantois.[62] Ney and Friedenberg postulated that the urachus arose from the allantois and the bladder from the urogenital sinus (ventral part of cloaca).[74] Tyler[84] considered the possibility that the epithelium of the bladder originated from the mesonephric ducts and ureters rather than from the cloaca that initially lined the bladder with intestinal epithelium, which would be displaced later by transitional epithelium from metaplasia. Begg believed that the bladder was derived from the entoderm of the ventral cloaca, except for a small segment which arose from the mesonephric ducts, and he further postulated that the cloaca grew upward to the level of the umbilicus, narrowed, and formed the urachus.[39] Following birth, the bladder descends into the pelvis, thus increasing its distance from the umbilicus. Begg stated that in the adult the urachus is only about 5 cm. long and that it is separated from the umbilicus by a distance of 12 cm. On the other hand, Hammond, Yglesias, and Davis have offered evidence that the urachus can extend to the umbilicus in the adult.[56]

DEMONSTRATION

Anomalies of the urachus can be demonstrated best by radiography. The method used depends upon the type of anomaly. The completely patent urachus can be injected at the umbilical opening with radiopaque material, or a cystogram can be performed, a procedure that demonstrates the patency to the umbilicus. The partially patent type may be demonstrated by using the proper procedure, depending on the location of its opening. The difficult ones to demonstrate are the urachal cysts, which are closed at both ends and must be injected directly.

FREQUENCY AND COMPLICATIONS

The so-called acquired type of umbilical urinary fistula (type 1C) is seen more commonly than the congenital types. It is usually associated with obstructing lesions of the lower urinary tract. Actually, no abnormality of the umbilicus may be noted at birth, but dribbling of urine from the umbilicus occurs later. It has been postulated that the lower tract obstruction forces urine back through the incompletely obliterated canal.

Various complications of urachal anomalies have been reported. Some of these have been infection, abscess formations, stones, and tumors, especially carcinomas and adenocarcinomas. Echinococcus cyst can simulate a urachal cyst (Fig. 24–20).[44]

EXSTROPHY OF THE BLADDER

There are many variations of exstrophy of the bladder, the most common being classic exstrophy, with inferior vesical fistula being next in frequency. In the male the exstrophy complex varies from spade penis through epispadias with continence to epispadias with incontinence to classic exstrophy associated with anal and rectal abnormalities to cloacal exstrophy to ectopic viscera abdominalis. In the female, exstrophy varies from patulous urethra through epispadias to classic exstrophy and then through the course described previously for the male.

In the classic exstrophy (Figs. 24–22, 24–23), there is absence of the anterior wall of the bladder and the corresponding portion of the anterior abdominal wall with the inner surface of the posterior bladder wall protruding upon the abdomen. Bilateral inguinal hernias are often present, and the testes may be undescended. The penis is short, upturned, and the epispadic mucosa covers the dorsal surface. In the female, the urethra is short, clitoris bifid, and labia minor widely separated.

In the exstrophy—epispadic complex, the pubic bones are separated more than the normal (no more than 10 mm. at any age).[105, 110] In this complex, this distance ranges from 12 to 170 mm.; the wider the separation, the more severe the complex. Muecke and Currarino found congenital widening of the pubic symphysis as follows[113]: 66 per cent in classic exstrophy or its variants; 24 per cent in epispadias without exstrophy; and the remaining 10 per cent

occurring with other unusual entities such as anorectal anomalies, urethral duplication, duplicated phallus, and pseudoexstrophy.

Adenocarcinoma is the most common malignancy occurring in cases of exstrophy, in both the unclosed variety and after vesicoplasty.[107a 110a, 114]

Roentgenographic Findings. Plain film of the pelvis: Muecke and Currarino have described the following three anatomic features related to pubic separation[113]:

1. Outward rotation of the innominate bones is seen relative to the sagittal plane of the body, along the sacroiliac joints.
2. There is an eversion or outward rotation of the pubic bone at its junction with the ischium and ilium.
3. In the most severe cases there may be some degree of lateral separation of the innominate bones inferiorly, with the fulcrum at the iliosacral joint.

Intravenous urogram may show normal upper tracts, but usually there is some dilatation, unilateral or bilateral, with obstruction at the ureterovesical junction from prolapse of the ureter and possibly from metaplasia or fibrosis of the bladder mucosa. The bladder may appear as an irregular globular mass.

Exstrophy (epispadic variety) has been reported with skeletal changes. Also, the musculoskeletal deformity has been reported without exstrophy.

SPECIFIC TYPES

Certain specific types of exstrophy have been described that should be clarified.

Cloacal Exstrophy (Intestinal Vesical Fissure)

In this type there is an extensive variation of exstrophy of the bladder, including eversion of the ileum and the colon; absence of the large intestine, the rectum, and the anus; undescended gonads; spina bifida; and hydromyelomeningoceles or meningoceles.

Superior Vesical Fissure

There is an opening in the upper portion with musculoskeletal deformity, but continence is present. Campbell states that the pubes are closed in superior vesical fissure.[106]

Duplicate Exstrophy

There is a normal internal urinary tract, but a rudimentary exstrophy is present externally.

Inferior Vesical Fissure

This term is used differently by different authors. Campbell considers this to be complete exstrophy, whereas others consider this to be only penopubic epispadias.[106]

Classic Exstrophy

See the preceding section.

Epispadias Not Associated with Exstrophy

This anomaly is extremely rare, occurring in 1 in 95,000 births. Boys are affected 4:1. Balanitic, penile, penile-pubic, or complete types have been described. Incontinence varies, but the persons with the complete type are always incontinent. On examination, the urethral mucosal groove is dorsally placed, creating a depression in the penis. The corpus spongiosum is absent. The penis is foreshortened and the testes are undescended in 40% of cases.

In girls, the lesion is usually of the complete type. Sphincteric involvement is present in almost 100%. There can be partial or incomplete forms in which the patient may be totally incontinent; however, stress incontinence is not uncommon. There is bifid clitoris, with anterior displacement of the labia majora and minora. The vaginal orifice is stenotic in two-thirds of cases. There may be absent vagina and bicornuate uterus. The urethra is wide and short; the bladder is usually small, and there may be vesicoureteral reflux with lateral displacement of ureteral orifices.

CHAPTER 24, ILLUSTRATIONS

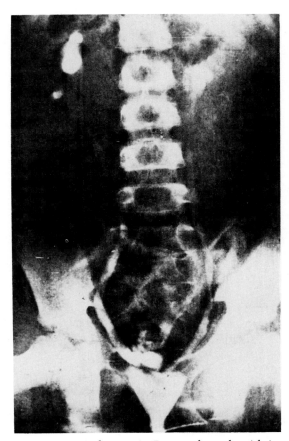

FIG. 24–1. Vesical agenesis. Retrograde study with incidental vaginogram. The bladder and urethra were absent. The ureters joined in the midline and drained into the vagina. (Vakili, B.F.: J. Urol., *109*:510, 1973)

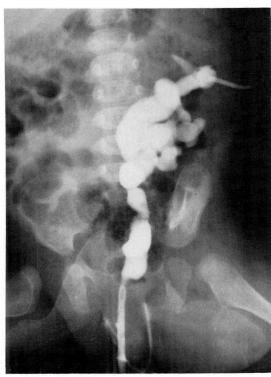

FIG. 24–2. Agenesis of the bladder. Pyeloureterourethrogram reveals tortuous ureters extending to urethra. No bladder. Catheter is in distal portion of normal urethra. (Graham, S.D.: J. Urol., *107*:660, 1972)

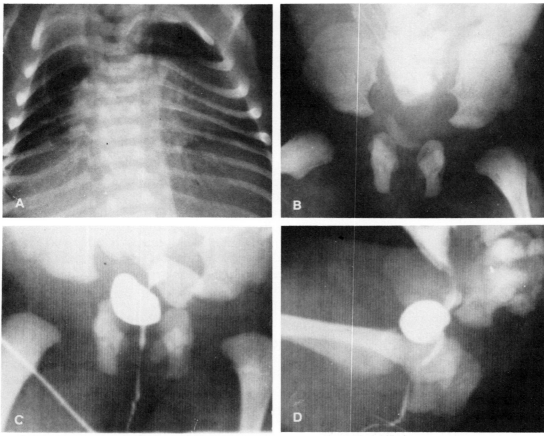

FIG. 24–3. Hypoplasia (dwarf bladder). **(A)** Chest, frontal roentgenogram, showing mediastinal emphysema. **(B)** Pelvis frontal roentgenogram, showing a contracted bladder outlet. **(C and D)** Retrograde urethrogram, in frontal and lateral projections, showing a minute urethra and bladder and a vesicorectal communication; the sacrum is defective. (Currarino, G.: Am. J. Roentgenol., *109*:399–1970)

FIG. 24–4. Hypoplasia (dwarf bladder). **(A)** Chest, frontal roentgenogram, showing tension pneumothorax on the left. **(B)** Pelvis, frontal roentgenogram, showing a contracted pelvic outlet. **(C and D)** Retrograde urethrogram, in frontal and lateral projections, showing a minute urethra and bladder. In lateral projection **(D)** the vesicorectal communication is well demonstrated, as is the urachus. The sacrum is defective. (Currarino, G.: Am. J. Roentgenol., *109*:399–1970)

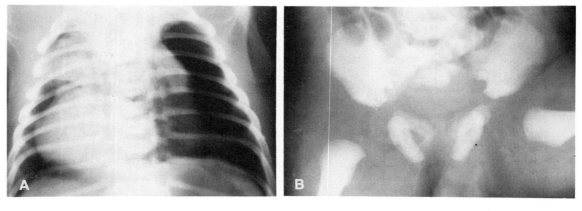

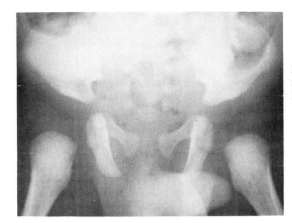

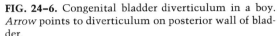

FIG. 24–5. Frontal roentgenogram of the pelvis of a normal full-term newborn. (Currarino, G.: Am. J. Roentgenol., *109*:399, 1970)

FIG. 24–6. Congenital bladder diverticulum in a boy. *Arrow* points to diverticulum on posterior wall of bladder.

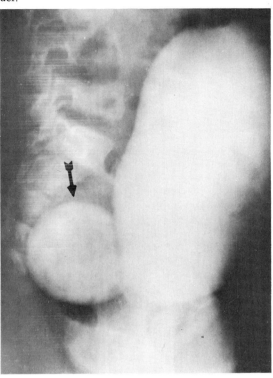

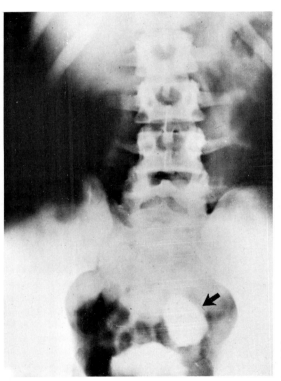

FIG. 24–7. Congenital bladder diverticulum in a 14-year-old boy. *Arrow* points to diverticulum. Bladder is slightly trabeculated due to bladder neck obstruction.

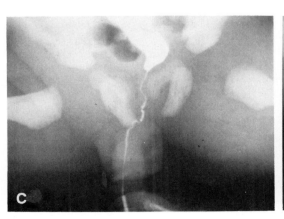

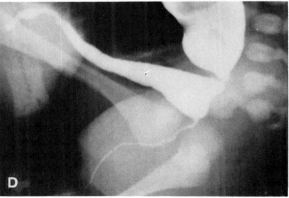

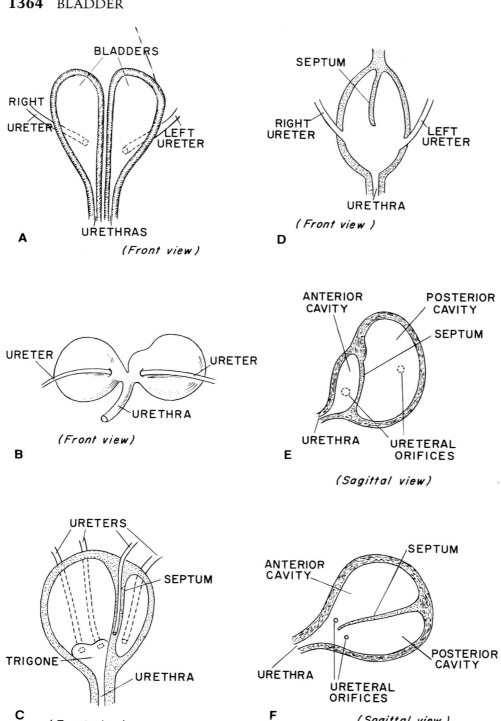

FIG. 24–8. Diagrams illustrating the various types of divisions of the bladder. **(A)** Complete reduplication of bladder. **(B)** Incomplete reduplication of bladder. **(C)** Complete sagittal septum of bladder. **(D)** Incomplete sagittal septum of bladder. **(E)** Complete frontal septum of bladder. **(F)** Incomplete frontal septum of bladder. (Burns, E., Cummins, H., and Hyman, J.: J. Urol., 57:257, 1947)

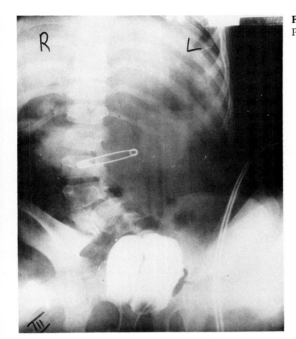

FIG. 24–9. Double bladder; double urethra. (Courtesy of Prof. C. Servadio, Beilinson Med. Center, Israel)

FIG. 24–10. Double bladder, one urethra. **(A)** Intravenous urogram, two bladders. Ureters enter each bladder. **(B)** Voiding cystourethrogram. Bladder joins at distal end; one urethra.

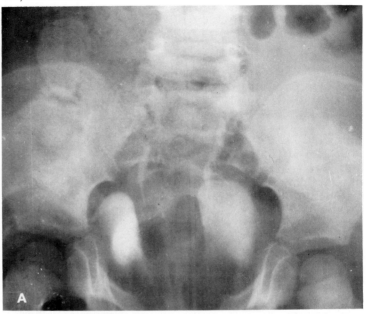

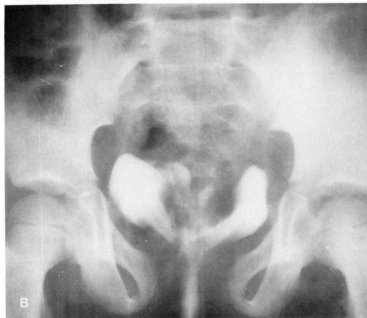

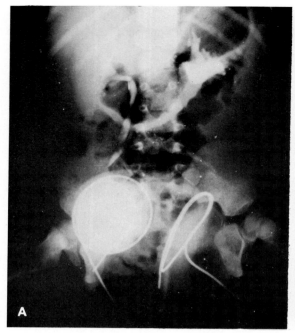

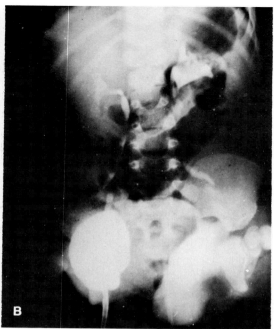

FIG. 24–11. Congenital bladder. Double bladder and double urethra in a girl. Each bladder has one ureter and kidney. Intestine was exstrophied between the two bladders. **(A)** Ureteral catheters were put into each bladder as well as contrast material. **(B)** Only contrast material can be seen in each bladder. (Courtesy of W.E. Goodwin, M.D.)

FIG. 24–12. Double bladder and double urethra in a boy. Left nephrectomy had been performed previously. Contrast medium has been injected into left bladder through a catheter passed down left ureter *(upper arrow)*. The left bladder and the urethra *(lower arrow)* are outlined. Air has been injected into the right bladder through a catheter passed into the right urethra (catheter is still in place). There is no communication between the two bladders or the two urethras. (Ravitch, M.M., and Scott, W.W.: Surgery, *34*:843, 1953)

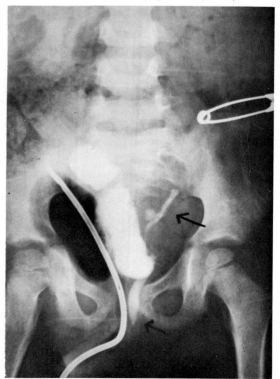

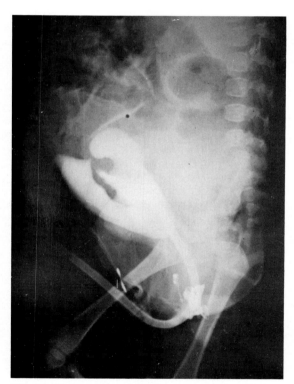

FIG. 24–13. Incomplete frontal septum dividing bladder into anterior and posterior segments. Only one urethra is present. (Burns, E., Cummins, H., and Hyman, J.: J. Urol., *57*:257, 1947)

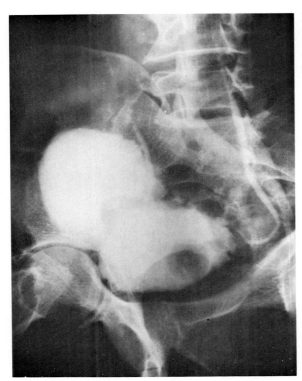

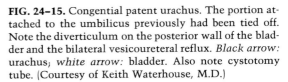

FIG. 24–14. Hourglass bladder. Case of prostatic hypertrophy. The upper structure was thought to be a diverticulum of the bladder, but the slight irregularity of its wall would be in favor of hourglass bladder. Note that the ureteral orifices enter the lower structure.

FIG. 24–15. Congential patent urachus. The portion attached to the umbilicus previously had been tied off. Note the diverticulum on the posterior wall of the bladder and the bilateral vesicoureteral reflux. *Black arrow:* urachus; *white arrow:* bladder. Also note cystotomy tube. (Courtesy of Keith Waterhouse, M.D.)

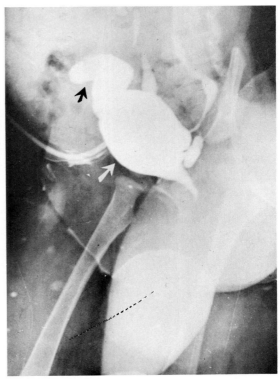

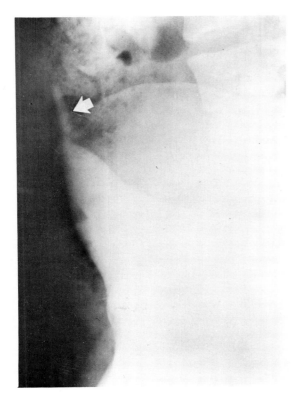

FIG. 24–16. Acquired urachal fistula (type IC) in a 24-year-old man with urinary drainage from umbilicus. Bladder neck obstruction was present. Cystogram demonstrates the fistulous tract (*arrow*).

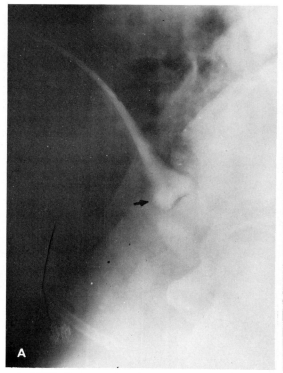

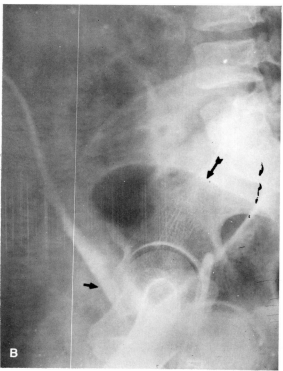

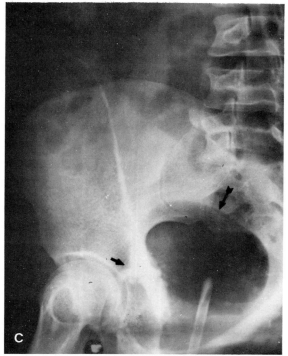

FIG. 24–17. Urachal cyst connecting with umbilicus but not with bladder. Three views of one case. **(A)** Lateral view. *Arrow* points to cyst. **(B)** Lateral view. *Small arrow* points to urachal cyst. *Large arrow* points to bladder outlined by air. Note that the cyst is adjacent to the lower anterior surface of the bladder. **(C)** Oblique view. *Small arrow* points to urachal cyst. *Large arrow* points to bladder outlined by air. The lower portion of the tract from the umbilicus and the cystic structure are adjacent to the anterior wall of the bladder. (Courtesy of J.J. Arnold, M.D.)

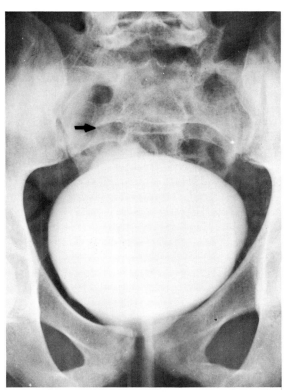

FIG. 24–18. Partially patent urachus. Cystogram reveals urachal structure opening into bladder but closed at umbilical end.

FIG. 24–19. Partially patent urachus; cystogram reveals urachal structure closed at umbilical end and opened into bladder.

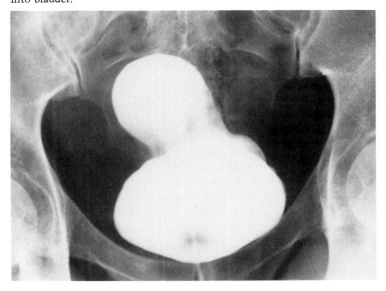

FIG. 24–20. Echinococcus cyst simulating urachal cyst. Cystogram after abdominal cyst had been aspirated and injected with contrast medium. No connection to bladder. (A, B) Anterior-posterior and oblique views. (Constantian, H.M., and Bolduc, R.A.: J. Urol., 99:755, 1968)

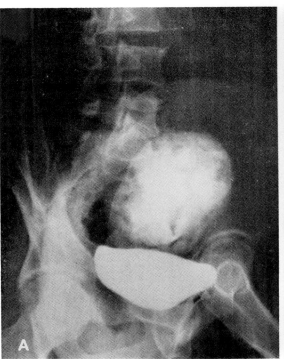

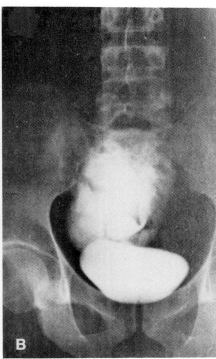

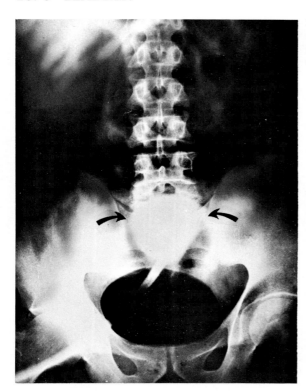

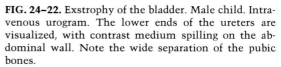

FIG. 24–21. Urachal cyst (*arrows*). There is no communication with the bladder or the umbilicus. A tube was put directly into the cyst and the contrast injected. Air in bladder. (Courtesy of Herbert Kenyon, M.D.)

FIG. 24–22. Exstrophy of the bladder. Male child. Intravenous urogram. The lower ends of the ureters are visualized, with contrast medium spilling on the abdominal wall. Note the wide separation of the pubic bones.

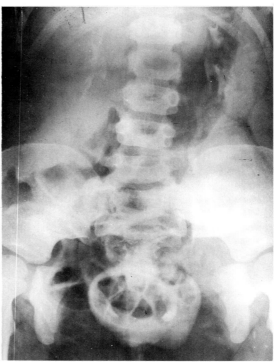

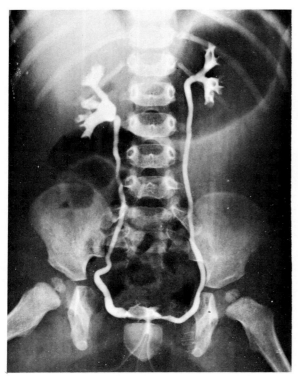

FIG. 24–23. Exstrophy of the bladder. Retrograde pyelogram in a 22-month-old boy. Note the wide separation of the symphysis pubis.

BIBLIOGRAPHY

Vesical Agenesis

1. Glenn, J.F.: Agenesis of the bladder. J.A.M.A., *196*:2016–2018, 1959.
2. Gould, G.M., and Pyle, W.L.: Anomalies of the bladder. *In* Gould, G.M., and Pyle, W.L.: Anomalies and Curiosities of Medicine. p. 205. New York, Sydenham Publ., 1937.
3. Graham, S.D.: Agenesis of bladder. J. Urol., *107*:660–661, 1972.
4. Huber, H.G.: Nabelkoliken bei Doppelbildung und Verengung des Ureters. Kinderärztl. Praxis, *7*:254–256, 1936.
5. Miller, H.L.: Agenesis of the urinary bladder and urethra. J. Urol., *59*:1156–1163, 1948.
6. Palmer, J.M., and Ruggi, M.F.: Persistent congenital sinus with absence of bladder and urethra. J. Urol., *102*:590–594, 1969.
7. Vakili, B.F.: Agenesis of the bladder: a case report. J. Urol., *109*:510–511, 1973.

Hypoplasia

8. Campbell, M.F.: Pediatric Urology. New York, Macmillan, 1937, p. 294.
9. Currarino, G.: Association of congenitally small pelvic outlet with hypoplasia of bladder and absent kidneys. Am. J. Roentgenol., *109*:399–402, 1970.

Reduplication

10. Abrahamson, J.: Double bladder and related anomalies: clinical and embrological aspects and case report. Br. J. Urol., *33*:195–214, 1961.
11. Bates, R.C.: A case of double vagina and bladder. Rhode Island Med. J., *14*:192–193, 1931.
12. Boissonnat, P.: Vessie double (vesical duplex) avec uretre unique chez un garcon de 4 ans. J. Urol. (Paris), *59*:883–886, 1953.
13. Boulgakow, B., and Malek, S.A.: Vesica urinaria bipartita Asymetrica. J. Egypt. Med. Assoc., *23*:185–191, 1940.
14. Burns, E., Cummins, H., and Hyman, J.: Incomplete reduplication of the bladder with congenital solitary kidney: report of a case. J. Urol., *57*:257–269, 1947.
15. Cacciarelli, A.A., Lucas, B., and McAlister, W.H.: Multichambered bladder anomalies. Am. J. Roentgenol., *126*:642–646, 1976.
16. Cathelin, F., and Sempe, C.: La Vessie Double. Ann. d. Mal. des Organes Genito-Urinaires, *21*:339–358, 1903.
17. Caulk, J.R.: Remarks on the resection of the base of the bladder for transverse septa. Ann. Surg., *71*:22–27, 1920.
18. Edwards, C.: Congenital multilocular bladder. Med. J. Aust., *2*:443–448, 1933.
19. Greenberg, G.: Vesica duplex with gangrenous cystitis. Urol. Cut. Rev., *40*:175–178, 1936.
20. Kohler, H.H.: Septal bladder. J. Urol., *44*:63–66, 1940.
21. Lanman, T., and Mahoney, P.J.: Intravenous urography in children. Am. J. Dis. Child., *42*:611–636, 1931.
22. Lee, H., Davis, J.E., and Beneventi, F.: Reduplication of bladder by incomplete frontal septum and associated anomalies. J. Urol., *102*:635–639, 1969.

23. Marshall, V.F., and Muecke, E.C.: Congenital abnormalities of the bladder. *In* Encyclopedia of Urology. VII. Malformations. pp. 172–184, 195–197. Berlin, Springer-Verlag, 1968.
24. Nesbit, R.M., and Bromme, W.: Double penis and double bladder. Am. J. Roentgenol., *30*:497–502, 1933.
25. Ravitch, M.M., and Scott, W.W.: Duplication of the entire colon, bladder and urethra. Surgery, *34*:843–858, 1953.
26. Robson, M.C., and Ruth, E.B.: Bilocular bladder: an anatomical study of a case, with a consideration of urinary tract abnormalities. Anat. Rev., *142*:63–68, 1962.
27. Satter, E.J., and Mossman, H.W.: Case report of double bladder and double urethra in female child. J. Urol., *79*:274–278, 1958.
28. Senger, F.L., and Santare, V.J.: Congenital multilocular bladder: a case report. Trans. Am. Assoc. Genitourin. Surg., *43*:114–119, 1951.
29. Singh, J.P., and Nagabhushanam, S.: Complete duplication of bladder and urethra: case report with review of literature. J. Urol., *109*:512–514, 1973.
30. Swenson, O., and Oeconomopoulos, C.T.: Double lower genitourinary systems in a child. J. Urol., *85*:540–542, 1961.
31. Takaha, M., Nakarai, K., and Ikoma, F.: Complete reduplication of the urinary bladder associated with hindgut duplication: report of a case. Acta Urol. Jap., *17*:401–414, 1971.
32. Wehrbein, H.L.: Double kidney, double urethra and bilocular bladder in a child. J. Urol., *43*:804–810, 1940.
33. Young, H.H., and Davis, D.M.: Young's Practice of Urology. Philadelphia, Saunders, 1926.

Abnormalities of the Urachus

Urachal Anomalies Including Cysts

34. Aleman, O.: Operated case of cyst of urachus. Hygeia Stockholm, *78*:952–955, 1916.
35. Arey, L.B.: Developmental Anatomy: A Textbook and Laboratory Manual of Embryology. Philadelphia, Saunders, 1965.
36. Atcheson, D.W.: Patent urachus with a report of two additional cases. J. Urol., *51*:424–430, 1944.
37. Baldwin, J.F.: Large cysts of the urachus. Surg. Gynecol. Obstet., *14*:636, 1912.
38. Begg, R.C.: The urachus and umbilical fistulae. Surg. Gynecol. Obstet., *45*:165–178, 1927.
39. Begg, R.C.: The urachus: its anatomy, histology, and development. J. Anat., *74*:170–183, 1930.
40. Benton, B.F., Lanford, H.G., and Hardy, J.O.: Patent urachus. Am. J. Surg., *85*:513–515, 1954.
41. Carreau, E.P., and Higgins, G.A.: Diseases of the urachus. Am. J. Surg., *84*:205–211, 1952.
42. Cherry, J.W.: Patent urachus: review and report of a case. J. Urol., *63*:693–697, 1950.
43. Constantian, H.M., and Amaral, E.L.: Urachal cyst: case report. J. Urol., *106*:429–431, 1971.
44. Constantian, H.M., and Bolduc, R.A.: Echinococcus cyst simulating urachal cyst. J. Urol., *99*:755–758, 1968.
45. Cullen, T.S.: The Umbilicus and Its Diseases. Philadelphia, Saunders, 1916.
46. Cullen, T.S.: Further notes on diseases of the umbilicus. Surg. Gynecol. Obstet., *35*:257–283, 1922.

47. Dailey, U.G.: Patent urachus. Ann. Surg., *81*:1047–1049, 1925.

48. Davis, B.F.: Cyst of the urachus. Surg. Clin. Chicago, *3*:521–529, 1919.

49. Douglass, M.: Urachal cysts and fistulae. Am. J. Surg., *22*:557–560, 1933.

50. Dudgeon, H., Jr.: Patent urachus. Texas J. Med., *34*:401–404, 1938.

51. Edington, G.H.: Case of large urachal cyst. Lancet, *1*:791, 1922.

52. Felix, W.: The development of the urogenital organs. *In* Keibel, G.F., and Moll, F.P., eds.: Manual of Human Embryology. p. 752. Philadelphia, Lippincott, 1912.

53. Fox, P.F.: Uncommon umbilical anomalies in children. Surg. Gynecol. Obstet., *92*:95–100, 1951.

54. Garvin, E.J.: Patent urachus. J. Int. Coll. Surg., *11*:511–516, 1948.

55. Gayet, G., and Verriere, P.: Kyste de l'ouraque. Lyon Chir., *33*:253–256, 1936.

56. Hammond, G., Yglesias, L., and Davis, J.E.: The urachus, the anatomy and associated fascia. Anat. Rec., *80*:271–287, 1941.

57. Hinman, F., Jr.: Urologic aspects of the alternating urachal sinus. Am. J. Surg., *102*:339–343, 1961.

58. Hinman, F., Jr.: Surgical disorders of the bladder and umbilicus of urachal origin. Surg. Gynecol. Obstet., *113*:605–614, 1961.

59. Howard, A.H., Bodner, H., and Lerner, M.: Patent urachus, case report. Ann. West. Med. Surg., *6*:669–671, 1952.

60. Jacoby, A.: A case of cyst of the urachus. Urol. Cut. Rev., *20*:383–384, 1916.

61. Kantor, H.I.: Cysts of the urachusL report of two cases. Ann. Surg., *109*:277–285, 1939.

62. Kjellberg, S.R., Ericsson, N.O., and Rudhe, U.: The Lower Urinary Tract in Childhood: Some Correlated Clinical and Roentgenological Observations. Chicago, Year Book, 1957.

63. Koch, F., and Nielsen, O.V.: Anatomic variants of the urachus related to clinical appearance and surgical treatment of urachal lesions. Surg. Gynecol. Obstet., *137*:51, 1973.

64. Lavand'homme, P.: Du diagnostic der tumeurs kystiques abdominales volumineuses et des kystes de l'ouraque en particulier. Bruxeller Med., *17*:820–823, 1937.

65. Leitch, N.: Patent urachus. Urol. Cut. Rev., *54*:656–657, 1950.

66. Lloyd, F.A., and Pranke, O.: Patent urachus. Urol. Cut. Rev., *55*:734, 1951.

67. Long, L.: Cysts of urachus. J. Okla. Med. Assoc., *24*:388–391, 1931.

68. Lowman, R.M., Waters, L.L., and Stanley, H.W.: The roentgen aspects of the congenital anomalies in the umbilical region. Am. J. Roentgenol., *70*:883–910, 1953.

69. Lubash, S.: Congenital cyst of urachus. Am. J. Surg., *7*:851–853, 1929.

70. MacDonald, T.L.: An enormous cyst of the urachus. Ann. Surg., *44*:230–232, 1907.

71. Mahoney, P.J., and Ennis, O.: Congenital patent urachus. N. Engl. J. Med., *215*193–195, 1936.

72. Mast, W.H., Streamer, C.W., and Unfug, G.A.: Patent urachus. Am. J. Surg., *23*:210–214, 1933.

73. Means, J.W.: Cysts of the urachus with report of a case. Ann. Surg., *64*:53–57, 1916.

74. Ney, C., and Friedenberg, R.M.: Radiographic findings in anomalies of the urachus. J. Urol., *99*:288–291, 1968.

75. Nichols, R.W., and Lowman, R.M.: Patent urachus. Am. J. Roentgenol., *52*:615–619, 1944.

76. Nix, J.T., Menville, J.G., Albert, M., and Wendt, D.L.: Congenital patent urachus. J. Urol., *79*:264–273, 1958.

77. Perrin, M.G.: A case of patent urachus. Br. J. Urol., *9*:179, 1937.

78. Powell, R.E.: Cyst of the urachus. Can. Med. Assoc. J., *10*:675–676, 1920.

79. Rives, J.D.: Cysts of urachus. U.S. Nav. Med. Bull., *32*:205–207, 1934.

80. Ronald, A.: Cyst of urachus. Br. Med. J., *2*:771–772, 1930.

81. Sterling, J.A., and Goldsmith, R.: Lesions of urachus which appear in the adult. Ann. Surg., *137*:120–128, 1953.

82. Tassouatz, S.: Des kystes de l'ouraque. Strasbourg Med., *93*:783–786, 1933.

83. Trimingham, H.L., and McDonald, J.R.: Congenital anomalies in the region of the umbilicus. Surg. Gynecol. Obstet., *80*:152–163, 1945.

84. Tyler, D.E.: Epithelium of intestinal type in the normal urachus: a new theory of vesical embryology. J. Urol., *92*:505–507, 1964.

85. Weiser, W.R.: Cysts of the urachus. Ann. Surg., *44*:529–552, 1906.

86. Williams, C.: Unusual surgical lesions of the umbilicus. Ann. Surg., *124*:1108–1124, 1946.

87. Wilmoth, C.L.: Persistent urachus in the adult. J.A.M.A., *106*:526–529, 1936.

88. Wutz, J.B.: Uber Urachus und Urachuscysten. Virchow Arch. Path. Anat., *92*:387–423, 1883.

Infections, Including Tuberculosis

89. Arrou, M.: Kipte suppure de l'ouraque. Bull. et mem. Soc. Chir. (Paris), *36*:832–836, 1910.

90. DeCastro, B.R.: Cisto supperado de Uraco. Arch. Brasil Med., *16*:210–212, 1926.

91. Deneen, E.V., and Margold, A.: Urachus cyst abscess rupturing into peritoneal cavity. J. Urol., *25*:457–459, 1931.

92. Gramen, K.: Ein fall von infizierto Urachuseyste. Hygeia Stockholm, *78*:1460–1467, 1916.

93. McClelland, J.C., and Davis, K.F.: Patent urachus associated with urinary tuberculosis. J. Urol., *57*:270, 1947.

94. Morone, G.: Di una grossa cisti supperata dell'uraco. Pensiero Med., *5*:174–178, 1915.

95. Pearse, H.E., and Miller, E.L.: Hematuria from tuberculosis of a patent urachus. J.A.M.A., *58*:1684, 1912.

96. Powell, R.E.: Abscess in a patent urachus in a child nine months old. Canad. Med. Assoc. J., *10*:675–676, 1920.

97. Powers, H.J.: Patent urachus with chronic suppuration. Med. Bull. Vet. Admin., *18*:446–448, 1942.

98. Squier, J.B., and Cahill, G.F.: Chronic infection of the urachus. J. Urol., *28*:607–617, 1932.

Stones in the Urachus

99. Dreyfuss, M.L., and Fliess, M.M.: Patent urachus with stone formation. J. Urol., *46*:77–81, 1941.

100. Dyres, C.: Patent urachus and encysted urinary calculi. Lancet, *1*:566–567, 1910.

101. Siddall, A.C.: Cyst of urachus with calculus formation. Chin. Med. J., *46*:894–898, 1932.

102. Vasburgh, R.: Patent urachus with calculus. Med. Rec., *12*:606–607, 1877.

103. Ward, W.G.: Supporting cyst of urachus with concretion. Ann. Surg., *59*:329–330, 1919.

104. Wyatt, G.M., and Lanman, T.H.: Calculus in urachus. Am. J. Roentgenol., *43*:673–675, 1940.

Exstrophy of the Bladder

105. Abramson, D., Roberto, S.M., and Wilson, P.D.: Relaxation of the pelvic joints in pregnancy. Surg. Gynecol. Obstet., *55*:595–613, 1934.
106. Campbell, M.F.: Exstrophy of the Bladder in Urology. vol. 1, pp. 377–388. Philadelphia, Saunders, 1954.
107. Engel, R.M.: Exstrophy of the bladder and associated anomalies. Birth Defects, *10*:146–149, 1974.
107a. Engel, R.M., and Wilkinson, H.A.: Bladder exstrophy. J. Urol. *104*:699–704, 1970.
108. Gross, R.E., and Cresson, S.L.: Exstrophy of bladder; observations from 80 cases. J.A.M.A., *149*:1640–1644, 1952.
109. Gross, R.E., and Cresson, S.L.: Treatment of epispadias: a report of 18 cases. J. Urol., *68*:477–488, 1952.
110. Heyman, J., and Lundquist, A.: The symphysis pubis in pregnancy and parturition. Acta Obst. Gynecol. Scand., *12*:191–226, 1932.
110a. Kandzari, S.J., Majid, A., and Orteza, A.O.: Exstrophy of urinary bladder complicated by adenocarcinoma. Urology *3*:496–498, 1974.
111. Maloney, F.R., Jr., Gleason, D.M., and Lattimer, J.R.: Ureteral physiology and exstrophy of the bladder. J. Urol., *93*:588–592, 1965.
112. Marshall, V.F., and Muecke, E.C.: Variations in exstrophy of the bladder. J. Urol., *88*:766–796, 1962.
113. Muecke, E.C., and Currarino, G.: Congenital widening of the pubic symphysis, associated clinical disorders and Roentgen anatomy of affected bony pelvis. Am. J. Roentgenol., *102*:179–185, 1968.
114. O'Kane, H.O.J., Megaw, J. McI.: Carcinoma of the exstrophic bladder. Br. J. Surg. *55*:631–635, 1968.

Epispadias

115. Ambrose, S.S.: Epispadias with vesicoureteral reflux. South Med. J. *63*:1193–1194, 1970.
116. Burkholder, G.V., and Williams, D.I.: Epispadias and incontinence: Surgical treatment of 27 children. J. Urol., *94*:673, 1965.
117. Dees, J.E.: Congenital epispadias with incontinence. J. Urol. *62*:512–522, 1949.
118. Higgins, C.C.: An evaluation of cystectomy for exstrophy, for papillomatosis and for carcinoma of the bladder. J. Urol. *80*:274–292, 1958.
119. Jones, H.W., Jr.: An anomaly of the external genitalia in female patients with exstrophy of the bladder. Am. J. Obstet. Gynecol. *117*:748–755, 1973.
120. Muecke, E.C., and Marshall, V.F.: Subsymphyseal epispadias in the female patient. J. Urol. *99*:622–628, 1968.
121. Stanton, S.L.: Gynecologic complication of epispadias and bladder exstrophy. Am. J. Obstet. Gynecol, *119*:749–754, 1974.
122. Weed, J.C., and McKee, D.M.: Vulvoplasty in cases of exstrophy of the bladder. Obstet. Gynecol. *43*:512–516, 1974.
123. Williams, D.I.: Epispadias and exstrophy. Proc. R. Soc. Med. *62*:1079–1081, 1969.
124. Young, H.H.: Exstrophy of the bladder. Surg. Gynecol. Obstet. *74*:729–737, 1942.

The bladder can be displaced in any direction, but posterior displacement is extremely rare. Deviation of the bladder, as in neurogenic lesions, is not considered in this section.

A mass must attain considerable size before producing displacement of the bladder, although small masses may cause changes in bladder configuration. The most common causes of bladder displacement are fibroid uterus (Figs. 25–1, 25–2), ovarian tumors (Fig. 25–3), perivesical abscesses (Figs. 25–4, 25–5), fecal impaction (Figs. 25–6, 25–7, 25–8), lymph nodes (Fig. 25–9), and presacral or retrorectal tumors (Figs. 25–10 to 25–28). (Prostatic deviation of the bladder is considered in Chapter 34.)

Presacral tumors have also been called Middeldorph tumors. They are extraperitoneal, often displacing or obstructing the ureters, displacing the bladder, or obstructing the vesical outlet and the urethra. Symptoms consist of lower abdominal pain or pain referred to the low back, the perineum, the buttocks, or the legs. There may be urinary retention, frequency, dysuria, and rarely hematuria; or there may be pain in one or both kidney areas from ureteral obstruction. Bowel dysfunction and difficulty in walking have been reported. The symptoms may be caused by actual tumor mass or result from nerve involvement. When symptoms occur, the tumor usually can be palpated rectally.

The cases have been summarized in excellent reviews by Jackman, Clark, and Smith[4]; Mayo, Baker, and Smith[6]; and Werner.[8]

CLASSIFICATION

A composite classification is as follows:

1. Congenital tumors
   Chordoma
   Teratoma
   Dermoid cyst
   Meningocele
2. Inflammatory lesions

25

Displacement of the Bladder

3. Neurogenic tumors
   Ependymoma
   Neurofibroma
   Neurilemoma
4. Osseous tumors
   Osteogenic sarcoma
   Chondroma
   Giant cell tumor
   Osteoma
5. Miscellaneous tumors
   Neuroblastoma
   Metastatic tumors
   Lipoma
   Plasma cell myeloma
   Hemangioendothelioma
   Fibrosarcoma
   Leiomyosarcoma
   Chondromyxosarcoma
   Lymphomas

The most common presacral tumors are the congenital variety (32–39%), with chordoma being the predominant lesion. Inflammatory lesions represent 11 to 22 per cent of all presacral masses.[4, 6] Neurogenic tumors represent between 11 and 15 per cent; osseous tumors, 6 to 9 per cent; and miscellaneous tumors, 7 to 18 per cent.

Causes of lateral displacement of the bladder have been summarized by Korobin[2]:

Aneurysm
Hematoma
Lymphadenopathy
Lymphocele
Bladder diverticulum
Soft tissue tumor
Fecal impaction
Inguinal hernia
Prostate tumor
Adrenal cyst or tumor
Innominate bone tumor
Rheumatoid cyst
Hip arthroplasty
Abscess
Urachal remnants
Extension of thigh or retroperitoneal abscess or tumor
Sacral meningocele or myelocele

DIAGNOSIS OF PELVIC MASSES, INCLUDING PRESACRAL TUMORS

Plain Film. Calcification is seen in teratomas and dermoid cysts. Changes in the bones of the pelvis are seen in chordomas, ependymomas, neurofibromas, neurilemomas, and anterior meningoceles. Displacement of the coccyx may be produced by dermoid cysts and teratomas.

Intravenous urography may demonstrate the following:

1. Displacement, usually laterally, of the ureter
2. Obstruction of ureter by direct pressure of mass, or, rarely, secondary to bladder obstruction.
3. Anterior and lateral displacement of the bladder
4. Flattening and indentation of posterior and lateral walls of bladder
5. Distention of bladder from vesical neck or urethral obstruction

Barium enemas may reveal pressure and displacement of rectum.

Ultrasonography differentiates cysts and solid tumor structures and has the added advantage of wider choice of planes for sectioning, including sagittal, transverse, and oblique. It provides an advantage in localizing lesions for biopsy and aspiration. It is most useful in pregnant women and in repeated studies in children and young adults.

Computed tomography (CT) scan gives clear delineation of anatomy and permits identification of soft tissue structures and bone and calcified structures.

Individual Considerations. Chordomas (Fig. 25–10) arise from remnants of the fetal notochord and are found most commonly in the sacrococcygeal region (54 per cent). Of these, 35 per cent are found in the sphenooccipital area, and the remainder appear along the rest of spine. They are slow-growing malignant tumors that are definitely invasive, but metastases are late, occurring by the blood in 43 per cent of cases.[13] Radiographically they destroy the sacrum by expansion best seen on AP view but also by erosion and invasion. Remnants of bone may be seen free in the tumor.

Teratomas. These are encapsulated cystic or solid tumors in which usually more than one germ layer is represented (Figs. 25–11, 25–12). Lung, bone, cartilage, muscle, teeth, nerve tissue, fat, hair, intestinal mucosa, adrenal, thyroid, and pancreas have been demonstrated in these tumors. They are usually benign, and the incidence of malignancy varies (11 per cent,[23] 20 per cent,[20] 22 per cent[21] and 25 per cent[25]). They are commonly found in the sacrococcygeal area, but only 12.5 per cent of these are presacral.[26]

Metastases and recurrence of the malignant variety are common. Teratomas often obstruct the rectum and displace and obstruct the bladder. Female infants and children are most frequently involved (females 2:1).[25]

ROENTGENOGRAPHIC FINDINGS. Calcification occurs in 44 per cent.[26] These tumors may become extremely large before producing any bone change. There is a large soft tissue mass anterior to the sacrum, producing anterior displacement of the rectum and posterior tilting of the coccyx. Erosion of sacrum or coccyx is rare.

Dermoid Cysts. These (Figs. 25-13 to 25-15) are really a cystic form of teratoma and are caused by a faulty inclusion of ectoderm when the embryo coalesces. The epithelial lining continually secretes and desquamates. Hair and teeth may be present in these dermoid cysts. They rarely give rise to symptoms unless infection has occurred, in which case they may result in fistula formation or a chronic inflammatory process.

ROENTGENOGRAPHIC FINDINGS. The soft tissue mass can usually be visualized on plain film and may be surrounded by radiolucent fat. On CT scan, Carter and co-workers found the cystic teratomas to be more radiolucent than muscle with a delta value of 25 (compared to 40).[1] The surrounding fat had a delta value of −250. The coccyx may be displaced posteriorly without erosion.

Lipoma. Lipoma is a benign tumor, often continuous with the spinal cord, filum terminale, or cauda equina.[8] There may be associated neural defects. They are studied by plain radiography, myelography, ultrasonography, and CT scan. Plain radiography reveals the spina bifida and occasionally enlargement of a sacral foramen. A myelogram may demonstrate a deformity of the sacral sac. Ultrasonography shows a solid but relatively transsonic mass. CT scan confirms the primary fat content and is informative concerning the osseous structures.

Anterior Meningocele. These are herniations of the meninges through an anterior defect in the sac produced by failure of fusion of laminae (Figs. 25-16 to 25-21). They are uncommon, only 69 cases up to 1969.[32] They appear usually in women but can occur in men.[35] Neurologic problems related to bladder and bowel are common.

ROENTGENOGRAPHIC DIAGNOSIS. The sacrum usually has a characteristic scimitar configuration.

The defect is anterior, smooth, oval, and well marginated. The bladder may be displaced anteriorly and to either side. Sonography clearly defines the mass. CT scan may add validity to the diagnosis.[1]

Ependymoma. This is a benign primary tumor of the central nervous system occurring in approximately equal numbers intracranially and intraspinally.[38] The intracranial tumors are seen more commonly in children, whereas in the intraspinal group patients over 15 years predominate. There is no sex predilection. In the intraspinal group the tumor is usually situated in the conus region, filum terminale, or cauda equina. They may present posterior to sacrum. Metastases are extremely rare.[37, 39] Ependymomas can produce sharp or well-defined erosions of sacrum and lumbar bodies. There may be multiloculated areas of destruction in the sacrum.

Neurofibroma. This tumor is benign and characterized by diffuse proliferation of peripheral nerve elements. It may cause erosion of the sacral canal, sacral foramen, and external surface of sacrum.

Neurilemoma (Schwannoma). This is an encapsulated, benign tumor that arises from the sheath of Schwann in peripheral, cranial, and sympathetic nerves (Fig. 25-22). Bony changes are unusual, and displacement of any part of the urinary tract is rare. Deming reported a case displacing the upper two-thirds of left ureter in a pregnant woman.[40]

Rhabdomyosarcoma. This (Figs. 25-23 to 25-25) is the most common soft tissue sarcoma in children,[48] 15 per cent arising from bladder or prostate. Embryonic sarcoma of the bladder and urogenital sinus probably accounts for 10 per cent of malignant tumors in childhood. Intravenous urogram, voiding cystourethrogram, and ultrasonography plus cystoscopy establish the diagnosis.

Retrorectal Cysts. Retrorectal cysts of developmental origin are rare. There are several histologic types, such as squamous-lined (dermoid or epidermoid) cysts; postanal gut (tail gut) cysts, which are lined by cuboidal to columnar epithelium and contain mucus-secreting goblet cells; and rectal duplications (enteric or enterogenous cysts, enterocystomas) lined by squamous or glandular epithelium of intestinal type plus one or more layers of smooth muscle.

Radiographically there is a soft tissue mass in the retrorectal region. Barium enema reveals a smooth indentation on the posterior wall of the rectum.

Sacrum and coccyx are normal. Often they become infected and develop a sinus to perineum or skin or fistulize to anus, rectum, or vagina.

Inflammatory Lesions. These are chronic, internal abscesses appearing as walled-off accumulations of pus. Occasionally, fistulization occurs to bowel. Rarely, foreign body abscesses (i.e., oleomas) occur secondary to injections or trauma. These inflammatory lesions usually do not produce changes in the sacrum or coccyx.

Neuroblastomas. Neuroblastomas (Figs. 25–27, 25–28) are a common lesion of the presacral area.

DIFFERENTIAL DIAGNOSIS OF PELVIC MASSES

Presacral tumors must be differentiated from müllerian duct cysts, hydrocolpos, hematocolpos, ectopic kidney, bladder diverticula, bladder tumors, and seminal vesicle cysts.

Müllerian duct cysts may be identified by catheterization of the utricular opening or needle aspiration through perineum or rectum, followed by injection of contrast.

Vaginal obstructions producing hydrocolpos and hematocolpos may be diagnosed by needle aspiration and injections of contrast medium. The dilated vagina and occasionally the dilated uterus may be visualized.

Ectopic kidney should be recognized on intravenous urography.

Bladder diverticula may on occasion not fill on intravenous urography, and a mass be misdiagnosed, but retrograde cystography and cystoscopy usually demonstrate the lesion.

Bladder tumors extending outside the bladder may produce a mass, which at times can be extremely confusing. However, cystoscopic examination, biopsies, cystography, and further investigations such as arteriography, endoperivesical gas and CT scans should permit one to make the diagnosis.

Seminal vesicle cysts must be considered at times. Diagnosis requires injection of the ejaculatory duct or vas deferens with contrast medium.

CHAPTER 25, ILLUSTRATIONS

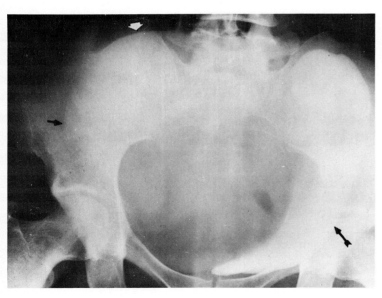

FIG. 25–1. Displacement of the bladder to the left and anteriorly with marked compression and partial obstruction by an interligamentous fibroid of the uterus. *Large arrow* points to bladder. *Small arrows* indicate right edge of fibroid.

FIG. 25–5. Displacement of the bladder by a perivesical abscess in a 4½-year-old boy. **(A)** Intravenous urogram shows displacement of the bladder to the right by a perivesical abscess. Child had a suprapubic tube in preparation for a hypospadias repair. On attempts to replace the tube it was pushed extravesically toward the left side, and an abscess developed in this area. *Arrow* points to gas formation in the area of the abscess. **(B)** Intraveous urogram 12 days later, showing normal position of bladder.

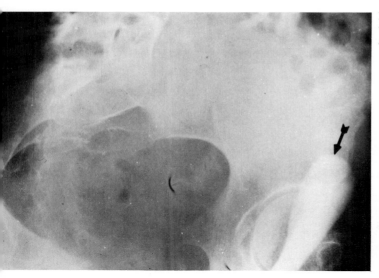

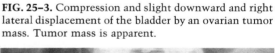

FIG. 25–2. Anterior displacement of the bladder by uterine fibroid. Left oblique view. *Arrow* demonstrates anteriorly displaced bladder.

FIG. 25–3. Compression and slight downward and right lateral displacement of the bladder by an ovarian tumor mass. Tumor mass is apparent.

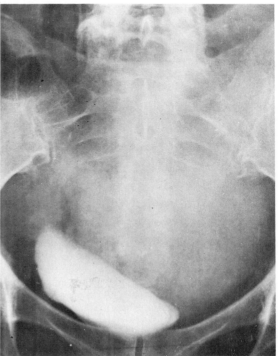

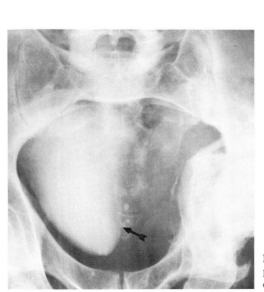

FIG. 25–4. Pelvic abscess from osteomyelitis of the left pelvis in a 53-year-old man. Bladder is compressed and displaced to the right (*arrow*).

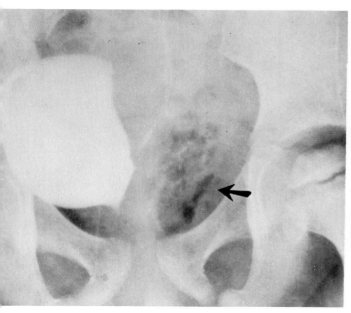

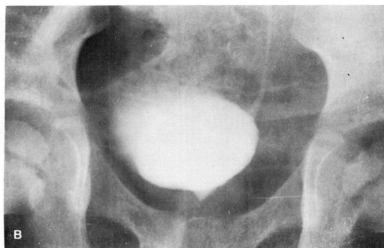

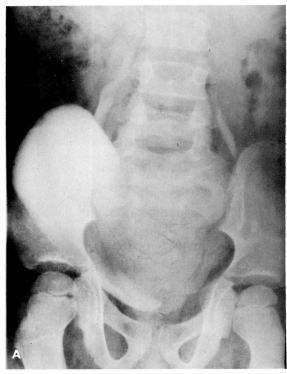
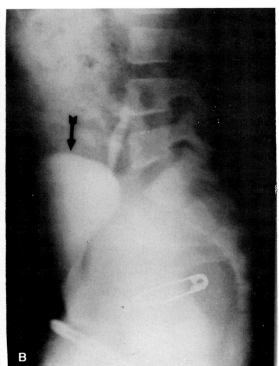

FIG. 25–6. Displacement of the bladder in a boy by a large fecal impaction. **(A)** AP view. Intravenous urogram shows the bladder to be compressed and deviated to the right. The upward extension is caused by compression by the large mass. There is slight lateral deviation of the ureters. **(B)** Lateral view. *Arrow* points to bladder. The bladder is slightly anterior. The bladder returned to normal position after bowel evacuation.

FIG. 25–7. Compression and left lateral displacement of the urinary bladder by large fecal impaction in a young man with stricture of the anus.

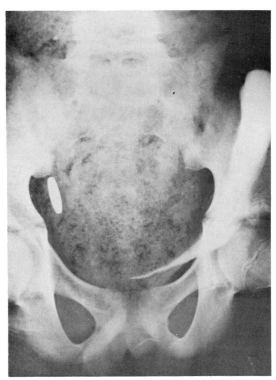

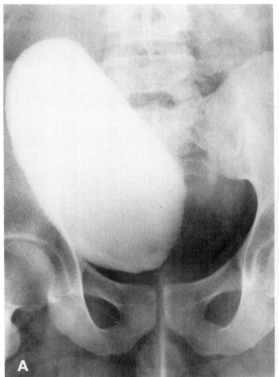

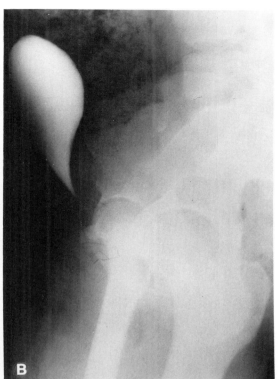

FIG. 25–8. Fecal impaction. (A) Elongated bladder deviated to right. (B) Lateral view; indentation of posterior wall of bladder.

FIG. 25–9. Hodgkin's disease deviating bladder; solitary nodal metastasis.

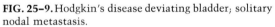

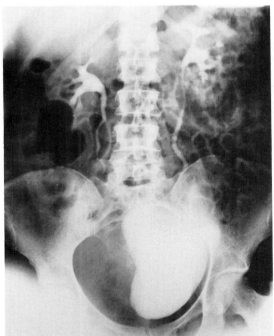

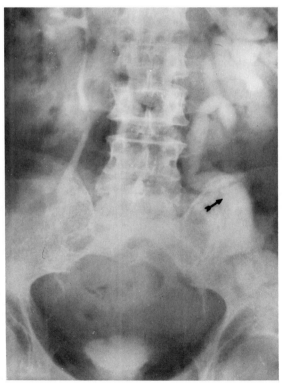

FIG. 25–10. Chordoma. Mass in presacral region. Lower sacrum and coccyx previously had been removed. Left hydroureter (*arrow*) and hydronephrosis due to compression by the mass. Small bladder, slightly compressed on upper surface. (Courtesy of Arthur Tessler, M.D.)

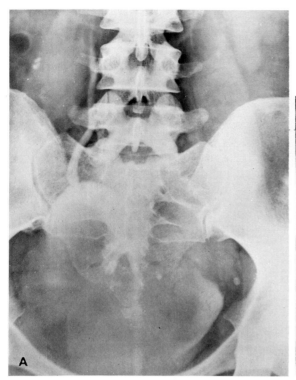

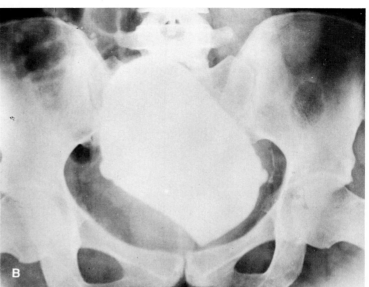

FIG. 25–11. Teratoma, presacral. **(A)** Intravenous pyelogram. Huge pressure defect on the bladder. Bladder appears to be somewhat enlarged. **(B)** Retrograde cystogram. Large pressure defect on the right inferior side of the bladder by extrinsic mass. (Courtesy of A. Balsamo, M.D.)

FIG) 25–12. Sacrococcygeal teratoma in a 2½-year-old girl. **(A)** Supine film. Tumor contained piece of mandible with teeth in sacrococcygeal area. Both ureters seem to be somewhat dilated, and there is right hydronephrosis. **(B)** Prone film. Bladder is elevated markedly, and right ureter is deviated laterally. Child had great difficulty in bowel movements.

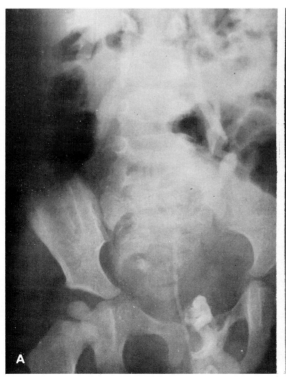

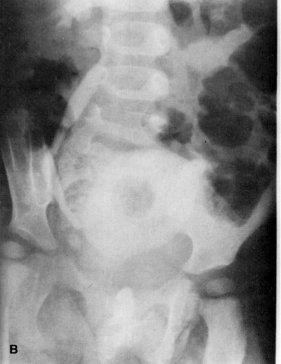

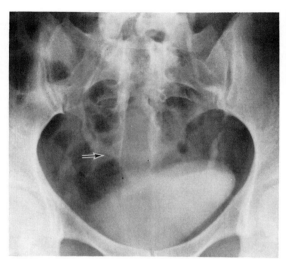

FIG. 25–13. Presacral cystic teratoma. The right ureter is deviated medially (*arrow*), and there is an extrinsic pressure defect against the superior aspect of the bladder on the right side. A spina bifida is present at L-5 through the entire sacrum. (Carter, B.L., Kahn, P.C., Wolpert, S.M., et al.: Radiology, *121*:383, 1976)

FIG. 25–14. Same case as shown in Figure 25–13. Ultrasound studies through the horizontal axis (**A**) and the longitudinal axis (**B**) demonstrate a sonarlucent mass (*arrows*) posterior to the floor of the bladder, displacing the uterus cephalad. (Carter, B.L., Kahn, P.C., Wolpert, S.M., et al.: Radiology, *121*:383, 1976)

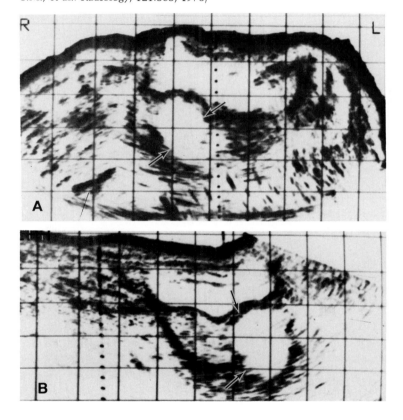

FIG. 25–15. Same case as shown in Figure 25–13. CT scan. A relatively radiolucent soft tissue mass (*horizontal arrow*) extends from the tip of the coccyx to the floor of the bladder (filled with contrast medium). The rectangular outline (*vertical arrow*) is a reference area for direct reading of the Delta value. (Carter, B.L., Kahn, P.C., Wolpert, S.M., et al.: Radiology, *121*:383, 1976)

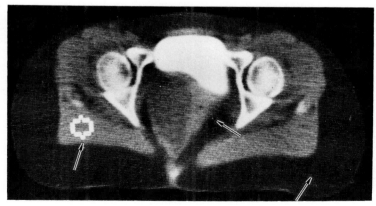

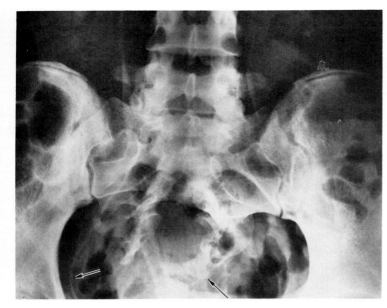

FIG. 25–16. Anterior meningocele. An excretory urogram reveals a scimitar sacrum (*vertical arrow*) and lateral displacement of the right ureter (*horizontal arrow*). A cystotomy tube is draining the bladder. (Carter, B.L., Kahn, P.C., Wolpert, S.M., et al.: Unusual pelvic masses: Radiology, *121*:383, 1976)

FIG. 25–17. Same case as shown in Figure 25–16. Uterus didelphys is present; the left cervix, uterus, and tube are outlined by hysterosalpingography. (Carter, B.L., Kahn, P.C., Wolpert, S.M., et al.: Radiology, *121*:383, 1976)

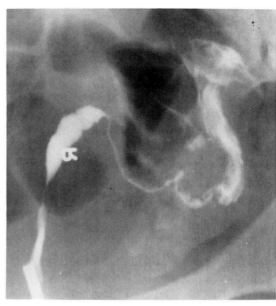

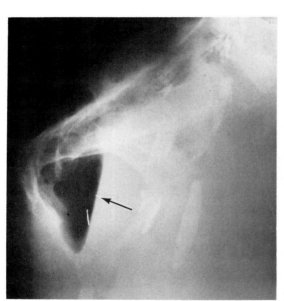

FIG. 25–18. Same case as shown in Figure 25–16. An air-fluid level is present in the anterior meningocele (*arrow*). (Carter, B.L., Kahn, P.C., Wolpert, S.M., et al.: Radiology, *121*:383, 1976).

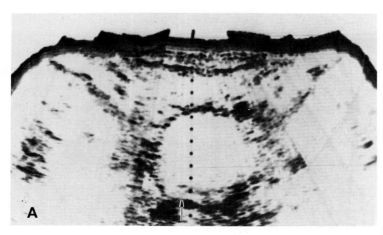

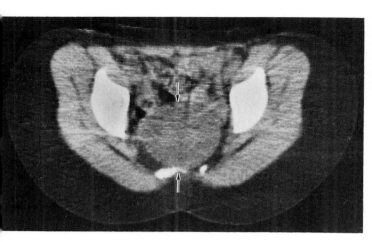

FIG. 25–20. Same case as shown in Figure 25–16. CT scan. A relatively radiolucent mass (*downward arrow*) just anterior to the sacrum displaces bowel loops anteriorly. Spina bifida of the sacrum (*upward arrow*) is evident. (Carter, B.L., Kahn, P.C., Wolpert, S.M., et al.: Radiology, *121*:383, 1976)

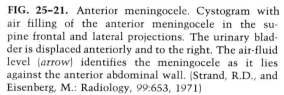

FIG. 25–21. Anterior meningocele. Cystogram with air filling of the anterior meningocele in the supine frontal and lateral projections. The urinary bladder is displaced anteriorly and to the right. The air-fluid level (*arrow*) identifies the meningocele as it lies against the anterior abdominal wall. (Strand, R.D., and Eisenberg, M.: Radiology, *99*:653, 1971)

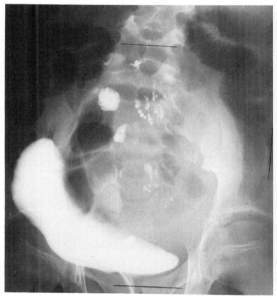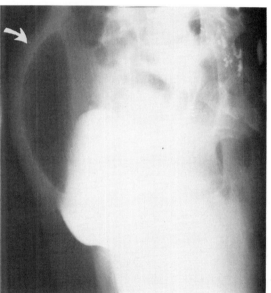

FIG. 25–22. Neurilemoma. Left oblique view of cystogram showing displacement of bladder upward and to the left. (Roberts, L.C., Coppridge, W.M., and Hughes, J.: J. Urol., *79*:159, 1958)

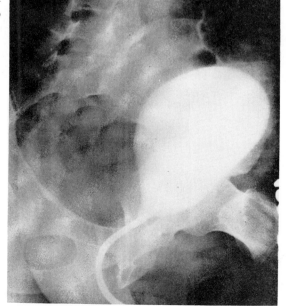

FIG. 25–19. Same case as shown in Figure 25–16. Ultrasound studies through the horizontal axis (**A**) and the longitudinal axis (**B**). A transsonic mass (*arrows*) is clearly visualized within the pelvis anterior to the sacrum. (Carter, B.L., Kahn, P.C., Wolpert, S.M., et al.: Radiology, *121*:383, 1976)

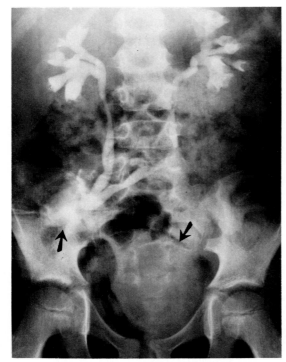

FIG. 25–23. Recurrent rhabdomyosarcoma. A mass (*downward arrow*) in the pelvis displaces the bowel. Both ureters are draining into an ileostomy (*upward arrow*). (Carter, B.L., Kahn, P.C., Wolpert, S.M., et al.: Radiology, *121*:383, 1976)

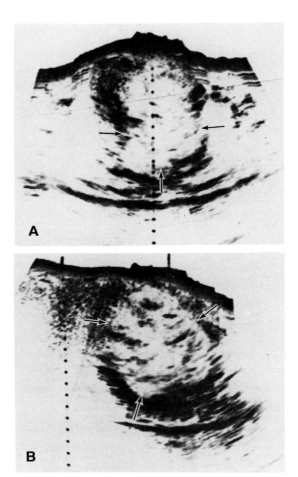

FIG. 25–24. Same case as shown in Figure 25–23. Horizontal (**A**) and longitudinal (**B**) scans obtained by ultrasonography outline the total extent of a solid mass (*arrow*) within the pelvis. (Carter, B.L., Kahn, P.C., Wolpert, S.M., et al.: Radiology, *121*:383, 1976)

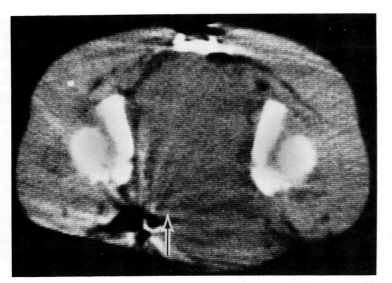

FIG. 25–25. Same case as shown in Figure 25–23. CT scan. A large soft tissue mass (*arrow*) in the pelvis displaces the bowel. (Carter, B.L., Kahn, P.C., Wolpert, S.M., et al.: Radiology, *121*:383, 1976)

FIG. 25–26. Displacement and indentation of posterior wall of bladder by a mass in the rectovesical pouch. Primary carcinoma of the pancreas, metastatic.

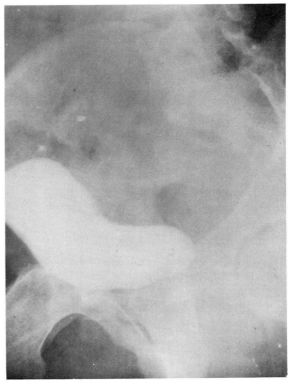

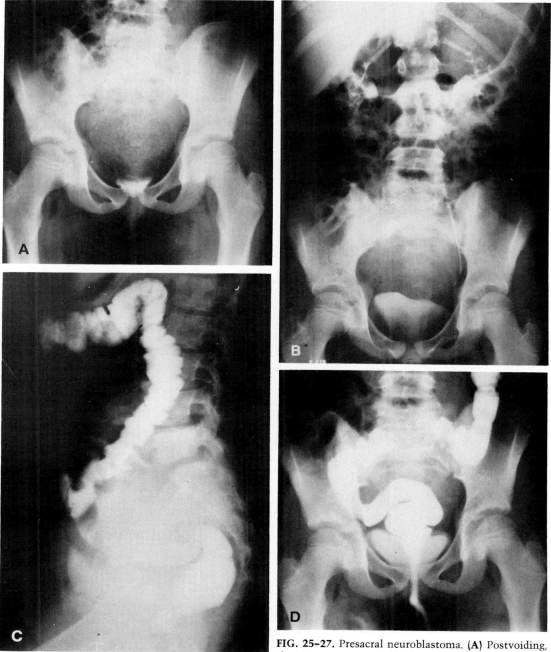

FIG. 25–27. Presacral neuroblastoma. (**A**) Postvoiding, showing mass presacrally. (**B**) Lateral deviation of left ureter by mass. (**C**) Lateral view; compression of sigmoid. (**D**) Barium enema; compression of sigmoid colon. (Courtesy of Walter Berdon)

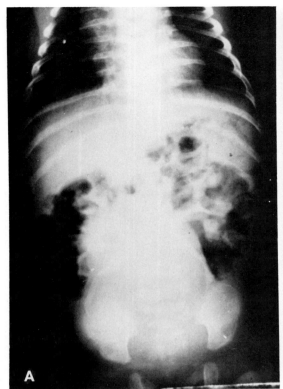

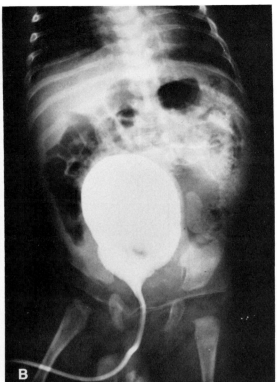

FIG. 25–28. Neuroblastoma: 6-week-old boy. **(A)** Intravenous urogram: large mass deviating ureter. **(B)** AP cystogram: defective bladder. **(C)** Lateral view: flattening of posterior wall of bladder. (Courtesy of Sandra Fernbach, M.D. and Leonard Bouras)

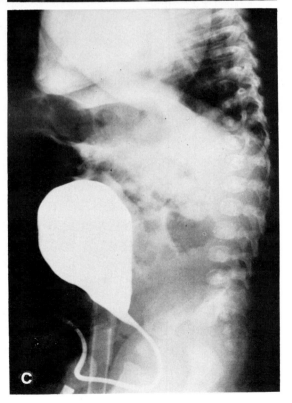

BIBLIOGRAPHY

General

1. Carter, B.L., Kahn, P.C., Wolpert, S.M., et al.: Unusual pelvic masses: a comparison of computed tomographic scanning and ultrasonography. Radiology, *121*:383–390, 1976.
2. Korobin, M., Minagi, H., and Palubinskas, A.J.: Lateral displacement of the bladder. Am. J. Roentgenol., *125*:337–344, 1975.

Presacral Tumors

3. Camp, J.B., and Good, C.A.: The roentgenologic diagnosis of tumors involving the sacrum. Radiology, *31*:348–403, 1938.
4. Jackman, R.J., Clark, P.L., and Smith, N.D.: Retrorectal tumors. J.A.M.A., *145*:956–962, 1951.
5. MacCarty, C.S., Waugh, G.M., Mayo, C.W., and Coventry, M.B.: The surgical treatment of presacral tumors: a combined problem. Proc. Mayo Clin., *27*:73–84, 1952.
6. Mayo, C.W., Baker, G.S., and Smith, L.R.: Presacral tumors: differential diagnosis and report of a case. Proc. Mayo Clin., *28*:616–622, 1953.
7. Middledorpf, K.: Zur Kenntniss do angeboren Sacralgeschwulste. Arch. Pathol. Anat., *101*:37–44, 1885.
8. Werner, J.L., and Taubi, H.: Presacral masses in childhood. Am. J. Roentgenol., *109*:403–410, 1970.
9. Whitaker, L.D., and Pemberton, J. de J.: Tumors ventral to the sacrum. Ann. Surg., *107*:96–106, 1938.

Chordomas

10. Adson, A.W., Moersch, F.P., and Kernohan, J.W.: Neurogenic tumors arising from the sacrum. Arch. Neurol. Psychiatry, *41*:535–555, 1939.
11. Dahlin, D.C., and MacCarty, C.S.: Chordoma: a study of 59 cases. Cancer, *5*:1170–1178, 1952.
12. Harvey, W.F., and Dawson, E.K.: Chordoma. Edinburgh Med. J., *48*:713–730, 1941.
13. Higinbotham, N.L., Phillips, R.F., Farr, H.W., et al.: Chordoma. Thirty-five year study at Memorial Hospital. Cancer, *20*:1841–1850, 1967.

Teratomas

14. Altman, R.R., Randolph, J.G., and Lilly, J.R.: Sacrococcygeal teratoma: American Academy of Pediatric Surgical Section Survey–1973. J. Pediatr. Surg., *9*:389–398, 1974.
15. Ashcraft, K.W., and Holder, T.M.: Hereditary presacral teratoma. J. Pediatr. Surg., *9*:691–697, 1974.
16. Carney, J.A., Thompson, D.P., Johnson, C.L., et al.: Teratoma in children. Clinical and pathological aspects. J. Pediatr. Surg., *7*:271–282, 1972.
17. Dillard, B.M., Mayer, J.H., McAlister, W.H., et al.: Sacrococcygeal teratomas in children. J. Pediatr. Surg., *5*:53–59, 1970.
18. Eklof, O.: Roentgenologic findings in sacrococcygeal teratoma. Acta. Radiol., *3*:41–48, 1965.
19. Exelby, P.R.: Sacrococcygeal teratomas in children. Calif. Cancer J. Clin., *22*:202–225, 1972.
20. Gross, R.E., Clatsworthy, H.W., Jr., and Meeker, I.A., Jr.: Sacrococcygeal teratoma in infants and children: a report of 40 cases. Surg. Gynecol. Obstet., *92*:341–354, 1951.

21. Gwinn, J.L., Dockerty, M.B., and Kennedy, R.L.J.: Presacral teratoma in infancy and childhood. Pediatrics, *16*:239–249, 1955.
22. Hanbery, J.W., Senz, E.H., and Jeffrey, R.A.: Sacrococcygeal teratoma in infants and childhood. Stanford Med. Bull., *16*:154–168, 1958.
23. Hatteland, K., and Knutrud, O.: Sacrococcygeal teratomata in children. Acta Chir. Scand., *119*:444–452, 1960.
24. Head, H.D., Gerstein, J.D., and Muir, R.W.: Presacral teratoma in the adult. Am. Surg., *41*:240–248, 1975.
25. Mahour, G.H., Woolley, M.M., Trivedi, S.N., et al.: Teratomas in infancy and childhood: experience with 81 cases. Surgery, *76*:309–316, 1974.
26. Mahour, G.H., Woolley, M.M., Trivedi, S.N., et al.: Sacrococcygeal teratoma: a 33-year experience. J. Pediatr. Surg., *10*:183–188, 1975.

Lipomas

27. Lassman, L.P., and James, C.L.M.: Lumbosacral lipoma: critical survey of 26 cases submitted to laminectomy. J. Neural Neurosurg. Psychiatr., *30*:174–181, 1967.

Anterior Meningocele

78. Abbott, K.H., Retter, R.H., and Leimbach, W.H.: The role of perineural sacral cysts in the sciatic and sacrococcygeal syndrome: a review of the literature and report of 9 cases. J. Neurosurg., *14*:5–21, 1957.
29. Amacher, A.L., Drake, C.G., and McLachlin, A.D.: Anterior sacral meningocele. Surg. Gynecol. Obstet., *126*:986–994, 1968.
30. Barlow, D., and Gracey, L.: Anterior sacral meningocele causing urinary retention. Br. J. Surg., *50*:732–734, 1963.
31. Chovnick, S.D.: Anterior sacral meningocele as a cause of urinary retention. J. Urol., *106*:371–374, 1971.
32. Cohn, J., and Bay-Nielsen, E.: Hereditary defect of the sacrum and coccyx with anterior sacral meningocele. Acta Paediatr. Scand., *58*:268–274, 1969.
33. Haddad, F.S.: Anterior sacral meningocele: report of two cases and review of the literature. Canad. J. Surg., *1*:230–242, 1958.
34. Ivamoto, H.S., and Wallman, L.J.: Anterior sacral meningocele. Arch. Neurol., *31*:345–346, 1974.
35. Klenerman, L., and Merrick, M.V.: Anterior sacral meningocele occurring in a family. J. Bone Joint Surg., *55*:331–334, 1973.
36. Strand, R.D., and Eisenberg, H.M.: Anterior sacral meningocele in association with Marfan's syndrome. Radiology, *99*:653–654, 1971.

Ependymoma

37. Fragoyannis, S., and Yallin, S.: Ependymomas with distant metastases. Report of 2 cases and a review of the literature. Cancer, *19*:246–356, 1966.
38. Mork, S.J., and Loken, A.L.: Ependymoma. A follow-up study of 101 cases. Cancer, *40*:907–915, 1977.
39. Wolff, M., Santiago, H., and Duly, M.M.: Delayed distal metastases from a subcutaneous sacrococcygeal ependymoma. Cancer, *30*:1046–1067, 1972.

Neurilemoma

40. Deming, C.L.: Tumors of the urogenital tract. *In* Campbell, M.: Urology. vol. 2, pp. 969, 1004–1005. Philadelphia, Saunders, 1954.
41. Krekeler, A.: Über ein Neurinoma in der Wand des Mastdorms. Inaug-Diss, Bonn, 1928.
42. Krumbien, C.: Über die "Band- oder Pallisadenstellung" der Kerne, eine Wuchsform des feinfibrillaren mesenchymalen Gewebes: Zugleich eine Ableitung der Neurinoma (Verocay) vom feinfibrillaren Bindegewebe (Fibroma tenuifibrillare). Arch. Pathol. Anat., *225*:304–331, 1925.
43. Pava, C.: Neurinoma del Piccolo Bucino con Amiloidose Generalizzata. Osp. Maggione, *19*:741–747, 1931.
44. Roberts, L.C., Coppridge, W.M., and Hughes, J.: Tumors and cysts of the male pelvis which interfere with urination. J. Urol., *79*:159–164, 1958.
45. Stout, A.P.: Peripheral manifestations of the specific nerve sheath tumor (neurilemoma). Am. J. Cancer, *24*:751–796, 1936.
46. Young, H.B.: Neurilemoma of pelvis presenting with acute manifestations. Br. J. Surg., *41*:315–316, 1953.

Rhabdomyosarcoma

47. Bretagne, M.C., Chabet, B., L'Hermite, J., et al.: Embryonic sarcomas of the urogenital sinus: five cases in infants and adolescents (abstr.). Radiology, *117*:507, 1975.
48. Clatsworthy, H.W., Jr., Braren, V., and Smith, J.P.: Surgery of bladder and prostatic neoplasms in children. Cancer, *32*:1157–1160, 1973.
49. Ghazali, S.: Embryonic rhabdomyosarcoma of the urogenital tract. Br. J. Surg., *60*:124–128, 1973.
50. Tefft, M., and Jaffe, N.: Sarcoma of the bladder and prostate in children. Cancer, *32*:1161–1177, 1973.

Retrorectal Cyst

51. Campbell, W.L., and Wolff, M.: Retrorectal cysts of developmental origin. Am. J. Roentgenol., *117*:307–313, 1973.

Miscellaneous

52. Cunningham, J.J., and Winningham, D.G.: Retroperitoneal cystic lymphangioma presenting as an unusual pelvic mass. J. Urol., *108*:717–718, 1972.

Inflammations of the bladder are varied and extremely difficult to diagnose roentgenographically. Diagnosis usually depends on history, culture, cystoscopic examination, and biopsy.

Most cases of cystitis occur in adult women and are usually a combination of urethritis and cystitis. *Escherichia coli* is the predominant organism. Symptoms may persist even when the bladder is sterile. It has been suggested that female patients with recurrent urinary infection have a higher percentage of pathogenic bacteria within the urethra than female patients with a negative urologic history.[1] It has been pointed out that the urethral and bladder infections may be influenced by the introital bacteria.[2] Cystitis in men is usually secondary to prostatitis or prostatic hypertrophy. In children, urinary infection is usually more serious and should be thoroughly investigated with intravenous urograms and voiding cystourethrograms.

CYSTOTRIGONITIS

Cystotrigonitis (Figs. 26-2 to 26-4) can be diagnosed by an irregularity of the trigone. Diagnosis by this means may occur more frequently than is supposed, but the area is obscured by the contrast medium as it gradually fills the bladder on intravenous urography.

HEMORRHAGIC CYSTITIS

Hemorrhagic cystitis is a special form of cystitis with multiple hemorrhages in the mucosa and lamina propria (Figs. 26-5, 26-7). It is often part of the signs and symptoms of "honeymoon cystitis," a syndrome following sexual intercourse. Intercourse may cause transient increases of bacteria in the urine.[2a] Postcoital hemorrhagic cystitis in the el-

26

Inflammation of the Bladder

1391

derly woman may be caused by atrophic vaginitis. *E. coli* is probably the most common cause of hemorrhagic cystitis in adults. In children, it is often associated with the adenoviruses[2g] and possibly sometimes with papovirus-like particles.[2c] It can also be a complication of the management of pediatric neoplasms.[2h] Epidemics due to influenza A virus have occurred.[2d] On excretory cystogram, there is a marked irregularity of the bladder with bleeding, V-shaped, marginal indentations. In both cystotrigonitis and hemorrhagic cystitis, retrograde cystograms usually obscure the foregoing findings. Reflux and sterile hemorrhagic cystitis has been reported.[2i]

BULLOUS EDEMA

Bullous edema is an inflammatory change of the bladder macroscopically seen in acute cystitis.[3-5] The mucosa appears irregularly thickened, inflamed, rigid, and covered by rounded cystlike elevations varying in size and often appearing like grapes.

The bullous edema may be widespread (Fig. 26–8) as a part of an acute generalized cystitis. It is most commonly seen as a result of irritation of the bladder mucosa by indwelling catheters. This irritation produces the bullous edema of the superior lateral part of the dome, posterior wall, and trigone. It may become polypoid in appearance.[3a] Acute obstruction of ureters has been reported.[5a]

CHRONIC CYSTITIS

Irregularities of the bladder wall associated with trabeculations and often a somewhat smaller bladder capacity are the roentgenographic characteristics of chronic cystitis (Figs. 26–1, 26–2). Reflux may occur.

INTERSTITIAL CYSTITIS

Interstitial cystitis is a chronic disease of the bladder occurring especially in women and characterized cystoscopically by a localized reddened area or scar formation with ulceration in the vault of the bladder (Figs. 26–9 to 26–12). There may be single or multiple lesions. The bladder gets progressively smaller, averaging 100–150 cc., but in the late stages it may hold only an ounce of fluid. Frequently it is accompanied by intractable symptoms, such as frequency of urination, pain when bladder is full, and strangury. Emptying the bladder often relieves the symptoms. The urine is usually clear and sterile but may contain red cells. Attempts to dilate the bladder may lead to bleeding of involved mucosa in the vault (Hunner's ulcer). Histologically the entire thickness of the bladder is involved, and there is marked infiltration by lymphocytes, plasma cells, and leukocytes with edema and hypertrophy of muscle. The peritoneal surface may be thickened, and a chronic ulcer may be present on the mucosal side. Fibrosis of the musculature occurs later with a small-capacity bladder completely resistant to attempts at dilatation.

The incidence of interstitial cystitis is 0.23 per cent of hospital admissions.[15]

ETIOLOGY

Bacteria, viruses, and fungi are probably not direct causes of interstitial cystitis.[10a]

Neurosis has been considered related to interstitial cystitis,[11] because so many of the patients have neurotic symptoms.

In rabbits, an inflammation similar to interstitial cystitis has been produced by injection of *Streptococcus pyogenes* Group A, Type 12 (a causative factor in glomerulonephritis and rheumatic fever).[11a]

Autoimmune disease: Oravisto et al. found antinuclear antibodies in 85 per cent of cases, allergy of reagin type in 13 per cent, and hypersensitivity reaction to drugs in 35 per cent.[18a] Jokinen et al. concluded that interstitial cystitis is an autoimmune disease in which the disease is restricted to one organ but in which the autoantibodies are non-organ specific.[14a] In 1973 they reported a drop in the antibody titers against cell nuclei and crude kidney homogenate after cystectomy in three patients.[14b] Silk[20] and Gordon et al.[8] also considered immune responses in this disease.

The disease may be caused by vascular or possibly neurovegetative vascular disturbances.[20a]

Radiographically, the bladder is smaller than normal. It may or may not be trabeculated. Often there is an associated vesicoureteral reflux. The ureter may be obstructed at the ureterovesical junction without reflux. Tuberculosis, abacteria pyuria, radiation cystitis, and hypertonic neurogenic bladder must be differentiated from interstitial cystitis. Many cases have been diagnosed as interstitial cystitis that may later be proven to be carcinoma in situ.[18, 22] Carcinoma of the bladder has also been confused and associated with interstitial cystitis.[17, 21, 23] Carcinoma arising in Hunner's ulcer has been reported.[9, 19]

EOSINOPHILIC CYSTITIS

Eosinophilic cystitis (Figs. 26–13, 26–14) is a form of cystitis represented by infiltration of eosinophils into mucosa, lamina propria, muscularis, and around blood vessels.[25-40]

The presenting symptoms are frequency, urgency, dysuria, and nocturia. Gross hematuria or microhematuria is frequent. The disease may become chronic, and recurrences and exacerbations are not unusual. Eosinophilia and eosinophilic pyuria may be present; heavy proteinuria is common. Culture of the urine is occasionally sterile, but usually the common pathogens are cultured. No ova or parasites have been demonstrated in the urine, stool, or tissues, although one patient has been reported with serum antibodies to *Toxocara cati*.[37] The victims are usually young, children representing nearly 50 per cent of cases (75% of the children have been black). Hydronephrosis and hydroureter have been reported[26, 27, 29] and can improve on therapy. Progression to renal failure may occur.[31]

Frenzelli,[28] Goldstein,[29] Kindall,[33] and Pastinszky[36] suggested an allergic reaction may be responsible for eosinophilic cystitis, but no definite allergens have been found. The ileum and the colon have also shown eosinophilic infiltration in association with eosinophilic cystitis.[35]

Cystoscopy. The following variable descriptions have been reported on cystoscopy: (1) no mucosal abnormalities may be seen; (2) ulcerations; (3) polypoid projections; (4) edema, often bullous; (5) nonerythematous cobblestone appearance; (6) raised yellowish and erythematous plaques; and (7) nodular areas.

Roentgenographic Findings. The bladder wall may be greatly thickened (Fig. 26–14). Hydronephrosis and hydroureter have been reported. Vesicoureteral reflux may occur. The usual finding is nodularity of the bladder from indentations of bladder wall or multiple rounded grapelike defects (Fig. 26–13).

DIFFERENTIAL DIAGNOSIS

Eosinophilic cystitis may be confused with carcinoma, but the lesions are more likely to be multiple in the former. In addition, infiltrative defects are rare in eosinophilic cystitis.

Eosinophilic granulomatous prostatitis may produce eosinophilic lesions in the bladder, but the finding of definite granulomas should differentiate these two entities.

GRANULOMATOUS CYSTITIS

Granulomatous cystitis is a rare disease occurring under the following conditions:[41-56]

1. A complication of chronic granulomatous disease of childhood
2. Secondary to granulomatous disease of the bowel as a result of direct extension
3. Secondary to granulomatous prostatitis
4. Isolated primary disease of the bladder

Type 1. Granulomatous cystitis as a complication of granulomatous disease of childhood. Chronic granulomatous disease of childhood is characterized by granulomatous and suppurative destruction involving lymph nodes, cutaneous abscesses, hepatosplenomegaly, pulmonary infiltrates, and eczematoid rash. It is usually a fatal disease. Chronic granulomatous disease of childhood is probably a sex-linked genetically inherited condition. Boys are involved much more frequently than girls. In both instances the defect appears to be within the polymorphonuclear leukocytes. In the male, the phagocytic cells in patients with granulomatous disease lack the peroxidase-myeloperoxidase halide antimicrobial system,[51] and they are therefore unable to produce H_2O_2.[52] Thus the amount of H_2O_2 produced is decreased, and the intracellular viability of the bacteria continues. In girls, the leukocytes are deficient in glutathione peroxidase.

The disease has rarely involved the urinary tract, but reports by Kontras and co-workers,[53] Cyr and co-workers,[46] and Bloomberg and co-workers[44] have included cases involving the bladder. Bloomberg's case also involved the kidney, and one case of kidney involvement was reported by Carson at postmortem examination.[45]

Type 2. Secondary to granulomatous disease of bowel as a result of direct extension. Vesical involvement by granulomatous colitis or ileitis is usually above the trigone near the dome of the bladder or on the lateral wall. The mass infiltrating the bladder can be large, and fistulization is common.

Type 3. Secondary to granulomatous prostatitis. Several instances of involvement of the bladder from granulomatous prostatitis of the eosinophilic variety have been reported.[56] The involvement is differentiated from eosinophilic cystitis by the presence of granulomas.

Type 4. Isolated primary disease of bladder. This is an extremely rare condition of involvement of bladder by granulomatous lesions; it is nontuberculous (Figs. 26–17, 26–18).

Cystoscopic findings vary from edematous, elevated fronds to large infiltrating appearing masses, easily confused with carcinoma.

ROENTGENOGRAPHIC FINDINGS

Roentgenographic findings vary somewhat with the type of granulomatous cystitis:

Type 1. There is an irregular indentation of the bladder wall appearing like an extravesical lesion (Fig. 26–15).[44]

Type 2. This presents a large mass appearing as an infiltrating lesion often with fistula formation. The mass is irregular, bulging, and is similar to the infiltrating type of carcinoma of the bladder (Fig. 26–16).

Type 3. There are no characteristic findings, because the lesion is on the floor of the bladder and does not visualize well, although an irregular base can be seen.

Type 4. This type may give a bubbly appearance to the mucosa on double contrast study (Fig. 26–18) or nodular irregularity (Fig. 26–17).

CYSTITIS EMPHYSEMATOSA

Cystitis emphysematosia[57-79] is an inflammatory lesion of the bladder associated with gas vesicles in the bladder wall (Figs. 26–19 to 26–22). (Generalized gas-producing infection with secondary bladder involvement usually is excluded from this group.) The condition usually is caused by gas-forming bacilli of the colon group and often is associated with diabetes mellitus or hyperglycemia due to intravenous fluid therapy. Rarely, diabetes without infection can production this entity. Marks reported two cases, one on corticosteroid therapy and one on hyperalimentation that developed pneumaturia.[83] Both cases, however, had glycosuria with infection. The disease is usually transient and benign. The radiographic picture varies with the stage of the disease.

The following three stages are described by Boijsen and Lewis-Johnson[60]:

Stage 1. A clear zone 1 mm. wide may be seen around the contrast medium. There is no free gas in the lumen. The gas vesicles are so small that they cannot be distinguished radiographically.

Stage 2. The bladder wall is irregular, swollen, and thicker owing to increased intramural gas production. The gas-filled vesicles can now be made out clearly in the wall of the bladder. There is no gas in the bladder lumen. Bladder capacity has diminished.

Stage 3. The vesicles have ruptured, and free gas appears in the lumen of the bladder, with less gas demonstrable in the wall. The capacity of the bladder returns to normal but later increases in size. Still later, the amount of free gas diminishes, and the bladder returns to normal. Twenty-one days apparently have been the upper limit of the extent of the duration of this disease.[79] However, the duration depends on the type of infection, the degree and the presence of hyperglycemia, and the speed with which the infection is brought under control.

Roentgenographic Appearance. Following are the characteristic roentgenographic findings in cystitis emphysematosa:

1. Small gas-filled vesicles, usually on one side of the bladder and giving a cobblestone effect (Fig. 26–19). We believe that this may be the earliest picture of cystitis emphysematosa.
2. A ring of gas lying outside the mucosa in the lamina propria or musculature going around the bladder in a horseshoe-type fashion (Figs. 26–20 to 26–23).
3. Gas in the bladder lumen, with or without the gas appearing in the wall (Figs. 26–23 to 26–25).
4. A collection of gas in the region of the urinary bladder, forming the shape of the bladder and divided into small compartments.[67]

PNEUMATURIA

Pneumaturia (Figs. 26–23 to 26–25), the finding of free gas in the lumen of the urinary bladder, is caused by the following factors:[80-87] (1) instrumentation of the genitourinary tract; (2) fistula formation between the intestinal or the genital tracts, or both, and the urinary tract; (3) fermentation (primary pneumaturia), with or without glycosuria; and (4) cystitis emphysematosa.

The formation of gas in the urinary bladder in diabetes is caused by the fermentation of sugars by an infecting organism. The most frequent organisms are *Escherichia coli*, *Aerobacter aerogenes*, and yeast. The gas is composed of carbon dioxide, hydrogen, nitrogen, and methane. Obstruction is the usual prerequisite for the persistence of gas in the bladder lumen.

PROLIFERATIVE LESIONS OF THE BLADDER

CYSTITIS CYSTICA

Cystitis cystica (Figs. 26–26, 26–27) is an inflammatory lesion of the bladder included in the general classification of proliferative cystitis, a term used to include a variety of inflammatory lesions of the bladder characterized by granulomatous nodular cystic cavities.[88-95] Other lesions included in this group are cystitis follicularis, cystitis granulosa and polyposa, and cystitis glandularis. In cystitis cystica there are superficial sessile polypoid or, rarely, pedunculated small rounded cysts varying in size, often translucent, but occasionally hemorrhagic. The accompanying mucosa is inflamed.

Cystitis cystica is found more commonly on the trigone and base of the bladder. It is seen more frequently in women. Kaplan and King found an incidence of 2.4 per cent in a group of children with urinary tract infection.[88] Uehling and King believe that the associated submucosal glandular cysts and lymphoid follicles raise the possibility of an immunologic role in cystitis cystica.[93] Uehling and Steihm found elevated levels of secretory IgA in children with urinary tract infection and speculated that cyst formation may be related to an immune response whereby the lymphoid follicles attempt to produce antibodies.[94] It is seen with great frequency in otherwise normal bladders.[95a]

Roentgenographic Appearance. The most common appearance of cystitis cystica is irregular indentation of the contrast-filled lumen by cysts of varying size, usually on the floor but occasionally occurring on the lateral and the posterior walls.

Marked irregularity of the entire bladder is seen, with the irregularities projecting into the bladder lumen. The cysts often are coated with the contrast material, which therefore is not evenly distributed. This type of roentgenographic appearance may be confused with that of carcinoma.

CYSTITIS GLANDULARIS

Cystitis glandularis (Figs. 26–28 to 26–30a)[96-119] is characterized by the proliferation of glands (usually mucus-producing) in the mucosa and lamina propria of the bladder.[109] Two forms have been recognized cystoscopically and pathologically: (1) Cystoscopically, (a) there is an irregular, villous appearance, usually at the dome or (b) mammillated, bleblike elevations with a sharp demarcation between normal and abnormal mucosa found on the floor of the bladder. (2) Pathologically, (a) there is a single layer of mucus-producing goblet cells resembling mucosa of large bowel or (b) multilayered, usually mucus-producing cells that resemble prostate gland.

Although each of these cell types has been found in both bladder dome and trigone area, the first type is more likely to be found in the dome in the region of the urachus, and the second type more likely on the trigone.

Cystitis glandularis is often associated with cystitis cystica,[99, 109, 110] pelvic lipomatosis,[119a] extrophy of the bladder, and urachal remnants.[97a, 100] Symptoms include dysuria, frequency, and hematuria[101, 104, 114] but ureteral obstruction may draw the attention of the urologist.[97, 112, 113]

Etiology. Numerous causes have been championed in the literature:

1. Embryonic rests displaced in the separation of rectum and urogenital sinus[101, 108]
2. An inflammatory process obstructing von Brunn's nests causing either cystic degeneration or secretory activity[107]
3. Metaplasia of bladder from inflammation[118]
4. Cataplasia: reversal to a type through which it has passed in its previous development[100]
5. The lesion at the dome may arise from the urachus[102]

Sterling and Ash found no glandular elements in the bladder of the newborn infant,[116] and because similar lesions are found in the ureter and renal pelvis, the embryonic rest theory in relation to the bladder may be untenable.

Cystitis glandularis usually runs a benign course, but several well-documented cases of transformation to an adenocarcinoma have been reported.[115, 117] It may be a precancerous lesion leading to adenocarcinoma.[109]

Roentgenographic Findings. Multiple defects or a single defect, rounded in shape, and not infiltrating the bladder wall, may be seen. A large, irregular single defect (usually seen at the dome) or multiple, smooth "cobblestone" filling defects (usually on floor) may be seen. Occasionally hydroureter and hydronephrosis may occur, suggesting infiltration and thus being confused with malignancy. It must be differentiated from blood clots, nonopaque stones, and bullous edema; the latter may be especially difficult to differentiate except by biopsy.

CYSTITIS FOLLICULARIS

Cystitis follicularis is a condition of indefinite etiology and obscure pathogenesis. It has been associated with malacoplakia and cancer of the bladder.[119b] It is characterized by a study of the mucosa, which exhibits discrete, closely packed nodules. The lamina propria contains lymph follicles surrounded by edema, engourgement of capillaries, lymphocytes, plasma cells, and monocytes. There has been no definite cystographic finding.

ABACTERIAL PYURIA
(ACUTE INTERSTITIAL CYSTITIS, STERILE PYURIA, ABACTERIAL CYSTITIS, AMICROBIC PYURIA, AMICROBIC CYSTITIS)

Abacterial pyuria (Fig. 26-31) is an unusual disorder of the bladder of unknown etiology.[120-123] The onset is acute, and its symptoms vary from mild to severe. There may be mild urethral irritation with gradations to disabling diurnal and nocturnal frequency, strangury, and gross hematuria. Suprapubic pain is usually present. There is no evidence of generalized illness. A mucopurulent urethral discharge may occur. The distinguishing sign is the absence of bacteria in the urine despite the usual finding of pyuria; cultures for l-form bacteria and tuberculosis are negative. Young adults, 20 to 30 years of age, are the common victims. It is much more common in men but may occur in women. It has been suggested that it may be related to Reiter's disease,[121] or it may be similar to sterile hemorrhagic cystitis secondary to cyclophosphamide (Cytoxan) therapy.[120]

Cystoscopic findings are considered characteristic. The mucosa of the bladder is velvety red, usually with exudate, and with or without ulcerations. Improvement may be spontaneous or secondary to treatment. Recurrences, however, are common.[121]

Roentgenographic Findings. The bladder is small and irregular, and the lower ureter may be dilated (Fig. 26-31A). However, the condition is reversible as evidenced by the posttreatment intravenous urogram showing a normal bladder (Fig. 26-31B).

DIFFERENTIAL DIAGNOSIS

Bacterial Infections. In this entity the culture is positive, there may be systemic symptoms, and the cystoscopic findings do not show the velvety appearance of abacterial pyuria.

Tuberculosis. Here cultures of tuberculosis are positive, and there are abnormal upper tracts. The onset is less acute in tuberculosis.

Carcinoma In Situ. The cystoscopic findings disclose multiple hemorrhagic areas in the mucosa.[123] They have a granular or cobblestone appearance and are slightly raised. Conspicuous white or yellow excrescence within the hemorrhagic areas can be seen. However, exfoliative urine cytology studies are positive, and biopsies may be diagnostic.

Interstitial Cystitis. This is usually progressive, being more common in women.

Radiation Cystitis. This is differentiated by history and persistence of lesions.

Neurogenic Bladder. This is usually associated with neurologic findings.

CYCLOPHOSPHAMIDE CYSTITIS

The use of cyclophosphamide (Cytoxan),[124-132] may produce severe bladder symptoms and changes in the bladder. There are two types (Figs. 26-32, 26-33). The acute type may occur 24 to 48 hours after the massive intravenous infusion or months after the initiation of daily small oral doses. The symptoms are burning on urination, urgency, frequency, and hematuria. Cystoscopically there is hyperemic, edematous mucosa with hemorrhagic areas. This form usually subsides 4 to 5 days after cessation of the drug, but it may persist for 2 months after its discontinuance.[126, 127] The chronic form (Fig. 26-32) occurs after prolonged use of large amounts of cyclophosphamide. Severe bleeding may be resistant to treatment. Mucosal telangiectasia is frequently present. The bladder can become contracted and fibrotic. Calcification has been reported (Fig. 26-34).

Roentgenographic Findings. Nodular defects may represent the early findings. Later appearance reveals contracture of bladder with a thickened, fibrotic wall. Dilated upper tracts may be the result of vesicoureteral reflux.[125, 128, 131]

RADIATION CYSTITIS

Radiation cystitis occurs any time after a few months to 14 years after completion of irradiation.[132c] It occurs more frequently after intracavitary irradiation and is infrequent after super voltage techniques.

On cystoscopy, the mucosa is pale and edematous. Petechiae, telangiectasis, and dilated and tortuous vessels may be visualized. Necrotizing arteriolitis has been reported. Fibrosis occurs in the lamina propria and muscularis. Ulcerations and incrustations[132c] may be present.

The roentgenographic findings show a small contracted bladder that may be either smooth or irregular (Fig. 26–35).

FUNGUS BALLS OF THE URINARY BLADDER

Fungus balls in the urinary bladder are the result of infection by a fungus, especially *Candida albicans*.[133-143] Organisms most likely invade the bladder through the urethra, although involvement from the blood route or regional spread from contiguous organisms is a possibility. Under less favorable conditions for growth, that is, semianaerobic, the organisms take on a multicellular mycelial thread form. These collect in large sheets or colonies.[133] The fungus balls are composed of layers of mycelia separated by air and proteinaceous material giving a laminated appearance.

Several factors play a role in the transformation of *Candida* to a pathogen. These include prolonged antibiotic therapy, protracted use of steroids, immunosuppressive medication, and severe debilitating disease.[142] Stasis may play an important additional role.

Uncontrolled diabetes has been an important factor in many cases of fungus balls in the urinary tract.[134, 135, 138] Air within the fungus balls has been reported by Margolis,[138] Chisholm and Hutch,[134] and McDonald and Fagan.[139] Air is the result of action of bacteria or fungi on glucose in the urine, producing CO_2 and butyric and lactic acid. The gas formed can accentuate the layered colonies of fungi, forming a laminated appearance of the fungus balls. There may be a single large fungus ball or multiple small fungus balls.

Roentgenographic Diagnosis: KUB. Fungus balls (Figs. 26–36, 26–37) may be visualized because of gas within them and occasionally around them.[139] The contrast-filled bladder reveals filling defects within the lumen. Occasionally, the contrast medium may enter the fungus balls, further accentuating the laminated appearance.

Differential Diagnosis. Neoplasia, blood clots, nonopaque calculi, bullous edema, and various forms of cystitis—eosinophilic, glandularis—must be differentiated. A history of diabetes, prolonged use of antibiotics or steroid therapy, or immunosuppressive therapy is extremely helpful in making the diagnosis. The appearance of gas-filled, laminated, rounded masses would be diagnostic.

Aspergillosis (Fig. 26–36) is a rare mycosis that is considered to be ubiquitous and a facultative pathogen for man.[140] These infections are usually associated with host debilitation as a result of tuberculosis, diabetes mellitus, Hodgkin's disease, acute leukemia, chemotherapy or radiotherapy for malignant disease. There is a possibility of the entry of aspergillosis as a result of multiple injections in addicts.[140]

TUBERCULOSIS

Tuberculosis (Figs. 26–38 to 26–41) has marked effects on the urinary bladder.[144-147] In the early stages, there may be only trabeculations with irregularity of the bladder and a slight decrease in capacity. As the disease progresses, the bladder becomes smaller and tends to become more smooth-walled. In the late stages, the bladder may disappear nearly completely, with the ureters practically entering the urethra directly. At all stages, there may be reflux. Occasionally, dilatation of the upper tract may be secondary to bladder muscular hypertrophy, producing constriction of the intramural portion of the ureters. Tuberculosis of the bladder is almost always associated with renal tuberculosis.

MALACOPLAKIA

Malacoplakia (Fig. 26–42) is an unusual inflammatory condition especially affecting the bladder and lower urinary tract, where it is generally considered to be benign.[148-157] Renal malacoplakia is neither a benign nor a self-limiting disease and can be fatal, especially if bilateral. The histologic features consist predominantly of a submucosal infiltrate of histiocytes by multinucleated giant cells; lymphocytes, plasma cells, and polymorphonuclears are usually present. The characteristic features are Michaelis-Gutmann bodies that are located usually within the cytoplasm of histiocytes. The bodies are composed of salts that are embedded in an organic matrix. The condition occurs predominantly in women, and most cases are found in the sixth decade of life, although it may occur in children. Urinary tract infection, especially with *E. coli*, often is associated with malacoplakia. The disease has been reported in debilitated persons or in those compromised immunologically. The relationship of sarcoidosis and tuberculosis to malacoplakia has not been clarified.[149, 155]

Malacoplakia in the majority of cases involves the bladder. The lesions are usually scattered throughout and are described as raised, soft plaques. They may be single or multiple, rounded, and rarely pedunculated. They are usually smooth, centrally unfilicated plaques raised slightly above the surface of the mucosa. The color is yellowish-gray to brown, and the adjacent mucosa may or may not reveal congestion.

Roentgenographic Appearance. There will be a smooth oval or rounded filling defect in the bladder lumen. The defects usually are small but may be 1 cm. or more in diameter; they may be single or multiple. The most common location is on the floor of the bladder. It has a tendency to recur.

SCHISTOSOMIASIS

Schistosomiasis[158-176] is a parasitic disease caused by a fluke. There are three forms of flukes: (1) *Schistosoma japonicum*, involving mainly lungs and liver; (2) *S. mansoni*, involving chiefly rectum and liver; and (3) *S. haematobium*, involving primarily the urinary tract.

LIFE CYCLE OF THE PARASITE
1. The egg is passed with the urine from humans.
2. In water, the egg ruptures and forms a miracidium.
3. The miracidium enters a snail (*Physopsis africana*) and becomes a spore cyst.
4. After several generations of spore cysts, cercariae are formed.

5. The latter leave the snail, swim free in water, and enter the skin or mucous membrane of the human being.
6. They enter the venous or lymphatic system, pass to the heart, and then to lung capillaries.
7. From here, by way of an arterial route, they finally enter the portal system.
8. Some weeks later, the maturing worms enter superior mesenteric, inferior mesenteric, and spermatic veins and gain access to pelvic, vesical, and ureteral plexuses by going against the blood stream.
9. In the vesical plexus, the female migrates to smaller vessels and deposits eggs in venules beneath the vesical mucosa. Their spines engage the vessel wall, which permits extrusion into perivenous spaces. The ova can then enter lumen as a result of muscular contraction or lytic enzymes.
10. They are then voided with the urine.[173]

In the bladder, the ova stimulate hyperemia and edema. They may break through the mucosa, producing bleeding. The lesion later appears as yellowish granules surrounded by hyperemia. They appear similar to tubercles and are produced by proliferative changes and hyperplasia. These lesions enlarge and become nodular. If the nodules coalesce, they form bilharzial nodes (bilharziomata). These latter can become necrotic, ulcerate, or calcify. Histologically, the primary lesion is a granuloma containing macrophages, foreign body giant cells, lymphocytes, plasma cells, and occasionally eosinophils in the periphery.

The result of this infection takes the following forms in the bladder:

1. Hyperemia and edema
2. Granular stage simulating tuberculosis
3. Hyperplastic lesions: nodules, polyps. There are three types of polyps according to El-Badawi:[162] (a) granulomatous polyp: developing during active phase; (b) fibrocalcific polyp: associated with chronic bilharzial cystitis; (c) villous polyp: resembling neoplastic papillomas.
4. Atrophic lesions (fibrosis of bladder) and calcification; may be associated with fibrocalcific polyps
5. Ulceration of bladder mucosa

ROENTGENOGRAPHIC DIAGNOSIS

KUB. The roentgenographic findings, especially in the late stages, may be characteristic. A calcification (Figs. 26–43, 26–44) of the bladder wall may surround the bladder completely in a 1 to 3 mm.-wide band. This is situated usually in the lamina propria or muscularis. The calcification is fairly dense and homogeneous but may appear in layers. The calcification in the bladder may vary with the degree of filling. In the collapsed bladder the calcification may give a laminated appearance, whereas in the distended bladder the calcification may appear as a narrow, well-defined, circumferential dense line. Calculi can appear in the bladder but, of course, are not diagnostic. (See Figure 28–14.)

Cystography. A single, spherical defect with sharp festooned outline at one side of bladder shadow and multiple discrete separate filling defects are the usual findings.

When there is diffuse involvement, the spherical filling defects produce a honeycomb appearance. Occasionally, irregular papillomatous lesions resembling carcinoma of bladder are visualized.

Intravenous urography may show unilatreal or bilateral dilatation of ureter, usually limited to pelvic ureter, but hydronephrosis may occur. The cause of the dilatation is either stricture, polyps of ureter, or reflux.

Complications. Infection, lithiasis, contracted bladder, contracted bladder neck, ureteral stones, reflux, dilatation of upper tracts, and carcinoma may occur. The last named is usually of squamous variety, but transitional cell and adenocarcinoma may occur.[161, 165] Origin on trigone is rare. Squamous metaplasia and carcinoma in situ may be associated.

GANGRENE OF THE BLADDER

Gangrene of the bladder, representing necrosis of the entire bladder except trigone, also includes cases involving only mucosa (diphtheritic or dissecting gangrenous cystitis) or in a localized part of the bladder. In the generalized form, the symptoms can be severe with abdominal pain, chills, vomiting, abdominal distention with tenderness and rebound and total gross hematuria. Rupture has been reported.[178] There may be necrosis of the mucosa, lamina propria, or muscularis. Regeneration has been described.[179, 180]

On cystoscopy, there may be erythema and discrete ulcerated necrotic areas. Possible etiologic factors are (1) trauma (labor and delivery, vesical stone, prostatic or extensive pelvic operation); (2) generalized infection, such as diphtheria or typhoid; (3) obstruction; (4) iatrogenic, that is, radiation, intracavitary chemicals; and (5) miscellaneous factors, such as pelvic thrombophlebitis.

ALKALINE-ENCRUSTED CYSTITIS

Alkaline-encrusted cystitis is a form of chronic cystitis characterized by phosphatic encrustations on an inflamed bladder mucosa or on a tumor base and by the passage of gritty (calcareous) material in the urine. It is more common in women.

It is produced by an organism that converts urea to ammonia, producing an alkaline medium in which calcium, magnesium, and ammonia phosphate are precipitated. It often follows fulguration of the bladder mucosa, radiation, or drug-induced cystitis.[182a] Cystoscopically, there are patches of whitish encrustations attached to the mucosa. They may be few in number or cover almost all of the surface. On roentgenographic examination, the calcific deposits are sometimes confused with stones (Fig. 26–45).

CHAPTER 26, ILLUSTRATIONS

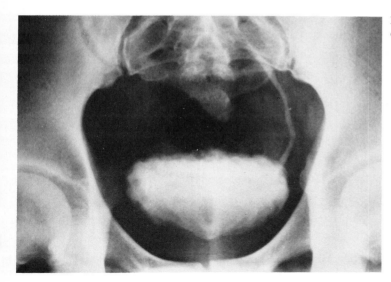

FIG. 26–1. Chronic cystitis. Irregular bladder, few trabeculations.

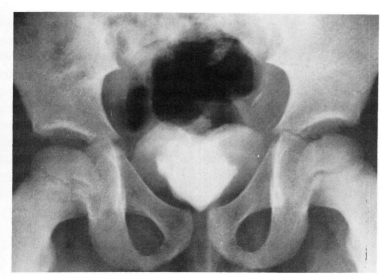

FIG. 26–2. Chronic cystitis. Irregular bladder and trigone. The size of the bladder was misinterpreted as interstitial cystitis, but intravenous urogram revealed a larger bladder.

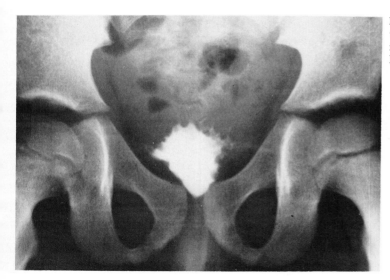

FIG. 26–3. Trigonitis. Irregular trigone.

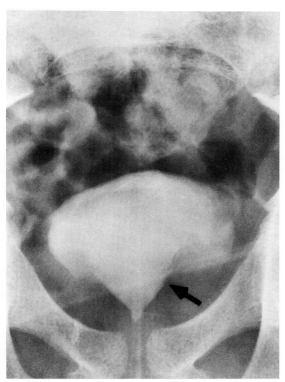

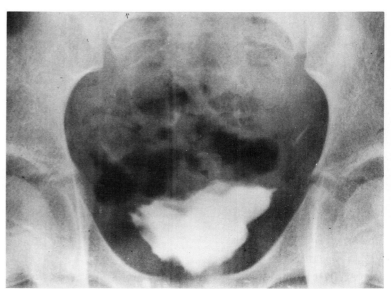

FIG. 26–5. Hemorrhagic cystitis proved by biopsy and cystoscopic examination. Note the irregularity of the bladder with broad V-shaped indentations along the bladder margins.

FIG. 26–4. Cystotrigonitis. *Arrow* points to irregular edge of the trigone.

FIG. 26–6. Hemorrhagic cystitis. Intravenous urogram; irregular bladder, V-shaped indentations, dilated lower ureters.

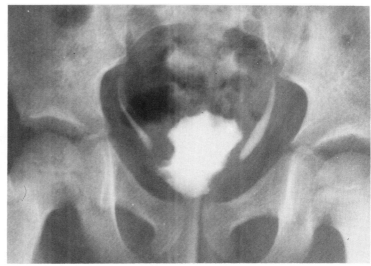

FIG. 26–7. Hemorrhagic cystitis. Intravenous urogram; irregular bladder with V-shaped indentations.

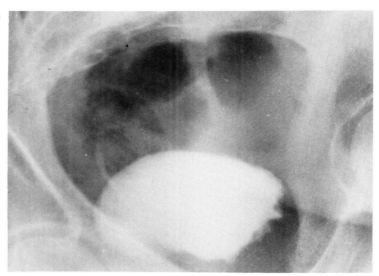

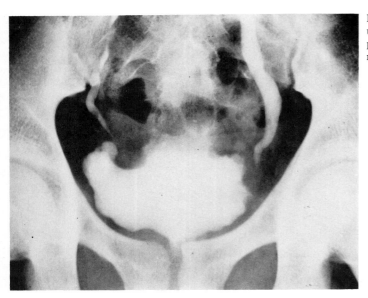

FIG. 26-8. Bullous edema. Intravenous urogram; irregular bladder with multiple rounded indentations on practically all surfaces. Bladder slightly smaller than normal.

FIG. 26-9. Interstitial cystitis. Bladder is slightly less than normal size. Note the marked irregularity. The clear zone around the bladder is perivesical fat. Woman, 36-years old. No bladder neck obstruction.

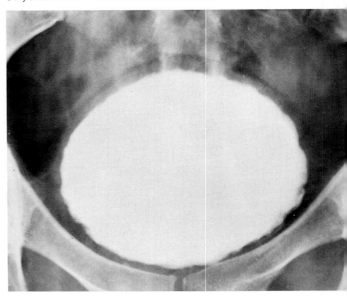

FIG. 26-10. Interstitial cystitis associated with mild contracture of the bladder neck. Small-capacity bladder. Note the mild trabeculation.

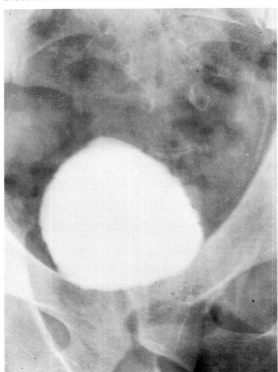

FIG. 26-11. Interstitial cystitis. Marked contracture of the bladder. Bilateral vesicoureteral reflux with dilatation of the lower ureters. (Courtesy of A. Uson, M.D.)

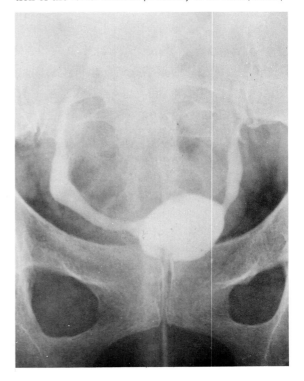

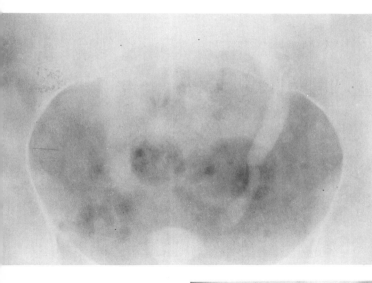

FIG. 26-12. Interstitial cystitis. Markedly contracted bladder. Intravenous pyelogram. Ureters are dilated moderately. Late tuberculosis of bladder may present same findings.

FIG. 26-13. Eosinophilic cystitis. **(A)** Intravenous urogram. Bilateral hydroureteral nephrosis. **(B)** Voiding cystourethrogram. Multiple oval and rounded filling defects in bladder. At dome, irregularities similar to those of bullous edema but not as severe. Its side shows irregularities of chronic cystitis. **(C)** Intravenous urogram shows resolution of dilated upper tracts. After therapy with antibiotics and Prednisone, some mucosal edema. **(D)** Voiding cystourethrogram. Filling defects nearly completely gone. (Kessler, W.D., Clark, P.L., Kaplan, G.S.: Eosinophilic cystitis. Urology, 6:499, 1975)

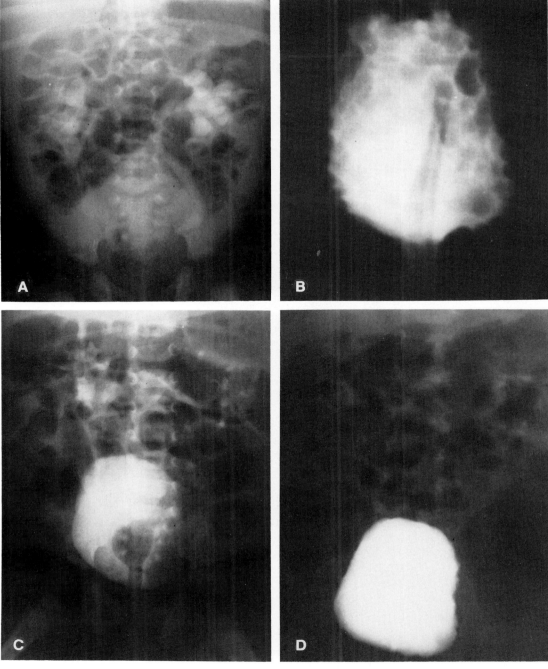

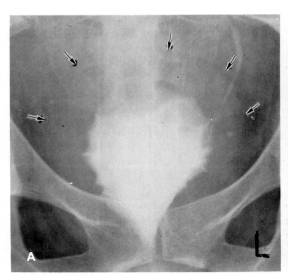

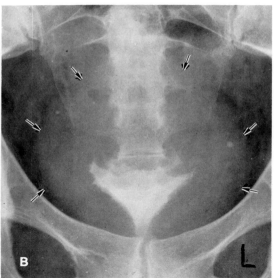

FIG. 26–14. Eosinophilic cystitis. **(A)** Anteroposterior view of urinary bladder with patient erect. Intravenous cystogram obtained 30 minutes after injection of contrast medium. Peripheral bladder outlined by *arrows*. **(B)** Postvoiding film of bladder taken at termination of intravenous urogram. Note considerable thickening of bladder wall. (Palubinskas, A.J.: Radiology, 75:589, 1960)

FIG. 26–15. Granulomatous cystitis as a complication of granulomatous disease of childhood. **(A)** Intravenous urogram showing hydroureteral nephrosis on left and large irregular filling defect on right side of bladder. **(B)** Two weeks later intravenous urogram reveals no visualization on left side. **(C)** Two months after insertion of nephrostomy tube, complete obstruction of left ureter. Note decrease in bladder deformity. (Bloomberg, S.D., Ehrlich, R.M., Neu, H.C., et al.: Urology, 4:193, 1974)

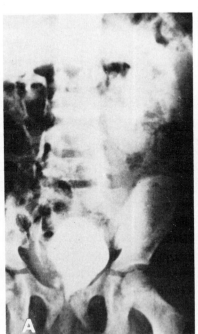

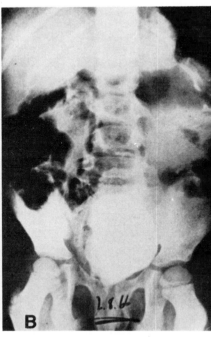

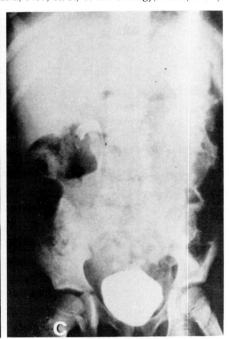

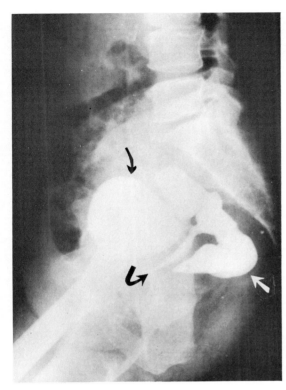

FIG. 26–16. Rectovesical and rectovaginal fistula from granulomatous colitis. Barium enema. *White arrow* points to rectum, *U-shaped arrow* to vagina and *upper arrow* to bladder.

FIG. 26–17. Primary granulomatous cystitis. Retrograde cystogram; markedly irregular bladder. Note large nodular areas on right side of bladder. (Courtesy of Erich Lang, M.D.)

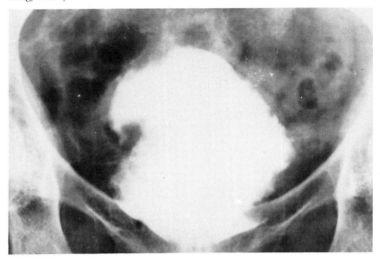

FIG. 26–18. Primary granulomatous cystitis. Barium air cystogram. Note the coarse, bubbly appearance. (Courtesy of Erich Lang, M.D.)

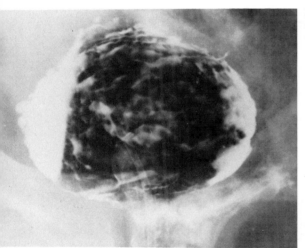

FIG. 26–19. Cystitis emphysematosa in a diabetic. *Arrow* points to an area containing discrete gas-filled vesicles. There is no free gas in the lumen, and there is no clear zone or ring of gas in the wall of the bladder. (Courtesy of S. Simon, M.D.)

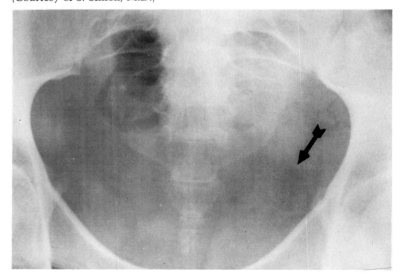

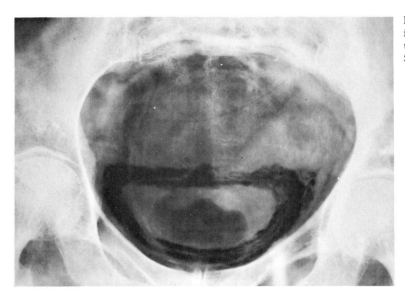

FIG. 26–20. Cystitis emphysematosa in a diabetic. Gas is apparent in wall of the bladder. There is no free gas in the lumen. (Donner, M.W., McAfee, J.G.: Am. J. Med. Sci., *239*:622, 1960)

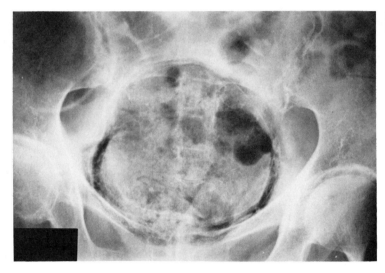

FIG. 26–21. Cystitis emphysematosa: gas in wall of bladder.

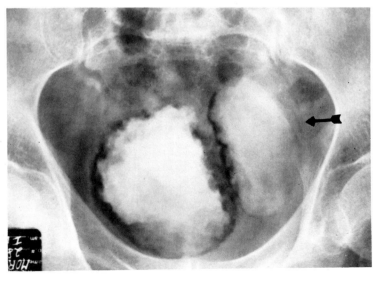

FIG. 26–22. Cystitis emphysematosa in a chronically infected bladder. Cystitis granularis also present. Note gas in wall of bladder and extending around diverticulum (*arrow*).

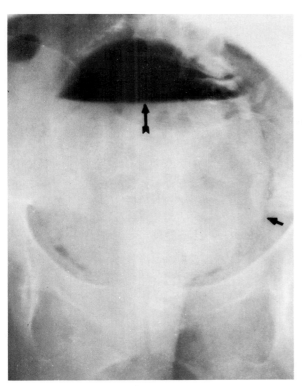

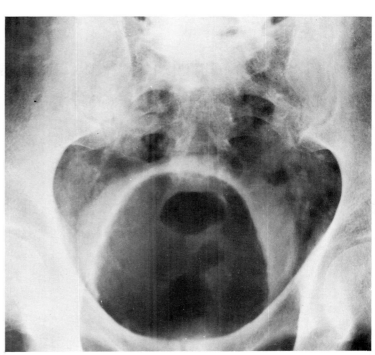

FIG. 26–24. Pneumaturia in a diabetic. Gas in the lumen of the bladder. (Courtesy of Samuel Madell, M.D.)

FIG. 26–23. Cystitis emphysematosa with free gas in the lumen of the bladder. Nondiabetic. *Escherichia coli* infection. *Small arrow* points to gas in the wall of the bladder. *Large arrow* indicates free gas in the lumen.

FIG. 26–25. Pneumaturia in a nondiabetic. Severe *Escherichia coli* and streptococcus infection. Gas can be seen in the upper part of the bladder.

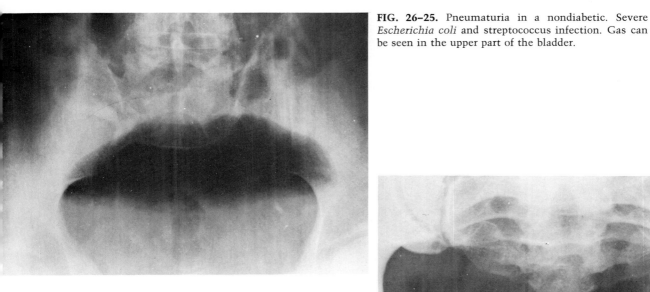

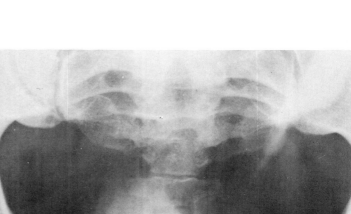

FIG. 26–26. Cystitis cystica. Irregularity of bladder floor and lateral and posterior walls due to numerous cysts of varying size. Note dilated left ureter. (Courtesy of Sol Unger, M.D., Veterans Administration)

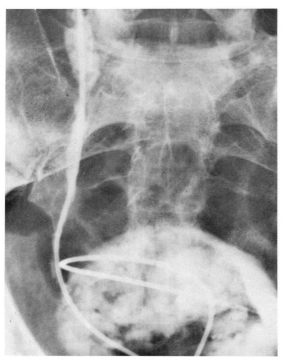

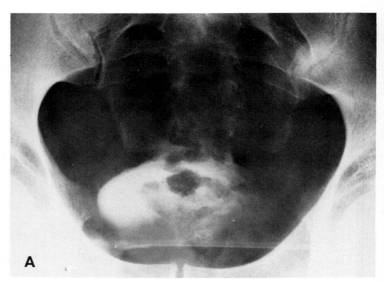

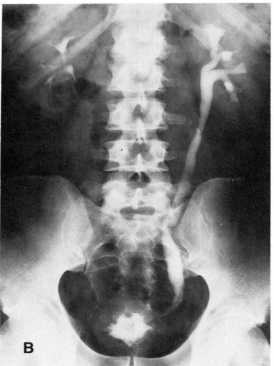

FIG. 26–27. Cystitis cystica. Marked irregularity of the luminal content due to large cystic masses covering nearly the entire bladder surface. Present also is ureteritis cystica. This was a man, 53 years old, with a long-standing history of pyelonephritis and renal lithiasis. (Courtesy of Bernard Loitman, M.D.)

FIG. 26–28. Cystitis glandularis. **(A)** Cystogram during excretory urography shows multiple defects in trigonal area. Large mass obscured left ureteral orifice. **(B)** Post-voiding film obtained several minutes after removal of compression bag demonstrates partial obstruction of left collecting system by the trigonal mass. (Brogdon, D.G., Silbiger, M.L., Colston, J.A.C., Jr.: Radiology, *85*:470, 1965)

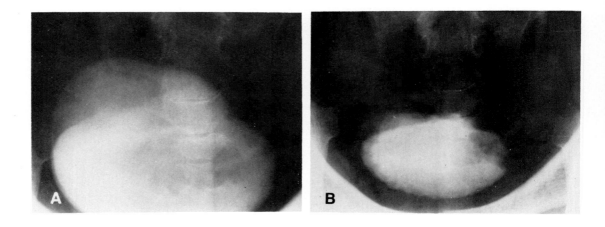

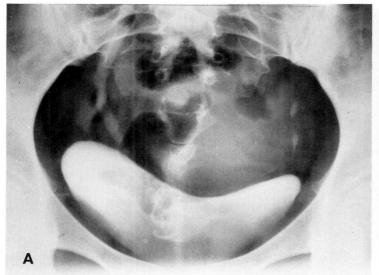

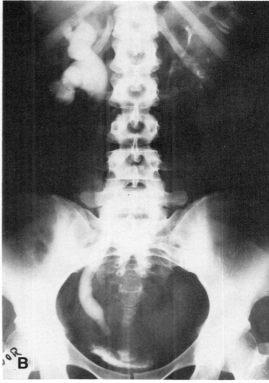

FIG. 26–29. Cystitis glandularis. **(A)** Multiple rounded filling defects in the bladder wall seen extending superiorly and laterally from region of right ureteral orifice. Note slightly dilated right ureter (plastic fastener superimposed on bladder is part of an external belt supporter). **(B)** Postvoiding film demonstrates the right ureteropyelocalyectasis. (Brogdon, D.G., Silibiger, M.L., Colston, J.A.C., Jr.: Radiology, *85*:470, 1965)

FIG. 26–30. Cystitis glandularis. Multiple defects on floor and posterior wall of bladder. Moderate obstruction of both ureters due to cystitis glandularis. (Courtesy of F. Lopez)

FIG. 26–30a. Cystitis glandularis. **(A)** Multiple, rounded filling defects are seen on trigonal area of distended bladder during excretory urography. **(B)** Partial emptying of bladder better demonstrates mass lesion on left. (Brogdon, D.G., Silibiger, M.L., Colston, J.A.C., Jr.: Radiology, *85*:470, 1965)

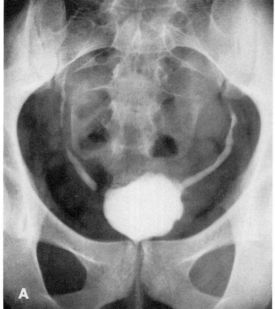
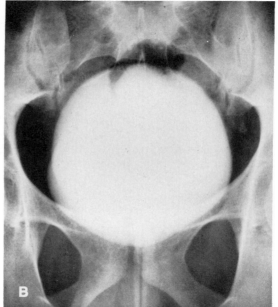

FIG. 26–31. Abacteria pyuria. **(A)** Pretreatment intravenous urogram reveals small, irregular bladder and slight dilatation of ureter. **(B)** Post-treatment intravenous urogram shows normal bladder (treated with Mapharsen). (Hewitt, C.B., Stewart, B.H., and Kiser, W.S.: J. Urol., *109*:86, 1973)

FIG. 26–32. Cyclophosphamide cystitis, chronic form. Four-year-old girl with neuroblastoma. Postvoiding film shows irregular nodular defects ("thumb-printing") in bladder wall; ecchymoses and telangiectasia on cystoscopy. (Renert, W.A., Berdon, W.E., and Baker, D.H.: Am. J. Roentgen., *117*:664, 1973)

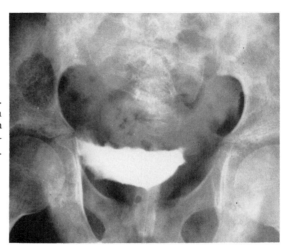

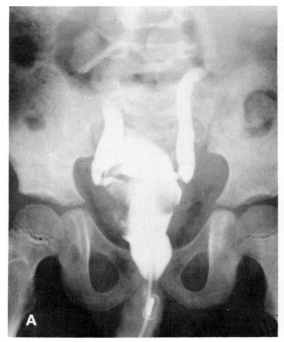
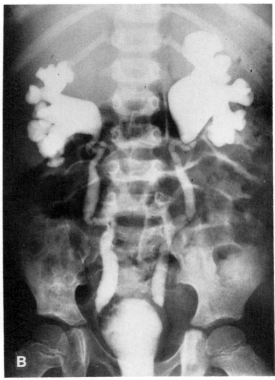

FIG. 26–34. Calcification of bladder wall following cyclophosphamide (Cytoxan) therapy.

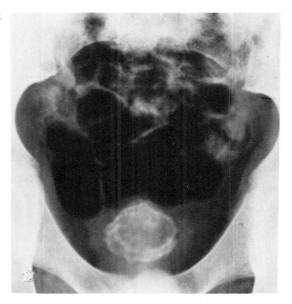

FIG. 26–35. Irregularly contracted bladder from radiation. Patient had carcinoma of prostate.

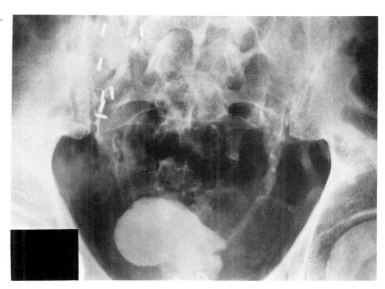

FIG. 26–36. Fungus balls in urinary bladder; aspergillosis. Air in lumen; large fungus ball with air and coating of contrast medium.

FIG. 26–33. Cyclophosphamide cystitis. Three-year-old boy with metastatic retinoblastoma—hematuria. **(A)** Cystogram shows bilateral vesicoureteral reflux, a contracted bladder with large contour defects, and elevation of trigone. Cystoscopy: bullous edema. Intravenous urogram showed bilateral hydronephrosis. **(B)** One week after discontinuing cyclophosphamide: Intravenous urogram shows good visualization of dilated upper tracts, showing improvement; bladder elongated, possibly mildly contracted, defects gone. (Renert, W.A., Berdon, W.E., Baker, D.H.: Am. J. Roentgenol., *117*:664, 1973)

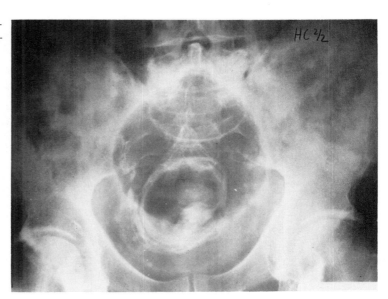

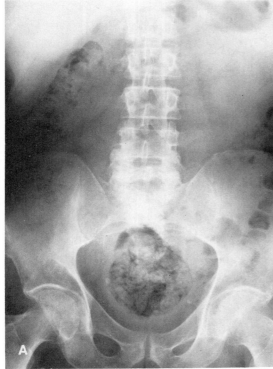

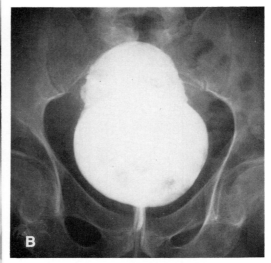

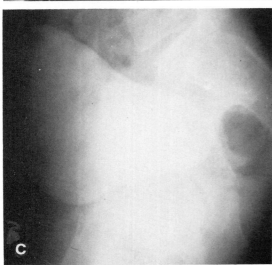

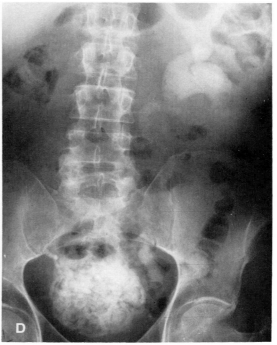

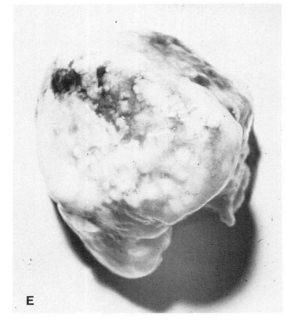

FIG. 26–37. Fungus balls in urinary bladder. *Candida albicans.* (A) Roentgenogram of urinary tract demonstrates air in lumen of bladder, allowing identification of numerous air-containing laminated fungus balls. Frontal (B) and lateral (C) cystograms reveal numerous round regular defects (fungus balls) in contrast medium outlining lumen of urinary bladder. Ureteral reflux on right. (D) 20-minute excretory urogram demonstrates hydroureter and hydronephrosis on the left. Right kidney surgically absent. Contrast medium from previous cystogram has impregnated the walls of the fungus balls demonstrating their air-containing laminated structure. (E) One of the 36 fungus balls removed from the bladder. (McDonald, D.F., and Fagon, C.J.: Am. J. Roentgenol. Radium Ther. Nucl. Med., *4*:753, 1972)

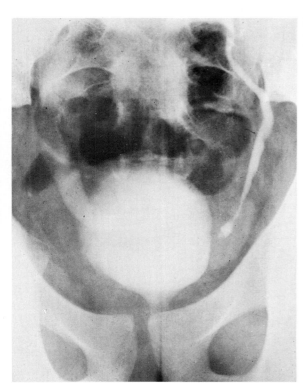

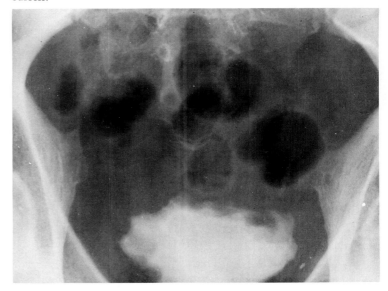

FIG. 26–38. Tuberculosis of the bladder. Small-capacity, slightly irregular bladder. Bilateral vesicoureteral reflux with dilated right ureter.

FIG. 26–39. Tuberculosis of the bladder. Small contracted bladder with marked irregularity due to tuberculosis.

FIG. 26–40. Tuberculosis of the bladder with marked right vesicoureteral reflex. Contracted, small, irregular bladder. Hydroureter and hydronephrosis.

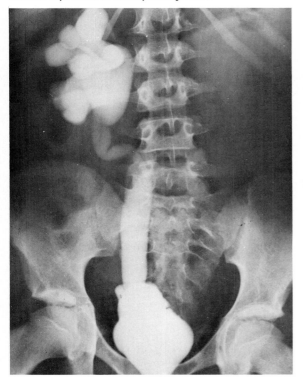

FIG. 26–41. Tuberculosis of bladder; cystogram shows small irregular bladder, round nodular defects.

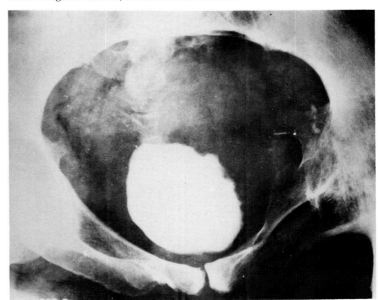

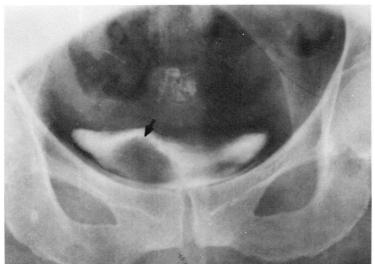

FIG. 26–42. Malacoplakia of the bladder. Woman, 65 years old. *Arrow* points to a large rounded mass that was situated in the region of the right ureteral orifice, preventing the passage of a catheter up the right ureter. Patient complained of right renal colic, and there was poor function of the right kidney with right hydronephrosis on intravenous urogram. Repeated specimens were taken by biopsy, and patient was treated with antibiotics. Mass disappeared, kidney returned to normal size and function, and patient has remained well. Now catheter can be gotten up the right ureter easily.

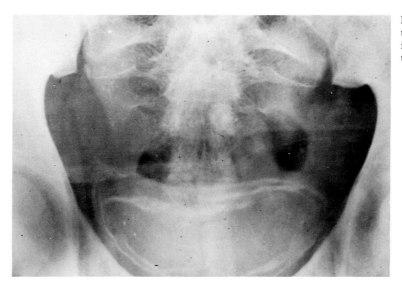

FIG. 26–43. Schistosomiasis of the bladder. Calcification in the wall of the bladder in layers. This appearance is more characteristic of a collapsed bladder. On filling, the laminated appearance may disappear.

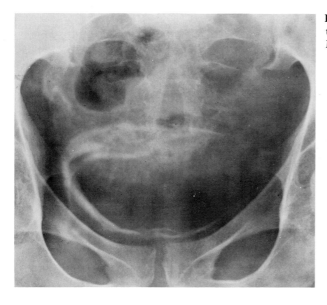

FIG. 26–44. Schistosomiasis of bladder. Calcification in the wall of the urinary bladder. (Courtesy of P. Jamison, M.D., Tanta, Egypt)

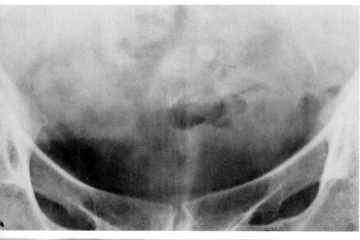

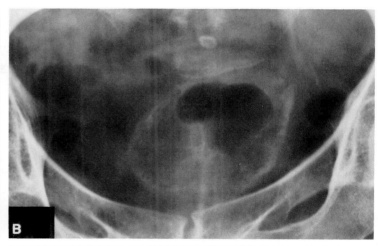

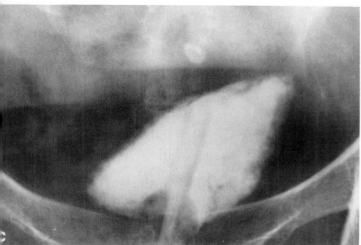

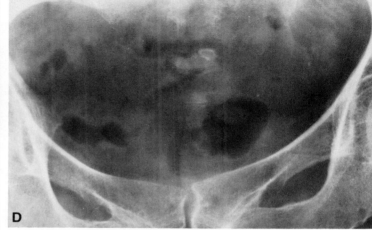

FIG. 26–45. Alkaline-encrusted cystitis. **(A)** Films of the pelvis show no evidence of bladder calcification in August of 1976. The rounded calcification in the pelvis is presumed to be in a uterine fibroid and has been present since 1970. **(B)** Plain films of the pelvis in December of 1976 revealed the bladder to be outlined with calcium. **(C)** The bladder outline is confirmed by cystogram. The triangular configuration of the bladder is due to the left ureteroneocystostomy in 1971. **(D)** Films of the pelvis in January 1977 following urinary diversion and bladder irrigation reveal almost complete disappearance of bladder calcification. (Harrison, R.B., Stier, F.M., and Cochrane, J.A.: Alkaline encrusting cystitis. Am. J. Roentgenol., *130*:575–577, 1978).

BIBLIOGRAPHY

General

1. Cox, C.E., Lacy, S.S., and Hinman, F., Jr.: The urethra and its relationship to urinary tract infection. II. The urethral floor of the female with recurrent urinary infection. J. Urol., 97:632–638, 1968.
2. Stamey, T.A., Timothy, M., Millar, M., et al.: Recurrent urinary infections in adult women. The role of introital enterobacteria. Calif. Med., 115:1–19, 1971.

Hemorrhagic Cystitis

2a. Buckley, R.M., Jr., McGuckin, M., and MacGregor, R.R.: Urine bacterial counts after sexual intercourse. N. Engl. J. Med., 298:321–324, 1978.
2b. Chang, T.W.: Identification of viral particles in acute hemorrhagic cystitis (letter). J. Pediatr., 90:667–668, 1977.
2c. Hashida, A.V., Gaffney, P.C., and Yunis, E.J.: Acute hemorrhagic cystitis of childhood and papovirus-like particles. J. Pediatr., 89:83–87, 1976.
2d. Kharpour, M., and Nik-Akhtar, B.: Epidemic of hemorrhagic cystitis due to influenza A virus. Postgrad. Med. J., 53:251–253, 1977.
2e. Kunim, C.M.: Sexual intercourse and urinary infection. N. Engl. J. Med., 298:336–337, 1978.
2f. Macklin, M.: "Honeymoon cystitis." (letter) N. Engl. J. Med., 298:1035, 1978.
2g. Mufson, M.A., Belshe, P.B., Horrigan, T.J. et al.: Causes of acute hemorrhagic cystitis in children. Am. J. Dis. Child., 126:605–609, 1973.
2h. Texter, J.H., Koontz, W.W., Jr., and McWilliams, N.B.: Hemorrhagic cystitis as a complication of the management of pediatric neoplasms. Urol. Surv., 29:47–48, 1979.
2i. Uy, G., Khani, A.J., and Evans, H.E.: Vesicoureteral reflux complicating sterile hemorrhagic cystitis: a case report. J. Urol., 115:612, 1976.

Bullous Edema

3. Beard, E.E., Goodyear, W.F., and Weens, H.S.: Radiologic Diagnosis of the Lower Urinary Tract. Springfield, Ill., Charles C Thomas, 1952.
3a. Ekelund, P., and Johansson, S.: Polypoid cystitis: a catheter associated lesion of the human bladder. Acta Pathol. Microbiol. Scand. (A) 87A:179–184, 1979.
4. Kerr, H.D., and Gillies, C.L.: The Urinary Tract: A Handbook of Roentgen Diagnosis. Chicago, Year Book Publishers, 1949.
5. Pittari, J.J., and May, R.E.: Bullous edema of the bladder simulating tumor. Am. J. Roentgenol., 86:863–865, 1961.
5a. Shackleford, G.D., and Manley, C.B.: Acute ureteral obstruction secondary to bullous cystitis of the trigone. Radiology, 132:351–354, 1979.

Interstitial Cystitis

6. Badenoch, A.W.: Chronic interstitial cystitis. Br. J. Urol., 43:718–721, 1971.
7. Burford, E.H., and Burford, C.E.: Hunner ulcer of the bladder. A report of 187 cases. J. Urol., 79:952–955, 1958.
8. Gordon, H.L., Rossen, R.D., Hersh, E.M., et al.: Immunologic aspects of interstitial cystitis. J. Urol., 109:228–233, 1973.
9. Hagner, F.R.: Malignancy of bladder occurring in a Hunner ulcer. Trans. Am. Assoc. Genitourin. Surg., 30:197–198, 1937.
10. Hamilton, M.: Cancer of bladder presenting as "cystitis" or "prostatism." Med. J. Austr., 2:89–91, 1969.
10a. Hanash, K.A., and Pool, T.L.: Interstitial and hemorrhagic cystitis: viral, bacterial, and fungal studies. J. Urol., 104:705–708, 1970.
11. Hand, J.R.: Interstitial cystitis: report of 223 cases (204 women and 19 men). J. Urol., 61:291–310, 1949.
11a. Harn, S.D., and Keutel, H.J.: Bladder cystitis following focal infection of Group A Streptococcus. Nature, 241:131–132, 1973.
12. Howard, T.L.: My personal opinion on interstitial cystitis (Hunner's ulcer). J. Urol., 51:526–534, 1944.
13. Hunner, G.L.: Elusive ulcer of the bladder. Further notes on a rare type of bladder ulcer, with a report of twenty-five cases. Am. J. Obstet., 78:374–395, 1918.
14. Hunner, G.L.: Necrosis of the bladder. J. Urol., 24:567–585, 1930.
14a. Jokinen, E.J., Alfthan, O.S., and Oravisto, K.J.: Antitissue antibodies in interstitial cystitis. Clin. Exp. Immunol., 11:333–339, 1972.
14b. Jokinen, E.J., Oravisto, K.J., and Alfthan, O.S.: The effect of cystectomy on antitissue antibodies in interstitial cystitis. Clin. Exp. Immunol., 15:457–460, 1973.
15. Kinder, C.H., and Smith, R.D.: Hunner's ulcer. Br. J. Urol., 30:338–343, 1958.
16. Kretschmer, H.L.: Elusive ulcer of the bladder. A report of 138 cases. J. Urol., 42:385–395, 1939.
17. Lamn, D.L., and Gittes, R.F.: Inflammatory carcinoma of bladder and interstitial cystitis. J. Urol., 117:49–51, 1977.
18. Moloney, P.J., Elliott, G.B., McLaughlin, M., and Sinclair, A.B.: In situ transitional cell carcinoma and the non-specifically inflamed contracting bladder. J. Urol., 111:162–164, 1974.
18a. Oravisto, K.J., Alfthan, O.S., and Jokinen, E.J.: Interstitial cystitis: clinical and immunological findings. Scand. J. Urol. Nephrol., 4:37–42, 1970.
19. Rusche, C.F., and Hager, B.H.: Further observations on the development of malignancy in Hunner ulcer. Trans. Am. Assoc. Genitourin. Surg., 32:203–210, 1939.
20. Silk, M.R.: Bladder antibodies and interstitial cystitis. J. Urol., 103:307–309, 1971.
20a. Skoluda, D., Wegner, K., and Lemmel, E.M.: Kritische Bemerkungen zur Immunpathogenese der interstitiellen Cystitis. Urologe (A), 13:15–23, 1974.
21. Smith, J.C., and Badenoch, A.W.: Carcinoma of the bladder simulating chronic cystitis. Br. J. Urol., 37:93–99, 1965.
22. Utz, D.C., and Zincke, H.: The masquerade of bladder cancer in situ as interstitial cystitis. J. Urol., 111:160–161, 1974.
23. Vose, S.N., and Dixey, G.M.: Coincidence of carcinoma of the bladder and interstitial cystitis. J. Urol., 59:580–582, 1948.
24. Weaver, R.G., Doughterly, T.F., and Natoli, C.A.: Recent concepts of interstitial cystitis. J. Urol., 89:377–383, 1963.

Eosinophilic Cystitis

25. Brown, E.W.: Eosinophilic granuloma of the bladder. J. Urol., 83:665–668, 1960.

26. Champion, R.H., and Ackles, R.C.: Eosinophilic cystitis. J. Urol., 96:729–732, 1966.
27. Farber, S., and Vawter, G.F.: Clinical Path. Conf. J. Pediatr., 62:941–945, 1963.
28. Frenzelli, F.J., Sacher, E.L., and Keegan, G.T.: Eosinophilic cystitis observations on etiology. J. Urol., 107:595–596, 1972.
29. Goldstein, M.: Eosinophilic cystitis. J. Urol., 106:854–857, 1971.
30. Gregg, J.A., and Utz, D.C.: Eosinophilic cystitis associated with cystitis. Mayo Clin. Proc., 49:185–187, 1974.
31. Horowitz, J., Slavin, S., and Pfau, A.: Chronic renal failure due to eosinophilic cystitis. Ann. Allergy, 30:502, 1972.
32. Kessler, W.O., Clarke, P.L., and Kaplan, G.W.: Eosinophilic cystitis. Urology, 6:499–501, 1975.
33. Kindall, L., and Nickels, T.T.: Allergy of pelvic urinary tract in females: preliminary report. J. Urol., 61:222–236, 1949.
34. Marshall, F.F., and Middleton, A.W., Jr.: Eosinophilic cystitis. J. Urol., 112:335–337, 1974.
35. Palubinskas, A.J.: Eosinophilic cystitis: case report of eosinophilic infiltration of the urinary bladder. Radiology, 75:589–591, 1960.
36. Pastinszky, I.: The allergic diseases of the male genitourinary tract with special reference to allergic urethritis and cystitis. Urol. Int., 9:288–305, 1959.
37. Perlmutter, A.D., Edlow, J.B., and Kevy, S.V.: Toxacaro antibodies in eosinophilic cystitis. J. Pediatr., 73:340–344, 1965.
38. Rubin, L., and Pincus, M.B.: Eosinophilic cystitis: the relationship of allergy in the urinary tract to eosinophilic cystitis and the paraphysiology of eosinophils. J. Urol., 112:457–460, 1972.
39. Wenzl, J.E., Greene, L.F., and Harris, L.E.: Eosinophilic cystitis. J. Pediatr., 64:746–749, 1964.
40. Zeitlhofer, J., and Bibus, B.: Zur Klinik und Pathologie der eosinophilen Hornblaseninfiltrates. Wien. Klin. Wschr., 79:958–961, 1967.

Granulomatous Cystitis

41. Azimi, P.H., Bodenbender, J.G., Hintz, R.L., and Kontras, S.B.: Chronic granulomatous disease in three sisters. Lancet, 7:208–209, 1968.
42. Bannatyne, R.M., Skowron, P.N., and Weber, J.L.: Job's syndrome—a variant of chronic granulomatous disease. J. Pediatr., 75:236–242, 1969.
43. Berendes, H., Bridges, R.A., and Good, R.A.: A fatal granulomatosis of childhood: the clinical study of a new syndrome. Minn. Med., 40:309–312, 1957.
44. Bloomberg, S.D., Ehrlich, R.M., Neu, H.C., and Blanc, M.A.: Chronic granulomatous disease of childhood with renal involvement. Urology, 4:193–197, 1974.
45. Carson, M.S., Chadwick, D.L., Brubaker, C.A., et al.: Thirteen boys with progressive septic granulomatosis. Pediatrics, 35:405–412, 1965.
46. Cyr, W.L., Johnson, H., and Balfour, J.: Granulomatous cystitis as a manifestation of chronic granulomatous disease of childhood. J. Urol., 110:357–359, 1973.
47. Holmes, B., Quie, P.G., Windhorst, D.B., et al.: Protection of phagocytized bacteria from the killing action of antibiotics. Nature, 210:1131–1132, 1966.
48. Holmes, B., Page, A.R., and Good, R.A.: Studies of the metabolic activity of leukocytes from patients with a genetic abnormality of phagocytic function. J. Clin. Invest., 46:1422–1432, 1967.
49. Holmes, B., Poole, B.H., Malawista, S.E., et al.: Chronic granulomatous disease in females: a deficiency of leukocyte glutathione peroxidase. N. Engl. J. Med., 283:217–221, 1970.
50. Holmes, B. Quie, P.G., Windhorst, D.B., et al.: Fatal granulomatous disease of childhood. An inborn abnormality of phagocytic function. Lancet, 1:1225–1228, 1966.
51. Klebanoff, S.J.: Myeloperoxidase-halide-hydrogen peroxide antibacterial system. J. Bacteriol., 95:2131–2138, 1968.
52. Klebanoff, S.J., and White, L.R.: Iodination defect in the leukocytes of a patient with chronic granulomatous disease of childhood. N. Engl. J. Med., 280:460–466, 1969.
53. Kontras, S.B., Bodenbender, J.G., McClave, C.R., and Smith, J.P.: Interstitial cystitis in chronic granulomatous disease. J. Urol., 105:575–578, 1971.
54. Quie, P.G., Kaplan, E.L., Page, A.R., et al.: Defective polymorphonuclear leukocyte function and chronic granulomatous disease in two female children. N. Engl. J. Med., 278:976–980, 1968.
55. Quie, P.G., White, J.G., Holmes, B., and Good, R.A.: In vitro bactericidal capacity of human polymorphonuclear leukocytes: diminished activity in chronic granulomatous disease of childhood. J. Clin. Invest., 46:668–679, 1967.
56. Towfighi, J., Sadeghee, S., Wheeler, J.E., et al.: Granulomatous prostatitis with emphasis on the eosinophilic variety. Am. J. Clin. Path., 58:630–641, 1972.

Cystitis Emphysematosa

57. Antoine, T.: Zur klinik, der Cystitis Emphysematosa. Zbl. Gynack, 38:2230–2235, 1934.
58. Bailey, H.: Cystitis emphysematosa. Am. J. Roentgenol., 86:850–862, 1961.
59. Bastecky, J., Holy, S., and Poch, R.: Cystitis and peri-cystitis urinaria emphysematosa. Acta Radiol. Cancerol. Bohemoslov., 4:120–128, 1949.
60. Boijsen, E., and Lewis-Jonsson, J.: Emphysematous cystitis. Acta Radiol. (Stockholm), 41:269–276, 1954.
61. Burns, R.A.: Cystitis emphysematosa: a case report. J. Urol., 49:808–814, 1943.
62. Burrell, N.L.: Cystitis emphysematosa: case report and review of the literature. J. Urol., 36:690–693, 1936.
63. Donner, M.W., and McAfee, J.G.: Roentgenographic manifestations of diabetes mellitus. Am. J. Med. Sci., 239(5):622–641, 1960.
64. Faingold, J.E., Hansen, C.O., and Rigler, L.G.: Cystitis emphysematosa: four cases. Radiology, 61:346–354, 1953.
65. Ganem, E.J., Calitri, E.J., and Glidden, H.S.: The roentgenographic diagnosis of cystitis emphysematosa. J. Urol., 78:245–251, 1957.
66. Hall, E.R.: Cystitis emphysematosa (report of three cases). Canad. Med. Assoc. J., 43:585–587, 1940.
67. Lane, J.W., and Francke, E.P.: Cystitis emphysematosa: case report. J. Urol., 75:256–260, 1956.
68. Lee, J.B.: Cystitis emphysematosa: review of literature and report of case with disseminated inflammatory emphysema. Arch. Intern. Med., 105:618–626, 1960.
69. Lund, H.G., Zingale, F.G., and O'Dowd, J.A.: Cystitis emphysematosa: report of a case found at cystoscopy and followed by recovery. J. Urol., 42:684–688, 1939.
70. Marquardt, C.R.: Cystitis emphysematosa. Urol. Cut. Rev., 44:295–296, 1940.
71. Maurer, J.E., Lich, R., and Burdon, S.: Cystitis emphysematosa: a report of the fourteenth human case diagnosed at cystoscopy. Urol. Cut. Rev., 53:530–531, 1949.

72. Mills, R.G.: Cystitis emphysematosa, report of three cases in men. J. Urol., 23:289–306, 1930.

73. Mills, R.G.: Cystitis emphysematosa; report of three additional cases in women. Surg. Gynecol. Obstet., 51:545–551, 1930.

74. Milner, W.A., Garlick, W.B., and Mamonas, C.: Cystitis emphysematosa: case report with clinical diagnosis and review of the literature. N. Engl. J. Med., 246:902–905, 1952.

75. Ortmayer, M.: Cystitis emphysematosa: with a report of the twelfth human case diagnosed at cystoscopy. J. Urol., 60:757–762, 1948.

76. Packard, D.R., Beazlie, F.S., Jr., and Creecy, A.A.: Unusual Complications in Diabetes Mellitus. Case Report. Virginia Med. Monthly, 80:557–559, 1953.

77. Ravich, A., and Katzen, P.: Cystitis emphysematosa: review of the literature. Report of an authentic case terminating in recovery. J.A.M.A., 98:1256–1259, 1932.

78. Teasley, G.H.: Cystitis emphysematosa: case report with review of the literature. J. Urol., 62:48–51, 1949.

79. Wheeler, L.D.: Cystitis emphysematosa: case report. J. Urol., 71:43–48, 1954.

Pneumaturia

80. Fineman, S., Ferber, W.L., and Roginsky, D.N.: Primary pneumaturia, with report of 2 cases. Radiology, 59:63–69, 1952.

81. Foord, R.D., Nabarro, J.D., and Riches, E.W.: Diabetic pneumaturia. Br. Med. J., 1:433–434, 1956.

82. Kent, H.P.: Gas in urinary tract. J. Fac. Radiologists, 7:57–65, 1955.

83. Marks, M.I.: Iatrogenic pneumaturia. J. Urol., 106:407–408, 1971.

84. Marsh, A.P.: Primary diabetic pneumaturia, diagnosed radiographically. N. Engl. J. Med., 262:666–667, 1960.

85. Olsson, O.: Spontanes gaspyelogramm. Acta Radiol., 20:578–584, 1939.

86. Spring, M., and Hymes, J.J.: Pneumaturia: report of a case in diabetes with review of literature. Diabetes, 1:378–382, 1952.

87. Thomas, R.G., and Sandler, A.: Primary pneumaturia. S. Afr. Med. J., 32:309–311, 1958.

Cystitis Cystica

88. Kaplan, G.W., and King, L.R.: Cystitis cystica in childhood. J. Urol., 103:657–659, 1970.

89. Kopp, J.H.: Pyelitis, ureteritis and cystitis cystica. J. Urol., 56:28–34, 1946.

90. Morse, H.D.: Etiology and pathology of pyelitis cystica, ureteritis cystica and cystitis cystica. Am. J. Pathol., 4:33–50, 1928.

91. Patch, F.S.: Pyelitis, ureteritis and cystitis cystica. N. Engl. J. Med., 220:979–987, 1939.

92. Patch, F.S., and Rhea, L.J.: Genesis and development of Bruno's nests and their relation to cystitis cystica, cystitis glandularis, and primary adenocarcinoma of the bladder. Canad. Med. Assoc. J., 33:597–606, 1935.

93. Uehling, D.T., and King, L.R.: Secretory immunoglobulins — and excretion in cystitis cystica. Urol., 1:305–306, 1973.

94. Uehling, D.T., and Steihm, F.R.: Elevated urinary secretory IgA in children with urinary tract infection. Pediatrics, 47:40–46, 1971.

95. Warrick, W.D.: Cystitis cystica; bacteriological studies in 28 cases. J. Urol., 45:835–843, 1941.

95a. Wiener, D.P., Koss, L.G., Sablay, B. et al.: The prevalence and significance of Brunn's nests, cystitis cystica, and squamous metaplasia in normal bladders. J. Urol., 122:317–321, 1979.

Cystitis Glandularis

96. Bell, T.E., and Wendel, R.G.: Cystitis glandularis: benign or malignant. J. Urol., 100:462–465, 1968.

97. Blum, J.A.: Cystitis glandularis causing bilateral upper urinary tract obstruction. Chicago Med. Sch. Quarterly, 25:250–252, 1966.

97a. Bourne, C.W., and May, J.E.: Urachal remnants: Benign or malignant? J. Urol. 118:743–747, 1977.

98. Brogdon, D.G., Silbiger, M.L., and Colston, J.A.C., Jr.: Cystitis glandularis. Radiology, 85:470–473, 1965.

99. Coppridge, W.M., Roberts, L.C., and Culp, D.A.: Glandular tumors of the bladder. J. Urol., 65:540–549, 1951.

100. Culp, D.A.: The histology of the exstrophied bladder. J. Urol., 91:538–548, 1964.

101. Emmett, J.L., and McDonald, J.A.: Proliferation of glands of the urinary bladder simulating malignant neoplasm. J. Urol., 48:257–265, 1942.

102. Foot, N.C.: Glandular metaplasia of the epithelium of the urinary tract. South. Med. J., 37:137–142, 1944.

103. Immergut, J., and Cottler, Z.R.: Mucin-producing adenocarcinoma of the bladder associated with cystitis follicularis and glandularis. Urol. Cutan. Rev., 54:531–534, 1950.

104. Kittredge, W.E., and Brannon, W.: Cystitis glandularis. Trans. Am. Assoc. Genitourin. Surg., 50:136–147, 1958.

105. Kittredge, W.E., Collett, A.J., and Morgan, C., Jr.: Adenocarcinoma of the bladder associated with cystitis glandularis: a case report. J. Urol., 91:145–150, 1964.

106. Lowry, E.C., Hamm, F.C., and Blood, D.E.: Extensive glandular proliferation of urinary bladder resembling malignant neoplasm. J. Urol., 52:133–138, 1944.

107. Morse, H.D.: The etiology and pathology of pyelitis cystica, ureteritis cystica and cystitis cystica. Am. J. Pathol., 4:33–50, 1928.

108. Patch, F.S.: Epithelial metaplasia of the urinary tract. J.A.M.A., 136:824–827, 1948.

109. Patch, F.S., and Rhea, L.J.: The genesis and development of Brunn's nests and their relation to cystitis cystica, cystitis glandularis, and primary adenocarcinoma of the bladder. Canad. Med. Assoc. J., 33:597–606, 1935.

110. Porter, C.: Cystitis cystica and glandularis. Proc. Roy. Soc. Med., 63:239–242, 1970.

111. Pund, E.R., Yount, H.A., and Blumberg, J.M.: Variations in morphology of the urinary bladder epithelium. Special reference to cystitis glandularis and carcinomas. J. Urol., 68:242–251, 1952.

112. Rao, K.G.: Cystitis glandularis causing bilateral ureteric obstruction and hydronephrosis. Br. J. Urol., 47:398, 1975.

113. Roll, W.A.: Cystitis glandularis cause of lymphoma. J. Urol., 84:76–78, 1960.

114. Sauer, H.R., and Bliele, M.S.: Cystitis glandularis: a consideration of symptoms, diagnosis and clinical course of the disease. J. Urol., 60:446–458, 1948.

115. Shaw, J.L., Gislason, G.J., nad Imbriglia, J.E.: Transition of cystitis glandularis to primary adenocarcinoma of the bladder. J. Urol., 79:815–822, 1958.

116. Stirling, W.C., and Ash, J.E.: Chronic proliferative lesions of the urinary tract. J. Urol., 45:342–360, 1941.

117. Susmano, D., Rubenstein, A.B., Dakin, A.R., et al.: Cystitis glandularis and adenocarcinoma of the bladder. J. Urol., 105:671–674, 1971.

118. Wheeler, J.D., and Hill, W.T.: Adenocarcinoma involving the urinary bladder. Cancer, 7:119–135, 1954.
119. Winter, C.C., and Goodwin, W.E.: Mucus-secreting adenocarcinoma of the urinary bladder simulating carcinoma of the gastrointestinal tract. Am. Surg., 25:875–882, 1959.
119a. Yalla, S.V., Ivker, M., Burros, H.M. et al.: Cystitis glandularis with perivesical lipomatosis: frequent association of two unusual proliferative conditions. Urology 5:383–386, 1975.

Cystitis Follicularis

119b. Bleisch, V.R., and Konikov, F.: Malakoplakia of the urinary bladder—report of 4 cases and discussion of etiology. Arch. Pathol., 56:388–397, 1952.
119c. Brownstein, P.K., Mannes, H., and Bogaev, J.H.: Sarcoidosis and malakoplakia. Urology, 6:249–251, 1975.
119d. Sarma, K.P.: The role of lymphoid reaction in bladder cancer. J. Urol., 104:843–849, 1970.

Abacteria Pyuria

120. Hewitt, C.B., Stewart, B.H., and Kiser, W.S.: Abacteria pyuria. J. Urol., 109:86–89, 1973.
121. Landes, R.R., and Ransom, C.L.: Abacterial pyuria: possible relationship to Reiter's syndrome. J. Urol., 60:666–677, 1948.
122. Sillar, S.R.: Abacterial cystitis. Urol. Digest, 9:12–20, 1970.
123. Utz, D.C., and Farrow, G.M.: Carcinoma in situ of the bladder. Urol. Digest, 16:19–32, 1977.

Cytoxan Cystitis

124. Anderson, E.E., Cobb, O.E., and Glenn, J.: Cyclophosphamide hemorrhagic cystitis. J. Urol., 97:857–858, 1967.
125. Gellman, E., Kissane, J., Frech, R., et al.: Cyclophosphamide cystitis. J. Can. Assoc. Radiol., 20:99–101, 1969.
126. George, P.: Haemorrhagic cystitis and cyclophosphamide. Lancet, 2:942, 1963.
127. Johnson, W.H., and Meadows, D.C.: Urinary bladder fibrosis and telangiectasia associated with long-term cyclophosphamide therapy. N. Engl. J. Med., 284:290–294, 1971.
128. Marsh, F.B., Vince, F.D., and Pollack, D.J.: Cyclophosphamide necrosis of bladder causing calcification, coatracture and reflux: treated by colocystoplasty. Br. J. Urol., 43:324–332, 1971.
129. Pearlman, C.K.: Cystitis due to Cytoxan: case report. J. Urol., 95:713–715, 1966.
130. Philips, F.S., Sternberge, S.S., Cronin, A.P., et al.: Cyclophosphamide and urinary bladder toxicity. Cancer Res., 21:1577–1589, 1961.
131. Renert, W.A., Berdon, W.E., and Baker, D.H.: Hemorrhagic cystitis and vesicoureteral reflux secondary to Cytoxan therapy for childhood malignancies. Am. J. Roentgenol., 117:664–669, 1973.
132. Rubin, S.S., and Rubin, R.T.: Cyclophosphamide hemorrhagic cystitis. J. Urol., 96:313–316, 1966.

Radiation Cystitis

132a. Goldstein, A.G., D'Escrivan, J.C., and Allen, S.D.: Hemorrhagic radiation cystitis. Br. J. Urol., 40:475–478, 1968.
132b. Lapides, J.: Treatment of delayed intractable hemorrhagic cystitis following radiation or chemotherapy. J. Urol., 104:707–708, 1970.
132c. Pool, T.L.: Irradiation cystitis; diagnosis and treatment. Surg. Clin. North Am., 39:947–951, 1959.

Fungus Balls in Urinary Bladder

133. Burrows, W.: Textbook of Microbiology. ed. 6. Philadelphia, W.B. Saunders, 1955.
134. Chisholm, E.R., and Hutch, J.A.: Fungus ball (Candida albicans) formation in bladder. J. Urol., 86:559–562, 1961.
135. Felson, B., and Wirt, J.: Case of the Day. ed. 1. Springfield, Ill., Charles C Thomas, 1967.
136. Goldman, H.J., Littman, M.L., Oppenheimer, G.D., et al.: Monilial cystitis: effective treatment with instillations of amphotericin B. J.A.M.A., 175:359–361, 1960.
137. Guze, L.B., and Haley, L.D.: Fungus infections of urinary tract. Yale J. Biol. Med., 30:292–305, 1958.
138. Margolis, H.N.: Fungus infection of urinary tract. Seminars in Roentgenology, 6:323–330, 1971.
139. McDonald, D.F., and Fagan, C.J.: Fungus balls in the urinary bladder. Am. J. Roentgenol. Radium Ther. Nucl. Med., 4:753–757, 1972.
140. Melchior, J., Mebust, W.K., and Volk, W.L.: Ureteral colic from a fungus ball—unusual presentation of a systemic aspergillosis. J. Urol., 108:698–699, 1972.
141. Sauer, H.R., and Metzner, W.T.: Thrush infections of urinary bladder: case report. J. Urol., 59:38–41, 1948.
142. Schwarz, J., and Baum, G.L.: Fungus disease of lungs. Seminars in Roentgenology, 5:73–76, 1970.
143. Woods, J.W., Manning, I.H., and Patterson, C.N.: Monilial infections complicating therapeutic use of antibiotics. J.A.M.A., 145:207–211, 1951.

Tuberculosis

144. Alton, B.H.: Spontaneous intraperitoneal rupture of a tuberculous bladder. N. Engl. J. Med., 205:1177–1181, 1931.
145. Bowen, J.A., and Bennett, G.A.: Solitary tuberculoma of bladder. Surg. Gynecol. Obstet., 50:1015–1017, 1930.
146. Dakin, W.A.: Cutaneous ureterostomy as a means of relief in contracted tuberculous bladder. Can. Med. Assoc. J., 47:207–212, 1942.
147. Wear, J.B.: End results of tuberculous cystitis. Arch. Surg., 37:821–826, 1938.

Malacoplakia

148. Bleisch, V.R., and Konikov, N.F.: Malacoplakia of urinary bladder: report of 4 cases and discussion of etiology. Arch. Pathol., 54:388–397, 1952.
149. Brownstein, P.K., Mannes, H., and Rogaev, J.H.: Sarcoidosis and malacoplakia. Urology, 6:249–251, 1975.
150. Elliott, G.B., Moloney, P.J., and Clement, J.G.: Malacoplakia of the urinary tract. Am. J. Roentgenol., 116:830–837, 1971.
151. Gibson, T.E., Bareta, J., and Lake, G.C.: Malacoplakia: report of a case involving the bladder and one kidney and ureter. Urol. Int., 1:5–14, 1955.
152. Kolodny, G.M.: Ureteral dilatation with pyuria. J.A.M.A., 197:577–578, 1966.
153. McDonald, S., and Sewell, W.T.: Malacoplakia of the bladder and kidneys. J. Pathol. Bacteriol., 18:306–318, 1913.
154. O'Dea, M.J., Malek, R.S., and Farrow, G.M.: Malacoplakia of the urinary tract: challenges and frustrations with 10 cases. J. Urol., 118:739–742, 1977.

155. Redewill, F.H.: Malacoplakia of urinary bladder and generalized sarcoidosis, striking similarity of their pathology, etiology, gross appearance and methods of treatment. J. Urol., 49:401–407, 1943.

156. Smith, B.H.: Malacoplakia of the urinary tract: a study of twenty-four cases. Am. J. Clin. Pathol., 43:409–417, 1965.

157. Terner, J.Y., and Lattes, R.: Malacoplakia of colon and retroperitoneum: report of a case with a histochemical study of the Michaelis-Gutmann inclusion bodies. Am. J. Clin. Pathol., 44:20–31, 1965.

Schistosomiasis

158. Al-Ghorab, M.M.: Radiological manifestation of genitourinary Bilharziasis. Clin. Radiol., 19:100–111, 1968.

159. Al-Ghorab, M.M., El-Badawi, A.A., and Effat, H.: Vesicoureteral reflux in urinary Bilharziasis. A clinico-radiological study. Clin. Radiol., 14:42–47, 1966.

160. Cheynet, M.: Radiological study of urinary bilharziasis. J. Urol. Med. Chir. (Paris), 66:237–253, 1960.

161. Dimmette, R.M., Sproat, H.F., and Sayegh, E.S.: The classification of carcinoma of the urinary bladder associated with Schistosomiasis and metaplasia. J. Urol., 75:680–686, 1956.

162. El-Badawi, A.A.: Bilharzial polyps of the urinary bladder. Br. J. Urol., 38:24–35, 1966.

163. Gelfand, M.: Bilharzial affections of the ureter. A study of 110 consecutive necropsies showing vesical Bilharzia. Br. Med. J., 1:1228–1230, 1948.

164. James, W.B.: Urological manifestations in Schistosoma hematobium infestations. Br. J. Radiol., 36:40–45, 1963.

165. Khafagy, M.M., El-Bolkainy, M.N., and Monsour, M.A.: Carcinoma of the Bilharzial urinary bladder. A study of the associated mucosal lesions in 86 cases. Cancer, 30:150–159, 1972.

166. Kirkkaldy-Willis, W.H.: Cystoscopy in the diagnosis and treatment in Bilharzia haematobium infection. Br. J. Surg., 34:189–194, 1946.

167. Makar, N.: Urological aspects of Bilharziosis in Egypt. Cairo Societe Orientale de Publicite. p. 125. 1955.

168. Maker, N.: A note on the pathogenesis of cancer of the bilharzial bladder. Fouad I. Cairo, Cairo Univ. Press, 1950.

169. Ockuly, E.A.: Bilharziosis of the bladder. J. Urol., 54:39–45, 1945.

170. Phillips, J.F., Cockrill, H., Jorge, E., et al.: Radiographic evaluation of patients with Schistosomiasis. Radiology, 114:31–37, 1975.

171. Sayegh, E.S.: Late complication of urinary bilharziosis. J. Urol., 63:353–371, 1950.

172. Smith, J.H., Torky, H., Kelada, A.S., et al.: Schistosomal polyposis of the urinary bladder. Am. J. Trop. Med. Hyg., 26:83–88, 1977.

173. Vermooten, V.: Bilharziasis of the ureter and its pathognomonic roentgenographic appearance. J. Urol., 38:430–441, 1937.

174. Young, S.W., Khalib, K.H., Farid, Z., et al.: Urinary-tract lesions of Schistosomal haemotobium with detailed radiographic consideration of the ureter. Radiology, 111:81–84, 1974.

175. Zaher, M.F., and Atala, A.: Experience with treatment of 450 cases of Bilharzial ulcer of bladder. J. Urol., 97:859–861, 1967.

176. Zaher, M.F., Badr, M.M., and Fawzy, R.M.: Bilharzial urinary fistula with report on 50 cases. J. Egypt Med. Assoc., 41:412–419, 1959.

Gangrene of Bladder

177. Cristol, D.S., and Greene, L.F.: Gangrenous cystitis. Surgery, 18:343–346, 1945.

178. Daines, S.L., and Hodgson, N.B.,: Spontaneous rupture of a necrotic bladder. J. Urol., 102:431–433, 1969.

179. Garrett, R.A., and Vaughn, W.R.: Regeneration of bladder: case report. J. Urol., 77:718–723, 1957.

180. McCallum, D.C.: Gangrene of the bladder with subsequent regrowth. J. Urol., 94:669–670, 1965.

181. Stirling, W.C., and Hopkins, G.A.: Gangrene of the bladder: review of two hundred seven cases; report of two personal cases. J. Urol., 31:517–525, 1934.

Alkaline-Encrusted Cystitis

182. Hager, R.B., and Magath, T.B.: The etiology of encrusted cystitis with alkaline urine. J.A.M.A., 85:1352, 1926.

182a. Harrison, R.B., Stier, F.M., and Cochrane, J.A.: Alkaline encrusting cystitis. Am. J. Roentgenol., 130:575–577, 1978.

183. Randall, A., and Campbell, E.W.: Alkaline encrusted cystitis. J. Urol., 37:284–299, 1937.

HERNIA OF THE BLADDER

True herniation of the bladder into inguinal or femoral rings is not uncommon. Koontz[7] found the bladder to be involved in 1 to 3 per cent of all inguinal hernias and in 10 per cent of men over 50 years of age. Wakely[13] reported 75 instances in 5000 cases of hernia. The inguinal type (Fig. 27–1, *B*) is more frequent and usually occurs in males, whereas the femoral type is predominant in females. The scrotal variety (Figs. 27–2 to 27–4) (scrotal cystocele, Levine[8]) is rare. Herniation of the bladder is seen in children[4] but is probably more common in the older age group. There are very likely many causes, but bladder neck obstruction should not be overlooked. In females the pressure of a gravid uterus may be an etiologic factor.

Bladder herniation may present as part of an obturator, ischiorectal, suprapubic or Gironcoli hernia, but these are rare. Papilloma, carcinoma, and stones have been associated with herniation of the bladder.

Inguinal hernias of the bladder are classified according to their relationship with the peritoneum.

TYPES

Extraperitoneal. This is a direct inguinal hernia in which there is a protrusion of the anterior or the lateral walls of the bladder (often with large amounts of prevesical fat) into the inguinal or the femoral canals. The peritoneum does not protrude. This is the least common variety.

Intraperitoneal. This type is usually indirect. The hernial sac may contain the entire bladder with the exception of the trigone, or a portion of the bladder, a vesical diverticulum, or prevesical fat alone, but in all instances it is covered by peritoneum. The sac may contain loops of small intestine and the ureters or, in females, the uterus, the ovaries, and the fallopian tubes.

27

Herniation and Diverticula of the Bladder

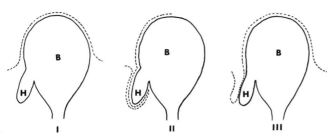

Classification of inguinal herniation of the bladder. The solid line represents bladder wall. The dashed line represents peritoneum.

  I. Extraperitoneal
 II. Intraperitoneal
III. Paraperitoneal

Paraperitoneal. This type can be direct or indirect. The bladder is situated on the inner side of the hernial sac, the inner wall of which is formed by the serous covering (peritoneum) of the superior surface of the bladder. This is the most common type.

Symptoms. The reduction in the size of the mass after voiding and the effects of two-stage micturition (i.e., initial spontaneous urination followed by manual compression of the hernia with further urination) are diagnostic features.[41]

ROENTGENOGRAPHIC DIAGNOSIS

Intravenous urogram:

1. Medial displacement of the ureter on the side opposite the hernia
2. Occasional lateral displacement of the ureter on the same side as the hernia
3. A small, asymmetric bladder
4. Incomplete filling of bladder base when associated with an inguinal or femoral hernia
5. Deviation of the trigone to the side of the hernia (Fig. 27-4)

Retrograde cystograms definitely delineate hernias of the bladder, which appear as dilated sacs outside the bladder developing in the region of the inguinal canal. The neck and upper part of the herniation are much narrower than the peripheral portion.

BLADDER EARS

These occur in 9 per cent of infants under 12 months of age and are seen mostly in those under 6 months of age. The relaxed bladder protrudes into the inguinal ring to form a transitory extraperitoneal hernia, usually bilateral. They are associated in 20 per cent of the cases with inguinal hernia and are more common in males. These "ears" disappear on complete filling of the bladder and probably represent a normal variance (Figs. 27-5, 27-6).

BLADDER DIVERTICULA

Diverticula of the urinary bladder are outpocketings of the bladder wall between interlacing bundles of muscle, usually hypertrophic but occasionally normal (Figs. 27-7 to 27-13).[28] Diverticula may be single or multiple, small or large. Males are affected more frequently than females (Fig. 27-9).[38, 39] It is possible that the production and the distention of diverticula may protect the kidney from severe back pressure. The openings of the diverticula occur most frequently at the base and the lower halves of the lateral walls of the bladder, often in the region of the ureteral orifices. In uncomplicated cases the walls are thin, consisting of stretched mucosa, small amounts of elastic and fibrous tissue, and a few attenuated muscle fibers.

The causes of diverticula are not entirely clear. It has been suggested that embryologic defects or obstruction or both are the etiologic agents, although infravesical obstruction seems to be the primary factor. Burns found diverticula to be of clinical importance in about 6 per cent of obstructions of the vesical neck.[30] Prostatic hypertrophy is the single most important cause. The pathology of excised diverticula is as follows[41]: chronic inflammation, 62.5 per cent; squamous cell metaplasia plus chronic inflammation, 9.0 per cent; squamous cell metaplasia, 3.0 per cent; fibrosis, 9.0 per cent; no disease, 16.9 per cent.

CLASSIFICATION

There are two groups in the classification of bladder diverticula.

Congenital Diverticula. These are rare, usually single, and found primarily in children, usually in juxtaposition to the ureteral orifice, most commonly posterolateral (Fig. 27-7; see also Chapter 24, Congenital Anomalies of the Bladder). Most vesical diverticula in childhood are not associated with bladder outflow obstruction,[15, 16, 19, 20] and they are possibly the result of congenitally weak areas in the detrusor muscle.[25, 29] Burns and co-workers found only 3 diverticula in 81 cases of obstruction of the bladder neck in children.[17] They occur usually between the ages of 3 and 10 years. They are more common in males, and urinary infection is the most frequent symptom. Over 93 per cent have vesicoureteral reflux and this is the cause of upper tract changes in most cases, but occasionally obstruction of the ureter may result from a large diverticulum pressing directly on this structure. Urinary retention secondary to urethral compression has occurred.

Differential Diagnosis.

URACHAL DIVERTICULUM This is present at the dome of the bladder and may show trabeculations owing to the muscle layer.

BLADDER EARS. The position is related to the inguinal ring; they are not visualized on complete filling of the bladder and disappear in time.

THE WIDE-MOUTH DIVERTICULUM. This is seen in females with large atonic bladders.[26] It is a saucer-shaped depression posterolateral to the ureteral orifice. It does not remain full when the bladder is empty. It appears similar to recesses in adult females (Chapter 23, see Normal Bladder).

Acquired Diverticula. These occur later in life, and obstruction plays the predominant role. Acquired diverticula are often multiple and differ from the congenital in that they may occur in areas other than the posterior angle of the trigone. Rupture of a diverticulum of the bladder is rare.[47, 48]

DIAGNOSIS

Diverticula are diagnosed often by cystoscopy and are seen on the cystogram of the intravenous urogram, but retrograde cystography, sometimes including pneumocystography, is the most accurate method. In many instances it may be difficult to differentiate bladder and diverticulum, as the latter may be even larger than the former.

Two cardinal points aid in the differentiation of the diverticulum and the bladder:

1. Introduction of an opaque urethral catheter points out the true bladder.

2. The diverticulum is smooth-walled, whereas the bladder in these cases is irregular owing to trabeculation. Congenital diverticulum may be irregular because of muscle present in the wall.

PERTINENT FACTORS

Merely diagnosing that a diverticulum exists is not sufficient. The following factors must be ascertained.

Does the diverticulum empty? This information is ascertained by evacuating the bladder of its contrast medium with a catheter and then making another roentgenogram (Figs. 27-13, 27-20).

Is the diverticulum infected?[20, 36, 38] Infection is evaluated better by cystoscopy.

Does the diverticulum contain stones (Figs. 27-14, 27-18)? The nonopaque variety must be differentiated from tumors and blood clots. Dumbbell-shaped stones, with the isthmus at the neck of the diverticulum, have been reported.

Is there a carcinoma in the diverticulum (see Figs. 27-15 to 27-18)? Carcinoma in a diverticulum of the bladder is probably not as rare as previously thought. Substantial literature describing such cases now has been presented. Actually the incidence of tumor in a bladder diverticulum is 4 per cent,[62] 7 per cent,[61] and so forth. The incidence of tumor occurring in the bladder proper when there is an associated diverticulum is only 2.4 per cent. Thus, whenever a tumor and diverticulum are in the same bladder, the tumor will most likely be in the diverticulum. Prognosis for these cases depends to a great extent upon the differentiation of the tumor.[62] The well-differentiated tumor had a good prognosis, but patients with anaplastic tumors rarely survived beyond 2 years. Transitional cell carcinomas are the most frequent type, but squamous cell carcinoma is found not infrequently. Carcinoma in diverticula of the bladder must be differentiated from nonopaque stone and blood clot (Fig. 27-19). The presence of stone and carcinoma (Fig. 27-18) in the same diverticulum is unusual. The stone may so fill the diverticulum that the malignancy is overlooked. Sarcoma in a diverticulum of the bladder has been reported only rarely.

Does the diverticulum affect the ureter? The ureter can enter the diverticulum (Figs. 27-21, 27-22). This may or may not be the cause of the obstruction of the ureter. The diverticulum can deviate the ureter (Figs. 27-17, 27-20) and in some instances can cause hydroureter and hydronephrosis (Fig. 27-23). The deviation usually is medial, but exceptions occur.

HUTCH DIVERTICULUM

Hutch described a saccule or diverticulum near the ureteral orifice, most frequently in neurogenic lesions, especially in paraplegics (Figs. 27-24, 27-25).[81] The out-pocketing had certain characteristics.

1. It lay above and lateral to the ureteral orifice. It involved the bladder wall just beyond the lateral perimeter of the trigone but never involved the trigone itself.

2. A catheter would outline the ureter passing under the floor of the saccule.

3. The saccule involves the detrusor muscle (lying in the region of intramural ureter), weakening and destroying it. Thus, there is a lack of firm muscle under the intramural ureter, and the ureter therefore has no firm backing to be compressed against when the intravesical pressure rises, and reflux may occur. The ureter tended to fall extravesically.

4. Often there appeared to be an obstructed area in the ureter just above the bladder, producing a defect called the "notch sign."

These diverticula are seen more commonly in children and are more prevalent in males. They may be missed on intravenous urogram, and cystography is the best method for demonstration. Urinary infection is the most common type of presentation. These diverticula can be associated with vesicoureteric reflux and duplication of the pelvicalyceal collecting system. This has suggested to some authors that the reflux is primary in some cases and is related to lateral ectopia of the ureteric orifice. This whole syndrome complex may be inherited.[80] The diverticula tend to enlarge over a period of time but may not persist. If obstruction distally or infection, or both are corrected, both the reflux and the outpocketing may disappear.

CHAPTER 27, ILLUSTRATIONS

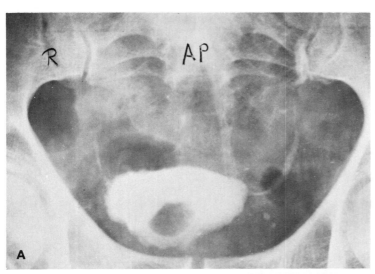

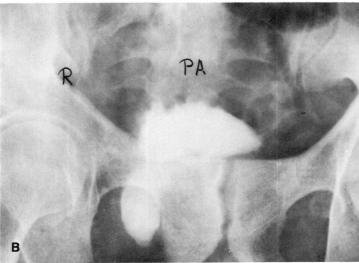

FIG. 27-1. Herniation of the bladder. (A) Supine view. Essentially normal bladder except for some trabeculation. Foley bag in bladder. (B) Prone view. Herniation of the bladder into the inguinal ring on right now can be visualized. This emphasizes the importance of the prone film. (Courtesy of M. Elkin, M.D.)

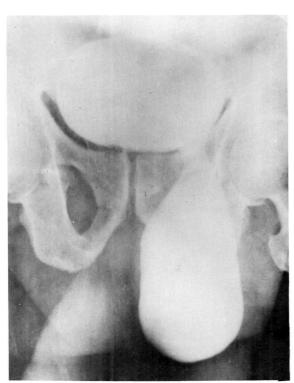

FIG. 27–2. Scrotal herniation of the bladder. Large scrotal hernia on left owing to herniation of bladder.

FIG. 27–3. Scrotal herniation of the bladder. Note the stone (*arrow*) present in the scrotal cystocele.

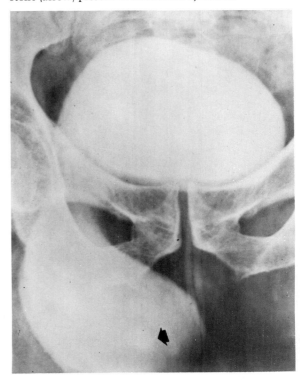

FIG. 27–4. Bladder in scrotal hernia. **(A)** Retrograde cystogram. **(B)** Intravenous pyelogram. *Arrow* points to trigone, which is pulled markedly to the right. Note the deviation of the left ureter secondary to the hernia.

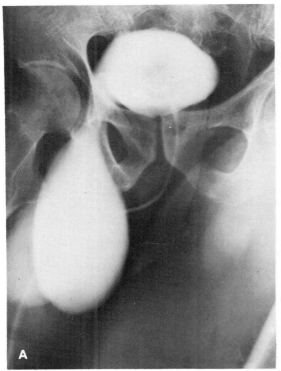

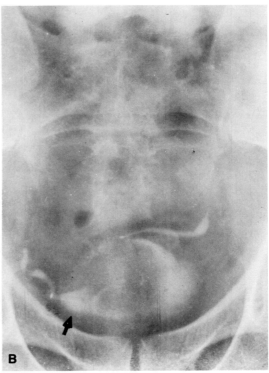

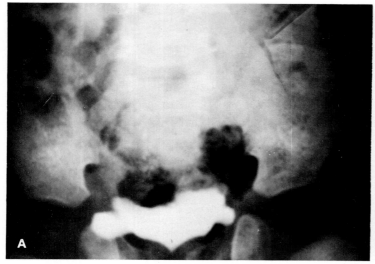
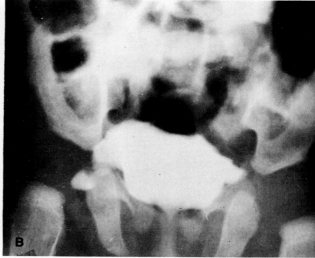

FIG. 27–5 (A,B) Bilateral "bladder ears." These occur in 9 per cent of infants under 12 months of age and are seen mostly under 6 months of age. The relaxed bladder protrudes into the inguinal ring to form a transitory extraperitoneal hernia, usually bilateral. They are associated in 20 per cent of the cases with inguinal hernia (**A**) and are more common in males. These "ears" disappear on complete filling of the bladder and probably represent a normal variation. (Allen, R.P., and Condon, V.R.: Radiology, 77:979, 1961)

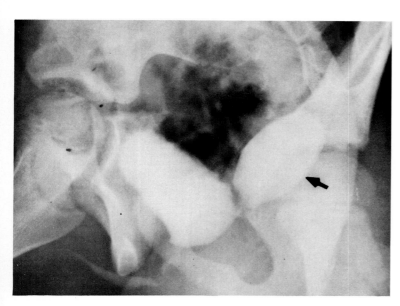

FIG. 27–6. Bladder ears in a 10-year-old girl.

FIG. 27–7. Congenital bladder diverticulum (*arrow*) in a male. Right oblique view. The bladder neck can be seen easily, the diverticulum is smooth-walled, and the bladder is trabeculated. (Courtesy of Keith Waterhouse, M.D.)

FIG. 27–8. Bladder saccules and small diverticula in a case of prostatic hypertrophy. Filling defect in the bladder is caused by Foley bag.

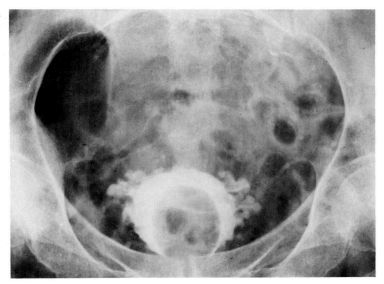

FIG. 27–9. Bladder diverticulum in a female with bladder neck obstruction. *Arrow* points to diverticulum. Bladder is trabeculated; diverticulum is smooth. (Courtesy of Herbert Kenyon, M.D.)

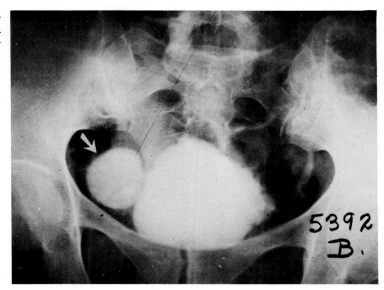

FIG. 27–10. Diverticulum of a bladder secondary to contracture of bladder neck. *Arrow* points to the smooth-walled diverticulum. This looks like an hourglass bladder and should be compared with it (see Fig. 24–14). Note that in the present case the bladder proper is irregular, whereas the diverticulum is smooth-walled. In hourglass bladder both compartments would show trabeculation if obstruction or infection has taken place.

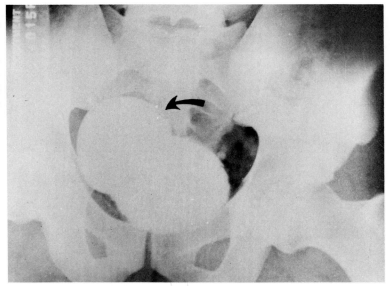

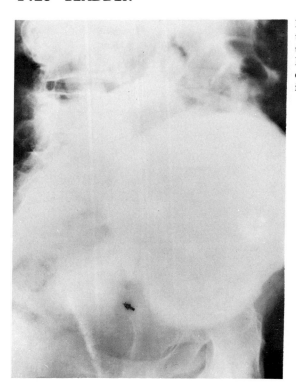

FIG. 27–11. Diverticulum of the bladder. The diverticulum is on the left, and it is much larger than the true bladder (*arrow*). The bladder is identified by the following two points: (1) it is more irregular than the diverticulum, and (2) the outline of the urethra going into the bladder can be seen.

FIG. 27–12. Diverticulum of the bladder in a case of prostatic hypertrophy. **(A)** AP view. *Arrow* points to a diverticulum on right side of bladder. Note how easily this can be overlooked. **(B)** Right oblique view. *Arrow* points to diverticulum, now clearly separated from the bladder.

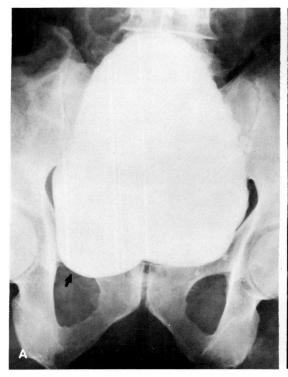

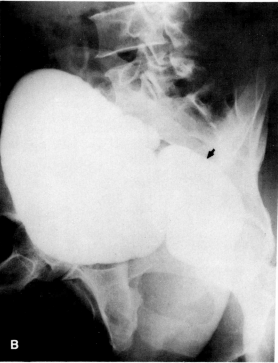

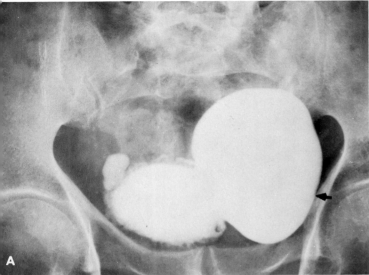

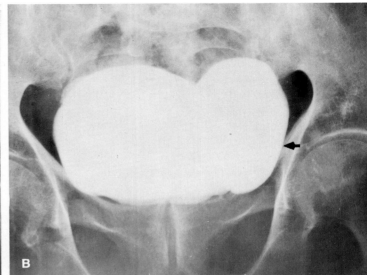

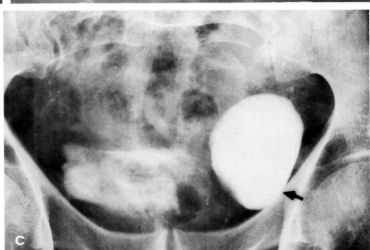

FIG. 27–13. Diverticula of bladder due to fibrous contracture of bladder neck. (**A**) Bladder is irregular and trabeculated, with a small diverticulum on the right and a large diverticulum on the left (*arrow*). (**B**) Overdistention of bladder with contrast material, showing obliteration of trabeculations. (**C**) Postevacuation film. Small amount of contrast material is present in the bladder, but the large diverticulum on the left (*arrow*) still retains a large amount of its contrast material.

FIG. 27–14. Stone in diverticulum of bladder. (**A**) Scout film. Stone situated considerably above symphysis pubis. There are also prostatic calculi. (**B**) Cystogram following intravenous pyelogram. Note numerous diverticula and stone in upper right diverticulum.

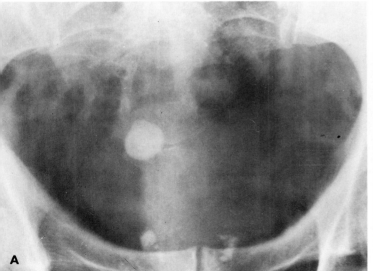

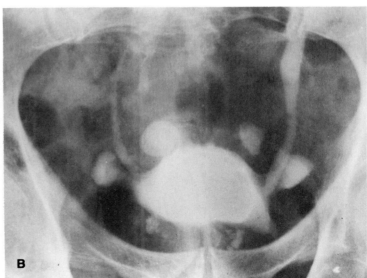

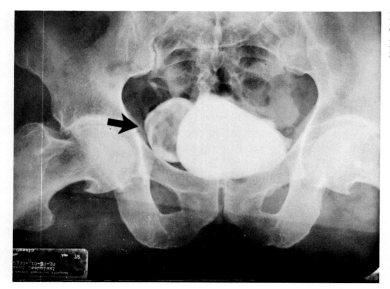

FIG. 27–15. Carcinoma in a diverticulum of the bladder. Diverticulum on right side of the bladder incompletely filled due to the carcinoma (*arrow*). (Courtesy of S.M. Marcus, M.D.)

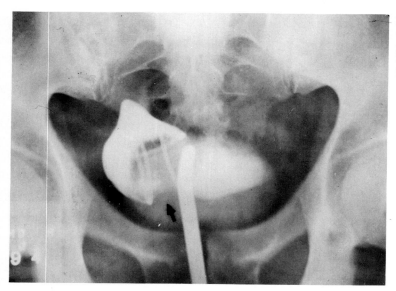

Fig. 27–16. Carcinoma in a diverticulum of the bladder (*arrow*). A catheter has been coiled up in the diverticulum, and contrast material has been injected. The large filling defect noted is caused by the carcinoma. (Courtesy of Peter Ross, M.D.)

FIG. 27–17. Carcinoma in a diverticulum of the bladder. **(A)** Ureteral catheter in a diverticulum, essentially normal. **(B)** Three years later. *Arrow* points to a large defect in the diverticulum corresponding to malignancy. Note the medial deviation of the left ureter.

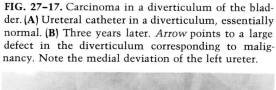

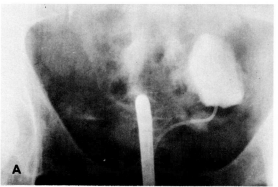

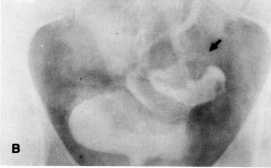

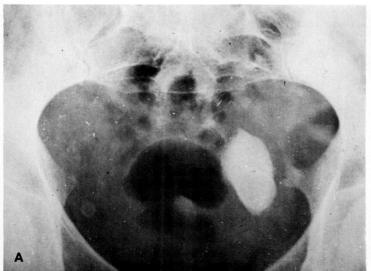

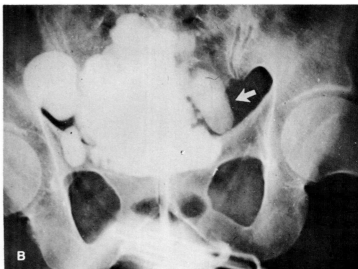

FIG. 27–18. Carcinoma and stone in the same diverticulum of the bladder. **(A)** Scout film. Calculus seen lying just outside bladder. **(B)** Cystogram. Irregular trabeculated bladder with many saccules and cellules and multiple diverticula. *Arrow* points to stone in a diverticulum on the left side. No evidence of neoplasm can be seen, but on exploration a large infiltrating carcinoma of the diverticulum completely surrounding the stone was found. Perivesical tissues were involved, but the bladder was free of tumor. (Ney, C., and Adlerman, E.J.: N.Y. State J. Med., *53:*1782, 1953)

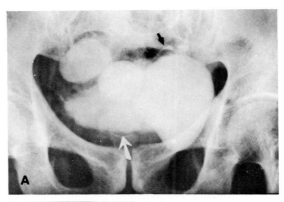

FIG. 27–19. Bladder diverticula. Case of prostatic obstruction. **(A)** *Arrows* point to the two diverticula with filling defects due to blood clots. Retrograde cystogram. **(B)** Six days later blood clots have been evacuated.

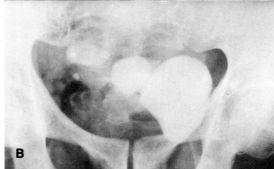

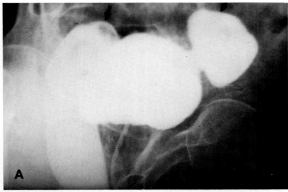

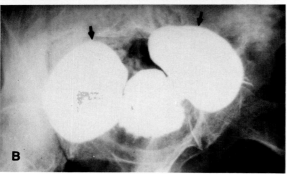

FIG. 27–20. Diverticula of the bladder associated with benign prostatic hypertrophy. **(A)** Cystogram revealing irregular bladder (*white arrow*) and three smooth-walled diverticula. *Black arrow* points to ureter, which has been deviated medially by the large diverticulum on the left. **(B)** Postevacuation of bladder by urethral catheter. Contrast material still is retained in the three diverticula.

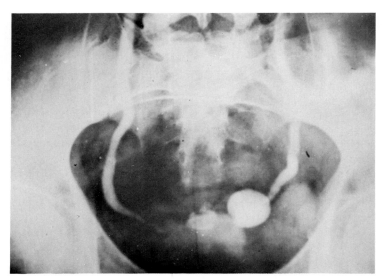

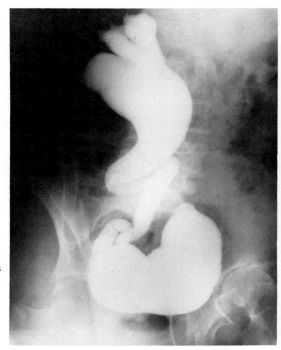

FIG. 27–21. Left ureter entering a diverticulum of the bladder.

FIG. 27–22. Ureter entering a diverticulum of the bladder. Retrograde cystogram; notice that catheter enters into bladder. On the right is a moderate-sized diverticulum, with the ureter from the right kidney entering the diverticulum and showing a huge hydroureter and hydronephrosis secondary to reflux.

FIG. 27–23. Bladder diverticulum. **(A)** Catheter coiled in diverticulum of bladder secondary to prostatic obstruction. **(B)** Contrast medium inserted in diverticulum during intravenous pyelogram. *Small arrow* points to diverticulum. *Large arrow* shows compression of ureter by diverticulum with dilatation of the proximal ureter. Patient also had hydronephrosis. (Courtesy of J.J. Arnold, M.D.)

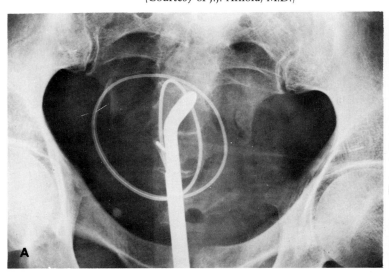

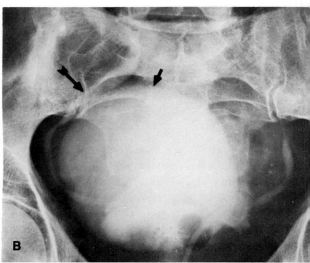

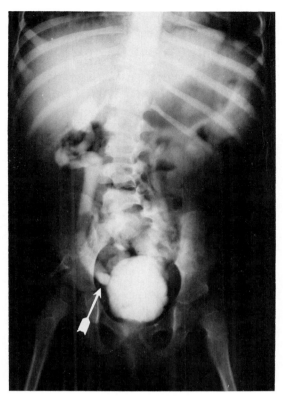

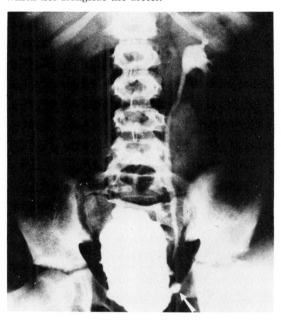

FIG. 27–24. Hutch diverticulum. *Arrows* point to the diverticulum in the region of the right refluxing ureter in a case of spina bifida with a neurogenic bladder.

FIG. 27–25. Hutch diverticulum in a urogenic bladder caused by spina bifida. *Arrow* points to diverticulum, which lies alongside the ureter.

BIBLIOGRAPHY

Hernia of the Bladder

1. Barquin, O.P., and Madsen, P.O.: Scrotal herniation of the lower urinary tract. J. Urol., *98*:508–511, 1967.
2. Becker, J.A.: A hernia of the urinary bladder. Radiology, *84*:270–273, 1965.
3. Bierhoff, A., and Unger, A.S.: Inguinal hernia of bladder. Am. J. Surg., *30*:506–507, 1935.
4. Campbell, M.F.: Urology. p. 1604. Philadelphia, W.B. Saunders, 1954.
5. Heineck, A.P.: Hernia of the urinary bladder. Surg. Gynecol. Obstet., *22*:592–602, 1916.
6. Kollberg, S.: Bladder hernia survey and case report. Acta Chir. Scand., *105*:407–413, 1953.
7. Koontz, A.R.: Sliding hernia of diverticulum of bladder. Arch. Surg., *70*:436–438, 1955.
8. Levine, B.: Scrotal cystocele. J.A.M.A., *147*:1439–1441, 1951.
9. Liebeskind, A.L., Elkin, M., and Goldman, S.H.: Herniation of the bladder. Radiology, *106*:257–262, 1973.
10. Ray, B., Darwish, M.E., Baker, R.J., et al.: Massive inguino-scrotal bladder herniation. J. Urol., *118*:330–331, 1977.
11. Reardon, J.V., and Lowman, R.M.: Massive herniation of the bladder: "the roentgen findings." J. Urol., *97*:1019–1020, 1967.
12. Soloway, H.M., Portney, F., and Kaplan, A.: Hernia of the bladder. J. Urol., *84*:539–543, 1960.
13. Wakely, C.P.G.: Treatment of certain types of external herniae (Hunterian Lecture). Lancet, *1*:822–826, 1940.

Bladder Ears

14. Allen, R.P., and Condon, V.R.: Transitory extraperitoneal hernia of the bladder in infants (bladder ears). Radiology, *77*:979–983, 1961.

Diverticula of the Bladder

Congenital

15. Barrett, D.M., Malek, R.S., and Kelalis, P.P.: Observations on vesical diverticulum in childhood. J. Urol., *116*:234–236, 1975.
16. Bauer, S.B., and Retik, A.B.: Bladder diverticula in infants and children. Urology, *3*:712–715, 1974.
17. Burns, E., Pratt, A.M., and Hendon, R.G.: Management of bladder neck obstruction in children. J.A.M.A., *157*:570–574, 1955.
18. Campbell, M.F.: Clinical Pediatric Urology. p. 257. Philadelphia, W.B. Saunders, 1951.
19. Cendron, J., and Alain, J.L.: Diverticule vésical chez l'enfant sans obstacle du bas apareil urinarire. J. Urol. Néphrol., *78*:793–807, 1972.
20. Forsythe, I.W., and Smyth, B.T.: Diverticula of the bladder in children. Pediatrics, *24*:322–329, 1959.
21. Hyman, A.: Diverticula of the bladder in children. Surg. Gynecol. Obstet., *36*:27–35, 1923.

22. Judd, E., and Scholl, A.: Diverticulum of urinary bladder. Surg. Gynecol. Obstet., 38:14–26, 1924.

23. Kjellberg, S.R., Ericsson, H.O., and Rudle, U.: The Lower Urinary Bladder in Childhood. p. 180. Chicago, Year Book Publishers, 1957.

24. Kretschmer, H.L.: Diverticula of bladder in infancy and childhood. Am. J. Dis. Child., 48:842–857, 1934.

25. Mackellar, A., and Stephens, F.D.: Vesical diverticula in children. Austr. N.A. J. Surg., 30:20–31, 1960.

26. Stephens, F.D.: Congenital Malformations of the Rectum, Anus, and the Genitourinary Tract. London, Livingstone, 1963.

27. Watson, E.M.: Developmental bases for certain vesical diverticula. J.A.M.A., 75:1473–1474, 1920.

28. Williams, D.I.: Congenital bladder-neck obstruction and megaureter; clinical observation. Br. J. Urol., 29:389–392, 1957.

29. Williams, D.I., ed. Urology in Childhood. pp. 202–206. New York, Springer Verlag, 1974.

Acquired

30. Burns, E.: Diverticula of the urinary bladder. Ann. Surg., 119:656–664, 1944.

31. Crenshaw, J.L., and Crompton, B.R.: Coincident calculus and diverticulum of the bladder. Collect. Papers Mayo Clin., 13:358–367, 1921.

32. Day, R.V., and Martin, H.W.: Diverticula of urinary bladder. J.A.M.A., 84:268–272, 1925.

33. English, J.: Isolirte Emtzunoung der Blasen-divertikel und Perforations peritonitis. Arch. Klin. Chir., 73:1–67, 1904.

34. Harris, A.: Carcinoma in diverticulum of the bladder. Urol. Cut. Rev., 28:143–145, 1924.

35. Joly, J.S.: Congenital diverticula of the bladder. Am. J. Urol., 10:486–499, 1914.

36. Judd, E.S.: Diverticula of the bladder. Ann. Surg., 68:298–305, 1918.

37. Kimbrough, J.C.: The treatment of bladder diverticulum. J. Urol., 48:368–381, 1941.

38. Kretschmer, H.L.: Diverticula of the urinary bladder. Surg. Gynecol. Obstet., 71:491–502, 1940.

39. Kutzmann, A.A.: Diverticulum of the urinary bladder in women. Am. Surg., 29-30:102–114, 1935.

40. Miller, A.: The aetiology and treatment of diverticulum of the bladder. Br. J. Urol., 30:43–56, 1958.

41. Peterson, L.J., Paulsan, D.F., and Glenn, J.F.: The histopathology of vesical diverticula. J. Urol., 110:62–64, 1973.

42. Pugh, W.S.: Diverticulum of bladder. Med. J. Rec., 130:203–209, 1929.

43. Rathbun, N.P.: Notes on vesical diverticula: Modified technique of surgical attack. Surg. Gynecol. Obstet., 29:28–32, 1919.

44. Rose, D.K.: Stages in formation of bladder diverticula. South. Med. J., 19:206–212, 1926.

45. Ward, R.O.: A clinical study of 11 cases of vesical diverticula. Br. J. Surg., 13:144–157, 1925.

46. Young, H.H., and Davis, D.M.: Practice of Urology. Philadelphia, W.B. Saunders, 1924.

Rupture of a Bladder Diverticulum

47. Creekmur, R.L.: Diverticula of bladder; report of case of spontaneous rupture. J. Urol., 37:363–366, 1937.

48. Magoun, J.A.H.: Vesical diverticula. J. Urol., 33:474–482, 1935.

Dumbbell-Shaped Stones and Bladder Diverticulum

49. Cassanetto, R.: Singuliere assoc. de lithiase vesicale. J. d'urol. Med. Chir., 10:223–228, 1920.

50. Crenshaw, J., and Crompton, B.: Coincident calculus and diverticula of the bladder. Collect. Papers Mayo Clin., 13:358–367, 1921.

51. Davis, D.: Preliminary diverticulectomy. J.A.M.A., 89:192–194, 1927.

52. Martin, S.P.: Dumbbell stones in diverticula of the bladder. Ann. Surg., 67:94–95, 1918.

Carcinoma in a Bladder Diverticulum

53. Abeshouse, B.S., and Goldstein, A.E.: Primary carcinoma in a diverticulum of the bladder. A report of 4 cases and a review of the literature. J. Urol., 49:534–557, 1943.

54. Boylan, R.N., Greene, L.F., and McDonald, J.R.: Epithelial neoplasms arising in diverticula of the urinary bladder. J. Urol., 65:1041–1050, 1951.

55. Briggs, W.T.: Carcinoma in diverticulum of the bladder. J. Urol., 24:517–520, 1930.

56. Deming, C.L.: Primary carcinoma of diverticulum of bladder. J. Urol., 18:73–84, 1927.

57. Gill, R.D.: Carcinoma in diverticulum of the bladder. J. Urol., 24:521–529, 1930.

58. Hicks, J.B.: Carcinoma in diverticulum of the bladder. J. Urol., 24:205–209, 1930.

59. Higgins, C.C.: Neoplasms primary in diverticula of urinary bladder. Am. J. Surg., 33:78–84, 1936.

60. Hunt, V.C.: Malignant disease in diverticulum of bladder. J. Urol., 22:1–12, 1929.

61. Kelalis, P.P., and McLean, P.: The treatment of diverticulum of the bladder. J. Urol., 98:349–352, 1967.

62. Knappenberger, S.T., Uson, A.C., and Melicow, M.M.: Primary neoplasm occurring in vesical diverticula: a report of 18 cases. J. Urol., 83:153–159, 1960.

63. Kretschmer, H.L.: Diverticula of the urinary bladder. Surg. Gynecol. Obstet., 71:491–503, 1940.

64. Kretschmer, H.L., and Barber, K.E.: Carcinoma in a bladder diverticulum. J. Urol., 21:381–395, 1929.

65. LeComte, R.M.: Neoplasms primary in the bladder diverticula. J. Urol., 27:667–684, 1932.

66. Lower, W.E., and Higgins, C.C.: Diverticula of the urinary bladder. J. Urol., 20:635–661, 1928.

67. Mayer, R.F., and Moore, T.D.: Carcinoma complicating vesical diverticulum. J. Urol., 71:307–315, 1954.

68. Montague, D.K., and Boltuch, R.L.: Primary neoplasms in vesical diverticula: report of 10 cases. J. Urol., 116:41–42, 1976.

69. Moore, T.D.: Carcinoma of the bladder. J. Urol., 51:496–504, 1944.

70. Ney, C., and Adlerman, E.J.: Calculus and primary carcinoma in a diverticulum of the bladder. N.Y. State J. Med., 53:1782–1784, 1953.

71. Ostroff, F.B., Alperstein, J.B., and Young, J.D., Jr.: Neoplasm in vesical diverticulum; report of 4 patients including a 21-year old. J. Urol., 110:65–69, 1973.

72. Petkovic, S.: Tumor in a diverticulum of the bladder. Urol. Cut. Rev., 54:333–337, 1950.

73. Smith, P.G., and Suder, G.L.: Primary carcinoma in bladder diverticula. Urol. Cut. Rev., 54:321–324, 1950.

74. Spence, H.M., and Baird, S.S.: Vesical diverticula: a clinical study with reference to treatment. J. Urol., 58:327–343, 1947.

Involvement of the Ureter

75. Fox, M., Power, R.F., and Bruce, A.W.: Diverticulum of the bladder. Presentation and evaluation of treatment of 115 cases. Br. J. Urol., *34*:286–298, 1962.
76. Hinman, F.: The etiology of vesical diverticula. J. Urol., *3*:207–246, 1919.
77. Hinman, F.: Vesical diverticula. Surg. Gynecol. Obstet., *29*:150–172, 1919.
78. Judd, E., and Scholl, A.: Diverticulum of urinary bladder. Surg. Gynecol. Obstet., *38*:14–26, 1924.
79. Paschkis, R.: Zur Kenntnis der Anomalien der Harnblase. Ztschr. Urol. Chir., *4*:365–381, 1919.

Hutch Diverticulum

80. Atwell, J.D., and Allen, N.H.: The interrelationship between paraureteric diverticula, vesicoureteric reflux, and duplication of the pelvicaliceal collecting system: a family study. Br. J. Urol. *52*:269–273, 1980.
81. Colodny, A.H., Bauer, S.B., and Retik, A.B.: Spontaneous disappearance of vesico-ureteric reflux associated with para-ureteral diverticula. Read at New England Section AUA, September 16, 1980, Whitefield, N.H.
82. Hutch, J.H.: Vesico-ureteral reflux in the paraplegic. Cause and correction. J. Urol., *68*:457–467, 1952.

Bladder calculi can arise primarily as a result of stasis, infection, foreign body, immobilization, or secondarily from the kidneys. Following operations on the bladder, stones may appear, probably as a result of tissue necrosis along the line of the incision but not as the result of suture material itself.[6] Bladder calculi are found predominantly in males, although they have been found in females as a result of bladder obstruction (Figs. 28-1, 28-11, 28-12) or foreign bodies (Fig. 28-13).

Vesical calculi are observed most frequently in adults, especially in Western countries, although they are common in children in endemic areas.

Stasis is probably the most common cause of bladder calculi (Figs. 28-2 to 28-7). Examples are strictures of the urethra, benign prostatic hypertrophy, diverticula of the bladder, a contracture of the bladder neck, and spinal cord injury. Frequently calculi are associated with foreign bodies and infections caused by urea-splitting organisms. Schistosomiasis (Fig. 28-14) is frequently associated with bladder calculi, especially in Egypt. The type of stone found in the bladder varies according to the type of infection, pH of the urine, and probably other factors. The components of bladder calculi are usually magnesium ammonium phosphate-apatite mixtures[7] or uric acid mixed with urates. Although foreign bodies can be the core on which salts are deposited to form calculi, it is interesting to note that some foreign bodies are not necessarily encrusted and may have been present in the bladder for many years.[18, 19] The stones found in the bladder may be single, multiple, small, or large.

Complications of bladder calculi are reflux,[10, 16] anuria,[12] infection, and retention of urine.

Endemic calculi refers to urinary stone formation in certain countries—India, Thailand, Turkey, usually occurring in children, and generally in the bladder (Fig. 28-15). It is believed to be a deficiency

28

Bladder Calculi

disorder because of its occurrence in children belonging to poor socioeconomic groups.[3] It is prevalent in boys under 5 years of age and is essentially a neonatal disease.[17] In an analysis of Ubol Province in Thailand, where the city dwellers rarely had vesical calculi and the villagers had a high incidence, Valyasevi[17] summarized the findings as follows:

1. Village mothers supplement breast feeding with glutinous rice feedings during the first week of life, probably resulting in lower consumption of breast milk.

2. Village women did not increase their intake of proteins and other foods during pregnancy and lactation.

3. The 24-hour urine volumes were frequently less in village newborn infants, in those under 1 year of age, and in children 2 to 10 years of age than in those of comparable ages in the city.

4. The urine of the infants from the rural areas had significantly lower concentrations and 24-hour excretion values of phosphate than did urine from city infants up to 1 year of age. However, the urinary concentrations and 24-hour excretion values of calcium were higher in the village children.

5. Total inorganic sulfate and free inorganic sulfate in the urine were lower in samples from village boys up to 1 year of age when compared with urban dwellers of similar age.

6. Oxalate crystalluria was more common in the village children.

It is thought that the mineral and protein intakes were lower in rural areas, and that this may play a role in the formation of stone. Ammonium acid urate and calcium oxalate are the two main components of bladder stones in Thailand.

Roentgenographic Findings. Bladder calculi are often missed on the plain film of the abdomen because many are nonopaque (Figs. 28–7, 28–8). Even the calcified stones can be missed because of bony structures, phleboliths, and calcification in vessels. Therefore, it is important that the plain film be compared carefully with the cystogram.

CHAPTER 28, ILLUSTRATIONS

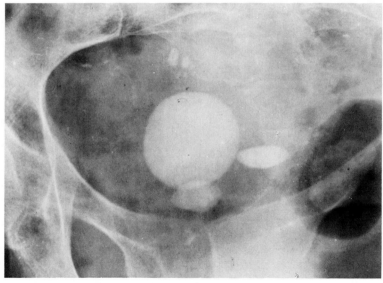

FIG. 28–1. Three large bladder calculi seen on right oblique view. Female with bladder neck obstruction.

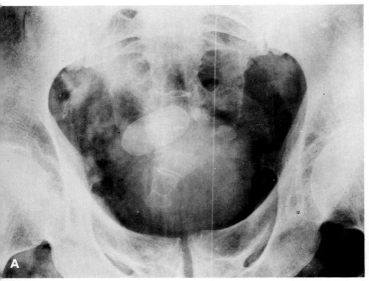
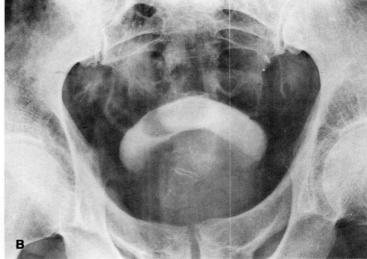

FIG. 28–2. Bladder calculus in prostatic hypertrophy. **(A)** Plain film. Stone visible. **(B)** Cystogram on intravenous urogram. Filling defect in bladder produced by stone.

FIG. 28–3. Mulberry-shaped stone in bladder. Prostatic obstruction. (Courtesy of Sol Unger, M.D., Veterans Administration, Bronx, N.Y.)

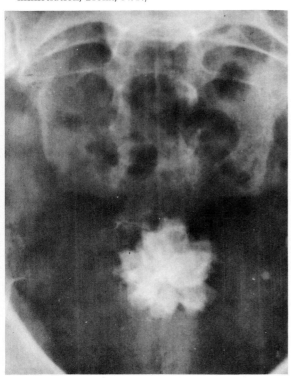

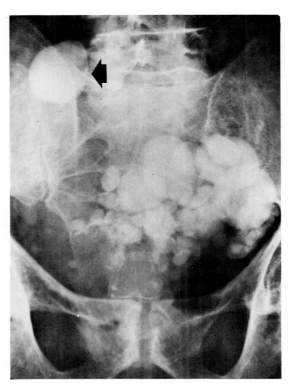

FIG. 28–4. Bladder calculi with prostatic hypertrophy. The isolated stone (*arrow*) is in a diverticulum of the bladder.

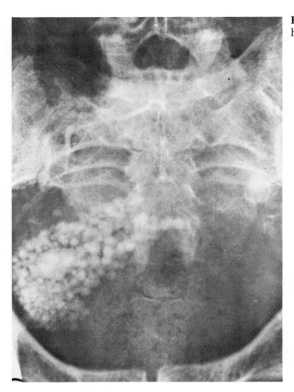

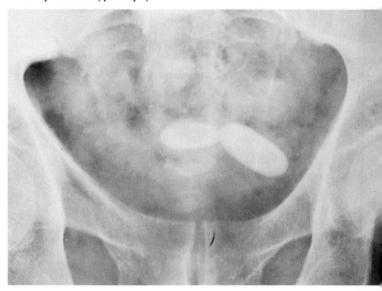

FIG. 28–5. Multiple bladder calculi in a case of prostatic hypertrophy.

FIG. 28–6. Bladder stones with translucent center in a case of prostatic hypertrophy.

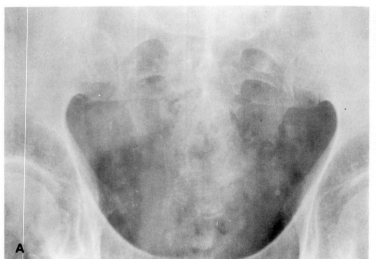

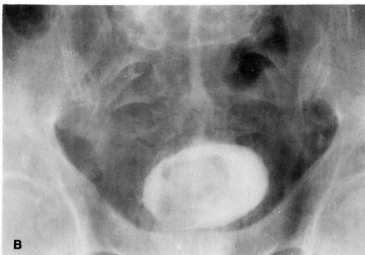

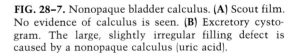

FIG. 28–7. Nonopaque bladder calculus. (A) Scout film. No evidence of calculus is seen. (B) Excretory cystogram. The large, slightly irregular filling defect is caused by a nonopaque calculus (uric acid).

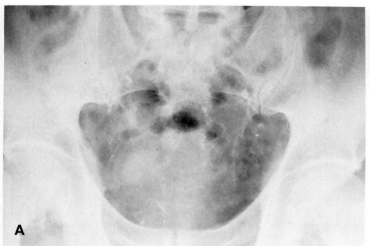

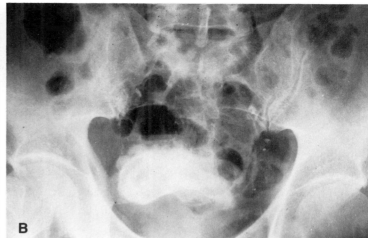

FIG. 28–8. Nonopaque bladder calculi. **(A)** Plain film of the pelvis showing a faint calcification in the right side of the bladder but no other areas of calcification seen. **(B)** On cystogram of the intravenous urogram, the faintly calcified stone on the right side is now seen as a filling defect, but several other stones are visualized as defects that could not be seen on the plain film.

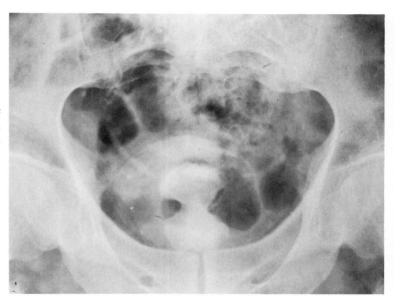

FIG. 28–9. Dumbbell-shaped calculus with the neck of the calculus at the bladder neck. The upper part of the calculus is in the bladder proper, and the lower part is in the prostatic cavity following a prostatectomy.

FIG. 28–10. Dumbbell-shaped calculus (postprostatectomy). *Arrow* points to region of bladder neck.

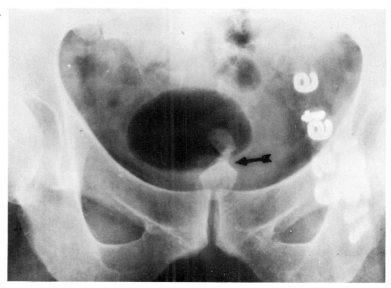

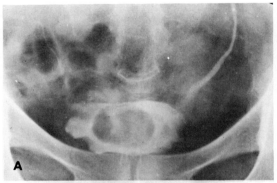

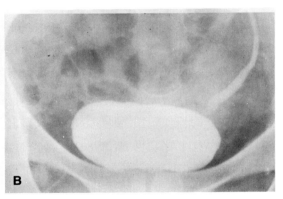

FIG. 28–11. Bladder calculus. Female with bladder neck contracture. **(A)** Defect in bladder owing to stone. Excretory cystogram. **(B)** Stone is obscured as more contrast material fills bladder. (Courtesy of J.J. Arnold, M.D.)

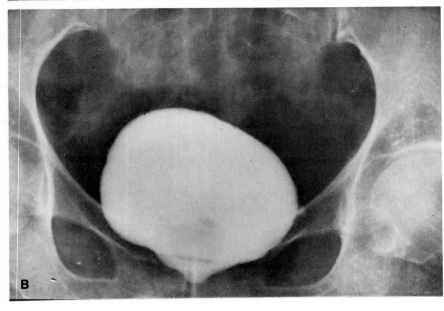

FIG. 28–12. Calculus in bladder. Female with mild cystocele and contracture of the bladder neck. **(A)** Scout film. Calculus seen above symphysis pubis. **(B)** Retrograde cystogram. Filling defect in bladder produced by calculus.

FIG. 28-13. Bladder calculus developing on foreign body. Female. Sponge apparently left in bladder 1 year previously. Stone formation now can be seen around the sponge. **(A)** Scout film revealing sponge impregnated with and surrounded by calcific material. **(B)** Cystogram reveals large defect in bladder corresponding to stone.

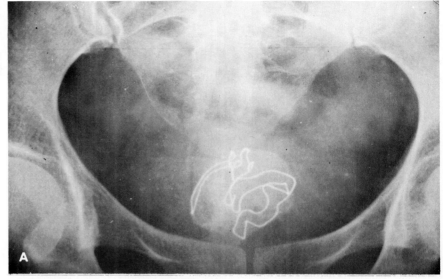

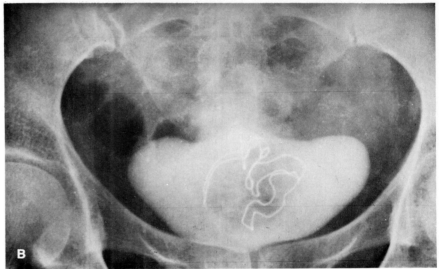

FIG. 28-14. Large bladder calculus in a case of schistosomiasis. (Courtesy of P. Jamison, M.D., Tanta, Egypt)

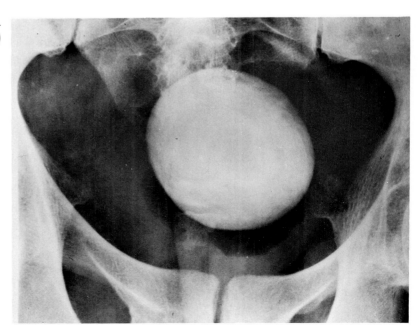

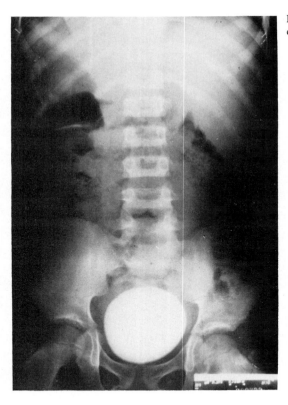

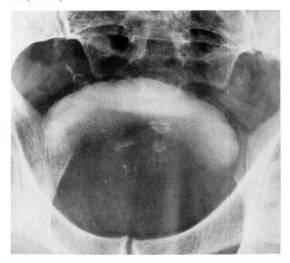

FIG. 28–15. Large bladder calculus in a Thai child. Endemic calculus.

FIG. 28–16. Scout film. Numerous fine calculi of the bladder in a case of hypertrophy of the prostate. Note nearly homogeneous character that gives appearance of milk of calcium stones. (Courtesy of Lennart Andersson, M.D.)

BIBLIOGRAPHY

1. Anderson, D.A.: Relationship between malnutrition and bladder stones. J. Christ. M.A. India, 34:154–161, 1959.
2. Anderson, D.A.: Nutritional significance of primary bladder stone. Br. J. Urol., 34:160, 1962.
3. Aurora, A.L., Tanejo, O.P., and Gupta, D.N.: Bladder stone disease of childhood. I. Epidemiological study. II. A clinicopathological study. Acta Paediatr. Scand., 59:177–184; 585–598, 1970.
4. Chutikorn, C., Valyasevi, A., and Halstead, S.B.: Studies of bladder stone disease in Thailand. II. Hospital Experience. Urolithiasis at Ubol Provincial Hospital, 1956–1962. Am. J. Clin. Nutr., 20:1320–1328, 1967.
5. Eckstein, H.B.: Harnsteine im Kindesalter. Z. Kindercher Grenzgsh, 2:451, 1965.
6. Kronberg, O., Ostergaard, A., Steven, K., et al.: Polyglycolic acid versus chromic catgut in bladder surgery. Br. J. Urol., 50:324–327, 1978.
7. Lagergren, C.: Biophysical investigations of urinary calculi, x-ray crystalographic and microdiagraphic study. Acta Radiol. (Stockholm) Suppl., 133:1–71, 1956.
8. Loutfi, A., and VanReen, R.: Studies of bladder stone disease in Egyptian children. I. Prospectus. J. Egypt. Med. Assoc., 57:89–95, 1974.
8a. Loutfi, A., VanReen, R., and Abdel-Hamid, G.: Studies of bladder stone disease in Egyptian children. II. Methodology and general aspects of the disease. J. Egypt. Med. Assoc., 57:96–108, 1974.
9. Lowsley, O.S., and Kirwin, T.J.: Clinical Urology. ed. 3, pp. 534–536. Baltimore, Williams and Wilkins, 1956.
10. Marks, L.S.: Vesico-ureteral reflux from foreign body calculus in the bladder. J. Urol., 112:516–518, 1974.
11. Naysan, P., Shulman, V., Pochaczevsky, R., et al.: Bladder stones in children. N.Y. State J. Med., 75:1288–1289, 1975.
12. Nygaard, E., and Terjesen, T.: Giant vesical calculi and anuria. Scand. J. Urol. Nephrol., 10:88–90, 1976.
13. Passmore, R.: Observations on the epidemiology of stone in the bladder in Thailand. Lancet, 1:638–640, 1953.
14. Potter, W.M., Greene, L.F., and Keating, F.R., Jr.: Vesical calculi and hyperparathyroidism. J. Urol., 96:203–206, 1966.
15. Squire, F.H., and Kretschmer, H.L.: Limitations of roentgen rays in diagnosis of bladder stones. J.A.M.A., 145:81–82, 1951.
16. Taneja, O.P.: Pathogenesis of ureteric reflux in vesical calculous disease of childhood. A clinical study. Br. J. Urol., 47:625–629, 1975.
17. Valyasevi, A., and VanReen, R.: Pediatric bladder stone disease; current status of research. J. Pediatr., 72:546–553, 1968.
18. VanRavenswaay, A.: Steel pin inserted into neck of femur found in bladder. Am. J. Surg., 31:566, 1936.
19. Walker, A.S., and Kaufman, D.R.: Spontaneous migration of a bullet into the urinary bladder after a 5-year interval. Urol. Cut. Rev., 46:217–219, 1942.
20. Williams, J.P.: Massive bladder stone. Br. J. Urol., 49:51–56, 1977.
21. Wishard, W.N., and Nourse, M.H.: Vesical calculus: report of a gigantic stone in female bladder. J. Urol., 63:794–801, 1950.

TRAUMA TO THE BLADDER

CLASSIFICATION

Injuries to the bladder may be produced by the following:

1. External penetrating agents, such as bullets, shell fragments, stab wounds, and bone fragments
2. Internal agents such as cystoscopes, resectoscopes, lithotrites, sounds, filiforms and followers, and catheters
3. Lower abdominal surgery including gynecologic procedures
4. Nonpenetrating agents:
   Blows to the lower abdomen, especially when the bladder is distended
   Fractures of the pelvis
5. Obstetric injuries
6. Spontaneous rupture

EXTERNAL PENETRATING AGENTS

These represent 10 to 25 per cent of cases of trauma to the urinary bladder.[18, 21] They often are associated with other abdominal visceral injuries. High-velocity missiles can produce extensive tissue injury.

INTERNAL AGENTS

The cystoscopes and resectoscopes are probably the most common causes of urinary bladder trauma. The injury in resections is usually caused by direct perforation, but explosions can occur secondary to hydrogen gas (formed from electrolytic or thermolytic decompression of tissue) mixed with air.[17] Indwelling Foley catheters can produce bladder perforation.[9, 20]

29

Trauma and Foreign Bodies of the Bladder

LOWER ABDOMINAL SURGERY INCLUDING
GYNECOLOGIC OPERATIONS

Gynecologic operations are not a common cause of bladder injury, but radical pelvic surgery for carcinoma and operations for endometriosis and pelvic inflammatory disease may result in bladder injury directly or secondary to impairment of the vasculature.

NONPENETRATING AGENTS

Most bladder injuries secondary to blunt trauma have associated pelvic fractures but only about 10 per cent of patients with pelvic fractures have ruptured bladders. Extraperitoneal rupture is often caused by fractured pelvis, but intraperitoneal rupture can occur in a distended bladder without pelvic fracture.

OBSTETRIC INJURIES

There are various types of obstetric injuries to the bladder: (1) injuries resulting from fetal head compressing bladder base against pubis in prolonged labor[30]: (2) cesarean section, a common cause of bladder injury; and (3) bladder rupture secondary to uterine rupture.[31] This is a common cause in the less-developed countries. The injury can be complete (through all layers of the bladder) or partial. Simultaneous rupture of the bladder and uterus may allow escape of fetus into bladder.[28, 29]

SPONTANEOUS RUPTURE

Rupture of the bladder without obvious cause, such as instrumentation or external trauma, is an unusual occurrence. It occurs under the following three conditions:[35] (1) disease of bladder, such as malignancy or cystitis; (2) obstruction of bladder; and (3) drugs such as carbachol (a parasympathomimetic agent).[49]

Spontaneous rupture, therefore, should not be called "spontaneous," because it is secondary to disease.[59] Rupture of a bladder diverticulum has been reported.[59]

The sequelae of ruptured bladder are hemorrhage, shock, and sepsis. Acute vesicoureteral reflux has followed trauma to bladder and urethra.[61] Another complication that has been reported is ureteral and periureteral fibrosis.[62]

TYPES AS DISTINGUISHED BY RADIOLOGIC TECHNIQUES

The types of injury recognizable by radiologic techniques are (1) contusions (only if associated with blood clots in the bladder); (2) intraperitoneal rupture (Figs. 29-1, 29-2); (3) extraperitoneal rupture (Figs.

29-3 to 29-5); (4) combined intraperitoneal and extraperitoneal rupture (Figs. 29-6 to 29-8); and (5) perivesical hemorrhage ("tear drop" bladder; Figs. 29-9 to 29-11).

The diagnosis of injuries of the bladder is made best by cystograms. First, a scout film is taken of the bladder area, including the pelvic bones. Second, AP and oblique films are made following injection of contrast material. Third, the contrast medium is removed from the bladder by means of urethral catheter, and another film is obtained.

CONTUSIONS

There is no break in the continuity of the bladder, and so there is no escape of urinary contents or injected contrast material from the bladder. This is a clinical diagnosis, but a roentgenogram will confirm it if blood clots are seen in the bladder when there is no injury to the rest of the genitourinary tract.

INTRAPERITONEAL RUPTURE

There is a tear in the bladder, with communication to the peritoneal cavity.

Radiologic Diagnosis. The contrast material accumulates in the peritoneal cavity near the dome of the bladder. The medium appears in a smooth, regular manner and not in streaks, a feathery, or a patchy fashion. Commonly, it extends laterally on either side from the dome of the bladder in a bandlike fashion. When it encloses the bowel, gas-filled defects are seen, surrounded by circular or partially circular segments of contrast medium. Along the paracolic recesses the small and the large bowels may give a scalloped effect to the bandlike patterns of contrast material. Occasionally, the contrast material can be seen around the liver margins.

EXTRAPERITONEAL RUPTURE OF THE BLADDER

There is a break in the bladder wall communicating with the extraperitoneal space.

Radiologic Diagnosis. The contrast medium overlies the lower half of the bladder and spreads distally in an irregular, occasionally feathery, and often streaky manner along fascial planes. The contrast medium usually extends upward and spreads out as it extends distally from the bladder. A subserosal extravasation presents an elliptical appearance (Fig. 29-12).

COMBINED INTRAPERITONEAL AND
EXTRAPERITONEAL RUPTURE.

This type of injury is a combination of the second and third types described previously. It has been stated that this particular injury represents 50 per cent of all bladder injuries, but we have found it to be much rarer.

Radiologic Diagnosis. The characteristics of both intraperitoneal and extraperitoneal rupture are seen in the same cystogram. At times the diagnosis is difficult because the contrast medium in the intraperitoneal portion may be obscured by extraperitoneal extravasations.

PERIVESICAL HEMORRHAGE

The extravesical hemorrhage can produce a "tear drop" bladder[19] without causing an actual rupture of the bladder, although in many instances the two are combined.

Radiologic Diagnosis. The bladder has a "tear drop" shape, is vertically elongated, and narrowed. It appears to be elevated above the symphysis pubis, and there may be a considerable space between the symphysis pubis and the base of the bladder. When the condition is combined with rupture of the bladder, the contrast material on cystograms appears in the extravesical space in the same manner as was described in extraperitoneal rupture of the bladder.

FOREIGN BODIES IN THE BLADDER

CLASSIFICATION BY ROUTE OF ENTRY

Foreign bodies may enter the bladder by any of the routes described in the following sections.

THE URETHRA

The introduction of the foreign body may be purposeful or accidental (Figs. 29–13, 29–14, 29–16). Purposeful introductions of an enormous variety of objects have been seen in intoxicated individuals, malingerers, the insane, and sexual perverts.

THE BOWEL

Occasionally, foreign bodies have passed through the wall of the bowel into the lumen of the bladder (Fig. 29–17). In most cases it is assumed that the bowel is adherent to the bladder. Cases have been reported in which swallowed foreign bodies have entered the bladder after an interval of 3 months. Young reported a case in which a needle migrated from the small intestine into the bladder.[77] Bond reported a case of a fistula of the ileum connecting with the bladder, in which numerous foreign bodies passed through the fistula and into the bladder.[76]

MIGRATION FROM TISSUES OUTSIDE THE BLADDER

The migration into the bladder may take place over a period of months or years. Usually, the foreign body is in the tissues adjacent to the bladder. The most common types of foreign bodies entering the bladder by this route are bullets, needles, or shrapnel fragments. Metallic pins utilized in hip pinning reportedly have migrated into the bladder.

DIRECT ENTRANCE

Through puncture wounds, such objects as bullets[92] and a wood splinter[91] have entered the bladder directly.

SURGICAL FOREIGN BODIES

This group consists of foreign bodies left at the time of surgery, such as sponges, needles, radon seeds, or fragments of indwelling catheters (Figs. 29–15, 29–18 to 29–20).

URETER AND KIDNEY

Foreign bodies in the kidney and the ureter (usually from instrumental catheters) may pass into the bladder.

RADIOLOGIC APPEARANCE

If the foreign body is opaque, identification is simple on a routine roentgenogram. Nonopaque foreign bodies are identified best following injection of air or dilute contrast medium. Oblique and, rarely, lateral views are essential for localization. If a foreign body has been present in the bladder for any length of time, it frequently forms the nidus for a bladder calculus. However, foreign bodies have been present in the bladder for a considerable length of time without encrustation.

CHAPTER 29, ILLUSTRATIONS

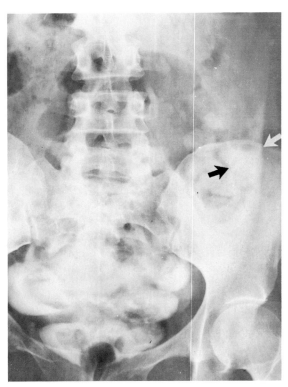

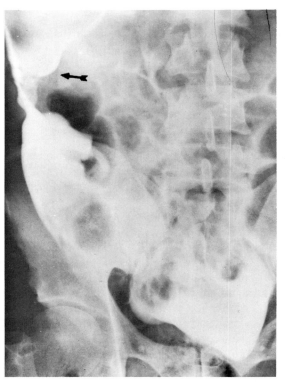

FIG. 29–1. Intraperitoneal rupture of the bladder. Young woman fell from a high building. Cystogram reveals contrast material escaping from upper part of bladder and appearing in a smooth, regular bandlike fashion. Where the contrast material encircles bowel, there are gas-filled defects surrounded by partially circular segments. *Arrows* outline contrast medium in paracolic recesses. There is a fracture of the pelvic ring in the region of the right obturator foramen.

FIG. 29–2. Intraperitoneal rupture of the bladder. Automobile accident. Contrast medium is escaping from dome of bladder in bandlike fashion. On right, a circular segment with a gas-filled central portion is visualized. Notice contrast medium along paracolic recesses. *Arrow* points to contrast medium under liver edge.

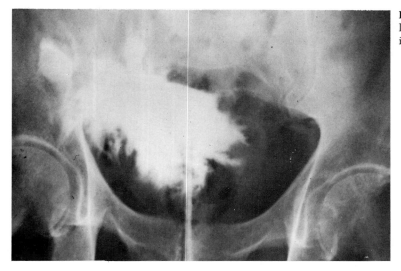

FIG. 29–3. Extraperitoneal rupture of the bladder following cystoscopy. Contrast medium is spreading out irregularly from bladder area.

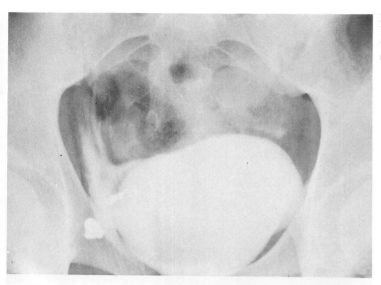

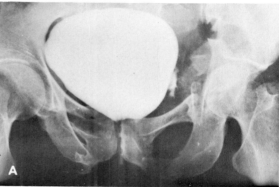

FIG. 29–4. Retroperitoneal rupture of the bladder from a bullet injury. There is diffuse spread of the contrast material into the extraperitoneal space. Note the pieces of schrapnel. (Courtesy of Keith Waterhouse, M.D.)

FIG. 29–5. Extraperitoneal rupture of the bladder. Automobile accident. (**A**) Retrograde cystogram. The contrast material can be seen outside the bladder on the left, adjacent to a fragment of bone which had penetrated the bladder. (**B**) Postevacuation film. Note contrast medium outside the bladder. *Arrow* points to the bone fragment.

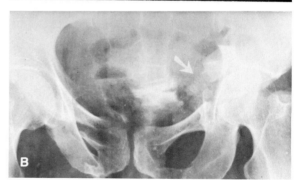

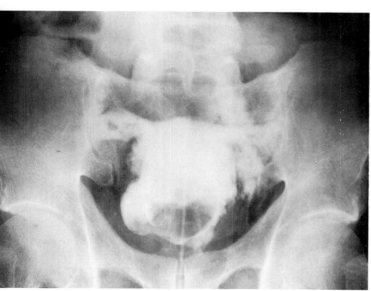

FIG. 29–6. Intraperitoneal and extraperitoneal rupture of the bladder as a result of transurethral prostatic resection. Contrast medium is seen above the bladder on either side, spreading laterally; on the left side there is some extraperitoneal leakage. On the right side at the dome contrast medium is escaping intraperitoneally. At exploration an opening was found in the peritoneal cavity.

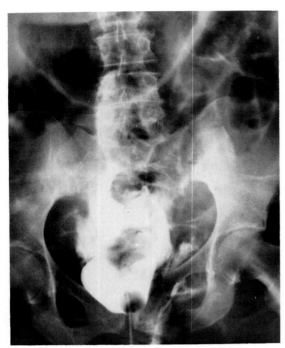

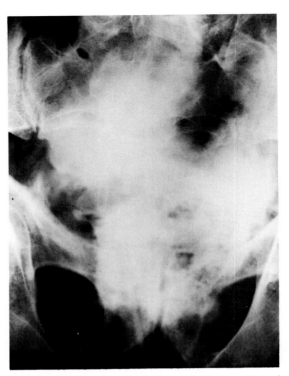

FIG. 29–7. Intra- and extraperitoneal rupture of the bladder. Note extravasation retroperitoneally on the left side of the bladder and the intraperitoneal rupture directly above the bladder.

FIG. 29–8. Rupture at the bladder neck. Extraperitoneal extravasation of contrast medium (left side of bladder) following a transurethral resection of the bladder neck. In addition there is an intraperitoneal collection of contrast material (at dome), most likely owing to rupture caused by overdistention of the bladder.

FIG. 29–9. "Tear drop" bladder. Extravesical hemorrhage but no rupture of bladder. The bladder is elongated and elevated. Note fractures of pubic rami. (Courtesy of George Prather, M.D.)

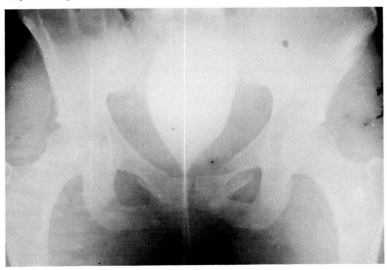

FIG. 29–10. Extraperitoneal rupture of the bladder due to an automobile accident. *Arrow* points to contrast medium that has extravasated on the right side. The bladder is elongated and elevated ("tear drop"). There are bilateral severe pelvic fractures.

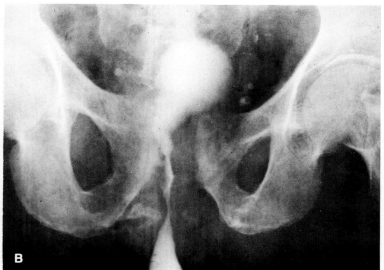

FIG. 29–11. Rupture of the bladder at the bladder neck following an automobile accident. **(A)** Marked retroperitoneal extravasation of contrast material with a "tear drop" bladder. There is a wide separation of the symphysis pubis. **(B)** Three months later, showing marked distortion of the posterior urethra and marked contraction of the bladder. The symphysis now is improved greatly.

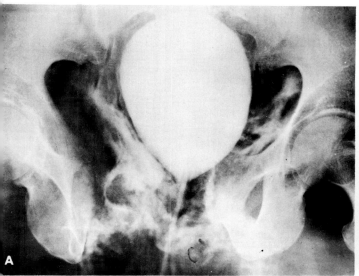

FIG. 29–12. Subserosal rupture of the bladder. Notice collection of contrast under the serosal surface of the bladder, producing a more or less smooth elliptic shape.

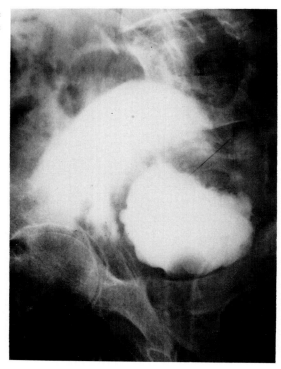

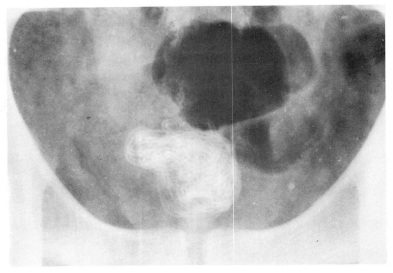

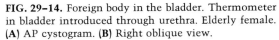

FIG. 29–13. Foreign body in the bladder. Wire insulation in the bladder. Man. The foreign body was introduced through the urethra.

FIG. 29–14. Foreign body in the bladder. Thermometer in bladder introduced through urethra. Elderly female. **(A)** AP cystogram. **(B)** Right oblique view.

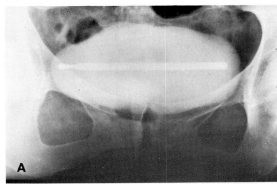

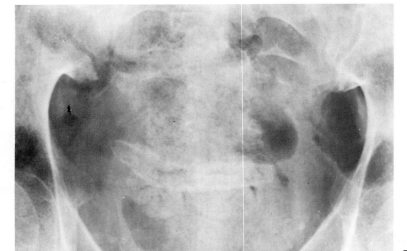

FIG. 29–15. Foreign body in the bladder. Portion of broken Foley catheter left in bladder. Female.

FIG. 29–16. Foreign body in the bladder. Stone formed around nail in bladder. Man. Nail was introduced through the urethra. (Courtesy of F.C. McClellan, M.D.)

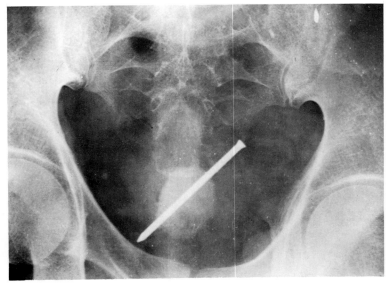

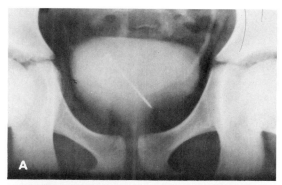

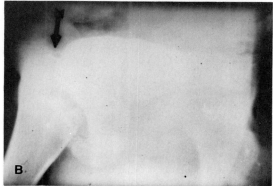

FIG. 29–17. Foreign body in the bladder. **(A)** Pin in urinary bladder. Seven-year-old boy who had swallowed a pin 3 months previously. **(B)** Oblique view reveals the head of pin is outside bladder (*arrow*). At operation small bowel was adherent to bladder, and head of pin was still present in the bowel, with the body of the pin in the bladder lumen.

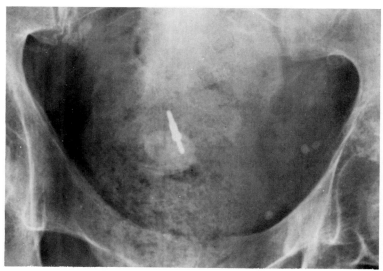

FIG. 29–18. Foreign body in the bladder. Stone formation around a broken extractor. Man.

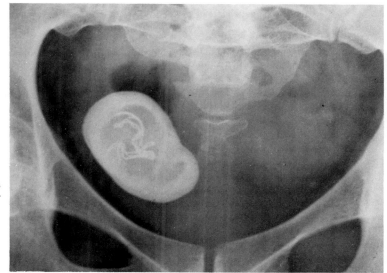

FIG. 29–19. Foreign body in the bladder. Calculus formed around gauze. Cystocele was repaired 1 year previously.

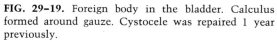

FIG. 29–20. Foreign body in the bladder. Stone formation around a surgical needle left in wall of urinary bladder. Hysterectomy had been performed 20 years previously, and there had been three subsequent operations for vesicovaginal fistula. (Courtesy of A.A. Solomon, M.D.)

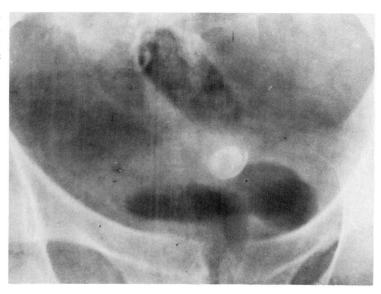

BIBLIOGRAPHY

Trauma to the Bladder

1. Bacon, S.K.: Rupture of the urinary bladder. J. Urol., *49*:432–435, 1943.
2. Cahill, G.F.: Rupture of bladder and urethra. Am. J. Surg., *36*:653–662, 1937.
3. Campbell, M.F.: Rupture of the bladder. Surg. Gynecol. Obstet., *49*:540–546, 1929.
3a. Carswell, J.W.: Intraperitoneal rupture of the bladder. Br. J. Urol., *46*:425–429, 1974.
4. Cohen, M.S., Warner, R.S., Fish, L., et al.: Bladder perforation after orthopedic hip surgery. Urology, *9*:291–293, 1977.
5. Coplan, M., Woods, F.M., and Melvin, P.D.: Surgical repair of the lower ureters and bladder which had been injured during pelvic surgery. J. Urol., *73*:790–793, 1953.
6. Crane, J., and Schenck, G.: Rupture of the urinary bladder. Urol. Cut. Rev., *36*:614–619, 1932.
7. DeWeerd, J.H.: Management of injuries to the bladder, urethra and genitalia. Surg. Clin. North Am., *39*:973–987, 1959.
8. Holm, O.: Rupture of bladder. Diagnosis of injury. Acta Radiol., *24*:198–205, 1943.
9. Hughes, P., Gambee, J., and Edwards, C.: Perforation of the bladder: a complication of long-dwelling Foley catheter. J. Urol., *109*:237, 1973.
10. Kenyon, H.R.: Perforations in transurethral operations: technique for immediate diagnosis and management of extravasations. J.A.M.A., *142*:798–802, 1950.
11. Kicklighter, J.E.: Traumatic rupture of the urinary bladder. South. Med. J., *47*:837–841, 1954.
12. Lynch, K.M., Jr.: Traumatic urinary injury: pitfalls in their diagnosis and treatment. J. Urol., *77*:90–95, 1957.
13. McCague, E.J., and Semans, J.H.: The management of traumatic rupture of the urethra and bladder complicating fracture of the pelvis. J. Urol., *52*:36–41, 1944.
14. Michels, L.M.: Wounds of the urinary bladder: an analysis of 155 cases. Ann. Surg., *123*:999–1002, 1946.
15. Miller, G.: Catheter-induced hemorrhagic pseudopolyps of the urinary bladder. J.A.M.A., *193*:968–969, 1965.
16. Montie, J.: Bladder injuries. Urol. Clin. North Am., *4*:59–67, 1977.
17. Ning, T.C., Jr., Atkins, D.M., and Murphy, R.C.: Bladder explosions during transurethral surgery. J. Urol., *114*:536–539, 1975.
18. Ochsner, T.G., Busch, F.M., and Clarke, R.L.: Urogenital wounds in Vietnam. J. Urol., *101*:224–225, 1969.
19. Prather, G.C., and Kaiser, T.F.: The bladder in fracture of the bony pelvis; significance of "tear drop bladder." J. Urol., *63*:1019–1030, 1950.
20. Rubinstein, A., Benaroya, Y., and Rubinstein, E.: Foley catheter perforation of the urinary bladder. J.A.M.A., *136*:822, 1976.
21. Salvatierra, O., Jr., Rigdon, W.O., Morris, D.M., et al.: Vietnam experience with 252 urological war injuries. J. Urol., *101*:615–630, 1969.
22. Stevens, A.R., and Delzell, W.R.: Traumatic injuries of the bladder. J. Urol., *38*:475–485, 1937.
23. Stirling, W.C., and Belt, N.: Traumatic rupture of the bladder, with perivesical extravasations. J.A.M.A., *92*:2006–2009, 1929.
24. Van Buskirk, K.E., and Kimbrough, J.C.: Urological surgery in combat. J. Urol., *71*:639–646, 1954.
25. Weens, H.S., Newman, J.H., and Florence, T.J.: Trauma of the lower urinary tract. N. Engl. J. Med., *234*:357–366, 1946.

Rupture of the Bladder in the Newborn and Children

26. Donahue, J.P.: Ureteral and bladder injuries in children. Ped. Clin. North Am., *22*:393–399, 1975.
27. Miller, A.L., Jr., Sharp, L., Anderson, E.V., and Emlet, J.R.: Rupture of the bladder in the newborn. J. Urol., *83*:630–633, 1960.

Obstetrical Causes of Rupture of the Bladder

28. Davis, N.S.: A case of rupture of the uterus and bladder with escape of foetus into the bladder. J. Obstet. Gynaecol. Br. Commonw., *69*:140–141, 1962.
29. Hassim, A.M., Lucas, C., and Acharya, R.J.: Fetal survival after partial extrusion into the bladder. Br. Med. J., *1*:286–287, 1972.
30. Linke, C.A., Linke, C.L., and Worden, A.C.: Bladder and urethral injuries following prolonged labor. J. Urol., *105*:679–682, 1971.
31. Raghavaiah, N.V., and Devi, A.I.: Bladder surgery associated with rupture of the uterus. Obstet. Gynecol., *46*:573–576, 1975.
32. Rous, S.N., Major, F., and Gordon, M.: Rupture of the bladder secondary to uterine vacuum curettage: a case report and review of the literature. J. Urol., *186*:685–686, 1971.
33. Sarkar, A.N.: Spontaneous intraperitoneal rupture of the bladder in association with displaced gravid uterus. J. Ind. Med. Assoc., *13*:113–114, 1944.
34. Torpin, R.: Spontaneous rupture of the bladder in labor. Urol. Cut. Rev., *44*:553–557, 1940.

Spontaneous Rupture

35. Altman, B., and Horsburgh, A.G.: Spontaneous rupture of the bladder. Br. J. Urol., *38*:85–88, 1966.
36. Bacon, S.K.: Rupture of the urinary bladder. J. Urol., *49*:432–435, 1943.
37. Barnes, R.W., and Steele, A.A.: Spontaneous intraperitoneal rupture of the normal urinary bladder. J.A.M.A., *105*:1758, 1935.
38. Bastable, J.R.G., DeJode, L.R., and Warren, R.P.: Spontaneous rupture of the bladder. Br. J. Urol., *31*:78–86, 1959.
39. Beresford-Jones, A.B.: Spontaneous rupture of the bladder in the female. Br. J. Surg., *29*:154–156, 1941.
40. Clinton-Thomas, C.L.: Idiopathic spontaneous rupture of bladder. Br. J. Urol., *27*:235–238, 1955.
41. Crastnopol, P., Artz, R., and Rosett, L.: Recurrent spontaneous rupture of the urinary bladder. Arch. Surg., *60*:1093–1101, 1950.
42. Daines, S.L., and Hodgson, N.B.: Spontaneous rupture of a necrotic bladder. J. Urol., *102*:431–433, 1969.
43. Feigal, W.N., and Polzak, J.A.: Spontaneous rupture of the urinary bladder. J. Urol., *56*:196–199, 1946.
44. Hammar, B.: Spontaneous rupture of the bladder. Br. J. Urol., *33*:289–291, 1961.
45. Hershman, H., and Allen, H.L.: Spontaneous rupture of the normal urinary bladder. Surgery, *35*:805–808, 1954.

46. Innis, C.: Spontaneous intraperitoneal rupture of the urinary bladder. Br. J. Surg., 49:173–174, 1961.

47. Jones, A.: Spontaneous rupture intraperitoneally of the urinary bladder. N. Engl. J. Med., 210:1262–1264, 1934.

48. Lipow, E.G., and Vogel, J.: Spontaneous rupture of the bladder. J. Urol., 47:277–282, 1942.

49. Macalister, C.L.O.: Spontaneous rupture of urinary bladder. Proc. Roy. Soc. Med., 48:693–697, 1955.

50. Marbury, W.B., and Fry, W.: Spontaneous rupture of urinary bladder. Ann. Surg., 117:760–765, 1943.

51. Moroney, J.: A case of spontaneous rupture of tuberculous bladder. Br. J. Surg., 31:98, 1943.

52. Nemser, M.A., and Weinberger, H.A.: Spontaneous rupture of the urinary bladder in the male. J. Urol., 68:603–607, 1952.

53. Oppenheimer, G.D., and Druckerman, L.J.: Recurrent nontraumatic intraperitoneal rupture of the urinary bladder. J. Urol., 57:238–241, 1941.

54. Pole, F.: Recurrent non-traumatic rupture of the urinary bladder. Va. Med. Mon., 71:477–478, 1944.

55. Saphir, O., and Shapiro, I.J.: Fatty infiltration of urinary bladder with spontaneous rupture. Am. J. Surg., 29:263–267, 1935.

56. Stone, E.: Spontaneous rupture of the bladder. Arch. Surg., 23:129–144, 1931.

57. Taylor, R.A.: Spontaneous rupture of urinary bladder. Br. J. Urol., 20:117–120, 1948.

58. Thomas, G.K.: Spontaneous rupture of bladder. Br. J. Surg., 44:328–330, 1956.

59. Thompson, I.M., Johnson, E.L., and Ross, G., Jr.: The acute abdomen of unrecognized bladder rupture. Arch. Surg., 90:371–374, 1965.

60. Yarwood, G.R.: Spontaneous rupture of normal urinary bladder. Br. J. Urol., 31:87–88, 1959.

Complications of Bladder Trauma

61. Marshall, V.R., Paris, A.M., Flynn, N.J., et al.: Acute vesicoureteral reflux following vesicourethral trauma. J. Urol., 112:593–594, 1974.

62. Rao, M.S., Bapna, B.C., and Vaidyanathan, S.: Ureteral and periureteral fibrosis as delayed sequelae to lower urinary tract injury. J. Urol., 113:610–613, 1975.

Foreign Bodies in the Bladder

General

63. Herwig, K.R., and Hubbard, H.: Iatrogenic foreign bodies of the urinary bladder. J.A.M.A., 210:1589–1590, 1969.

64. Lee, L.W.: Vesical foreign bodies I have known. Nebr. Med. J., 48:219–221, 1963.

65. Prasad, S., Smith, A.M., Uson, A., et al.: Foreign bodies in urinary bladder. Urology, 2:258–264, 1973.

Entering the Bladder From the Urethra

66. Bors, E.: The removal of a broken glass catheter from the female bladder. J. Urol., 49:658–659, 1943.

67. Brewer, A.C., and Marcus, R.: Foreign bodies in urinary bladder: an unusual case. Br. J. Surg., 35:324–325, 1948.

68. Dakin, W.B.: Urological Oddities. Privately printed, 1948.

69. Grossman, S.L., and Hottenstein, H.F.: Foreign bodies in the bladder: report of 3 cases. Urol. Cut. Rev., 41:788–791, 1937.

70. Katzen, P.: Paraffin foreign body in the bladder. J.A.M.A., 105:1422–1423, 1935.

71. Krugman, P.I., and Reiser, C.: Thermometer in the urinary bladder. Fertil. Steril., 3:263–265, 1952.

72. Schloss, W.A., and Solomkin, M.: Foreign body in bladder: removal of thermometer with Stern-McCarthy resectoscope. J.A.M.A., 143:804–805, 1950.

73. Turner, J.H.: Two unusual foreign bodies in male urinary bladder. J. Urol., 11:581–585, 1924.

74. Zeitlin, A.B., Cottrell, T.L., and Lloyd, F.A.: Hair as a lower urinary tract foreign body. J. Urol., 77:840–842, 1957.

Entering the Bladder From the Bowel

75. Baron, S., and Lipshutz, F.: Unusual foreign body ulcerating into bladder from the bowel. J. Urol., 58:112–113, 1947.

76. Bond, S.P.: Foreign bodies in the bladder. J.A.M.A., 83:1163, 1924.

77. Young, H.H.: Removal from bladder, through the cystoscope, of a needle which had been swallowed 9 years before. Am. Med., 3:63–64, 1902.

Migrating into the Bladder From Tissues Outside the Bladder

78. Alpers, D.D.: Migration of broken hip pin into urinary bladder. J.A.M.A., 212:2123–2124, 1970.

79. Branham, D.W., and Richey, H.M.: Foreign body (Kirschner wire) removed from bladder. J. Urol., 57:869, 1947.

80. Bors, E., and Bowie, C.F.: Migration of foreign bodies with report of case of migration of a shell fragment into the bladder. J. Urol., 55:358–362, 1947.

81. Fitzpatrick, R.J.: Unusual foreign body (Steinman pin) in bladder. J.A.M.A., 170:671–672, 1959.

82. Floyd, E., and Pittman, J.L.: Transmigration of the head of the femur into the urinary bladder. Urol. Cut. Rev., 45:303–304, 1941.

83. Fullerton, A.: Observations on bladder injury in warfare. A study of 53 cases. Br. J. Surg., 6:24–56, 1918.

84. Grant, O.: An unusual foreign body (bone peg) in the bladder. J.A.M.A., 107:1632–1633, 1936.

85. Jalundhwala, J.M.: An unusual foreign body (guide wire) in bladder. Br. J. Urol., 34:335–337, 1962.

86. Lattimer, J.K.: Late erosion of shell fragment into the bladder. J. Urol., 55:483–485, 1946.

87. Saronwala, K.C., Ravindersingh, M.S., and Dass, H.: Lippes loop perforation of the uterus and urinary bladder with stone formation. Obstet. Gynecol., 44:424–427, 1974.

88. Van Ravenswaay, Alex: Steel pin inserted into neck of femur found in bladder. Am. J. Surg., 31:566, 1936.

89. Walker, A.S., and Kaufman, D.R.: Spontaneous migration of a bullet into the urinary bladder, after a five-year interval. Urol. Cut. Rev., 46:217–219, 1942.

90. Wells: Quoted by Thomson-Walker. In Disease of the Genito-Urinary System. ed. 2, p. 553. Baltimore, Wood, 1936.

Direct Entrance into the Bladder Through Puncture Wounds

91. Crane, J.J., and Moody, E.E.: A splinter of wood lodged in the urinary bladder. J.A.M.A., 104:1702–1703, 1935.

92. Luys, G.: Extraction of a rifle bullet from the bladder, from a natural route. N.Y. State J. Med., 111:181–183, 1920.

Foreign Bodies Left in the Bladder as a Result of Surgical Procedure

93. Chute, R.: Bladder calculi formed around retained fragments of ruptured foley catheter balloons. J. Urol., 87:355–358, 1962.

94. Marconis, J.T.: Foreign body in bladder with unusual aspects. J. Urol., 86:400–402, 1951.

A fistula is an abnormal communication between two epithelial surfaces. A sinus is a blind tract connecting a cavity with the skin or a mucous surface.

CLASSIFICATION

Sinus
    Vesicocutaneous
    Vesicoretroperitoneal
Fistula
    Males
        Vesicointestinal (vesicoenteric)
            Vesico–small bowel
            Vesicocolonic
            Vesicorectal
            Vesicoappendiceal
    Females
        Vesicointestinal
            Vesico–small bowel
            Vesicocolonic
            Vesicorectal
            Vesicoappendiceal
        Vesicouterine
        Vesicovaginal
        Vesicovaginal–intestinal

The vesicocutaneous sinus in both sexes is usually secondary to an operative procedure. It is rarely congenital except in cases of patent urachus. Vesicoretroperitoneal sinuses result from operations, inflammations, and malignancies of bladder and bowel.

Vesicointestinal Fistulas. The congenital variety is associated with imperforate anus and the cloacal process.

In acquired vesicointestinal fistulas, diverticulitis (Figs. 30–1, 30–2) represents 51 per cent, colorectal carcinoma (Figs. 30–3 to 30–6) 16 per cent, Crohn's disease (Figs. 30–7 to 30–9) 12 per cent, and bladder

30

Vesical Fistulas

carcinoma (Figs. 30–10 to 30–13) 5 per cent.[9] Additional causes are surgical injury (transurethral or open prostatectomy), irradiation (Figs. 30–16, 30–22, 30–23), foreign bodies, and abscesses (Figs. 30–14, 30–15), such as prostatic or pelvic. In general, small-bowel–vesical fistulas are secondary to inflammation such as granulomatous disease of the ileum (Crohn's disease) or foreign bodies. Large-bowel-vesical fistulas are most commonly the result of diverticulitis, with carcinoma of the colon second.

In the majority of intestinal-vesical fistulas, regardless of etiology, there is usually abscess formation (Figs. 30–3, 30–7) with final breakthrough into the bladder. There are two routes of involvement: (1) actual adherence to the bladder by abscess formation and later rupture into the bladder, and (2) extension of an inflammatory process along the ureter or the mesosigmoid to the bladder base and then to the bladder. The most common site of fistula formation is on the left side of the posterior wall of the bladder, with the next most common site being the bladder dome. Neoplastic diseases producing vesicointestinal fistulas are primarily carcinomas of the intestinal tract and less commonly carcinomas of the bladder.

Vesicoappendiceal Fistulas. A fistulous tract between the appendix and bladder has been reported in as high as 5 per cent of enterovesical fistulas (described in the surgical literature[40]) but is probably much rarer (Figs. 30–17, 30–18). Males predominate 5 to 1. This type has been found in children.[37, 50, 50a] The opening is usually on the right side of the bladder and may not be visualized because of a mass of granulomatous tissue or a depressed necrotic area that may be the only sign of a fistula.[49] Prolapse of appendiceal mucosa into the bladder may simulate neoplasm.[41, 48] Pneumaturia has occurred. Occasionally, feces, pus, or a small wormlike mass may be seen protruding from the opening.[41a]

ROENTGENOGRAPHIC FINDINGS. Roentgenograms rarely depict the fistula.

Vesicouterine Fistulas. Vesicouterine fistulas are rare (Figs. 30–19, 30–19a). The most common single cause is cesarean section. In underdeveloped areas, rupture of the uterus and bladder has occurred during pregnancy, and connections have occurred (see Chapter 29, Trauma and Foreign Bodies of the Bladder). There are two types of vesicouterine fistulas: (1) The fistula is below the internal os. In this case, the patient experiences urinary incontinence through the cervical canal plus normal menses but may have blood through the urethra. (2)

The fistula is above the uterine isthmus. In this case, there is menstrual discharge through the urethra in the presence of a patent cervical canal without involuntary loss of urine.

The explanation for the phenomenon is a sphincteric action at the uterine isthmus preventing the passage of urine or menstrual blood.[67] It is a high-pressure sphincter, which is normally opened by distention of the uterine cavity by menstrual blood. Contrast medium injected into the bladder in this type does not often leak through the cervix.

Vesicovaginal Fistula. Vesicovaginal fistula (Figs. 30–20, 30–21) may be caused by injury, such as pelvic fractures, penetrating injuries, obstetric injuries, gynecologic operations, radium therapy, or malignant disease of the bladder, the cervix, the uterus, and, rarely, the vagina. The most common cause today is gynecologic surgery, particularly total hysterectomy for benign disease and radical hysterectomy for carcinoma of the uterus, the cervix, or the ovary. The fistulas almost always are high up in the vaginal vault in the anterior wall and at the level of or slightly above the vesical trigone.

Vesicovaginal–intestinal fistulas (Figs. 30–22, 30–23) are complicated fistulas, often the result of radical gynecologic surgery plus irradiation.

ROENTGENOGRAPHIC DIAGNOSIS

Cystograms are important in demonstrating a fistula between the bladder and any other organ. Frontal, both oblique, and even lateral views may be necessary. In cases of vesicointestinal involvement there may be a prodromal stage in which an abscess or a tumor or both may be diagnosed before fistulization has taken place.[18] The earliest sign of such prodromal involvement may be a crescent-shaped defect ("herald" sign[24]) in the upper margin of the bladder. This sometimes is seen best on oblique films. This defect may represent a perivesical abscess.[17] Later, one may see an actual intraluminal mass on air cystogram or a filling defect intraluminally when contrast medium is used. At this stage there has been involvement of the bladder wall. Actual fistulization can be diagnosed by the appearance of gas in the bladder or by demonstration of a connection between the bladder and the bowel by contrast medium.

Barium enemas may occasionally add information on the presence of a vesicointestinal fistula, but they actually may be positive in only about 20 per cent of cases. Proctoscopy also may be positive in only 14 per cent of cases.[9]

CHAPTER 30, ILLUSTRATIONS

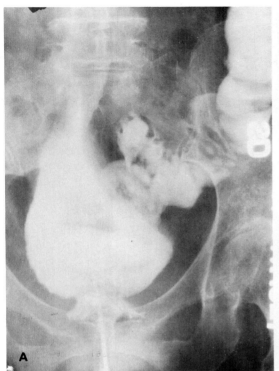

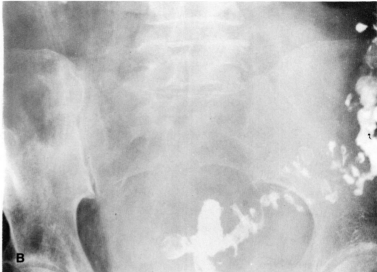

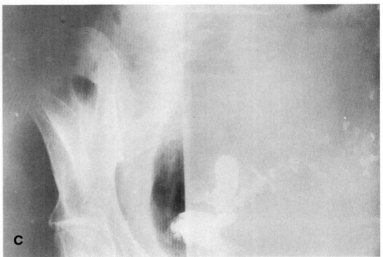

FIG. 30-1. Vesicocolonic fistula secondary to diverticulitis of colon. **(A)** Retrograde cystogram showing fistulous tract between bladder and sigmoid colon. Bladder is compressed on the left superior surface by an extravesical mass (abscess formation). **(B)** Showing diverticula of bowel. Gas-filled bladder is displaced to right by pelvic mass. **(C)** Left lateral decubitus film showing fluid level in bladder. Gas entered bladder from the bowel.

FIG. 30-2. Vesicocolonic fistula caused by diverticulitis. Cystogram shows contrast medium entering sigmoid colon.

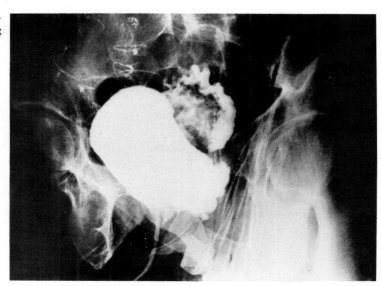

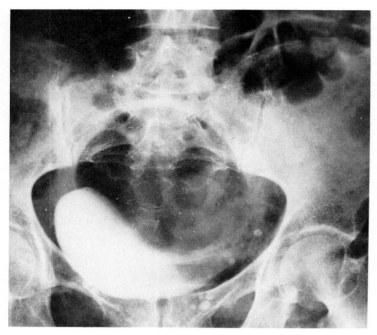

FIG. 30–3. Gas-filled abscess from carcinoma of sigmoid. Note small amount of gas in bladder.

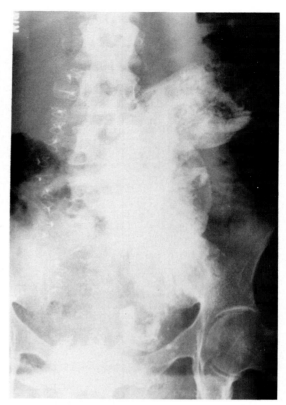

FIG. 30–4. Vesicocolonic fistula from carcinoma of colon. Cystogram shows contrast medium entering large bowel.

FIG. 30–5. Carcinoma of sigmoid with extension to bladder. (A) Cystogram shows fistula to bowel. (B) Later increased amount of contrast medium.

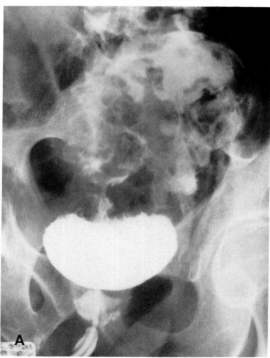

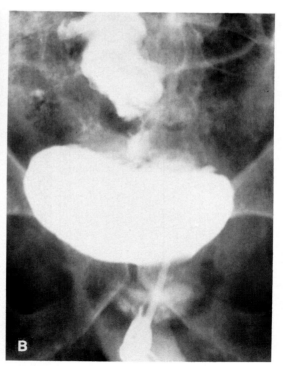

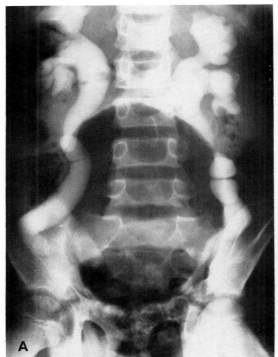
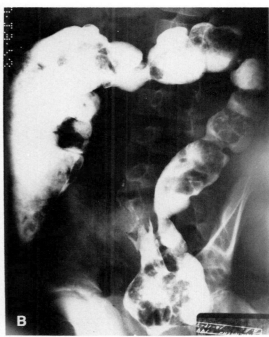

FIG. 30–6. Vesicosigmoid fistula from carcinoma of sigmoid. **(A)** Intravenous urogram; dilated upper tracts, gas-filled bladder. **(B)** Barium enema; contrast medium enters bladder.

FIG. 30–7. Perivesical abscess from regional ileitis. **(A)** Bladder is essentially normal. **(B)** Same case 5 days later showing a huge perivesical abscess causing a pressure defect in the upper surface of the bladder. (Courtesy of Mt. Sinai Hospital, New York, N.Y.)

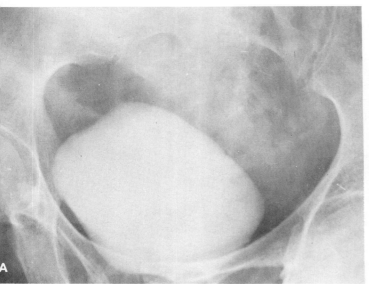
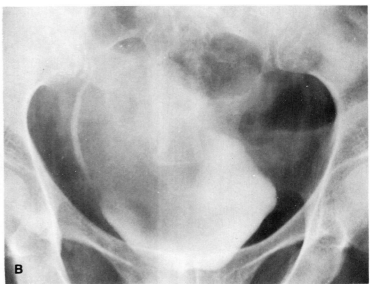

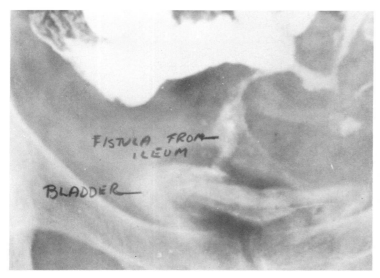

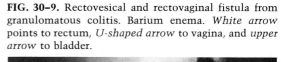

FIG. 30–8. Fistula from ileum into bladder secondary to regional ileitis. (Courtesy of Mt. Sinai Hospital, New York, N.Y.)

FIG. 30–9. Rectovesical and rectovaginal fistula from granulomatous colitis. Barium enema. *White arrow* points to rectum, *U-shaped arrow* to vagina, and *upper arrow* to bladder.

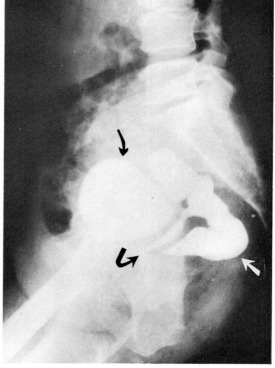

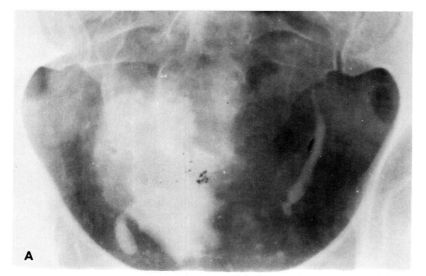

FIG. 30–10. Vesicorectosigmoid fistula from carcinoma of bladder. (A) Intravenous urogram showing extensive filling defect left side of bladder. (B) Retrograde cystogram showing fistulous tract between bladder (over symphysis) and rectosigmoid. The contrast medium in the colon is from cystourethrogram. (Courtesy of Sol Unger, M.D.)

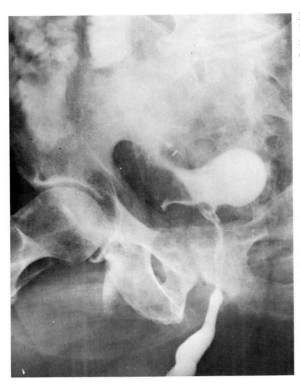

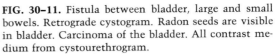

FIG. 30–11. Fistula between bladder, large and small bowels. Retrograde cystogram. Radon seeds are visible in bladder. Carcinoma of the bladder. All contrast medium from cystourethrogram.

FIG. 30–12. Carcinoma of bladder invading sigmoid colon. Barium enema; contrast medium entering bladder (*arrow*).

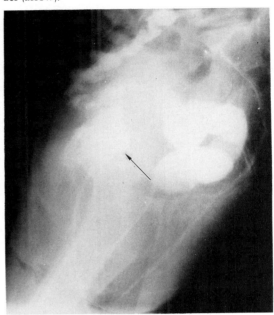

FIG. 30–13. Vesico-ileal fistula. Carcinoma of the bladder. Fistula occurred following fulguration. (**A**) Cystogram. AP view. *Arrow* points to contrast material entering ileum. (**B**) Oblique view. *Arrow* points to ileum filled with contrast material.

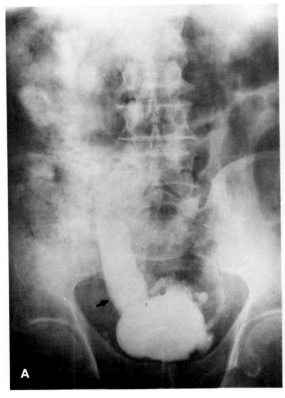

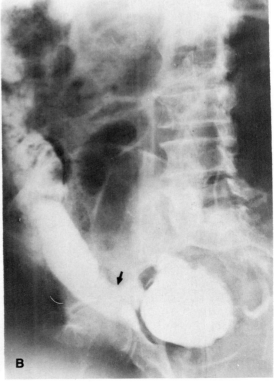

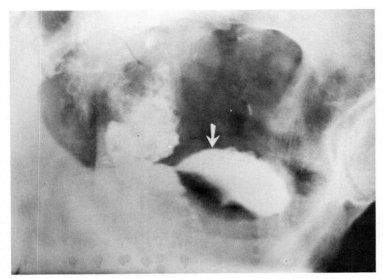

FIG. 30–14. Vesicorectal fistula following prostatic abscess. Abscess ruptured into the bladder and the rectum, thereby producing a fistula. Left oblique view. *Arrow* points to bladder. Fistulous tract between bladder and rectum is visualized. (Courtesy of Sol Unger, M.D., Veterans' Adminstration)

FIG. 30–16. Vesicocolonic fistula secondary to irradiation for carcinoma of cervix.

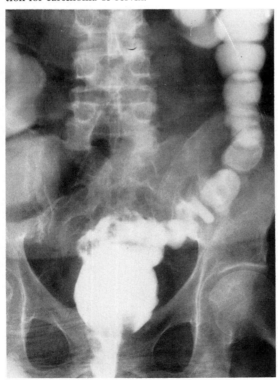

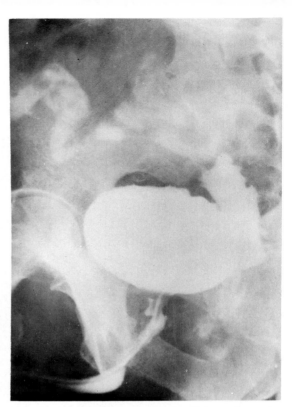

FIG. 30–15. Vesicoenteric fistula. Retrograde cystogram. Right oblique view. Repeated pelvic abscesses following rupture of large bowel while irrigating colostomy. Previous abdominal perineal excision of rectum for carcinoma. Contrast medium can be seen entering small bowel at posterior surface of bladder.

FIG. 30–17. Appendiceal vesical fistula. *Arrow* points to bladder, filled on a barium enema. Actual point of fistulation is not visualized. Confirmed at operation. (Courtesy of Mt. Sinai Hospital, New York, N.Y.)

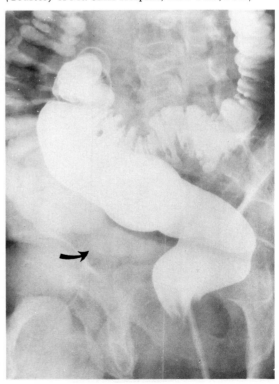

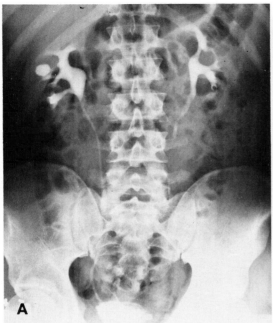

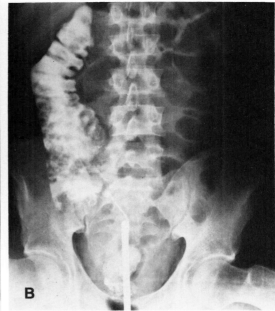

FIG. 30–18. Appendicovesical fistula. **(A)** Intravenous pyelogram demonstrates calyceal diverticulum in right kidney. Remainder of upper tracts and bladder outline are normal. **(B)** In retrograde study, injection of urographic contrast medium through a ureteral catheter passed transurethrally into appendicovesical fistula filling cecum and ascending colon. (Carson, C.C., Malek, R.H., and Remine, W.H.: J. Urol., *119*:744, 1978)

FIG. 30–19a. Vesicouterine fistula post cesarean section. The bladder is indicated by the *large arrow*, the fistulous tract, by the *small arrow*. (Courtesy of M. Leon Tancer, M.D.)

FIG. 30–19. Vesical uterine fistula following a cesarean section. Cystogram reveals contrast material entering the uterine cavity (*arrow*).

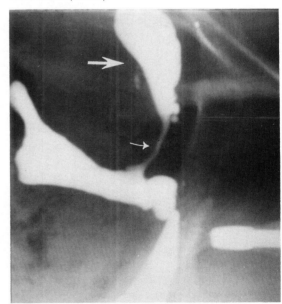

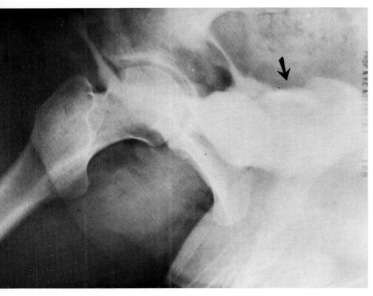

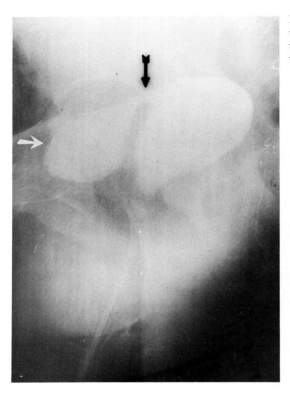

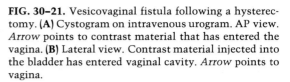

FIG. 30–20. Vesicovaginal fistula following a hysterectomy. Lateral view. *Black arrow* points to fistulous tract between bladder and vagina. *White arrow* points to bladder.

FIG. 30–21. Vesicovaginal fistula following a hysterectomy. (**A**) Cystogram on intravenous urogram. AP view. *Arrow* points to contrast material that has entered the vagina. (**B**) Lateral view. Contrast material injected into the bladder has entered vaginal cavity. *Arrow* points to vagina.

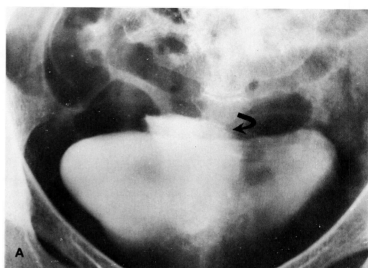

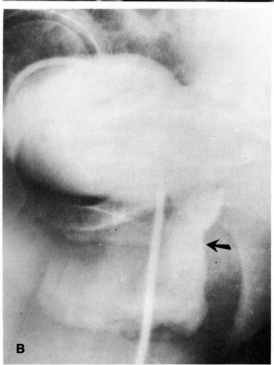

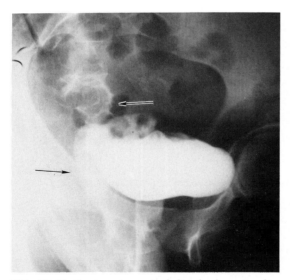

FIG. 30–22. Rectovesicovaginal fistula from irradiation for carcinoma of cervix. *Black arrow* points to the vagina, *white arrow* to the sigmoid.

FIG. 30–23. Carcinoma of cervix: operation, radiation therapy, and radium. Vesicovaginal, vesicocolonic, and vesico–small-bowel fistulas. *Straight black arrow* points to bladder; *curved black arrow* to small bowel; *straight white arrow* to rectum; and *curved white arrow* to vagina.

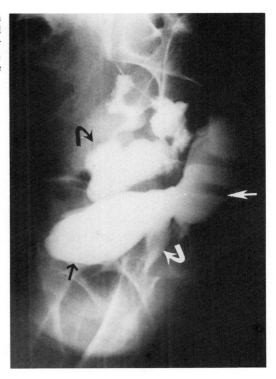

BIBLIOGRAPHY

Bladder Fistula

1. Abeshouse, B.S., Robbins, M.K., Gann, M., and Salik, J.O.: Intestino-vesical fistulas. J.A.M.A., *164*:251–257, 1957.
2. Aldrete, J.S., and Remine, W.H.: Vesico-colic fistula: a complication of colonic cancer. Long-term results of its surgical treatment. Arch. Surg., *94*:627–737, 1967.
3. Bailey, H.: Acquired vesico-intestinal and urethro-intestinal fistulae. Br. J. Urol., *1*:175–181, 1929.
4. Barambon, J., Laughlin, V.C., Dreyfuss, W., and Boyd, P.F.: Acquired vesico-colic fistulas. J. Int. Coll. Surg., *32*:276–286, 1959.
5. Best, J.W., and Davis, R.M.: Vesico-intestinal fistulas. J. Urol., *101*:62–65, 1969.
6. Black, W.R., and Bolt, D.E.: Ileovesical fistula. Review of literature and report of a case. Br. J. Surg., *42*:265–267, 1954.
7. Bors, E., and Kudish, H.G.: Intestinal vesical fistula: report of 6 cases. J. Urol., *72*:365–373, 1954.
8. Bramon, R.T., Carson, R.B., Wells, D., and Williams, J.I.: Vesicointestinal fistulas: a study and report of ten cases. Trans. Southeast Sect. Am. Urol. Assoc., *30*:30–34, 1960.
9. Carson, C.C., Malek, R.S., and Remine, W.H.: Urologic aspects of vesico-enteric fistula. J. Urol., *119*:744–746, 1978.
10. Cornes, J.S., and Stecker, M.: Primary Crohn's disease of colon and rectum. Gut, *2*:189–201, 1961.
11. Counseller, V.S.: Vesical and enterovesical fistulas. Surg. Clin. North Am., *30*:1223–1234, 1950.
12. Crohn, B.B.: Indications for surgical intervention in regional ileitis. A.M.A. Arch. Surg., *74*:305–311, 1957.
13. Crohn, B.B., Ginsberg, L., and Oppenheimer, G.O.: Regional ileitis; a pathological and clinical entity. J.A.M.A., *99*:1323–1329, 1932.
14. Ewell, G.H.: Intestinovesical fistula. J. Urol., *71*:603–607, 1954.
15. Ginzburg, L., and Oppenheimer, G.D.: Urological complications of regional ileitis. J. Urol., *59*:948–952, 1948.
16. Goodwin, W.E., Turner, R.D., and Winter, C.C.: Recto-urinary fistula: principles of management and a technique of surgical closure. J. Urol., *80*:246–254, 1958.
17. Goodwin, W.E., Winter, C.C., and Turner, R.D.: Fistulas between bowel and urinary tract. J. Urol., *84*:95–105, 1960.
18. Gray, F.W., and Newman, H.R.: Granuloma of the bladder associated with regional enteritis: case report. J. Urol., *78*:393–397, 1957.
19. Hafner, L.D., Ponka, J.L., and Brock, E.B.: Genitourinary manifestation of diverticula of the colon. A study of 500 cases. J.A.M.A., *179*:76–78, 1962.
20. Higgins, C.C.: Vesico-intestinal fistula. J. Urol., *36*:694–709, 1936.
21. Lidner, A.E., Marshak, R.H., Wolf, B.S., and Janowitz, H.D.: Granulomatous colitis. A clinical study. N. Engl. J. Med., *269*:379–385, 1963.
22. Mayfield, L.H., and Waugh, J.M.: Sigmoidovesical fistulae resulting from diverticulitis of sigmoid colon. Ann. Surg., *130*:186–199, 1949.
23. Mayo, C.W., and Blunt, C.P.: Vesicosigmoidal fistulas complicating diverticulitis. Surg. Gynecol. Obstet., *91*:612–616, 1950.
24. Melicow, M.M., and Uson, A.C.: The "herald" lesion of the bladder: a lesion which portends the approach of cancer or inflammation from outside the bladder. J. Urol., *85*:543–551, 1961.

25. Oppenheimer, G.D.: Late invasion of the bladder and prostate in carcinoma of the rectum or recto-sigmoid following abdomino-perineal resection. Ann. Surg., *117*:456–467, 1943.
26. Perri, A.J., Feldman, A.E., Kendall, A.R., et al.: Vesico-enteric fistula due to rupture of bladder carcinoma into bowel. Urol., *6*:762–763, 1975.
27. Peters, H.R., and Sacks, M.S.: Vesico-intestinal fistula. Int. Abstr. Surg., *69*:582–588, 1939.
28. Pugh, J.I.: On the pathology and behavior of acquired non-traumatic vesico-intestinal fistula. Br. J. Surg., *51*:644, 1964.
29. Rankin, F., and Brown, P.W.: Diverticulitis of Colon. Surg. Gynecol. Obstet., *50*:836–847, 1930.
30. Robinson, R.H.O.B.: Vesico-intestinal fistula, with special reference to Crohn's disease. Br. J. Urol., *25*:127–131, 1953.
31. Sutton, G.D.: Vesicosigmoidal fistulae. Surg. Gynecol. Obstet., *32*:318–327, 1921.
32. Ward, J.N., Lavengood, R.W., Jr., Nay, H.R., et al.: Diagnosis and treatment of colovesical fistulas. Surg. Gynecol. Obstet., *130*:1082–1090, 1970.
33. Williams, R.J.: Vesico-intestinal fistula and Crohn's disease. Br. J. Surg., *42*:179–182, 1954.
34. Winter, C.C., Turner, R.D., and Goodwin, W.E.: Urinary fistulas. Postgrad. Med., *26*:450–456, 1959.
35. Wolf, B.S., and Marshak, R.H.: Granulomatous colitis (Crohn's disease of colon). Roentgen features. Am. J. Roentgenol., *88*:662–670, 1962.

Appendicovesical Fistula

36. Abu-Dalu, J. Urca, I., and Meiraz, D.: Appendicovesical fistula—a rare complication of acute appendicitis. Br. J. Urol., *46*:586, 1974.
37. Castleman, B., and Toune, V.W.: Case records of the Massachusetts General Hospital. N. Engl. J. Med., *254*:1238–1240, 1956.
38. Edelman, S.: Appendico-vesical fistula. J. Mt. Sinai Hosp. N.Y., *31*:424–429, 1964.
39. Fitzpatrick, P.J.: Vesico-intestinal fistulas: case report of vesico-appendiceal and vesico-intestinal fistula. J. Urol., *85*:580–583, 1961.
40. Forbes, K.A., and Rose, R.J.: Appendico-vesico fistula. Ann. Surg., *160*:801–803, 1964.
41. Goldstein, A.E.: Rupture of urinary bladder following fulguration of protruding intravesical vermiform appendix thought to be bladder tumor. Am. J. Surg., *41*:96–102, 1938.
41a. Gross, M., and Peng, B.: Appendicoversic fistula. J. Urol., *102*:697–698, 1969.
42. Higgins, C.C.: Vesico-intestinal fistula. J. Urol., *36*:694–709, 1936.
43. Hyman, S., and Capos, N.J.: Appendiceal-vesical fistula. J.A.M.A., *170*:2177–2181, 1959.
44. Jaffe, J., and Evans, A.T.: Appendiceal-vesical fistula. J. Urol., *92*:295–296, 1964.
45. Kahn, F.A.: Appendico-vesical fistula with stone in the appendix. Br. J. Urol., *46*:345, 1974.
46. Kellogg, W.A.: Vesico-intestinal fistula. Am. J. Surg., *41*:135–186, 1938.
47. Marchail, V.R., Molland, E., and Blandy, J.P.: Appendico-vesicocolic fistula. Br. J. Urol., *47*:544, 1975.
48. Parton, L.I.: Appendico-vesical fistula. Br. J. Surg., *45*:583–588, 1958.
49. Pemberton, J. de J., Pool, T.L., and Miller, J.M.: Vesico-appendiceal fistula. J. Urol., *44*:274–278, 1940.

50. Rizin, B.K., Itzig, C., Jr., and Quinn, P.J., III: Appendicovesical fistula in childhood. Am. J. Dis. Child., *130*:530–531, 1976.
50a. Zvara, V., and Bruch-Acova, V.: A-V fistula in 2 children. Cesk. Pediatr., *19*:705–706, 1964.

Vesicouterine Fistula

51. Bond, W., and Rogers, G.: Unusual vesico-uterine fistula. Am. J. Obstet. Gynecol., *63*:215–216, 1952.
52. Bourgeois, G.A.: Cure of bladder fistulas. Am. J. Surg., *83*:671–673, 1952.
53. Brodhead, G.L.: Spontaneous closure of large uterovesical fistula. Med. Rec., *98*:437, 1920.
54. Falk, H.C., and Tancer, M.L.: Management of vesical fistulas after cesarean section. Am. J. Obstet. Gynecol., *71*:97–106, 1956.
55. Frankel, T., and Buchsbaum, H.J.: Vesico-corporeal fistula with menouria. J. Urol., *106*:860–861, 1971.
56. Herrmann, R.W., Tarr, N., and Stier, H.A.: Vesicouterine fistula. An unusual entity. J. Urol., *89*:826–828, 1963.
57. Kafetsoulis, A.A.: A case of vesicouterine fistula. Br. J. Urol., *46*:587, 1974.
58. Magri, J.: An unusual case of uterovesical fistula. Br. J. Surg., *48*:69–72, 1960.
59. Nourse, M.H., and Wishard, W.N., Jr.: Uterovesical fistula with fetal parts presenting in external urethral meatus. J. Urol., *72*:374–377, 1954.
60. Rauch, R.J., and Rodgers, M.W.: Spontaneous closure of vesicouterine fistula following cesarean section. J.A.M.A., *181*:997–999, 1962.
61. Rossi, D., Gargilo, F., and Nappi, E.: La sindrome menuria—amenorrea nella fistola utero-vesicale post cesarea. Russ. Int'l. Clin. Ter., *46*:561–566, 1966.
62. Sammour, M.B.: Cystouterine fistula following cesarean section with discharge of menstrual blood per urethram. Am. J. Obstet. Gynecol., *107*:321–322, 1970.
63. Sims, G.K.: Spontaneous healing in vesico-uterine fistulas following labor: report of a case. J.A.M.A., *90*:759–760, 1928.
64. Williams, R.J., and Shaw, A.F.B.: Utero-vesical fistula. Br. J. Surg., *31*:404–406, 1944.
65. Willson-Pepper, J.K.: Vesicouterine fistula. Br. J. Urol., *37*:433–436, 1965.
66. Youssef, A.F.: "Menouria" following lower segment cesarean section. Am. J. Obstet. Gynecol., *73*:759–767, 1957.
67. Youssef, A.F.: The uterine isthmus and its sphincter mechanism: a radiographic study. I. The uterine isthmus under normal conditions. Am. J. Obstet. Gynecol., *75*:1305–1314, 1958.

Vesicovaginal Fistula

68. Greene, L.F., and Litin, R.B.: Diagnosis of urinary vaginal fistulas. Surg. Clin. North Am., *39*:1047–1052, 1959.
69. Moir, J.C.: Injuries of the bladder. Am. J. Obstet. Gynecol., *82*:124–131, 1961.
70. Moir, J.C.: The Vesico-vaginal Fistula. London, Bailliere, Tindall & Cox, 1961.
71. Valk, W.L., and Foret, J.D.: The problem of vesicovaginal and ureterovaginal fistulas. Med. Clin. North Am., *43*:1769–1777, 1959.

Although there are many neurogenic lesions affecting the bladder, the most common are trauma with damage to the spinal cord or the cauda equina, syphilis, diabetes mellitus, multiple sclerosis, various neoplasms affecting the cord and the cauda equina, and congenital lesions such as spina bifida. Of course, the clinical picture varies, depending on the severity of the lesion and its level.

Radiographic Findings. The radiographic findings associated with a neurogenic bladder are caused directly by the neuromuscular effects of the neurogenic lesions on the bladder and the sphincters and indirectly by the resulting obstruction. The roentgenographic picture is confused also by secondary infection and calculi formation. The major abnormalities in the various roentgenographic pictures reflect changes in the shape, the size, and the position of the bladder, the configuration of the urethra, the status of the external urethral sphincter, and the competence of the ureteral orifices.

Vertebral Defects. Spina bifida is a failure of fusion of the laminae of the vertebra. If a cystic lesion appears on the surface of the body, the combination lesion is called spina bifida cystica. These lesions are designated as (1) meningocele, if the cyst includes only the spinal membrane; (2) meningomyelocele, if it includes portions of the meninges and the spinal cord; (3) myelocele, if the cord itself is exposed.

Spina bifida occulta refers to the failure of the fusion of the lamina, but there is no external swelling over the defect to indicate its presence. However, there may be thickening or dimpling of the skin, abnormal growth of hair, abnormal pigmentation, or the presence of a lipoma or fibroma. The laminal defect is nearly always posterior and is usually filled in by a fibrofatty pad, which has been

31

Neurogenic Bladder

described as an intermedullary lipoma.[1] Ventral spina bifida is rare.

The incidence of neural tube defects, of which myelomeningocele is one, varies greatly from 0.8 per cent to 9 per cent affected patients per 1000 live births, varying among different populations. There have been various anomalies of the urinary tract associated with myelomeningocele, such as horseshoe kidney, cystic disease, renal agenesis, exstrophy, and cloacal exstrophy.[18] Forbes found renal dysplasia in 12 per cent of myelomeningocele patients at autopsy.[6]

It is impossible to correlate the data of spina bifida with the severity of the neurologic defect. Spina bifida in some form is frequently seen on routine roentgenographic examinations of the lumbar spine. Karlin estimated that it is seen in more than 50 per cent of "normal" children.[9]

Agenesis of the sacrum is a general term used when any or all of the segments of the sacrum are missing. True sacral agenesis implies that two or more sacral segments are absent (Figs. 31-1, 31-2).[20] Sacral agenesis is often associated with anorectal anomalies, such as imperforate anus and atresia, and rectourethral fistula.[20] Of infants with the syndrome, 16 per cent are born of diabetic mothers, and 1 per cent of infants born of diabetic mothers have agenesis of the sacrum.[17]

EFFECTS ON THE BLADDER

SHAPE OF BLADDER

The shape of the bladder varies widely, depending on many factors not clearly understood. It may be rounded or oval, have a smooth wall, or be irregular from trabeculations, cellules, saccules, and diverticula.

Pine-Tree Bladder. This (Fig. 31-1) is a descriptive term applied to certain bladders, usually of the hypertonic type. It is wide at the base, gradually tapering as the dome is approached. Its outline commonly is serrated and irregular. This form usually is considered to be most characteristic of neurogenic bladders, but differentiation must be made from other conditions, especially patent urachus or bladder neck obstruction.

Hourglass Bladder. This (Fig. 31-3) is seen also in hypertonic lesions. It has been used in the literature in two senses: first, as a descriptive term applied to those bladders which give the appearance of an hourglass; second, as a definitive term limited to congenital lesions, the so-called true hourglass bladder. In any particular instance the attempt to differentiate congenital hourglass bladder and hourglass bladder due to other causes may be extremely difficult, if not impossible. In neurogenic bladder, for example, unless the patient has been studied prior to the development of the neurogenic lesion the exact cause of the hourglass appearance may not be ascertained. Caulk believed that most hourglass bladders have a congenital basis in the form of preexisting hypertrophic bands.[2]

Trabeculations, cellules, saccules, and diverticula, which usually are not prominent, are the result of both obstructive and neurogenic factors.

SIZE OF BLADDER

The size of the neurogenic bladder varies from a capacity of only a few milliliters of urine (Fig. 31-5) to many liters. For the most part, the size depends on the type and the level of the lesion. Large atonic bladders (Fig. 31-4) are the result primarily of the lesion and secondarily of the obstruction. Large atonic bladders are seen in spina bifida, diabetes, tabes dorsalies, syringomyelia, idiopathic primary atony, and hysteria. Rarely, obstruction can cause such extensive decompensation of the bladder that the bladder wall is thinned out, producing a bladder somewhat similar to the atonic neurogenic bladder. Large hypertonic bladders probably are caused entirely by outlet obstruction, which causes a gradual increase in residual urine.

POSITION OF BLADDER

The frequency of lateral deviation of the bladder (Fig. 31-4) is impressive.[16] Most of the deviations are to the right. Change in position is not a direct result of bladder size but is probably caused by the sigmoid colon, although an asymmetric effect of the neurologic disturbance on the innervation of the bladder or its supporting structures may be the etiologic factor.

EFFECTS ON THE URETHRA

FUNNEL URETHRA

This (Figs. 31-3, 31-7, 31-9) is a dilatation of the prostatic urethra of the shape suggested by this designation. The wider portion is at the bladder neck, with gradual distal tapering. There has been a great difference of opinion on the significance and the cause of this phenomenon. A survey of the literature has been presented elsewhere.[11, 14]

SACCULAR DILATATION OF THE POSTERIOR URETHRA

This condition (Fig. 31-8) is a rare observation in neurogenic bladders. It may be related to funnel urethra, but it has a distinctive appearance, the dilatation being widest at the midportion rather than proximally. It has been found only in hypertonic bladders.

PSEUDOSPHINCTER FORMATION

This term is applied to a sphincterlike structure lying between the internal and the external sphincters (Fig. 31-7).[3a] Although its exact significance has not yet been established, we have found it to be an important obstructive factor in some of our cases.

SPASTIC EXTERNAL SPHINCTER

Spasticity of the external urethral sphincter is not unusual in neurogenic lesions and may be suspected during the passage or the withdrawal of a catheter (Figs. 31-8 to 31-10). In many instances the spasticity of the external sphincter does not prevent complete emptying of the bladder, but certainly it is a primary obstructing factor in some cases in which emptying is incomplete.

RELAXED EXTERNAL SPHINCTER

Relaxation of the external sphincter is more common than one would gather from the literature (Fig. 31-11). It has been found both in flaccid and spastic cases and apparently is not related to the level of the lesion. In general, the volume of residual urine is small, but this is not invariably true.

Emmett and co-workers have presented an excellent discussion of the ectopic sphincter problem, especially in relation to those cases with small residuals and incontinence.[5]

EFFECTS ON THE URETER

Vesicoureteral reflux (Figs. 31-3, 31-4, 31-6, 31-12, 31-13) is common in neurogenic lesions. It is visualized radiographically when contrast material is injected into the bladder through a suprapubic tube or catheter and enters either or both ureters. Often a complete ureteropyelogram is obtained.

MISCELLANEOUS EFFECTS

Calculus formation (Fig. 31-6) is common in neurogenic lesions. It is the result of many factors, including stasis, infection, prolonged immobilization, and bone injury.

OCCULT NEUROGENIC BLADDER

It is now generally recognized that a neurogenic bladder can occur without detectable neurologic signs and no gross spinal anomaly. These cases can have trabeculated bladder, residual urine, hydronephrosis, vesicoureteral reflux, enuresis, diurnal incontinence, and repeated urinary tract infections without anatomic obstruction. Various terms, such as non-neurogenic neurogenic bladder,[23] subclinical neurogenic bladder,[24] isolated neurogenic dysfunction,[26] and occult neurogenic bladder,[27, 28] have been used to describe the condition. There may be associated constipation and fecal soiling and personality disorders.[23, 25]

Urodynamic studies have revealed good detrusor tone but a discoordination between the detrusor and the sphincter.[23] This type of occult neurogenic bladder is considered by many to be functional, not organic.[23, 25]

However, some cases of neurogenic bladder apparently occur affecting the bladder but in which careful radiologic work-up might reveal intraspinal lipomas, cysts, or tethered cord. Williams separates these two concepts, but certainly in many instances the distinction may be too finely drawn.[28] It is possible that in many cases anatomic changes in the spinal region will be discovered.

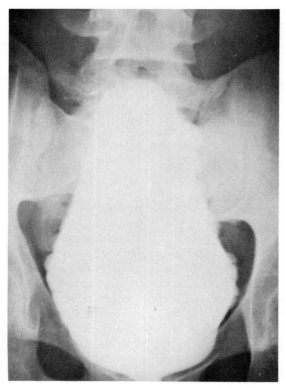

FIG. 31–1. Hypertonic bladder of "pine-tree" shape. Marked trabeculations and sacculations. Congenital neurogenic bladder with absence of lower three sacral segments and the entire coccyx.

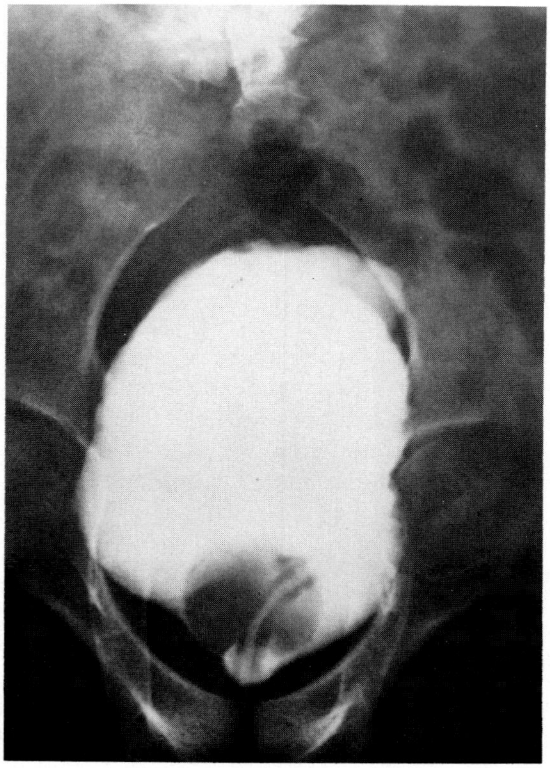

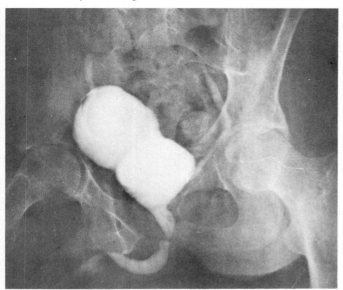

FIG. 31–3. Hourglass bladder. Paraplegic due to injury at L-1 as a result of an automobile accident. There are vesicoureteral reflux, funnel urethra, and a spastic external sphincter. The basis of the hourglass configuration may be congenital owing to hypertrophic bands, or it may be neurogenic.

FIG. 31–2. Absence of sacrum. Large irregular bladder. Foley bag in bladder.

FIG. 31–4. Large hypotonic bladder with vesicoureteral reflux and lateral deviation of the bladder to the right. The bladder is very smooth walled. At operation the muscle fibers were found to be greatly attenuated, and in places they appeared to be absent. Four-and-a-half-year-old girl with neurogenic bladder as a complication of spina bifida in the lumbosacral area.

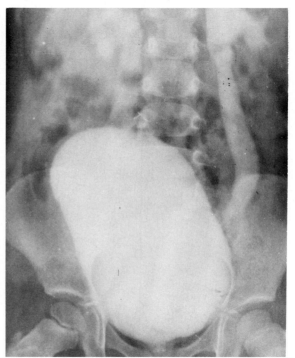

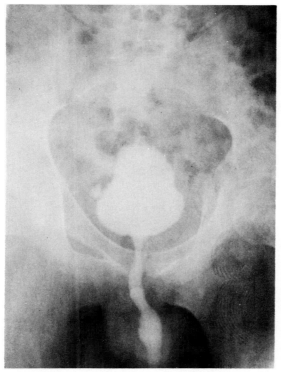

FIG. 31–5. Severe hypertonic contracted bladder with sacculations but without vesicoureteral reflux or a spastic external sphincter. Total bladder capacity, 100 ml. Paraplegic with lesion at T-11 to T-12.

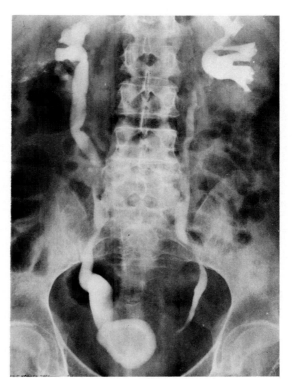

FIG. 31–6. Large calculus nearly completely filling a contracted spastic bladder. There is bilateral vesicoureteral reflux present. Both ureters are dilated. There is atrophy of the right kidney. Multiple sclerosis.

FIG. 31–7. Paraplegic with incomplete lesion at L-3 due to a shell fragment. Bladder is slightly trabeculated; present are a funnel urethra and a spastic external sphincter. Right oblique view. *Arrows* point to region of pseudosphincter formation.

FIG. 31–8. Saccular dilatation of the posterior urethra. Hypertonic bladder with spastic external sphincter and a small diverticulum of the anterior urethra due to the wearing of an incontinence clamp. Bladder is trabeculated. Complete paraplegic due to injury at C-7. Saccular dilatation is differentiated from funnel urethra, since the dilatation is widest at the midportion of the dilated posterior urethra rather than proximally, as it is in funnel urethra.

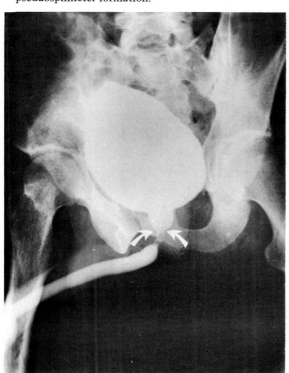

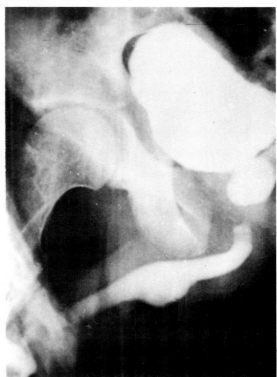

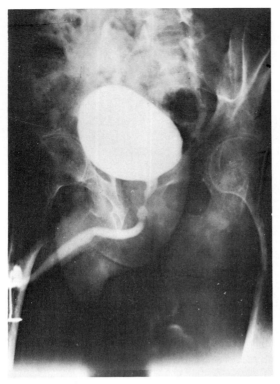

FIG. 31-9. Spastic external sphincter with a mild degree of hypertonicity of the bladder. Bladder is fairly smooth walled. Paraplegic with complete lesion at T-11 owing to a schrapnel injury.

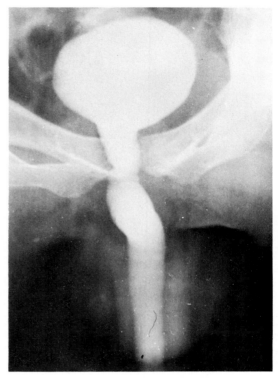

FIG. 31-10. Spastic external sphincter in a case of spina bifida, lumbosacral area. (A) Injecting cystourethrogram showing spastic external sphincter (*arrow*). (B) Following bilateral internal pudendal nerve blocks. *Arrow* points to relaxed external sphincter, as shown by dilated urethra.

FIG. 31-11. Hypertonic bladder with a dilated relaxed external sphincter. Patient dribbled urine nearly continuously. Paraplegic with complete lesion at T-10.

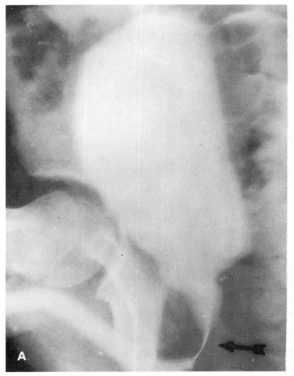

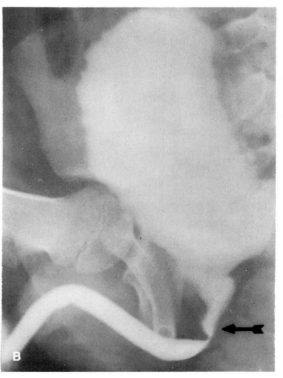

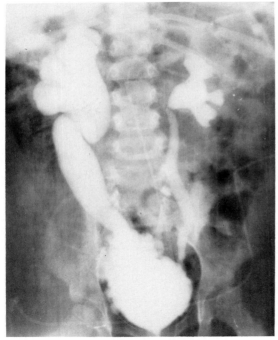

FIG. 31–12. Spina bifida of the lumbosacral area. Hypertonic irregular, small capacity bladder. Bilateral vesicoureteral reflux.

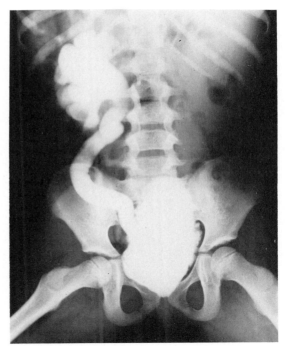

FIG. 31–13. Spina bifida. Female. Elongated, irregular bladder. Right vesicoureteral reflux.

BIBLIOGRAPHY

1. Campbell, J.B.: Neurosurgical treatment of bladder and bowel dysfunction resulting from anomalous development of the sacral neural axis. Clin. Neurosurg., 8:133–156, 1960.
2. Caulk, J.R.: Hour-glass bladder; remarks on the resection of the base of the bladder for transverse septa. Ann. Surg., 71:22–27, 1950.
3. Check, W.: Epidemiology of spina bifida is unique. J.A.M.A., 238:1442–1456, 1977.
4. Cohn, J., and Bay-Neilsen, E.: Hereditary defect of the sacrum and coccyx with anterior sacral meningocele. Acta Ped. Scand., 58:268–274, 1969.
5. Emmett, J.L., Daut, R.V., and Dunn, J.H.: Role of external urethral sphincter in the normal bladder and cord bladder. J. Urol., 59:439–454, 1948.
6. Forbes, M.: Renal dysplasia in infants with neurospinal dysraphism. J. Pathol., 107:13–19, 1972.
7. Gunterberg, B.: Effects of major resection of sacrum. Clinical studies on urogenital and anorectal function and a biomechanical study on pelvic strength. Acta Orthopaedica Scand. Suppl., 162:9–38, 1976 (Munksgaard Copenhagen).
8. Kaplan, G.W.: Myelomeningocele and related disorders. J.C.E. Urol., 17:15–27, 1978.
9. Karlin, I.W.: Incidence of spina bifida occulta in children with and without enuresis. Am. J. Dis. Child., 49:125–134, 1935.
10. Koontz, W.W., Jr., and Prout, G.R., Jr.: Agenesis of sacrum and neurogenic bladder. J.A.M.A., 203:481–486, 1968.
11. MacAlpine, J.B., and Wilson, D.S.P.: Funnel neck deformity of bladder. Br. J. Surg., 24:501–528, 1937.
12. Naggan, L.: Anencephaly and spina bifida in Israel. Pediatrics, 47:577–586, 1971.
13. Naggan, L., and MacMahon, B.: Ethnic differences in the prevalence of anencephaly and spina bifida in Boston, Massachusetts. N. Engl. J. Med., 227:1119–1123, 1967.
13a. Ney, C., Auerbach, O., and Hoen, T.I.: Pseudo-sphincter formation in neurogenic bladder. J. Urol., 57:858–868, 1947.
14. Ney, C., and Duff, J.: Cystourethrography: its role in diagnosis of neurogenic bladder. J. Urol., 63:640–652, 1950.
15. Ney, C., and Friedenberg, R.M.: The radiographic findings in neurogenic bladder. Radiology, 76:795–800, 1961.
16. Ney, C., Tausend, M.E., and Friedenberg, R.M.: Deviation of the bladder in neurogenic lesions. J. Urol., 81:659–662, 1959.
17. Passorge, E., and Lenz, W.: Syndrome of caudal regression in infants of diabetic mothers. Observation of further cases. Pediatrics, 37:672–675, 1966.
18. Roberts, J.B.M.: Congenital anomalies of the urinary tract and their association with spina bifida. Br. J. Urol., 33:309–315, 1961.
19. Thompson, I.M., Kirk, R.M., and Dale, M.: Sacral agenesis. Pediatrics, 54:236–238, 1974.
20. Williams, D.I., and Nixon, H.H.: Agenesis of the sacrum. Surg. Gynecol. Obstet., 105:84–88, 1957.
21. Young, H.H., and Wesson, M.B.: The anatomy and surgery of the trigone. Arch. Surg., 3:1–37, 1921.
22. Zellermayer, J., and Carlson, H.E.: Congenital hour-glass bladder. J. Urol., 51:24–30, 1944.

Occult Neurogenic Bladder

23. Allen, T.D.: The non-neurogenic neurogenic bladder. J. Urol., 117:232–238, 1977.
24. Dorfman, L.E., Bailey, J., and Smith, J.B.: Subclinical neurogenic bladder in children. J. Urol., 101:48–54, 1969.
25. Hinman, F., and Baumann, F.W.: Vesical and ureteral damage from voiding dysfunction in boys without neurological or obstruction disease. J. Urol., 109:727–732, 1973.
26. Kamhi, B., Horowitz, M.I., and Kovetz, A.: Isolated neurogenic dysfunction of the bladder in children with urinary tract infection. J. Urol., 106:151–153, 1971.
27. Martin, D.C., Datta, N.S., and Schweitz, B.: The occult neurological bladder. J. Urol., 105:735–738, 1971.
28. Williams, D.I., Hirst, G., and Doyle, D.: The occult neuropathic bladder. J. Ped. Surg., 9:35–41, 1974.

CLASSIFICATION

Epithelial tumors of the bladder
  Papillary transitional cell tumor
    Papillary carcinoma grade I
    Papillary carcinoma grades II and III
  Nonpapillary carcinoma
    Invasive transitional cell carcinoma
    Squamous cell carcinoma
    Adenocarcinoma
    Spindle cell carcinoma
    Carcinoma mixed type
  Cancer of bladder associated with other conditions: lithiasis, diverticula, inverted papilloma
  Precancerous lesions of the urothelium: carcinoma in situ
Nonepithelial tumors of the bladder
  Benign: leiomyoma, rhabdomyoma, fibroma
  Malignant
    Leiomyosarcoma
    Embryonal rhabdomyosarcoma
    Rhabdomyosarcoma in adult
Other tumors of bladder
  Pheochromocytoma
  Hemangioma
  Polyp
  Endometriosis
  Neurofibroma
  Nephrogenic adenoma
  Leukoplakia
  Lymphoma
  Leukemia
  Carcinosarcoma
Secondary tumors of the bladder

32

Tumors of the Bladder

PRIMARY TUMORS OF THE BLADDER

Primary bladder tumors are principally epithelial in origin, less than 10 per cent arising from non-epithelial sources. The epithelial tumors are essentially malignant, although the term "benign papilloma" is still used by some authors. The gross appearance of these tumors may be papillary, sessile, or a combination of both. Occasionally there is a submucosal variety in which the mucosa appears intact.

The majority of primary bladder epithelial tumors are of the transitional cell types (Figs. 32–1 to 32–17).; squamous cell and adenocarcinomas are relatively uncommon. Papillary tumors (the most common type) occur most frequently on the lateral walls and trigone. They may be multifocal, which appears to convey a greater chance of recurrence.[35] Males predominate 2:1 to 5:1, depending upon the investigator. The tumors occur usually in the sixth to seventh decades. Epithelial tumors in children are of lower grade malignancy and show no evidence of invasion and no tendency to recur.[7]

Broders divided tumors of the bladder into four grades, depending on the degree of cellular differentiation.[6] He considered that the degree of malignancy could be correlated directly with the extent to which the cell had differentiated from normal. Mostofi and co-workers,[41] Friedell and colleagues,[17] and Koss[33] have classified transitional cell tumors of the bladder into three grades: I, II, and III. According to Koss, papillary grade I tumors, if recurrent, may appear as similar tumors or tumors with high-grade abnormalities. The recurrence rate is 65 to 75 per cent. Invasion has occurred usually with recurrences. Grade II carcinoma is invasive and tends to carry a poorer prognosis than grade I. The epithelium adjacent to the tumor may show hyperplasia or atypical hyperplasia. Occasionally nonpapillary carcinoma in situ may occur. Grade III tumors are extremely invasive, prognosis is poor, and recurrences are common. The bladder epithelium adjacent to the tumor is abnormal with atypical hyperplasia or nonpapillary carcinoma in situ.

Nonpapillary transitional cell invasive carcinoma probably originates from nonpapillary carcinoma in situ and frequently has a squamous or glandular component. In their past history, a majority have had papillary neoplasia. The prognosis is poor. However, from the standpoint of prognosis and possible treatment, the depth to which the tumor has infiltrated the bladder wall is of paramount importance (Fig. 32–18). Infiltrating carcinoma of the bladder includes those cases in which the carcinoma has penetrated the basement membrane and is present in the stroma of the pedicle or has invaded the bladder wall, or both. Jewett and colleagues[24, 29, 30] and Marshall[35] divided bladder epithelial tumors into two groups:

Noninfiltrating: localized to the mucosa
Infiltrating: divided into four stages, as follows:

Stage A: The tumor cells have invaded the lamina propria but have not extended to the muscle.

Stage B: The tumor cells can be divided into two separate stages.

B_1 The invasion is less than halfway through the muscle.

B_2 The tumor has extended halfway through the muscle or more.

Stage C: The tumor cells have invaded the perivesical fat or the lymphatics.

Stage D: Known metastases of the tumor cells are present.

D_1 The metastases are localized to the pelvis.

D_2 The metastases extend beyond the pelvis.

The newer TNM classification has not been adopted universally but is an attempt to standardize the staging of bladder tumors.

Metastases occur from both hemantogenous and lymphogenous spread. Autopsy figures on the occurrence of metastases are reported as follows: Spooner, 30 per cent[107]; Jewett and Strong, 50 per cent[30]; and Franksson, 54 per cent.[113] Metastases occur to lymph nodes, liver, and lungs. Jewett has emphasized that metastases and extravesical extension, and therefore prognosis, are related primarily to the depth to which a tumor has penetrated the bladder wall, the critical point being the halfway mark. However, some superficial, well-differentiated papillary tumors may produce metastases.[106]

There appears to be a close correlation between the absence of A, B, and O blood group antigens on the surface of initially low-grade, noninvasive transitional cell carcinoma cells of the bladder and subsequent invasion.[54a] Also, Fabor and Ward, in cytogenetic studies of bladder cancer, have found chromosomal abnormalities that correlate well with recurrence and tumor invasion.[14a]

Cancer of the bladder has been produced by the aromatic amines,[33] cyclophosphamides,[2, 11, 48, 51] possibly smoking,[9] artificial sweeteners,[39] and coffee.[8]

Squamous cell carcinoma (Figs. 32–19, 32–20) is an uncommon tumor varying in frequency according to the observer: Pugh, 1.5 per cent[60]; Sarma, 3 per cent[62]; Kovetz, 4.5 per cent[57]; and Melicow, 11.5 per cent.[58] These tumors are associated with squamous metaplasia in practically all instances and are the bladder tumors most frequently associated with schistosomiasis haematobia, 55 per cent.[73] Tumors are graded I to IV on a gradual scale, with I described as pearl-forming tumors with only slight nuclear abnormalities and IV as a poorly differentiated squamous cell carcinoma.

Forty per cent occur in females and the tumor appears in a younger age group than do other carcinomas of the bladder.[55, 57] More than two-thirds of patients have a history of chronic urinary tract disorders such as stricture, calculi, or chronic infection.[55] Many of the patients present with symptoms such as weight loss, back or pelvic pain, or obstructive symptoms suggestive of adnexal disease. At the time of diagnosis, about 65% of patients have abnormal intravenous urograms and about 99% have infiltrating lesions. The mortality rate is usually quoted as high. Approximately 65% die within 1 year of diagnosis and only 7.4 per cent survive 5 to 10 years.

Because these lesions are infiltrating, they have the roentgenographic characteristics of any infiltrating tumor.

Primary adenocarcinoma of the bladder (including urachal carcinoma) (Figs. 32–21, 32–22) is rare, comprising only 1% of all bladder malignancies.[72] In view of the embryologic derivation of the bladder, the tumor can either arise from islands of mucus-containing hindgut epithelium persisting in the bladder during development or result from the potential of transitional epithelium of the bladder, which is derived chiefly from the cloaca to change into mucous and glandular epithelium.

In general, vesical adenocarcinoma is usually but not always mucus-producing and varies from papillary to solid (60%). Males predominate 3:1. The tumor occurs primarily in the fifth to sixth decades but the teens are not exempt. It occupies essentially the dome and trigone, but the anterior, posterior, and lateral walls may be involved. The tumors are usually single (63%) especially those at the dome that represent 57 per cent of all single lesions.[86] They are the most common tumors of the exstrophied bladder and may arise from cystitis glandularis.[65, 71] There are two categories, depending upon position and origin.

Type 1 is situated on the trigone and represents nearly 65 per cent of all adenocarcinomas. Patients with these tumors are reported to have a survival rate paralleling that of patients with papillary and infiltrative transitional cell carcinoma, but there is some evidence that the prognosis is far worse (Fig. 32–21).[78]

Type 2 arises in the dome and is of urachal origin, if the following criteria are met[86]:

1. Situated in dome or anterior wall of bladder
2. Mostly intramural
3. Deep ramifications in bladder wall
4. Intact or ulcerated surface epithelium overlying the tumor, with a sharp demarcation between tumor and a surface epithelium devoid of glandular and polypoid proliferation
5. Demonstrated not to be a secondary tumor

These tumors represent approximately 35 per cent of adenocarcinomas of the bladder. Urachal remnants (epithelial lined areas) often associated with glandular metaplasia are common, occurring in 70 per cent of autopsy specimens, especially prepared.[68] Adenocarcinomas developing in these remnants are rare, but more than 132 cases have been reported.[78] The 5-year survival rate is 16 per cent, but those reported to be free of tumor at this time represent only 5 per cent (Fig. 32–22).[86]

Since these are infiltrating tumors, they have the same characteristics as the usual infiltrating tumors (Fig. 32–22). The urachal tumors show a mass in the region of the dome, and it may be calcified.

DIFFERENTIAL DIAGNOSIS OF BLADDER TUMORS

Steps necessary to assess bladder tumors properly include history, physical examination, urinalysis, intravenous urogram, cystoscopy, biopsy, and careful bimanual examination under anesthesia. However, in differentiating the noninfiltrating from the infiltrating types, the following radiologic techniques can be utilized:

1. Plain film
2. Conventional cystogram
3. Fractionated cystography
4. Double contrast cystography
5. Endoperivesical gas
6. Angiography with endoperivesical gas
7. CT scan

Calcification within bladder tumors is an unusual roentgenographic finding (see Figs. 32–1 to 32–5) and usually indicates malignancy.[110] The incidence varies as follows: Miller and Pfister, 0.43 per cent[111]; Braband, 0.69 per cent[112]; and Ferris and O'Connor, 6.7 per cent.[110] The calcification occurs either on the surface (usually with an alkaline urine) or subepithelially (usually in necrotic areas). The appearance is either (1) finely punctate or granular; (2) grossly nodular; or (3) a mixture of both.

The differential diagnosis includes the following conditions:

1. Tuberculous cystitis may have calcific deposits but no mass.
2. Schistosomiasis. At an early stage, there may be multiple small nodular filling defects but no definite mass. Later there may be circumferential calcification.
3. Bladder tumor calcification must be differentiated from phleboliths, uterine fibroid calcification, ovarian dermoid, and calcification in vas deferens and arterial walls.

A cystogram usually locates the lesion and separates phleboliths, fibroid calcification, and vas deferens calcification. Ovarian dermoids may have a clear, fatty envelope. Arterial calcification may be difficult, but gas studies in various positions usually help separate these two entities.

CONVENTIONAL CYSTOGRAM

Pedunculated Noninfiltrating Carcinoma. In cases of pedunculated noninfiltrating tumor there is a well-demarcated circumscribed filling defect, usually rounded in shape, with a serrated margin (Figs. 32–6 to 32–11). The contrast material may surround the filling defect completely. Peripherally, the contrast material is intact, although occasionally a view may be obtained in which a stalk produces a break in the peripheral margin. In large pedunculated masses, the entire bladder may appear to be filled with the tumor, with only a rim of contrast material. Too heavy a concentration of contrast material may obscure the noninfiltrating tumor. In cases of sessile noninfiltrating tumor, the cystogram may give the appearance of an infiltrating lesion, because the contrast medium cannot surround the tumor completely as it does in the pedunculated type. However, by using the other modalities that are described later, the separation of this type from the infiltrating type should be possible.

Infiltrating Carcinoma. The normal luminal pattern is distorted (Figs. 32–11 to 32–17, 32–19 to 32–22). The bladder wall may appear to be irregular at the tumor site, and there may be an indentation as well. Usually, the edge of the defect is serrated or irregular. The contrast material cannot surround the involved area completely, because it cannot get between the bladder wall and the tumor itself.

Obstruction of a ureter can appear on an IVU as

lower segmental dilatation, ureteropyelectasia, or complete absence of function. Marked lower segmental dilatation (Figs. 32–13, 32–17), ureteral pyelectasia (Fig. 32–14), or nonfunction (Fig. 32–15) is more common with infiltrating tumors than with the noninfiltrating type. However, Smith reported bilateral hydronephrosis in papillomatosis.[116] Of 82 cases of papillomata, only 4 had advanced upper tract changes. Reflux has been the cause of ureteral dilatation in some instances.

Other indications of infiltration include the following conditions:

1. *Increased thickness of bladder wall* (Fig. 32–13) in the region of the tumor generally means an infiltrating tumor. This is determined by the distance between the contrast medium in the bladder and the perivesical fat.[113-115] In cases in which the contour formed by the perivesical fat against the bladder wall cannot be followed across the entire tumor, an increase in thickness of the bladder wall in the peripheral edge (Fig. 32–13) of the tumor-bearing area is an indication of infiltration.[113, 115]

2. *Sloping contour of the edge of the tumor* as opposed to an acute angular junction with the adjacent bladder wall represents an infiltrating tumor. A roentgenographic diagnosis of infiltration usually can be made by examining the internal contour adjacent to the tumor. If this outline is elevated and then gradually returns to normal, a definite sign of at least submucosal infiltration probably is present.[114]

3. *Displacement of the lumen of the bladder* to the opposite side in cases of a tumor that does not bulge to any marked degree into the bladder is a sign of extensive involvement of the wall.[114] In such cases edema or a diverticulum must be ruled out.

FRACTIONATED CYSTOGRAMS

The use of fractionated cystograms (Figs. 32–25 to 32–27) is an additional method for determining the extent of a bladder tumor by demonstrating the fixation or the mobility of the bladder wall at the site of the tumor. Possible sources of error include the presence of blood clots, which may be mistaken for superficial tumors; previous operations rendering the bladder wall fixed; and local fixation produced by perivesical inflammation or peridiverticulitis. This method cannot be used in small-capacity, severely inflamed bladders.

The method consists of instilling contrast medium into the bladder in increments of 40 ml. On a single film an exposure is made after each instillation, the patient's position remaining unchanged. The method is of value in determining the degree of infiltration of the bladder tumor as shown by the immobility of the bladder wall. Cobb and Anderson modified the technique by using normal saline solution for increments.[117]

DOUBLE CONTRAST CYSTOGRAPHY

The method is as follows (Figs. 32–28, 32–29):

1. A barium suspension is prepared by mixing 5 ounces of micronized barium sulfate (previously sterilized by dry heat in a hot-air oven) with 120 ml. of saline solution. This suspension is introduced into the bladder by means of a No. 16 or 18 Foley catheter.
2. Conventional filled bladder films are taken.
3. The bladder is partially emptied, and pure carbon dioxide is insufflated with a three-way stopcock.
4. Double contrast films are taken. They should include right and left lateral decubitus views.
5. The bladder is emptied and irrigated with isotonic sterile saline solution to remove residual barium sulfate.

ENDOPERIVESICAL GAS INSUFFLATION

The method of endoperivesical gas insufflation (Figs. 32–30 to 32–33) of the urinary bladder has been used over the years to delineate tumors of the bladder and to determine accurately the bladder wall thickness in the region of the tumor.[121, 122, 123, 125] (The technique is described under Arteriography of Bladder Tumors in this chapter.)

This method is excellent for evaluating the wall thickness at the site of the bladder tumor. However, no information regarding the depth of tumor infiltration into the perivesical space can be obtained from this method, because not infrequently there is some nonuniformity in the distribution of the perivesical gas.

ASSESSMENT AND STAGING OF BLADDER TUMORS BY ROENTGENOGRAPHIC TECHNIQUES

ERICH K. LANG

A definitive relationship between curability of bladder carcinoma and the degree of invasiveness has been established by Jewett.[135, 136] Although the histologic grade of the neoplasm provides another important parameter for prognosis, there is no direct correlation between pathologic stage and histologic grade of the tumor.[139, 151, 154] The stage of a tumor depends on the growth rate and the duration of disease.[135, 151]

Clinical staging of bladder tumors by bimanual examination, cystoscopy, and biopsy achieves an accuracy varyingly reported from 20 to 80 per cent.[135, 136, 139, 140, 162] To improve the accuracy of staging of bladder tumors, a variety of roentgenologic procedures have been advocated in the recent past.

Computed tomography is currently favored because it provides criteria allowing assessment of contiguous extension of bladder neoplasms into the perivesical fat or adjacent organs and for its ability to detect enlarged regional or para-aortic nodes suspected of harboring metastases.[157a, 158]

Ultrasound has likewise been proven to be of value in identifying extension of tumor into the perivesical space and to adjacent organs.[133a] However, although both of these modalities are reasonably sensitive for detection of a mass, they lack specificity and offer no criteria for confident differentiation between neoplastic and inflammatory components of such a mass.

The propensity of 90 per cent of all bladder neoplasms to exhibit a striking neovascularity offers an opportunity for demonstrating the tumor itself.[137, 140–142, 144, 153, 165] The relative specificity of tumor neovascularity and existence of criteria allowing differentiation of neoplastic from inflammatory neovascularity assure a continued position of importance for arteriography within the armamentarium of staging examinations.

However, the combination of computed tomography and guided thin-needle biopsy promises to eliminate uncertainties of inflammatory versus neoplastic causes of a demonstrated mass and once established as a reliable technique might well obviate the use of arteriograms.

The cystograms, superimposition cystogram and double contrast barium gas cystogram, do not provide reliable criteria for staging of bladder neoplasms.

VASCULAR ANATOMY

The principal supply of the bladder is derived from the superior and inferior vesical arteries, the artery of the ductus deferens, and occasionally small branches from the internal pudendal, obturator, and medial rectal arteries (Fig. 32–34).[129, 132, 142, 144, 153]

The superior vesical arteries are branches of the partially obliterated umbilical artery and supply the dome and portions of the lateral bladder wall. The inferior vesical arteries supply the floor of the bladder, portions of the lateral bladder wall, and have branches to the prostate, the seminal vesicles, or the vagina. Additional supply to the floor of the bladder may be derived from the artery of the ductus deferens, the uterine artery, and the medial rectal artery.

TECHNIQUE

Percutaneous transfemoral catheterization (Seldinger technique) is advocated. The peculiarity of the arterial supply of the urinary bladder dictates either selective injection of the anterior division of the hypogastric arteries or flush injection into the distal abdominal aorta.

Selective injections into the anterior division of the hypogastric arteries offer the advantage of an unimpaired view of the area of interest. However, in older patients with extensive arteriosclerotic disease, flush injection into the distal aorta or common iliac arteries may be the procedure of choice.[144-146, 153] Moreover, even if selective arteriography of the anterior divisions of the hypogastric artery is carried out, an additional aortic flush injection is advocated to assess cannibalization of the arterial system of adjacent organs and/or supply derived from the medial rectal artery (Fig. 32–35A).

Twelve milliliters of contrast medium injected over 2 seconds assure optimal opacification of the branches of the anterior division of the hypogastric artery, whereas flush injections into the distal aorta call for the injection of 40 to 60 ml. of contrast medium at a rate of 20 to 25 cc. per second.

The documentation of small tumor vessels can be improved by using a low-kilovoltage technique that in turn is facilitated by introduction of gas into the bladder and into the perivesical space (Fig. 32–36B). The perivesical gas insufflation facilitates identification of the perivesical cleavage plane, an important reference point to establish the degree of permeation by a bladder neoplasm (Figs. 36B-D, 38A,B). To dissect satisfactorily the perivesical plane, 400 to 700 ml. of nitrous oxide or carbon dioxide are injected through 20-gauge needles advanced from a suprapubic approach into the space of Retzius and through a transperineal approach to a point just below the prostate or bladder floor.

Arteriograms should be recorded on serial roentgenograms at an exposure rate of two per second for the first 4 seconds, and one per second for the ensuing 10 seconds.

Unless the precise position of the bladder tumor is known from prior cystoscopic examination, multiple contrast medium injections may be necessary to document the tumor in a tangential projection. As a rule, the staging examination can be completed by one flush injection into the aorta and a selective injection into the anterior division of the hypogastric artery principally supplying the tumor, and recorded in an obliquity in order to document the tumor in tangential projection.

ARTERIOGRAPHIC CHARACTERISTICS OF BLADDER NEOPLASMS

The arteriograms may show the following angiographic findings in bladder tumors:[127-129, 140-142, 144, 153, 162]

1. The vesical artery supplying the bladder tumor is enlarged and tortuous, reflecting increased flow (Figs. 32–35A, 32–37).
2. Tumor vessels, that is, atypical vessels with rapidly changing caliber (corkscrew vessels), are identified within the tumor and therefore can be used to delineate the tumor (Figs. 32–35A, 32–36B).
3. Tumor vessels fill earlier and more rapidly than vessels supplying normal segments of the bladder (Fig. 32–35A).
4. Premature opacification of draining veins may be noted (attributable to arteriovenous shunts within the tumor) (Figs. 32–35B, 32–36C).
5. Lacunar dye-filled structures or puddling of contrast medium may be present (particularly in undifferentiated tumors, indicating necrosis and extravasation of contrast medium).
6. The staining quality of a tumor, homogeneous or inhomogeneous, reflects to some degree histologic differentiation, growth rate, and particularly areas of central necrosis (Figs. 32–35B, 32–36D).

The preceding criteria permit identification of tumor or tumors of the bladder; however, assessment of the depth of infiltration (staging) necessitates presentation of the arteriographically delineated tumor in a tangential fashion.[140, 142-146, 162, 165] Optimally, the bladder should be distended with air or nitrous oxide and the perivesical fat plane accentuated by perivesical gas dissection.[144-146] Depth of infiltration into the muscularis or permeation into the perivesical fat or adjacent tissues by a tumor is then readily assessable (Figs. 32–35A, 32–36C,D, 32–38B). It is, however, emphasized that the diagnosis hinges upon identification of abnormal tumor vessels, since the rich vascular stalk of a benign papilloma could otherwise mimic an infiltrating tumor (Fig. 32–37).

DIAGNOSTIC ACCURACY

The recent literature credits staging by pelvic arteri-

TABLE 32-1
A Comparison of the Accuracy of Staging by Clinical Modalities and Arteriography

Surg.-Path.		Arteriography/Clin. Stage						%-Accuracy
		T1	T2	T3	T3	T4	T4	
Submucosal	T1	2/4	1/0	1/1	0/0	0/0	1/0	40/80
Muscularis 1/2	T2	2/3	17/17	1/1	1/0	0/0	1/1	77/77
All muscularis	T3	1/3	1/2	20/18	2/2	1/0	1/1	77/69
Perivesical fat	T3	1/4	1/11	3/10	68/50	2/1	3/2	87/64
Lateral pelvic wall	T4	0/0	0/2	1/5	2/5	32/25	3/1	84/65
Distant meta	T4	0/0	0/2	2/4	3/7	3/3	60/52	88/76

ography with greater accuracy than staging by clinical means, including TUR biopsy.[126-129, 132, 135, 139-146, 150, 160, 162-165] When they analyze arteriographic accuracy for different stages, the authors of all large series concur that the method is most reliable for more advanced stages (stages C and D) and least reliable for less invasive lesions (stage A).[140, 145, 146, 150, 152, 155, 162, 164, 165] Conversely, clinical staging is considered most accurate for less invasive lesions.[135, 136, 139] Hence, the two modalities appear to complement each other (Table 32–1).

The triple cystogram (bladder arteriogram with endo- and perivesical gas study) has been combined with lymphangiography to provide criteria for staging bladder tumors according to the TNM system.[126, 127, 134, 149, 155, 165] The "T" stage is assigned on the basis of the arteriographically delineated tumor.[154] Pedal lymphangiography is recommended to ascertain the presence of lymph node metastases.[134, 137, 149, 154, 163] Because regional lymph nodes are not opacified by pedal lymphangiography, the earliest identifiable lesion is an "N-2" lesion.

To eliminate or decrease the known high rate of false positives, thin-needle biopsy of nodes showing a defect on lymphangiogram has been advocated.[130a] To validate the authenticity of the biopsy site, biopsies are best performed under biplane fluoroscopic guidance and documented on radiographs exposed in anteroposterior and cross-table lateral projections (Fig. 32–39A, B).

COMPUTED TOMOGRAPHY AND ULTRASONOGRAPHY

Computed tomography and ultrasonography have been advocated for assessment of direct extension of neoplasms as well as for identification of metastases to lymph nodes or to the liver (Figs. 32–40, 32–42 to 32–45).[133a, 157a, 158] The demonstration of pelvic structures in cross-sectional anatomic array lends itself to scrutinization of extravesical extension of a neoplasm (Figs. 32–40, 32–42, 32–47a).[157a, 158] Even though fluid-filled bowel loops fortuitously positioned adjacent to segments of the bladder wall harboring a tumor have resulted in erroneous overstaging, this problem can be eliminated by authenticating the origin of the mass on computerized tomograms obtained in different positions (fortuitously abutting soft tissue structures tend to separate in decubitus positions).[158] Moreover, the administration of oral contrast medium should opacify such small-bowel loops and permit their positive identification.

Computed tomography has been found reliable for differentiation of early lesions (A, B-1, B-2) and advanced C and D lesions.[158] Direct tumor extension into the seminal vesicles is diagnosable on computed tomograms with confidence; in the past this diagnosis hinged on retrograde vesiculography (Figs. 32–40, 32–41).[157a]

Computed tomography permits one readily to identify enlarged regional, external, or common iliac, and/or enlarged para-aortic lymph nodes (Figs. 32–45 to 32–47a).[157a, 158] Although computed tomography is highly sensitive for the detection of enlarged lymph nodes, it lacks criteria to differentiate inflammatory from neoplastic masses. To affirm the diagnosis of metastatic involvement of nodes, CT-guided, thin-needle biopsy of suspect nodes is advocated (Fig. 32–47). The combination of computed tomography—proven to be highly sensitive in detecting direct extension of neoplasm into the perivesical fat, seminal vesicals, and other adjacent structures and in detecting abnormally enlarged lymph nodes — and CT-guided, thin-needle biopsy affirming the histologic etiology of any documented mass, promises greatly to improve the accuracy of staging of bladder neoplasms.

Transrectal sonography has been advocated to ascertain spread of the neoplasm into the perivesical fat or into adjacent structures.[133a] Because of frequent bladder deformity and wall irregularities, attendant fulguration, biopsy, and/or radiation therapy, sonographic assessment of extension of the neoplasm into the muscularis is fraught with difficulty, and only extension of a mass into the perivesical fat or into adjacent structures can be documented with reasonable accuracy (Figs. 32–47a to 32–47c).[133a] However, once again sonography does not permit differentiation of a neoplastic from an inflammatory condition.

Distant metastases can be assessed by radionuclide scans, computed tomography, and arteriography.[126, 154, 157] Technetium polyphosphate bone scans are probably the most sensitive method for identifying early bone metastases.

The precise etiologic diagnosis of certain benign and highly vascularized tumors of the bladder such as hemangiomas, hemangiopericytomas, and pheochromocytomas is possible on the basis of characteristic angiographic features.[130, 133] The combination of computed tomography and arteriography is, hence, particularly useful in the diagnosis of nonepithelial benign bladder neoplasms.

Pelvic angiography has been expanded to serve therapeutic purposes. Superselective catheterization of pelvic arteries can be exploited for delivery of chemotherapeutic agents and radioactive infarct particles into tumors or for embolization of bleeding sites with autologous blood clot or inert embolic material to effect hemostatis.[138, 143, 148, 156] Intractable hemorrhage from the bladder attributable to invasion by pelvic neoplasms can be readily controlled by transcatheter embolization with inert embolic material such as Gelfoam.[143] Superselective embolization of the anterior division of the hypogastric arteries with particles of a size prone to lodge in arterioles effectively controls hemorrhage, yet permits some continued collateral perfusion of tissues through the precapillary plexus, thus precluding necrosis of the bladder (Fig. 32–48A, B).[143] Limitation of embolization to branches of the anterior division of the hypogastric artery assures unimpaired vascular supply to the gluteal muscles, which have been found intolerant to deprivation of their vascular supply. This method has also been found useful in the management of intractable hemorrhage from telangiectatic vessels caused by radiation therapy to bladder tumors (Fig. 32–49A, B).

SPINDLE CELL AND GIANT CELL CARCINOMA

These are rare varieties of invasive transitional cell or squamous cell carcinoma of the bladder. The prognosis is poor.

CARCINOMA MIXED TYPE

This term refers to various combinations of tumor types that have been described previously. It is usually a combination of papillary urothelial tumors, whether noninfiltrating or infiltrating, with nonpapillary variants of urothelial carcinoma in situ or infiltrating. Squamous cell and adenocarcinomas may occur in association with other tumor types.

CARCINOMA OF THE BLADDER ASSOCIATED WITH OTHER CONDITIONS

LITHIASIS

Lithiasis is often associated with bladder carcinoma, and Wynder and co-workers consider lithiasis to be a major epidemiologic factor in carcinoma of the bladder.[167] In many instances the diagnosis of cancer of the bladder in the presence of lithiasis may be extremely difficult. Koss has pointed out that, in the presence of stones, the urinary sediment may show considerable atypia that may be mistaken for cancer and that even bladder biopsies may be difficult to interpet because of the severe inflammatory changes.[166]

DIVERTICULA

See Chapter 27, Herniation and Diverticula of the Bladder.

INVERTED PAPILLOMA OF THE BLADDER

Inverted papilloma of the bladder is a benign, usually pedunculated or sessile tumor that appears usually on the trigone. The unique histologic feature is the inversion of the usual structure of a bladder papilloma, the fronds being surrounded by the fibromuscular stroma. The entire lesion is covered by relatively normal-appearing transitional epithelium; the fronds appear to arise from the epithelium. The cords have peripheral basal cells arranged perpendicular to the long axis and central cells arranged horizontal to the long axis.

Roentgenographic appearance: There is an irregular, polypoid, noninvasive defect.[170]

CARCINOMA IN SITU

The precancerous lesions of the bladder are simple hyperplasia, atypical hyperplasia, and carcinoma in situ. In the latter, the epithelium is composed of cells with obvious nuclear abnormalities and disorderly patterns of growth. Carcinoma in situ may either progress directly to invasive nonpapillary carcinoma or to a papillary carcinoma that may in time become invasive.[33] Many of the multifocal carcinomas of the bladder are a result of carcinoma in situ. It is frequently found with recurrent carcinoma and may accompany synchronous or metachronous papillary or nonpapillary tumors of the bladder. The lesion can involve the ureteral orifices, the terminal ureteral mucosa, the prostatic urethra, and prostatic ducts. It has been found in 15 per cent of lower ureters in the cystectomy specimens for carcinoma of the bladder.

Urinary exfoliative cytologic study is a valuable method for diagnosis. Specimens taken by cystoscopic biopsy can be diagnostic.

With the cystoscope, the lesions are usually seen as multiple hemorrhagic areas. They have a slightly raised, granulomatous or cobblestone appearance. Conspicuous white or yellow excrescences within erythematous areas are often seen.

Roentgenograms of the bladder usually are not helpful. There may be a diminution in size of the bladder and interstitial cystitis may be the primary diagnosis. In 23 per cent of men and 1.3 per cent of women treated for interstitial cystitis at the Mayo Clinic, carcinoma in situ was ultimately diagnosed.[184]

NONEPITHELIAL TUMORS OF THE BLADDER

LEIOMYOMA OF THE BLADDER

Leiomyoma of the bladder is an uncommon tumor usually found on the trigone (Figs. 32–50, 32–51).[187-191] It is slow growing and may become large. Small tumors are sessile; the larger ones are globular and pedunculated. Patients may have hematuria, infection, and obstructive symptoms. They are usually found in families.

Roentgenographic Findings. There is a filling defect in the bladder, but no infiltration.

RHABDOMYOMA OF THE BLADDER

Although the malignant variety is not unusual, the benign type is practically unknown.

LEIOMYOSARCOMA OF THE BLADDER

Leiomyosarcoma of the bladder is an uncommon tumor of malignant smooth muscle cells (Figs. 32–53, 32–54).[192-201] It occurs usually after 40 although it has been seen in children and young adults. Females are involved as often as males, usually in a distensible part of the bladder.[192] The lower grade tumors present as an intramural nodule beneath the normal mucosa. High-grade lesions may be large and ulcerated. The prognosis is better than that of rhabdomyosarcoma. Spindle cell sarcoma is an unusual infiltrating tumor of the bladder (Fig. 32–55).

EMBRYONAL RHABDOMYOSARCOMA OF THE BLADDER (BOTRYOID SARCOMA)

Embryonal rhabdomyosarcoma of the bladder (botryoid sarcoma) is a rare tumor found usually in the first few years of life, occurring occasionally in older children and rarely in adults. In children, especially, it may be difficult to ascertain accurately the actual point of origin, whether bladder or prostate (see Part IX, Pediatric Urology). The lesion's actual origin is generally believed to be the urogenital sinus and mesonephric duct remnants represented by the trigone, bladder neck, and prostatic urethera in the male and the entire urethra and lower vagina in the female.

Various explanations for its histogenesis have been presented: embryonal tumors of dysontogenetic origin,[208] embryonal heterotopia occurring in anomalous development of the wolffian duct system,[205, 212] embryonic tissue with the potential of developing into striated muscle,[209, 213] heterotopic displacement of vagrant rhabdomyoblasts into vesical submucosa from sites containing striated muscles such as urogenital diaphragms, prostatic capsule, or from mesenchyme of the urogenital region.[211]

Approximately 75 per cent of children with sarcoma of the bladder present before 5 years of age. Boys predominate 2:1.[214] Botryoid sarcoma of the bladder has a multicentric origin and is broad-based but gives the appearance of being polypoid. It lies superficially in the bladder, usually at the trigone and bladder neck and infiltrates and metastasizes late in contrast to the prostatic variety, which metastasizes early. The lesion in girls arising from vagina or urethra gives a similar polypoid appearance (see Fig. 12–80). Symptoms are usually the result of obstruction of the bladder neck and include poor stream, dysuria, and frequency. Later there may be hematuria, obstipation, and suprapubic pain. Strangury may differentiate this lesion from sarcoma of the prostate.[214] Ureteral obstruction leads to renal failure. In the infant and children there may be a large, palpable, suprapubic mass that may not disappear after catheterization.

Roentgenographic Findings: On excretory or retrograde cystograms, there are multiple, smooth, rounded defects in the lumen of the bladder that when situated in the lower part of the bladder and posterior urethra in the infant or child usually are diagnostic. The ureter may be angulated as in prostatic hypertrophy. The bladder may be elevated, but this is usually characteristic of prostatic sarcoma. Prognosis is usually poor; survivors have been treated by cystectomy.

Differential Diagnoses: Ectopic ureteroceles with a waistlike defect in the bladder could be confused with rhabdomyosarcoma, but the double collecting systems and cystoscopic findings should differentiate the two.

RHABDOMYOSARCOMA IN THE ADULT

According to the review articles of Evans and Bell[202] and Joshi,[204] rhabdomyosarcoma in the adult is rare (Fig. 32–56).[203, 206, 207] Clinically, it is similar to the carcinoma of the bladder. It may occur anywhere in the bladder, and it usually presents as large ulcerated nodules. Rarely has a true botryoid appearance been described. They occur in adults over 20 years of age and the prognosis is poor.

OTHER TUMORS OF THE BLADDER

PRIMARY BENIGN NONEPITHELIAL TUMORS

Primary benign nonepithelial tumors include fibroma (Fig. 32–52), myxoma, fibromyxoma, leiomyoma, nephrogenic adenoma, neurofibroma, neurofibromatosis, xanthoma, osteoma, hemangioma, endometriosis, and pheochromocytoma.[215-309] Some heterotopic types are rhabdomyoma, chondroma, and dermoid cysts. Amyloid tumors of the bladder are not in a strict sense neoplastic. Leukoplakia is a tumorlike condition, unclassified.

PHEOCHROMOCYTOMA

Pheochromocytoma is a rare tumor of the bladder representing 0.5% of bladder tumors (Figs. 32–57 to 32–59).[215-233] It is more common in the second and fourth decades; women predominate 1.6 to 1. It is a slow-growing tumor with long duration of symptoms.

Hematuria, frequency of urination, nocturia, and tenesmus may occur but about half of cases had signs and symptoms produced by catecholamine secretions such as headaches, sweats, pallor, and paroxysmal or sustained hypertension. These findings are diagnostic if associated with voiding. Distention of the bladder by cystogram or manipulation at cystoscopy may induce an attack.[215, 231] Studies of blood and urine for catecholamines are necessary. Pheochromocytomas may involve any part of the bladder and are light brown to yellow-brown in color. They are rarely multicentric. Metastases to lymph nodes and distant sites have been reported.[216, 222, 223, 225, 226] The malignant variety (Fig. 32–59) has been reported as being capable of secreting 3.4-dehydroxyphenylalanine (dopa and dopamine).[216]

Paragangliomas are usually designated as pheochromocytomas and chemodectomas. The pheochromocytomas are chromaffin positive, humorally active, and arise in adrenal medulla. Chemodectomas[32-58] (Fig. 32–58) are represented by carotid body, aortic pulmonary bodies, and glomus jugulare. These are chromaffin-negative and usually but not always hormonally inactive. Popular usage designates pheochromocytoma as limited to the adrenal medulla and paragangliomas as in extra-adrenal sites, with chemodectomas representing the nonchromaffin variety in special locations.

Roentgenographic Diagnosis. An irregular filling defect in the bladder is the usual appearance on cystograms. Arteriography reveals a highly vascular tumor with abnormal vessels, dense stain, and occasional early venous filling. Distention of the bladder by cystogram, manipulation at cystoscopy, or injection of contrast material into the vascular supply of the tumor may induce an attack.[215, 229, 231]

HEMANGIOMA

Hemangioma is an unusual bladder tumor although Ganem and Ainsworth[236] considered it the most common benign connective tissue tumor of that organ (Figs. 32–60, 32–61).[47, 234-251] Seventy cases have been reported up to 1971,[240] 32 occurring in the first two decades of life. The earliest age reported is 5 weeks.[249] Approximately half occur under 20 years of age.[242] It is generally considered a congenital lesion. About one-third of the cases have hemangiomas elsewhere in the body, usually on the skin of the lower abdomen, external genitalia, or thighs. The vesical lesion is solitary in two-thirds of the cases involving, according to Ray and colleagues, the upper half of the bladder.[47] In one-third of the cases, there are multiple lesions present anywhere in the bladder. The tumor is usually cavernous in type, but plexiform and capillary varieties occur. They are usually sessile, elevated tumors, but the pedunculated type is not rare. Recurrent, painless hematuria is a common finding.

Roentgenographic Diagnosis. There is a slightly irregular, usually nonpedunculated filling defect in the bladder. Such finding in a young individual would increase the possibility of diagnosis of hemangioma, although there is no characteristic roentgenographic appearance. The tumor is readily compressible and may be obliterated on retrograde cystogram.

POLYP

A polyp is a not uncommon tumor that consists of a fibrous stalk with a covering of normal transitional epithelium. It produces a defect in the bladder that can move in any direction (Fig. 32–62).

ENDOMETRIOSIS

Endometriosis of the bladder (Fig. 32–63) is an uncommon involvement of the bladder with uterine endometrium. It was first described by Judd in 1921, and approximately 120 cases have been reported up to 1960.[252] There is no unanimity of opinion concerning its pathogenesis, but apparently it arises by (1) direct invasion, (2) implantation, or (3) metastasis.

Pain or cyclic urinary symptoms are the most common features. Hematuria occurs in about 25 per cent of cases and may be cyclic. Previous gynecologic or abdominal operations have been reported in 60 to 70 per cent of the cases. A majority of the patients have no abnormalities of female reproductive organs that are demonstrated by palpation or operations, although pelvic endometriosis and "chocolate cyst" of the ovary have been described as occurring with vesical endometriosis.

Diagnosis. Cystoscopy generally is considered to be the most accurate method of diagnosis, but the appearance of the lesion varies with the menstrual cycle. Histologic confirmation by biopsy is essential. The location of the tumor is usually on the posterior wall between the trigone and the dome, although it may be on the trigone proper and even overlie an ureteric orifice. Cystographic descriptions are sparse in the literature. The filling defect, when seen, is smooth, rounded, and occasionally multilobular and gives the impression of an indentation produced by an extrinsic lesion.

NEUROFIBROMA

Neurofibroma rarely involves the urinary system (Figs. 32–64, 32–65).[261-268] In adults multiple areas of skin pigmentation associated with tissue overgrowth of nerve sheaths and fibrous tissue elements are usually seen. In children, the pedunculated skin tumors are less common but cafe-au-lait spots may be present. Symptoms vary from none to urinary frequency, incontinence, hematuria, and abdominal pain. Rectal examination can sometimes be useful. Localized clitoral hypertrophy has been reported. Generalized Von Recklinghausen's disease is seen in about 55 per cent of the cases.

Roentgenographic Findings. These include (1) intrinsic mass; (2) external mass; (3) diffuse infiltrative process. The intrinsic mass appears similar to carcinoma; the external mass produces indentations that are usually rather regular and rounded; the diffuse infiltrative process gives an irregular apearance to most of the bladder.

NEPHROGENIC ADENOMA

Nephrogenic adenoma is a slow-growing, generally benign lesion associated with previous bladder trauma and chronic infection and occurring in young men (Fig. 32–66).[269-282] The typical lesion consists of epithelium tubules lined by a single layer of columnar or cuboidal epithelium. Most authors have emphasized the strong similarity to proximal distal and collecting tubules, as well as loop of Henle, but Molland and colleagues found no evidence for this resemblance on ultrastructural studies.[281] There have been several references to malignant change.[270, 281] These tumors may progress and often recur, can be single or multiple, and have been seen in the urethra.

Diagnosis. Biopsy is essential. The symptoms can be severe but are similar to those of cystitis. The roentgenographic feature is nonspecific, showing only a filling defect in the bladder.

LEUKOPLAKIA OF THE BLADDER

Leukoplakia is an uncommon bladder lesion often confused in former years with squamous metaplasia of the trigonal type seen in females (Fig. 32–67).[283-292] They appear as discrete, white, flat areas with sharp, well-demarcated edges. They are only slightly raised above the mucosal level. Most cases are associated with chronic infection. Large masses are rare in the bladder. The ratio of male to female is 3:1 but in cases developing carcinoma, the ratio is 6 males to 1 female.[283] Leukoplakia can apparently undergo malignant transformation to squamous carcinoma or be associated with squamous carcinoma.[283-285, 287a, 288, 292] Witherington's patient (Fig. 32–67) developed squamous cell carcinoma 8 years after the diagnosis of leukoplakia.[291, 292] Cholesteatoma of the bladder is an extremely rare finding.[289a]

Roentgenographic Diagnosis. The usual leukoplakic patch cannot be diagnosed by roentgenographic means. The large mass lesion produces a negative filling defect on cystography that is not diagnostic. Witherington's patient showed irregular, broad, frondlike projections into the bladder lumen.[291]

PRIMARY LYMPHOMA OF BLADDER

Primary lymphoma of bladder[293-301a] is a rare disease; only 39 cases have been reported since 1931 (Fig. 32–68).[293] The etiology is not known, and investigators do not agree whether lymphoid tissue can be found in normal bladder, [294, 298] although it is found in chronic cystitis cases.

The tumors arise in a single focus in the bladder and may metastasize to regional or distal sites. It is a disease of middle age, and families are not frequently involved.

Hematuria, frequency, and dysuria are the common symptoms.[298] The cystoscopic appearance of a round, nodular, solid mass below the mucosa but retrojecting into the bladder may be a clue to the diagnosis. The mucosa is usually normal but ulceration may occur. The base and trigone appear to be the common sites but any area can be involved.

A comparison of clinical and urologic aspects of primary and secondary vesical lymphomas made by Sufrin and co-workers, is shown in Table 32–2.[299]

SECONDARY INVOLVEMENT OF THE BLADDER BY MALIGNANT LYMPHOMA

Secondary vesical involvement by malignant lymphoma was found in 13 per cent of cases (Fig. 32–69).[293] Vesical involvement with non-Hodgkin's lymphoma was more common than with Hodgkin's disease. Males and females are affected equally. Involvement of the bladder with malignant lymphoma apparently does not affect survival.

Non-Hodgkin's lymphoma of the bladder frequently is associated with kidney or ureteral foci. In Hodgkin's disease the vesical involvement in the absence of renal or ureteral involvement occurred in 45 per cent of the cases.[299] Involvement may be anywhere in the bladder and may be either multiple or single. Microscopic changes were more common than macroscopic. The latter, however, is more likely to be symptomatic. Watson and co-workers suggested the following routes of involvement of the bladder[301a]:

1. Circumscribed single or multiple foci limited to the bladder wall
2. Direct invasion of bladder by perivesical tumor
3. Vesical extension from prostatic foci

Extrinsic infiltrates have been considered the most common routes of invasion but Sufrin considered hematogenous dissemination the primary route and found no extension into or continuity with perivesical foci. Symptoms consist of urgency, frequency (in absence of infection), and hematuria only with mucosal involvement. Transitional cell carcinoma may accompany the lymphatic involvement but is unrelated in position.[299]

ROENTGENOGRAPHIC FINDINGS

One sees multiple large, rounded, smooth-appear-

TABLE 32-2
Comparison of Primary and Secondary Vesical Lymphomas

	Primary Lymphoma	Secondary Lymphoma
Age at diagnosis	More than 50	Less than 50
Sex incidence	Women more than men	Men more than women
Histologic type	Invariably non-Hodgkin's; usually lymphosarcoma	All histologic types involved about equally
Bladder site involved	Base and trigone	All sites equally
Clinical symptoms of involvement	Common	Uncommon
Prognosis	Good	Poor

ing masses distending the bladder lumen. Lobulations may occur.

LEUKEMIA

Although leukemia involves the urinary tract in 63 per cent of cases, vesical infiltration is rare (Fig. 32–70).[302-309] There may be hemorrhage as the main symptom. The bladder may be diffusely infiltrated or demonstrate localized masses.

Roentgenographic Findings. The filling defects that may be localized or more diffuse are not diagnostic.

CARCINOSARCOMA

Carcinosarcoma is a rare variety of invasive transitional or squamous cell carcinoma of the bladder often associated with giant tumor cells. It may occur spontaneously or as a pattern of recurrence after radiotherapy.

SECONDARY TUMORS OF THE BLADDER

Secondary tumors of the bladder may be classified according to the following types[310-322]:

1. Those that arise by direct extension from primary growths in the prostate gland (Figs. 32–71, 32–72), the uterus (Fig. 32–73), the bowel (Fig. 32–74), the cervix, and the ovary
2. Those that are secondary to tumors of the kidney or the ureter
   Papillary tumors of the kidney or the ureter
   Clear cell adenocarcinoma of the kidney
3. Those that are true metastatic lesions of the bladder from such areas as lung, breast, stomach, and malignant melanoma of the skin (see Fig. 32–29).
4. Involvement by lymphoma and leukemic infiltrations

Metastatic lesions to the bladder (type 3) are unusual. Their frequency is one-tenth of all vesical tumors. Symptoms related to bladder involvement are unusual because the lesions are small and do not ulcerate the mucosa.[311, 316] Metastatic tumors to the bladder associated with primary bladder carcinoma have been reported.[321]

CHAPTER 32, ILLUSTRATIONS

FIG. 32–1. Calcified carcinoma of the bladder. (A) Scout film showing rim of calcification on right side of bladder around margins of large papillary tumor. (B) Excretory cystogram more clearly outlines the large mass in the bladder, with contrast medium completely surrounding the tumor. In general, there are three types of calcification in bladder eipthelial neoplasms: (1) hazy opacity with dense rim, (2) speckled irregular stippling, and (3) nodular dense calcification.

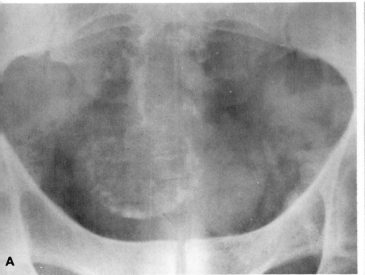

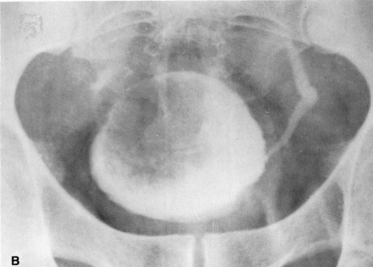

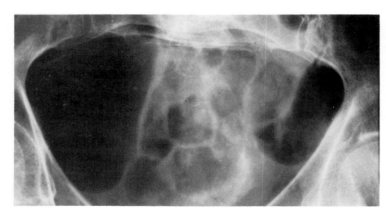

FIG. 32–2. Calcification in bladder tumor. Wide band of finely granular calcification on the surface (encrusted) of squamous cell carcinoma. (Miller, S.W., Pfister, R.C.: Am. J. Roentgenol., *121*:827–831, 1974)

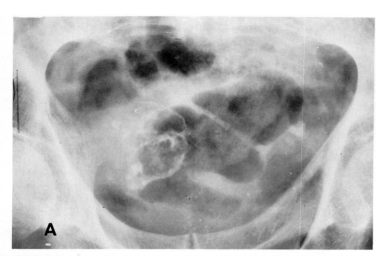

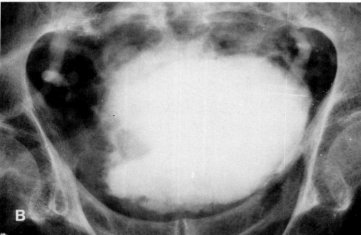

FIG. 32–3. Calcification in bladder tumor. **(A)** Nodular calcification on the surface of large transitional cell neoplasm. **(B)** Corresponding opacified bladder showing correlating tumor size. (Miller, S.W., Pfister, R.C.: Am. J. Roentgenol., *121*:827–831, 1974)

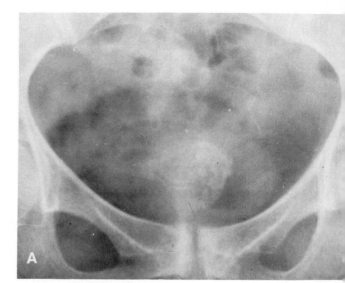

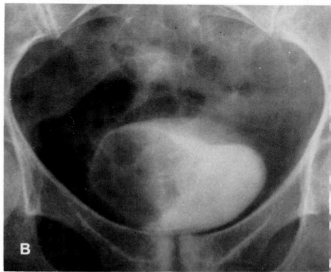

FIG. 32–4. (A) Mixed granular and nodular calcifications involving left side of transitional cell carcinoma. **(B)** Only a portion of the large neoplasm is calcified. (Miller, S.W., Pfister, R.C.: Am. J. Roentgenol., *121*:827–831, 1974)

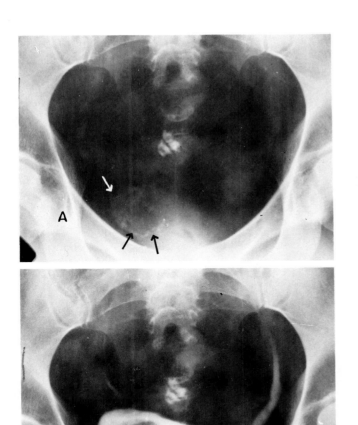

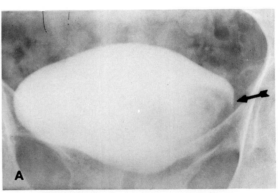

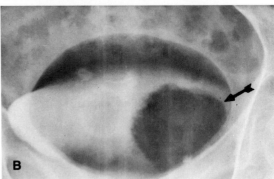

FIG. 32–6. (A) Conventional cystogram. Papillary carcinoma of the bladder, noninfiltrating. *Arrow* points to filling defect in bladder completely surrounded by contrast material. **(B)** Double contrast air cystogram better delineates tumor mass (*arrow*).

FIG. 32–5. (A) Mixed soft granular–nodular calcification (*arrows*) in subepithelial portion of transitional cell neoplasm. **(B)** Larger tumor volume readily apparent. Note unassociated supravesical calcifications. (Miller, S.W., Pfister, R.C.: Am. J. Roentgenol., *121*:827–831, 1974)

FIG. 32–7. Conventional cystogram. Noninfiltrating carcinoma of bladder. *Arrow* points to small filling defect.

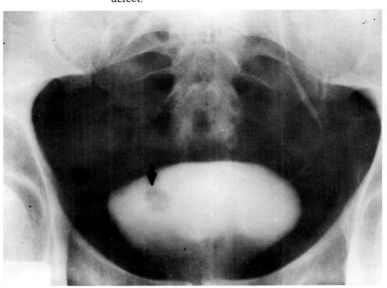

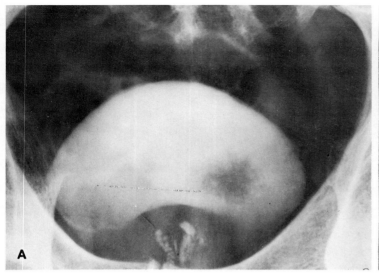

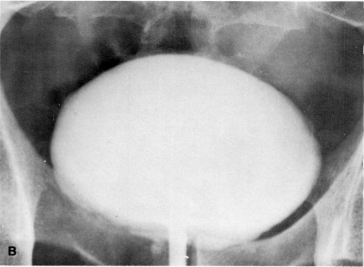

FIG. 32–8. Conventional cystogram. Noninfiltrating bladder carcinoma. (A) Filling defect on left side of bladder. Note enlarged prostate with prostatic calculi. (B) Tumors obscured by dense contrast material.

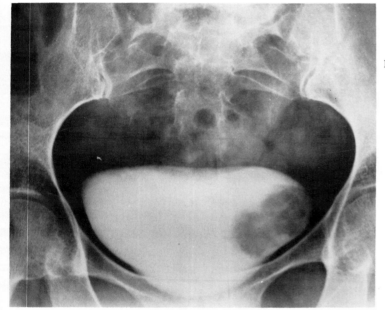

FIG. 32–9. Large transitional cell carcinoma of bladder.

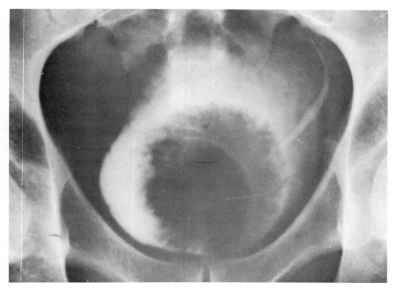

FIG. 32–10. Conventional cystogram. Noninfiltrating bladder carcinoma. Note extension of the contrast material around the tumor except in the region of the pedicle on the left bladder floor.

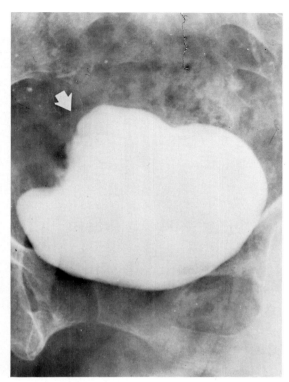

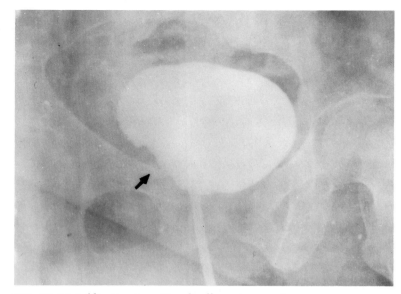

FIG. 32–12. Infiltrating transitional cell carcinoma of bladder. Conventional cystogram showing an irregular filling defect on right lower lateral wall of bladder (*arrow*).

FIG. 32–11. Infiltrating transitional cell carcinoma of the bladder. Conventional cystogram showing an irregular filling defect of the upper side of the right bladder wall. *Arrow* points to perivesical fat at the edge of the tumor-bearing area. The beginning thickening of the bladder wall in this area is an indication of infiltration.

FIG. 32–14. Infiltrating transitional cell carcinoma. Intravenous urogram. The cystogram shows an irregularly contracted bladder. On the right side there is an extensive deformity of the bladder wall with flattening and indentations. The dilatation of the right ureter indicates an infiltrating tumor. There was also pyelectasis.

FIG. 32–13. Infiltrating transitional cell carcinoma of the bladder. Conventional cystogram showing irregular deformity of left bladder wall (*black arrow*). The dilated left ureter is indicative of infiltration. There is a great increase in thickness of the bladder wall in the area of the tumor. This wall is measured between the contrast medium and the perivesical fat (*white arrow*). Note small, irregularly contracted bladder.

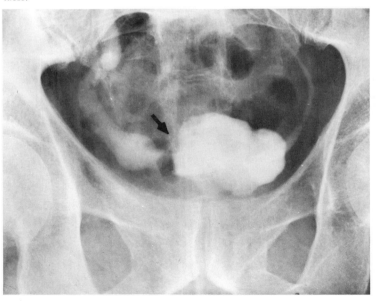

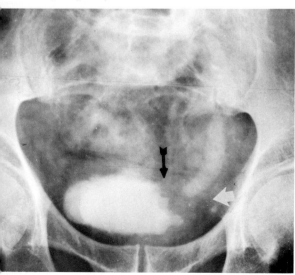

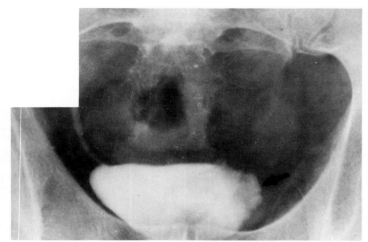

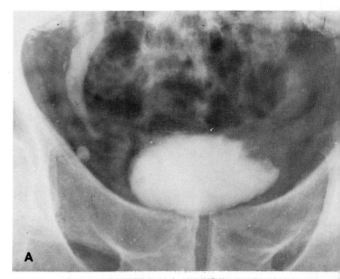

FIG. 32–15. Infiltrating transitional cell carcinoma of bladder. Cystogram on intravenous urogram. *Arrow* points to infiltrating lesion of left wall of the bladder. There is a fuzzy appearance with uneven distribution of the contrast material. Note nonvisualization of the left ureter. The left kidney was nonfunctioning due to tumor obstruction in the bladder. This is another indication of infiltrating tumor.

FIG. 32–16. Rapid growth of a transitional cell carcinoma. **(A)** Intravenous urogram showing moderately sized filling defect on the left side of bladder. Wall intact, ureter normal. **(B)** Three months later, large infiltrating lesion on left side of bladder producing irregularity and displacement of left lateral wall and dilated lower ureter.

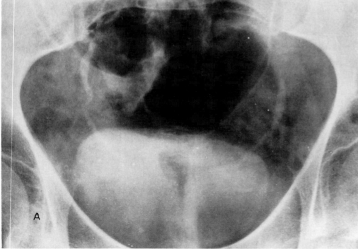

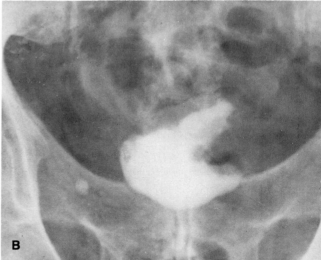

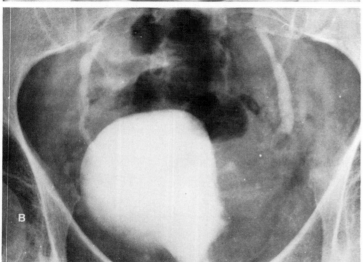

FIG. 32–17. Conventional cystogram showing progression of infiltrating transitional cell carcinoma of bladder in a 6-month interval. **(A)** Excretory cystogram. There is an irregular area in the left lateral wall of the bladder. The left ureter is seen faintly but is dilated; the right ureter also is dilated. **(B)** Increase in the size of the tumor on retrograde cystogram taken 6 months later.

FIG. 32–18. Staging of carcinoma of the bladder. This diagram shows the clinical and pathologic staging of carcinoma of the bladder according to Jewett and the International Union Against Cancer (U.I.C.C.). T = tumor; T.I.S. = tumor confined to epithelium; $N^{\pm}$ = lymph node metastases present or absent. (Courtesy of Willet Whitmore, M.D.)

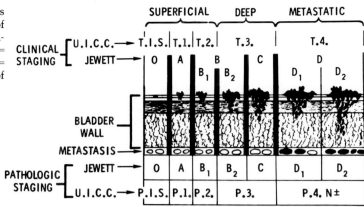

FIG. 32–19. Excretory urogram. Squamous cell carcinoma of the bladder. *Arrow* points to an irregularity on the floor of the bladder, right side, due to an infiltrating squamous cell carcinoma.

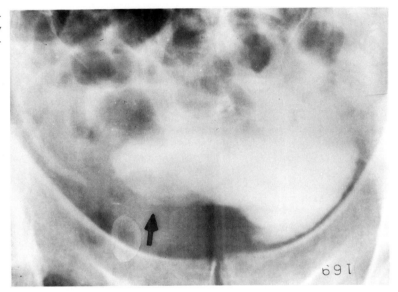

FIG. 32–20. Squamous cell carcinoma: infiltrating tumor at dome. Large defect in wall of bladder.

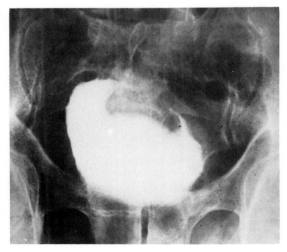

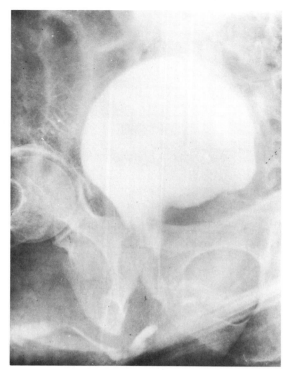

FIG. 32-21. Voiding cystourethrogram. Adenocarcinoma of the bladder. Cystogram shows that the floor of the bladder on the left side is elevated irregularly by a mass in the region. (Adenocarcinoma commonly arises here.) In the dome it would probably arise from an urachal remnant. (Courtesy of Keith Waterhouse, M.D.)

FIG. 32-23. Pitfalls in diagnosis of bladder tumors. Importance of multiple views. Infiltrating transitional cell carcinoma of the bladder. Conventional cystogram. (A) Small contracted bladder, showing slight flattening of bladder on right side, upper border. This is not diagnostic of tumor. (B) Right oblique view. Arrow points to an indentation at posterolateral wall of bladder, which is smooth in contour at the tumor site. Note slight dilatation of right ureter and straight course of left ureter.

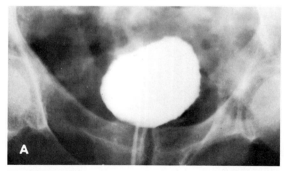

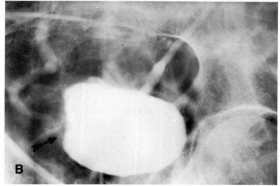

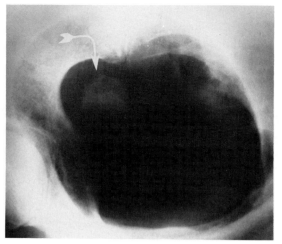

FIG. 32-22. Urachal mucinous adenocarcinoma. Air cystogram. Arrow points to tumor at dome.

FIG. 32-24. Pitfalls in diagnosis of bladder tumors. The importance of repeated studies. (A) Excretory cystogram. Multiple areas of decreased densities simulating tumor. (B) Retrograde cystogram showing smooth, evenly distributed contrast material. The defects in the top film were due to gas and fecal material in the rectum. This is a common error and must be evaluated carefully.

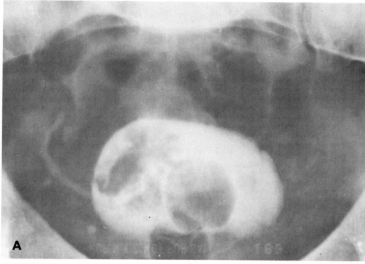

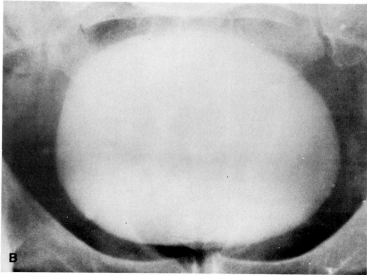

FIG. 32–25. Fractionated cystogram. Normal-appearing bladder with this technique. Note expanding bladder outlines with each increment of contrast material. On a single film four exposures were taken, one after each increment of 40 cc. of contrast material. There is a pseudodiverticulum at the right lower lateral wall. (Courtesy of D.M. Wallace, M.D., and J.G. Connolly, M.D.)

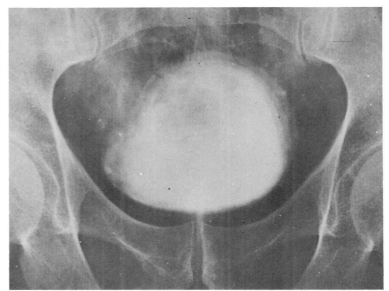

FIG. 32–26. Fractionated cystogram technique revealing fixation of the right lower wall of the bladder by infiltrating tumor. The expansion of bladder contour is clearly demonstrated along the left bladder margin. In the area of tumor the four exposures are superimposed, appearing as a single bladder margin indicating fixation.

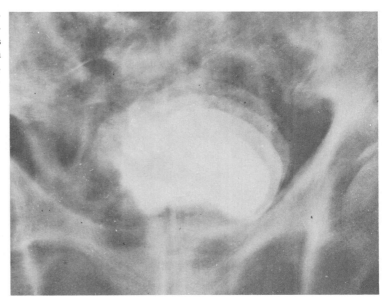

FIG. 32–27. Fractionated cystogram technique revealing fixation of the right wall of the bladder by infiltrating carcinoma (Courtesy of D.M. Wallace, M.D., and J.G. Connolly, M.D.)

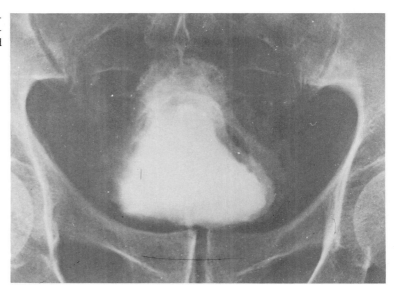

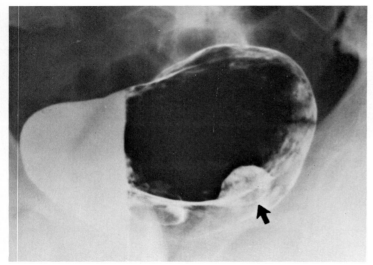

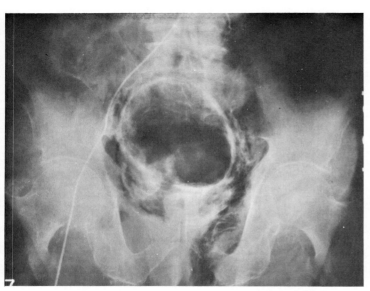

FIG. 32–30. A preliminary film revealing guide wire in place in right iliac artery with combined endoperivesical gas completely outlining the bladder wall. Note the large tumor extending along the base of the bladder to the right lateral wall.

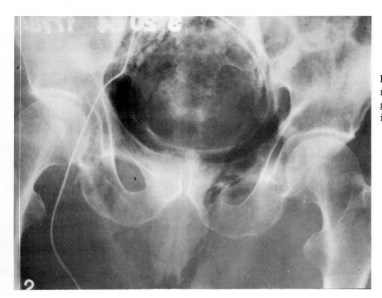

FIG. 32–28. Double contrast barium cystogram uses carbon dioxide. Right lateral decubitus view. A polypoid lesion well coated with barium is demonstrated at the left base (*arrow*). Cystoscopy and biopsy revealed a papilloma with in situ carcinoma. (Pochaczevsky, R., Grabstald, H.: Am. J. Roentgenol., *92*:365–373, 1964)

FIG. 32–29. Double contrast barium carbon dioxide cystogram. Left lateral decubitus view. Note excellent coating of the polypoid lesions (*single arrow*) with barium. The larger tumor on the right infiltrated the muscular wall. Note "bladder horns" above and below the lesion (*double arrow*). Metastatic melanoma. The presence of "bladder horns" is a sign that is described as presumptive evidence of muscular involvement. The following is a description of this sign:

> An odd-shaped localized ballooning out of the bladder wall was a frequently encountered sign. This was felt to be direct evidence of muscular infiltration by tumor, and presumably secondary to nonuniform distention of the uninvolved portion of the bladder adjacent to the tumor. This ballooning phenomenon was felt to be best described as a "bladder horn."

(Pochaczevsky, R., Grabstald, H.: Am. J. Roentgenol., *92*:365–373, 1964)

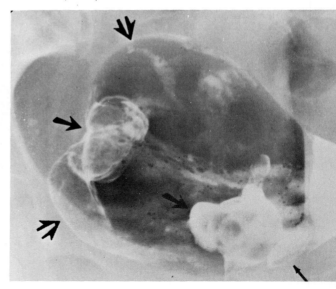

FIG. 32–31. Endoperivesical gas insufflation. Preliminary film. Note the uneven distribution of perivesical gas along the right lateral bladder wall. The bladder wall is being pushed medially in the region of the tumor.

FIG. 32–32. Preliminary film revealing endoperivesical gas and nonuniform dissection of gas along the right inferior margin of the bladder. A guide wire is seen in place in right iliac artery.

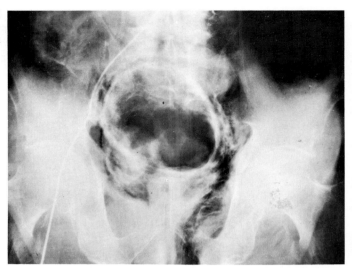

FIG. 32–33. Transitional cell carcinoma of the bladder. **(A)** Intravenous urogram: cystogram. *Arrow* points to filling defect, left posterior wall. Wall looks intact. Slight dilatation left ureter. **(B)** Endoperivesical gas. Mass left side of bladder. Thickening of wall indicates infiltration.

FIG. 32–34. Schematized diagram of the triple contrast study (combined endoperivesical gas and pelvic arteriography) for the diagnosis of bladder tumors. L.S. = Lumbosacral artery; S.G. = superior gluteal artery; Um. = umbilical artery; I.G. = inferior gluteal artery; Ut. = uterine artery; Va. = vaginal artery; S.V. = superior vesical artery; I.V. = inferior vesical artery; Ob. = obturator artery; I.P. = internal pudendal artery)

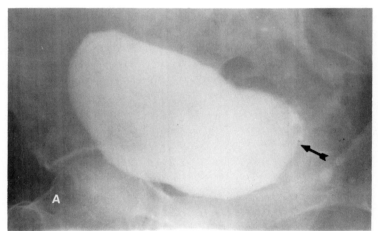

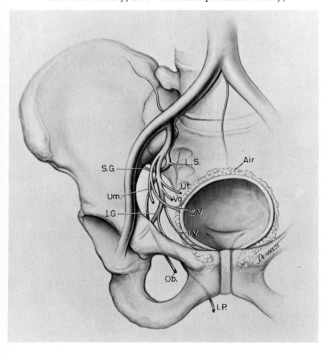

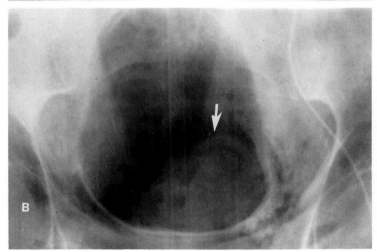

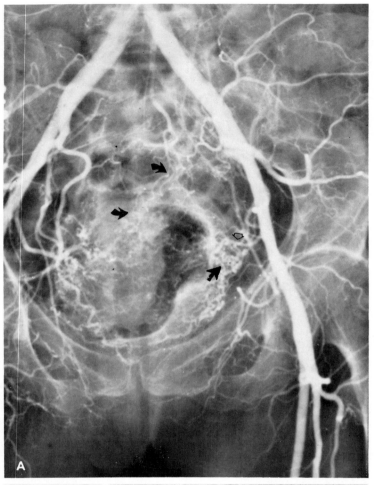

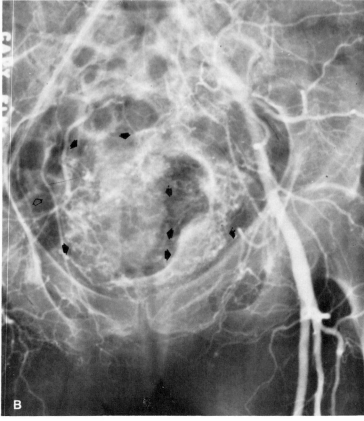

FIG. 32–35. (A) Corkscrew vessels (vessels of rapidly changing caliber) clearly identify a huge tumor involving the entire bladder. Note the unusually large vesical arteries (*lucent arrow*). Increased flow is reflected by early filling of tumor vessels. Cannibalization of the vascular supply of the midhemorrhoidal artery (*curved arrows*) indicates direct tumor extension into the recum. (Lang, E.K.: Roentgenographic Diagnosis of Bladder Tumors. Springfield, Ill.: Charles C Thomas, 1968.) **(B)** An inhomogeneous staining quality of different sections of this tumor is noted. This may reflect different vascular patterns found in areas of different histologic grade and differentiation of this tumor. Note premature opacification of draining veins (*lucent arrow*), indicating the presence of arteriovenous shunts within the tumor.

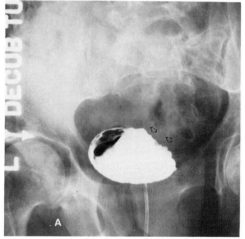

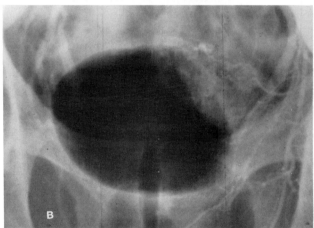

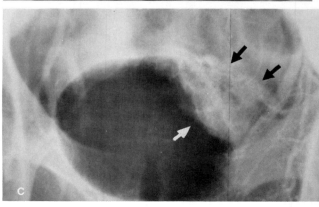

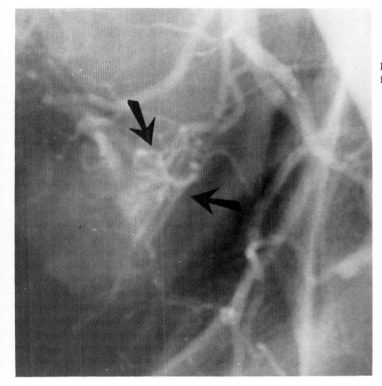

FIG. 32–37. A papillary tumor of the bladder is supplied from a hypertrophied vesical artery.

FIG. 32–38. (A) A combined barium air cystogram and perivesical gas study documents multiple lobulated tumors originating from the right lateral bladder wall and the floor of the bladder (*arrows*). Normal thickness of the bladder wall and the dome segment and clear dissectability of the perivesical fat plane along the right lateral bladder wall (in apposition to the tumor) appear to exclude permeation of the tumor into the perivesical space (*solid arrows*). (Lang, E.K.: J.A.M.A., *207*:342–344, 1969.) **(B)** An arteriogram combined with endo- and perivesical gas insufflation documents the intravesical tumor (*arrows*) but also a huge staining tumor metastasis along the right lateral pelvic wall (*arrows*). The fact that the perivesical dissection plane is intact suggested metastases to external iliac nodes rather than direct tumor extension. Exploration confirmed this impression.

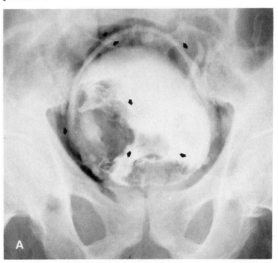

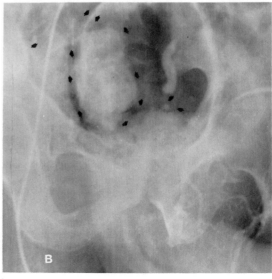

FIG. 32–36. (A) Lack of distensibility of the left lateral bladder wall and dome segment seen on a barium air cystogram suggests neoplastic or inflammatory fixation (*lucent arrows*). **(B)** A pelvic arteriogram, in conjunction with endo- and perivesical gas study, demonstrates an "iceberg" tumor involving the dome of the bladder and extending into the perivesical fat. **(C)** The extravesical circumference of the tumor is best defined on a 1½-second phase arteriogram. Prematurely opacifying draining veins splayed around the outer circumference of the lesion facilitate identification (*solid arrows*). **(D)** A 2½-second parenchymal phase arteriogram documents continued homogeneous staining of the tumor (indicative of a histologically well-differentiated neoplasm). Note the characteristic displacement of the perivesical gas around the tumor extension into the perivesical fat.

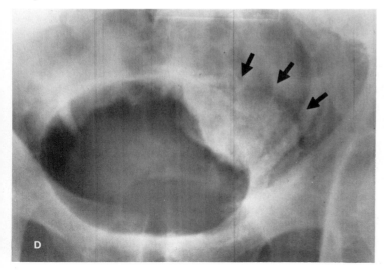

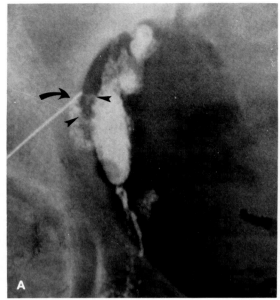

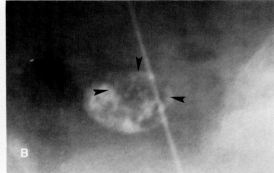

FIG. 32–39. (A) An ominous defect is noted in an external iliac node on this pedal lymphangiogram (arrows). Note position of a 23-gauge shiba needle advanced into the incriminated node (curved arrow). (B) Proper position of the biopsy needle through the involved portion of the node is documented on a cross-table lateral projection. In this particular case, the defect in the node proved to be attributable to inflammatory disease, later confirmed by examination of the specimen of the node dissection.

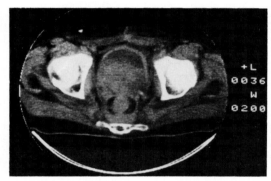

FIG. 32–40. A computed tomogram demonstrates a large transitional cell carcinoma of the bladder with invasion of seminal vesicles and prostate. B = bladder, P = prostate, SV = seminal vesicles. (Courtesy of Dr. Robert R. Hattery, Mayo Clinic Rochester, Minnesota)

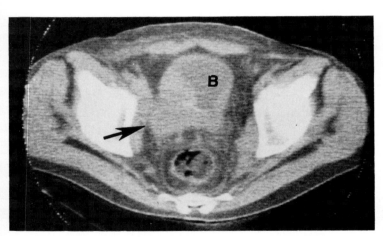

FIG. 32–41. CT scan. Carcinoma of bladder invading seminal vesicles (arrow). B = bladder

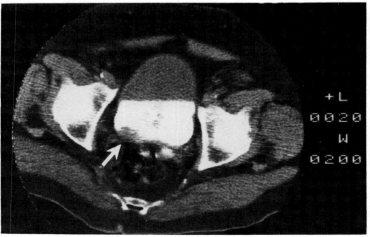

FIG. 32–42. Transitional cell carcinoma of the bladder with invasion just to the outer wall of the bladder shown on computed tomogram (arrow). (Courtesy of Dr. Robert R. Hattery, Mayo Clinic Rochester, Minnesota)

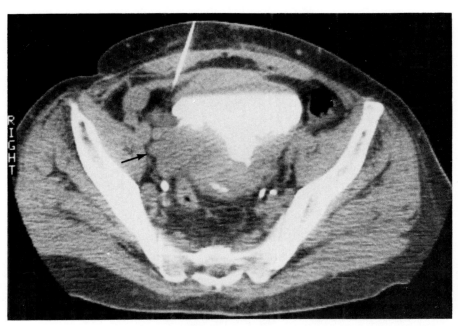

FIG. 32–43. A computed tomogram demonstrates a huge bladder tumor involving the posterior wall of the bladder. Note a rounded mass presenting in the region of the right hypogastric nodes (*arrow*).

FIG. 32–44. A computed tomogram (patient in supine position) demonstrates an extensive bladder tumor involving the left anterior, lateral, and posterior bladder wall with extension into the perivesical fat left laterally and posteriorly. The tumor abuts but does not appear to extend into the vagina (identified by the spherical shape of a low-density Tampax: *arrowhead*). A separate mass along the left lateral pelvic wall suggests enlarged nodes (*arrow*). (Courtesy Dr. Priskin, Barnes Hospital and Washington Medical School, St. Louis, Missouri)

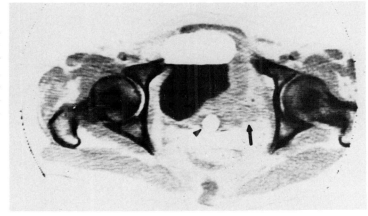

FIG. 32–45. A computed tomogram with the patient in prone position shows separation of the tumor extending contiguously into the perivesical fat and the spherical mass. This identifies the spherical mass as an enlarged node of the hypogastric group. (Courtesy of Bruce Mc-Clennan, M.D., Mallinckrodt Institute of Radiology, St. Louis, Missouri)

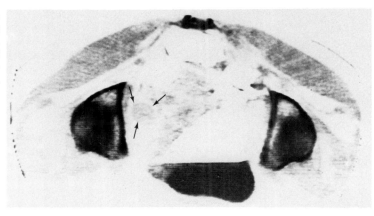

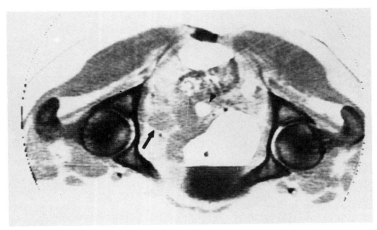

FIG. 32–46. The computed tomogram in the prone position identifies the tumor extension along the left lateral bladder wall and posteriorly into the perivesical fat. The enlarged node is now clearly separated from the primary tumor and enveloped by fat (*arrow*). Histopathologic examination confirms a grade III transitional cell carcinoma of the bladder extending into the perivesical fat anteriorly, left laterally and posteriorly. Though the prone view suggested separation of the bladder and vaginal wall (*arrowhead*), microscopic sections demonstrated superficial invasion of the myometrium. Metastatic carcinoma was proved in one of two lymph nodes identified at surgical resection as "left pelvic lymph nodes." (Courtesy of Dr. Priskin, Barnes Hospital and Washington University Medical School, St. Louis, Missouri)

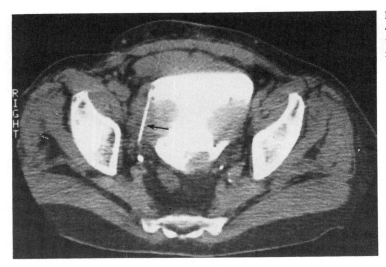

FIG. 32–47. A CT cut 5 mm lower than that in Fig. 32–43 demonstrates a 22-gauge sheeba biopsy needle through the suspect nodes. The specimen confirmed neoplastic involvement of these nodes.

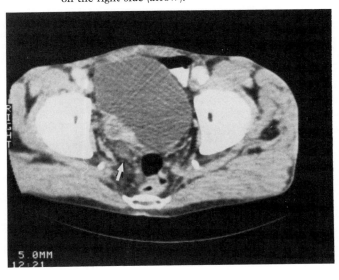

FIG. 32–47a. Dynamic computed tomogram demonstrates a neoplasm involving the right posterolateral bladder wall. The tumor clearly extends into the perivesicle fat and shows enhancement on this dynamic study. Note a prominent node of the hypogastric group on the right side (*arrow*).

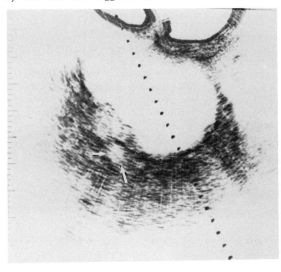

FIG. 32–47b. A transverse sonographic cut demonstrates the bladder tumor in an almost identical fashion to the computed tomogram, again suggesting extension into the perivesicle fat. Moreover, the presence of a large node with homogeneous transmission surrounded by fat is likewise suggested (*arrows*).

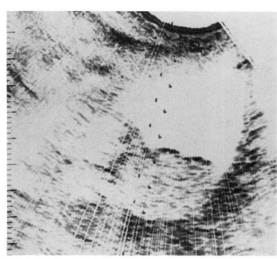

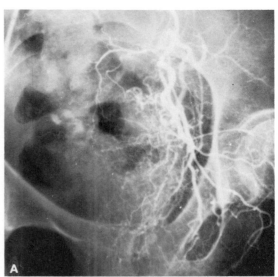

FIG. 32–47c. A parasagittal sonographic cut best demonstrates the thickness of the tumor involving the right posterior lateral bladder wall exceeding 2.5 cm.

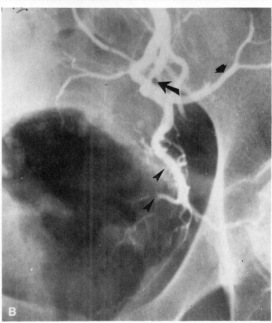

FIG. 32–48. (A) A superselective arteriogram of the anterior division of the left hypogastric artery demonstrates extensive tumor neovascularity in the lateral and posterior bladder wall with predominant supply from the superior and inferior vesical arteries and branches of the internal pudendal group. **(B)** Intractable hemorrhage from the bladder was readily controlled by transcatheter embolization of the anterior division of the hypogastric artery with 3.5 cc. of absorbable gelatin sponge suspension. Note successful occlusion of all branches of the anterior division (*arrowheads*), yet unimpaired flow into the superior gluteal, posterior division (*arrows*). (**A & B:** Long, E.K., et al.: J. Urol., *121*:30–36, 1979)

FIG. 32–49. (A) An initial arteriogram performed for staging documents a multilobulated tumor in the floor of the bladder (*arrows*). Note displacement of the Foley balloon. **(B)** The tumor has all but disappeared 6 weeks after completion of external ^{60}Co therapy delivering 6000 rads.

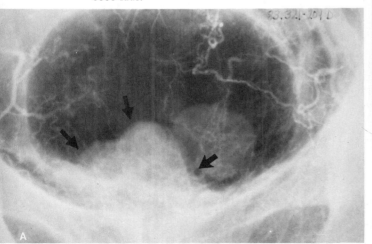

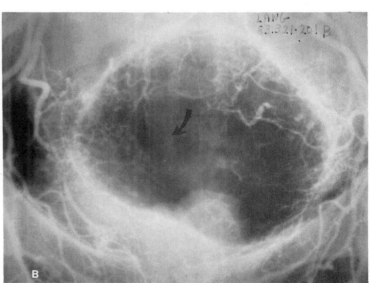

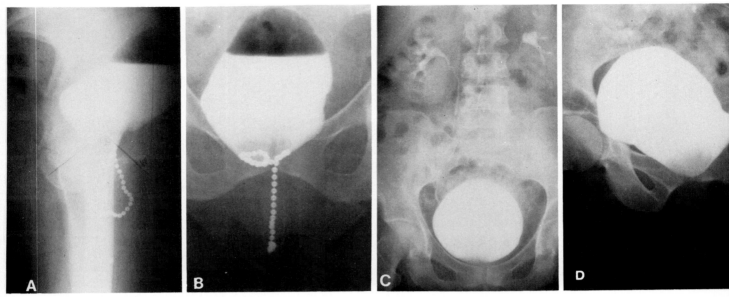

FIG. 32–50. Leiomyoma of bladder. **(A)** Direct lateral view of chain cystogram demonstrates type 2 stress incontinence. **(B)** Chain cystogram showing deviation of chain at bladder neck by mass. **(C)** Intravenous urogram revealing normal upper tracts and mass at base of bladder. **(D)** Voiding cystogram showing mass obstructing bladder neck. (Katz, R.B., Waldbaum, R.S.: Urology, 5:236–238, 1975)

FIG. 32–51. Leiomyoma of bladder. Intravenous urogram revealing 3 × 3 cm. filling defect in bladder. (O'Connell, K., Edson, M.: Urology, 6:114–115, 1975)

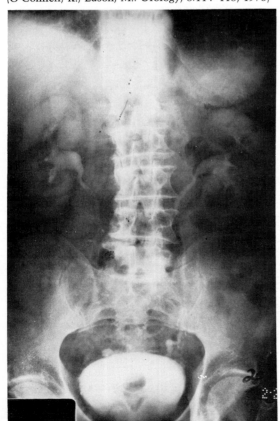

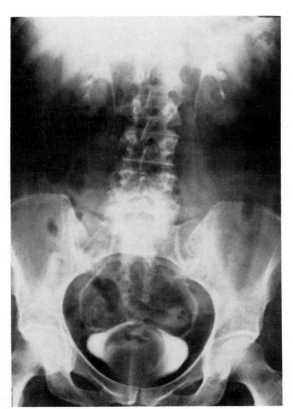

FIG. 32–52. Fibroma. Intravenous urogram with large filling defect of bladder relatively unchanged in 15 years. (Katz, R.B., Waldbaum, R.S.: Urology, 5:236–238, 1975)

FIG. 32–53. Leiomyosarcoma of the bladder. Large mass involving most of the posterior wall, right lateral wall, and floor of the bladder. The irregularity of the bladder wall is demonstrated by the bizarre appearance of the contrast. (Courtesy of A. Balsamo, M.D.)

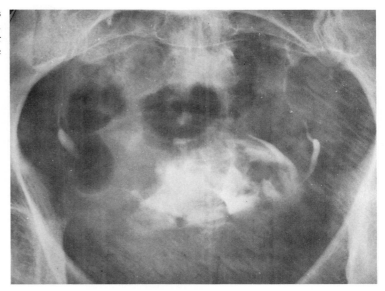

FIG. 32–54. Leiomyosarcoma of bladder. Intravenous urogram showing large nodular defect in bladder with apparent invasion of left lateral wall. (Tara, H.H., Mentur, N.L.: Urology, 2:460–462, 1973)

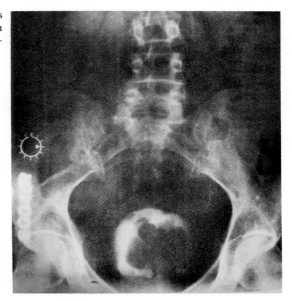

FIG. 32–55. Spindle cell sarcoma of the bladder in an adult, producing a regular filling defect at the base on the right side. (Courtesy of Hans Goldmann, M.D.)

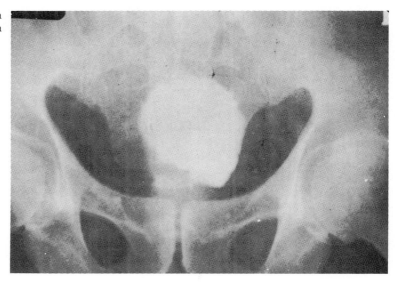

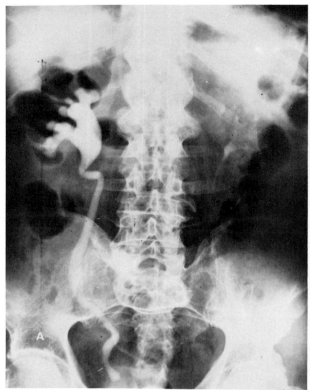

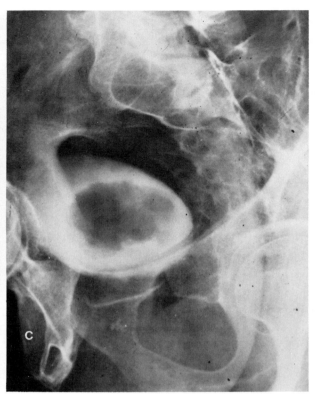

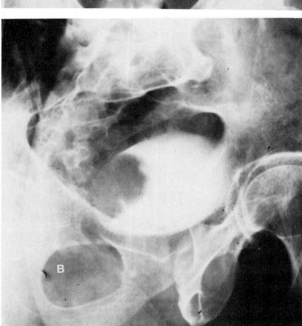

FIG. 32–56. Rhabdomyosarcoma in 60-year-old man. (A) Intravenous urogram: dilated right kidney and ureter; defect of right side of bladder. (B) Left oblique: large infiltrating tumor, right posterior wall. (C) Right oblique: large polypoid mass producing a defect.

FIG. 32–57. Pheochromocytoma of the bladder. Filling defect on right side of bladder produced by a pheochromocytoma. (Tan, T.L., Young, B.W.: J. Urol., 87:63–67, 1962)

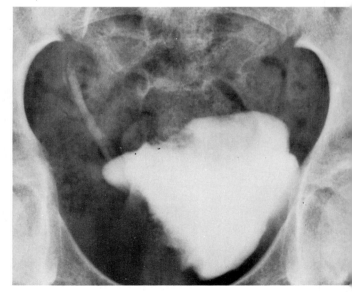

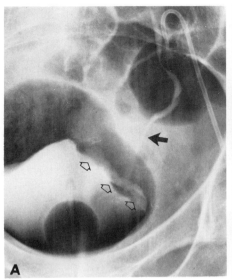
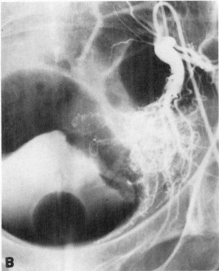
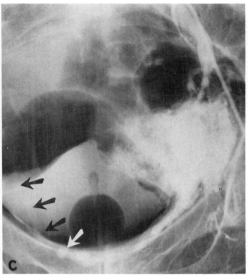

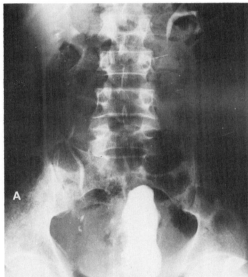

FIG. 32–58. Functioning nonchromaffin paraganglioma (chemodectoma) of the urinary bladder. Selective left hypogastric arteriogram. **(A)** Injected CO_2 distends and outlines bladder. A small amount of excreted contrast material outlines an irregular mass infiltrating the left bladder wall (*open arrows*). The distal left ureter is deviated medially. **(B)** Arterial phase: Vesical branches supply a highly vascular tumor with extension of "pathologic" vessels along base of bladder. **(C)** Tissue phase: Dense tumor stain outlines the full extent of the mass. An early draining vein is seen to the right of midline (*arrows*). (Spitzer, R., Borrison, R., Castellino, R.A.: Radiology, *98*:577–578, 1971)

FIG. 32–59. Malignant pheochromocytoma of bladder, metastases to lymph nodes. **(A)** Large filling defect of right side of bladder. **(B)** Few abnormal vessels present. **(C)** Abnormal vessels with dense tumor stain. (Javaheri, P., Raafat, J.: Br. J. Urol., *47*:401–404, 1975)

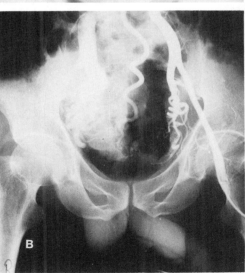
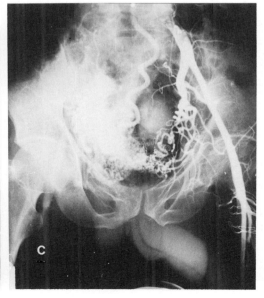

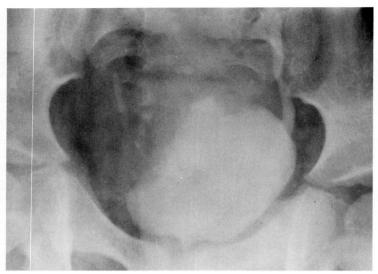

FIG. 32–60. Hemangioma in a child. Large filling defect in right side of bladder. The appearance is similar to that of infiltrating tumor on conventional cystogram. (Courtesy of H.W. Dargeon, M.D.)

FIG. 32–61. Hemangioma bladder. Seven-year-old boy with hematuria and melena. **(A)** *Arrows* at right lumbar area demonstrate phleboliths characteristic of vascular tumor. Patient had cavernous hemangioma of lower half of trunk and right leg. Note defect of midbladder. **(B)** Retroperitoneal hemangioma, right side. Multiple small hemangiomas involving bladder. (Tucker, A.S., Persky, L.: Am. J. Roentgenol., *109*:390–398, 1970)

FIG. 32–62. Bladder polyp in a 2-year, 5-month-old (29 month) boy. **(A)** Small defect, base of bladder. **(B)** Voiding film—prolapse of mass into urethra—polyp on a stalk. Diagnosis: angiohamartomatous malformation. (Tucker, H.S., Persky, L.: Am. J. Roentgenol., *109*:390–398, 1970)

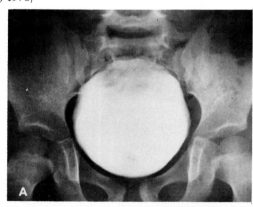

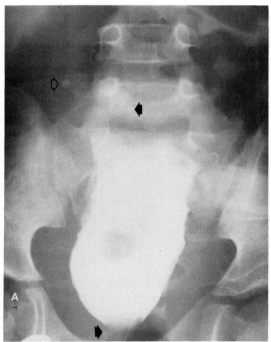

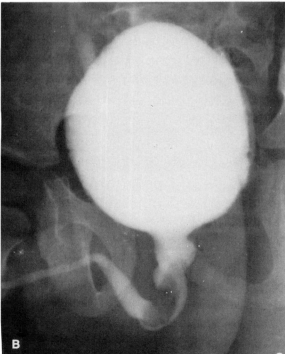

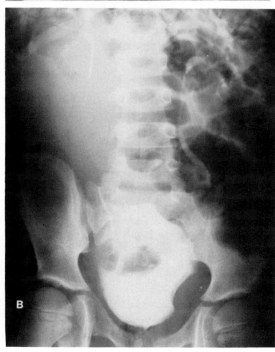

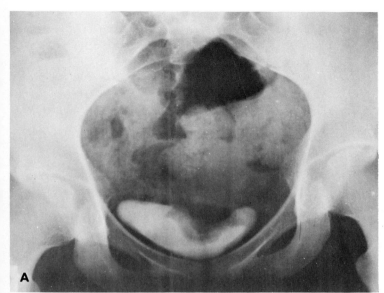

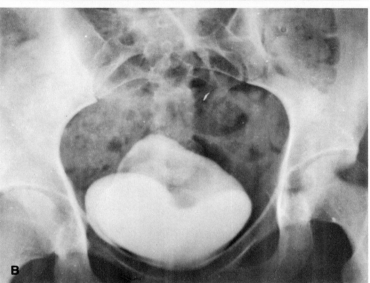

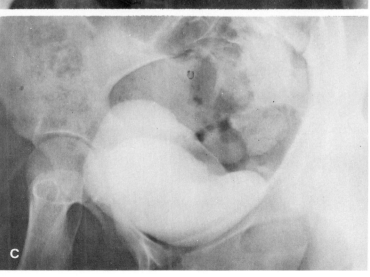

FIG. 32–63. Endometriosis of the bladder. Cystograms taken 2 years after a curettage. Patient was thought to have pelvic endometriosis and was treated over this interval. **(A)** Smooth filling defect of upper surface of bladder, giving the appearance of an extrinsic lesion indenting the bladder. **(B)** More adequate filling showing a defect in the upper part of the bladder and indentation on the more dense contrast medium at the base. **(C)** Right oblique view confirming the mass in the upper posterior surface of the bladder. (Courtesy of B.F. Horton, M.D., and R.L. Fein, M.D.)

FIG. 32–64. Neurofibroma. Eleven-year-old boy with café-au-lait spots. Family history of fibromatosis. Excretory urogram of bladder shows an irregular lobulated tumor involving most of the left lateral wall of the bladder. (Carlson, D.H., Wilkinson, R.H.: Radiology, *105*:401–404, 1972)

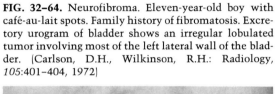

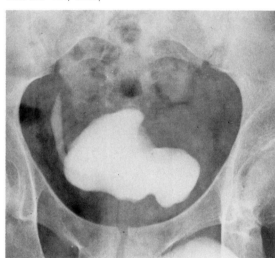

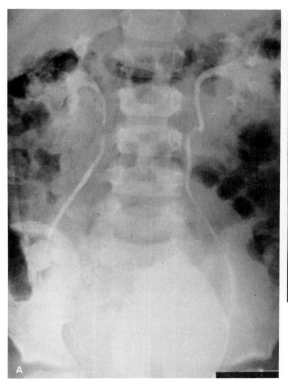

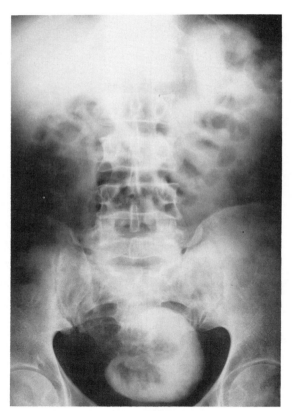

FIG. 32-65. Neurofibroma of bladder. Six-year-old boy with café-au-lait spots. (A) Excretory urogram. Anteroposterior view showing lateral displacement of lower half of ureter by mass. The bladder is displaced to the left; irregular right side. (B) Bladder displaced anteriorly by presacral mass. Irregular dome. Tumor in dome extending into sacral promontory. (Carlson, D.H., Wilkinson, R.H.: Radiology, *105*:401–404, 1972)

FIG. 32-66. Nephrogenic adenoma. Intravenous urogram showing irregular, lobular filling defect in right side of dome or bladder. (Kaany,E., Werner, S.L.: Urology, *4*:343–345, 1974)

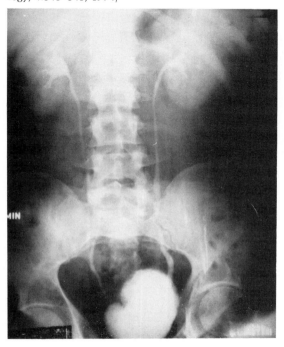

FIG. 32-67. Leukoplakia of bladder. Intravenous urogram, 25-minute film, reveals a 4-cm. irregular lobulated filling defect on right side of bladder (this patient later developed squamous cell carcinoma). (Witherington, R.: J. Urol., *98*:206–208, 1967)

1512

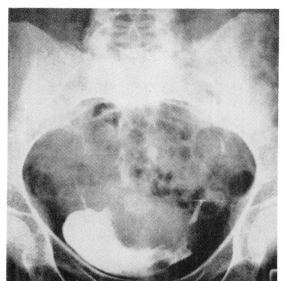

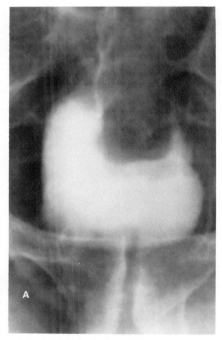

FIG. 32–68. Primary lymphoma of bladder. Excretory cystogram shows a large bosselated filling defect in left side of posterolateral and superior portion of bladder. (Pontius, E.E., Nourse, M.H., Paz, L., et al.: J. Urol., *90*:58–61, 1963)

FIG. 32–69. Secondary lymphoma of bladder. **(A)** Cystogram: large, irregular, lobulated mass in left side of dome of bladder and posterior wall. **(B)** Left oblique view showing distinct lobulation. **(C)** Air cystogram: mass pushing into bladder lumen (*arrow*).

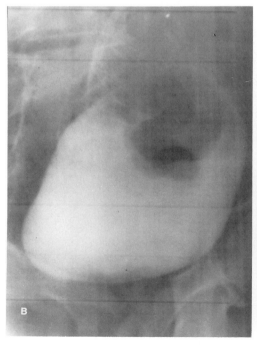

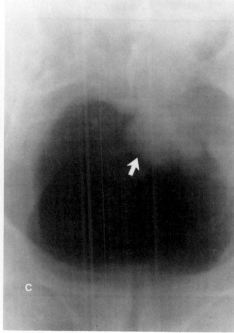

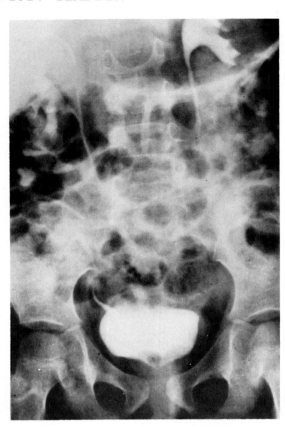

FIG. 32–70. Leukemia (acute lymphoblastic). Excretory cystogram reveals a mottled appearance of base of bladder with a filling defect involving floor at midline and extending over to left side. (Troup, C.W., Thatcher, G., Hodgson, N.B.: J. Urol., *107*:314–315, 1972)

FIG. 32–71. Carcinoma of the prostate invading the bladder. Excretory cystogram. Entire floor of bladder is raised by an enlarged prostate. The irregularity of the outline of the contrast medium is due to direct invasion of the bladder by carcinoma of the prostate.

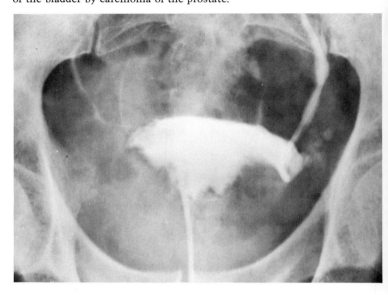

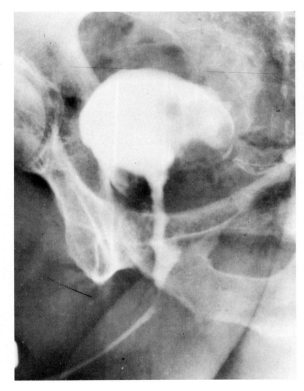

FIG. 32–72. Leiomyosarcoma of prostate invading bladder. Voiding cystourethrogram. The base of the bladder is elevated by the enlarged prostate. There is irregularity of the floor of the bladder, especially on the left side. The prostatic urethra has a scalloped effect, especially on the right side proximally, indicating invasion by the tumor. (Courtesy of Sol Unger, M.D., Veterans Administration)

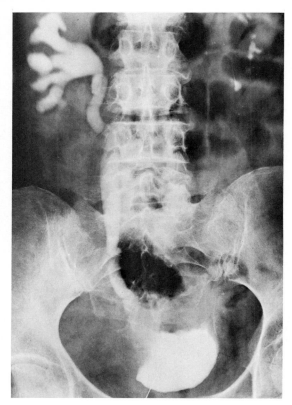

FIG. 32–73. Carcinoma of uterus invading bladder. Intravenous urogram and retrograde cystogram. There is right hydronephrosis and hydroureter. The lower end of the right ureter is not filled completely by contrast due to tumor involvement. The bladder is contracted, and the upper border is irregular with serrations, produced by a mass irregularly outlined above. The right side of the bladder is involved similarly.

FIG. 32–74. Carcinoma of sigmoid invading bladder. Retrograde cystogram. *Arrows* outline an irregularly indented area in superior surface of bladder, caused by carcinoma of sigmoid extending to bladder. The ureters are outlined from an intravenous urogram. There is a Foley balloon in the bladder.

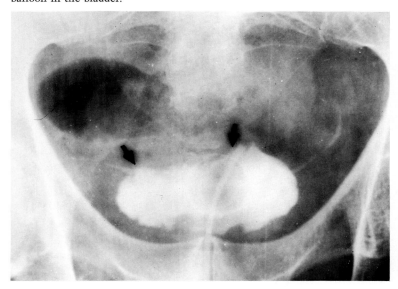

BIBLIOGRAPHY

Tumors of the Urinary Bladder

General

1. American Joint Committee (American College of Surgeons) for Cancer Staging and End Results Reporting: Clinical Staging System for Carcinoma of the Urinary Bladder. American Cancer Society, Publication 7, 1967.
2. Ansell, I.D., and Castro, J.E.: Carcinoma of the bladder complicating cyclophosphamide therapy. Br. J. Urol., 47:413–415, 1975.
3. Aschner, P.W.: Pathology of vesical neoplasms. J.A.M.A., 91:1697–1704, 1928.
4. Ash, J.F.: Epithelial tumors of the bladder. J. Urol., 44:135–145, 1940.
5. Bowles, W.T., and Cordonnier, J.J.: Total cystectomy for carcinoma of the bladder. J. Urol., 90:731–735, 1963.
6. Broders, A.C.: Epithelioma of genito-urinary organ. Ann. Surg., 75:574–604, 1922.
7. Castellanos, R.D., Wakefield, P.B., and Evans, A.T.: Carcinoma of bladder in children. J. Urol., 113:261–263, 1975.
8. Cole, P.: Coffee drinking and carcinoma of the lower urinary tract. Lancet, 1:1335–1337, 1971.
9. Cole, P., Monson, R.R., Haning, H., et al.: Smoking and carcinoma of the lower urinary tract. N. Engl., J. Med., 284:129–134, 1971.
10. Conway, J.F., and Broders, A.C.: Submucous extension of squamous cell epithelioma of the urinary bladder. J. Urol., 47:461–471, 1942.
11. Dale, G.A., and Smith, R.B.: Transitional cell carcinoma of the bladder associated with cyclophosphamide. J. Urol., 112:603–604, 1974.
12. Dean, A.L.: Tumors of the bladder, tumors of the genito-urinary tract. *In* Christopher, Frederick (ed.): A Textbook of Surgery, 5th ed. Saunders, Philadelphia, 1949.
13. Dean, A.L., Mostofi, F.K., Thomson, R.V., et al.: A restudy of the first 1,400 tumors in the Bladder Tumor Registry, Armed Forces Institute of Pathology. J. Urol., 71:571–590, 1954.
14. Deming, C.L.: Biological behavior of transitional cell papilloma of bladder. J. Urol., 63:815–820, 1950.
14a. Fabor, W.H., and Ward, R.M.: Prognosis of early carcinoma of the bladder based on chromosomal analysis. J. Urol., 119:44–48, 1978.
15. Ferguson, R.S., and Committee: Cancer of the bladder. A study of the 5 year end results in 658 epithelial tumors of the bladder in the Carcinoma Registry of the American Urological Association. J. Urol., 35:481–490, 1936.
16. Ferguson, R.S., and Committee: Grading of epithelial tu-

mors of the urinary bladder. J. Urol., 36:651–668, 1936.

17. Friedell, G.H., Bell, J.R., Burney, S.W., et al.: Histopathology and classification of urinary bladder carcinoma. Urol. Clin. North Am., 3:53–70, 1976.

18. Ganem, E.J., and Batal, J.T.: Secondary malignant tumors of the urinary bladder metastatic from primary foci in distant organs. J. Urol., 75:965–972, 1956.

19. Geraghty, J.T.: Treatment of malignant disease of the prostate and bladder. J. Urol., 7:33–63, 1922.

20. Hovenanian, M.S., and Deming, C.L.: Heterologous transplantation of uro-epithelial tumors. II. Transplantation of bladder tumors. Yale J. Biol. Med., 19:149–153, 1946.

21. International Union Against Cancer: TNM classification of malignant tumours. 2nd ed., p. 79. Geneva, I.U.C.C. 1974.

22. Jewett, H.J.: Infiltrating carcinoma of bladder; application of pathologic observations to clinical diagnosis and prognosis. J.A.M.A., 134:496–500, 1947.

23. Jewett, H.J.: Carcinoma of bladder; treatment and prognosis. South. Med. J., 43:661–666, 1950.

24. Jewett, H.J.: Carcinoma of bladder; influence of depth of infiltration on 5 year end results following complete extirpation of primary growth. J. Urol., 67:672–676, 1952.

25. Jewett, H.J.: Carcinoma of the bladder, diagnosis and staging. Cancer, 32:1072–1074, 1973.

26. Jewett, H.J., and Blackman, S.S.: Infiltrating carcinoma of bladder: Histologic pattern and degree of cellular differentiation in 97 autopsy cases. J. Urol., 56:200–210, 1946.

27. Jewett, H.J., and Eversole, S.L., Jr.: Carcinoma of the bladder; characteristic modes of local invasion. J. Urol., 83:383–389, 1960.

28. Jewett, H.J., King, L.R., and Shelley, W.M.: A study of 365 cases of infiltrating bladder cancer. Relation of certain pathological characteristics to prognosis after extirpation. J. Urol., 92:668–678, 1964.

29. Jewett, H.J., and Strong, G.H.: Infiltrating carcinoma of urinary bladder; diagnosis and clinical evaluation of curability. South. Med. J., 39:203–208, 1946.

30. Jewett, H.J., and Strong, G.H.: Infiltrating carcinoma of bladder; relation of depth of penetration of bladder wall to incidence of local extension and metastases. J. Urol., 55:366–372, 1946.

31. Kaplan, J.H., McDonald, J.R., and Thompson, G.J.: Multicentric origin of papillary tumors of the urinary tract. J. Urol., 66:792–804, 1951.

32. Kenny, G.M., Hardner, G.J., and Murphy, G.P.: Clinical staging of bladder tumors. J. Urol., 104:720–723, 1970.

33. Koss, L.G.: Tumors of the urinary bladder. In Armed Forces Institute of Pathology: Atlas of Tumor Pathology, Fascicle 11. Washington, D.C., 1975.

34. Marshall, V.F.: Relation of preoperative estimate to pathologic demonstration of extent of vesical neoplasms. J. Urol., 68:714–723, 1952.

35. Marshall, V.F.: Current clinical problems regarding bladder tumors. Cancer, 9:543–550, 1956.

36. Marshall, V.F., and Whitmore, W.F., Jr.: Radical total cystectomy for cancer of the bladder; 230 consecutive cases five years later. J. Urol., 87:853–868, 1962.

37. McDonald, J.R., and Thompson, G.J.: Carcinoma of urinary bladder; pathological study with special reference to invasiveness and vascular invasion. J. Urol., 60:435–445, 1948.

38. Melicow, M.M.: Tumors of the urinary bladder: A clinicopathological analysis of over 2,500 specimens and biopsies. J. Urol., 74:498–521, 1955.

39. Morgan, R.W., and Jain, M.G.: Bladder cancer: Smoking, beverages, and artificial sweeteners. Can. Med. Assoc. J., 111:1067–1070, 1974.

40. Mostofi, F.K.: Pathological aspects and spread of carcinoma of the bladder. J.A.M.A., 206:1764–1769, 1968.

41. Mostofi, F.K., Sobin, L.H., and Torioni, H. (eds.): Histological Typing of Urinary Bladder Tumours. International Histological Classification of Tumours #10. W.H.O., Geneva, 1973.

42. Murphy, G.P.: The current status of bladder carcinoma. Surg. Annu., 7:175–218, 1975.

43. Nilson, A.E.: The palpability of infiltrative bladder tumours: a diagnostic comparison with roentgenographic findings. Acta Chir. Scand., 115:132–137, 1958.

44. Novak, D., Hilweg, D., and Haug, H.P.: The role of roentgenographic procedures in staging of carcinoma of the urinary bladder by TNM system. Urol. Int'l., 26:149–160, 1971.

45. Prout, G.R., Jr.: Current concepts of bladder carcinoma. N. Engl. J. Med., 287:86–90, 1973.

46. Prout, G.R., Jr.: Bladder carcinoma and a TNM system of classification. J. Urol., 117:583–590, 1977.

47. Ray, B., Grabstald, H., Exelby, P.R., et al.: Bladder tumors in children. Urology, 2:426–435, 1973.

48. Seltzer, S.E., Benazzi, R.M., and Kearney, G.P.: Cyclophosphamide and cancer of the bladder. Urology, 11:352–356, 1978.

49. Skinner, D.G.: Current state of classification and staging of bladder carcinoma. Cancer Res., 37:2838–2842, 1977.

50. Stirling, W.C., and Ash, J.E.: Tumors of the bladder. J.A.M.A., 141:1036–1039, 1949.

51. Wall, R.L., and Clausen, K.P.: Carcinoma of the urinary bladder in patients receiving cyclophosphamide. N. Engl. J. Med., 293:271–273, 1975.

52. Wallace, D.M.: Tumors of the Bladder. Williams & Wilkins, Baltimore, 1959.

53. Wallace, D.M.: Urothelial neoplasia. Causes, assessment, and treatment. Ann. R. Coll. Surg. Engl., 51:91–102, 1972.

54. Wallace, D.M.: Classification of bladder tumours. Eur. Urol., 1:65–67, 1975.

54a. Young, A.K., Hammond, E., and Middleton, A.W., Jr.: The prognostic value of cell surface antigen in low grade, non-invasive transitional cell carcinoma of the bladder. J. Urol., 122:462–464, 1979.

Squamous Cell Carcinoma

55. Bessette, R.L., Abell, M.R., and Herwig, K.R.: A clinicopathological study of squamous cell carcinoma of the bladder. J. Urol., 112:66–67, 1974.

56. Conway, J.F., and Broders, A.C.: Submucous extension of squamous cell epithelioma of urinary bladder. J. Urol., 47:461–471, 1942.

57. Kovetz, A., and Weinberg, S.R.: The management of bladder tumors in a community hospital. J. Urol., 105:92–96, 1971.

58. Melicow, M.M.: Terminology in uropathology; a plea for consensus, including a discussion of retroplasia versus metaplasia. J. Urol., 105:714–719, 1971.

59. Newman, D.M., Brown, J.R., Jay, A.C., et al.: Squamous cell carcinoma of the bladder. J. Urol., 100:470–473, 1968.

60. Pugh, R.L.B.: The pathology of bladder tumors, pp. 116–156. In Wallace, D.M., Edinburgh, E., S. Livingstone, Ltd. (eds.): Tumors of the Bladder. Neoplastic diseases of various sites, vol. 2. Williams & Wilkins, Baltimore, 1959.

61. Sakkas, J.L.: Clinical pattern and treatment of squamous cell carcinoma of the bladder. Int. Surg., 45:71–76, 1966.

62. Sarma, K.P.: Squamous cell carcinoma of the bladder. Int. Surg., 53:313–319, 1970.

63. Shivers, C.H. de T., and Henderson, K.P.: Tumors of the bladder; review of 101 cases. J. Urol., 42:761–777, 1939.

64. Vose, S.N., and Dixey, G.M.: Coincidence of carcinoma of the bladder and interstitial cystitis. J. Urol., 59:580–582, 1948.

Adenocarcinoma

65. Abeshouse, B.S.: Exstrophy of the bladder complicated by adenocarcinoma of the bladder and renal calculi. A report of a case and a review of the literature. J. Urol., 49:259–289, 1943.

66. Allen, T.D., and Henderson, B.W.: Adenocarcinoma of the bladder. J. Urol., 93:50–56, 1965.

67. Begg, R.E.: Colloid adenocarcinomata of bladder vault arising from epithelium of urachal canal with survey of tumors of urachus. Br. J. Surg., 18:422–466, 1931.

68. Bourne, C.W., and May, J.E.: Urachal remnants: Benign or malignant? J. Urol., 118:743–747, 1977.

69. Butler, D.B., and Rosenberg, H.S.: Sarcoma of the urachus. Arch. Surg., 79:724–728, 1959.

70. Coppridge, W.M., Roberts, L.C., and Culp, D.A.: Glandular tumors of the bladder. J. Urol., 65:540–549, 1951.

71. Culp, D.A.: The histology of the exstrophial bladder. J. Urol., 91:538–548, 1964.

72. Dean, A.L., and Ash, J.E.: Study of the bladder tumors in the American Urology Association. J. Urol., 63:618–621, 1950.

73. Dimmette, R.M., Sproat, H.F., and Sayegh, E.S.: The classification of carcinoma of the urinary bladder, associated with schistosomiasis and metaplasia. J. Urol., 75:680–686, 1956.

74. Elliott, G.B., and Greigang, B.: Observations on the nature of mucin secreting urachal cystadenoma. Ann. Surg., 157:613–617, 1963.

75. Hayes, J.J., and Segal, A.D.: Mucinous carcinoma of the urachus invading the bladder. J. Urol., 53:659–669, 1945.

76. Helsby, R.: Ruptured infected urachal cyst. Br. Med. J., 2:603, 1955.

77. Hurwitz, S.P., Jacobson, C.B., and Ottenstein, H.H.: Mucoid adenocarcinoma of urachus. J. Urol., 65:87–92, 1951.

78. Jacobo, E., Loening, S., Schmidt, J.D., et al.: Primary adenocarcinoma of the bladder: a retrospective study of 20 patients. J. Urol., 117:54–56, 1977.

79. Johnson, D.E., Hogan, J.M., and Ayala, A.G.: Primary adenocarcinoma of the urinary bladder. South. Med. J., 65:527–530, 1972.

80. Kittredge, W.E., Collett, A.J., and Morgan, C., Jr.: Adenocarcinoma of bladder associated with cystitis glandularis. J. Urol., 91:141–150, 1964.

81. Kretschmer, H.L.: Primary mucous secreting adenocarcinoma of the bladder. J. Urol., 61:754–765, 1949.

82. Learoyd, H.M.: Carcinoma of the urachus. Br. J. Urol., 46:114–120, 1974.

83. McCloy, T.J., and Lewis, C.W., Jr.: Mucinous adenocarcinoma of the urachus. J. Urol., 96:317–319, 1966.

84. McIntosh, J.F., and Worley, G., Jr.: Adenocarcinoma arising in exstrophy of the bladder; report of 2 cases and review of the literature. J. Urol., 73:820–829, 1955.

85. Melicow, M.M.: Tumors of the urinary bladder: a clinico-pathological analysis of over 2500 specimens and biopsies. J. Urol., 74:498–521, 1958.

86. Mostofi, F.K., Thomson, R.U., and Dean, A.L., Jr.: Mucous adenocarcinoma of the urinary bladder. Cancer, 8:741–758, 1955.

87. Nadjmi, B., Whitehead, E.D., McKiel, C.F., Jr., et al.: Carcinoma of the urachus: report of two cases and review of the literature. J. Urol., 100:738–743, 1968.

88. Ohman, U., von Garrelts, B., and Moberg, A.: Carcinoma of the urachus. Scand. J. Urol. Nephrol., 5:91–95, 1971.

89. Patch, F.S., and Pritchard, J.E.: Mucinous adenocarcinoma of the bladder. J. Urol., 57:126–132, 1947.

90. Patch, F.S., and Rhea, L.J.: The genesis and development of Brunn's nests and their relation to cystitis cystica, cystitis glandularis, and primary adenocarcinoma of the bladder. Can. Med. Assoc. J., 33:597–606, 1935.

91. Pollack, A.V.: A case of adenocarcinoma of the urachus storing extreme calcification. Br. J. Surg., 40:187–188, 1952.

92. Powley, P.H.: Sarcoma of the urachus. Br. J. Surg., 48:649–650, 1961.

93. Ransom, H.R.: Sarcoma of the urachus. Am. J. Surg., 22:187–191, 1933.

94. Saphir, O., and Kurland, S.K.: Adenocarcinoma of the urinary bladder. Urol. Cutan. Rev., 43:709–719, 1939.

95. Shaw, J.L., Gislason, G.J., and Imbriglia, J.E.: Transition of cystitis glandularis to primary adenocarcinoma of the bladder. J. Urol., 79:815–822, 1958.

96. Shaw, R.E.: Sarcoma of the urachus. Br. J. Surg., 37:95–98, 1949.

97. Slater, G.S., and Torassa, G.L.: Mucinous adenocarcinoma of urachus connected to urinary bladder. Stanford Med. Bull., 11:19–29, 1957.

98. Thomas, D.G., Ward, A.M., and Williams, J.L.: A study of 52 cases of adenocarcinoma of the bladder. Br. J. Urol., 43:4–15, 1971.

99. Thomford, N.R., Knight, P.R., and Nusbaum, J.W.: Urachal abnormalities in the adult. Am. Surg., 37:405–407, 1971.

100. Wheeler, J.D., and Hill, W.T.: Adenocarcinoma involving the urinary bladder. Cancer, 7:119–135, 1954.

101. Williams, J.I., Godwin, M.C., and Cross, R.R.: Adenocarcinoma of the urinary bladder. J. Int. Coll. Surg., 25:461–470, 1956.

102. Yu, H.H., and Leong, C.H.: Carcinoma of the urachus: Report of one case and a review of the literature. Surgery, 77:726–729, 1975.

Metastases from Carcinoma of the Bladder

103. Cooling, C.E.: Review of 150 post mortems of carcinoma of the urinary bladder. pp. 171–186. *In* Wallace, D.M., Edinburgh, E. and S. Livingstone, Ltd. (eds.): Tumors of the Bladder. Neoplastic Disease at Various Sites. Vol. 2. Williams and Wilkins Co., Baltimore, 1959.

104. Fetter, T.R., Bogaev, J.H., McCuskey, B., et al.: Carcinoma of the bladder. Site of metastases. J. Urol., 81:746–748, 1959.

105. Jewett, H.J., and Strong, G.H.: Infiltrating carcinoma of bladder; relation of depth of penetration of bladder wall to incidence of local extension and metastases. J. Urol., 55:366–372, 1946.

106. Seymour, J.E., Malin, J.M., and Pierce, J.M., Jr.: Late metastases of a superficial transitional cell carcinoma of the bladder: Report of a case. J. Urol., 108:277–278, 1972.

107. Spooner, A.D.: Metastasis in epithelioma of the urinary

bladder. Trans. Am. Assoc. Genitourin. Surg., 27:81–89, 1934.

Calcification

108. Bartholomew, L.G.: Cain, J.C., Davis, G.D., et al.: Misleading calcific shadows in abdomen. Post. Grad. Med., 30:51–66, 1961.
109. Davidson, H.G., Witten, D.M., and Culp, O.S.: Roentgenologically demonstrable calcifications in tumors of bladder: report of 3 cases. Am. J. Roentgenol., 95:450–454, 1965.
110. Ferris, E.J., and O'Connor, S.J.: Calcification in urinary bladder tumors. Am. J. Roentgen., 95:447–449, 1965.
111. Miller, S.W., Pfister, R.C.: Calcification in uroepithelial tumors of the bladder. Report of 5 cases and survey of the literature. Am. J. Roentgenol., 121:827–831, 1974.

Conventional Cystogram

112. Braband, H.: The incidence of urographic findings in tumours of the urinary bladder. Br. J. Radiol., 34:625–629, 1961.
113. Franksson, C.: Tumors of the urinary bladder. A pathological and clinical study of 434 cases. Acta Chir. Scand. (Suppl.), 151:4–203, 1950.
114. Franksson, C., and Lindblom, K.: Roentgenographic signs of tumor infiltration of the wall of the urinary bladder. Acta Radiol., 37:1–7, 1952.
115. Franksson, C., Lindblom, K., and Whitehouse, W.: The reliability of roentgen signs of varying degrees of malignancy of bladder tumors. Acta Radiol., 45:266–271, 1956.
116. Smith, W.H.: The reliability of excretion urography in the diagnosis of bladder tumours. J. Fac. Radiologists, 6:48–54, 1954.

Fractionated Cystograms

117. Cobb, O.E., and Anderson, E.E.: Superimposition cystography in the diagnosis of infiltrating tumors of the bladder. J. Urol., 94:569–572, 1965.
118. Connolly, J.E., Challis, T.W., Wallace, D.M., et al.: An evaluation of the fractionated cystogram in the assessment of infiltrating tumors of the bladder. J. Urol., 98:356–360, 1967.

Double Contrast Barium Cystography Utilizing Carbon Dioxide

119. Bartley, O., and Helander, C.G.: Double-contrast cystography in tumors of the urinary bladder. Acta Radiol., 54:161–169, 1960.
120. Pochaczevsky, R., and Grabstald, H.: Double contrast barium cystography utilizing carbon dioxide. Am. J. Roentgenol., 92:365–373, 1964.

Combined Endoperivesical Gas Insufflation

121. Bartley, O., and Eckerbom, H.: Peri-vesical insufflation of gas for determination of bladder wall thickness in tumors of the bladder. Acta Radiol., 54:241–250, 1960.
122. Gosalby, R., and Gil-Vernet, J.M.: Bladder tomography: The use of air intra- and perivesically in the radiologic study of bladder tumors. J. Urol., 88:312–317, 1962.

123. Luzzatti, G., and Goldini, S.: La pneumocitrografia associata a pneumo-retzius vella diagnosi dei tumori della vesica. Chir. Milano, 12:239, 1947.
124. Soifer, E., and Margulies, M.: Visualization of infiltrating tumors by perivesical gas insufflation. J. Urol., 89:759–762, 1963.
125. Wuerdinger, H.: Combined endoperivesical double contrast cystography of the urinary bladder. Fortschr. Roentgenstr., 95:676, 1961.

Assessment and Staging of Bladder Tumors by Roentgenologic Techniques

126. Alberti, C., and Ghisleri, G.: Carcinoma Vescicale: Criteri Classificativi Anatomopatologici T.N.M. (P) E Angiografici: Arteriografia Pelvica, Flebografia Ipogastrica, Linfografia. Urologia (Treviso), 39:472–481, 1972.
127. Anacker, H., and Heun, J.M.: Abgrenzung der Harnblasentumoren im Angiogramm, pp. 52–59. In Glauner, R.: Radiologische Diagnostik und Therapie Bei Malignen Tumoren im Becken. Thieme, Stuttgart, 1970.
128. Bachmann, D., and Taenzer, V.: Methodik und Ergebnisse der Harnblasenarteriographie, pp. 60–63. In Glauner, R.: Radiologische Diagnostik und Therapie Bei Malignen Tumoren im Becken. Thieme, Stuttgart, 1970.
129. Baudisch, E., and Arndt, J.: Atlas Angiographischer Befunde bei Nierenerkrankungen und Malignen Blasentumoren. Fischer, Jena, 1969.
130. Esguerra, A., Carvajal, A., and Mouton, H.: Pelvic Arteriography in the diagnosis of hemangioma of the bladder. J. Urol., 109:609–611, 1973.
130a. Farah, R.N., and Cerny, J.C.: Lymphangiography in staging of patients with carcinoma of the bladder. J. Urol., 119:40–41, 1978.
131. Fujita, K., Nakauchi, K., and Matsumoto, K.: A simple and useful method of double contrast cystography in the diagnosis of bladder tumors. J. Urol., 107:396–398, 1972.
132. Glauner, R.: Radiologische Diagnostik und Therapie bei Malignen Tumoren im Becken. Thieme, Stuttgart, 1970.
133. Hakala, T.R., Page, D., and Fleischli, D.J.: Paravesical Hemangiopericytoma. J. Urol., 103:436–440, 1970.
133a. Harada, K., Igari, D., Tanahashi, Y., et al.: Staging of bladder tumors by means of transrectal ultrasonography. J. Clin. Ultrasound, 5:338–392, 1977.
134. Hilweg, D., Novak, D., and Haug, H.P.: Inclusion of lymphography in the classification of malignant bladder tumors according to the TNM system. Strahlentherapie, 142:521–526, 1971.
135. Jewett, H.J.: Cancer of the bladder: Diagnosis and staging. Cancer, 32:1072–1074, 1973.
136. Jewett, H.J.: Carcinoma of the bladder: Development and evaluation of current concepts of therapy. J. Urol., 82:92–100, 1959.
137. Jochem, W., Buchelt, L., and Bichler, K.H.: Der Aussagewert Lymphographischer Veranderungen bei Harnblasenkarzinomen, pp. 83–86. In Glauner, R.: Radiologische Diagnostik und Therapie Bei Malignen Tumoren im Becken. Thieme, Stuttgart, 1970.
138. Kadish, L.J., Stein, J.M., Kotler, S., et al.: Angiographic diagnosis and treatment of bleeding due to pelvic trauma. J. Trauma, 13:1083–1085, 1973.
139. Kenny, G.M., Hardner, G.J., and Murphy, G.P.: Clinical staging of bladder tumors. J. Urol., 104:720–723, 1970.

140. Lacy, S.S., Whitley, J.E., and Cox, C.E.: Vesical arteriography: An adjunct to staging of bladder tumors. Br. J. Urol., *42*:50–55, 1970.
141. Lang, E.K., Wishard, W.M., Jr., Nourse, M., et al.: Retrograde arteriography in the diagnosis of bladder tumors. Trans. Am. Assn. Genitourin. Surg., *54*:15–19, 1962.
142. Lang, E.K.: The use of arteriography in the demonstration and staging of bladder tumors. Radiology, *80*:62–68, 1963.
143. Lang, E.K., Deutsch, J.S., Goodman, J.R., et al.: Transcatheter embolization of hypogastric branch arteries in the management of intractable bladder hemorrhage. J. Urol., *121*:30–36, 1979.
144. Lang, E.K.: Roentgenographic Diagnosis of Bladder Tumors. Charles C Thomas, Springfield, 1968.
145. Lang, E.K.: The roentgenographic assessment of bladder tumors (a comparison of diagnostic accuracy of roentgenographic techniques). Cancer, *23*:717–724, 1969.
146. Lang, E.K.: Triple cystogram and selective arteriography (Current Cancer Concepts). J.A.M.A., *207*:342–344, 1969.
147. Lang, E.K.: Double contrast gas barium cystography in the assessment of diverticula of the bladder. Am. J. Roentgenol., *107*:769–775, 1969.
148. Lang, E.K.: Superselective arterial catheterization as a vehicle for delivering radioactive infarct particles to tumors. Radiology, *98*:391–399, 1971.
149. Liebscher, J., Schadeberg, A., Kohler, K., et al.: Lymphographic diagnosis of metastases in bladder carcinoma. Z. Urol. Nephrol., *66*:1–11, 1973.
150. Matsumoto, K., Fujita, K., Nakuchi, K., et al.: Accurate roentgenographic diagnosis of vesical tumors with double contrast cystography and arteriography. J. Urol., *107*:46–48, 1972.
151. Mostofi, F.K.: Pathological aspects and spread of carcinoma of the bladder. J.A.M.A., *206*:1764–1769, 1968.
152. Murphy, G.P.: Developments in preoperative staging of bladder tumors. Urology, *9*:109–115, 1978.
153. Nilsson, J.: Angiography in tumors of the urinary bladder. Acta Radiologica (Stockholm) (Suppl.) pp. 1–130, 1967.
154. Novak, D., Hilweg, D., and Haug, H.P.: Die Rolle der Beckenangiographie, Peripneumozystographie, Tomographie sowie Lymphographie zur Stadieneinteilung maligner Harnblasentumoren nach dem TNM-System, pp. 108–113. *In* Glauner, R.: Radiologische Diagnostik und Therapie Bei Malignen Tumoren im Becken. Thieme. Stuttgart, 1970.
155. Novak, D., Hilweg, D., and Haug, H.P.: The role of roentgenographic procedures in staging of carcinoma of the urinary bladder by TNM system. Urol. Int., *26*:149–160, 1971.
156. Ring, E.J., Athanasoulis, C., Waltman, A.C., et al.: Arteriographic management of hemorrhage following pelvic fracture. Radiology, *109*:65–70, 1973.
157. Schenck, P., Maier-Borst, W., Lorenz, W.J., et al.: Erfahrungen mit szintigraphischen Untersuchungen bei Beckentumoren, pp. 99–108. *In* Glauner, R.: Radiologische Diagnostik und Therapie Bei Malignen Tumoren im Becken. Thieme, Stuttgart, 1970.
157a. Seidelmann, F.E., Cohen, W.N., and Bryan, P.J.: CT staging of bladder neoplasms. Radiologic Clin. North Am., *15*:419–440, 1977.
158. Seidelmann, F.E., Cohen, W.N., Bryan, P.J., et al.: Accuracy of CT staging of bladder neoplasms using the gas-filled method: A report of 21 patients with surgical confirmation. Am. J. Roentgenol., *130*:735–739, 1978.
159. Taylor, D.A., Macken, R.L., Veenema, R.J., et al.: A preliminary report of a new method for the staging of bladder carcinoma by a triple contrast technique. Br. J. Radiol., *38*:667–672, 1965.
160. Vogler, E.: Moglichkeiten und Grenzen der Angiographie in der Diagnostic von Tumoren der Harnblase, pp. 3–13. *In* Glauner, R.: Radiologische Diagnostik und Therapie Bei Malignen Tumoren im Becken. Thieme, Stuttgart, 1970.
161. Winterberger, A.R., Jennings, E.C., and Murphy, G.P.: Arteriography in metastatic tumors to the bladder. J. Urol., *108*:577–580, 1972.
162. Winterberger, A.R., Kenny, G.M., Choi, S.A., et al.: Correlation of selective arteriography in the staging of bladder tumors. Cancer, *29*:332–337, 1972.
163. Winterberger, A.R., and Murphy, G.P.: Correlation of B-scan ultrasonic laminography with bilateral hypogastric arteriography and lymphography in bladder tumors. Vasc. Surg., *8*:169–176, 1974.
164. Wise, H.M., Jr., and Fainsinger, M.H.: Angiography in the evaluation of carcinoma of the bladder. J.A.M.A., *192*:1027–1031, 1965.
165. Zedgenidze, G.A., Dunchik, V.N., Tysb, A.F., et al.: Clinical and roentgenographic criteria of the extent of a carcinomatous process in the urinary bladder (notes and suggestions on International Classification). Vestn. Roentgenol. Radiol., *48*:72–77, 1973.

Carcinoma of the Bladder Associated with Other Conditions

Lithiasis

166. Koss, L.G.: Diagnostic Cytology and Its Histopathologic Basis, 2nd Ed. J.B. Lippincott, Philadelphia, 1968.
167. Wynder, E.L., Onderdonk, Jr., and Mantel, N.: An epidemiologic investigation of cancer of the bladder. Cancer, *16*:1388–1407, 1963.

Inverted Papilloma

168. Assor, D., and Taylor, J.N.: Inverted papilloma of the bladder. J. Urol., *104*:715–717, 1970.
169. Cameron, K.M., and Lupton, C.H.: Inverted papilloma of the lower urinary tract. Br. J. Urol., *48*:567–577, 1976.
170. DeMeester, L.J., Farrow, G.M., and Utz, D.C.: Inverted papilloma of the urinary bladder. Cancer, *36*:505–512, 1975.
171. Pienkos, F.J., Iglesias, F., and Jablokow, V.R.: Inverted papilloma of bladder. Urology, *2*:178–179, 1973.
172. Potts, I.F., and Hirst, E.: Inverted papilloma of the bladder. J. Urol., *90*:175–179, 1963.
173. Trites, A.E.W.: Inverted urothelial papilloma; report of two cases. J. Urol., *101*:216–219, 1969.

Carcinoma In Situ

174. Culp, O.S., Utz, D.C., and Harrison, E.G., Jr.: Experiences with ureteral carcinoma in situ detected during operations for vesical neoplasms. J. Urol., *97*:679–682, 1967.
175. Koss, L.G., Nakanishi, I., and Freed, S.Z.: Nonpapillary carcinoma in situ and atypical hyperplasia in cancerous bladders. Urology, *11*:442–455, 1977.
176. Koss, L.G., Tiamson, E.M., and Robbins, M.A.: Mapping cancerous and precancerous bladder changes. J.A.M.A., *227*:281–286, 1974.

177. Melamed, M.R., Voutsa, N.G., and Grabstald, H.: Natural history and clinical behavior of in situ carcinoma of the human urinary bladder. Cancer, 17:1533–1545, 1964.

178. Melicow, M.M.: Histologic study of vesical uroepithelium intervening between gross neoplasms in total cystectomy. J. Urol., 68:261–278, 1952.

179. Melicow, M.M., and Hollowall, J.W.: Intraurothelial cancer. Carcinoma in situ. Bowen's disease of the urinary system. Discussion of 30 cases. J. Urol., 68:763–772, 1952.

180. Schade, R.O.K., and Swinney, J.: Precancerous changes in bladder epithelium. Lancet, 2:943–946, 1968.

181. Seemayer, T.A., Knaack, J., Thelmo, W.L., et al.: Further observations on carcinoma in situ of the urinary bladder: silent but extensive intraprostatic involvement. Cancer, 36:514–520, 1975.

182. Utz, D.C., and Farrow, G.M.: Carcinoma in situ of the bladder. Urol. Digest, 16:19–31, 1977.

183. Utz, D.C., Hanash, K.A., and Farrow, G.M.: The plight of the patient with carcinoma in situ of the bladder. J. Urol., 103:160–164, 1970.

184. Utz, D.C., and Zincke, H.: The masquerade of bladder cancer in situ as interstitial cystitis. J. Urol., 111:160–161, 1974.

185. Voutsa, N.G., and Melamde, M.R.: Cytology of in situ carcinoma of the human urinary bladder. Cancer, 16:1307–1316, 1963.

186. Yates-Bell, A.J.: Carcinoma in situ of the bladder. Br. J. Surg., 58:283–288, 1973.

Nonepithelial Tumors of the Bladder

Leiomyoma

187. Katz, R.B., and Waldbaum, R.S.: Benign mesothelial tumors of bladder. Urology, 5:236–238, 1975.

188. Mutchler, R.W., Jr., and Gorder, J.L.: Leiomyoma of the bladder in a child. Br. J. Radiol., 45:528–540, 1972.

189. O'Connell, K., and Edson, M.: Leiomyoma of bladder. Urology, 6:114–115, 1975.

190. Sarma, K.P.: Tumours of the Urinary Bladder, p. 88. Appleton-Century-Croft, New York, 1964.

191. Thompson, I.M., and Balfour, J.: Leiomyomatous vesical neck obstruction. Urology, 3:92–93, 1974.

Leiomyosarcoma

192. Brown, H.E.: Leiomyoma of the bladder: Follow-up report of two cases with 4 and 10 years' survival. J. Urol., 94:247–251, 1965.

193. Cibert, J., and Durand, L.: Results of surgical treatment of 10 cases of myosarcoma of bladder. J. Urol., 71:58–62, 1954.

194. Kretschmer, H.L., and Doehring, P.: Leiomyosarcoma of the urinary bladder. Arch. Surg., 38:274–286, 1939.

195. Lev, M., and Bell, W.E.: Leiomyosarcoma of the urinary bladder: Report of a case. J. Urol., 57:251–256, 1947.

196. MacKenzie, A.R., Whitmore, W.F., Jr., and Melamed, M.R.: Myosarcoma of the bladder and prostate. Cancer, 22:833–844, 1968.

197. Ramey, W.P., Ashburn, L.L., Grabstald, H., and Haines, J.S.: Myosarcoma of the urinary bladder. J. Urol., 70:906–913, 1953.

198. Samuel, E.: Radiological features of vesical leiomyoma and leiomyosarcoma: case report. Br. J. Radiol., 20:423–425, 1947.

199. Silbar, J.D., and Silber, S.J.: Leiomyosarcoma of bladder; three case reports and a review of literature. J. Urol., 73:103–111, 1955.

200. Tara, H.H., and Mentur, N.L.: Leiomyosarcoma of urinary bladder. Urology, 2:460–462, 1973.

201. Weyerbacher, A.F., and Balch, J.F.: Leiomyosarcoma of the bladder. J. Urol., 38:278–287, 1937.

Rhabdomyosarcoma

202. Evans, A.T., and Bell, T.E.: Rhabdomyosarcoma of the bladder in adult patients: Report of three cases. J. Urol., 94:573–575, 1965.

203. Jones, C.B., Jr., Oberman, H.T.: Rhabdomyosarcoma of the bladder — occurrence in childhood and advanced age. J. Urol., 91:533–537, 1964.

204. Joshi, D.P., Wessely, Z., Seery, W.H., et al.: Rhabdomyosarcoma of the bladder in an adult: Case report and review of the literature. J. Urol., 96:214–217, 1966.

205. Khoury, E.N., and Speer, F.E.: Rhabdomyosarcoma of the urinary bladder. J. Urol., 51:505–516, 1944.

206. Legier, J.F.: Botryoid sarcoma and rhabdomyosarcoma of the bladder: Review of the literature and report of 3 cases. J. Urol., 86:583–590, 1961.

207. Longley, J.: Sarcoma of prostate and bladder. J. Urol., 73:417–423, 1955.

208. McFarland, J.: Dysontogenetic and mixed tumors of the urogenital region. Surg. Gynecol. Obstet., 61:42–57, 1935.

209. Mostofi, F.K., and Morse, W.H.: Polypoid rhabdomyosarcoma (sarcoma botryoides) of bladder in children. J. Urol., 67:681–687, 1952.

210. Ober, W.B., and Edgcomb, J.H.: Sarcoma botryoides in female urogenital tract. Cancer, 7:75–91, 1954.

211. Ober, W.B., Smith, J.A., and Rouillard, F.C.: Congenital sarcoma botryoides of the vagina: report of 2 cases. Cancer, 11:620–623, 1958.

212. Smith, J.A., Jr.: Sarcoma botryoides — rhabdomyosarcoma of the bladder. J. Urol., 82:101–104, 1959.

213. White, L.L.R.: Embryonic sarcoma of the urogenital system. Thesis: Univ. of Wales, 1955. Cited by Williams, D.I. and Schistad, G.

214. Williams, D.I., and Schistad, G.: Lower urinary tract tumours in children. Br. J. Urol., 36:51–65, 1964.

Other Tumors of the Bladder

Pheochromocytoma

215. Albores-Saavedro, J., Maldonado, M.E., Ibarra, J., et al.: Pheochromocytoma of the urinary bladder. Cancer, 23:1110–1118, 1969.

216. Anton, A.H., Greer, M., Sayre, D.F., et al.: Dehydroxyphenylalanine secretion in a malignant pheochromocytoma. Am. J. Med., 42:469–475, 1967.

217. Berry, K.W., Jr., and Scott, E.V.Z.: Pheochromocytoma of the bladder. J. Urol., 85:156–158, 1961.

218. Bourne, R.B., and Beltaos, E.: Pheochromocytoma of the bladder: A case report and summary of literature. J. Urol., 98:361–364, 1967.

219. Cabanas, V.Y., Faulconer, R.J., and Fekete, A.M.: Pheochromocytoma presenting as ureterocele. J. Urol., 110:389–390, 1973.

220. Doctor, V.M., Phadke, A.G., and Sirsat, M.V.: Pheochromocytoma of the urinary bladder. Br. J. Urol., 44:351–355, 1972.

221. Farley, S.E., and Smith, C.L.: Unusual location of pheochromocytoma in the urinary bladder. J. Urol., *81*:130–132, 1959.
222. Higgins, P.M., and Tresidder, G.C.: Phaeochromocytoma of the urinary bladder. Br. Med. J., 2:274–277, 1966.
223. Javaheri, P., and Raafat, J.: Malignant phaeochromocytoma of the urinary bladder—report of two cases. Br. J. Urol., *47*:401–404, 1975.
224. Leetsma, J.E., and Price, E.B., Jr.: Paraganglioma of the urinary bladder. Cancer, *28*:1063–1073, 1971.
225. Moloney, G.E., Cowdell, R.H., and Lewis, C.L.: Malignant phaeochromocytoma of the bladder. Br. J. Urol., *38*:461–470, 1966.
226. Pugh, R.C.B., Gresham, G.A., and Mullaney, J.: Pheochromocytoma of the urinary bladder. J. Pathol. Bacteriol., *79*:89–107, 1960.
227. Rosenberg, L.M.: Pheochromocytoma of the urinary bladder. N. Engl. J. Med., *257*:1212–1215, 1957.
228. Scott, W.W., and Eversole, S.L.: Pheochromocytoma of the urinary bladder. J. Urol., *83*:656–664, 1960.
229. Spitzer, R., Burrison, R., and Castellino, R.A.: Functioning nonchromaffin paraganglioma (chemodectoma) of the urinary bladder. Radiology, *98*:577–578, 1971.
230. Tan, Toh-Leong, and Young, B.W.: Pheochromocytoma of the bladder. Case report. J. Urol., *87*:63–67, 1962.
231. Van Buskirk, K.E., O'Shaughnessy, J.E., Hano, J., et al.: Pheochromocytoma of the bladder. J.A.M.A., *196*:293–294, 1966.
232. Zimmerman, I.J., Biron, R.E., and MacMahon, H.E.: Pheochromocytoma of urinary bladder. N. Engl. J. Med., *249*:25–66, 1953.
233. Zornow, D.H., Bentrovato, D.A., Olson, H.W., et al.: Vesical-related paraganglioma. J. Urol., *118*:247–250, 1977.

Hemangioma

234. Ferulano, O.: Study of vascular tumors of the bladder; clinical case of cavernous angioma. Gior. ital. chir., *11*:1131–1152, 1955.
235. Fuqua, F., Alexander, J.C., King, K.B., et al.: Cavernous hemangioma of the bladder in a child: A case report. J. Urol., *74*:82–84, 1955.
236. Ganem, E.J., and Ainsworth, L.B.: Benign neoplasma of the urinary bladder in children. Review of the literature and report of a case. J. Urol., *73*:1032–1038, 1955.
237. Graham, J.B., and Bulkley, G.J.: Angioma of bladder. J. Urol., *74*:777–779, 1956.
238. Hamer, H.G., and Mertz, H.O.: Angioma of the bladder. Surg. Gynecol. Obstet., *51*:541–544, 1930.
239. Hamsher, J.B., Farrar, T., and Moore, T.D.: Congenital vascular tumors and malformation involving urinary tract: Diagnosis and surgical management. J. Urol., *80*:299–310, 1958.
240. Hendry, W.F., and Vinnicombe, J.: Hemangioma of bladder in children and young adults. Br. J. Urol., *43*:209–216, 1971.
241. Hyams, J.A., and Silberblatt, J.M.: A case of hemangioma coincident with papillary carcinoma of the urinary bladder. J. Urol., *46*:271–277, 1941.
242. Kahle, P.J., Maltry, E., and Vickery, G.: Hemangioma of the bladder. J. Urol., *47*:267–269, 1942.
243. Karris, Z., and Cammenos, A.: Hemangioma of bladder in an 8 year old girl. Urol. Int., *1*:43–46, 1955.
244. Liang, D.S.: Hemangioma of the bladder. J. Urol., *79*:956–960, 1958.
245. Litin, R.B., Donohue, C.D., Overstreet, R.M., et al.: Hemangioma of the bladder; report of two cases. J. Urol., *85*:556–558, 1961.

246. Morales, A.: Hemangioma of the bladder. Portugal Med. J., *48*:117–118, 1972.
247. Rathbun, N.P.: Primary bladder tumors in infants and children; with report of case of hemangioma in male child 27 months of age. Surg. Gynecol. Obstet., *64*:914–918, 1937.
248. Riches, E.W.: Case of cavernous hemangioma of bladder. Br. J. Urol., *23*:204–208, 1951.
249. Sarma, K.P.: Tumor of the Urinary Bladder, pp. 90–93, 95–101, 105–111. Appleton-Century-Crofts, London, 1969.
250. Segal, A.D., and Fink, H.: Cavernous hemangioma of bladder. J. Urol., *47*:453–460, 1942.
251. Staple, T.W., and McAlister, W.H.: Hemangioma of the bladder. Am. J. Roentgenol., *92*:375–377, 1964.

Endometriosis

252. Abeshouse, B.S., and Abeshouse, G.: Endometriosis of the urinary tract: A review of the literature and a report of four cases of vesical endometriosis. J. Int. Coll. Surg., *34*:43–63, 1960.
253. Ajamil, L.F., Pernas, E., and Valverde, M.: Vesical endometriosis. J. Urol. *72*:833–836, 1956.
254. Counsellor, V.S., and Crenshaw, J.L., Jr.: A clinical and surgical review of endometriosis. Am. J. Obstet. Gynecol., *52*:930–942, 1951.
255. Judd, E.S.: Adenomyomata presenting as tumor of the bladder. Surg. Clin. North Am., *1*:1271, 1921.
256. Kahle, P.J., Vickery, G.W., and Maltry, E.: Endometriosis of the bladder, report of 2 additional cases. J. Urol., *46*:52–56, 1941.
257. Kretschmer, H.: Endometriosis of bladder. J. Urol., *53*:459–465, 1945.
258. Moore, T.D., Herring, A.L., and McCannel, D.A.: Some urological aspects of endometriosis. J. Urol., *49*:171–177, 1943.
259. O'Connor, V.J., and Greenhill, J.P.: Endometriosis of the bladder and ureter. Surg. Gynecol. Obstet., *80*:113–119, 1945.
260. Phillips, R.B.: Endometriosis vesicae. J. Obstet. Gynaecol. Br. Emp., *41*:165–189, 1934.

Neurofibroma

261. Barbalias, G.A.: Neurofibroma of the pelvis and bladder. Case report and review of the literature. Del. Med. J., *45*:33–37, 1973.
262. Bernstein, W.C.: Neurofibroma of the bladder presenting as a perirectal hernia: report of a case. Dis. Colon Rectum, *6*:457–458, 1963.
263. Burghele, T., Joachim, H., and Goldstein, J.: Recklinghausen's disease with urinary manifestations; neurofibroma of the bladder. Am. J. Surg., *97*:108–112, 1959.
264. Carlson, D.H., and Wilkinson, R.H.: Neurofibromatosis of the bladder in children. Radiol., *105*:401–404, 1972.
265. Deniz, E., Shimkus, G.J., and Weller, C.G.: Pelvic neurofibromatosis: localized von Recklinghausen's disease of the bladder. J. Urol., *96*:906–909, 1966.
266. Gold, B.M.: Neurofibromatosis of the bladder and vagina. Am. J. Obstet. Gynecol., *113*:1055–1056, 1972.
267. Labardini, M.M., Kallet, H.A., and Cerny, J.C.: Neurogenital neurofibromatosis simulating an intersex problem. J. Urol., *98*:627–632, 1967.
268. Van Buskirk, K.E., Clark, P.K., Snoga, J.R., et al.: Neurofibroma of the bladder; case report and review of the literature. J. Urol., *91*:241–245, 1964.

Nephrogenic Adenoma

269. Allan, E.: Nephrogenic adenoma of the bladder. J. Urol., 113:35–41, 1975.
270. Christoffersen, J., and Miller, J.E.: Adenomatoid tumour of the urinary bladder. Swed. J. Urol. Nephrol., 6:295–298, 1972.
271. Colby, F.H.: Embryonic rests of urinary bladder. Surg. Gynecol. Obstet., 40:528, 1925.
272. Davis, T.A.: Hamartoma of the urinary bladder. Northwest Med., 48:182, 1949.
273. Dow, J.A., and Young, J.D., Jr.: Mesonephric adenocarcinoma of the bladder. J. Urol., 100:466–469, 1968.
274. Friedman, N.B., and Kuhlenbeck, H.: Adenomatoid tumors of the bladder reproducing renal strictures (nephrogenic adenomas). J. Urol., 64:657–670, 1950.
275. Friedman, N.B., and Ash, J.E.: Tumors of the urinary bladder. In Atlas of Tumor Pathology, Washington, D.C., Armed Forces Institute of Pathology, 1959, Section 8, Part 31A.
276. Goldman, R.L.: Nephrogenic metaplasia (nephrogenic adenoma, adenomatoid tumor) of the bladder. J. Urol., 108:565–567, 1972.
277. Hasen, H.B.: Nephrogenic adenoma of the bladder. J. Urol., 88:629–630, 1962.
278. Kaany, E., and Werner, S.L.: Nephrogenic adenoma of bladder. Urology, 4:343–345, 1974.
279. Kaswick, J.A., Waisman, J., and Goodwin, W.E.: Nephrogenic metaplasia (adenomatoid tumor) of the bladder. Urology, 8:283–286, 1976.
280. Leonard, S.A., Silverman, A.J., Langston, J.W., et al.: Postoperative nephrogenic adenoma of bladder. Urology, 7:327–328, 1976.
281. Molland, E.A., Trott, P.A., Paris, A.M., et al.: Nephrogenic adenoma: A form of adenomatous metaplasia of the bladder. A clinical and elective microsurgical study. Br. J. Urol., 48:453–462, 1976.
282. Mostofi, F.K.: Potentialities of bladder epithelium. J. Urol., 71:705–714, 1954.

Leukoplakia

283. Connery, D.B.: Leukoplakia of the urinary bladder and its association with carcinoma. J. Urol., 69:121–127, 1953.
284. Holley, P.S., and Melligo, G.T.: Leukoplakia of the bladder and carcinoma. J. Urol., 86:235–241, 1961.
285. Kelalis, P.P., Emmett, J.L., and DeWeerd, J.H.: Leukoplakia of the urinary bladder: report of a case with unusual features. Proc. Staff Meet. Mayo Clin., 38:517–518, 1963.
286. Marion, G.: Leukoplakia of bladder. J. Urol., 9:257–261, 1920.
287. Melicow, M.M.: Tumors of the urinary drainage tract. Urothelial tumors. J. Urol., 54:186–193, 1945.
287a. O'Flynn, J.D., and Mullaney, J.: Vesical leukoplakia progressing to carcinoma. Br. J. Urol., 46:31–37, 1974.
288. Robson, S.M.: Leukoplakia and carcinoma: Report of a case with review of the listerature. J. Urol., 35:321–341, 1936.
289. Stevens, A.R.: Leukoplakia in bladder diverticulum. J. Urol., 21:689–694, 1929.
289a. Thomas, S.D., Sanders, P.W., III, and Sanders, P.W., Jr.: Cholesteatoma of the bladder. J. Urol., 112:598–599, 1974.
290. Thompson, G.J., and Stein, J.J.: Leukoplakia of the urinary bladder: A report of 34 clinical cases. J. Urol., 44:634–649, 1940.
291. Witherington, R.: Leukoplastic keratinizing tumor of the bladder. J. Urol., 98:206–208, 1967.
292. Witherington, R.: Leukoplakia of the bladder: An 8-year follow-up. J. Urol., 112:600–602, 1974.

Primary Lymphoma

293. Aquilina, J.N., and Bugeja, T.J.: Primary malignant lymphoma of the bladder: Case report and review of the literature. J. Urol., 112:64–65, 1974.
294. Borski, A.A.: Lymphosarcoma of the bladder. J. Urol., 84:551, 1960.
295. Boyd, H.L.: Lymphomatous involvement of the genitourinary tract. N.Y. State J. Med., 52:197–204, 1952.
296. Givler, R.C.: Involvement of the bladder in leukemia and lymphoma. J. Urol., 105:667–670, 1971.
297. Pontius, E.E., Nourse, M.H., Paz, L., and McCallum, D.L.: Primary malignant lymphoma of the bladder. J. Urol., 90:58–61, 1963.
298. Santino, A.M., Shumaker, E.J., and Garles, J.: Primary malignant lymphoma of the bladder. J. Urol., 103:310–313, 1970.
299. Sufrin, G., Keogh, B., Moore, R.H., et al.: Secondary involvement of the bladder in malignant lymphoma. J. Urol., 118:251–253, 1977.
300. Tremann, J.A., Norris, H.T., and McRoberts, J.W.: Lymphoproliferative disease of the bladder. J. Urol., 106:687–691, 1971.
301. Wang, C.C., Scully, R.E., and Leadbetter, W.F.: Primary malignant lymphoma of the urinary bladder. Cancer, 24:772–776, 1969.
301a. Watson, E.M., Sauer, H.R., and Sadugor, M.G.: Manifestations of the lymphoblastomas in the genitourinary tract. J. Urol., 61:626–645, 1949.

Leukemia

302. Barney, J.D., Hunter, F.T., and Mintz, E.R.: The urologic aspects of radiosensitive tumors of blood-forming organs. J.A.M.A., 98:1145–1250, 1932.
303. Grooms, A.M.: Hematuria and leukemic infiltration of the bladder. J.A.M.A., 223:193–194, 1973.
304. Hermann, H.B., Goldberg, M.M., and Salerno, F.M.: Leukemic infiltration of the bladder neck in a female patient. J. Urol., 83:51–53, 1960.
305. Kirshbaum, J.D., and Preuss, F.S.: Leukemia. A clinical and pathologic study of one hundred and twenty-three fatal cases in a series of 14,400 necropsies. Arch. Int., Med., 71:777–792, 1943.
306. Pentecost, C.L., and Pizzolato, P.: Involvement of the genitourinary tract in leukemia with report of case of involvement of urinary bladder. J. Urol., 53:725–731, 1945.
306a. Persky, L., Neidman, A.J., and Tucker, A.S.: Urologic manifestations of leukemia. J. Urol., 107:1073–1077, 1972.
307. Tribedi, B.D., and Banerjee, S.K.: An unusual manifestation of lymphatic leukemia. J. Indiana Med. Assn., 12:139–140, 1943.
308. Troup, C.W., Thatcher, G., and Hodgson, N.B.: Infiltrative lesion of the bladder, presenting as gross hematuria in child with leukemia. J. Urol., 107:314–315, 1972.
309. Tucker, A.S., and Persky, L.: Cystography in childhood. Tumors and pseudotumors. Am. J. Roentgenol., 109:390–398, 1970.

Secondary Tumors of the Bladder

310. Dean, A.L., and Ash, J.E.: Study of bladder tumors in the registry of the American Urological Association. J. Urol., 63:618–621, 1950.
311. Ganem, E.J., and Batal, J.T.: Secondary malignant tumors of the urinary bladder metastatic from primary foci in distant organ. J. Urol., 75:965–972, 1956.

312. Goldstein, A.G.: Metastatic carcinoma to the bladder. J. Urol., *98*:209–215, 1967.
313. Goldstein, H.M., Kaminsky, S., Wallace, S., et al.: Urographic manifestations of metastatic melanoma. Am. J. Roentgenol., *121*:801–805, 1974.
314. Heslin, J.E., Milner, W.A., and Garlick, W.B.: Lower urinary tract implants or metastases from clear cell carcinoma of the kidney. J. Urol., *73*:39–46, 1955.
315. Hovenanian, M.S.: Implantation of renal parenchymal carcinoma. J. Urol., *64*:188–192, 1950.
316. Klinger, M.E.: Secondary tumors of the genitourinary tract. J. Urol., *65*:144–153, 1951.
317. Meyer, J.E.: Metastatic melanoma of the urinary bladder. Cancer, *34*:1822–1824, 1974.
318. Piva, A.E., and Koss, L.G.: Cytologic diagnosis of metastatic malignant melanoma in urinary sediment. Acta Cytol., *8*:398–402, 1964.
319. Shaw, R.E.: Metastasis to bladder from carcinoma of the kidney. Br. J. Surg., *48*:420–422, 1960–1961.
320. Sheehan, E.E., Greenberg, S.D., and Scott, R., Jr.: Metastatic neoplasms of the bladder. J. Urol., *90*:281–284, 1963.
321. Ward-McQuad, J.N.: Carcinoma of bladder and multiple unrelated malignancies. Br. J. Urol., *35*:169–172, 1963.
322. Weston, P.A.M., and Smith, B.J.: Metastatic melanoma in bladder and urethra. Br. J. Surg., *51*:78–79, 1964.

PELVIC (PERIVESICAL) LIPOMATOSIS

Pelvic lipomatosis (Figs. 33–1 to 33–11) is a disease of dense infiltration of benign fatty tissue in the bony pelvis. It is primarily confined to males; only three females have been reported.[14, 23] It usually occurs in the 20 to 30 year age group, and blacks predominate (49 per cent black, 33 per cent white, 18 per cent not specified).[33] It may be asymptomatic, but 43 per cent have lower-urinary-tract symptoms such as frequency of urination, dysuria, nocturia, perineal and suprapubic discomfort, and decreased size of stream. The prostate gland is found in a high position in 20 per cent, normal position in 22 per cent, and not specified in 58 per cent.[33] A palpable suprapubic fullness is present in 29 per cent of the patients, with no comment concerning this in other reports.[33]

DIAGNOSIS

Cystoscopic examination has been extremely difficult in these cases owing to the high position of the bladder and prostate. However, in those examined cytoscopically, various types of proliferative cystitis have been found, especially cystitis glandularis.[8, 29, 36]

Specimens obtained by exploratory laparotomy have revealed some form of infiltrative benign fatty tissue (normal fat, benign lipoma, fibrofatty tissue, and fatty tissue of varying degrees of inflammation).

Although obesity has been recorded in this syndrome, it was not until recently that fat reduction was shown to relieve the radiographic appearance of pelvic lipomatosis; and, conversely, a relatively minor weight gain produces a recurrence of the syndrome with subsequent radiographic changes (Figs. 33–9 to 33–11).[33]

ROENTGENOGRAPHIC FINDINGS

1. Radiolucent areas in pelvis
2. Elevation and vertical elongation of bladder with an inverted "tear drop" or gourd, or pear-

33

Miscellaneous Conditions of the Bladder

shaped appearance, which is the characteristic finding. However, elongation and narrowing of the bladder without the gourd or "tear drop" appearance is not unusual. Occasionally the bladder maintains its usual shape except for slight narrowing and elevation. The bladder is usually displaced anteriorly.

3. Straightening, elongation, and elevation of the rectosigmoid with or without extrinsic compression

4. Medial displacement of the lower ureter and lateral displacement of midureter and dilatation of ureters and kidneys have been reported.[9, 11, 29]

Operations for the removal of the fatty components have been generally unsuccessful, although Carpenter reported a patient successfully treated with extirpation of the lipomatous masses.[8] Rarely uremia and death may ensue.[21]

DIFFERENTIAL DIAGNOSIS

Several conditions can give practically the same appearance of the bladder as perivesical lipomatosis:

1. *Perivesical hemorrhage secondary to trauma.* In this instance there is usually an increased density of the pelvic area and the fractures are usually easily recognized, if present. History, of course, is an important aid to diagnosis.

2. *Pelvic neoplasm.* Nussbaum reported a case in which the radiographic findings were similar to pelvic lipomatosis, but the cause was metastasis to the lymph nodes of the pelvis from an adenocarcinoma of the prostate (Fig. 33–12).[27]

3. *Obstruction of the vena cava.* This condition can sometimes produce similar findings (Fig. 33–13).[3, 16] However, several cases of obstruction of the vena cava have been reported in which there was an associated pelvic lipomatosis.[1, 34] In these instances the radiographic findings were probably the result of the pelvic lipomatosis rather than of the venous obstruction. In cases of inferior vena cava obstruction, if lower extremity edema is present, it is suggestive of the diagnosis, but edema can be variable and transitory. Collaterals are also seen in the lower abdominal wall in many instances.[24] In these cases the bladder may be compressed bilaterally and displaced superiorly and anteriorly, probably secondary to the collaterals produced by the obstruction. Notching of the ureter below L-3 can sometimes be visualized. An inferior venacavogram would substantiate the diagnosis. Schechter has reported obstruction of one external iliac vein and compression of the other (Fig. 33–8).[34]

4. *Lymphocysts.* They are essentially lymph-filled spaces in the retroperitoneum without a distinct epithelial lining (Fig. 33–14). They are caused by the division of afferent lymph channels during a lymphadenectomy. They may be unilateral or bilateral and are usually small. The incidence appears to be in direct proportion to the extent of the lymph node dissection. Lymphocysts, if large enough, can compress the bladder to produce a similarity to pelvic lipomatosis. Lymphography shows pooling in the lymphocyst.[35]

5. *Lipoplastic lymphadenopathy.* This condition can simulate pelvic lipomatosis with elevation and elongation of the bladder and elevation and straightening of the sigmoid colon. In these cases no definite radiolucencies are seen, and it is more likely to occur in females than is pelvic lipomatosis.

LIPOPLASTIC LYMPHADENOPATHY

Lipoplastic lymphadenopathy is a rare, benign disorder of lymphoid tissue[38] that represents replacement of lymph follicles with fat with enlargement of the same nodes. The enlarged nodes are characteristically found in the axillae, but cases involving pelvic and retroperitoneal nodes have been described.[37, 38]

Radiographically the disease simulates perivesical lipomatosis; there is elevation and elongation of the bladder and elevation and straightening of the sigmoid colon. Differentiating points of lipoplastic lymphadenopathy are the following:

1. No definite radiolucencies are seen.
2. There tends to be a lateral deviation of the left ureter.
3. It is seen in females, whereas pelvic lipomatosis usually affects males.

Lymphangiograms appear like non-Hodgkin's lymphoma, but the [67]gallium scintiscan is negative.[37] The course is benign, and operation is usually not necessary except for diagnosis.

THE UNSTABLE BLADDER

The unstable bladder (Fig. 33–15) refers to spontaneous and induced bladder instability as demonstrated by the accompanying of a desire to void by an involuntary detrusor contraction. It has been considered part of urgency incontinence,[42] stress incontinence,[41] and the persisting symptoms after prostatectomy.[46] The term probably should include the uninhibited bladder.

Apparently filling rate and filling position (supine, sitting, erect) have no effect on spontaneous detrusor contraction, although the erect position does reduce mean bladder capacity.[45] Arnold believed that 58 per cent of patients with instability were not detected by the supine filling alone, and certainly the erect position does add some cases.[40]

The unstable bladder may be divided into two groups: (1) idiopathic instability and (2) secondary instability, which in turn is classified as outflow obstruction, associated neurologic abnormality, urinary infection, and others.

DEFUNCTIONALIZED URINARY BLADDER

The urinary bladder may be defunctionalized (Figs. 33–16 to 33–18) under two circumstances:

1. Completely defunctionalized bladder after urinary diversion in which the bladder is left in (Fig. 33–16)
2. Partially defunctionalized bladder in those cases of end-stage kidney disease in which there is little or no urine production (Figs. 33–17, 33–18)

Both types are similar in that the bladder tends to become smaller and the cystometric readings give a hypertonic appearance (really myotonic owing to small capacity). They differ in that type 1 appears to develop vesicoureteral reflux more commonly than type 2. The incidence of vesicoureteral reflux in type 2 may be as high as 30 per cent.[49a] Bladder dysfunction in uremic patients is supposed to be the reason for this high incidence of reflux.[54a, 54b] However, it is most likely that the diminution in efflux is the primary cause. Type 1 in our experience has had a higher incidence of reflux, probably as high as 50 per cent. After reconstruction in type 1, the reflux disappears (see Vesicoureteral Reflux).

Empyema cystis means an accumulation of purulent material in a defunctionalized bladder. It is characterized by urethral discharge, fever, and suprapubic discomfort. Severe pain may occur when the discharge is expelled. The majority of patients with empyema cystis develop the complication in the first year following diversion.[50] Children develop this complication in only 8 per cent of the cases, whereas 26 per cent of women and 14 per cent of men with defunctionalized bladders develop empyema cystis.[50] Proteus seems to be the most significant organism producing this problem. Cases with sterile urine before diversion do not usually develop the empyema. Defunctionalization of a normal bladder does not limit its ability for expansion after refunctionalization.[61]

Roentgenographic Findings. The defunctionalized bladder is a small, usually smooth-walled bladder in which reflux can occur either in the completely or partially defunctionalized type. Trabeculations may occur if there is a neurogenic element present. In cases of empyema cystis, the bladder is small and irregular but this complication is difficult to visualize radiographically.

URINARY INCONTINENCE

True Incontinence is caused by loss of sphincteric action as the result of improper innervation or by direct injury as a result of prostatic operations, resections of bladder neck in females, excisions of diverticula of the urethra, hysterectomies, and others.

Paradoxical Incontinence. The bladder is unable to empty itself because of a large residual urine. Any increase in pressure can cause voiding. Usually there is dribbling or frequent voiding in small amounts. The usual causes are obstructions of the bladder such as prostate and strictures. Impaired voiding contractions of the bladder may simulate this condition.

Stress Incontinence. Urinary incontinence on coughing, sneezing, lifting, or laughing, with good control without stress, is characteristic. The pressures in the bladder under straining conditions are high enough to produce voiding that usually would not occur because of proper resistance in the urethra.

Extrasphincteric Incontinence. Ectopic ureters entering the vagina or distal urethra in females may cause a continual leaking. This gives the same effect as vesicovaginal or ureterovaginal fistulas as a result of operative injury, and the latter should be included in this category.

Urgency Incontinence. This is related to the unstable bladder, which is described in a separate portion of this section.

Incontinence Due to Mental Deterioration. This is an ill-defined condition that occurs often in mentally disturbed or deteriorated patients who are not conscious of their desire to void and therefore void at inopportune times.

Enuresis. This is the inappropriate or involuntary voiding of urine at an age when control should be present. Nocturnal enuresis is defined as night wetting beyond the age of 3 years. Primary enuresis refers to those patients who have never achieved control. Secondary enuresis refers to those patients who have had a dry period for an indefinite period of time and then recommence wetting. Most enuretics wet only at night, but a few wet day and night, and a rare few only by day.

Although there have been many hypotheses regarding the causes of primary enuresis, the best one seems to be the maturational lag,[64] delayed functional maturation of the central nervous system. Theories that have had some prominence regarding the causes of primary enuresis are genetic,[66] environmental, sleep disorders,[63] psychologic,[70] allergic reactions,[65] urinary infections, and various urinary tract lesions, including obstructions.

It is noted that there is reduction in capacity of the bladder[65, 69] which appears to be functional, the cystometrograms showing a hypertonic curve, uninhibited contractions, and a small capacity.[68]

AMYLOIDOSIS OF BLADDER

Amyloidosis of the bladder may occur under the following circumstances:

1. As part of secondary amyloidosis in which there are recognizable predisposing causes
2. As part of primary systemic amyloidosis (with diffuse involvement of various organs). No cause has been found.
3. As a localized primary amyloidosis of the bladder with tumefactive or diffuse involvement

Briggs reported that the lower urogenital system was involved in 50 per cent of cases of primary amyloidosis and only 25 per cent of cases of secondary.[75] Sexes are affected equally, and 50 to 60 years of age is the predominant group.

The symptoms are intermittent gross painless hematuria, which is usually mild but can be severe,[79] frequency, dysuria, and nocturia.[73, 76] These symptoms apply to all types of the disease, but severe hemorrhage is more common in the secondary type of amyloidosis.[72, 81, 82]

Recurrences are unusual after transurethral resection and electrocoagulation, except in some cases of secondary amyloidosis.

Cystoscopically the appearance resembles an infiltrating neoplasm. There is usually a solid circumscribed, elevated, sessile mass. Diffuse involvement is rare.[76] There may be a hemorrhagic irregular surface, yellowish in tint, and frequently oozing blood.[80]

It may occur in any part of the bladder, but the right lateral wall seems to be the most frequent site; the trigone is generally spared.[79]

Roentgenographic Findings. Cystograms have rarely been reported. There may be an irregular, lobulated defect in the bladder without involvement of the perivesical fat (Fig. 33–19).[84]

Differential Diagnosis. Tumor, endometriosis, cavernous hemangioma, cystitis cystica, and cystitis glandularis must all be considered in a differential diagnosis. Roentgenographic findings probably do not in most cases differentiate amyloidosis from other entities.

CONDYLOMATA ACCUMINATA

Condylomata accuminata is a proliferative lesion of squamous epithelium shown to be of viral etiology, probably by the papova virus group.[90] It usually appears on the moist mucocutaneous surface of the penis, labia, vaginal mucosa, urethral meatus, perianal skin, anal canal, perineum, and scrotum. The urethra is involved in 5 per cent of cases—always the anterior urethra, occasionally the entire urethra, including the posterior urethra, but never the posterior urethra alone (see Condylomata of the Urethra). The bladder is involved along with the urethra in most cases,[87, 88, 91] but Kleiman and Lancaster's case did not involve the urethra but only a suprapubic sinus and the bladder.[89] The lesion appears as papillomatous projections in the bladder and urethra. Obstruction of the ureter has been reported.[88]

Roentgenographic Findings. Roentgenograms of the bladder with condylomata accuminata have not been published, but urethral involvement has been visualized by cystourethrography. (See Chapter 43, Miscellaneous Conditions of the Urethra.)

CAUSES OF CONTRACTED BLADDERS

A small or a contracted bladder (Figs. 30–20 to 30–25) may be produced by or be one of the following:

1. Interstitial cystitis (Fig. 33–20)
2. Tuberculosis (Fig. 33–21)

3. Neurogenic bladder (Fig. 33–22)
4. Contracted bladder with obstruction, such as prostatic hypertrophy (Fig. 33–23)
5. Infiltrating carcinoma of the bladder (Fig. 33–24)
6. Radium cystitis (Fig. 33–25)
7. Defunctionalized bladder
8. Abacteria pyuria (Fig. 26–31)
9. Total incontinence, preventing filling of bladder (Fig. 33–25a)

LARGE BLADDERS

Large bladders (Figs. 33–26 to 33–34) are defined as bladders having an increased capacity that usually is visualized on cystogram as beyond the limits of normal (defined under Normal Bladder). In adults large bladders fall into the following categories:

1. Bladders affected by obstruction, such as prostatic hypertrophy, contracture of the bladder neck (Fig. 33–26)
2. Neurogenic bladders, including those affected by congenital lesions, trauma to the spinal cord (Fig. 33–28), tumors, and diabetes
3. Idiopathic atony of the bladder (Fig. 33–29)
4. Hysterical bladders (Fig. 33–30)

In children large bladders fall into the following categories:

1. Bladders affected by obstruction, such as contracture of the bladder neck (Fig. 33–31), strictures of the urethra, valves
2. Neurogenic bladders (Figs. 33–32)
3. Megacystis syndrome (Figs. 33–33, 33–39 to 33–42)
4. Absence of the abdominal musculature (Fig. 33–34)

Most of these categories have been discussed in their respective sections. Atony of the bladder is observed with mechanical obstruction, congenital malformations, neurologic lesions, and psychoneurosis. However, there is an idiopathic atony, seen more commonly in females in our experience, which is characterized by a large atonic bladder without reflux and a normal upper tract. Psychoneurosis also may produce a large hypotonic or atonic bladder and may be at times difficult to differentiate from idiopathic atony, but a careful psychiatric evaluation should distinguish these two conditions.

OTHER CONDITIONS OF THE BLADDER

Figures 33–35 to 33–38 represent miscellaneous conditions of the bladder that are not considered elsewhere.

MEGACYSTIS SYNDROME

Megacystis syndrome refers to a large, smooth-walled bladder with a large trigone and vesicoureteral reflux. The syndrome was first described by Marcel[111] and was investigated further by Williams[114] and then by Paquin and co-workers.[112]

It occurs more frequently in girls than in boys and is seen more commonly in childhood. Cystoscopically the bladder wall is smooth, although occasionally fine trabeculations may be noted. The bladder trigone is characteristically two or more times larger than normal. The ureteral orifices are gaping.

Roentgenographic Findings. Intravenous urogram may demonstrate bilateral hydronephrosis and hydroureter, but in others the upper tracts are dilated only mildly or moderately or are entirely normal in appearance. The cystourethrogram reveals an abnormally large but smooth-walled bladder. There is bilateral or unilateral ureteral reflux occurring either at low pressure or only during voiding. The bladder neck and proximal urethra may be entirely normal in appearance, but more commonly these structures fail to funnel and distend normally during voiding. The postvoiding films demonstrate no significant true bladder residual.

ELECTRIC STIMULATION

Electric stimulation to the bladder has been used to aid in emptying it, and stimulation to the pelvic floor has been used to produce or assist in gaining continence.[115-119]

DYSSYNERGIA

Successful voiding depends upon intact coordinated activity between the detrusor muscle, bladder neck, proximal urethra, and external sphincter. Dyssynergia, or loss of coordination, occurs at two levels

—between the detrusor and internal sphincter and proximal urethra, or between detrusor and external sphincter. In the first type, there may be uninhibited sympathetic discharge that produces constriction of the proximal urethra (usually associated with other manifestations, such as piloerection, hypertension, and reflex bradycardia). Thus increased difficulty with bladder emptying occurs secondary to proximal urethral contraction. This usually occurs in neurogenic lesions above T-7. This destroys the inhibition of the sympathetic outflow below this level.

Type two usually occurs in hyper-reflexic bladders with high postvoiding residuals. These are associated with upper motor lesions, and the external sphincter is the most common cause of the obstruction. The detrusor-external sphincter dyssynergia is less common in the lower motor neuron lesion (areflexic bladder) but occurs because the pudendal nerve is spared.

It should be emphasized that voiding difficulties with dyssynergia can result from various drugs (anticholinergic drugs producing decreased bladder activity), and pro-alpha sympathetic drugs, such as decongestants can increase urethral tone and cause retention of urine. In addition, some cases of active or passive dysfunctional bladder neck obstruction may occur without definite neurologic abnormalities.

GARTNER'S DUCT CYST

The wolffian duct becomes the male sexual duct (vas deferens) after the ureters have budded from their distal ends. In the female, the wolffian duct atrophies and is called Gartner's duct, a vestigial structure that lies along the anterolateral margin of the vagina and terminates near the orifice of Bartholin's gland. Retention cysts occur when a small segment of the canal remains unobliterated and subsequent secretory activity develops.[129] The majority of vaginal cysts arise from Gartner's duct.[125] The cysts can involve the ureter, producing obstruction, and can actually form a dilated portion in the region of the bladder of an ectopic ureter from the upper segment of a double collecting system. Some have been implicated in the formation of urethral diverticula and periurethral cysts.[124, 126]

ROENTGENOGRAPHIC DIAGNOSIS

1. The cystic mass may produce a rounded, smooth, or irregular defect in the bladder (Figs. 33–44).
2. It can deviate and obstruct the ureter (Fig. 33–44).
3. If it becomes part of an ectopic ureter, it may actually be an ectopic ureterocele or be representative of a cecoureterocele.[128]
4. Direct injection of the cyst may show a somewhat irregular mass that may have a projection downward that might represent the terminal part of the original duct (Fig. 33–45).

DIFFERENTIAL DIAGNOSIS

1. The true vaginal retention cysts lie in the posterior vaginal wall and are squamous inclusions with sebaceous characteristics. In contrast, Gartner's duct cysts lie in the anterolateral wall of the vagina near the proximal end.[125] They contain clear amber fluid or mucinous material.[127]
2. Endometrial cysts becomes bluish and tender in the premenstrual and menstrual phases.
3. Urethral diverticula and periurethral cysts may be confusing but generally seem to arise from periurethral infection, although the congenital variety may be part of Gartner's duct.

MISLEADING FILMS

Many entities can cause changes in the bladder contour, which can be very confusing (Figs. 33–46 to 33–51). The most common, however, are gas and feces in the rectum.

CHAPTER 33, ILLUSTRATIONS

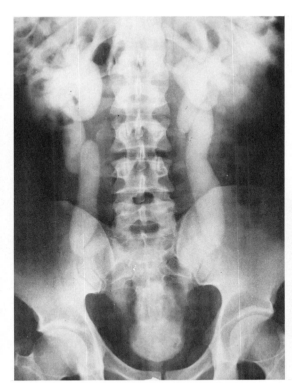

FIG. 33–1. Pelvic lipomatosis. Narrowed, elongated bladder with radiolucent areas on either side. Bilateral hydronephrosis. (Pepper, H.W., Clement, A.R., Drew, J.E.: Br. J. Radiol., *44*:313, 1971)

FIG. 33–2. Same case as in Fig. 33–1. Injecting cysto-urethrogram. The posterior urethra is elongated, and bladder is elevated. Markedly thickened mucosal folds on the posterolateral aspect of the partially filled bladder. (Pepper, H.W., Clement, A.R., Drew, J.E.: Br. J. Radiol., *44*:313, 1971)

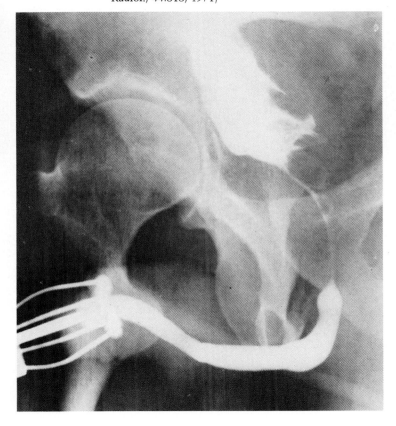

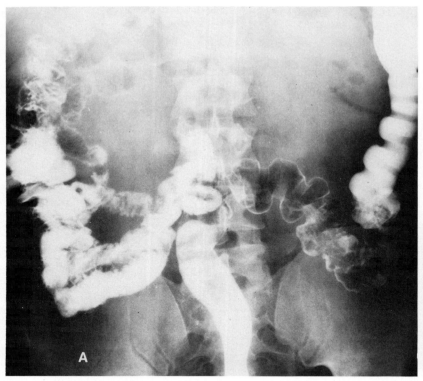

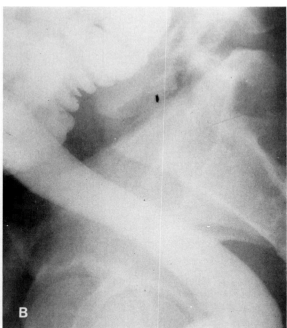

FIG. 33–3. Same case as in Fig. 33–1. **(A)** The rectum and distal sigmoid are narrowed and tubular in configuration. The sigmoid is elevated out of the true pelvis. **(B)** Lateral view. There is an increase in the retrorectal space. (Pepper, H.W., Clement, A.R., Drew, J.E.: Br. J. Radiol., *44*:313, 1971)

FIG. 33–4. Pear-shaped bladder due to pelvic lipomatosis. Bladder floor is elevated and compressed by radiolucent fat. (Courtesy of J.W. Smyth, M.D., Johns Hopkins Medical School)

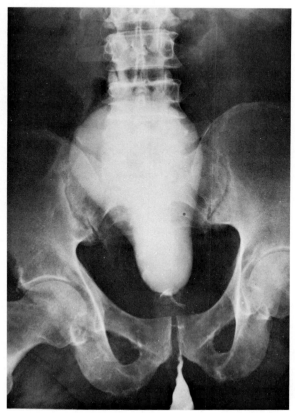

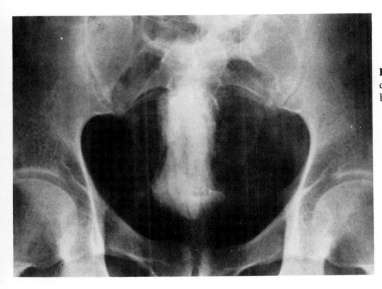

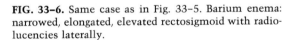

FIG. 33–5. Pelvic lipomatosis. Elevated, narrowed bladder. Note radiolucent areas below and on either side of bladder.

FIG. 33–6. Same case as in Fig. 33–5. Barium enema: narrowed, elongated, elevated rectosigmoid with radiolucencies laterally.

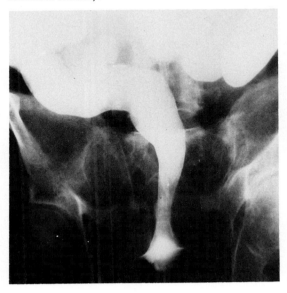

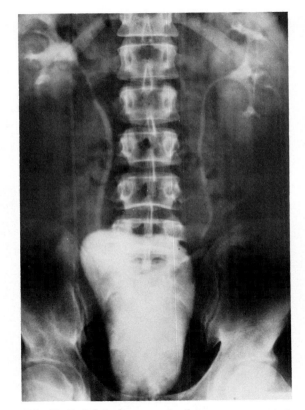

FIG. 33–7. Pelvic lipomatosis. Intravenous urogram reveals typically elevated, gourd-shaped bladder of pelvic lipomatosis. Clear areas are seen around the bladder. (Schecther, L.S.: J. Urol., *111*:757, 1974)

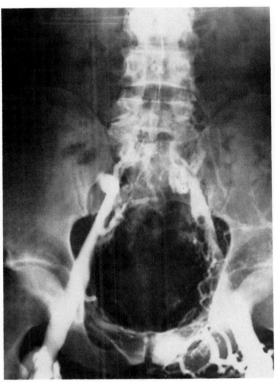

FIG. 33–8. Same case as in Fig. 33–7. Bilateral femoral venography shows complete obstruction of inferior vena cava and left external iliac vein with compression of medial aspect of right external iliac vein. Marked radiolucency of pelvic soft tissue represents fat. (Schechter, L.S.: J. Urol., *111*:757, 1974)

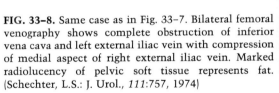

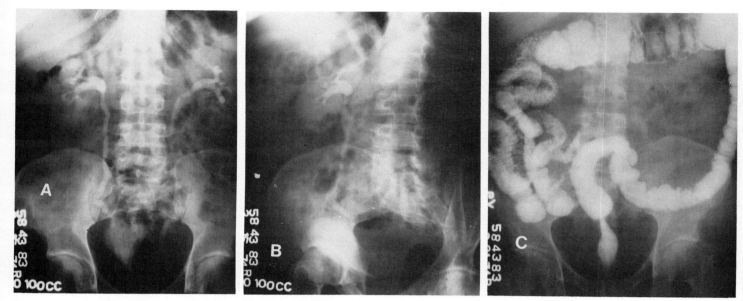

FIG. 33–9. (A–C) Anteroposterior and oblique excretory urograms taken at 10 minutes following injection of contrast medium show typical features of pelvic lipomatosis. Barium enema study shows narrowing of rectosigmoid colon. (Sacks, S.A., and Drenick, E.J.: Urology, 6:609, 1975)

FIG. 33–10. (A–C) Anteroposterior and oblique excretory urograms taken at 10 minutes following injection of contrast medium show external resolution of previous radiographic abnormalities. Patient has lost 45 pounds during a 40-day fast. Barium enema study shows less narrowing of rectosigmoid colon. (Sacks, S.A., and Drenick, E.J.: Urology, 6:609, 1975)

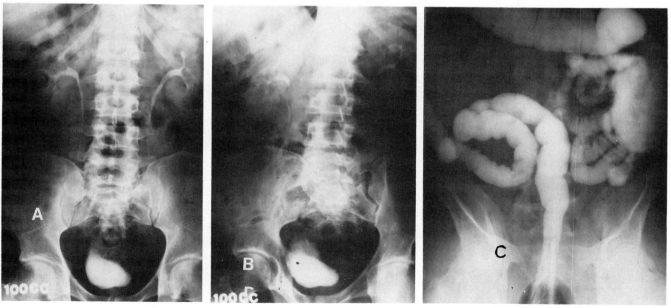

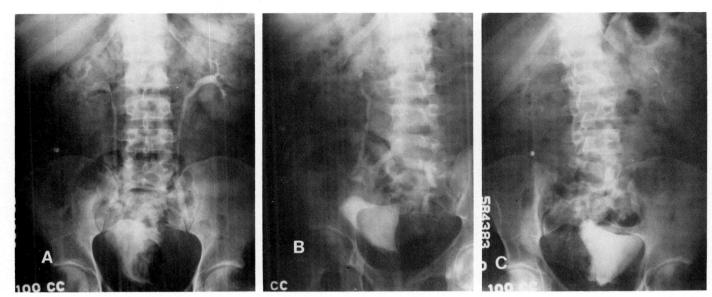

FIG. 33–11. (A–C) Anteroposterior and oblique excretory urograms taken at 10 minutes following injection of contrast medium show regressive changes approximating initial radiographic findings. Patient has regained 24 pounds in 30 days. (Sacks, S.A., and Drenick, E.J.: Urology, 6:609, 1975)

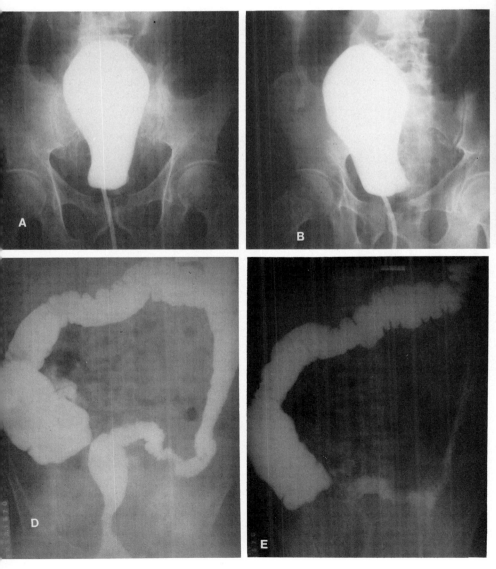

FIG. 33–12. Carcinoma of prostate with metastases resembling pelvic lipomatosis. (A) Anteroposterior cystogram; pear-shaped bladder, radiolucent areas in pelvis. (B) Oblique view. (C) Lateral view; bladder anteriorly displaced slightly. (D) Barium enema; markedly narrowed rectosigmoid rising vertically out of pelvis. (E) Postevacuation barium enema; narrowed rectosigmoid, poor emptying. (Nussbaum, P.S.: Surg. Clin. North Am., 52:405, 1972.

1535

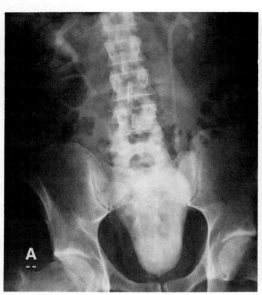
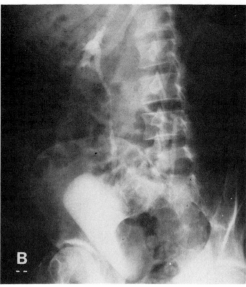
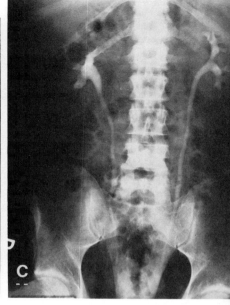

FIG. 33–13. Occlusion of inferior vena cava by metastatic testicular tumor. **(A)** Excretory urogram shows an inverted, pear-shaped bladder elevated out of pelvis. **(B)** Oblique view; the bladder is displaced anteriorly and superiorly. The lower ureter is displaced anteriorly. **(C)** Medial deviation of ureter. **(D)** Barium enema reveals symmetric narrowing of rectum consistent with extrinsic compression. The sigmoid colon has been elevated out of the pelvis. (Amoe, H.E., Jr., and Lewis, R.E.: Radiology, *108*:307, 1973)

FIG. 33–14. Two large pelvic lymphocysts (following radical Wertheim hysterectomy for squamous cell carcinoma of cervix) resembling pelvic lipomatosis. **(A)** Intravenous urogram 2½ months following the radical hysterectomy reveals bilateral hydronephrosis more marked on right side. Two large soft tissue masses in bony pelvis are obstructing ureters at pelvic brim. The bladder is narrowed and elongated. **(B)** Films of abdomen 24 hours after lymphangiogram demonstrate two large amorphous collections of contrast medium (*arrows*) accumulating in lymphocyst in body pelvis. Note some normal lymph nodes in right aortic chain. (Steinberg, A., Madayag, M.A., et al.: J. Urol., *109*:477, 1973)

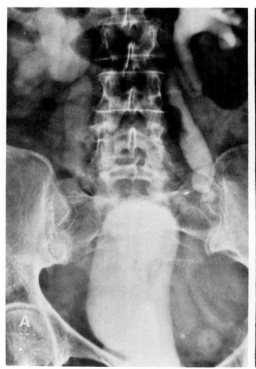
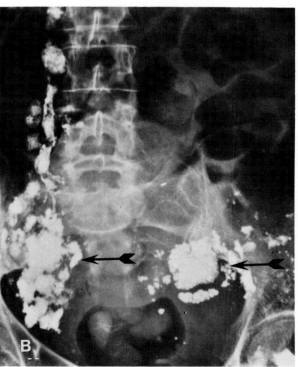

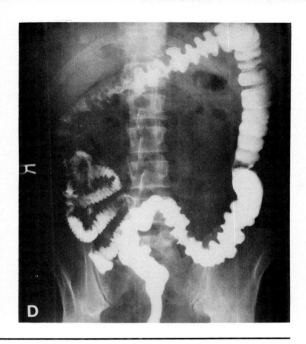

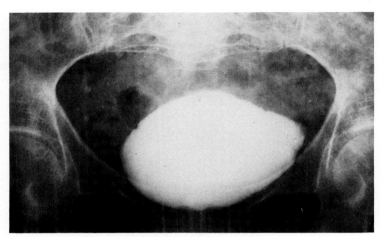

FIG. 33–15. Unstable bladder. Cystogram reveals a slightly irregular bladder of small capacity.

FIG. 33–16. Completely defunctionalized bladder; ureterosigmoidostomy performed. The patient had had a carcinoma in a diverticulum of the urethra, developed a recurrence in the urethra near the bladder neck, and following transurethral resection became totally incontinent. Cystogram reveals a small-capacity bladder with bilateral vesicoureteral reflux up to the cut end of the ureter.

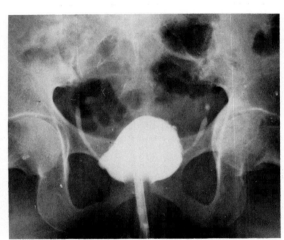

FIG. 33–17. Voiding cystourethrogram, oblique view. End-stage kidney, no diversion. Small-capacity bladder, no reflux.

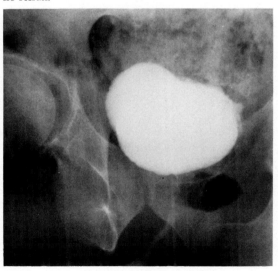

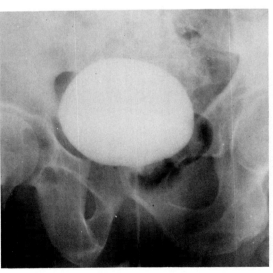

FIG. 33–18. Voiding cystourethrogram in an end-stage kidney. Small-capacity bladder, no reflux, no diversion.

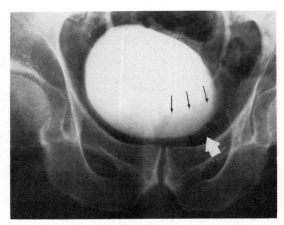

FIG. 33–19. Primary amyloidosis of bladder. Cystogram of intravenous urogram shows an irregular, lobulated mass near bladder neck (*arrow*). Upper tracts normal. (Strong, C.H., Kelsey, D., and Hoch, W.: J. Urol., *112*:463, 1974)

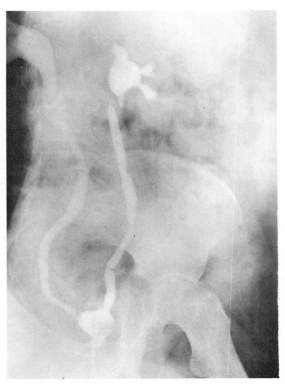

FIG. 33–20. Interstitial cystitis producing a contracted bladder with vesicoureteral reflux bilaterally.

FIG. 33–21. Tuberculous contracted bladder. Bladder is nearly absent (*arrow*). There is bilateral reflux. The left kidney shows marked involvement with a tuberculous process. There is a pyelostomy tube present. Note pipestem character of left ureter and dilatation of right ureter. Pelvis and calyces are dilated, although the right kidney is somewhat contracted. There is a large prostatic cavity secondary to tuberculous involvement.

FIG. 33–22. Neurogenic bladder. Small-capacity, trabeculated hypertonic bladder due to a level lesion at S-3 and S-4 as a result of a war injury. There is a spastic external sphincter.

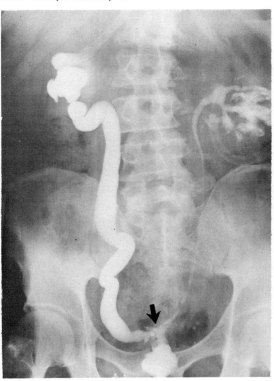

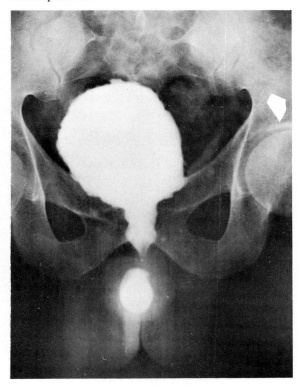

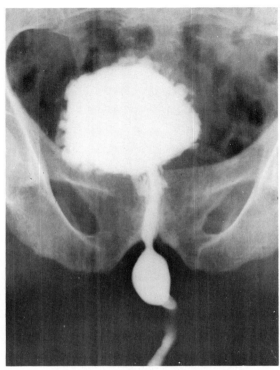

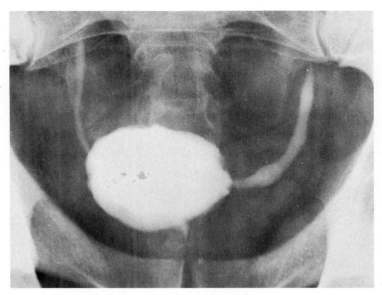

FIG. 33-24. Infiltrating carcinoma of the bladder, producing a small contracted bladder. The malignancy involves primarily the left lateral wall, producing left hydroureter. However, it spread through the muscularis and extended three-quarters of the way around the bladder.

FIG. 33-23. Contracted irregular bladder secondary to prostatic hypertrophy.

FIG. 33-25. Contracted bladder from radiotherapy. (Courtesy of A. Uson, M.D., and the Squier Urological Clinic, Columbia Presbyterian Medical Center)

FIG. 33-25a. Small-capacity bladder in a case of total incontinence following perineal prostatectomy. The continual leaking prevented adequate filling of bladder and it gradually diminished in size.

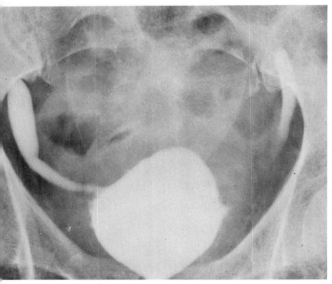

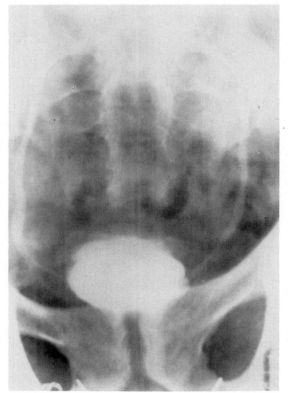

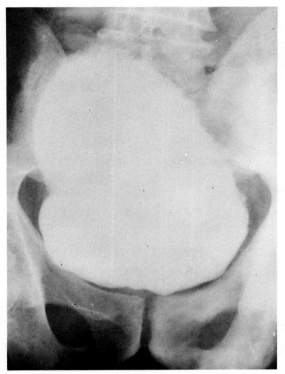

FIG. 33–26. Cystogram. Large-capacity hypotonic bladder secondary to prostatic hypertrophy.

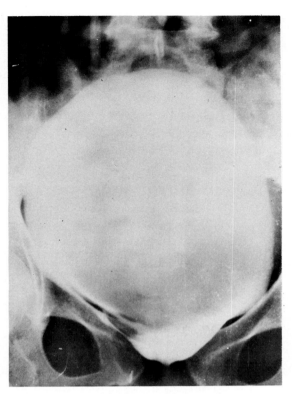

FIG. 33–27. Large bladder secondary to a large uterine fibroid. The compression of the bladder can be visualized by the clear areas in the bladder.

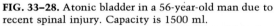

FIG. 33–28. Atonic bladder in a 56-year-old man due to recent spinal injury. Capacity is 1500 ml.

FIG. 33–29. Idiopathic atony of the bladder in a woman. Huge atonic bladder with no obstruction, holding 10,000 ml. (Courtesy of H. Bergman, M.D.)

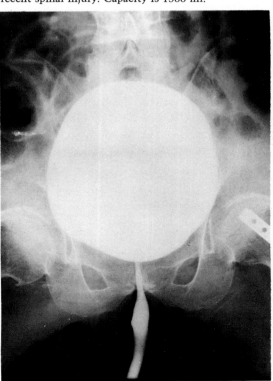

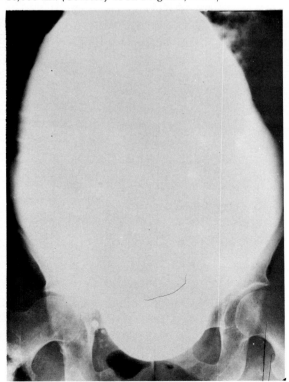

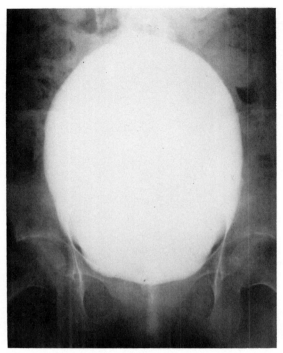

FIG. 33-30. Hysterical bladder. Large, smooth bladder of a young woman.

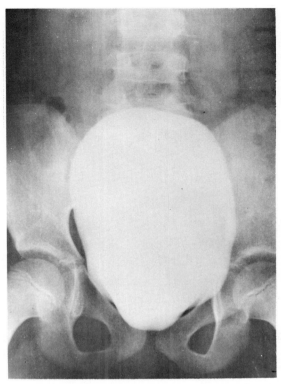

FIG. 33-31. Hypertrophy of bladder neck in a female child, producing a large-capacity bladder.

FIG. 33-32. Large atonic bladder. Neurogenic type. Lumbosacral spinal bifida in a 4½-year-old child. Retrograde cystogram showing bilateral reflux—hydroureter and hydronephrosis. Note atrophic right kidney.

FIG. 33-33. Megacystis in a 3½-year-old girl. Large smooth bladder. Bilateral reflux.

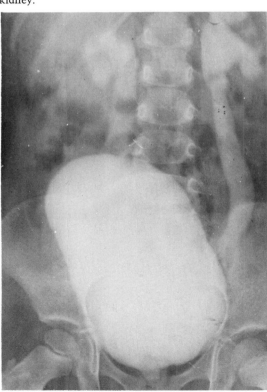

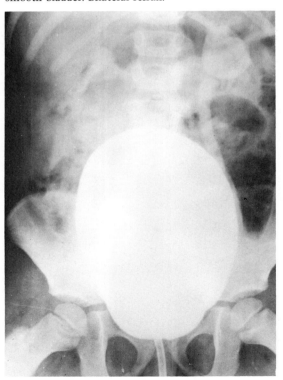

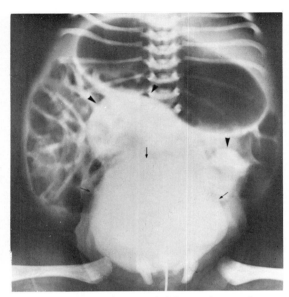

FIG. 33–34. Absence of abdominal musculature. *Small arrows* outline the bladder. *Large arrows* point to the dilated tortuous ureters. (Courtesy of G. Currarino, M.D. New York Hospital)

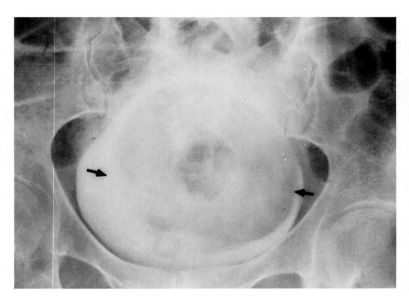

FIG. 33–35. Large filling defect in the bladder due to a blood clot secondary to kidney trauma. *Arrows* point to the large clot.

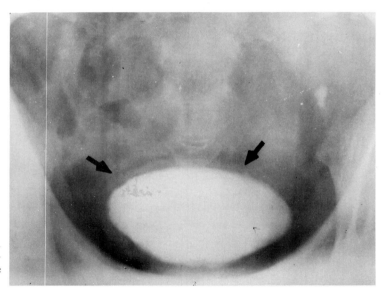

FIG. 33–36. Hypertrophy of bladder musculature. *Arrows* point to margins of hypertrophic muscle. Obstruction due to benign prostatic hypertrophy. The perivesical fat is outlined clearly.

FIG. 33–37. Contracture of bladder neck with marked thickening of the bladder wall. *Arrows* point to perivesical fat.

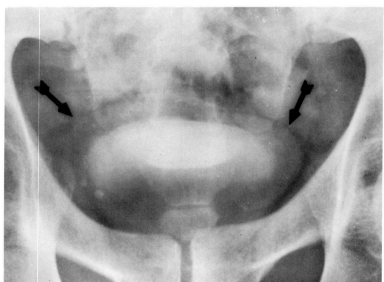

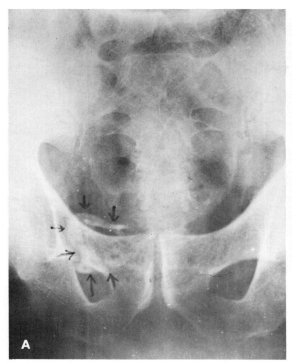

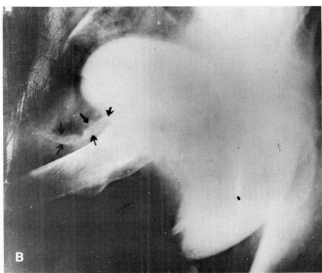

FIG. 33–38. Heterotypic bone formation in a suprapubic sinus. (Courtesy of B.S. Abeshouse, M.D.)

FIG. 33–39. Retrograde cystogram (15 mm. of water pressure) in a girl with megacystis syndrome. Note large smooth-walled bladder and vesicoureteral reflux.

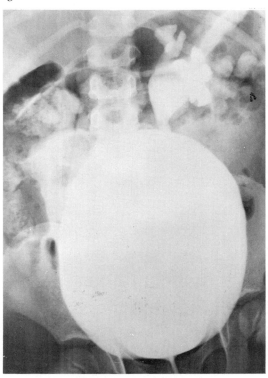

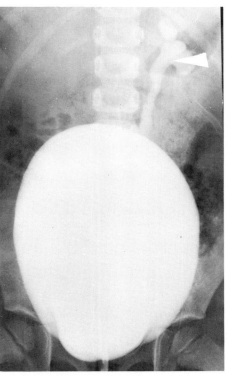

FIG. 33–40. Retrograde cystogram (15 mm. of water pressure) in a girl with megacystis syndrome. Note large smooth-walled bladder and vesicoureteral reflux on the left.

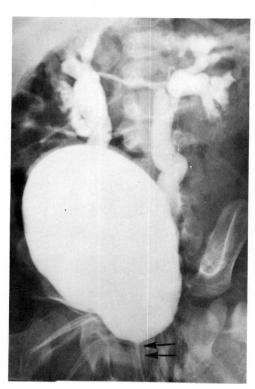

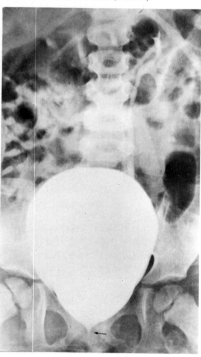

FIG. 33–41. Voiding cystourethrogram in a girl with megacystis syndrome. Note large smooth-walled bladder and bilateral ureteral reflux. Poor voiding with incomplete distention of the bladder neck and the urethra (*arrows*).

FIG. 33–42. Voiding cystogram in a girl with megacystis syndrome. Note large smooth-walled bladder and left ureteral reflux. Poor voiding with incomplete distention of the urethra (*arrow*).

FIG. 33–43. Electric stimulator of bladder. The bladder stimulator is above the bladder. The smaller device (*arrow*) is a pelvic floor stimulator. (Courtesy of Daniel C. Merrill)

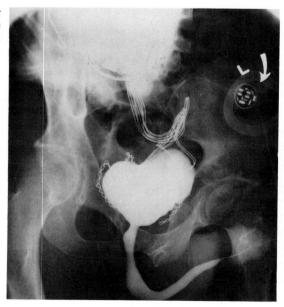

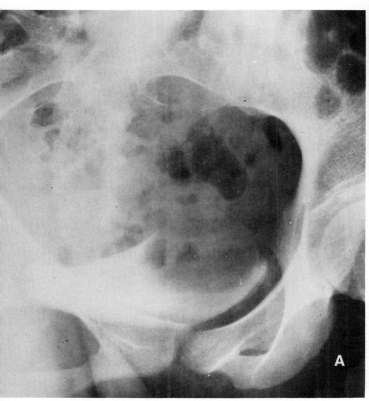

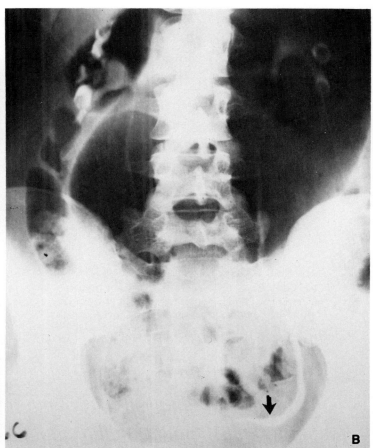

FIG. 33–44. Gartner's duct cyst. **(A)** Mass producing defect on left side of bladder on intravenous urogram. **(B)** Medial deviation of left ureter over mass (*arrow*). (Rhame, R.C., and Derrick, F.C., Jr.: J. Urol., *109*:60, 1973)

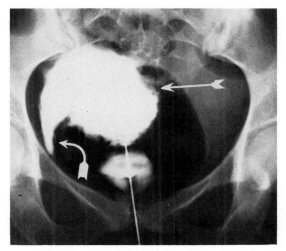

FIG. 33–45. Gartner's duct cyst. Contrast-filled, slightly irregular cystic mass (*straight arrow*) on right side of vagina and bladder. Air cystogram. The beak on the right side (*curved arrow*) is apparently the terminal end of the duct. Clear amber fluid obtained on aspiration.

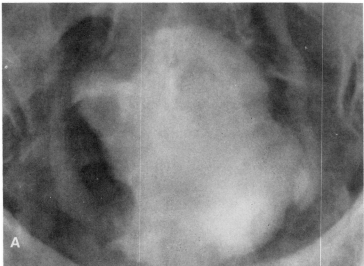
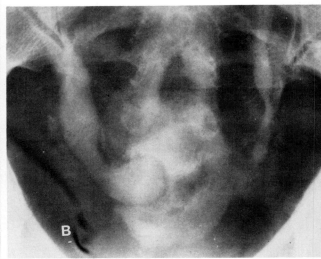

FIG. 33–46. Confusing bladder configuration. **(A)** Irregular defect on lateral aspect of right side of bladder with mild hydroureter could be confused with neoplasm. **(B)** Defect due to ureterocele. (Ney, C., and Miller, H.L.: Ill. Med. J., *144*:120–122, 1973)

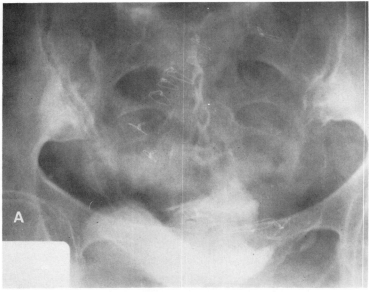

FIG. 33–47. Confusing bladder configuration. **(A)** Prone film showing irregular defect and protrusion of opaque material on superior aspect of the bladder. **(B)** Lateral view demonstrates defect to be caused by anterior abdominal wall bladder herniation. (Ney, C., and Miller, H.L.: Ill. Med., J., *144*:120–122, 1973)

FIG. 33–48. Confusing bladder configuration. **(A)** Displacement of bladder to right owing to extrinsic pressure on left side of bladder presenting as a smooth, regular defect. **(B)** The pressure defect shown to be caused by bowel incorporated in a huge scrotal hernia, which is only shown on an extended view of pelvis and hips. (Ney, C., and Miller, H.L.: Ill. Med. J., *144*:120–122, 1973)

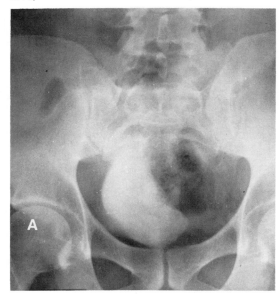

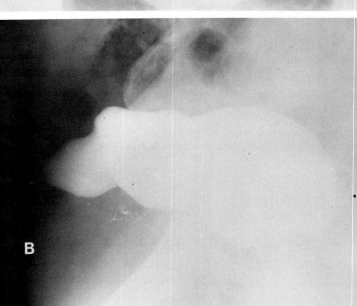

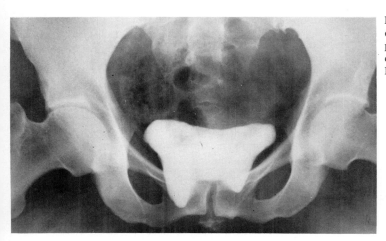

FIG. 33–49. Confusing bladder configuration. Bilateral elongation at base of bladder with straightening of mid-portion of base due to residual of a cystocele repair. This could be confused with herniation. (Ney, C., and Miller, H.L.: Ill. Med. J., *144*:120–122, 1973)

FIG. 33–50. Confusing bladder configuration. **(A)** Circular, well-defined lucency in bladder. **(B)** Defect due to subcervical lobe of prostate. (Ney, C., and Miller, H.L.: Ill. Med. J., *144*:120–122, 1973)

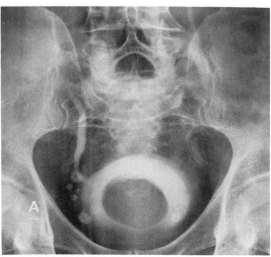

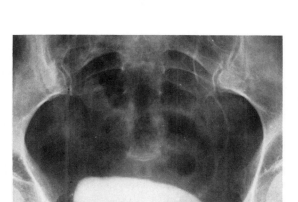

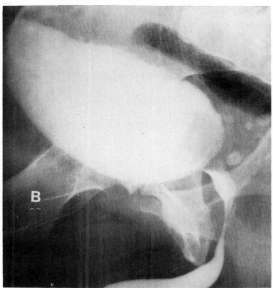

FIG. 33–51. Equal and bilateral impressions on inferior aspect of bladder owing to levator ani musculature. (Ney, C., and Miller, H.L.: Ill. Med. J., *144*:120–122, 1973)

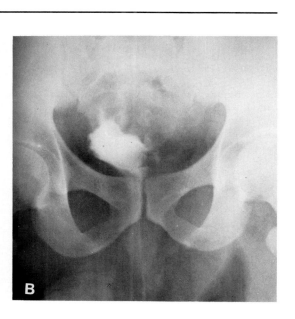

BIBLIOGRAPHY

Perivesical Lipomatosis

1. Abbott, D.A., and Skinner, D.G.: Congenital venous anomalies associated with pelvic lipomatosis (a case report). J. Urol., 112:739–742, 1974.
2. Ambos, M.A., Bosniak, M.A., Lafleur, R.S., et al.: The pear-shaped bladder. Radiology, 122:85–88, 1977.
3. Amoe, H.E., Jr., and Lewis, R.E.: Urographic and barium enema appearance in inferior vena cava obstruction. Radiology, 108:307–308, 1973.
4. Barry, J.M., Bilbao, M.K., and Hodges, C.V.: Pelvic lipomatosis: a rare cause of suprapubic mass. J. Urol., 109:592–594, 1973.
5. Becker, J.A., Weiss, R.M., Schiff, M., Jr., and Lytton, B.: Pelvic lipomatosis. A consideration in the diagnosis of intrapelvic neoplasms. Arch. Surg., 100:94–96, 1970.
6. Bender, L., and Kass, M.: Periureteral lipomatosis: case report. J. Urol., 103:293–295, 1970.
7. Blau, J.S., and Janson, K.L.: Pelvic lipomatosis. Consideration of the urinary tract complications. Arch. Surg., 105:498–500, 1972.
8. Carpenter, A.A.: Pelvic lipomatosis: successful surgical treatment. J. Urol., 110:397–399, 1973.
9. Engels, E.P.: Sigmoid colon and urinary bladder in high fixation: roentgen changes simulating pelvic tumor. Radiology, 72:419–422, 1959.
10. Flaherty, J.J., Kelley, R., Burnett, B., et al.: Relativity of pelvic bone fracture patterns to injury of the urethra and bladder. J. Urol., 99:297–300, 1965.
11. Fogg, L.B., and Smyth, J.W.: Pelvic lipomatosis: a condition simulating pelvic neoplasm. Radiology, 90:558–564, 1968.
12. Gellhorn, A., and Marks, P.A.: The composition and biosynthesis of lipid in human adipose tissue. J. Clin. Invest., 40:925–932, 1961.
13. Golding, P.L., Singh, M., and Worthington, B.: Bilateral ureteral obstruction caused by benign pelvic lipomatosis. Br. J. Surg., 59:69–72, 1972.
14. Goldstein, H.M., and Vargas, C.A.: Pelvic lipomatosis in females. J. Can. Assoc. Radiol., 25:65–68, 1974.
15. Grimmett, G.M., Hall, M.G., Jr., Aird, C.C., and Kurtz, L.H.: Pelvic lipomatosis. Am. J. Surg., 125:347–349, 1973.
16. Hall, R., and Jenkins, J.D.: Intravenous pyelography in acute idiopathic vena cava thrombosis. Br. J. Radiol., 43:781–786, 1970.
17. Harrow, B.R.: Retroperitoneal fibrosis following sclerosing injection for inguinal hernia and hemorrhoids. Am. J. Roentgenol., 99:90–95, 1967.
18. Hewett, A.L., and Headstream, J.W.: Pericystitis plastica. J. Urol., 83:103–107, 1960.
19. Leuzinger, D.E., Bahr, R.D., Miller, C.D., and Shipman, G.A.: Case report of high fixation of bladder and sigmoid colon. J. Urol., 85:163–165, 1961.
20. Long, W.W., Jr., Kellett, J.W., Gardner, W.A., and Lynch, K.M., Jr.: Perivesical lipomatosis. J. Urol., 109:238–241, 1973.
21. Lucey, D.T., and Smith, M.J.V.: Pelvic lipomatosis. J. Urol., 105:341–345, 1971.
22. Mahlin, M.S., and Dovitz, B.W.: Perivesical lipomatosis. J. Urol., 100:720–722, 1968.
23. Malter, I.J., and Omell, G.H.: Pelvic lipomatosis in a woman. A case report. Obstet. Gynecol., 37:63–66, 1971.
24. Missal, M.E., Robinson, J.H., and Tatum, R.W.: Inferior vena cava obstruction: clinical manifestations, diagnostic methods, and related problems. Ann. Intern. Med., 62:133–161, 1965.
25. Morretin, L.B., and Wilson, M.: Pelvic lipomatosis. Am. J. Roentgenol., 113:181–184, 1971.
26. Moss, A.A., Clark, R.E., Goldberg, H.I., and Pepper, H.W.: Pelvic lipomatosis: a roentgenographic diagnosis. Am. J. Roentgenol., 115:411–419, 1972.
27. Nussbaum, P.S.: Carcinoma of the prostate presenting as pelvic lipomatosis. Surg. Clin. North Am., 52:405–414, 1972.
28. O'Dea, M.J., and Malek, R.S.: Foreign body in bladder and perivesicular inflammation masquerading as pelvic lipomatosis. J. Urol., 116:669–670, 1976.
29. Pepper, H.W., Clement, A.R., and Drew, J.E.: Pelvic lipomatosis causing urinary obstruction. Br. J. Radiol., 44:313–315, 1971.
30. Puckette, S.E., Jr.: X-ray films of the month. J. Can. Med. Assoc., 66:248, 1970.
31. Radinsky, S., Cabal, E., and Shields, J.: Pelvic lipomatosis. Urology, 7:108–111, 1976.
32. Rosenberg, B., Hurwitz, A., and Hermann, H.: Dercum's disease with unusual retroperitoneal and paravesical fatty infiltration. Surgery, 54:451–455, 1963.
33. Sacks, S.A., and Drenick, E.J.: Pelvic lipomatosis: effect of diet. Urology, 6:609–615, 1975.
34. Schechter, L.S.: Venous obstruction in pelvic lipomatosis. J. Urol., 111:757–759, 1974.
35. Steinberg, A., Madayag, M., Bosniak, M.A., et al.: Demonstration of two unusually large pelvic lymphocysts by lymphography. J. Urol., 109:477–478, 1973.
36. Yalla, S.V., Ivker, M., Burros, H.M., and Dorey, F.: Cystitis glandularis with perivesical lipomatosis: frequent association of two unusual proliferative conditions. Urology, 5:383–386, 1975.

Lipoplastic Lymphadenopathy

37. Manning, L.G., Pischinger, R.J., and Bobroff, L.M.: Lipoplastic lymphadenopathy simulating malignant lymphoma and pelvic lipomatosis: report of a case and review of the literature. J. Urol., 114:788–790, 1975.
38. Morehead, R.P., and McClure, S.: Lipoplastic lymphadenopathy. Am. J. Pathol., 29:615, 1953.
39. Wolfel, D.A., and Smalley, R.H.: "Lipoplastic" lymphadenopathy. Am. J. Roentgenol., 112:610–612, 1971.

The Unstable Bladder

40. Arnold, E.P.: Cystometry—postural effects in incontinent women. Urologia Internationalis, 29:185–186, 1974.
41. Arnold, E.P., Webster, J.R., Loose, H., et al.: Urodynamics of female incontinence: factors influencing the results of surgery. Am. J. Obstet. Gynec., 117:805–813, 1973.
42. Bates, C.P.: Continence and incontinence. Ann. Roy. Coll. Surg., 49:18–35, 1971.
43. Farrar, D.J., Whiteside, C.G., Osbourne, J.L., and Turner Warwick, R.T.: A urodynamic analysis of micturition symptoms in the female. Surg. Gynecol. Obstet., 141:875–881, 1975.
44. Ramsden, P.D., Smith, J.C., Dunn, M., and Ardran, G.M.: Distension therapy for the unstable bladder: later results including an assessment of repeat distensions. Br. J. Urol., 48:623–629, 1976.
45. Ramsden, P.D., Smith, J.C., Pierce, J.M., and Ardran, G.M.: The unstable bladder—fact or artefact? Br. J. Urol., 49:633–639, 1977.

46. Turner Warwick, R.T., Whiteside, C.G., Arnold, E.P., et al.: A urodynamic view of prostatic obstruction and the results of prostatectomy. Br. J. Urol., *45*:631–645, 1973.
47. Turner Warwick, R.T., and Whiteside, C.G.: A urodynamic view of clinical urology. *In* Recent Advances in Urology. vol. 2, pp. 44–74. Edinburgh, Churchill Livingston, 1976.
48. Warrell, D.W., and Clow, W.M.: Critical appraisal of cystometry in evaluation of bladder function. Urologia Internationalis, *29*:187–189, 1974.
49. Whitfield, H.N., and Mayo, M.E.: Prolonged bladder distension in the treatment of the unstable bladder. Br. J. Urol., *47*:635–639, 1975.

Defunctionalized Bladder

49a. Bakshandeh, K., Lynne, C., and Carrion, H.: Vesico-ureteral reflux and end stage renal disease. J. Urol., *116*:557–558, 1976.
50. Dretler, S.P.: The occurrence of empyema cystis: management of the bladder to be defunctionalized. J. Urol., *108*:82–84, 1972.
51. Eckstein, B., and Mohindra, P.: The defunctioned neurogenic bladder: a clinical study. *In* Studies in Hydrocephalus and Spina Bifida. Developmental Medicine and Child Neurology (Suppl.), *22*:46–50, 1970.
52. Engel, R.M.: Complication of bilateral ureteric-ileocutaneous urinary diversion: a review of 208 cases. J. Urol., *101*:508–512, 1969.
53. Insoft, J., Gallagher, E.P., Jr., and Young, J.D., Jr.: Urinary diversion for neurogenic bladder: use of retroperitoneal ileal loop. J. Urol., *105*:211–213, 1971.
54. Kemp, D.R.: The forgotten bladder after urinary diversion. Br. J. Surg., *53*:236–239, 1966.
54a. Mosconi, C.E., Ianhez, L.E., Borelli, M., et al.: Bladder dysfunction in uremic patients. Acta Urol. Belg., *42*:418–420, 1974.
54b. Mosconi, C.E., Ianhez, L.E., Borelli, M., et al.: Vesico-ureteral reflux in patients in end stage chronic renal failure. Urol. Int., *30*:357–361, 1975.
55. Orecklin, J.R., and Goodwin, W.E.: Perineal vesicostomy: an alternative to cystectomy in male patients with a permanently defunctionalized bladder. J. Urol., *111*:151–153, 1974.
56. Ray, P., Tacuchi, Y., and McKinnon, K.J.: The pyocystis syndrome. Br. J. Urol., *43*:583–585, 1971.
57. Richie, J.P.: Intestinal loop urinary diversion in children. J. Urol., *111*:687–689, 1974.
58. Smith, D.: Follow-up study 150 ileal conduits in children. J. Ped. Surg., 7:1–10, 1972.
59. Spence, H.M., and Allen, T.D.: Vaginal vesicostomy for empyema of the defunctionalized bladder. J. Urol., *106*:862–864, 1971.
60. Stevens, P.S., and Eckstein, H.B.: The management of pyocystis following ileal conduit urinary diversion in children. Br. J. Urol., *47*:631–633, 1975.
61. Tanagho, E.A.: Congenitally obstructed bladder. Fate after prolonged defunctionalization. J. Urol., *111*:102–109, 1974.
62. Walker, W.C., and Wise, M.F.: Ureteroileostomy in management of neurogenic bladder in the adult. J. Urol., *102*:325–329, 1969.

Enuresis

63. Anders, T.F., Weinstein, P.: Sleep and its disorders in infants and children: a review. Pediatrics, *50*:312–324, 1972.
64. Bakwin, H.: Enuresis in children. J. Pediatr., *58*:806–819, 1961.
65. Esperanca, M., Gerrard, J.W.: Nocturnal enuresis: studies in bladder function in normal children and enuretics. Can. Med. Assoc. J., *101*:324–327, 1969A.
66. Frary, L.G.: Enuresis: a genetic study. Am. J. Dis. Child., *49*:557–578, 1935.
67. Hallgren, B.: Enuresis: a clinical and genetic study. Acta Psych. Neurol. Scand. (suppl.), *114*:1–159, 1957.
68. Linderholm, B.E.: The cystometric findings in enuresis. J. Urol., *96*:718–722, 1966.
69. Muellner, S.R.: Development of urinary control in children: some aspects of the cause and treatment of enuresis. J.A.M.A., *172*:1256–1261, 1960.
70. Werry, J.S.: Enuresis—a psychosomatic entity. Can. Med. Assoc. J., *97*:319–327, 1967.

Amyloidosis of Bladder

71. Au, K.K., and Gilbaugh, J.H., Jr.: Primary amyloidosis of the bladder. J. Urol., *114*:786–787, 1975.
72. Bender, L.I., and Kelly, C.E.: Secondary amyloidosis of the bladder: a case report. J. Urol., *102*:60–62, 1969.
73. Bergquist, D., and Westernmark, P.: Primary isolated amyloidosis of the urinary bladder: report of a case. Acta Chir. Scand., *137*:287–290, 1971.
74. Blath, R.A., and Bucy, J.G.: Localized primary amyloidosis of bladder. Br. J. Urol., *48*:219–220, 1976.
75. Briggs, G.W.: Amyloidosis. Ann. Intern. Med., *55*:943–957, 1961.
76. Grace, D.A., and Walton, K.N.: Primary localized amyloidosis of the bladder. J. Urol., *92*:655–658, 1964.
77. Hudson, H.C., and Tingley, J.D.: Primary amyloidosis of the bladder. J.A.M.A., *35*:353–355, 1965.
78. Kinzel, R.C., Harrison, E.G., Jr., and Utz, D.C.: Primary localized amyloidosis of the bladder. J. Urol., *85*:785–795, 1961.
79. Malek, R.S., Greene, L.F., and Farrow, G.M.: Amyloidosis of the urinary bladder. Br. J. Urol., *43*:189–200, 1971.
80. McDonald, J.H., and Heckel, N.J.: Primary amyloidosis of the lower genitourinary tract. J. Urol., *75*:122–132, 1956.
81. Missen, G.A.K., and Tribe, C.R.: Catastrophic haemorrhage from the bladder due to unrecognized secondary amyloidosis. Br. J. Urol., *42*:43–49, 1970.
82. Montie, J.E., and Stewart, B.H.: Massive bladder hemorrhage after cystoscopy in a patient with secondary systemic amyloidosis. J. Urol., *109*:49–50, 1973.
83. Nagel, R.: Localized amyloidosis of the bladder. J. Urol., *88*:56–59, 1966.
84. Strong, G.H., Kelsey, D., and Hoch, W.: Primary amyloid disease of the bladder. J. Urol., *112*:463–466, 1974.
85. Symmers, W.S.C.: Primary amyloidosis: a review. J. Clin. Pathol., *9*:187–211, 1956.
86. Tripathi, V.N.P., and Desautels, R.E.: Primary amyloidosis of the urogenital system: a study of 16 cases and brief review. J. Urol., *103*:96–101, 1969.

Condylomata Accuminata

87. Bissada, N.K., Cole, A.T., and Fried, F.A.: Extensive condylomata accuminata of the entire urethra and the bladder. J. Urol., *112*:201–203, 1974.
88. Hotchkiss, R.S., and Rouse, A.J.: Papillomatosis of the bladder and ureters, preceded by condyloma accuminata of the vulva: a case report. J. Urol., *100*:723–725, 1968.

89. Kleiman, H., and Lancaster, Y.: Condylomata accuminata of the bladder. J. Urol., 88:52–55, 1962.
90. Kovi, J., Tillman, M.A., and Lee, S.M.: Malignant transformation of condyloma accuminatum: a light microscopic and ultrastructural study. Am. J. Clin. Pathol., 61:702–710, 1974.
91. Lewis, H.Y., Wolf, P.L., and Pierce, J.M.: Condylomata accuminata of the bladder. J. Urol., 88:248–251, 1962.
92. Oriel, J.D., and Almeida, J.D.: Demonstration of virus particles in human genital warts. Br. J. Vener. Dis., 46:37–42, 1970.

Large Bladders in the Adult

93. Crabtree, E.G., and Muellner, S.R.: The bladder in prostatism: an operation for excessive bladder hypertrophy. J. Urol., 60:593–598, 1948.
94. Fish, G.W.: Surgery of dilated bladder. J. Urol., 63:802–851, 1950.
95. Fitzpatrick, R.J., Orr, L.M., Haywood, J.C., and Glanton, J.B.: Subtotal cystectomy for atonic bladder. J. Urol., 58:206–216, 1952.
96. Houtappel, H.C.E.M.: Subtotal cystectomy for atonic bladder. Br. J. Urol., 24:222–224, 1952.
97. Muellner, S.R.: Physiologic components of urinary bladder; their clinical significance. N. Engl. J. Med., 241:769–772, 1949.
98. Orr, L.M.: Management of the atonic bladder due to obstruction of vesical neck. South. Med. J., 30:519–524, 1937.
99. Ritter, J.S., and Sporer, A.: Physiologic principles governing therapy of neurogenic bladder. J. Urol., 61:528–544, 1949.
100. Trafford, H.S.: Atony of the female bladder. Br. Med. J., 1:149–151, 1959.

Psychogenic Bladders

101. Braasch, W.F., and Thompson, G.J.: Treatment of atonic bladder. Surg. Gynecol. Obstet., 61:379–384, 1935.
102. Bressler, B., Nyhus, P., and Magnussen, F.: Pregnancy fantasies in psychosomatic illness and symptom formation. Psychosom. Med., 20:187–202, 1958.
103. Chapman, A.H.: Psychogenic urinary retention in women. Psychosom. Med., 21:119–122, 1959.
104. Dunbar, H.F.: Emotions and Bodily Changes. New York, Columbia University Press, 1946.
105. Emmett, J.L., Hutchins, S.P.R., and McDonald, J.R.: Treatment of urinary retention in women by transurethral resection. J. Urol., 63:1031–1042, 1950.
106. Knox, S.J.: Psychogenic urinary retention after parturition, resulting in hydronephrosis. Br. Med. J., 2:1422–1424, 1960.
107. Larson, J.W., Swenson, W.M., Utz, D.C., and Steinhilber, R.M.: Psychogenic urinary retention in women. J.A.M.A., 184:697–700, 1964.
108. Margolis, G.J.: A review of literature on psychogenic urinary retention. J. Urol., 94:257–258, 1965.
109. Norden, C.W., and Friedman, E.A.: Psychogenic urinary retention: report of two cases. N. Engl. J. Med., 264:1096–1097, 1961.
110. Williams, G.E., and Johnson, A.M.: Recurrent urinary retention due to emotional factors: report of a case. Psychosom. Med., 18:77–80, 1956.

Megacystis Syndrome

111. Marcel, J.E.: Le syndrome mégavessie reflux cysto-pyélique. Presse Med., 60:1793–1796, 1952.
112. Paquin, A.J., Jr., Marshall, V.F., and McGovern, J.H.: The megacystis syndrome. J. Urol., 83:634–646, 1960.
113. Williams, D.I.: Urology in childhood. In Encyclopedia of Urology. vol. 15, pp. 57–61. Berlin, Springer, 1958.
114. Williams, D.I.: Megacystis and megaureter in children. Bull. N.Y. Acad. Med., 35:317–327, 1959.

Electric Stimulation

115. Grimes, J.H., Nashold, B.S., and Anderson, E.E.: Clinical application of electronic bladder stimulation in paraplegics. J. Urol., 113:328–340, 1975.
116. Halverstadt, D.B., and Parry, W.L.: Electronic stimulation of the human bladder: nine years later. J. Urol., 113:341–344, 1975.
117. Merrill, D.C.: Clinical experience with a mentor B stimulator. II. Meningomyelocele patients. J. Urol., 112:824–825, 1974.
118. Merrill, D.C.: Clinical experience with a mentor B stimulator. III. Patients with urinary vesical hypotonus. J. Urol., 113:335–337, 1975.
119. Merrill, D.C., and Conway, C.J.: Clinical experience with a mentor B stimulator. I. Patients with upper motor neuron lesions. J. Urol., 112:52–56, 1974.

Dyssynergia

120. Andersen, J.T., and Bradley, W.E.: The syndrome of detrusor-sphincter dyssynergia. J. Urol., 116:493–495, 1976.
121. Andersen, J.T., and Bradley, W.E.: Urethral pressure profilometry: assessment of urethral function by combined intraurethral pressure and electromyographic recording. J. Urol., 118:423–427, 1977.
122. Bright, T.C., III: Urethral pressure profile: Current concepts. J. Urol., 118:418–422, 1977.
123. Magee, M.C., and Fried, F.A.: Neurology for the urologist. J. Contin. Ed. Urol. 17:11–36, 1978.

Gartner's Duct Cyst

124. Hinman, F., Jr., and Cohlan, W.R.: Gartner's duct carcinoma in a urethral diverticulum. J. Urol., 83:414–415, 1960.
125. Jeffcoate, T.N.A.: Principles of Gynaecology. p. 493. London, Butterworth, 1967.
126. Johnson, C.M.: Diverticula and cyst of the female urethra. J. Urol., 39:506, 1938.
127. Rhame, R.C., and Derrick, F.C., Jr.: Gartner's duct cyst involving urinary tract. J. Urol., 109:60–61, 1973.
128. Stephens, D.: Caecoureterocele and concepts on the embryology and aetiology of ureteroceles. Aust. N.Z. Surg., 40:239–246, 1971.
129. TeLinde, R.W.: Operative Gynecology. p. 647. Philadelphia, J.B. Lippincott, 1948.

Misleading Films

130. Ney, C., and Miller, H.L.: Confusing bladder defects and configurations. Ill. Med. J., 144:120–122, 1973.

Part Six

PROSTATE, SEMINAL VESICLES,
EPIDIDYMIS, AND
VAS DEFERENS

BENIGN PROSTATIC HYPERTROPHY AND ITS EFFECTS ON THE GENITOURINARY TRACT

Benign prostatic hypertrophy or hyperplasia is a nodular enlargement of the prostate gland. Histologically, it may be composed mostly of stromal elements, mostly of glandular elements, or, most commonly, of a stromal-glandular mixture. It is generally considered to arise in the periurethral glands, the so-called inner groups of glands.[1, 2, 5, 9, 13]

However, some authors believe that the first changes take place in the periglandular stroma rather than in the glands proper.[3, 6, 10, 12]

Moore has emphasized that the earliest nodules are in the periurethral portions of the middle and the lateral lobes of the prostate between the bladder neck and the caudal limit of the verumontanum.[8] A recent redetermination of the origin and evolution of benign prostatic enlargement by McNeal emphasizes the importance of a transition zone that lies anterior to the large peripheral zone representing the lateral and posterior lobes and outside the periurethral area from which it is separated by a cylindrical sphincter muscle arising from the bladder neck.[7a] Clinical benign prostatic hyperplasia appears to arise essentially in the transition zone and for the most part is glandular in origin. Randall has given a gross anatomic description of the various types of hyperplasia depending on the topographic localization of the enlargement[11]:

1. Lateral lobes, producing intraurethral and infravesical enlargement (Figs. 34–4 to 34–9)
2. Posterior commissural (median lobe) lobe, which protrudes into the bladder, elevating the floor of the trigone. This lobe arises deep to the internal sphincter muscle (Figs. 34–10 to 34–12).

34

The Prostate

3. Lateral and median lobes that consist of both intraurethral and intravesical enlargements (Figs. 34–13 to 34–16)
4. Subcervical lobe, usually intravesical and pedunculated and covered only by mucous membrane (Figs. 34–17 to 34–20)
5. Lateral and subcervical lobes that protrude both intraurethrally and intravesically (Figs. 34–21 to 34–26)
6. Lateral, median, and subcervical lobes (same appearance on cysto-urethrography as Figs. 34–21 to 34–24)
7. Anterior commissural lobe (Fig. 34–27)
8. Subtrigonal lobe

Prostatic hypertrophy or hyperplasia has marked effects on the genitourinary tract. These effects are discussed under urethra, bladder, ejaculatory ducts and seminal vesicles, and the upper urinary tract, including the ureters and the kidneys.

EFFECTS ON THE URETHRA

LATERAL LOBES

The enlarged lateral lobes compress the urethra from either side, producing a slitlike appearance on cystourethrography when viewed from the frontal position. In the oblique position, the urethra appears to be widened and, usually, elongated (especially in the supracollicular portion), with a smooth contour. Occasionally, the lateral lobes do not tend to meet intraurethrally, and on the AP view the urethra does not appear to be especially narrowed. An oval filling defect in the posterior urethra may be produced by the touching of the lateral lobes. Large lateral lobe enlargement can produce a greatly increased concavity of the urethra anteriorly, with the urethra in this area displaced more posteriorly (Figs. 34–25, 34–26).

MIDDLE LOBE ENLARGEMENT

Angulation anteriorly (anterior tilting) in the region of the bladder neck usually is caused by middle lobe or subcervical enlargement. The angulation usually begins near the area of the verumontanum. A bifurcation or Y effect is the result of a subcervical enlargement (Figs. 34–17, 34–18, 34–21, 34–24).[67, 76] This is caused by the pedunculation characteristic of the subcervical lobe, allowing contrast medium to flow on either side.

In the typical appearance of prostatic enlargement, which includes both lateral and median and/or subcervical lobes, the urethra has a saberlike shape, is elongated, widened sagittally, and heavily curved.

EFFECTS ON THE BLADDER

FLOOR OF BLADDER

If the prostate enlarges intravesically, there may be a smooth filling defect in the bladder floor, which is readily discernible in the cystogram of the intravenous urogram or the retrograde cystogram. In general, the larger the prostate, the larger is the defect. Median and subcervical lobes tend to push intravesically and produce marked filling defects in the bladder floor (Figs. 34–2, 34–17, 34–18, 34–20, 34–23).

Subcervical lobe enlargement tends to produce a ball valve-type effect, and it often may present in the floor of the bladder a rounded defect, which may be confused with a Foley bag (Fig. 34–20). A Y effect at the bladder neck is characteristic.

The extravesically enlarged prostate (commonly associated with primary lateral lobe enlargement) elevates the floor of the bladder and pushes the trigone upward (Figs. 34–1, 34–3, 34–5, 34–6, 34–7, 34–8).

Anterior lobe enlargement is unusual and is rarely seen radiographically (Fig. 34–27). It mainly affects the urethra at the bladder neck.

POSITION OF BLADDER

The bladder may be displaced upward (Fig. 34–25) and laterally by an enlarged prostate.[21] This lateral displacement is uncommon.

SIZE OF BLADDER

Dilatation and decompensation of the bladder can occur in prostatic hypertrophy. The bladder wall first is thickened by muscular hypertrophy, but later it degenerates, becomes thin-walled, and finally may become fibrotic. Casper,[18] Sugimura,[23] Herman,[20] Crabtree and Muellner,[19] Binney,[15] Orr,[22] and Carter[17] have written on the atony that may occur in bladder neck obstructions, including prostatic hypertrophy. This atony may respond to removal of the obstruction, but occasionally resection of the bladder itself may be necessary (Figs. 34–10 to 34–12, 34–28).

OTHER EFFECTS

Trabeculation with cellule and saccule formation (Figs. 34–14, 34–29) is a result of obstruction at the bladder neck secondary to prostatic hypertrophy.

Prostatic hypertrophy is probably the most common vesical neck obstruction that causes bladder diverticula. There may be a single diverticulum or multiple diverticula, large or small. They may be larger than the bladder proper. Diverticula of clinical importance are found in 6 per cent of vesical neck obstructions.[16] Bladder calculi are a common result of prostatic hypertrophy. They are usually radiopaque, but occasionally nonopaque calculi are seen (uric acid stones). In some instances, uric acid may form the nonopaque nucleus for an opaque outer shell. Magnesium ammonium phosphate stones are the most common type. Xanthine calculi are rare.

EFFECTS ON THE KIDNEYS AND THE URETERS

Dilatation of the renal calyces, the pelvis, and the ureters (usually bilateral but occasionally unilateral) may be caused by hypertrophy of the prostate (Figs. 34–30 to 34–34).[25] There are many contributing factors leading to upper tract dilatation, but in any individual case the exact mechanisms are not always apparent. Some of the causes are as follows:

1. Back pressure
2. Reflux (Fig. 34–30)
3. Infection
4. The bladder muscular hypertrophy that occurs in prostatic obstruction can cause constriction of the ureter in its intramural position.
5. A large subtrigonal lobe can press directly on either or both ureters, causing obstruction.
6. Compression and obstruction of the ureters can occur at the point where they are crossed by the vasa deferentia.[28]
7. Hutch has described a type of ureteral obstruction in which the intravesical ureter becomes extravesical because of loss of support in the trabeculated bladder.[24] This may cause obstruction at the point where it joins the original extravesical ureter. Apparently, there may be a buckling in this area under the force of the advancing urinary stream.
8. A bladder diverticulum produced by an enlarged prostate can impinge on the ureter, causing obstruction (see Fig. 27–23).

EFFECTS ON THE URETER PROPER

The ureter may be deviated near its terminal end by the enlarged prostate. The deviation may take various forms,[27] but the common ones, in our opinion, are the fishhook variety (Fig. 34–33) and the right-angle turn (Fig. 34–34). A large diverticulum causes medial deviation of the ureter in most cases.

EFFECTS ON THE EJACULATORY DUCTS AND THE SEMINAL VESICLES

This subject is discussed in the chapter following and is not anticipated here. The usual characteristic of the ejaculatory ducts in benign prostatic hypertrophy is dilatation. Secondarily, the seminal vesicles are enlarged and dilated.

SILENT PROSTATISM

Silent prostatism is a well-defined entity of advanced bladder neck obstruction with moderate-to-severe injury to the bladder, ureters, and kidneys and few urinary complaints.[29, 30] It is often overlooked because such symptoms as abdominal discomfort, digestive disorders, symptoms of uremia, or coincidental diseases may direct attention away from the lower part of the urinary tract. Often the physician cannot palpate the distended bladder; the urine may be clear on urinalysis, and the prostate gland small on rectal examination. Some of these patients have progressed to severe uremia and huge dilatations of the ureters and kidneys without suspicion of prostatic obstruction (Fig. 34–35).

POSTPROSTATECTOMY ROENTGENOGRAMS

Figures 34–36 to 34–42 were taken post prostatectomy to demonstrate the normal prostatic cavity, incontinence, calculi, and patency of the ejaculatory ducts.

The female prostate (Fig. 34–43) is discussed under Normal Urethra.

CARCINOMA OF THE PROSTATE

Carcinoma of the prostate is one of the most common malignant conditions of males. Most authorities believe that it arises in the posterior lobe,[39, 41, 49, 51] although Kahler believes that it arises more commonly in the lateral lobes.[46] It metastasizes both by lymph and blood. Even in its earliest stages, the perineural spaces are found to be involved with tumor tissue. The most common sites of lymphatic spread are the obturator, hypogastric, and external iliac nodes. The osseous metastases (Fig. 34–44) result from the hematogenous route and in descending rate of occurrence are pelvic bones, lumbar spine, femurs, thoracic spine, and ribs. Spinal cord compression due to extradural metastases has been reported especially in the neurologic literature.[32, 33, 35, 36, 47, 56, 57] The most common sites for visceral metastases are the lungs, liver, and adrenal glands. Pulmonary metastases are pathologically lymphangitic, and pleural metastases are not uncommon.

Locally, prostatic carcinoma extends upward around the ejaculatory ducts, invading the perivesicular fascia and involving the seminal vesicles from without, usually affecting the medial portion of the gland first. It can spread into the lateral lobes of the prostate and sometimes directly through the capsule to the periprostatic system of lymphatics. The malignancy rarely extends beyond the membranous urethra and rarely invades the rectal mucosa, but may bulge into the rectum or produce an annular constriction. At times it has been known to invade the sigmoid (see Chapter 12). The urethra and the bladder mucosa are resistant to the growth. More than 95 per cent of prostatic malignancies are adenocarcinomas.[43, 46, 55] The remainder are transitional cell carcinomas, squamous cell carcinomas, and sarcomas. Most appear to be multifocal or extensive. Most adenocarcinomas arise from the tubuloalveolar glands, but ductal carcinomas do occur and appear to have a poor prognosis.

The incidence of histologic evidence of carcinoma of the prostate is high. Young found an incidence of 21 per cent in all cases of prostatic obstruction.[59] By the use of open perineal biopsy, Hudson found carcinoma in an incidence of 11.1 per cent in 686 older men with minimal or no prostatic symptoms.[44] In postmortem material, the incidence of carcinoma of the prostate has been reported by Rich at 14 per cent,[51] Moore at 16.8 per cent,[59] Gaynor at 21 per cent,[40] Baron and Angrist at 14.8 per cent for random sections and 46 per cent for multiple sections,[34] Vernet at 25 per cent,[42] Andrews at 16 per cent,[31] Starklint at 25.3 per cent,[53] Edwards and co-workers at 16.7 per cent,[38] and Franks at 38.7 per cent.[39]

GRADING OF PROSTATIC CARCINOMA

Grading of prostatic carcinoma has been reassessed against the background of patient survival.[49a] The four systems evaluated were the following:

Gleason system
Mostofi system
Gaeta system
Mayo Clinic system

In general, at present, grading systems do not reliably predict the lethal potential of a tumor or its responsiveness to treatment. However, poorly differentiated tumors generally have a greater likelihood of positive pelvic lymph nodes and probably of poor prognosis for the patient than do the better differentiated tumors.

STAGING OF PROSTATIC CARCINOMA

The following is the American system for staging of prostatic carcinoma (Fig. 34–45).

Stage A: Tumors are confined to the prostate and are neither suspected nor detected clinically; the diagnosis is made by histopathologic criteria from tissue obtained at operation or autopsy.

Stage A$_1$: Focal carcinoma involving only one lobe of the gland

Stage A$_2$: Multifocal or diffuse carcinoma

Stage B$_1$: The carcinoma is a distinct nodule less than 1.5 cm. in diameter confined within the capsule, limited to one lobe of the prostate, and with compressible prostatic tissue on two or three sides.

Stage B$_2$: Greater than 1.5 cm. in diameter or in more than one lobe

Stage C: Stage C carcinoma is a neoplasm that on digital rectal examination has extended beyond the confines of the prostatic capsule, usually into the seminal vesicles, but not to more distant sites. It may involve bladder neck or extend to the lateral side wall of the pelvis.

Patients with stages A, B, and C have normal radioisotopic bone scans and skeletal roentgenograms. Serum acid phosphatase levels are usually normal in stages A and B but may be elevated in stage C.

Stage D$_1$: Large tumors with invasion of local pelvic organs. Incidence of regional lymph node metastases may be as high as 100 per cent. Distal ureteral obstruction is common. Serum acid phosphatase levels may be elevated, but bone scans and skeletal roentgenograms are normal.

Stage D$_2$: Metastases to bone and areas outside the pelvis such as lung.

An elevated serum acid phosphatase level generally means that the lesion is beyond the prostate; however, approximately 22 per cent of patients with bone metastases have normal serum acid phosphatase levels.[54, 58] It would appear that improved methods for determining prostatic acid phosphatase, for example, solid-phase radioimmunoassay,[38a] would offer a more promising avenue for diagnosing prostatic carcinoma. Watson and Tang have summarized our knowledge of this subject.[57a]

The determination of bone marrow acid phosphatase levels and concomitant biopsy have been used as an additional modality for evaluating patients with carcinoma of prostate.[54] However, the usefulness of this modality is limited because of the incidence of false-positive results. Pontes and co-workers have summarized the subject of reliability of bone marrow acid phosphatase levels and concluded that it would be best to utilize all of the following methods[50a]—

Colorimetric assay
Immunochemical assays
    Counterimmunoelectrophoresis
    Radioimmunoassay

with emphasis on immunochemical methods. It

should be emphasized that, on digital examination, many so-called stage B tumors have metastases to lymph nodes and should be classified as stage D.[48]

Some authors have postulated *two* forms of prostatic carcinoma:

1. The obviously malignant and metastasizing form, which is the type just described.
2. The latent form. This type is potentially malignant and has the morphologic characteristics of the malignant type, but it remains localized to the prostate and clinically unrecognized.

Carcinoma and benign prostatic hypertrophy frequently are associated.[49, 60]

EFFECTS OF PROSTATIC CARCINOMA ON THE GENITOURINARY TRACT

The following descriptions apply only to carcinoma of the prostate. If benign prostatic hypertrophy is present along with the carcinoma, the findings of course are entirely different.

EFFECTS ON THE URETHRA

On cystourethrography (Figs. 34–46 to 34–49), the prostatic urethra is irregular and more likely not to be widened in the oblique view. The length of the supracollicular portion is less likely to be elongated in carcinoma. The saberlike shape of the prostatic urethra (with elongation, widening on oblique view, and a heavy curve) is much more characteristic of benign prostatic hypertrophy. A narrow posterior urethra in all views, with absence of angulation and presence of irregularity of the urethra and the floor of the bladder, is characteristic of carcinoma of the prostate. Edling stated that lateral displacement of the whole posterior urethra is suggestive of carcinoma of the prostate.[68]

EFFECTS ON THE BLADDER

The floor of the bladder may be pushed up in carcinoma of the prostate, exactly as it is in benign prostatic hypertrophy. However, the contour is usually more irregular in carcinoma (Fig. 34–50).

Increase in the size of the bladder, trabeculation, diverticula, and the like may occur in carcinoma of the prostate, but these are less common than in benign prostatic hypertrophy because the obstruction is of shorter duration.

EFFECTS ON THE KIDNEY AND THE URETER

Little has been written on the effects of carcinoma of the prostate on the upper urinary tract. Postmortem studies have been reported by Graves and Militzer[62] and Mintz and Smith.[64] Ganem in a clinical study found that the obstructed urinary tract in prostatic cancer gave a poor prognosis.[61] In his cases, 30 per cent had unilateral or bilateral hydronephrosis. The incidence and the degree of hydronephrosis were no different in the cases with metastases than in the cases without metastases. After adequate treatment, in 60 per cent of the cases the upper tracts deteriorated, and in 40 per cent they either remained the same, improved, or returned completely to normal. Aggressive treatment, including diversion, may prolong life.[60a, 63a]

Obstruction of the upper urinary tract may be caused by bladder neck obstruction in both benign prostatic hypertrophy and carcinoma; but in cases of carcinoma it may be produced by trigonal infiltration (Fig. 34–50) or obstruction of the ureters above the bladder by invasion of the fascia surrounding the seminal vesicles and secondarily involving the ureters (Fig. 34–51).

EFFECTS ON THE SEMINAL VESICLES AND THE EJACULATORY DUCTS

These effects (Fig. 34–52) are different from those produced by prostatic hypertrophy. (See the section on Seminal Vesicles in Chapter 35.) Carcinoma of the prostate causes the following:

1. Narrowing of the lumen of the ejaculatory ducts with decreased luminal dilatability and rigid and irregular contours
2. Decreased caliber of the median infiltrated portion of the seminal vesicles
3. Dilated lateral portions of the seminal vesicles
4. Depression of the vesiculo-ampullar junction (the junction between the ductus deferens and the excretory duct of the seminal vesicle)
5. Greater tendency of the contrast material entering the posterior urethra from the ejaculatory ducts to flow distally rather than back into the bladder, as in benign prostatic hypertrophy

SARCOMA OF THE PROSTATE

Sarcoma of the prostate can be classifed as follows:

Primary
Primary lymphoma
Fibrosarcoma
Collusion tumor—carcinoma plus sarcoma
Myosarcoma: embryonal rhabdomyosarcoma, rhabdomyosarcoma, and leiomyosarcoma

Malignant schwannoma
Unclassified (undifferentiated tumors)
Secondary
Usually lymphoma

They represent 0.1 to 0.2 per cent of malignant tumors of the prostate and are present essentially in the age groups of 0 to 10 years and 40 to 70 years, although a few in the teens and thirties have been reported.

Histologically, several reports have indicated the similarity to either benign or malignant breast fibroadenomatous tumors.[79, 82]

The myosarcomas are the most prominent group. The prognosis is especially poor with rhabdomyosarcoma.

Locally, sarcoma of the prostate tends to invade the bladder, rectum, and os pubis, metastasizing to brain, lungs, liver, and bones (osteoclastic).

Diagnosis. Sarcoma of the prostate is difficult to differentiate from benign prostatic hypertrophy, carcinoma, and abscess. In children, abscess is the essential differential diagnosis.

Radiographic Findings. (Figs. 34–53, 34–54) There is a large filling defect in the base of the bladder representing prostatic enlargement, but often there is actual invasion of the bladder; the prostatic urethra is elongated and compressed laterally.

PROSTATIC CALCULI

True or endogenous prostatic calculi develop in the acini and the ducts of the prostate gland and are to be differentiated from urinary calculi lodged in the prostatic urethra (migrant) and from exogenous calculi that form in preexisting abscess cavities in the prostate gland. They are common in the fifth decade[110] or the sixth to the seventh decades, as reported by Lund and Cordonnier,[106] and are extremely rare in children (Fig. 34–55). Thompson believed that corpora amylacea were the precursors of prostatic calculi.[109] The relationship of infection to prostatic calculi is not clear, whether absent,[98, 107] an important association,[97, 101] or secondary.[103, 104]

The relationship of prostatic calculi to various other affections of the prostate varies with the observer. Gentile reported that prostatic calculi were associated more commonly with benign prostatic hypertrophy and prostatitis than with prostatitis alone,[97] whereas Young[110] found them more frequently with chronic prostatitis than benign prostatic hypertrophy. Gentile[97] and Lund and Cordon-

nier[106] reported the infrequent association of calculi and prostatic carcinoma; yet Cristol and Emmett[95] found an incidence of 6.3 per cent of prostatic calculi in the presence of carcinoma of the prostate.

The occurrence of upper tract calculi and prostatic calculi has been studied from two viewpoints. Joly found 34 cases of prostatic calculi in 636 cases of urinary calculi (an instance of 5.3 per cent).[100] Fox reported 484 cases of prostatic calculi and found associated calculi in upper urinary tract in 18 per cent.[96] Interestingly, those cases with no infection and no prostatic enlargement were in the younger age group, and the younger the patient with prostatic calculi, the greater the chance of having upper urinary tract calculi.

Prostatic calculi usually are multiple, varying in size from 1 mm. to 3 to 4 cm. Moore and Hanzel found calcium phosphate of undetermined type to be the most common constituent of prostatic calculi.[107] Huggins and Bear reported apatite as the most common type of prostatic calculus.[99] The calculi are found in the ducts and the acini of the prostate and occasionally in the stroma, when they have sloughed through the epithelium. The calculi lie outside the adenomatous portion of the gland and, on removal of the adenoma, may adhere to it.

Roentgenologic Findings. These may be summarized as follows:

1. Diffuse shadows seen throughout the gland. The calculi are usually rather small.
   Ring type. The calculi surround a clear central urethra (Fig. 34–58).
   Horseshoe type. The stones are present on both sides and dorsally, but there is a clear space anteriorly (Fig. 34–57).
2. Large solitary calculus
3. Multiple, but localized on both sides of the prostate gland with a clear space anteriorly and posteriorly (Fig. 34–56)
4. Large multiple calculi completely replacing the prostate (Figs. 34–59, 34–60)
5. Few discrete small calculi on either side (Fig. 34–61)

ACUTE PROSTATITIS

Acute prostatitis (Fig. 34–63) is an acute inflammation of the prostate gland caused by the gonococcus, staphylococcus, streptococcus, and E. coli bacilli, and possibly viruses.[112] E. coli and Staphylococcus are the predominant organisms. The symptoms and signs include chills, fever, low back and perineal pain, decreased size and force of urinary stream, dysuria, urgency, frequency, retention of urine, and a swollen, tender prostate gland. Formerly very common, it has become rare because of adequate treatment. The infection usually reaches the prostate from the urethra.

The radiographic findings of acute prostatitis are narrowing, elongation, and straightening of the prostatic urethra due to swelling of the prostate gland. The prostatic urethra may be so narrowed that it will give only a threadlike appearance of contrast medium.

PROSTATIC ABSCESS

Prostatic abscess (Figs. 34–64, 34–65) is a localized prostatic suppuration that usually begins in one lateral lobe and may spread to the other. The diagnosis is made clinically on the basis of the history, urinary obstruction of recent onset, chills, fever, and perineal pain. In recent years the widespread use of antibiotics has changed the clinical picture somewhat so that fever is unusual or of mild character; pain occurs in only one out of three cases, acute retention in one out of three cases, and sterile urine may be present in half of the cases.[136] The prostate may be enlarged in one lateral lobe, but frequently there is symmetric enlargement. There may or may not be tenderness, and often there are no distinctly palpable characteristics, although fluctuation may be present.[132]

The majority of the nonmetastatic cases are the result of urinary tract infection with *E. coli* and *Proteus*[136] as the predominant organisms often associated with bladder neck obstruction.[136] The gonococcus was formerly the most common agent. Prostatic abscess has been reported with systemic infections[116, 119, 125, 129] such as typhoid fever, influenza, measles, mumps, pneumonia, or anthrax, but the usual organism is *Staphylococcus aureus*,[113, 122, 125, 127, 128, 133, 136] metastatic from skin infection. Prostatic abscess is rare in infants and children[120, 121, 123, 134] and is the result of metastatic infection in over half of the cases. Prostatic abscesses may rupture into the urethra,[115, 117, 118, 124, 131, 136] rectum,[115, 117, 136] perineum,[117, 136] and peritoneum.[130, 132] Fifty per cent of cases of prostatic abscess in adults have been reported to have diabetes mellitus.[131, 136]

In infants and children, prostatic abscesses can be confused with sarcoma clinically, palpably, and on urethrography. In adults, it may be impossible to differentiate from benign prostatic hypertrophy. On urethrography,[111, 119, 128, 134, 135] there is elongation of the prostatic urethra with narrowing on the AP view and widening in the oblique position. Occasionally, anterior tilting is observed but is probably the result of previous bladder neck or middle lobe changes. Lateral deviation of prostatic urethra may occur in unilateral cases (Fig. 34–64).

An accurate diagnosis can be made only when the abscess has opened into the urethra, allowing contrast material to enter the cavity. In this instance, the examiner sees prostatic cavitation, which can vary in size from several millimeters to several centimeters, indicating that the parenchyma has been destroyed and replaced by liquefaction. Most of these cavities are fairly smooth, but occasionally they may be irregular in outline.

CHRONIC PROSTATITIS

Chronic prostatitis (Figs. 34–66, 34–67), or prostatoseminal vasiculitis, is a common clinical entity affecting approximately 35 per cent of men over 35 years of age. The symptoms and signs include decreased potentia, premature ejaculation, low backache, perineal or scrotal pain, urethral discharge, frequency, burning on urination, hematospermia, nocturnal emissions, boggy prostate, often a smaller prostate than normal, occasionally indurated prostate, increased leukocytes (over 10 per high-power field), and numerous oval fat bodies in the prostatic secretion.

Young found 40 per cent of smears and 70 per cent of cultures of the prostatic fluid positive for organisms.[162] Hinman found 57 per cent of the cultures sterile. Delzell and Lowsley in 38 patients with chronic prostatis found the staphylococcus to be the most common organism,[145] followed by streptococcus and *E. coli*. Cummings and Chittenden,[144] Ritter and Lippow,[157] and Gardner[146] found approximately the same organisms. O'Shaughnessy, Parrino, and White[156] were able to obtain positive cultures from prostate fluid obtained endoscopically in only 3 of 68 men considered to have the disease. Based on a study of 760 men, these authors believe that the finding of pus cells in the prostatic fluid is not sufficient evidence to establish the diagnosis of prostatitis. Calams, who studied the vesicles in 161 autopsies, found that histopathologic evidence of such a disease is observed only rarely.[143] Robbins believes that if more stringent criteria for the histopathologic diagnosis of chronic prostatitis were observed, the diagnosis would be made less frequently.[158] Barnes,[140] Beilin,[141] and Smith[160] all considered noninfective congestion of the prostate as the main change in this disease, but predisposing to infection. Leader emphasizes that the disease is really a functional derangement of the prostate and seminal vesicles due to a failure of these structures to empty themselves of their secretions.[148] He prefers the term vesiculoprostatostasis. Further studies have clarified the problem somewhat.[150, 151, 159] There are two similar but distinct entities[150, 151, 161].

1. Chronic prostatitis — caused by aerobic bacteria and showing an inflammatory reaction in the prostate, with pus cells in the secretion.
2. Prostatosis — having a similar inflammatory tissue reaction[150] with pus cells in the secretion but absent positive cultures on biopsy,[155] prostatic secretion,[150] and urine studies.[150] The cause of the latter is obscure. Nielsen and Vestergaard's studies[155] indicate absence of aerobic bacteria, anaerobic bacteria, mycoplasmas, viruses, or fungi. It may be explained by an autoimmune disease; the presence of organ-specific antigens in prostatic tissue and prostatic secretion has been demonstrated.[137, 140]

Roentgenographic Findings. On roentgenograms, one sees narrowing and straightening of the prostatic urethra. Occasionally, filling of the dilated prostatic ducts and the acini is seen. Only a single duct may be visualized unilaterally, but usually many ducts are seen bilaterally (Figs. 34–66, 34–67).

GRANULOMATOUS PROSTATITIS

Granulomatous prostatitis is an inflammation of the prostate gland, containing granulomatous tissue.
There are two varieties:

1. Specific — prostatic granulomas produced by known etiologic agents, such as *M. tuberculosis, T. pallidum*,[198] various fungi, metazoa, *Brucella abortus*,[180] schistosomiasis, malacoplakia.[175, 178]
2. Nonspecific — the result of the escape of prostatic contents (secretions, seminal plasma, corpora amylacea, spermatozoa) and bacterial products or urine into prostatic tissue, secondary to obstruction produced by benign prostatic hypertrophy or inflammation, or disruption of ducts and acini by prostatic surgery. The incidence in operative specimens varies from 4.44 per cent to 3.3 per cent. There are two varieties[200]:

    Noneosinophilic (Figs. 34–68, 34–68a, 34–68b)
    Simple (without fibrinoid necrosis)

With fibrinoid necrosis only
With fibrinoid necrosis and vasculitis
Eosinophilic (Fig. 34–69)
    Simple (without fibrinoid necrosis)
    With fibrinoid necrosis only
    With fibrinoid necrosis and vasculitis

Clinically, the nonspecific variety has the usual symptoms of prostatism, associated with an enlarged prostate, but it is often characterized by an accelerated course. All cases of nonspecific granulomatous prostatitis have been reported to have prostatic hypertrophy, but rectal examination may give the impression of carcinoma (28.5 per cent). According to Towfighi, histologically, the granulomas vary from a fibrohistiocytic proliferation, with a mild mononuclear cell infiltrate and a few multinucleated giant cells, to typical granulomas with epitheloid cells and a moderate number of giant multinucleated cells.[200] The eosinophilic variety contains marked eosinophilic infiltrates. The granulomas may present as a small focus in a benign prostatic hypertrophy or as diffuse displacement of prostatic tissue. Previous prostatic surgery, especially transurethral resection, seems to be the most prominent causative factor of nonspecific granulomatous prostatitis, whether eosinophilic or not. The time interval following operation for development of a granulomatous lesion is 2 to 6 weeks in the eosinophilic variety and over 6 months in the noneosinophilic variety.[200] Clinically, 28 per cent of eosinophilic granulomatous prostatitis cases have peripheral eosinophilia, and associated allergies such as asthma or mucocutaneous lesions are frequently present, especially in the cases with fibrinoid necrosis. Drug allergy may be an important etiologic factor.[185]

The lesion can secondarily involve the bladder. Differentiation from eosinophilic cystitis may be difficult; in the latter, however, there are usually no real granulomatous masses in the bladder. On palpation the lesion may be confused with carcinoma of the prostate.[168, 181] A rapid clinical course is characteristic and might give a clue to the diagnosis. Melicow's patient developed an enlarged prostate within a year (Fig. 34–69).[185]

Roentgenologic Findings. There is elongation of the prostatic urethra especially in the inframontane portion (Figs. 34–68, 34–68a, 34–68b). There is narrowing in the anteroposterior view and some widening in the oblique view. The elongation of the inframontane portion differentiates it from benign prostatic hypertrophy and the widening on the oblique view differentiates it from carcinoma of the prostate. However, when benign prostatic hypertrophy is associated with granulomatous prostatitis, the cystourethrogram can become extremely confusing.

TUBERCULOSIS OF THE PROSTATE GLAND

Tuberculosis of the prostate (Figs. 34–71 to 34–74) is almost always secondary to tuberculosis elsewhere in the body and usually is associated with tuberculous infection of the urinary tract.[208, 209, 210] The infection most likely is from the kidney by way of the descending route. It is probably the original area of infection of the genital tract,[208, 209, 210] although the epididymis and the seminal vesicles have been championed as the primary site.[205, 211] Pathologically, tubercles form just beneath the mucosa and spread throughout the lateral lobe. Abscess formation follows with caseation, cavitation, and fibrosis. Rupture may occur in the periprostatic space, the urethra, or even the rectum. Occasionally fistulas form in the perineum. Lattimer believes there is a characteristic cystoscopic appearance of the prostatic urethra in tuberculosis (dilatation, trabeculated floor, and "golf-hole" prostatic ducts).[206]

Roentgenologic Findings. May has described clearly the roentgenographic diagnosis in tuberculosis of the prostate (Fig. 34–74).[207] The following descriptions are similar to his, but with modifications.

SCOUT FILM.   There may be calcification in the prostatic gland indistinguishable from ordinary calculi.

CYSTOURETHROGRAPHY.   In early cases of tuberculosis the roentgenologic appearance of the prostate gland is similar to that of nonspecific prostatitis. There is filling of the prostatic ducts without evidence of cavitation.

The ducts may be greatly dilated, usually more than in chronic prostatitis.

There can be varying degrees of destruction of prostatic parenchyma, with sloughing, producing irregular cavitation.

Later, the entire prostate seems to be occupied by a smooth-walled cavity (Figs. 34–71 to 34–74).

PROSTATIC CYSTS

Prostatic cysts are either congenital or acquired. Congenital prostatic cysts are rare and usually are observed in middle-aged adults. They are caused by failure of communication between the wolffian

ducts and vesicourethral anlage. Dees in 1947 reported a case in which there was absence of the right kidney with only a rudimentary right ureter.[212] It is possible that this case, however, was really a cyst of the seminal vesicle. (Roberts reported a somewhat similar case.[219] The cases of Huggins[214] and Way and Popper[220] should not be considered to be in this category.) Roentgenographically, there is nothing characteristic of congenital prostatic cysts unless contrast material has been injected directly into them (Fig. 34–75).

Acquired prostatic cysts are the result of inflammation, trauma, or new growths. The most common type is the retention cyst. This is an acinus dilated secondary to duct obstruction, usually caused by inflammation.

Retention cysts usually occur in middle age, rarely causing symptoms unless they are large enough to project into the posterior urethra or the bladder neck, in which cases they can give urinary symptoms, even complete retention.

Acquired cysts are classified as follows:

1. Retention cysts
2. As part of a benign neoplasm (cystic adenoma)[215]
3. As part of benign prostatic hypertrophy (often multiple) and as part of a degenerating carcinoma

They are usually found at necropsy but may be discovered on prostatectomy or diagnosed clinically.[213] Usually they are unilocular, but a multilocular variety has been reported.[217] Bilharzial and echinococcal cysts are extremely rare.

Roentgenologic Findings. Cysts of the prostate usually are diagnosed by cystoscopy or rectal palpation (usually one-sided). They rarely are visualized on cystourethrography. If they are large enough, they may produce changes in the prostatic urethra (Fig. 34–76).[218] Cystlike structures occasionally are visualized on cystourethrography when they connect with the urethra, but these are more likely to be abscesses that have ruptured. Deviation of the ejaculatory duct[218] may be of some value in diagnosis (Figs. 34–77, 34–78). Direct injection confirms the existence of a cyst (Fig. 34–75).

LEUKEMIC INFILTRATION OF THE PROSTATE

Leukemic infiltration of the prostate is rare. Most of the cases are examples of chronic lymphatic leukemia,[221] although acute monocytic leukemia has been reported.[225, 229, 233] There seems to be no difference in the clinical findings and response to surgery between patients with leukemic infiltration of the prostate and benign prostatic hyperplasia. Meyer stated there were two types of leukemic infiltration of the prostate: a symptomless variety with no obstructive features, usually observed in younger patients; and an obstructive variety occurring in older men in which the leukemic infiltration is associated with benign prostatic hyperplasia.[231] The latter appears to be the cause of the obstructive symptoms rather than leukemic infiltration. The course of the prostatectomy is apparently not affected by the infiltration.

The occurrence of leukemic infiltration of the prostate produces no specific symptom complex or characteristic physical findings. It is purely a histologic finding. The obstructive symptoms are treated on their merit, and the usual methods of treatment are utilized.

AMYLOID OF THE PROSTATE

Amyloid of the prostate has rarely been reported. Wilson and co-workers have emphasized the frequency of the finding.[235] A selected group of patients expected to have a high percentage of amyloidosis underwent transrectal needle biopsy of the prostate. Amyloid deposits in the prostate were found in 33 per cent of paraplegics, 38 per cent of myelomatous patients, and 100 per cent of the group with primary amyloidosis. In an unselected group studied similarly, 10 per cent revealed amyloid in the prostate. Interestingly, the amyloid was frequently associated with adenocarcinoma of the prostate.

ANGIOGRAPHY OF THE PROSTATE

Angiography of the prostate has been used to locate specific bleeding sites and selectively occlude the bleeding vessels.[238]

Severe hemorrhage following prostatic surgery is unusual. Usually irrigations, suprapubic drainage, or cystostomy with clot removal and ligation of bleeding sites is adequate therapy. Occasionally more radical steps may be required, such as ligation of the hypogastric arteries, radical prostatectomy, or open packing of the bladder, but these involve prolonged hospitalization and increased risk.[236, 237]

Mitchell and co-workers have emphasized the value of angiography.[238] They perform hypogastric arterial studies to evaluate prostatic bleeding. Unilateral angiography and embolization may be inadequate because of extensive collateral blood supply. They used either autologous clot or Gelfoam for the bilateral hypogastric embolization (Figs. 34–79, 34–80) and obtained excellent results. This method is offered as an alternative nonoperative procedure in the management of persistent, severe postoperative prostatic bleeding.

PROSTATIC INFARCTION

Infarction of the prostate is a rather frequent finding in middle-aged and elderly men.

The morphologic appearance varies with the age of the infarct.[245] In the acute stage, there is coagulation necrosis of both stromal and glandular elements. During the first 24 to 48 hours, leukocytic infiltrations are minimal, but they increase progressively during the following days. About the fourth day, parenchymal necrosis, stromal edema, and neutrophilic infiltration are at their maximum. Focal parenchymal hemorrhage and squamous glandular metaplasia peripheral to the infarct may be present. During the third to sixth weeks, resolution and organization take place. At completion of the reparative stage, squamous metaplasia and occasional lymphocytes may be the only stigmata in infarcted sites.

Infarction is most frequently associated with prostatic hypertrophy and is apparently closely related to urinary retention.[239, 241, 242, 243] Baird, McKay, and Kimmelstiel[240] questioned these findings, however. Spiro and co-workers compared two groups[245]: one, with large prostate and acute urinary retention, and the other with prostatic hyperplasia without urinary retention. In the first group, 85 per cent showed infarcts, in the latter 3 per cent, thus emphasizing the relationship of infarct to acute urinary retention.

The causes of infarction are trauma (including instrumentation), infection, stasis, thrombosis, atherosclerosis, embolism, and benign prostatic hypertrophy.

The infarct probably produces enlargement of the gland secondary to edema, but it may produce a neurogenic disturbance secondary to anoxia.[245]

Clinically, an infarct may be palpable rectally as a firm-to-hard nodule and histologically may be similar to carcinoma.[244]

ULTRASONOGRAPHY AND COMPUTED TOMOGRAPHY OF THE PROSTATE

Ultrasonographic images of the prostate have been obtained by transrectal,[249, 251, 284] transurethral,[247] and suprapubic routes (Figs. 34–81, 34–82).[246, 250, 252]

Computed tomography demonstrates involvement of seminal vesicles and bladder in cases of carcinoma of the prostate and is especially excellent for demonstrating lymph node enlargement. However, it appears to be inferior to ultrasonography in demonstrating changes in the prostate proper, whether carcinoma, infection, or hypertrophied from benign disease.

THE NORMAL GLAND

ULTRASONOGRAPHY

The gray-scale appearance is as follows (Fig. 34–81A,B): The glandular elements have a low-level gray tone. The periurethral glands are seen as an echogenic region around the urethra in the central portion of the converging lobes. The individual lobes are usually not visualized. The seminal vesicles are seen as tubular projections from the cephalolateral aspect of the prostate gland.

COMPUTED TOMOGRAPHY

The normal prostate has a uniform scan density (Fig. 34–81C,D). The urethra is visible because of a contrast-filled catheter. The periurethral glands and individual lobes are not recognized as discrete structures. Morphologic information concerning the seminal vesicles and bladder can be obtained.

BENIGN PROSTATIC HYPERTROPHY

ULTRASONOGRAPHY

With gray-scale instrumentation, the periurethral glands have a low-level echogenicity distinct from a surgical capsule but more echogenic than the adenomatous growth (Figs. 34–82, 34–84A,B). The gland appears enlarged.

COMPUTED TOMOGRAPHY

The gland is enlarged and has a homogeneous density. The surgical capsule cannot be recognized (Fig. 34–82a).

PROSTATITIS

ULTRASONOGRAPHY

Gray-scale criteria for acute prostatitis (Figs. 34–83, 34–84A,B) are an enlarged gland, decreased echogenicity, and increased through transmission of sound. In chronic prostatitis, the finding of calcification aids in the diagnosis (Fig. 34–85A).

COMPUTED TOMOGRAPHY

There are no morphologic or density changes to assist in diagnosing acute (Figs. 34–82A, 34–84C) or chronic prostatitis. The finding of calcification may be significant (Fig. 34–85B).

CARCINOMA

ULTRASONOGRAPHY

On an ultrasonogram, the carcinomatous area will have increased echo patterns (Fig. 34–86) and decreased sound transmission (Fig. 34–87B) and possibly loss of a discrete surgical capsule. Invasion of seminal vesicles and lymph nodes can be visualized.

COMPUTED TOMOGRAPHY

Computed tomography reveals no visual density differences (Fig. 34–87C,D) but visualizes loss of discreteness of seminal vesicles when invaded (Fig. 34–88). Bladder involvement can also be identified (Fig. 34–89). It is also extremely helpful in demonstrating metastatic nodes (Fig. 34–90).

CHAPTER 34, ILLUSTRATIONS

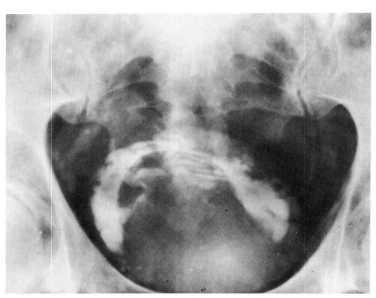

FIG. 34-1. Large prostate producing a huge filling defect in the bladder on the intravenous urogram. The bladder is trabeculated markedly with cellules and saccules. Small amount of residual urine.

FIG. 34-2. Irregular filling defect in an excretory cystogram, due to benign prostatic hypertrophy. (A) Excretory cystogram. (B) Air cystogram. *Arrows* point to the large subcervical lobe with an extra pedunculated lobe.

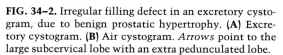

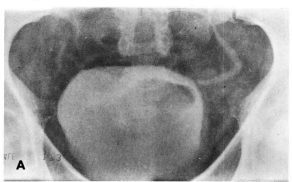

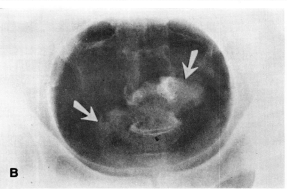

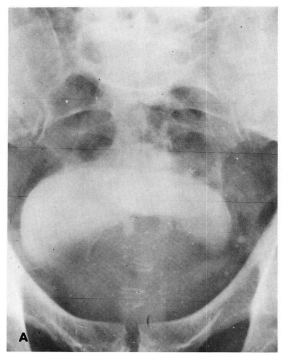

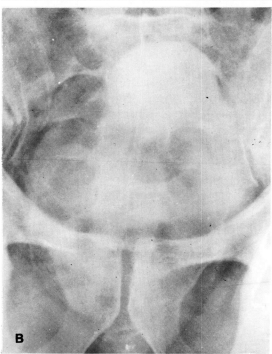

FIG. 34-3. Benign prostatic hypertrophy producing a large filling defect in the bladder on excretory cystogram. (A) Supine view. Floor of bladder is pushed upward by the enlarged prostate. (B) Prone view. Large filling defect in the floor of the bladder, with the bladder extending more cephalically as the contrast medium settles in the anterior portion of the bladder.

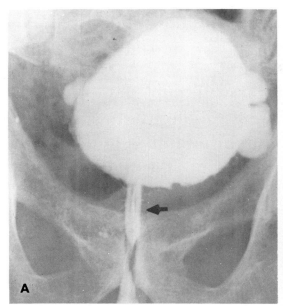

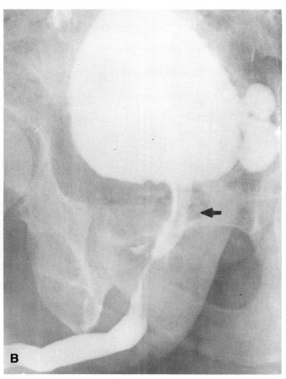

FIG. 34–4. Lateral lobe prostatic enlargement caused by 70-g. prostate. Injecting cystourethrogram. **(A)** AP view. *Arrow* points to prostatic urethra, which is not narrowed. Diverticula of the bladder are present. **(B)** Right oblique view. Slightly widened prostatic urethra (*arrow*). The slightly increased anterior concavity is due to lateral lobe enlargement.

FIG. 34–5. Large lateral lobes with pedunculated nodules in benign prostatic hypertrophy. Injecting cystourethrogram. **(A)** AP view. Large defect in bladder with an indentation between pedunculated nodules. **(B)** Right oblique view. Elongated prostatic urethra.

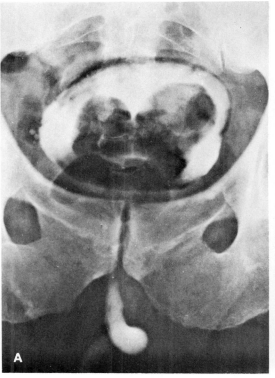

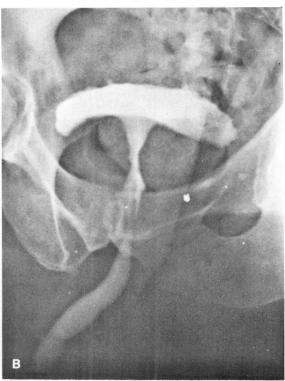

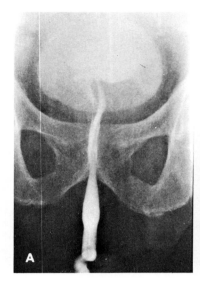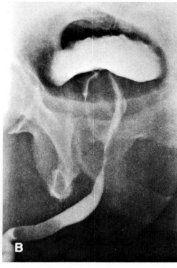

FIG. 34–6. Lateral lobe enlargement of prostate. Injecting cystourethrogram. **(A)** AP view. Elongated prostatic urethra. Note the column of contrast medium extending into the bladder, an indication of elongation of the urethra. **(B)** Oblique view. Air cystogram followed by injection of contrast material. Elongated prostatic urethra. The defect is due to a touching of the lateral prostatic lobes. The floor of the bladder neck was elevated slightly, but there was no distinct median lobe.

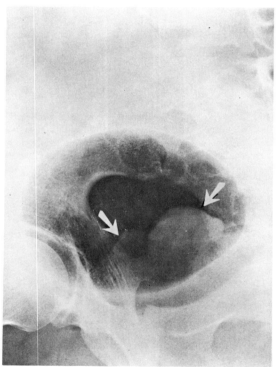

FIG. 34–7. Benign prostatic hypertrophy. Air cystogram. *Arrows* point to the lateral lobes projecting into the bladder.

FIG. 34–8. Lateral lobe enlargement in benign prostatic hypertrophy. Injecting cystourethrogram after air cystogram. Right oblique view. There is a markedly elongated prostatic urethra with a huge filling defect in the base of the bladder due to enlarged lateral lobes.

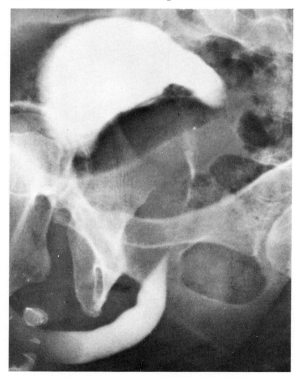

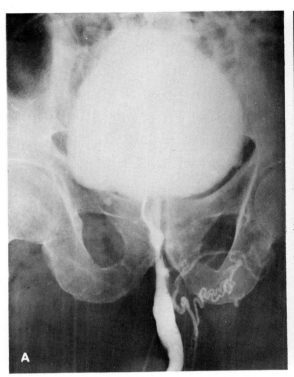

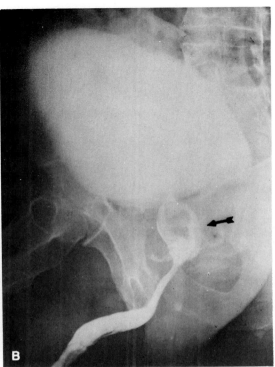

FIG. 34–9. Lateral lobe enlargement in benign prostatic hypertrophy. Injecting cystourethrogram. **(A)** AP view. The prostatic urethra is not elongated. There is urethro-cavernous reflux. **(B)** Oblique view. Widened prostatic urethra (*arrow*). This is called "spreading." The filling defect is due to touching of the lateral lobes, preventing an even distribution of contrast material. The lateral lobes have grown essentially intraurethral.

FIG. 34–10. Posterior commissural in benign prostatic hypertrophy. Large bladder having a capacity of 2200 ml. **(A)** AP view showing huge contour of a trabeculated bladder. Cystometric reading showed the bladder to be atonic. **(B)** Oblique view. Injecting cystourethrogram. Anterior tilting (*arrow*) of proximal urethra due to enlarged posterior commissural. Small lateral lobes.

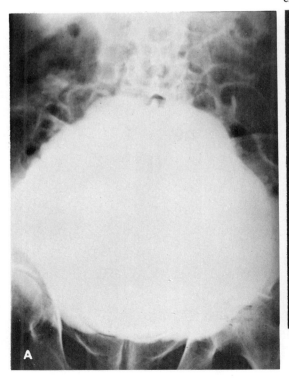

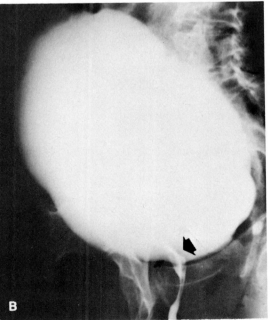

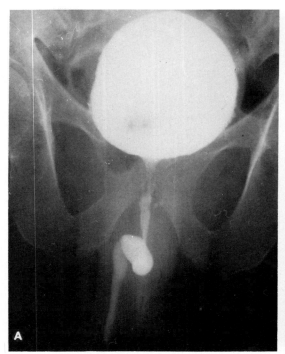

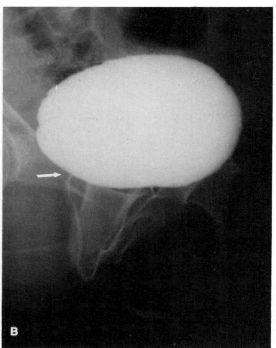

FIG. 34-11. Posterior commissural hypertrophy. Voiding cystourethrogram. **(A)** AP view. Normal-appearing urethra. **(B)** Left oblique view. *Arrow* points to anterior tilting at bladder neck representing posterior commissural hypertrophy.

FIG. 34–12. Large atonic bladder in benign prostatic hypertrophy. Capacity, 1800 ml., secondary to posterior commissural hypertrophy and possibly a neurogenic element. Patient was treated for syphilis 40 years previously. Spinal fluid equivocal. **(A)** Frontal view. Large irregular bladder. Notice the bismuth present in the buttocks. **(B)** Right oblique view. *Arrow* points to the anterior tilting of the proximal prostatic urethra. No enlarged lateral lobes present. Injecting cystourethrogram.

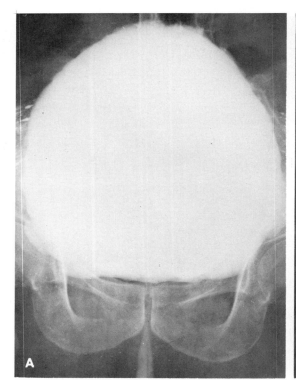

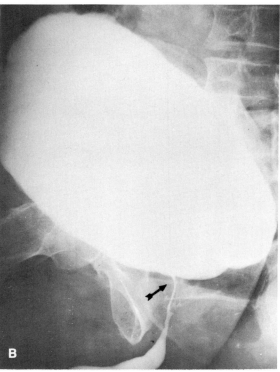

FIG. 34–13. Benign prostatic hypertrophy. Lateral lobe enlargement mainly with slight posterior commissural hypertrophy. **(A)** AP view. *Arrow* points to prostatic urethra, which is not narrowed. **(B)** Oblique view. Widened prostatic urethra *(arrow)*. The anterior tilting is due to mild posterior commissural hypertrophy.

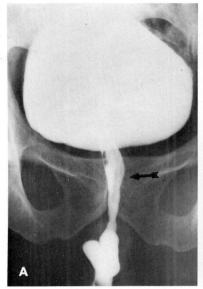
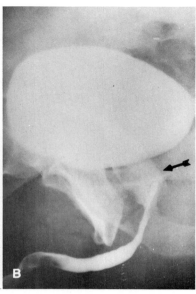

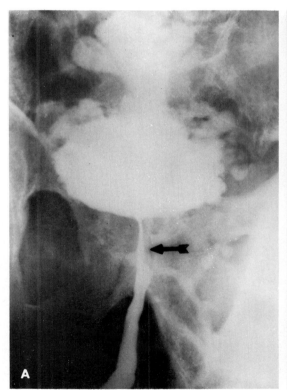
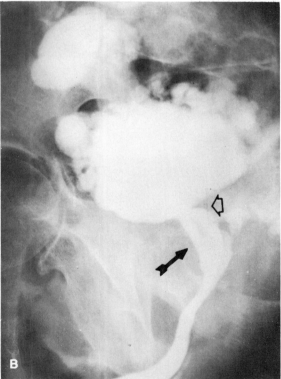

FIG. 34–14. Lateral and posterior commissural hypertrophy in benign prostatic hypertrophy. Injecting cystourethrogram. **(A)** AP view. *Arrow* points to elongated prostatic urethra. Bladder is irregular and trabeculated with cellules, saccules and diverticula. **(B)** Right oblique view. *Large arrow* points to widened, curved prostatic urethra. The anterior deviation at the bladder neck is due to posterior commissural hypertrophy *(open arrow)*.

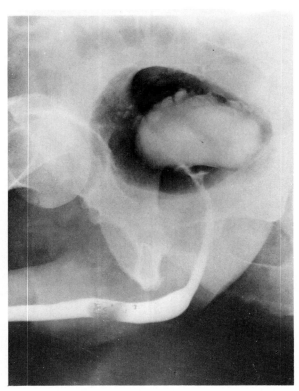

FIG. 34–15. Lateral and posterior commissural hypertrophy. Air cystogram with injecting cystourethrogram. Right oblique view. There is an elongated posterior urethra (lateral lobe enlargement) with some anterior tilting at the bladder neck (due to median lobe enlargement) (Post. Commissure).

FIG. 34–16. Lateral and posterior commissural hypertrophy. (A) Right oblique view. Injecting cystourethrogram. Elongated posterior urethra, which is due to lateral lobe enlargement, and there is some anterior tilting of the bladder neck due to median lobe enlargement. (B) Air cystogram with injecting cystourethrogram confirms the diagnosis.

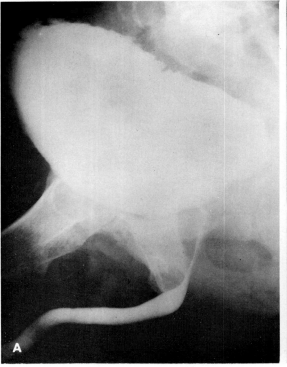

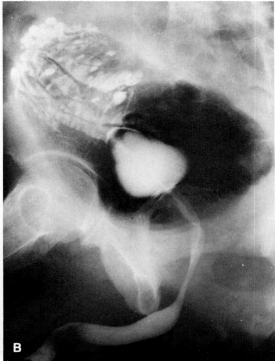

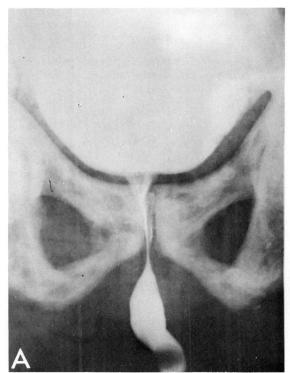

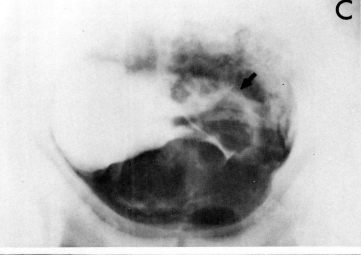

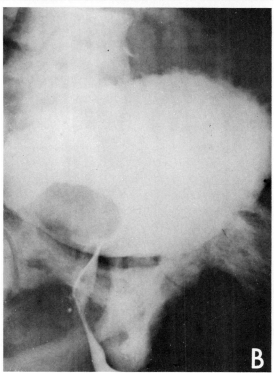

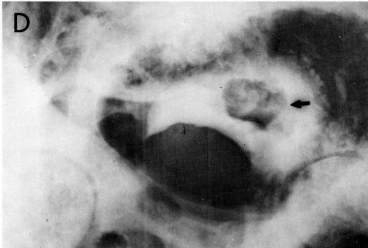

FIG. 34–17. Hypertrophied subcervical lobe with a pedunculated nodule in benign prostatic hypertrophy. Severe Paget's disease. **(A)** Injecting cystourethrogram. AP view. Y-effect seen at bladder neck. The large lobe is obscured by contrast medium. **(B)** Left oblique view. Injecting cystourethrogram. Anterior tilting of the prostatic urethra due to a large subcervical lobe. **(C)** Air cystogram with contrast medium. AP view. Large defect at floor due to a subcervical lobe. *Arrow* points to pedunculated nodule, arising from the subcervical lobe. **(D)** Left oblique view with air cystogram and contrast. Large rounded defect on floor of bladder represents the subcervical lobe. *Arrow* points to the pedunculated nodule.

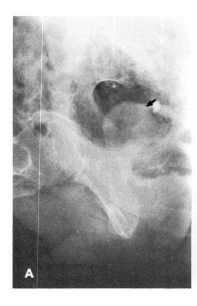
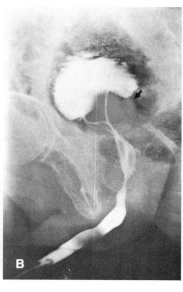

FIG. 34–18. Subcervical lobe in benign prostatic hypertrohy. **(A)** Right oblique view. Air cystogram. *Arrow* points to large subcervical lobe. **(B)** Contrast medium injected after air cystogram. There is an elongated prostatic urethra, indicating some lateral lobe enlargement. The Y-effect is due to subcervical lobe enlargement.

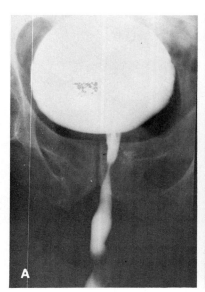
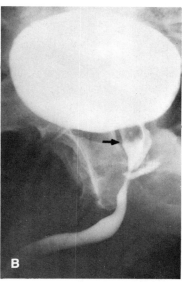

FIG. 34–19. Large subcervical lobe enlargement with slight lateral lobe enlargement in benign prostatic hypertrophy. Injecting cystourethrogram. **(A)** AP view. Essentially normal. **(B)** Right oblique view. *Arrow* points to defect at bladder neck, due to a ball valve type of subcervical lobe. Widening of prostatic urethra due to lateral lobe enlargement.

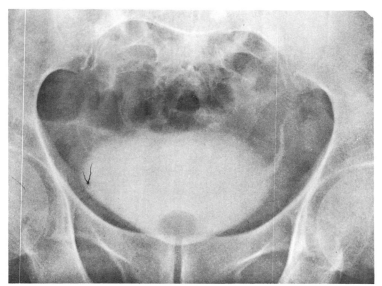

FIG. 34–20. Subcervical lobe in benign prostatic hypertrophy. The rounded defect on the floor of the bladder is due to subcervical lobe enlargement and easily could be confused with a Foley bag.

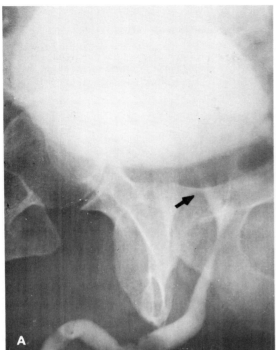

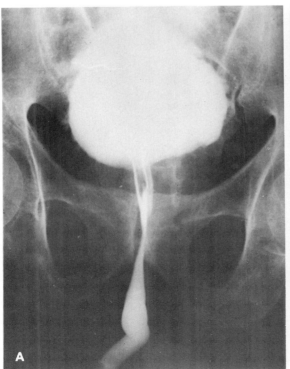

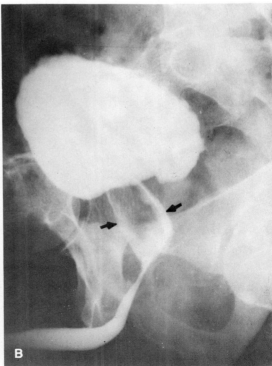

FIG. 34–21. Lateral and subcervical lobe prostatic enlargement. **(A)** Injecting cystourethrogram. Right oblique view. The defect in the floor of the bladder can be visualized. *Arrow* points to the elongated supracollicular portion of the prostatic urethra. Notice the Y-effect. **(B)** Air cystogram followed by injection of contrast material. Right oblique view. The elongated supracollicular urethra with some widening is due to lateral lobe enlargement. The slight anterior tilting is due to subcervical lobe enlargement.

FIG. 34–22. Lateral and subcervical prostatic enlargement. Injecting cystourethrogram **(A)** AP view. Elevated trabecular bladder. **(B)** Right oblique view. *Arrows* point to a widened prostatic urethra with a large filling defect, due to subcervical lobe enlargement of the bladder neck and touching of the lateral lobes more distally.

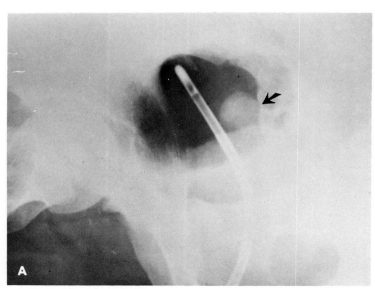

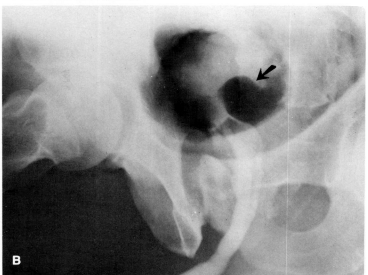

FIG. 34–23. Large lateral and subcervical lobe prostatic hypertrophy. **(A)** Oblique view. Air cystogram. *Arrow* points to large subcervical lobe. **(B)** Air cystogram and injection of contrast medium. Elongated, widened, curved prostatic urethra due to large lateral lobes. The rounded indentation producing anterior tilting is due to subcervical lobe enlargement (*arrow*).

FIG. 34–24. Benign prostatic hypertrophy. Right oblique view. Air cystogram with injecting cystourethrogram. Elongated posterior urethra indicating lateral lobe enlargement. The Y-effect at the bladder neck is due to subcervical lobe.

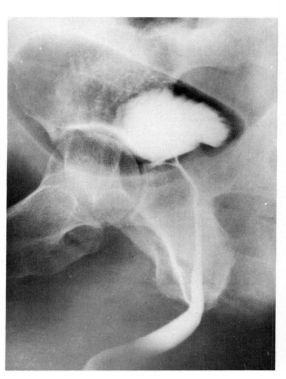

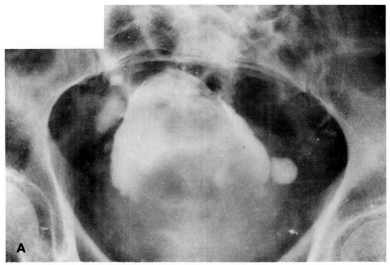

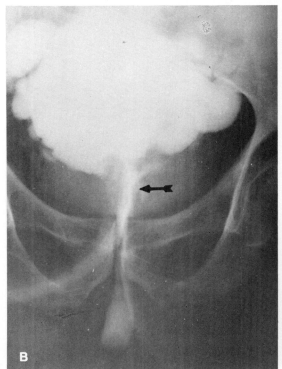

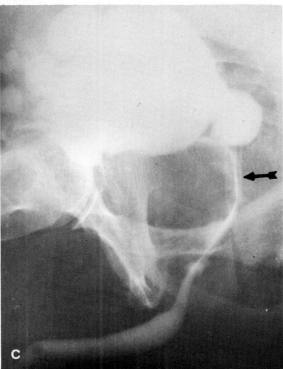

FIG. 34–25. Benign prostatic hypertrophy. Large prostate, 195 g. (A) Excretory cystogram. Huge filling defect in the bladder, which also has been elevated markedly. Several diverticula are present. (B) Injecting cystourethrogram. AP view. *Arrow* points to the elongated prostatic urethra. Bladder markedly elevated. (C) Right oblique view. Injecting cystourethrogram. Notice marked concavity anterior to the prostatic urethra. This is due to large lateral lobes. Marked anterior curvature at the bladder neck is due to a large subcervical lobe. A diverticulum at posterior surface of bladder is visualized.

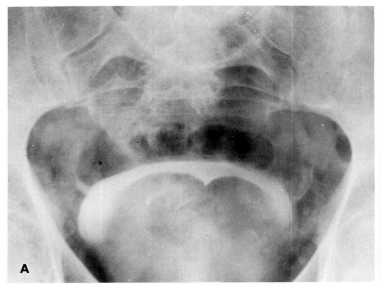

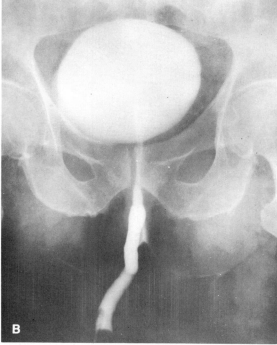

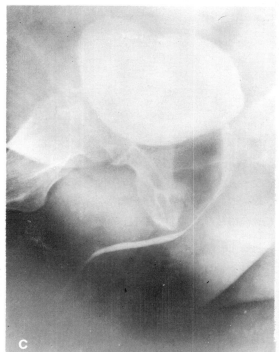

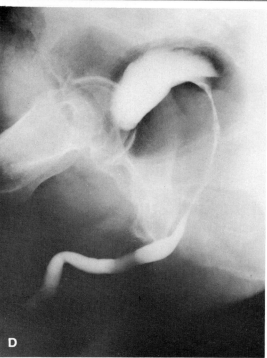

FIG. 34–26. Benign prostatic hypertrophy. Large prostate, 200 g. **(A)** Excretory cystogram reveals a large filling defect in the bladder. **(B)** Injecting cystourethrogram. AP view. Elongated prostatic urethra. Note the streak of contrast material in the bladder lumen, emphasizing the elongation of the urethra. **(C)** Voiding cystourethrogram. Right oblique view. Note widened elongated prostatic urethra. **(D)** Air cystourethrogram followed by injecting cystourethrogram. Note the lateral lobe enlargement projecting into the bladder floor. There is posterior commissure hypertrophy, but this is overshadowed by the lateral lobe enlargement. Marked increased concavity of urethra anteriorly.

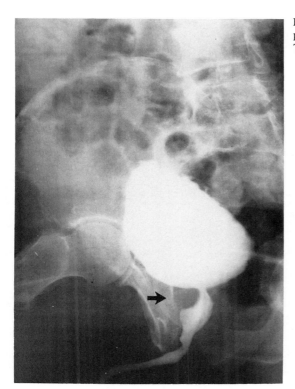

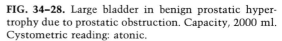
FIG. 34–27. Anterior commissural lobe; *arrow* points to pressure on anterior urethra produced by anterior lobe. This is a rare occurrence.

FIG. 34–28. Large bladder in benign prostatic hypertrophy due to prostatic obstruction. Capacity, 2000 ml. Cystometric reading: atonic.

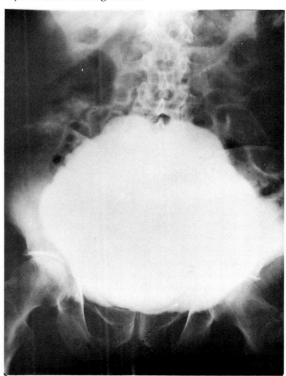

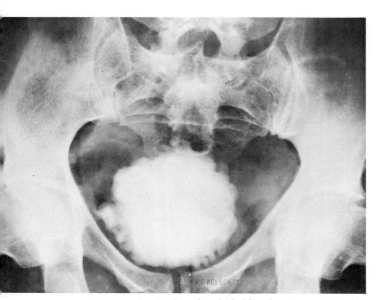

FIG. 34–29. Trabeculated bladder due to prostatic obstruction. Saccules and cellules are present.

FIG. 34–30. Double kidney with reflux secondary to prostatic obstruction.

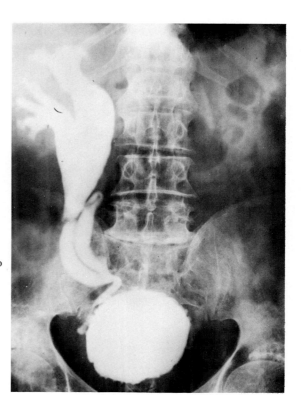

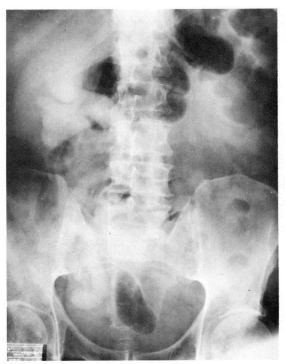

FIG. 34–31. Nonfunction of the left kidney. Right hydronephrosis and right hydroureter due to prostatic enlargement.

FIG. 34–32. Dilatation of ureters and kidneys secondary to prostatic obstruction.

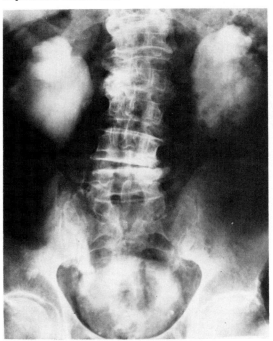

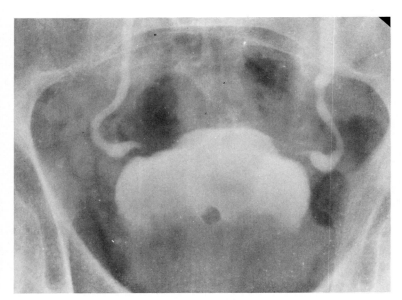

FIG. 34–33. Fishhook ureters secondary to prostatic enlargement.

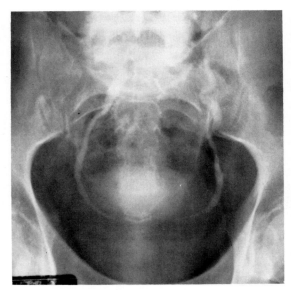

FIG. 34–34. Right-angle turn—lower ureters. This is the result of lateral lobe prostatic enlargement.

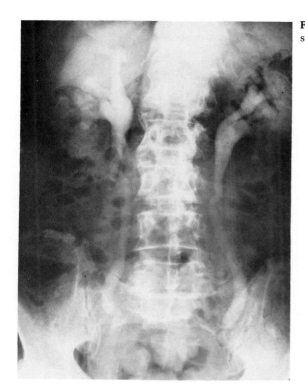

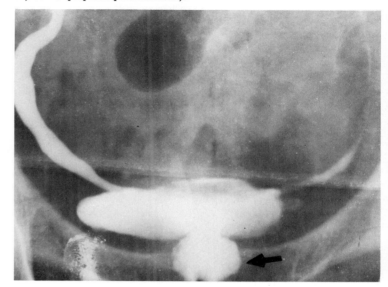

FIG. 34–35. Silent prostatism. Dilated upper tracts; unsuspected prostatic obstruction.

FIG. 34–36. Prostatic cavity seen on intravenous urogram. *Arrow* points to dilated prostatic cavity secondary to a suprapubic prostatectomy.

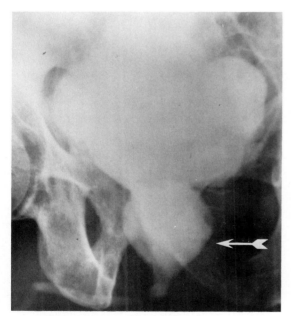

FIG. 34–37. Normal diluted prostatic cavity (*arrow*) secondary to a retropubic prostatectomy.

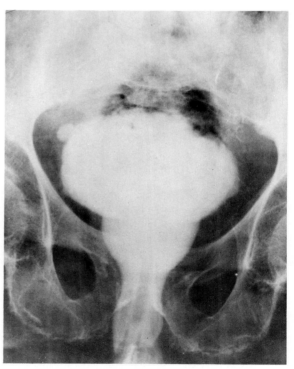

FIG. 34–38. Dilated prostatic and membranous urethra following suprapubic prostatectomy. Incontinence of urine.

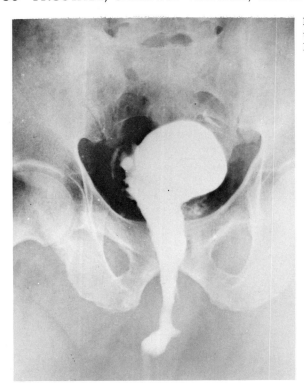

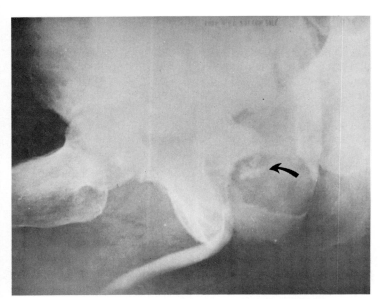

FIG. 34–39. Injecting cystourethrogram following a transurethral resection. Patient totally incontinent. Note loss of internal sphincter and external sphincter.

FIG. 34–40. Postoperative suprapubic prostatectomy. Right oblique view. Injecting cystourethrogram. Incontinence. Small-capacity bladder. Dilated prostatic urethra. The usual narrowing at the external sphincter is absent.

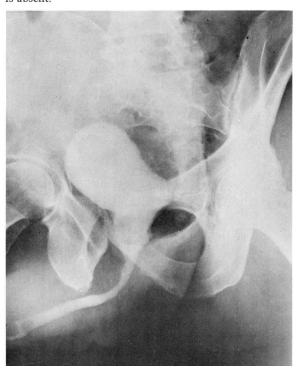

FIG. 34–41. Calculus (*arrow*) present in prostatic cavity, following a suprapubic prostatectomy.

FIG. 34–42. Seminal vesiculogram, performed by injection of contrast material into vas deferens, 4 years following suprapubic prostatectomy. *Arrow* points to dilated prostatic cavity. Notice the patency of the ejaculatory ducts.

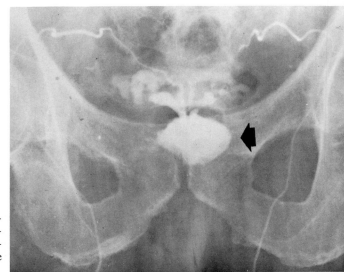

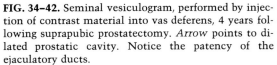

FIG. 34–43. Defect in the bladder produced by prostate in a female. Resected tissue revealed typical prostatic tissue. See Chapter 36, The Normal Urethra, for discussion of a female prostate.

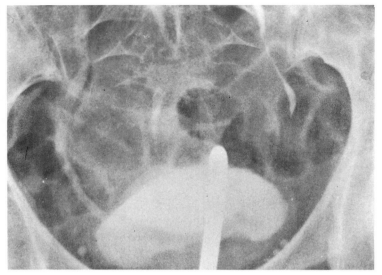

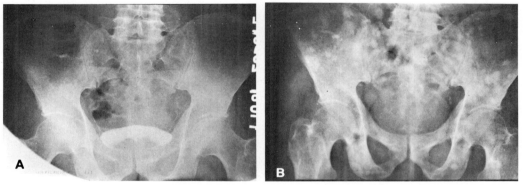

FIG. 34–44. Carcinoma of the prostate. **(A)** Intravenous urogram revealing essentially normal bone structure. **(B)** Six months later. Osteoblastic metastases from carcinoma of the prostate.

FIG. 34–45. American system for staging of prostatic cancer. **(A)** As described in text A_1 and A_2 are not diagnosed by rectal exam. B_1 and B_2 are localized to the prostate gland proper on rectal exam, whereas C is a direct extension beyond the prostate. D_1 and D_2 are associated with metastatic lesions. (Klein, L.A.: N. Engl. J. Med., *300*:824–833, 1979)

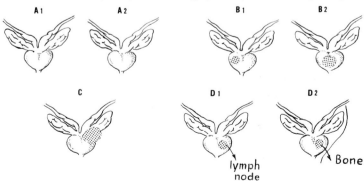

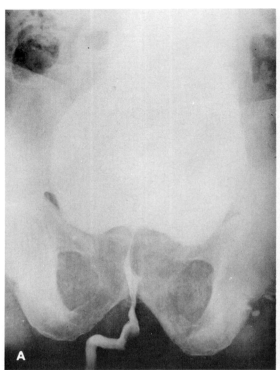

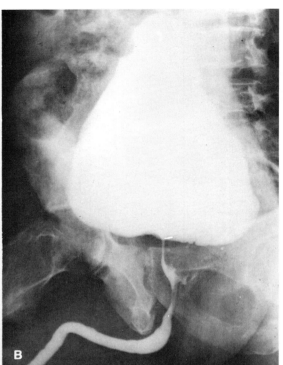

FIG. 34–46. Carcinoma of the prostate. Injecting cysto-urethrogram. **(A)** AP view. Narrowed posterior urethra. Slight right lateral deviation of the proximal portion. **(B)** Right oblique view. Posterior urethra still narrowed, especially in the supracollicular portion. Slight irregularity in floor of the bladder. Small utricle visible.

FIG. 34–47. Carcinoma of the prostate. Injecting cysto-urethrogram. Patient had had previous transurethral resection and had been intermittently on estrogen therapy for 2 years. **(A)** AP view. There is some widening of the proximal portion of the prostatic urethra with an irregular filling defect. **(B)** Right oblique view. The filling defect now can be seen more clearly. It was due to a nodule of tumor tissue.

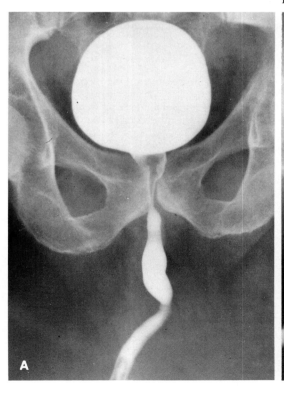

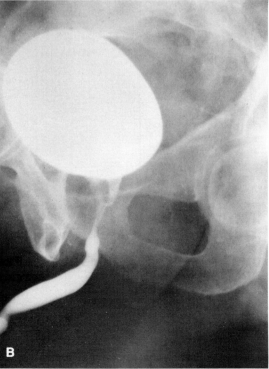

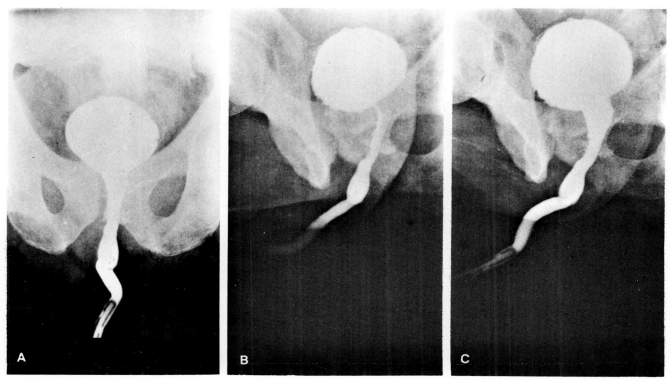

FIG. 34-48. Carcinoma of the prostate. **(A)** AP view. Injecting cystourethrogram. Posterior urethra is dilated. **(B)** Right oblique view; voiding. There is slight elongation of the posterior urethra, which is not narrowed. **(C)** Right oblique view. Injecting cystourethrogram. The widening and the lengthening of the posterior urethra now is seen clearly. This is a proved case of prostatic carcinoma, but there was no fixation of the urethra, and it was not narrowed.

FIG. 34-49. Carcinoma of the prostate with benign prostatic hypertrophy. Injecting cystourethrogram. **(A)** AP view. Narrow, elongated prostatic urethra. Floor of bladder is elevated slightly. **(B)** Right oblique view. Elongated, narrow posterior urethra. Subcervical lobe seen as defect in floor of the bladder with slight anterior tilting of the urethra.

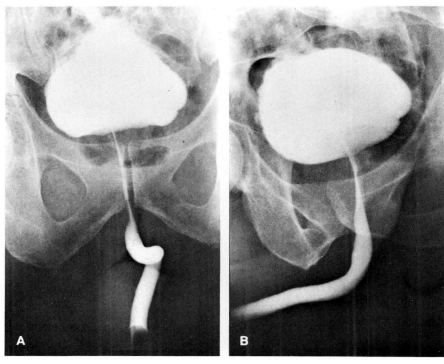

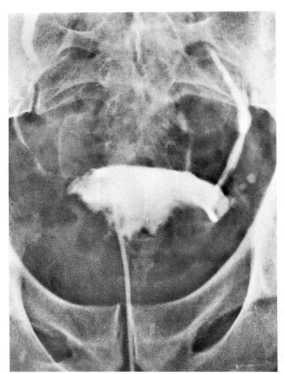

FIG. 34–50. Carcinoma of the prostate. Marked irregularity and elevation in the floor of the bladder from invasion by carcinoma of the prostate. (Courtesy of Dr. Sol. Unger, Vet. Ad.)

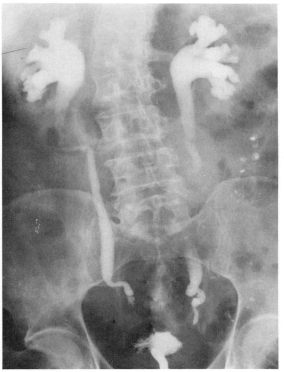

FIG. 34–51. Carcinoma of the prostate obstructing both ureters. Local extension of carcinoma of the prostate involved the base of the bladder but obstructed the ureters above the bladder in the region of the seminal vesicles. Catheters could be passed up each ureter, and retrograde pyelogram revealed bilateral hydronephrosis and hydro-ureter down to within several centimeters of the bladder, where there were constrictions of both ureters.

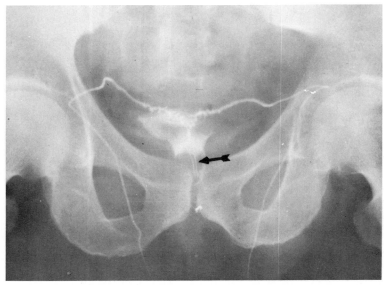

FIG. 34–52. Seminal vesiculogram in a case of carcinoma of the prostate proved 2 years previously by transurethral resection. Patient had been intermittently on estrogen therapy. *Arrow* points to narrow, straight, smooth ejaculatory ducts. (This is the same patient as Figure 34–47.)

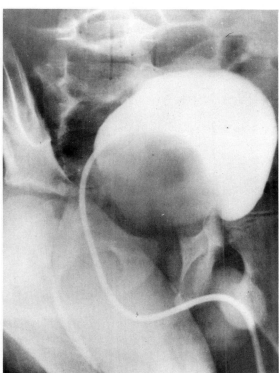

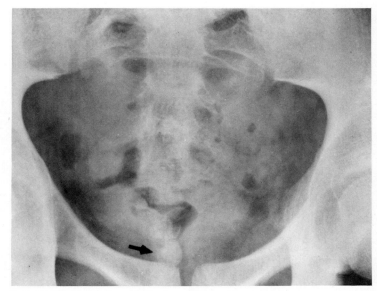

FIG. 34–53. Sarcoma of the prostate in a 4-year-old child. Left oblique view. Cystogram. There is a large, smooth filling defect in the base of the bladder.

FIG. 34–55. Prostatic calculus (*arrow*) in a 12-year-old boy. (Courtesy of W.F. Whitemore, M.D.)

FIG. 34–54. Rhabdomyosarcoma of prostate in a 3-year-old boy. IV urogram shows poor function of left kidney and a right mild hydronephrosis. Bladder displaced laterally and superiorly. Large defect at base of bladder. (Courtesy of Dr. N. Javadpour)

FIG. 34–56. Bilateral prostatic calcifications of moderate size in a patient who had tuberculosis of the left kidney. The calcifications could be tuberculous, but this was not proved.

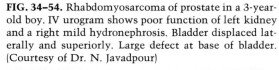

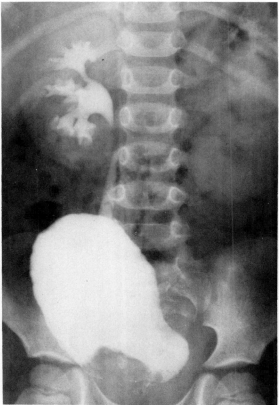

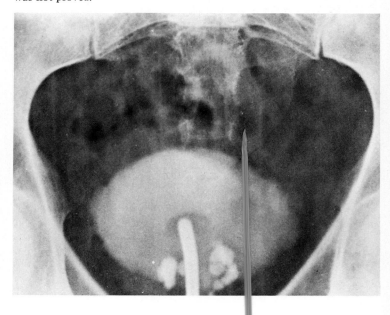

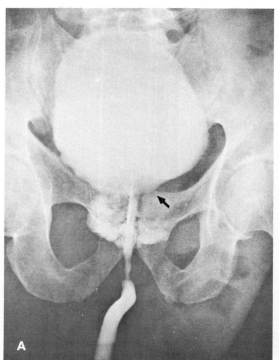

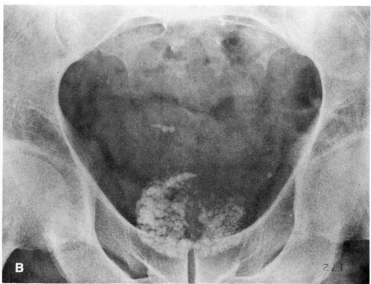

FIG. 34–57. Prostatic calculi. Horseshoe type of configuration. **(A)** Scout film. **(B)** Injecting cystourethrogram. AP view. Prostatic calculi visualized with the filling defect in the base of the bladder corresponding to the subcervical lobe.

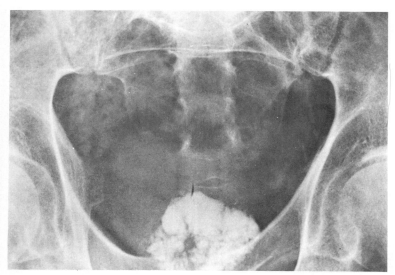

FIG. 34–58. Prostatic calculi. Ring type of configuration.

FIG. 34–59. Large distinct prostatic calculi. The lower one in the midline was not in the urethra but was found in the prostatic region. (Courtesy of L. Spivak, M.D.)

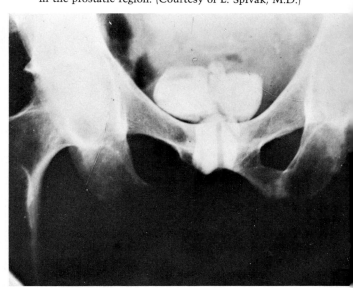

FIG. 34–60. Large prostatic calculi associated with benign prostatic hypertrophy. The prostate is well elevated into the bladder.

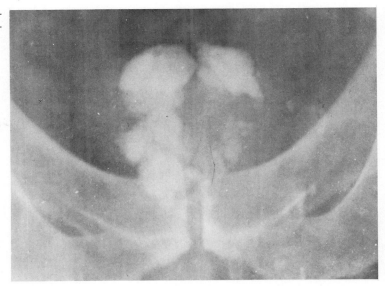

FIG. 34–61. Calculi of prostate (*arrow* points to small discrete calculi).

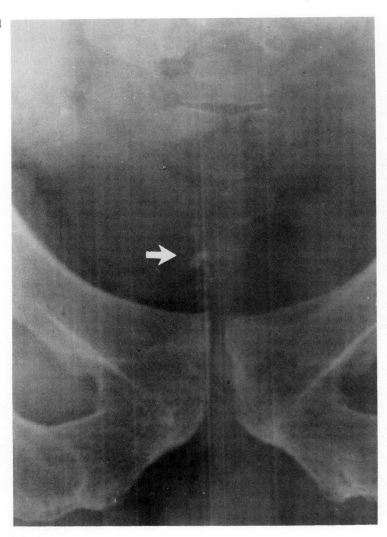

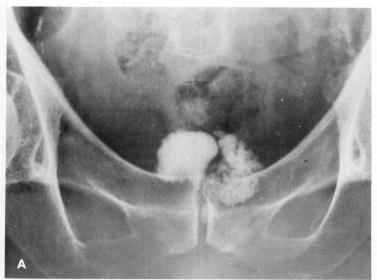

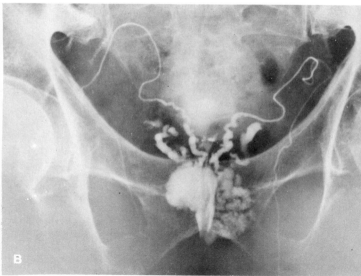

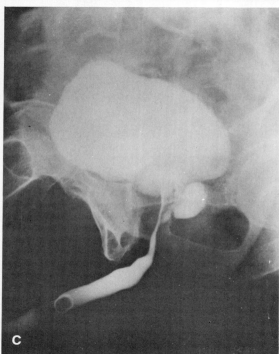

FIG. 34–62. Prostatic calculi. **(A)** Scout film. Large prostatic calculus on the right with several small calculi. Numerous distinct calculi in the left lobe. **(B)** Seminal vesiculogram. The ejaculatory ducts are essentially normal. There is bilateral interstitial seminal vesiculitis. **(C)** Injecting cystourethrogram. Right oblique view.

FIG. 34–63. Acute prostatitis. Elongation, diffuse narrowing and straightening of the posterior urethra. Patient, age 22, was in acute urinary retention at time of examination. (Beard, D.E., Goodyear, W.E., Weens, H.S.: Radiologic Diagnosis of the Lower Urinary Tract. Springfield, Charles C Thomas, 1952)

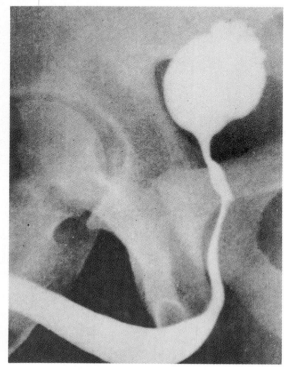

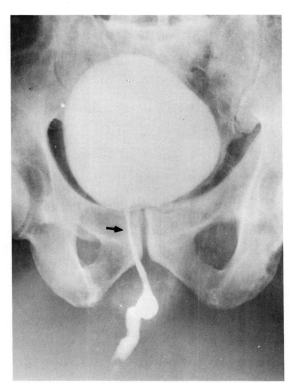

FIG. 34–64. Prostatic abscess, noncommunicating to urethra. AP view. Injecting cystourethrogram. *Arrow* points to elongated narrow posterior urethra with right lateral deviation, due to a large abscess in the left lateral lobe.

FIG. 34–65. Communicating prostatic abscess. Injecting cystourethrogram. (A) AP view. *Arrow* points to contrast-filled prostatic cavity. Patient had had a thick urethral discharge several weeks previous to the cystourethrogram. (B) Right oblique view confirms the prostatic cavity. There had been no previous prostatic surgery.

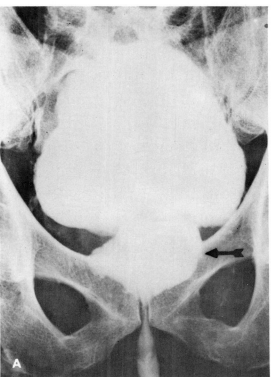

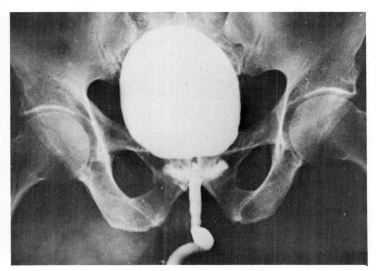

FIG. 34–66. Chronic prostatitis. Prostatic ducts visualized on injecting cystourethrogram. (Courtesy of Herbert Kenyon, M.D.)

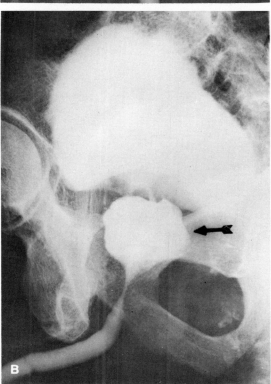

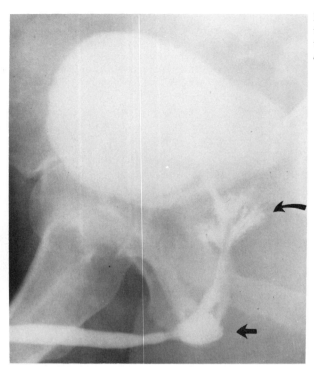

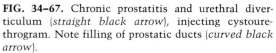

FIG. 34–67. Chronic prostatitis and urethral diverticulum (*straight black arrow*), injecting cystourethrogram. Note filling of prostatic ducts (*curved black arrow*).

FIG. 34–68. Noneosinophilic granulomatous prostatis. There is slight elongation of inframontane portion of prostatic urethra (*arrow*).

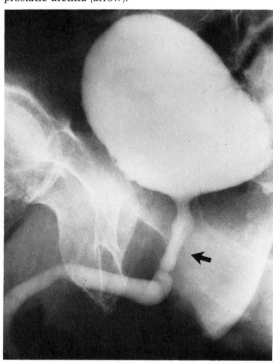

FIG. 34–68a. Anteroposterior (**A**) and oblique (**B**) cystourethrograms (injecting) in a case of noneosinophilic granulomatous prostatitis. There is narrowing of the prostatic urethra in **A** and widening in **B**. Note that the elongation is greater in the inframontane portion.

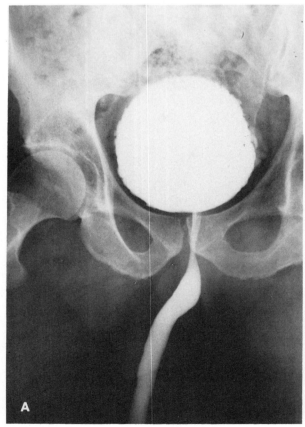

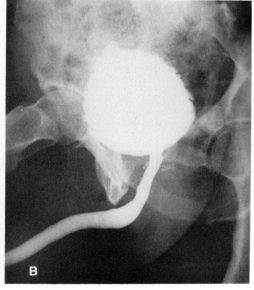

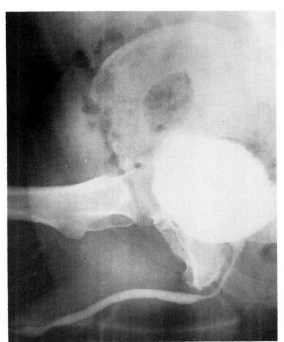

FIG. 34–68b. Voiding cystourethrogram, oblique view. Note the elongated urethra in the inframontane portion. (Same case as Fig. 34–68a)

FIG. 34–69. Eosinophilic granuloma of prostate. IVU — large filling defect at base of bladder. Enlarged prostate developed within 1 year. (Melicow, M.M.: J. Urol., 65:288, 1951)

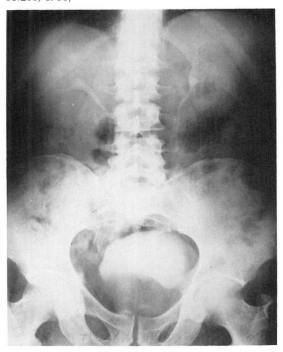

FIG. 34–70. Same as Figure 34–69. Eosinophilic infiltration in lung (Löffler syndrome). Radiographs of chest. **(A)** Note shadow in upper lung field (*arrow*). **(B)** Three weeks later. Note resolution of density (*arrow*). Eosinophiles 37 per cent. (Melicow, M.M.: J. Urol., 65:288, 1951)

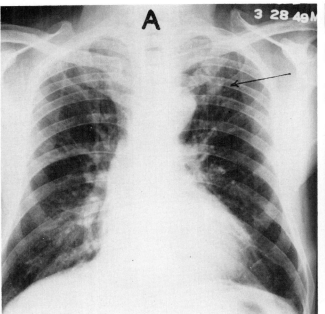

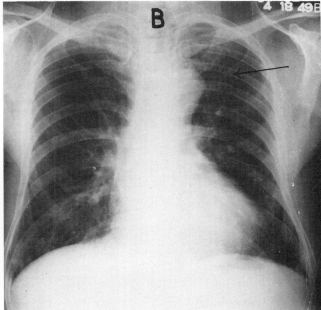

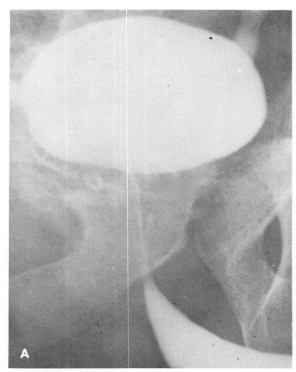

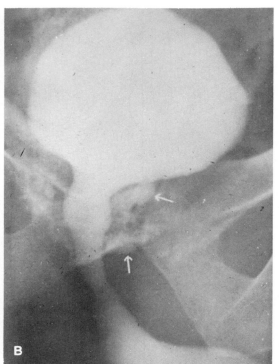

FIG. 34–71. Urogenital tuberculosis. Filling of prostatic cavity in a case of urogenital tuberculosis. **(A)** Injecting cystourethrogram, showing a few scattered prostatic cavities and left vesicoureteral reflux. **(B)** Voiding cystourethrogram. Filling of prostatic cavities now is more complete (*arrows*). (Edling, N.P.G.: Acta Radiol., *29*:461, 1948)

FIG. 34–73. Tuberculosis of the prostate. Marked irregular destruction of the prostate by tuberculosis. The contrast-filled cavity is seen easily. (Courtesy of Herman Wechsler, M.D.)

FIG. 34–72. Tuberculosis of the prostate. Injecting cystourethrogram. There is a stricture in the region of the membranous urethra with irregular prostatic excavation due to tuberculous involvement. Bilateral vesicoureteral reflux, more on the right. The bladder is contracted markedly and is scarcely visible (*arrow*). (Courtesy of Maxwell Malament, M.D.)

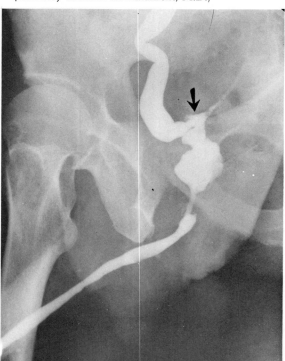

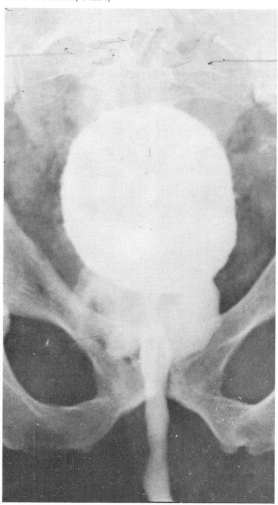

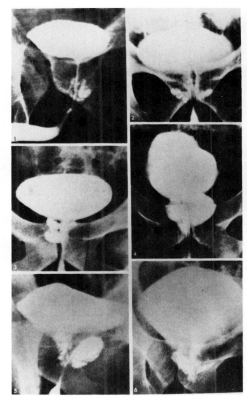

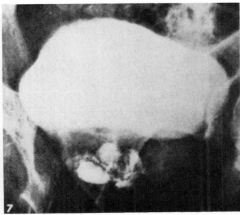

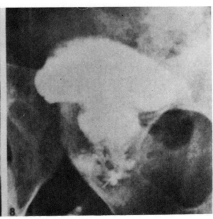

FIG. 34–74. Tuberculosis of prostate; retrograde cystourethrograms. 1. Bilateral periurethral cavities and beginning tuberculous contracture of bladder neck. 2. Symmetric extravasation of contrast medium in prostatic urethra. 3. Large prostatic cavity on right, small cavity on left. 4. Complete destruction of prostatic parenchyma. Formation of so-called anterior bladder. 5. Extensive cavernous prostatitis bilaterally. 6. Same patient as in 5 after transurethral prostatic resection. 7. Extensive cavernous prostatitis bilaterally. 8. Same patient as in 7 after 2 years. Complete liquefaction of prostatic parenchyma, marked "anterior bladder." (May, P., Hohenfellner, R., König, E., et al.: Urol. Int., *21*:329, 1966)

FIG. 34–75. Cyst of prostate. A-P roentgenogram after perineal aspiration of the cystic prostate and injection of contrast medium, demonstrating the large cysts in the lateral lobes of the prostate. (Fischelovitch, J. et al., Br. J. Urol., *47*:687, 1975)

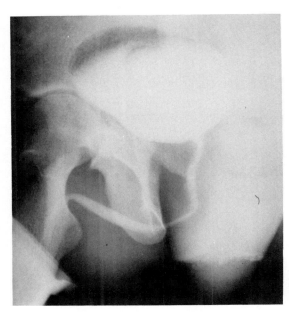

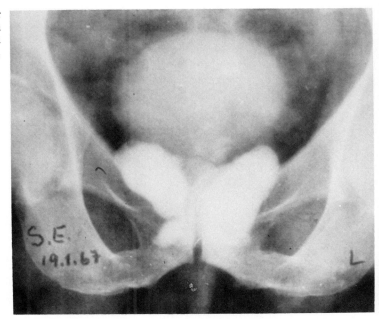

FIG. 34–76. Cyst of prostate. Voiding cystourethrogram shows anterior curvature of the prostatic urethra. (Reiser, C., Griffin, T.I.: J. Urol., *91*:282, 1964)

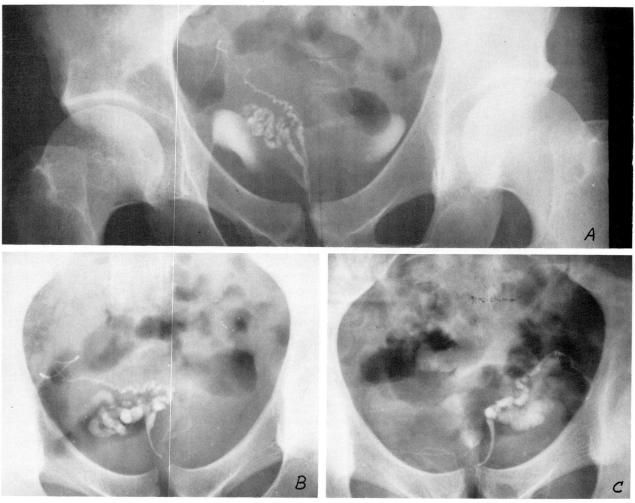

FIG. 34–77. Cyst of prostate (same case as shown in Fig. 34–76). (A) Right seminal vesiculogram in a normal man. (B) Right seminal vesiculogram illustrates convex course of ejaculatory duct. (C) Left seminal vesiculogram with similar convexity. (Reiser, C., Griffin, T.I.: J. Urol., *91*:282, 1964)

FIG. 34–78. Cyst of prostate (same case as shown in Fig. 34–76). (A) Right and (B) left retrograde seminal vesiculograms reveal curvilinear lateral deviation of ejaculatory ducts around margins of cysts. (Reiser, C., Griffin, T.I.: J. Urol., *91*:282, 1964)

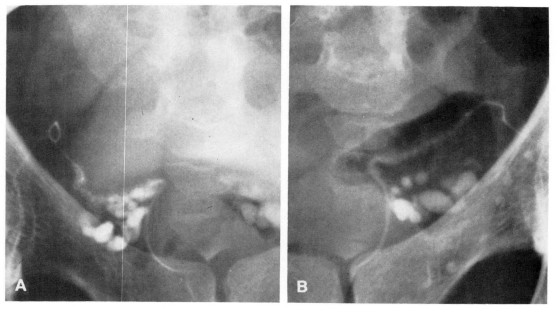

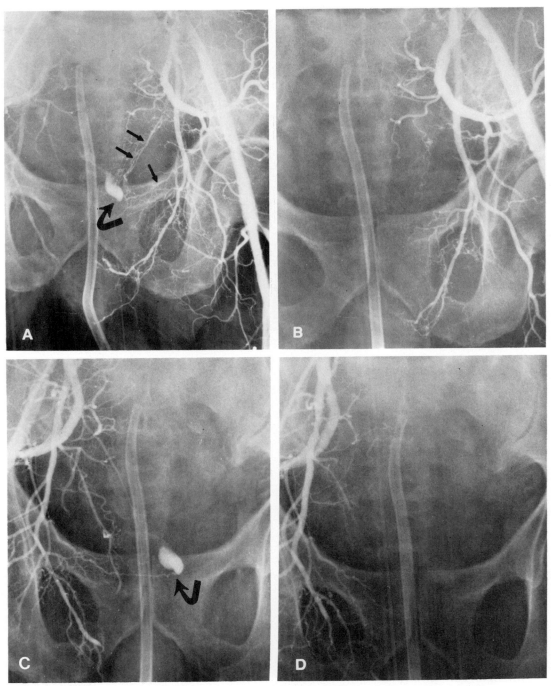

FIG. 34–79. A 67-year-old man bleeding after Vim–Silverman needle biopsy of the prostate. **(A)** Left hypogastric arteriogram demonstrates bleeding from a site in the prostate *(curved arrow)* supplied by both the superior vesical artery *(double arrow)* and the inferior vesical artery *(single arrow)*. There is a reflux of contrast medium to the external iliac and femoral artery. **(B)** A similar study after the introduction of autologous clot demonstrates no extravasation. The previously demonstrated superior and inferior vesical arteries are no longer visualized. **(C)** Right hypogastric arteriogram demonstrates extravasation of contrast medium at the same site *(curved arrow)* in **(A)** now supplied by the right inferior vesical artery. **(D)** After selective embolization the inferior vesical artery is now occluded, and there is no extravasation of contrast material on this repeat study. (Mitchell, M.E., Waltman, A.C., Athanasoulis, C.A., et al.: Am. Urol. Assoc., *1975*)

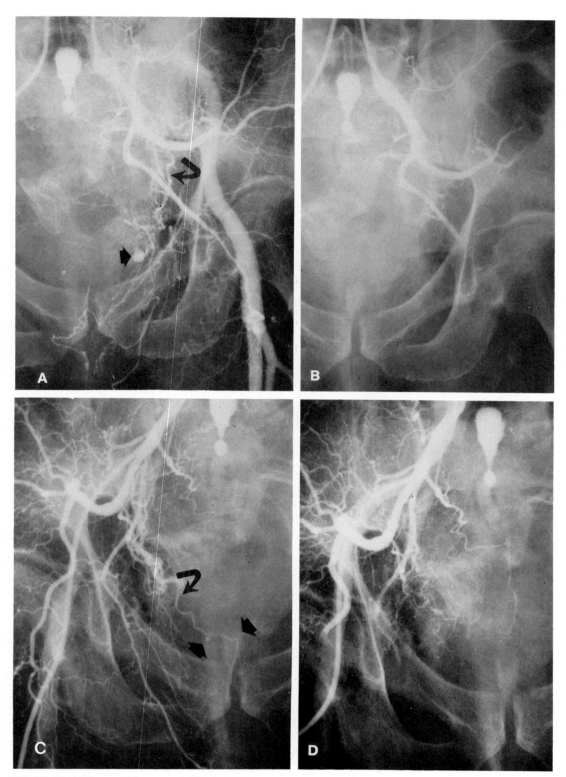

FIG. 34–80. A 70-year-old man with bleeding following transurethral resection of the prostate. **(A)** Selective left hypogastric arteriogram demonstrates bleeding (*straight arrow*) as extravasation of contrast medium from a branch of the left internal pudendal artery (*curved arrow*). There is reflux of contrast medium into the external iliac artery. **(B)** After selective embolization with Gelfoam clots extravasation of contrast medium is no longer visualized with repeat left hypogastric arteriogram. **(C)** Right hypogastric study demonstrates two different points of contrast extravasation (*straight arrows*) into the area of the prostate bed, both supplied by the superior vesical artery (*curved arrow*). **(D)** Repeat study on the right after Gelfoam embolization demonstrates no extravasation of contrast medium. (Mitchell, M.E., Waltman, A.C., Athanasoulis, C.A., et al.: Am. Urol. Assoc., 1975)

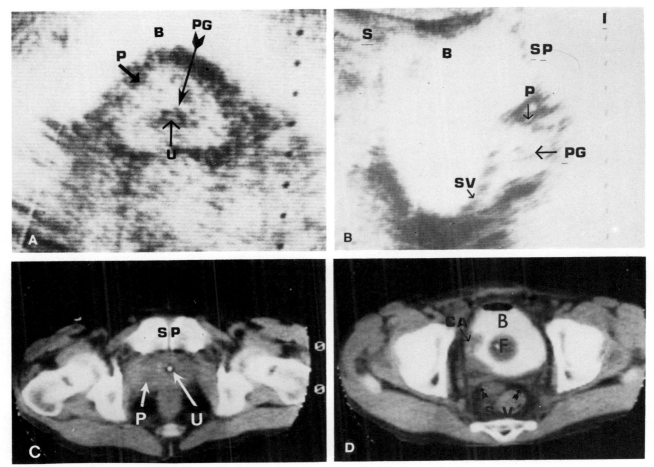

FIG. 34–81. (A) Transverse sonogram of triangularly shaped normal prostate. The deeply echogenic periurethral glands (PG) surround the urethra (U). **(B)** Longitudinal sonogram of normal prostate (P). The seminal vesicles (SV) extend from the superior (S) aspect. The scan is limited inferiorly (I) by the symphysis pubis (SP). **(C)** CT scan of normal prostate (P) with contrast-filled urethra (U). **(D)** CT scan performed 1 cm. cephalad shows contrast-filled bladder (B), Foley catheter (F), and transitional cell carcinoma (CA). (Sukov, R.J., Scardino, P.R., Sample, W.F. et al.: J. Comput. Assist. Tomogr. *1*:281–289, 1977)

FIG. 34–82. Transverse suprapubic ultrasonographic scan of patient with prostatic benign hyperplasia. B = bladder; A = adenoma; SC = surgical capsule. (Henneberry, M., Carter, M.F., Neuman, H.L.: J. Urol., *121*:615, 1979)

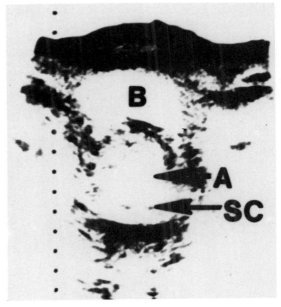

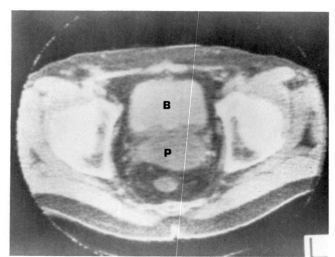

FIG. 34–82a. CT of an enlarged prostate due to benign prostatic hypertrophy. There are no distinguishing features except the enlarged prostate proved at surgery. *B* = bladder; *P* = prostate. (Courtesy of Mark Goldman, M.D.)

FIG. 34–83. Initial sonographic scan reveals acute prostatitis with a coexistent perineal abscess. These are demonstrated on both transverse (**A**) and longitudinal (**B**) scans. Note absence of echoes in the prostatic area. Follow-up sonograms 2 months later reveal resumption of normal prostate echogenicity and resolution of abscess. This can be seen on both the transverse (**C**) and longitudinal (**D**) scans. B = bladder; P = prostate; AB = abscess. (Courtesy of Richard J. Sukov)

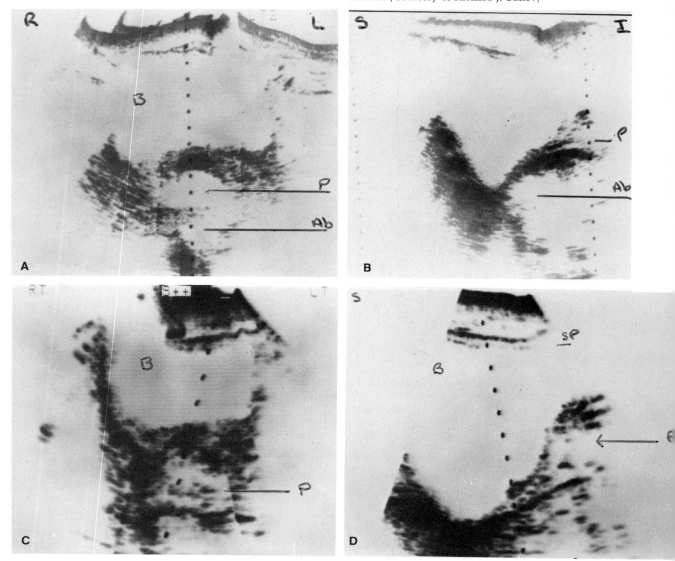

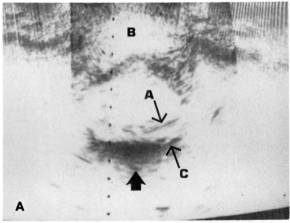

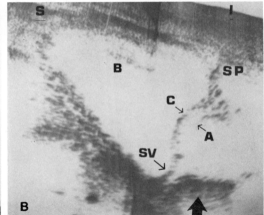

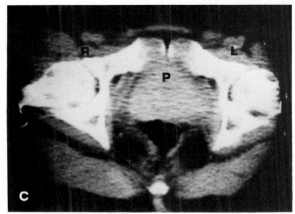

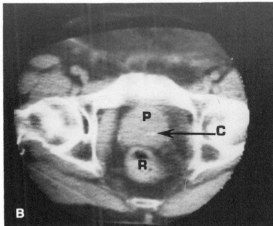

FIG. 34–84. (A) Transverse sonogram of patient with BPH and acute prostatitis. Note decreased echogenicity of the edematous adenoma **(A)** and striking increase in through transmission (*short thick arrow*). Width of surgical capsule (*C*) is indicated by the more echogenic area between the lipes of the two *thin arrows*. B = bladder. **(B)** Longitudinal sonogram of same patient with BPH and acute prostatitis again demonstrating decreased echogenicity of the edematous adenoma **(A)** and increase through transmission (*short arrow*). Width of surgical capsule (*C*) is indicated by the more echogenic area between the tips of the two arrows. SV = seminal vesicles. B = bladder; S = superior; I = inferior; SP = symphysis pubic. **(C)** CT scan of same patient with BPH and acute prostatitis. P = prostate; R = right; L = left. (Sukov, R.J., Scardino, P.R., Sample, W.F. et al.: J. Comput. Assist. Tomogr., *1*:281–289, 1977)

FIG. 34–85. (A) Transverse sonogram of patient with chronic prostatitis showing deeply echogenic foci of calcium **(C)**. Shadowing not present because of compound scanning. B = bladder; R = rectum. **(B)** CT scan of same patient with chronic prostatitis showing prostate **(P)** with foci of calcium **(C)**. R = rectum. (Sukov, R.J., Scardino, P.R., Sample, W.F., et al.: J. Comput. Assist. Tomogr., *1*:281–289, 1977)

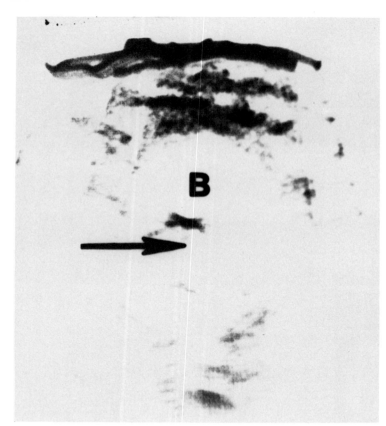

FIG. 34–86. Transverse suprapubic ultrasonographic scan of patient with bladder neck obstruction and diffuse adenocarcinoma of prostate. *Arrow* demonstrates increased echo patterns in periurethral prostatic tissue, consistent with pathologic diagnosis of carcinoma. **B** = bladder. (Henneberry, M., Carter, M.F., Neiman, H.L.: J. Urol., *121*:615, 1979)

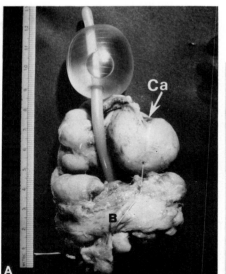

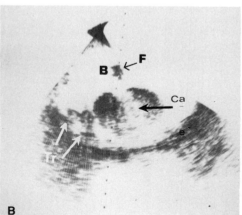

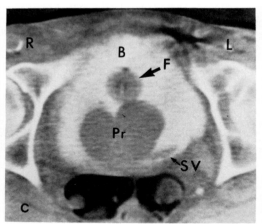

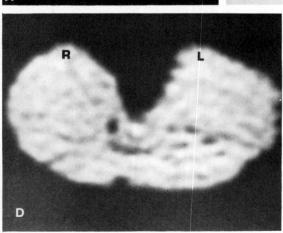

FIG. 34–87. (A) Anterior view of open prostatectomy specimen removed from patient who had a focus of well-differentiated adenocarcinoma **(Ca)** on the left at the apex. B = base. **(B)** Transverse sonogram of same patient with adenocarcinoma **(Ca).** Note the heavily trabeculated (Tr) bladder (B) and the Foley catheter (F). **(C)** CT scan at same level showing prostate (Pr), seminal vesicle (SV), and contrast-filled bladder (B) with Foley catheter (F). **(D)** CT scan of open prostatectomy specimen at level of the carcinoma. R = right; L = left. (Sukov, R.J., Scardino, P.R., Sample, W.F., et al.: J. Comput. Assist. Tomogr., *1*:281–289, 1977)

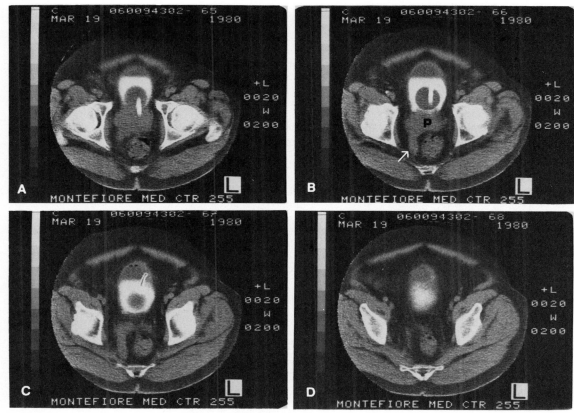

FIG. 34–88. Carcinoma of the prostate invading right seminal vesicle and pararectal area (*arrow*). P = prostate. (Courtesy of M. Goldman, M.D.)

FIG. 34–89. CT scan. Carcinoma of the prostate invading the bladder. *Arrow* indicates area of invasion. P = prostate; B = bladder. (Courtesy of M. Goldman, M.D.)

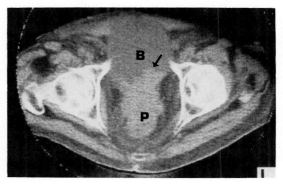

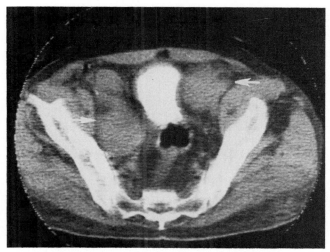

FIG. 34–90. Carcinoma of prostate. Lymph node metastases (*arrows*). (Courtesy of M. Goldman, M.D.)

BIBLIOGRAPHY

1. Adrion, W.: Ein Beitrag zu Etiologie der Prostata-hypertrophie. Beitr. Pathol. Anat., 70:179–202, 1922.
2. Albarran, J., and Motz, B.: Contribution a l'étude de l'anatomie macroscopic de la prostate hypertrophiée. Ann. d. mal. de org. genito-urin., 20:769–817, 1902.
3. Deming, C.L., and Neumann, C.: Early phases of prostatic hyperplasia. Surg. Gynecol. Obstet., 68:155–160, 1939.
4. Franks, L.M.: Benign nodular hyperplasia of the prostate: a review. Ann. Roy. Coll. Surg. Eng., 14:92–106, 1954.
5. Franks, L.M.: Atrophy and hyperplasia in the prostate proper. J. Pathol. Bact., 68:617–621, 1954.
6. Le Duc, J.E.: The anatomy of the prostate and the pathology of early benign hypertrophy. J. Urol., 42:1217–1241, 1939.
7. Lendorf, A.: Hvad foregaar der ved den suprapubiske Prostatektomi. Hvorfra udvikles den saskaldte Prostatahypertrofi. Hospitalstid ende: Raekke 5, vol. 4, pp. 1369–1389 and 1413–1420, 1911.
7a. McNeal, J.E.: Origin and evolution of benign prostatic enlargement. Invest. Urol., 15:340–345, 1978.
8. Moore, R.A.: Benign hypertrophy of the prostate: morphological study. J. Urol., 50:680–710, 1943.
9. Motz, B., and Perearnau, E.: Contribution a l'etude de l'évolution de l'hypertrophie de la prostate. Ann. d. mal. de org. genito-urin, 23:1521–1548, 1905.
10. Oberndorfer, S.: Handbuch der speciellen pathologischen Anatomie and Histologie. p. 457. Berlin, Henke und Lubarsch, 1931.
11. Randall, A.: Surgical Pathology of Prostatic Obstruction. Baltimore, William & Wilkins, 1931.
12. Reischauer, F.: Die Entstehung der sogenannten Prostatahypertrophie. Virchows Arch. Path. Anat., 256:357–389, 1925.
13. Tandler, J., and Zuckerkandl, O.: Studien zur Anatomie und Klinik der Prostatahypertrophie. Berlin, J. Springer, 1922.

Effects of Benign Prostatic Hypertrophy on the Bladder

14. Bernstein, R.G., Siegelman, S.S., Tein, A.B., and Bosniak, M.A.: Huge filling defect in the bladder caused by intravesical enlargement of the prostate. Radiology, 92:1447–1452, 1969.
15. Binney, H.: Bladder atony and prostatectomy. Trans. Am. Assoc. Genitourin. Surg., 6:98–112, 1911.
16. Burns, E.: Diverticula of the urinary bladder. Ann. Surg., 119:656–664, 1944.
17. Carter, R.G.: Vesical neck obstruction with over 8,000 cc. residual urine. J. Urol., 69:118–120, 1953.
18. Casper, L.: Ueber ungewohnliche Fälle dauernder Harnverhaultung. Berl. klin. Wschr., 47:425–426, 1910.
19. Crabtree, E.G., and Muellner, S.R.: The bladder in prostatism: an operation for excessive bladder hypertrophy. J. Urol., 60:593–598, 1948.
20. Herman, H.: Über de Substitution der Muskulatur der Harnblase durch Bindegewebe. Centralbl. allg. path. u. path. Anat., 35:417–426, 1925.
21. McGavran, H.G.: Giant prostate without symptoms: neurofibroma. J. Urol., 60:254–259, 1948.
22. Orr, L.M.: Management of the atonic bladder due to obstruction of vesical neck. South. Med. J., 30:519–524, 1937.
23. Sugimura, S.: Über die Entstehung der sogenannten echten Diverticel der Harnblase inbesondere des Blasengrundes,

nebst Beitragen zur Lehre von der Pathologie der Muskulatur und elastischen Gewebe in der Harnblase. Virchows Arch. (Pathol. Anat.), 204:349–372, 1911.

Effects of Benign Prostatic Hypertrophy on the Kidney and the Ureter

24. Hutch, J.A.: Nonobstructive dilation of the upper kidney tract. J. Urol., 71:412–420, 1954.
25. Kretschmer, H.L., and Squire, F.H.: The incidence and extent of hydronephrosis in prostatic obstruction. J. Urol., 60:1–6, 1948.
26. Pierce, J.M., Jr., and Braun, E.: Ureteral response to elevated intravesical pressure in humans. Surg. Forum, 11:482–484, 1960.
27. Squire, F.H., and Kretschmer, H.L.: A study of the ureters in bladder neck obstruction. Radiology, 46:32–35, 1946.
28. Young, H.H.: Practice of Urology. vol. 1, pp. 430–431. Philadelphia, Saunders, 1926.

Silent Prostatism

29. Dick, V.S.: Unrecognized prostatism. J.A.M.A., 148:925–928, 1952.
30. Dowd, J.B., and Ewert, E.E.: Silent prostatism (unrecognized bladder neck obstruction). J.A.M.A., 8:142–146, 1961.

Carcinoma of the Prostate

31. Andrews, G.S.: Latent carcinoma of prostate. J. Clin. Pathol., 2:197–208, 1949.
32. Arduino, L.J.: Unusual metastases of carcinoma of the prostate. Am. Surg., 21:1146–1153, 1955.
33. Barkin, M., Schachter, D., and Taranger, L.A.: Spinal cord compression due to metastatic carcinoma of the prostate. Read at Northeastern Section of A.U.A., Whitefield, N.H., September 28 to October 2, 1974.
34. Baron, E., and Angrist, A.: Incidence of occult adenocarcinoma of prostate after 50 years of age. Arch. Pathol., 32:787–793, 1941.
35. Brice, J., and McKissock, W.: Surgical treatment of malignant extradural spinal tumors. Br. Med. J., 1:1341–1344, 1965.
36. Clarke, B.G., and Viets, H.R.: Effect of diethylstilboestrol on neurological symptoms of carcinoma of the prostate. J.A.M.A., 121:499, 1943.
37. Edelman, I.S.: Paraplegia secondary to metastatic prostatic carcinoma treated with stilboestrol. Ann. Intern. Med., 31:1098–1102, 1949.
38. Edwards, C.N., Steinthorsson, F., and Nicholson, D.: Autopsy study of latent prostatic cancer. Cancer, 6:531–554, 1953.
38a. Foti, A.G., Cooper, J.F., Herschman, F. et al.: Detection of prostatic cancer by solid phase radioimmunoassay of serum prostatic acid phosphatase. N. Engl. J. Med. 297:1357–1361, 1977.
39. Franks, L.M.: Latent carcinoma of the prostate. J. Pathol. Bact., 68:603–616, 1954.
40. Gaynor, E.P.: Zur Frage des Prostatakrebses. Virchows Arch. (Pathol. Anat.), 301:602–652, 1938.

41. Geraghty, J.T., and Boyd, M.S., quoted in Lowsley, O.S.: Development of the human prostate gland. Am. J. Anat., *13*:299–350, 1912.

42. Gil-Vernet, S.: Cancer de prostata in Patologia Urogenital. vol. 1, Barcelone, Servet, 1944.

43. Hager, B.H., Hoffman, E.F.: Statistical data on 395 cases of carcinoma of the prostate observed at Los Angeles General Hospital from Jan. 1, 1923, to Jan. 1, 1936. J. Urol., *37*:180–185, 1937.

44. Hudson, P.B.: Prostatic cancer. XIV. Its incidence, extent and behavior in 686 men studied by prostatic biopsy. J. Am. Geriatr. Soc., *5*:338–350, 1957.

45. Huggins, C.: Prostatic cancer treated by orchiectomy. J.A.M.A., *131*:576–581, 1946.

46. Kahler, J.E.: Carcinoma of the prostate gland. Proc. Mayo Clin., *13*:589, 1938.

46a. Klein, L.A.: Prostatic carcinoma. N. Engl. J. Med., *300*:824–833, 1979.

47. Marshall, S., Tavel, F.R., and Schulte, J.W.: Spinal cord compression secondary to metastatic carcinoma of the prostate treated by decompression laminectomy. J. Urol., *88*:667–673, 1962.

48. McLaughlin, A.P., Saltzstein, S.L., McCullough, D.L., and Gittes, R.F.: Prostatic carcinoma; incidence and location of unsuspected lymphatic metastases. J. Urol., *115*:89–94, 1976.

49. Moore, R.A.: The morphology of small prostatic carcinoma. J. Urol., *33*:224–234, 1935.

49a. Murphy, G.P., and Whitmore, W.F., Jr.: A report of the workshops on the current status of the histologic grading of prostatic cancer. Cancer, *44*:1490–1494, 1979.

50. Nesbit, R.M., and Cummings, R.H.: Prostatic carcinoma treated by orchiectomy. J.A.M.A., *120*:1109–1111, 1942.

50a. Pontes, J.E., Choe, B., Rose, N., et al.: Reliability of bone marrow acid phosphatase as a parameter of metastatic prostatic cancer. J. Urol., *122*:178–179, 1979.

51. Rich, A.R.: On the frequency of occurrence of occult carcinoma of the prostate. J. Urol., *33*:215–223, 1935.

52. Rubin, P., et al.: Carcinoma of the urogenital tract: prostatic carcinoma. J.A.M.A., *209*:1695–1705, 1969.

53. Starklint, H.B.: Undersgelser over latent og Manifest Prostata-cancer (thesis). Copenhagen Munksgaard, 1950.

54. Sy, F.A., Gursel, E.O., and Veenema, R.J.: Positive random iliac bone biopsy in advanced prostatic cancer. Urology, *3*:125–127, 1973.

55. Thompson, G.J.: Transurethral resection of malignant lesions of the prostate gland. J.A.M.A., *120*:1105–1109, 1942.

56. Toulson, W.H., and Hawkins, C.W.: Paraplegia as a result of metastasis from carcinoma of the prostate gland. Bulletin of the School of Medicine, University of Maryland, *32*:159–162, 1948.

57. Vieth, R.G., and Odom, G.L.: Extradural spinal metastases and their neurosurgical treatment. J. Neurosurg., *23*:501–508, 1965.

57a. Watson, R.A., and Tang, D.B.: The predictive value of prostatic acid phosphatase as a screening test for prostatic cancer. N. Engl. J. Med. *303*:497–499, 1980.

58. Woodard, H.Q.: Factors leading to elevation of serum acid glycerophosphatase. Cancer, *5*:236–241, 1952.

59. Young, H.H.: Cancer of the prostate: a clinical pathological and postoperative analysis of 111 cases. Ann. Surg., *50*:1144–1233, 1909.

60. Young, H.H., and Davis, D.M.: Young's Practice of Urology. vol. 1, pp. 621–631. Philadelphia, Saunders, 1926.

Effects of Carcinoma of the Prostate on the Upper Urinary Tract

60a. Brin, E.N., Schiff, M., Jr., and Weiss, R.M.: Palliative urinary diversion for pelvic malignancy. J. Urol. *113*:619–622, 1975.

61. Ganem, E.J.: The upper urinary tract in advanced prostatic carcinoma. J. Urol., *78*:466–470, 1957.

62. Graves, R.C., and Militzer, R.E.: Carcinoma of the prostate with metastases. J. Urol., *33*:235–251, 1935.

63. Herbut, T.A.: Urological Pathology. vol. 2, p. 947. Philadelphia, Lea & Febiger, 1952.

63a. Khan, A.U., and Utz, D.C.: Clinical management of carcinoma of prostate associated with bilateral ureteral obstruction. J. Urol. *113*:816–819, 1975.

64. Mintz, E.R., and Smith, G.G.: Autopsy findings in 100 cases of prostatic cancer. N. Engl. J. Med., *211*:279–287, 1934.

65. Murka, L.S., et al.: Ureteral obstruction in the patient with prostatic carcinoma. Br. J. Urol., *44*:411–416, 1972.

Radiographic Appearance of Carcinoma of the Prostate and Benign Prostatic Hypertrophy

66. Crabtree, G., and Brodny, L.: An estimate of the value of urethrograms and cystograms in the diagnosis of prostatic obstruction. J. Urol., *29*:235–276, 1933.

67. Cuturi, L.: L'uretrografia (dissertazione). Padova, 1938.

68. Edling, N.P.C.: On the roentgen aspect of prostatic cancer by urethrocystography. Acta Radiol., *29*:461–474, 1948.

69. Edling, N.P.C.: Urethrocystography in the male with special regard to micturitions. Acta Radiol. (suppl.), *58*:5–144, 1945.

70. Flocks, R.H.: The roentgen visualization of the posterior urethra. J. Urol., *30*:711–736, 1933.

71. Kerr, H.D., and Gillies, C.L.: The Urinary Tract. Chicago, Year Book Publishers, 1944.

72. Knuttson, F.: On the technique of urethrography. Acta Radiol., *10*:437–441, 1929.

73. Knuttson, F.: Urethrography. Roentgen examination of male urethra and prostate after injection of contrast material into urethra. Acta Radiol. (suppl.), *28*:1–150, 1935.

74. Moulonguet, A.: Urethrographie retrograde et cancer prostatique. J. Urol. Nephrol., *59*:629–637, 1953.

75. Oravisto, K.J., and Schauman, S.: Urethrocystography in the differential diagnosis of prostatic carcinoma. J. Urol., *75*:995–999, 1956.

76. Pereira, A.: Importance of the roentgen examination in the diagnosis of adenoma of the prostate. Am. J. Roentgenol., *51*:600–613, 1944.

77. Vincent, P.G.A.: L'uretrographie par voie mictionelle. Paris, Vigot, 1935.

Sarcoma of the Prostate

78. Christoffersen, J.: Leiomyosarcoma of the prostate. Six new cases and a survey of the literature. Acta. Chir. Scand. (suppl.), *433*:75–84, 1973.

79. Cox, R., and Dawson, I.M.: A curious prostatic tumour: probably a true mixed tumour (cystadeno-leiomyofibroma). Br. J. Urol., *32*:306, 1960.

80. Danckers, U.F., et al.: Sarcomas of the prostate, periprostatic tissue, and bladder neck in children: report of a new case. Am. J. Roentgenol., *84*:555–561, 1960.

81. Graves, R.S., and Coleman, M.W.: Sarcoma of the prostate: an unusual survival. J. Urol., *72*:731–734, 1954.

82. Gueft, Boris, and Walsh, M.A.: Malignant prostatic cystosarcoma phyllodes. N.Y. State J. Med., 75:2226–2228, 1975.

83. Longley, J.: Sarcoma of prostate and bladder. J. Urol., 73:417–423, 1955.

84. Mackenzie, A.R., Whitmore, W., Jr., and Melamed, A.: Myosarcoma of the bladder and prostate. Cancer, 22:833–844, 1968.

85. Meeter, U.L., and Richards, J.N.: Osteogenic sarcoma of the prostate. J. Urol., 84:654–657, 1960.

86. Melicow, M.M., Pelton, T.H., and Fish, G.W.: Sarcoma of the prostate gland: review of literature; table of classification; report of four cases. J. Urol., 49:675–707, 1943.

87. Mostofi, F.K., and Price, E.B.: Tumors of the male genital system. In Atlas of Tumor Pathology. Second Series, no. 8, p. 310. Washington, D.C., Armed Forces Institute of Pathology, 1973.

88. Murphy, G., and Bradley, J.: Primary sarcoma of the prostate. J. Urol., 85:973–976, 1961.

89. Prince, C.L., and Vest, S.A.: Leiomyosarcoma of the prostate: report of a case and critical review. J. Urol., 46:1129–1143, 1941.

90. Scardino, P.L., and Prince, C.L.: Prostatic sarcoma: survival following radical perineal prostatectomy. J. Urol., 72:729–730, 1954.

91. Smith, B.H., and Dehner, L.P.: Sarcoma of the prostate gland. Am. J. Clin. Pathol., 58:43, 1972.

92. Stenram, U., and Holby, L-E.: A case of circumscribed myosarcoma of the prostate. Cancer, 24:803–806, 1969.

93. Stirling, W.C., and Ash, J.E.: Sarcoma of the prostate. J. Urol., 41:515–533, 1939.

94. Torres, L.F., Estrada, J.Y., and Esquivel, E.L., Jr.: Sarcoma of the prostate gland. J. Urol., 96:380–384, 1966.

Prostatic Calculi

95. Cristol, D.S., and Emmett, J.L.: The incidence of coincident prostatic calculi, prostatic hyperplasia and carcinoma of the prostate gland. J.A.M.A., 124:646, 1944.

96. Fox, M.: The association of stones in the upper urinary tract with prostatic calculi. Br. J. Urol., 32:458–463, 1960.

97. Gentile, A.: True prostatic calculus. J. Urol., 57:746–752, 1947.

98. Hinman, F.: Principles and Practice of Urology. Philadelphia, Saunders, 1935.

99. Huggins, C., and Bear, R.S.: The course of the prostatic ducts and the anatomy, chemical and x-ray diffraction analysis of prostatic calculi. J. Urol., 51:37–47, 1944.

100. Joly, J.S.: Stone and Calculus Disease of the Urinary Organs. St. Louis, Mosby, 1931.

101. Judd, E.S., and Crenshaw, J.L.: Prostatic calculi. Minnesota Med., 2:52–56, 1919.

102. Kretschmer, H.L.: True prostatic calculi: 76 cases. Surg. Gynecol. Obstet., 44:163–168, 1927.

103. Leader, A.J.: Prostatic calculi. South. Med. J., 51:600–604, 1958.

104. Leader, A.J., and Queen, D.M.: Prostatic calculous disease. Trans. South Cent. Sect. Am. Urol. Assoc., pp. 21–29, 1957.

105. Leader, A.J.: Prostatic calculous disease. J. Urol., 80:142–146, 1958.

106. Lund, H.G., and Cordonnier, J.J.: The incidence of prostatic calculi and the relationship of infection and carcinoma. Trans. South Cent. Sect. Am. Urol. Assoc., pp. 54–58, 1954.

107. Moore, R.A., and Hanzel, R.F.: Chemical composition of prostatic corpora amylacea and calculi. Arch. Path., 22:41–54, 1936.

108. Thomas, B.A., and Robert, J.T.: Prostatic calculi. J. Urol., 18:470–493, 1927.

109. Thompson, H.: The Diseases of the Prostate. ed. 4, pp. 308–325. Philadelphia, Henry C. Lea, 1873.

110. Young, H.H.: Prostatic calculi. J. Urol., 32:660–709, 1934.

Acute Prostatitis

111. Beard, D.E., Goodyear, W.E., and Weens, H.S.: Radiologic Diagnosis of the Lower Urinary Tract. p. 53, fig. 81. Springfield, Ill., Thomas, 1952.

112. Morrisseau, P.M., Phillips, C.A., and Leadbetter, G.W., Jr.: Viral prostatitis. J. Urol., 103:767–769, 1970.

Prostatic Abscess

113. Ball, W.G.: Metastatic staphylococcal prostatic abscesses. Br. J. Urol., 3:172–176, 1931.

114. Becker, L.E., and Harrin, W.R.: Prostatic abscess: a diagnostic and therapeutic approach. J. Urol., 91:582–585, 1964.

115. Bruce, A.W., and Fox, M.: Acute infection of the prostate gland. Br. J. Urol., 32:302–305, 1960.

116. Bugbee, H.G.: Infection of the genito-urinary tract complicating influenza. J.A.M.A., 73:1053–1056, 1919.

117. Chitty, K.: Prostatic abscess. Br. J. Surg., 44:599–602, 1957.

118. Dejani, A.M., and O'Flynn, J.D.: Prostate abscesses: a report of 25 cases. Br. J. Urol., 40:736–739, 1968.

119. Forsyth, W.E.: Prostatic abscess with particular reference to the use of the urethrogram in diagnosis. Urol. Cutan. Rev., 46:613–617, 1942.

120. Fox, C.P.: Gonorrheal prostatic abscess in a four year old boy. J.A.M.A., 103:748–749, 1934.

121. George, P.A.: Case of prostatic abscess in early infancy, Great Ormond St. J., pp. 58–60, 1953.

122. Herman, L., and Carp, J.: Prostatic abscess. Ann. Surg., 81:1115–1132, 1925.

123. Heyman, A., and Lombardo, L.J., Jr.: Metastatic prostate abscess with report of a case on a newborn infant. J. Urol., 87:174–177, 1962.

124. Jameson, R.M.: Prostatic abscess and carcinoma of the prostate. Br. J. Urol., 40:285–292, 1968.

125. Kickham, C.J.C.: Metastatic prostatic abscess. Urol. Cutan. Rev., 42:806–807, 1938.

126. Klotz, P.G.: Recent experience with abscess of the prostate. Can. J. Surg., 2:381–389, 1939.

127. Kretschmer, H.L.: Abscess of the prostate. Surg. Gynecol. Obstet., 32:259–268, 1921.

128. Last, S.F.: Non-specific prostatic abscess with an interesting prostatogram. Urol. Cutan. Rev., 43:206–209, 1939.

129. Lowsley, O.J.: Abscess of the prostate and seminal vesicle. Am. J. Surg., 46:662–668, 1939.

130. Mitchell, R.J., and Blake, J.R.S.: Spontaneous perforation of prostatic abscess with peritonitis. J. Urol., 107:622–623, 1972.

131. Persky, L., Austen, G., Jr., and Schatten, W.E.: Recent experience with prostatic abscess. Surg. Gynecol. Obstet., 101:629–633, 1955.

132. Sargent, J.C., and Irwin, R.: Prostatic abscess: clinical study of 42 cases. Am. J. Surg., 11:334–337, 1931.

133. Schwartz, J.: Metastatic abscess of the prostate. J. Urol., 43:108–115, 1940.

134. Szenkier, D.: Ein Prostataabzess bei einem zweieinhalbjährigen Knaben. Z. Urol., 23:119–121, 1929.

135. Thompson, G.J.: Chronic abscess of the prostate gland. Am. J. Surg., 38:96–100, 1937.

136. Trapnell, J., and Roberts, M.: Prostatic abscess. Br. J. Surg., 57:565–569, 1970.

Chronic Prostatitis

137. Ablin, R.J., Soanes, W.A., Benson, P., and Witebsky, E.: Precipitating antigens of the normal human prostate. J. Reprod. Fertil., 22:573–574, 1970.
138. Barnes, R.W.: Congested prostate and vesicles. Urol. Cutan. Rev., 33:661–665, 1929.
139. Barnes, R.W.: Experimental study of pharmacology of prostatic fluid. J. Urol., 42:1207–1216, 1939.
140. Barnes, K.W.: Toxic hyperplasia of prostate gland. J. Urol., 35:70–74, 1936.
141. Beilin, L.M.: Prostatic massage, facts and fallacies. Illinois Med. J., 62:164–169, 1932.
142. Buchert, W.I.: Chronic prostatitis in man past fifty. Penn. Med. J., 46:910–914, 1943.
143. Calams, J.A.: Histopathologic search for chronic seminal vesiculitis. J. Urol., 74:638–645, 1955.
144. Cummings, R.E., and Chittenden, G.E.: Pyogenic prostatitis. J. Urol., 39:118–122, 1938.
145. Delzell and Lowsley, quoted by Alyea, E.P. In Campbell, M.F.: Principles of Urology. ed. 2, vol. 1, p. 644. Philadelphia, Saunders, 1954.
146. Gardner, L.W.: Bacteriology of chronic prostatoseminal vesiculitis. Urol. Cutan. Rev., 44:278–281, 1940.
147. Hofstetter, A., and Schmidt, E.: Die abakterielle Prostatourethritis. Urologie, 11:80–81, 1972.
148. Leader, A.J.: Chronic vesiculo-prostatitis; a reorientation. J.A.M.A., 168:995–999, 1958.
149. Matilla, S.: Further studies on the prostatic tissue antigens. Separation of 2 molecular forms of amino-peptidase. Invest. Urol., 7:1–9, 1969.
150. Meares, E.M., Jr.: Bacterial prostatitis vs prostatism—a clinical and bacteriological study. J.A.M.A., 224:1372–1375, 1973.
151. Meares, E.M., Jr., and Stamey, T.A.: The diagnosis and management of bacterial prostatitis. Br. J. Urol., 44:175–179, 1972.
152. Moore, R.A.: Inflammation of prostate gland. J. Urol., 38:173–182, 1937.
153. Murnaghan, G.F., Tynan, A.P., Farnsworth, R.H., and Harvey, K.: Chronic prostatitis—an Australian view. Br. J. Urol., 46:55–59, 1974.
154. Nielsen, M.L., Asnaes, S., and Hattel, T.: Inflammatory changes in the noninfected prostate gland. A clinical, microbiological and histological investigation. J. Urol., 110:423–426, 1973.
155. Nielsen, M.L., and Vestergaard, B.F.: Virological investigation in chronic prostatitis. J. Urol., 109:1023–1025, 1973.
156. O'Shaughnessy, E.J., Parrino, P.S., and White, J.O.: Chronic prostatitis: fact or fiction? J.A.M.A., 160:540–542, 1956.
157. Ritter, J.S., and Lippow, C.: Symposium on pyogenic prostatitis: pathological and bacteriological processes present in prostatitis and tissue reaction to therapy. J. Urol., 39:111–117, 1938.
158. Robbins, S.L.: Textbook of Pathology with Clinical Application. pp. 993–994. Philadelphia, Saunders, 1957.
159. Schmidt, J.D., and Patterson, M.: Needle biopsy study of chronic prostatitis. J. Urol., 96:519–533, 1966.
160. Smith, R.L.: Non-specific prostatitis. Urol. Cutan. Rev., 38:469–470, 1934.
161. Stamey, T.A., and Pfau, A.: Urinary infections: a selective review and some observations. Calif. Med., 113:16–35, 1970.
162. Young, H.H.: Practice of Urology, Philadelphia, Saunders, 1926.

Granulomatous Prostatitis

163. Ablin, R.J., Soanes, W.A., and Gonder, M.J.: Immunologic studies of the prostate. A review. Int. Surg., 52:8–21, 1969.
164. Attah, E.B.: Non-specific inflammatory lesions of the prostate. Intern. Surg., 60:158–162, 1972.
165. Brown, H.E.: Granulomatous prostatitis: its clinical significance. J. Urol., 105:549–551, 1971.
166. Buddington, W.T.: Granulomatous prostatitis. J. Urol., 84:147–150, 1960.
167. Burckhardt, W., and Kartagener, M.: Fluchtige eosinophile Lungen-infiltrate beim fluchtiger eosinophiler (?) Epididymitis und Prostatitis. Schweiz Med. Wochenschr., 73:1550–1552, 1943.
168. Delaney, W.E., Burros, H.M., and Bhisitkul, I.: Eosinophilic granulomatous prostatitis simulating carcinoma. J. Urol., 87:169–173, 1962.
169. Dourov, N., and Sauvage, R.: Prostatic granulomateuse. Acta Urol. Belg., 35:412–419, 1967.
170. Dreyfuss, M.L., Simon, S., and Sommer, R.I.: Granulomatous prostatitis due to cryptococcus neoformans (Torula) with disseminated cryptococcosis and meningitis. N.Y. State J. Med., 61:1589–1592, 1961.
171. Epstein, W.L.: Granulomatous hypersensitivity. Progr. Allergy, 11:36–88, 1967.
172. Fox, H.: Nodular histocytic prostatitis. J. Urol., 96:372–374, 1966.
173. Goldman, R.L.: A case of malacoplakia with involvement of the prostate gland. J. Urol., 93:407–410, 1965.
174. Grimble, A., and Lessof, M.H.: Anti-prostate antibodies in arthritis. Br. Med. J., 2:263–264, 1965.
175. Gritti, E.J., Cook, F.E., Jr., and Spencer, H.B.: Coccidiodomycosis granuloma of the prostate: a rare manifestation of the disseminated disease. J. Urol., 89:249–252, 1963.
176. Gulianti, G.C., and Padocan, Q.: La prostatite granulomatosa aspecifica. Riv. Pathol. Clin. Sper., 6:19–44, 1965.
177. Harrison, F.G., and Neander, D.G.: Allergic granuloma of the prostate. J. Urol., 72:1218–1221, 1954.
178. Hoffman, E., and Garrido, M.: Malakoplakia of the prostate. Report of a case. J. Urol., 92:311–313, 1964.
179. Jacobs, T.P., and Garret, R.: Sinusitis, nodules in lungs, and hard prostate (CPC), N.Y. State J. Med., 65:2808–2815, 1965.
180. Kelalis, P.P., Greene, L.F., and Weed, L.A.: Brucellosis of the urogenital tract: a mimic of tuberculosis. J. Urol., 88:347–353, 1962.
181. Kelalis, P.P., Greene, L.F., and Harrison, E.G., Jr.: Granulomatous prostatitis: a mimic of carcinoma of the prostate. J.A.M.A., 191:287–289, 1965.
182. Kelalis, P.P., Harrison, E.G., Jr., and Greene, L.F.: Allergic granulomas of the prostate in asthmatics. J.A.M.A., 188:963–967, 1964.
183. Kelalis, P.P., Harrison, E.G., Jr., and Utz, D.C.: Allergic granulomas of the prostate: treatment with steroids. J. Urol., 96:573–577, 1966.
184. Malatinsky, E., et al.: Granulomatous prostatitis. Int. Urol. Nephrol., 4:179–181, 1972.
185. Melicow, M.M.: Allergic granulomas of the prostate gland. J. Urol., 65:288–296, 1951.
186. Miller, G., Bonenfant, J.L., and Coulonval, L.: La prostatite a eosinophiles. J. Urol. Nephrol. (Paris), 69:461–466, 1963.
187. Moore, M., and Halpern, L.K.: Blastomycosis involving the prostate: report of two cases. J. Urol., 60:612–622, 1948.

188. Moore, R.A.: Tuberculosis of the prostate gland. J. Urol., 37:372–384, 1937.
189. Nickey, W.M., and Montgomery, P.O.: Eosinophilic granulomatous prostatitis. J. Urol., 75:731–733, 1956.
190. Richards, H.G.H., and Rubin, J.: Eosinophilic granuloma of the prostate. Br. J. Urol., 30:70–73, 1958.
191. Sanchez-Lucas, J.G., Moragas, R.A.: Granulomatous giant cell prostatitis and eosinophilic granuloma of the prostate. Med. Clin. (Barc.), 43:229–234, 1964.
192. Schmidt, J.D.: Non-specific granulomatous prostatitis: classification, review and report of cases. J. Urol., 94:607–615, 1965.
193. Stewart, M.J., Wray, S., and Hall, M.: Allergic prostatitis in asthmatics. J. Pathol. Bacteriol., 57:423–430, 1954.
194. Symmers, W.: Non-specific granulomatous prostatitis. Br. J. Urol., 22:6–20, 1950.
195. Symmers, W.S.C.: Two cases of eosinophilic prostatitis due to metazoan infestation (with Oxyuris vermicularis, and with a larva of Linguatula serrata). J. Pathol. Bacteriol., 73:549–555, 1957.
196. Tanner, F.H., and McDonald, J.R.: Granulomatous prostatitis. A histologic study of granulomatous lesions collected from prostate glands. Arch. Pathol., 36:358–370, 1943.
197. Thompson, G.J., Albers, D.D.: Granulomatous prostatitis: a condition which clinically may be confused with cancer of prostate. J. Urol., 691:530–538, 1953.
198. Thompson, L.: Syphilis of the prostate. Am. J. Syphilis, 4:323–341, 1920.
199. Thybu, E., et al.: Granulomatous prostatitis. Scand. J. Urol. Nephrol., 7:111–114, 1973.
200. Towfighi, J., Sadeghee, S., Wheeler, J.F., and Enterline, H.T.: Granulomatous prostatitis with emphasis on the eosinophilic variety. Am. J. Clin. Pathol., 58:630–641, 1972.
201. Van De Pool, D.E., and De Ruiter, H.J.: Eosinophile granulomatous prostatitis. Arch. Chir. Neerl., 11:381–384, 1959.
202. Vondra, N.: Über die Rolle der eosinophilen Zellen bei den Erkrankungen der Prostata, mit besonderer Berucksichtigung ihrer Entzundungen. Z. Urol. Chir. Gynak., 44:357–362, 1938.
203. Yalowitz, P.A., Greene, L.F., Sheps, S.G., et al.: Wegener's granulomatosis involving the prostate gland: report of a case. J. Urol., 96:901–904, 1966.
204. Yamamoto, C.: Studies of non-gonococcal urethritis. Jap. J. Urol., 55:1223–1239, 1964.

Tuberculosis of the Prostate Gland

205. Barney, J.D.: In Cabot, H. (ed.): Modern Urology. vol. 1, p. 532. Philadelphia, Lea & Febiger, 1924.
206. Lattimer, J.K.: Tuberculous prostatic urethritis: a suggestive diagnostic sign. J. Urol., 59:326–327, 1948.
207. May, P., Hohenfellner, R., König, E., and König, K.: Diagnostik und Therapie der Prostata tuberkulose. Urol. Int., 21:329–337, 1966.
208. Medlar, E.M., Spain, D.M., and Holliday, R.W.: Post-mortem compared with clinical diagnosis of genito-urinary tuberculosis in adult males. J. Urol., 61:1078–1088, 1949.
209. Moore, R.A.: Tuberculosis of the prostate gland. J. Urol., 37:372–384, 1937.
210. Thomas, G.J., Stebbins, T.L., and Rigos, F.J.: Genital tuberculosis. Minnesota Med., 23:318–322, 1940.
211. Young, H.H.: A radical cure of tuberculosis of the seminal tract: brief survey of literature. Arch. Surg., 4:334–419, 1922.

Prostatic Cysts

212. Dees, J.E.: Congenital cyst of prostate communicating with right vas and rudimentary right ureter; case report. J. Urol., 57:304–309, 1947.
213. Emmett, J.L., and Braasch, W.F.: Cysts of prostate gland. J. Urol., 36:236–249, 1936.
213a. Fischelovitch, J., Meiraz, D., and Lazebnik, J.: Cysts of the prostate. Br. J. Urol., 47:687–689, 1975.
214. Huggins, C.B.: Syndrome of diverticulum of spermatic system in neighborhood of prostate, obstructing neck of urinary bladder. J. Urol., 24:100–111, 1930.
215. Kirkland, L.L., and Bale, P.M.: A cystic adenoma of the prostate. J. Urol., 97:324–327, 1967.
216. Magri, J.: Cysts of the prostate gland. Br. J. Urol., 32:295–301, 1960.
217. Melen, D.R.: Multilocular cyst of the prostate. J. Urol., 27:343–349, 1932.
218. Reiser, C., and Griffin, T.L.: Cysts of the prostate. J. Urol., 91:282–286, 1964.
219. Roberts, F.W.: Cysts of prostate gland with congenital absence of right kidney. Am. J. Surg., 4:221–222, 1928.
220. Way, R.A., and Popper, H.: Four urologic anomalies in one person. J. Urol., 55:454–459, 1946.

Leukemic Infiltration of Prostate

221. Butler, M.R., and O'Flynn, J.D.: Prostatic disease in the leukemic patient with particular reference to leukemic infiltration of the prostate—a retrospective clinical study. Br. J. Urol., 45:179–183, 1973.
222. Connor, J.J., Heinemann, S., and MacNish, J.M.: Prostatism complicated by chronic lymphatic leukemia. Urol. Cutan. Rev., 54:276–279, 1950.
223. Entz, F.H., and Kruse, R.F.: Complete retention of urine due to leukemic infiltration of the prostate. J. Urol., 86:127–129, 1961.
224. Fishman, A., and Taylor, W.N.: Leukemic infiltration of the prostate. J. Urol., 89:65–72, 1963.
225. Flaherty, S.A., Cope, H.E., and Shecket, H.A.: Prostatic obstruction as the presenting symptom of acute monocytic leukemia. J. Urol., 44:488–497, 1940.
226. Hare, D.M., Spence, H.M., and Fuqua, F.: Leukemic infiltration of the prostate. J. Urol., 62:845–848, 1949.
227. Jacobi, M., Panoff, C.E., and Herzlich, J.: Leukemic infiltration of the prostate. J. Urol., 38:494–499, 1937.
228. Johnson, N.A., and Gondersen, A.H.: Infiltration of the prostate by chronic lymphatic leukemia. J. Urol., 69:681–685, 1953.
229. Lubin, E.N., Fetter, T.R., and Erf, L.A.: Subacute monocytic leukemia presenting symptoms of prostatism: a case report. J. Urol., 58:272–276, 1947.
230. McCrea, L.E.: Leukemic infiltration of the prostate. Urol. Cutan. Rev., 44:694–696, 1940.
231. Meyer, L.M.: Pathology of the genito-urinary tract in leukemia. Urol. Cutan. Rev., 40:693–695, 1941.
232. O'Flynn, J.O.: Leukemic infiltration of the prostate. Urol. Digest., 5:15–17, 1966.
233. Tighe, J.R.: Leukemic infiltration of the prostate. Br. J. Urol., 47:658–660, 1960.
234. Vinnicombe, J.: Leukemic infiltration of the prostate. Br. J. Urol., 35:297–298, 1963.

Amyloid of the Prostate

235. Wilson, S.K., Buchanon, R.D., Stone, W.J., and Rhamy, R.K.: Amyloid deposition in the prostate. J. Urol., *110*:322–323, 1973.

Angiography of the Prostate

236. Binder, S.S., and Mitchell, G.A.: The control of the retractable pelvic hemorrhage of ligation of the lymphatic artery. South. Med. J., *53*:837–843, 1960.
237. Lapides, J.: Principles of treatment of persistent postprostatectomy hemorrhage. J. Urol., *106*:913–914, 1971.
238. Mitchell, M.B., Waltman, A.C., Athanasoulis, C.A., Kerr, W.S., Jr., and Dretler, S.P.: Control of massive prostatic bleeding using angiographic technique. Presented at Amer. Urol. Assn. Meeting, Miami Beach, Fla., May 15, 1975.

Prostatic Infarction

239. Abeshouse, B.S.: Infarct of the prostate. J. Urol., *30*:97–112, 1933.
240. Baird, H.H., McKay, H.W., and Kimmelstiel, P.: Ischemic infarction of the prostate gland. South. Med. J., *43*:234–240, 1950.
241. Hubly, J.W., and Thompson, G.J.: Infarction of the prostate: the clinical significance. Mayo Clin. Proc., *13*:401–403, 1938.
242. Hubly, J.W., and Thompson, G.J.: Infarction of the prostate gland and volumetric changes produced by the lesion: report of 3 cases. J. Urol., *43*:459–467, 1940.

243. Rogers, W.G.: Infarct of the prostate. J. Urol., *57*:484–487, 1947.
244. Roth, R.B.: Prostatic infarction. J. Urol., *62*:474–479, 1949.
245. Spiro, L.H., Labay, G., and Orkin, L.A.: Prostatic infarction. Role in acute urinary retention. Urology, *3*:345–347, 1974.

Ultrasonography and CT of the Prostate

246. Henneberry, M., Carter, M.F., and Neiman, H.L.: Estimations of prostatic size by suprapubic ultrasonography. J. Urol., *121*:615–617, 1979.
247. Hohn, H.H., and Northeved, A.: A Transurethral Ultrasonic Scanner. J. Urol., *111*:238–241, 1974.
248. King, W.W., Wilkiemeyer, R.M., and Boyce, W.H. et al.: Current status of prostatic echography. J.A.M.A., *226*:444–447, 1973.
249. Resnick, M.L., Willard, J.W., and Boyce, W.H.: Recent progress in ultrasonography of the bladder and prostate. J. Urol., *117*:444–446, 1977.
250. Sukov, R.J., Scardino, P.T., and Sample, W.F. et al.: Computed tomography and transabdominal ultrasound in the evaluation of the prostate. J. Comp. Assist. Tomography, *1*:281–289, 1977.
251. Watanabe, H., Igari, D., and Tanahashi, Y. et al.: Transrectal Ultrasonotomography of the prostate. J. Urol., *114*:734–739, 1975.
252. Whittingham, T.A., and Bishor, R.: Ultrasonic estimation of the volume of the enlarged prostate. Br. J. Radiol., *46*:68–70, 1973.

ANATOMY OF THE MALE GENITAL TRACT

The epididymis consists of a head, a body, and a tail. The head (globus major) is somewhat enlarged because of the 15 or 20 ductuli efferentes that are convoluted at this area, forming conical masses called "coni vasculosi." Each cone consists of a convoluted duct that opens, along with the others, into a single duct. The single duct by complex convolutions constitutes the body and the tail of the epididymis. The tail (globus minor) is continuous with the vas deferens.

The vas deferens is a thick-walled fibromuscular tube that extends from the globus minor of the epididymis to the ejaculatory duct. Beginning at its origin from the globus minor, the vas deferens is convoluted for a distance of 2 to 4 cm., but it quickly becomes a straight tube and extends upward in the posterior portion of the spermatic cord, traversing the inguinal canal. At the internal ring it separates from the other constituents of the cord, turns sharply posteriorly around the deep epigastric vessels, and ascends for a short distance in front of the external iliac artery. It then goes backward and slightly downward, crosses the external iliac vessels, and enters the pelvic cavity. Here it lies between the peritoneum and the lateral wall of the pelvis. It descends on the medial side of the obturator nerves and vessels and then crosses in front of the ureter to reach its medial side, where it bends acutely laterally behind the ureter and then again turns medially, passing between the fundus of the bladder and the upper medial edge of the seminal vesicle. In the vicinity of the trigone of the urinary bladder, and shortly before reaching the prostate, the vas undergoes a slight spindle-shaped dilatation to form the ampulla of the vas deferens. The ampulla gradually narrows, becomes more even again, and joins

35

Seminal Vesicles, Vas Deferens, and Epididymis

the excretory duct of the seminal vesicle to form the ejaculatory duct. The ductus deferens is 30 to 40 cm. long and 2 to 3 mm. thick, with a lumen having a diameter of about 0.5 mm. (0.16 mm., according to Bereira[14]; 0.85, Brueschke and co-workers[2]; and 0.55, Hulka and associates[8]).

The ampulla is 3 to 5 cm. long and 0.4 to 0.6 cm. thick, with a lumen approximately 0.8 to 1 mm. in diameter. It is a tortuous structure with multiple irregular recesses, giving the appearance of serrated margins.

The seminal vesicles are a pair of convoluted organs lying at the base of the bladder. Each seminal vesicle is about 4 to 6 cm. long and 8 to 12 mm. thick, with a lumen of about 0.5 cm. in diameter. Each vesicle has from 10 to 12 convolutions of uniform breadth and density. Usually, the seminal vesicles are set at an angle of 50° to 60° with the horizontal, and their upper ends or bases are approximately 7 to 8 cm. apart. The seminal duct is short and has a lumen of 1.5 mm. in diameter.

The ejaculatory duct is formed by a union of the vas deferens and a duct of the seminal vesicle. This juncture takes place at the upper surface or within the substance of the prostate. The ejaculatory ducts traverse about two-thirds of the gland, beginning at the posterior lateral aspects of the base at each side and opening into the urethra at each side of the prostatic utricle. The ejaculatory duct has a length of approximately 1.5 cm. and a lumen of 1.5 mm. in diameter. However, it gradually narrows, and at its orifice the diameter is about 0.5 mm. The outlines of the ejaculatory ducts are generally smooth and even, but there may be interruptions by five to seven circular folds projecting slightly into the lumen. The male genital tract is shown diagrammatically in Figure 35–1.

USE OF ROENTGENOLOGY

Roentgenology of the genital tract has not received widespread or extensive acceptance in the past, probably because of the limited diagnostic value considered attainable by its use. Seminal vesiculography has been performed in cases of infections of the seminal vesicles, in which it was combined with therapeutic drainage (by catheterization of the ejaculatory ducts), and in cases of sterility, when azoospermia was associated with spermatogenesis, to determine the point of occlusion (see Figs. 35–55, 35–56*A, B*).

More recently it has been used in the differentiation of benign prostatic hypertrophy and carcinoma of the prostate, in the diagnosis of secondary involvement of the seminal vesicles by other tumors, such as carcinoma of the bladder and the rectum, and in the visualization of cysts and tumors of the seminal vesicles.

SEMINAL VESICULOGRAPHY

Seminal vesiculography, or visualization of the seminal vesicles by injection of a contrast material, generally includes visualization of the ejaculatory ducts, the seminal ducts, the seminal vesicles, the ampullae, and the vasa deferentia.

TWO ACCEPTED METHODS

There are two accepted methods for performing seminal vesiculography:

1. *The ejaculatory ducts* may be catheterized from the urethral side by special catheters, usually No. 4 French with gold tips (but these are not essential). This catheterization may be performed either with a McCarthy instrument through a McCarthy endoscopic sheath or with the Lowsley-Peterson endoscope. Generally, the ducts are catheterized alternately, the catheter being withdrawn from one side before entering the opposite duct, although both ducts can be catheterized at the same time. Most investigators inject 1.5 to 5 ml. of contrast material (Diodrast, Hypaque, Renografin, iodized oil).

2. *The vas deferens* can be exposed by making a small incision in the scrotum, isolated and injected by one of several methods. The needle can be passed directly into the vas lumen without making an incision into the vas, or the vas can be incised either longitudinally or transversely and a needle or a polyethylene tube passed into the lumen, followed by the injection of contrast material.

There are advantages and disadvantages to each method. *Advantages* of the catheterization of the ejaculatory ducts include the following:

1. The passage of a catheter through the ejaculatory ducts has been used as a method of treatment in cases in which drainage has been necessary or dilatation of the ejaculatory duct has been required.
2. The vas is not opened by incision, and therefore there is less chance of stricture formation.
3. There is somewhat less chance of reflux into the bladder, and therefore there is less probability of obscuring the seminal vesicles.

Disadvantages of this method are as follows:

1. It is much more difficult to perform.
2. There is more chance of failure.
3. There is a greater percentage of epididymitis. Peterson believes that he eliminated this com-

plication by having the patient eliminate the seminal contents by ejaculation shortly after the procedure.[15]

Advantages of the scrotal incision method are the following:

1. It is easier to perform.
2. There is great chance of success.
3. Both sides can be injected simultaneously much more readily.
4. There is less chance of infection.

Disadvantages are as follows:

1. There is danger of injury to the vas, causing stricture formation.
2. There is greater chance of contrast material entering the posterior urethra and flowing into the bladder, thus obscuring the seminal vesicles.

NORMAL VESICULOGRAM

The normal seminal vesiculogram (Figs. 35–2, 35–3) shows 10 to 12 convolutions of uniform breadth and density. The gland has an oval or pyriform outline. The proximal portion appears to be slightly wider than the distal; however, Herbst and Merricks believe that the middle portion is the widest.[5] The physiologically distended seminal vesicles (Figs. 35–6, 35–7) present similar patterns to the normal, except that the convolutions are wider and the entire shadow may appear to be somewhat larger. There is some difference of opinion in the literature about whether physiologically distended glands filled with mucous secretion can be visualized clearly.

The vas deferens joins the seminal duct at an angle of 30° or greater to form the ejaculatory duct. In most cases the ejaculatory duct is in direct line with the vas deferens (Fig. 35–4, *A*), although the vas and the seminal duct may join dichotomously (Fig. 35–4, *B*) to form the ejaculatory duct. The ejaculatory duct and the seminal ducts are straight and well defined.

Isolated occlusions of the seminal ducts, either unilateral or bilateral, may occur secondary to infection (Fig. 35–5). Carcinoma of the prostate invading seminal vesicles does occlude these ducts but not as an isolated phenomenon.

IMPORTANT AFFECTIONS OF THE SEMINAL VESICLES

These are nonspecific seminal vesiculitis, gonococcal vesiculitis, tuberculosis of the seminal vesicles, calculi in the seminal vesicles, calcification of the seminal vesicles, cysts of seminal vesicles, benign tumors of the seminal vesicles, primary carcinoma of the seminal vesicles, sarcoma of the seminal vesicles, and secondary carcinoma of the seminal vesicles.

TYPES AND SUBDIVISIONS OF INFLAMMATORY DISEASES

Peterson has given a detailed description and classification of inflammatory diseases of the seminal vesicles.[15] In most of his cases nonspecific organisms predominated; however, it should be emphasized that, although in many instances the gonococcus may have been the primary organism, sooner or later secondary infection superseded it.

Peterson believes that the more severe pathologic changes were caused by nonspecific organisms.[15] He described two types: (1) the catarrhal and (2) the interstitial, each of which was subdivided into early, intermediate, and late stages.

Catarrhal Type. This is seen more frequently following nonvirulent infections, both specific and nonspecific.

EARLY CATARRHAL TYPE. The gland is well visualized and has excellent diffusion of the contrast material. The vesicle is somewhat distended, and its upper margin is raised close to or above the ampulla and the vas deferens, thus reducing the vesiculoampullar space. The capsule is intact (Fig. 35–8).

INTERMEDIATE CATARRHAL TYPE. There is definite dilatation of the terminal tubule or distal half of the vesicle, whereas the proximal portion appears to be normal. There may be disruption of the vesicular capsule at the point of dilatation. The terminal pole is raised to or above the level of the vas deferens (Figs. 35–9, 35–10).

LATE CATARRHAL TYPE. This presents dilatation of the entire gland and straightening of the convolutions. The organ resembles either a tortuous hydroureter or a row of circular or oval cavities (pyovesiculosis). The terminal pole rises high above the level of the vas and close to the ureter (Figs. 35–11 to 35–13).

Interstitial Type. This is the result of gonococcal infection or sudden mechanical closure of the duct.

EARLY INTERSTITIAL TYPE. There are few circular or spiral convolutions with localized distention and beginning obliteration of peripheral lumina (Fig. 35-14).

INTERMEDIATE INTERSTITIAL TYPE. This presents elongated and narrow tubular shadows with shallow, wavy convolutions (this type often has been confused with the normal) (Figs. 35-15, 35-16).

LATE INTERSTITIAL TYPE. This reveals a few irregular cavities that appear to be detached (Fig. 35-17).

In general, infection of the seminal vesicles affects the terminal part of the gland earlier and more severely than the proximal part of the gland. The ejaculatory ducts apparently are not affected early, but in the late stages they may develop strictures.

TUBERCULOSIS OF THE SEMINAL VESICLES

Tuberculosis produces much more destruction of the seminal vesicles than do the other inflammatory diseases. According to Auerbach, the disease may be bilateral or unilateral, the former being more common.[23] When it is unilateral, there is a predilection for the right side. The disease can be separated into interstitial and intracanalicular types, but in the late stages they are indistinguishable. Early there is a yellow exudate within the lumen and a slight increase in the thickness of the wall. Later there is dilatation, with the cavities filled with caseous material. The caseation extends outward, the seminal vesicles enlarge, and liquefaction of caseous material occurs. With further progression the partitions between the cavities break down, forming large, irregular communications with other portions of the seminal vesicles and also with similar cavities in the prostate. As healing occurs, there is an increasing firmness of the caseous material, followed by encasement with fibrous tissues and at times impregnation with calcium salts. An infrequent complication is rupture of a tubercular process of the seminal vesicles into the periprostatic spaces, the bladder, the urethra, or the rectum.

ROENTGENOGRAPHIC APPEARANCE

Tuberculosis of the seminal vesicles (Figs. 35-18 to 35-20) follows somewhat the course of other infections of the seminal vesicles but in a more severe form. The ejaculatory ducts first are dilated and later narrowed and obstructed. The seminal vesicles may become either more vertical or more horizontal, the former being the most common. At the onset, the peripheral portion of the glands is affected more severely than the proximal portion. There is disruption of the convolutions with areas of complete destruction. The convolutions actually become detached and irregularly dilated. The whole structure fills unevenly, and there may be destruction of the vesicular membrane. In the terminal stage, fibrosis may prevent contrast medium filling of the glands. Calcification occasionally is seen (see Figs. 35-24, 35-47).

CALCULI OF THE SEMINAL VESICLES

Calculi in the seminal vesicles are rare. They can vary in size from buckshot to cherrystone[31] and can be bilateral or unilateral (Fig. 35-21).

The scout film reveals a single calcification or multiple calcifications in the usual position of the seminal vesicles. Irregular small calcifications in the wall of the seminal vesicles may resemble calculi if they are not sufficiently linear in type. Occasionally, calculi in the upper part of an enlarged prostate can be confusing (Fig. 35-21).

CALCIFICATION OF THE SEMINAL VESICLES

Calcification of the seminal vesicles is an unusual phenomenon, one that rarely is reported in the literature. Most of the reports concern bilateral seminal vesicular calcification, although several cases of the unilateral variety have been reported. Calcification of the seminal vesicles has been seen in tuberculosis, schistosomiasis, diabetes, and nonspecific entities. Silber and McDonald reported calcification of the seminal vesicles and vas deferens in a uremic patient with secondary hyperparathyroidism.[47] There are certainly other nonspecific causes that have not been defined clearly. The calcification of the nonspecific variety (Fig. 35-22) usually involves the wall rather than the lumen, is more uniform, more dense, and better defined than the other types. This is similar to the diabetic type (Fig. 35-22a). The calcification in schistosomiasis (Fig. 35-23) also involves the wall and is mottled and lacy in appearance. It seems to involve the whole gland uniformly rather than being limited to one particular part. The calcification in tuberculosis (Figs. 35-24, 35-47) generally is rather limited, irregular, dense, and mottled. It rarely involves an entire gland and appears to be more intraluminal than the other types.

CONGENITAL ANOMALIES OF THE SEMINAL VESICLES

Congenital abnormalities of the seminal vesicles include (1) complete reduplication[67]; (2) absence (see vas deferens); (3) ectopia[58] (Fig. 35-25); (4) cysts (see below); (5) diverticula[67]; and (6) site of an ectopic ureteral opening (see congenital ureter).

ECTOPIA

There have been two cases of ectopia of the seminal vesicles reported, both associated with agenesis of the ipsilateral kidney (Fig. 35–25)[58, 65a] and one with an ectopic ureter entering the seminal vesicle.[65a]

CYSTS OF THE SEMINAL VESICLES

Cysts of the seminal vesicles (cystic seminal vesicles) are rare. They may represent localized dilatation of one or several convolutions or generalized dilatation of the entire gland. They usually are unilocular (Figs. 35–26, 35–28B), but the multilocular variety (Figs. 35–27, 35–28A) does occur.[51, 61, 62] The cysts may or may not be infected. Although most are unilateral, cases of the bilateral type (Fig. 35–28A, B) have been reported.[62, 71] This case was later diagnosed as neoplastic.

Seminal vesicle cysts are congenital or acquired. The congenital type has been associated with unilateral renal agenesis in many instances.[49, 52-56, 59, 60, 62, 65, 70, 73] The ureter and trigone on the same side may be absent,[54, 55, 62, 70] but a fibrous band[56] and a dilated blind-ending ureter[59] have been found. The acquired type is probably the result of partial or complete obstruction of the ejaculatory duct.

Symptoms of seminal vesicle cysts are dysuria, frequency of urination, difficult urination, perineal pain aggravated by defecation, and painful ejaculation. Hematospermia is rarely described.

Cystoscopically, the floor of the bladder may be elevated. The ureteral orifice on the affected side may be absent with unilateral trigone or impossible to visualize. The lower ureter on the affected side may be deviated medially.[61]

Roentgenographic diagnosis: Visualization by injection of the vas or ejaculatory duct is the preferred method, although direct puncture, suprapubically, transvesically, transrectally, or perineally, is a distinct possibility if the cyst is large. Spermatozoa are not necessarily found. The cyst is usually smooth-walled, regular, and unilocular. Rarely, a multilocular structure is discovered. Injection of the vas may reveal no drainage into the urethra, but catheterization of the ejaculatory duct may overcome an obstruction. An intravenous urogram should be performed to ascertain agenesis of the kidney.

BENIGN TUMORS OF THE SEMINAL VESICLES

Benign tumors of the seminal vesicles are extremely rare. These lesions for the most part contain smooth muscle and have been described under the terms leiomyoma,[75, 79] myoma,[82] fibromyoma,[76] cys-tomyoma,[80] fibroma, or cystadenoma.[78, 81] (Guelliot reported angiomas and lipomas.[77]) They are usually symptomless (hematospermia rarely occurs) and are discovered accidentally at autopsies, operations, or rectal examinations. Related structures appear to be displaced laterally, which substantiates to some extent the assumption that these tumors arise from the midportion of the müllerian duct and become manifest later in life. However, Bagley and co-workers reported a cyst containing a tumor, probably benign, which was considered mesonephric in origin (Fig. 35–29).[74]

Roentgenographic diagnosis: There are two few cases with seminal vesiculogram to describe the findings. Bagley's case, however, was a tumor within a cyst (Fig. 35–29).

PRIMARY CARCINOMA OF THE SEMINAL VESICLES

Primary carcinomas of the seminal vesicles are extremely unusual, and only a few of the cases reported have been proved with certainty to have arisen from that origin. By the time the tumor is discovered the seminal vesicles, prostate, and surrounding tissues are so involved that the exact origin is usually impossible to ascertain. However, the cytoplasmic finding of yellow-brown pigment or lipofuscin has been considered pathognomonic for seminal vesicular epithelium as opposed to prostatic origin.[105]

The tumors are predominantly adenocarcinoma, often papillary, although anaplastic and cuboidal cell lesions have been reported.

Carcinoma of the seminal vesicles occurs for the most part at 60 to 80 years of age. Symptoms resemble those of prostatic obstruction, often with hematuria; however, since benign prostatic hypertrophy has often been associated, it is difficult to ascribe these symptoms to the seminal vesicle lesion. Hematospermia and painful ejaculation are rarely noted. These tumors spread to neighboring regions, to viscera, and rarely to the bone, although osteolytic lesions have occurred. Carcinoma of the seminal vesicles appears to involve both vesicles,[109] but Awadella and co-workers reported a bilateral tumor that they considered to be two separate tumors arising simultaneously.[83] Massage of the tumor has produced neoplastic cells in urinary sediment.[101]

ROENTGENOGRAPHIC DIAGNOSIS

Cystogram. There may be an asymmetric upward displacement of the bladder floor. An actual defect can be visualized if the tumor has invaded the bladder.

Seminal Vesiculography. The seminal vesicle may be displaced medially and elevated; it may be irregularly elongated and dilated. Filling defects may be visualized (Figs. 35–30, 35–31).

Arteriography. This reveals irregular neoplastic vessels arising from superior and middle vesical branches with arteriovenous shunting (Fig. 35–32).[90]

SARCOMAS OF THE SEMINAL VESICLES

Primary sarcomas of the seminal vesicles are even rarer than carcinomas and possibly should be considered as primary malignant tumors of the rectovesical space, a concept postulated by Young.[111] Many of these cases have been small round cell sarcomas, but a fibrosarcoma,[75] a leiomyosarcoma,[110] a pleomorphic sarcoma,[109] and an alveolar cell sarcoma[108] have been reported.

SECONDARY CARCINOMA OF THE SEMINAL VESICLES

Secondary carcinoma of the seminal vesicles is nearly always an extension from the prostate (Figs. 35–33, 35–34, 35–40, 35–42), but it occasionally arises in the urinary bladder (Figs. 35–35, 35–41) or the rectum. The invasion is always from without inward, as the tumor spreads into the perivesicular tissue first.

The radiographic appearance of carcinoma of the prostate invading the seminal vesicles is as follows:

1. The ejaculatory ducts are narrowed, rigid, and of uniform size with decreased dilatability.
2. The invasion begins at the proximal part of the gland primarily, where there is a destructive process; there may be some dilatation of the terminal portion.
3. The affected seminal vesicles become more horizontal, and the vesiculo-ampullar angle seems to be depressed.
4. There is a tendency for the contrast material to go peripherally into the urethra, but this is not consistent. (For a comparison of the radiologic changes in carcinoma of the prostate and benign prostatic hypertrophy, see Chapter 34, The Prostate.)

In late cases there is obstruction of the ejaculatory ducts and the seminal duct, so that the seminal vesicles do not visualize. The vasa may be pushed to one side by asymmetric masses, as seen in Figure 35–40.

Carcinoma of the urinary bladder (Fig. 35–35) or the rectum invades the seminal vesicles by direct extension from the perivesicular tissue. Of course, it can invade at any point, but it appears to affect the terminal portion more frequently and more severely. The seminal vesicles are compressed, with destruction of the convolutions without terminal dilatation. The entire structure may appear to be depressed downward. The ejaculatory ducts rarely are affected. The entire picture could be confused with severe infection of the seminal vesicles, especially tuberculosis.

EFFECTS OF BENIGN PROSTATIC HYPERTROPHY ON EJACULATORY DUCTS AND SEMINAL VESICLES

In prostatic hypertrophy (Figs. 35–36, 35–37) the ejaculatory ducts usually are dilated to some extent. The dilatation appears to involve the whole duct, especially the middle and the lateral portions. The two ejaculatory ducts usually are symmetrically enlarged, but one side can be dilated greatly, whereas the other side is of nearly normal size. Usually, the dilatation of the ejaculatory ducts can be correlated with lateral lobe enlargement but not with median lobe enlargement. In general, the dilatation is greater on the side of the greater hypertrophy. The lumen of the ejaculatory duct usually is smooth and regular, even when there is marked dilatation.

Occasionally, the seminal vesicles are dilated secondary to the dilatation of the ejaculatory ducts. Vestby believes that the prostatic enlargement, especially of the lateral lobes, compresses the prostatic urethra from side to side, with compression and deformity of the verumontanum, which may hinder adequate drainage of the ejaculatory ducts.[122] He also states that, in obstruction of the posterior urethra by an enlarged prostate, there is hypertrophy of the trigonal muscle, whose contractile fibers arch around the ejaculatory ducts; tonic contractions of this muscle may compress the duct orifices.

Suprapubic prostatectomy does not necessarily injure the ejaculatory ducts. Figure 35–38 shows a seminal vesiculogram of a man who had a suprapubic prostatectomy four years previously. The ejaculatory ducts are patent, and contrast material outlines the prostatic cavity.

DISPLACEMENT OF THE SEMINAL VESICLES AND VASA DEFERENTIA

Displacement of the seminal vesicles and vasa deferentia may be produced by carcinoma of the prostate (Fig. 35–41), carcinoma of the bladder (Fig. 35–40), perivesicular abscess (Fig. 35–39), and possibly by other pelvic tumors. Congenital ectopia is rare (Fig. 35–25). The seminal vesicles and ampullary region of the vas are pushed medially and across the midline. The area between the inguinal vas and the ampulla is widened, and the pelvic portion may be elevated.

Carcinoma of the prostate is usually differentiated from other lesions, producing deviation on the basis of obliteration of the seminal or ejaculatory duct or both. Early deviation by invasion of carcinoma of the prostate, however, may occur without the diagnostic signs of obstruction to seminal duct and ejaculatory duct (Fig. 35–42). In these cases, the other criteria (see Secondary Carcinoma of Seminal Vesicles) must be recognized in order to make a diagnosis.

ANOMALIES OF THE VAS DEFERENS

Anomalies of the vas deferens include:

1. Absence (unilateral or bilateral)[124, 127-129, 131, 133, 134, 136, 138, 139, 142-149, 152]
2. Double[67, 125, 126, 130, 137, 141]
3. Incomplete duplication[151]
4. Separation from epididymis[185, 189, 190]
5. Diverticula[67]
6. Cysts[67, 132, 140]
7. Fistulization[135]
8. Direct attachment to ductuli efferentes
9. Fibrous strand, agenesis of short length, lack of canalization (normal external appearance), and a stump arising from the epididymal tract, all reported by Scorer and Farrington[189]

Absence of the vas deferens means absence of the body of epididymis, globus minor, vas deferens, seminal vesicle ampulla, and ejaculatory duct. These absent structures arise from mesonephric duct origin. A few instances of rudimentary[144] or cystic seminal vesicle[150] associated with absence of vas deferens have been reported. The globus major comprising ductuli efferentes, as well as epididymal duct, is present and continuous with the testis, as spermatozoa are found. Unilateral absence of the vas may be seen with absent kidney,[128, 134, 136, 145] ectopic kidney,[128] crossed ectopia,[138, 139] and pancake pelvic kidney.[128] Thus palpation of the cord for absent vas may lead to the diagnosis of kidney anomalies. There may be unilateral renal agenesis in bilateral absence of vasa deferentia.

Bilateral absence of the vas represents about 1.5 per cent of sterile men (13 per cent of obstructed aspermic men). Since the seminal vesicles are usually absent, there will be no fructose in the semen.[124]

Double vasa deferentia are extremely rare and may be associated with an absent ipsilateral kidney.[137, 141] It has been seen with polyorchidism.[130] Diverticula usually occur in the region of the ampulla. Cystic changes in the vas (Fig. 35–43) are probably congenital.

CALCIFICATION OF THE VAS DEFERENS

Calcification of the vas deferens is an unusual but not a rare condition, occurring most commonly in diabetics[178] (Figs. 35–22a, 35–45) but seen also in nondiabetics after inflammatory lesions such as nonspecific infection (Fig. 35–46), tuberculosis (Figs. 35–24, 35–47), gonorrhea, upper genitourinary infections, uremia with secondary hyperparathyroidism, and as a degenerative process (Figs. 35–22, 35–44).

The calcification usually occurs first in the intrapelvic segment medial to the ureters; it later often extends throughout the intra- and the extrapelvic portions of the vasa deferentia.

FORMS OF PATHOLOGIC INVOLVEMENT

There are two forms of pathologic involvement, the noninflammatory (diabetic and degenerative) and the inflammatory. The former has the calcification in the muscular elements of the vasa, and the lumens are widely patent. Culver and Tannenhaus have recognized three groups, varying in degree from faint or spotty calcification of one or both vasa deferentia, on one or both walls, to dense calcification of the vasa deferentia along the entire pelvic portions bilaterally.[158] However, the most usual form is a bilateral symmetric calcification (approximately 80 per cent of the cases), with an equal degree of density in nearly all cases.[178] At the most lateral portion of the calcification there may be a ring appearance due to the doubling over of the tube at its crossing of the ureter.

In the inflammatory form (Fig. 35–46) there may be either partial or complete thrombosis of the lumen of the vas deferens, with the result that the calcification is intraluminal. In this form the calcification is more likely to be unilateral than in the noninflammatory type.

CORRELATION

Culver and Tannenhaus found 11 cases of calcification of the vas deferens in 100 diabetics chosen at random.[158] They stated that there was no correlation between the duration and the severity of the diabetes and the degree of calcification of the vas deferens; furthermore, they said that there was no correlation between the degree of calcification of the vas and calcification of the pelvic arteries. However, Wilson and Marks stated that calcification of the vas apparently occurred much more quickly if the diabetes began after 40 years of age; in patients acquiring diabetes prior to 40, the disease usually had been present for 15 years before the calcification was noted.[178]

DIFFERENTIAL DIAGNOSIS

Differential diagnosis between calcification of the vas and calcification of an artery usually is not difficult. The intrapelvic portion of the vas deferens differs from that of any artery of the male pelvis in location and course. However, in the region of the obturator foramen, the internal pudendal arteries run the same course and must be differentiated from a calcified vas. Below the inguinal ring the testicular artery parallels the vas. In either case, if enough of the artery can be visualized, this differentiation should be comparatively easy.[178]

Differentiation between inflammatory and noninflammatory types of calcification should not be too difficult, but the calcification of the purely degenerative type may be impossible to separate from the calcification associated with diabetes.

TUMORS AND GRANULOMAS OF THE VAS DEFERENS

Tumors of the vas are rare. A ductal hyperplasia and a leiomyoma have been reported.[179, 181] Sperm granulomas of the vas—lesions peculiar to vasectomy—produce a tumor nodule in the area of the cut end of proximal vas and are caused by extravasation of sperm. They may also produce a pain resembling renal colic, or they may form a vasocutaneous fistula. They may occur years after the vasectomy and are the most probable cause of recanalization. Granulomas have resulted from injection of contrast medium.[183]

THE EPIDIDYMIS

CONGENITAL ANOMALIES OF THE EPIDIDYMIS

Congenital anomalies of the epididymis include the following (see Fig. 35–48, a normal epididymogram, for comparison):

Associated with cryptorchid testes:
1. Separated from testes, so-called detached epididymis.[185,189] Usually the whole epididymis lies at a distance from the testis. Not infrequently only the tail is detached. Rarely is the epididymal head pulled away from the testis.
2. Elongated or extended epididymis.[185, 189] Usually epididymis is no more than one and one-

half times the length of the testis, but in this type of abnormality it may be six times as long.
3. Angled epididymis—bent in midportion[189]
4. Absent epididymis—usually body plus tail and varying amounts of vas deferens[185, 186]
5. Presence of mesorchium. In about 10 per cent of cases of undescended testes, the testis and epididymis are lying on a mesentery, giving them unusual mobility.[189]

Not necessarily related to cryptorchidism:
1. Accessory epididymis[186]
2. Malposition in relation to testis[186]
3. Cystic changes in head[189]
4. Constriction of middle of body[189]
5. Complete separation of two halves of epididymis[189]
6. Absence of globus major and body of epididymis[186]
7. Direct anastomosis of ductuli efferentes to form vas (epididymis absent)
8. Absence of body of epididymis disconnecting vas and testis[186]

Windholz has described four types of abnormal testis–epididymal relationships[190]:

1. Congenital anorchism with descent of vas and epididymis
2. Undescended testis with descent of the epididymis, partially or completely, into scrotum, producing separation of epididymis and testis
3. Vas deferens alone present in the scrotum, with testis and epididymis undescended
4. Partial separation of the testis and epididymis (dislocation) most often seen when both are undescended

INFECTIONS OF THE EPIDIDYMIS

Epididymitis, an inflammation of the epididymis, is classified as follows:

1. Idiopathic (Fig. 35–49)
2. Nonspecific
3. Traumatic (Fig. 35–50)
4. Specific
   a. Metastatic
      Meningococcal septicemia, pneumococcal pneumonia, brucellosis
   b. Gonorrhea
   c. Tuberculosis (Fig. 35–51)
   d. Syphilis

See Chapter 43, Miscellaneous Conditions of the urethra, for radionuclide scan of epididymitis.

Idiopathic Epididymitis. This refers to epididymitis without a recent or concurrent infection. The same organisms are rarely isolated from both the urethra and epididymis. Organisms found in the epididymis are *Neisseria gonorrhea*, nonspecific urethral Corynebacterial species, mima polymorpha, and classic mycoplasma of an unknown species.[193]

Nonspecific Epididymitis. This includes those inflammations that cannot be ascribed to specific causes: tuberculosis, gonorrhea, undulant fever, mumps, influenza, and so on. It is nearly always caused by organisms such as staphylococcus, streptococcus, and *E. coli*. These can enter the epididymis by way of the prostate, seminal vesicles, or urethra,[195] or by blood from tonsils, carious teeth, or intestinal tract.[198] Some authorities[194, 196] believe that straining produces reflux into the vas and causes epididymitis, even with sterile urine.[194, 196]

Traumatic Epididymitis. This refers to a blow to the epididymis and might include reflux of sterile urine into the vas on straining, causing a chemical inflammation. Traumatic epididymitis is often associated with infection that can be lying dormant in the epididymis or be a secondary invader.

Specific Epididymitis. Of this group, gonorrhea and tuberculosis are the most common. Gonorrheal epididymitis occurs secondary to gonorrheal urethritis. The etiology of tuberculous epididymitis has not been entirely clarified. Ross and co-workers list the following three possible routes of infection[197]: (1) by way of the lumen of the vas from tuberculosis of prostate or kidney; (2) through the lymphatics; and (3) by way of the blood.

Sixty-five per cent of their cases had a positive urine for tuberculosis, and most authorities associate tuberculous epididymitis with renal tuberculosis. Thirty-four per cent of the cases are bilateral, and the globus minor is the most common site of involvement.

TUMORS OF THE EPIDIDYMIS

Tumors of epididymis are rare; they are classified as follows:

1. Benign
   Adenomatoid
   Papillary adenoma
   Vascular
2. Malignant
   Carcinoma
   Sarcoma

3. Metastatic
   Stomach, kidney, prostate, carcinoid

Benign. The most common benign tumor is the adenomatoid lesion (Fig. 35–52), which consists of irregular, glandlike spaces lined by cells, variously designated as endothelial, mesothelial, or epithelial. The cells are set in stroma of loose or dense fibrous tissue. However, a plexiform pattern may occur in which cells identical to the preceding are arranged singly, in small groups, or in solid cords.

These tumors are now generally considered to be mesothelial in origin. Hyaluronic acid has been found in cells of these tumors supporting the mesothelial origin. Mackey[199, 210] and co-workers found that the living cells of microscopic tumor channels contained microvilli and irregular cytoplasmic protrusions similar to mesothelial cells.[209]

Eighty per cent of adenomatoid tumors are in or adjacent to the epididymis. The rest are in the spermatic cord, tunica vaginalis, and testes. The globus minor is involved four times as often as the globus major. They occur usually in the fifth and sixth decades, but they have occurred in newborns.[201]

Kannenstein and Lustig[208] reported a case with hormone activity, positive Aschheim-Zondek test, gynecomastia, and loss of libido, all of which returned to normal after removal of the tumor. Malignancy in adenomatoid tumors has been reported.[204]

Papillary adenoma is a benign tumor situated within or close to the head of the epididymis. There is ectasia of efferent ducts, with papillary formation. It may be unilateral or bilateral. The lesion represents a component of von Hippel-Lindau disease. The unilateral variety may have no other changes, but the bilateral type often has lesions in other organs similar to those found in von Hippel-Lindau disease.

Malignant. Malignancy of epididymis is extremely rare, 50 per cent of them occurring between 20 and 40 years of age. Left and right epididymis are equally involved. Painful or painless swelling is present, and there may be a hydrocele. Varicocele is rare. There may be metastasis to the lungs. The patient rarely survives over 5 years. Histologic types reported have been papillary adenocarcinoma, seminomalike, and undifferentiated carcinoma.

VASOEPIDIDYMOGRAPHY

Vasoepididymography is the visualization of the proximal portion of the vas deferens and the epididymis by the injection of contrast medium. The vas is exposed in the scrotum or the inguinal area, and a

No. 26 hypodermic needle (we prefer a No. 50 polyethylene tubing) is inserted into the lumen of the vas deferens, with the needle pointed toward the epididymis. After 1 ml. of solution has been injected, the needle is withdrawn. The vas is then replaced in the scrotum, and the incision is closed. An x-ray exposure is made in the posteroanterior position[225] or the anteroposterior position,[231] with the film directly beneath the scrotum. Absehouse, Heller, and Salik make a second exposure after gently massaging the epididymis and rotating the testicle to another position.[225]

The anatomy of the vas deferens in this portion is as follows: The vas begins at the globus minor of the epididymis, where it forms an acute angle known as the vasoepididymal kink. The ascending portion of the vas begins with numerous convolutions for a distance of 2 to 4 cm., after which it straightens out. The globus minor of the epididymis begins at the vasoepididymal kink, and, on injection, there is a feathery appearance at this point. The body of the epididymis is forked. The globus major is not seen, because the contrast medium normally stops here.

Vasoepididymography is certainly of limited application, but it may be useful in sterility cases in determining the point of obstruction.

ASPERMIA

Aspermia is caused by testicular failure or failure of sperm to be ejaculated from the urethra. The latter is considered here.

Any disruption of the transport system can prevent the delivery of sperm. The most important are as follows:

1. Obstruction of distal part of epididymis and/or adjoining vas deferens (Fig. 35–54). This is the most common point of obstruction and represents approximately 58 per cent of azoospermic males. Two-thirds are congenital, one-third, postinflammatory or traumatic (fructose positive).[221]
2. Site of obstruction between testis and epididymis, usually congenital, representing 21 per cent (fructose positive)
3. Bilateral absence of vas — 13.4 per cent (fructose negative; absence of seminal vesicles)
4. Unilateral absence of vas with atrophic testicle on opposite side
5. Acquired vasal obstruction (fructose positive)
   a. Tuberculosis
   b. Postvaricocelectomy, hydrocelectomy, or herniorrhaphy
   c. Postvasectomy to produce sterility
   d. Obstruction from injection of vas
6. Bilateral obstruction of ejaculatory duct opening, secondary to inflammation (fructose negative)
7. Asymmetric obstruction — different on the two sides
   a. Vasal on one side, epididymal on the other
   b. Obstructed ejaculatory duct on one side and obstructed vas on the other (Fig. 35–55)
   c. Obstructed vas on one side, atrophic testicle on the other (Fig. 35–56).
8. Reflux ejaculation
   a. Postbladder-neck operations, including prostate
   b. Stricture of urethra
9. Neurogenic, failure to ejaculate

ASPERMIA AND CYSTIC FIBROSIS

Practically all postpubescent men with cystic fibrosis have been considered infertile.[240, 245] However, a few fertile men have been reported,[242, 249] and normal genital tracts have been found[246] on microdissection with serial section reconstruction. The genital defects found in cystic fibrosis consist of abnormal or absent bodies and tails of the epididymides, with the globus major usually remaining intact; abnormal, atretic, or absent vasa deferentia; and dilated or absent seminal vesicles. Whether the male genital abnormalities in patients with cystic fibrosis are caused by a genetic developmental abnormality[243, 244, 245, 247] or are secondary to obstruction by abnormal secretions with consequent atresia[241, 248, 249] is not known.

Infertility as a result of immotile sperm due to the absence of the dynein arms on the tail of spermatozoa may be associated with chronic infection of the upper and lower airways or with Kartagener's syndrome.[250]

CHAPTER 35, ILLUSTRATIONS

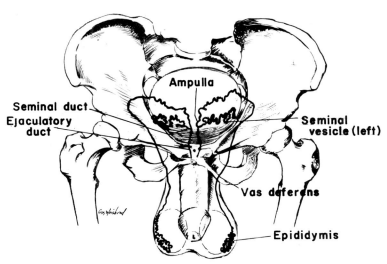

FIG. 35-1. Diagram of the genital tract.

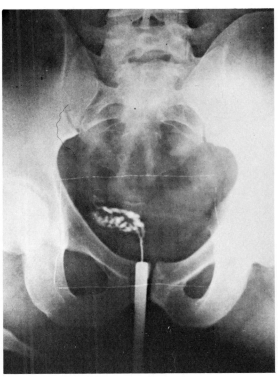

FIG. 35-2. Normal seminal vesicle (injected through ejaculatory duct). The convolutions are of uniform breadth and density. The gland is oval-shaped. The ampulla is distinct from the vesicle. The ejaculatory and the seminal ducts are straight. The vas deferens takes its lateral course high above the terminal pole. (Peterson, A.P.: J. Urol., 39:662, 1938)

FIG. 35-3. Seminal vesiculogram of a normal gland, obtained upon injection of 0.4 ml. of Diodrast before each exposure. Seminal vesicle, ampulla, and vas deferens perfectly outlined after third fraction (1.2 ml.). Regurgitation of the contrast material occurred upon filling of the vesicles. SV = seminal vesicles; A = ampulla; VD = vas deferens; R = regurgitation into bladder. (Courtesy of A.P. Peterson, M.D.)

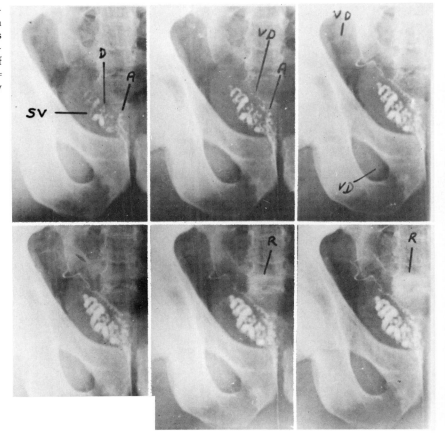

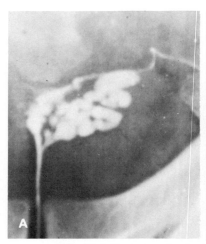
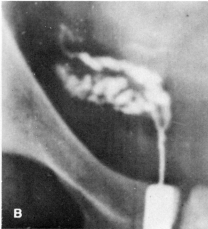
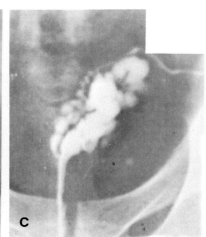

FIG. 35–4. Variations in the formation of the ejaculatory duct (injected through the ejaculatory duct). **(A)** The duct is a direct continuation of the vas. This is normal. **(B)** The vas and the seminal vesicular duct join dichotomously. This is normal. **(C)** The ejaculatory duct is a continuation of the seminal duct. This has been seen only in diseased cases. (Courtesy of A.P. Peterson, M.D.)

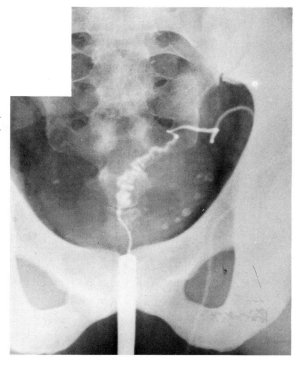

FIG. 35–5. Occlusion of seminal duct secondary to infection. Vas deferens is visualized. (Courtesy of A.P. Peterson, M.D.)

FIG. 35–6. Physiologically distended seminal vesicle. Injection through ejaculatory duct. This is similar to normal but presents larger shadows with wider convolutions and even distention. This is difficult to differentiate from an early catarrhal stage, but if pus is present and/or organisms in the ejaculate, the latter diagnosis is preferred. The physiologically distended vesicle is medium to large in size, soft to firm in consistency, easily palpable and usually tender. It is common in cases of prolonged sexual abstinence. (Courtesy of A.P. Peterson, M.D.)

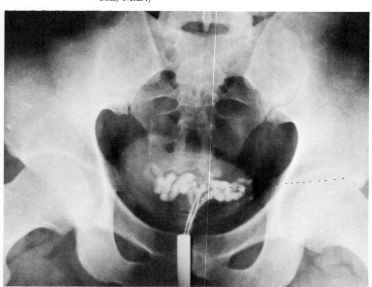

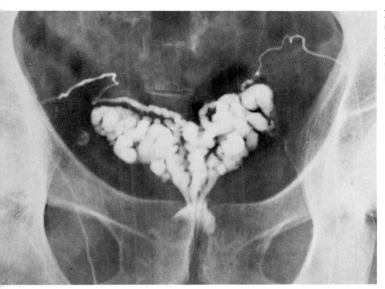

FIG. 35–7. Physiologically distended seminal vesicles (injected through the vasa deferentia). These are essentially normal seminal vesicles with moderate physiologic distention. Notice the clear-cut convolutions and the more or less oval shape of the seminal vesicles. (Courtesy of B.L. Stewart, M.D.)

FIG. 35–8. Early catarrhal vesiculitis. Injection through the ejaculatory duct. The diffusion of the contrast medium is distinct, and the details are clear. The vesicle is distended slightly, but there is no disruption of the capsule. The seminal and the ejaculatory ducts are narrow. The glands appear to be somewhat more vertical than normal. Often in this stage the upper margin is raised close to or above the ampulla and the vas deferens, reducing or entirely filling the vesicle-ampullar space. (Courtesy of A.P. Peterson, M.D.)

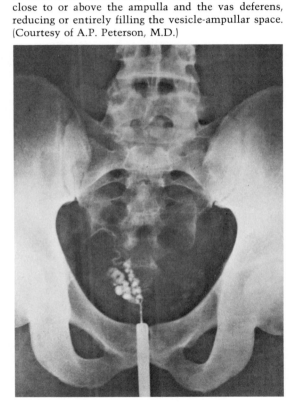

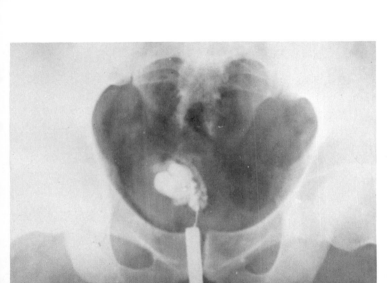

FIG. 35–9. Intermediate catarrhal seminal vesiculitis. Injection through the ejaculatory duct. There is definite dilatation of the terminal pole, whereas the proximal portion is practically normal. There is some disruption of the vesicular capsule at the point of dilatation. The terminal pole is raised to the level of the vas deferens. (Courtesy of A.P. Peterson, M.D.)

FIG. 35–10. Intermediate catarrhal vesiculitis. Injection through the ejaculatory duct. The seminal vesicle gives the same appearance as in the previous figure. There is a simultaneous prostatogram through an ejaculatory duct fistula into the prostate. (Courtesy of A.P. Peterson, M.D.)

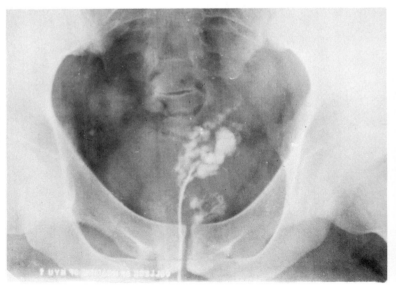

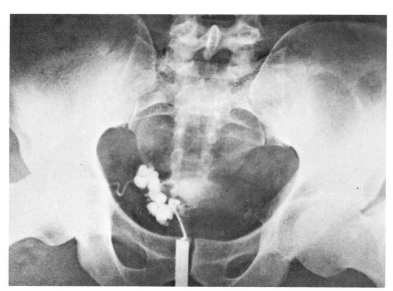

FIG. 35–11. Late catarrhal vesiculitis with generalized dilatation. Injection through ejaculatory duct. Dilatation of the entire gland and straightening of the convolutions are visualized. Notice that the terminal pole is above the level of the vas. (This causes it to be proximal to the ureter.) The vesicle is similar in appearance to a tortuous hydroureter. This type of gland will not return to normal. (Peterson, A.P.: J. Urol., *39*:662, 1938)

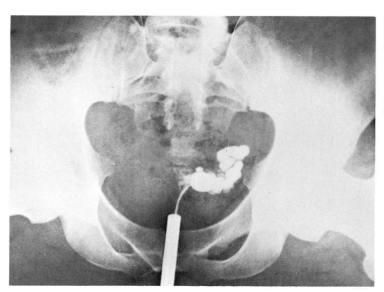

FIG. 35–12. Late catarrhal vesiculitis (pyovesiculosis). Injection through ejaculatory duct. There is dilatation of the entire gland and straightening of the convolutions. The organ appears as a row of circular or oval cavities. This type of gland is palpable and tender. The elasticity and the contractility are lost, and so the gland will not return to normal. (Peterson, A.P.: J. Urol., *39*:662, 1938)

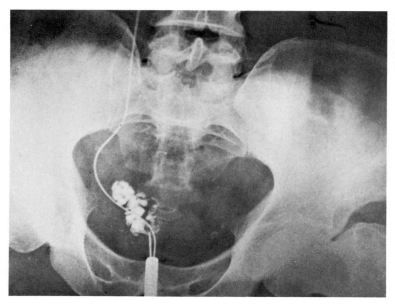

FIG. 35–13. Late catarrhal vesiculitis. Injection through ejaculatory duct with ureteral catheter in situ. This shows relationship to ureter. The seminal vesicle is more vertical. It is dilated, and the normal convolutions are lost. (Courtesy of A.P. Peterson, M.D.)

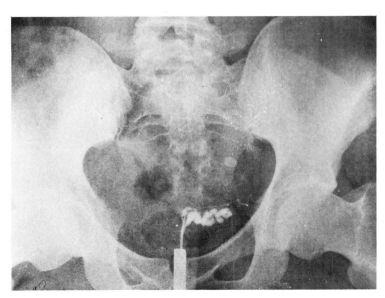

FIG. 35-14. Early interstitial vesiculitis. Injection through ejaculatory duct. This film shows a few circular or spiral convolutions with some localized distention. There appears to be a beginning obliteration of peripheral lumina. On palpation the gland was found to be small to medium in size, thickened, ovoid in shape, and nonsensitive. (Courtesy of A.P. Peterson, M.D.)

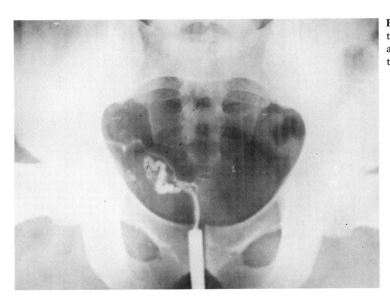

FIG. 35-15. Intermediate interstitial vesiculitis. Injection through the ejaculatory duct. Note the elongated and narrow tubal shadows with shallow, wavy convolutions. (Peterson, A.P.: J. Urol., *39*:662, 1938)

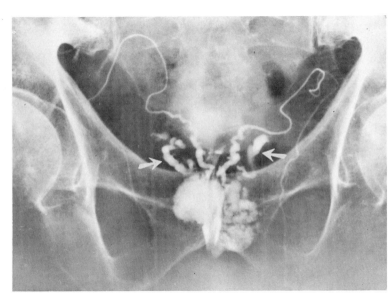

FIG. 35-16. Seminal vesiculogram in a case of prostatic calculi. Injection through both vasa deferentia. AP view. Both seminal vesicles (*arrows*) show the characteristics of intermediate interstitial vesiculitis. On the left side there is loss of the convolutions and dilatation of the terminal portion. On the right side there is some semblance of convolution formation, but essentially the convolutions have been obliterated. The ejaculatory ducts appear to be slightly dilated.

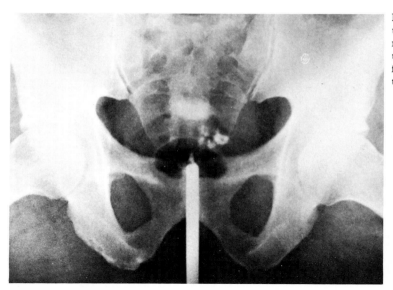

FIG. 35–17. Late interstitial vesiculitis. Injection through the ejaculatory duct. This film shows a few irregular cavities which may appear to be completely detached. The vesicle was nodular on palpation and easily felt. There were marked fibrosis and advanced obstructive changes. (Peterson, A.P.: J. Urol., 39:662, 1938)

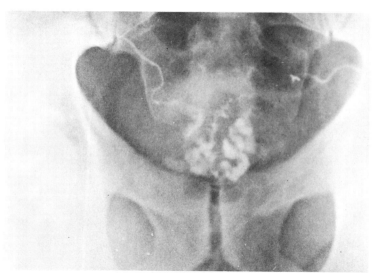

FIG. 35–18. Tuberculosis of the seminal vesicles. Seminal vesiculogram. Injection from vasa deferentia side. The structure on the right is partly destroyed. Notice the dilated, detached convolutions, which fill unevenly. On the left side there is a slight uneven distribution of the contrast material. The convolutions for the most part are nearly normal. Both seminal vesicles occupy a more vertical position than normal. (Courtesy of A.P. Peterson, M.D.)

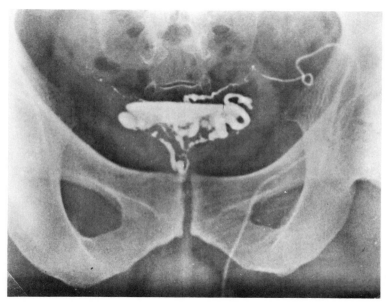

FIG. 35–19. Tuberculosis of right seminal vesicle (injected through the left vas deferens). There is reflux up the dilated right ejaculatory duct and also into the bladder. There is destruction of the right seminal vesicle with dilatation of the detached convolution. (This is somewhat similar to late interstitial vesiculitis.) On the left this type of gland has been considered to be normal but actually is similar to intermediate interstitial vesiculitis. (Wilhelm, S.F., Marks, R.: Sterility in the Male. New York, Oxford University Press, 1937.)

FIG. 35–20. Tuberculous abscess. **(A)** A vasoseminal vesiculogram showing complete retention in a case of tuberculosis of left seminal vesicle with ejaculatory duct occlusion. Injection through left vas deferens. **(B)** Vesiculogram 2 years after injection. Complete retention of iodized oil in abscess, stone in ureter (*arrow*). (Wilhelm, S.F., Marks, R.: Sterility in the Male. New York, Oxford University Press, 1937)

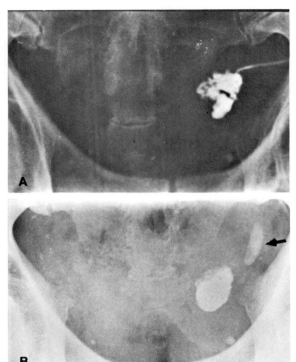

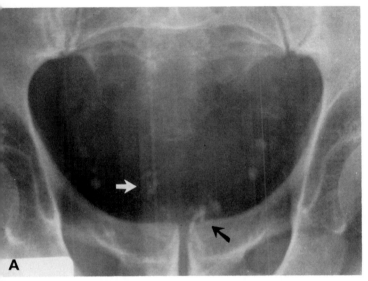

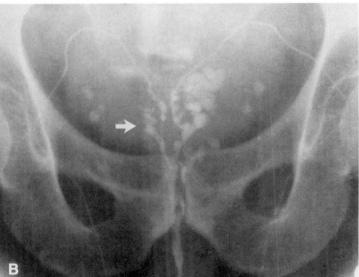

FIG. 35–21. Calculi of right seminal vesicle. **(A)** Plain film: *White arrow*—calculi in seminal vesicle. *Black arrow*—prostatic calculi. **(B)** Injection of contrast medium into vas on both sides outlining seminal vesicles. *White arrow*—seminal vesicle outlined by contrast medium obscuring calculi.

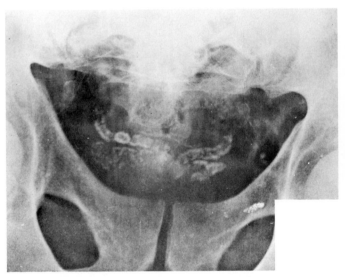

FIG. 35–22. Calcified vasa deferentia and seminal vesicle in a nondiabetic. This should be called nonspecific calcification of the seminal vesicles. Note that it is more uniform, more dense and more clear-cut than other types. The calcification is in the walls of the vasa deferentia and seminal vesicles. (Courtesy of J.J. Arnold, M.D.)

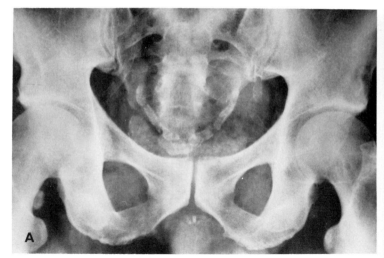

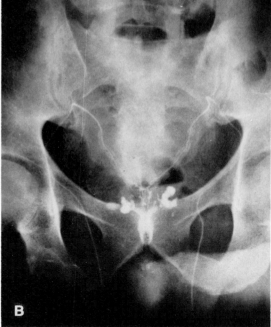

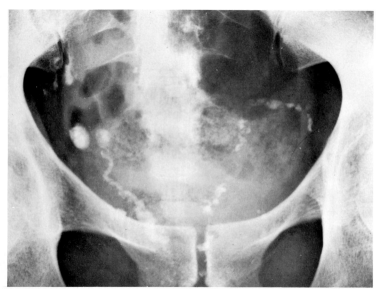

FIG. 35–22a. Calcified seminal vesicles and vasa deferentia in a diabetic. **(A)** Plain film. Calcification in seminal vesicles shows a diffuse, faint pattern with smaller, nodular densities. The vasa are calcified in the walls. **(B)** Seminal vesiculogram injected through vasa deferentia. The vasa are patent. Note the intermediate interstitial vesiculitis.

FIG. 35–23. Schistosomiasis. The seminal vesicles are diffusely calcified (*small arrows*). Note that the entire gland is involved in a mottled fashion. *Large arrow* points to the right calcified ureter. There is a laminated stone in the left ureter. (Courtesy of P. Jamison, M.D., Tanta, Egypt)

FIG. 35–24. Case of tuberculosis calcification of the vasa deferentia and the seminal vesicles, especially on the right. This shows intraluminal calcification of the vas on both sides and an irregular calcification of the right seminal vesicle involving only a portion of the gland. There may be a small calcification in the left seminal vesicle. (Courtesy of T. Leon Howard, M.D.)

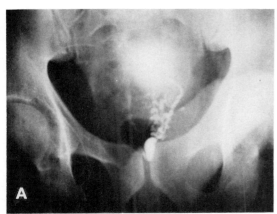

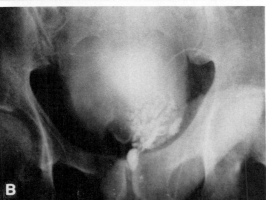

FIG. 35–25. Ectopia of seminal vesicle; bilateral seminal vesiculogram. **(A)** Proximal right vas deferens is normal, but distal vas crosses midline; seminal vesicle and ejaculatory duct are ectopic, entering posterior urethra on left. Dilatation of ejaculatory duct indicates partial obstruction. **(B)** Both vasa, seminal vesicles, and ejaculatory ducts are filled, left side normal. Right kidney was absent. (Holt, S.A., Peterson, N.E.: Urology, 4:322–324, 1974)

FIG. 35–26. Cyst of seminal vesicle. Ejaculatory duct was catheterized, catheter entered cyst, and contrast medium was injected. (Stewart, B.L., Nicoll, G.A.: J. Urol., 62:189, 1949)

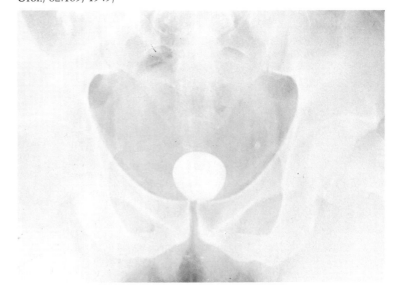

FIG. 35–27. Multilocular cyst of seminal vesicle. Left ampulla, vesicle, and ejaculatory duct entirely normal, allowing partial filling of the bladder. Right seminal vesicle shown and multilocular appearance is evident. No kidney found on right. Surgery revealed multilocular cyst of right seminal vesicle with no continuity with a normal ejaculatory duct, or any other visible structure that could have represented it. (Linhares-Furtado, A.J.: Br. J. Urol., 45:536, 1973)

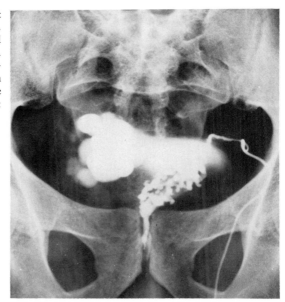

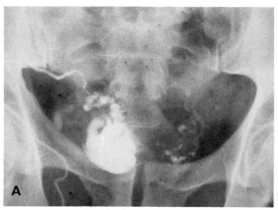

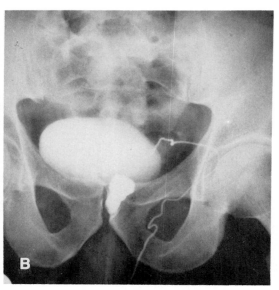

FIG. 35–28. Bilateral cysts of seminal vesicles; absence of left kidney and ureter. **(A)** Right cystic seminal vesicle, possibly multilocular; contrast medium did not pass into urethra. **(B)** Left cystic seminal vesicle. Free passage of contrast medium into urethra and bladder. (This cystic structure on left could be a dilated ejaculatory duct from its position.) (Linhares-Furtado, A.J.: Br. J. Urol., *45*:536, 1973)

FIG. 35–29. Mesonephroid tumor in a seminal vesicle cyst. **(A)** Excretory urogram showing compression over left superior border of bladder. **(B)** Left seminal vesiculogram demonstrating left vas deferens and the left seminal vesicle. The proximal left seminal vesicle is displaced upward by a large cystic mass in the seminal vesicle. **(C)** Post-drainage film showing retention of contrast medium in cystic structure. (Bagley, D.H., Javadpour, N., Witebsky, F.G., et al.: Urology, *5*:147, 1975)

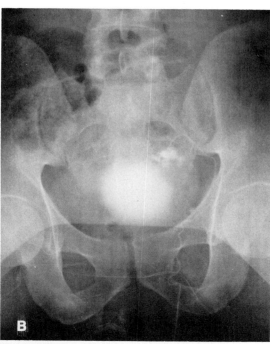

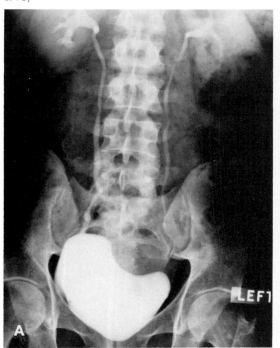

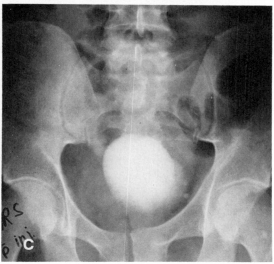

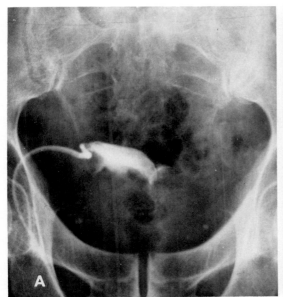 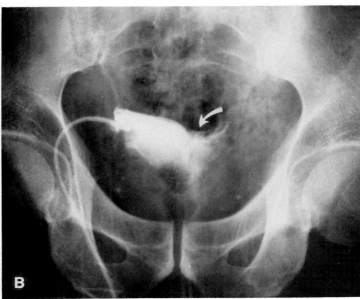

FIG. 35–30. Carcinoma of right seminal vesicle; contrast medium injected through right vas deferens. **(A)** Dilated right seminal vesicle with irregular inferior surface. The gland is elevated and displaced. **(B)** More contast medium injected, revealing rupture of capsule medially (*arrow*). (Smith, B.A., Jr., et al.: J. Urol., *97*:743, 1967)

FIG. 35–31. Carcinoma of left seminal vesicle. Right vas only was injected with contrast medium, yet both vasa and seminal vesicles are visualized. Note large filling defect in left seminal vesicle. There is displacement of the right seminal vesicle to left, with some distortion of its shape. (Smith, B.A., Jr., Webb, E.A., and Price, W.E.: J. Urol., *97*:743, 1967)

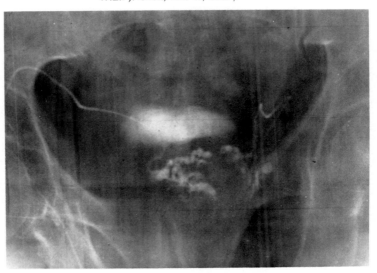

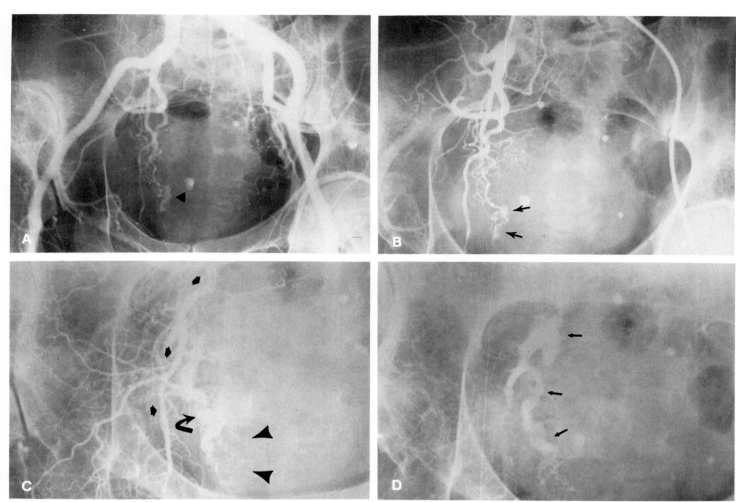

FIG. 35–32. Carcinoma of the right seminal vesicle. **(A)** Arterial phase of the pelvic aortogram performed by the left femoral route because of old fracture-dislocation of the right femur. The angiogram demonstrates extravasation and puddling of contrast medium within the pelvis (*arrowhead*). **(B)** Selective right hypogastric arteriogram performed by the left femoral arterial route demonstrates puddling of contrast medium (*arrows*) within the pelvis, with primary distribution from the middle vesical arteries. **(C)** Selective right hypogastric arteriogram slightly later in the injection demonstrates persistent opacification of the right hypogastric artery (*small arrows*) as well as small, irregular tumor vessels within the pelvis (*arrowheads*) and shunting of contrast medium into large pudendal and iliac veins (*curved arrow*). **(D)** Later film in the arterial phase of the selective hypogastric arteriogram demonstrates persistent capillary filling within the pelvis but vivid opacification of the dilated pudendal and iliac veins (*arrow*) noted on the earlier arterial phase of the examination. (Goldstein, A.G., Wilson, E.S.: Br. J. Urol., *45*:211, 1973)

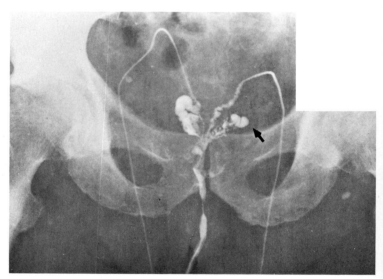

FIG. 35–33. Carcinoma of prostate invading left seminal vesicle. Injection through vasa deferentia. The left seminal vesicle lies more horizontal than the right. The vesiculo-ampullar junction (junction of the seminal duct with the ampulla) is somewhat lower than that on the right. The medial portion of the left seminal vesicle is compressed irregularly, and the terminal pole is dilated (*arrow*). The left ejaculatory duct is somewhat narrowed. Notice that contrast material in the urethra flows distally and does not enter the bladder.

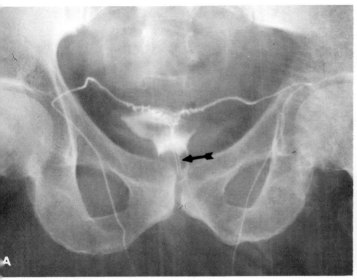
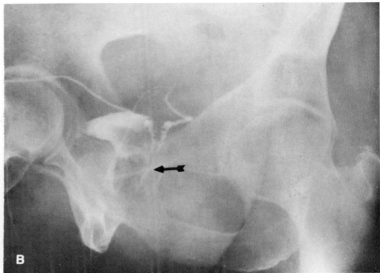

FIG. 35–34. Seminal vesiculogram in a case of carcinoma of the prostate. Diagnosis had been made 2 years previously by transurethral resection. Patient had been intermittently on female sex hormones. The ejaculatory ducts are greatly narrowed, straight, and rigid (*arrow*). The seminal ducts and the seminal vesicles are not visualized due to obliteration. Note that contrast material enters the bladder and does not go distally into the urethra. In patients with prostatic carcinoma who have been on female hormone, the ejaculatory ducts generally respond better than the seminal vesicle itself. (A) AP view. (B) Right oblique view.

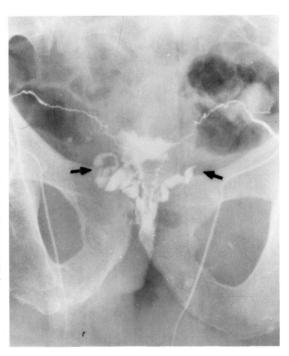

FIG. 35–35. Anaplastic carcinoma of the bladder invading the seminal vesicles (injected through the vasa deferentia). The terminal poles (*arrows*) are partially destroyed on the right and obliterated on the left. The appearance approaches that of intermediate interstitial vesiculitis. The convolutions are shallow, and the entire gland appears to be tubular. The ejaculatory ducts are dilated due to benign prostatic hypertrophy. Note that both seminal vesicles appear to be somewhat lower than normal.

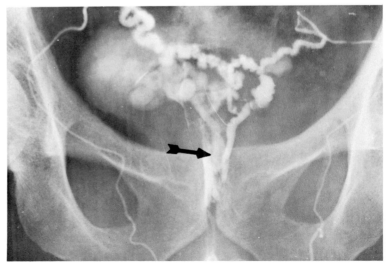

FIG. 35–36. Case of benign prostatic hypertrophy. Injection through the vasa deferentia. The ejaculatory ducts are dilated, especially the right (*arrow*), and are smooth and regular. The right seminal vesicle is dilated noticeably.

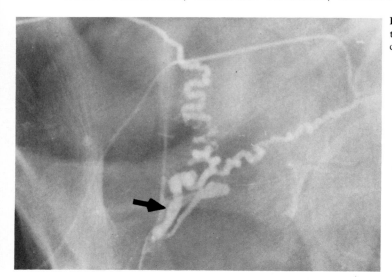

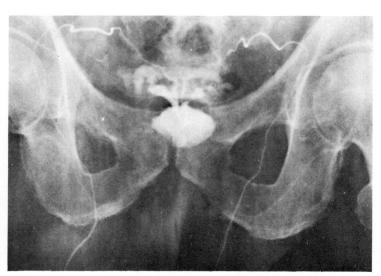

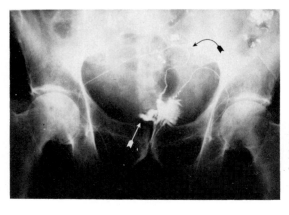

FIG. 35–37. Benign prostatic hypertrophy. Injection through vasa deferentia. Right oblique view. *Arrow* indicates a greatly dilated right ejaculatory duct.

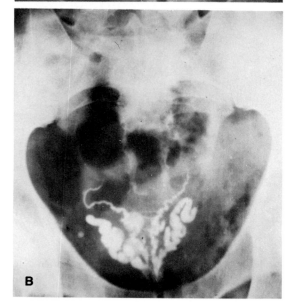

FIG. 35–38. Seminal vesiculogram 4 years after suprapubic prostatectomy. Injection through vas deferens bilaterally. The prostatic cavity is well defined, and the ejaculatory ducts are clearly present. This demonstrates that in many instances the ejaculatory ducts remain patent after a suprapubic prostatectomy.

FIG. 35–39. Perivesical abscess. **(A)** Seminal vesicles pushed to the right by a soft-tissue mass. **(B)** Two weeks postdrainage, showing the seminal vesicles in practically normal position. (Courtesy of S.F. Wilhelm, M.D., and Robert Marks, M.D.)

FIG. 35–40. Displacement of seminal vesicles by carcinoma of bladder. Right seminal vesicle (*white arrow*) has been pushed to left side by large carcinoma of bladder. Note position of right vas deferens (*black arrow*).

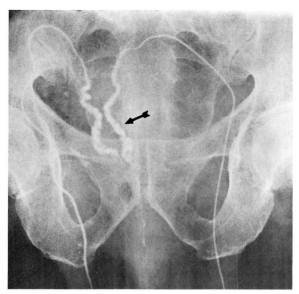

FIG. 35–41. Carcinoma of the prostate invading seminal vesicles. Injection through both vasa deferentia. The seminal and the ejaculatory ducts are obliterated. The seminal vesicles are not visualized. Note the great displacement of the ampulla of the left vas (*arrow*) to the opposite side by a mass that has invaded the left seminal vesicle.

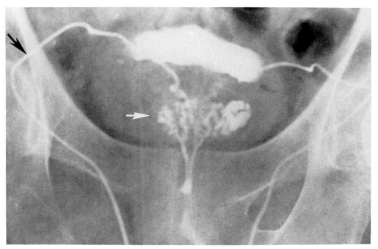

FIG. 35–42. Carcinoma of prostate invading seminal vesicles. There is widening of the course of the right vas deferens (*straight black arrow*). The right seminal vesicle (*white arrow*) is more vertical than usual, being pushed slightly to the left side. This is an early case, before obstruction of the seminal and ejaculatory ducts has taken place. There is dilatation of terminal portions of the left seminal vesicle. (Courtesy of B.S. Abeshouse, M.D.)

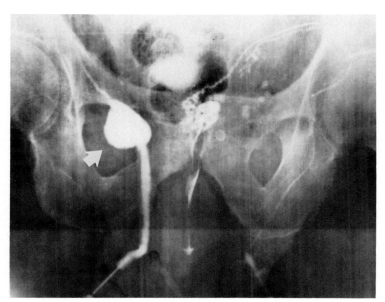

FIG. 35–43. Cyst of right vas deferens. *Arrow* points to cystic structure in right vas deferens. (Courtesy of Dr. F. Lopez, M.D.)

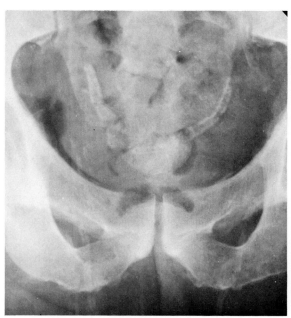

FIG. 35–44. Calcification of the vas deferens in a nondiabetic (degenerative form). The calcification is in the walls, and the lumina are patent.

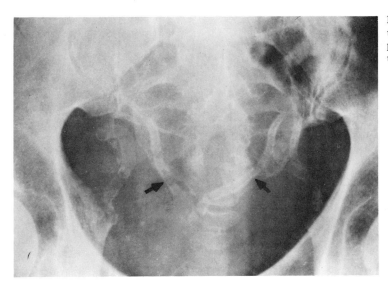

FIG. 35–45. Calcification of the vas deferens in a diabetic. The calcification is in the walls, and the lumina are patent. This cannot be differentiated from the degenerative form. The external iliac vessels also are calcified.

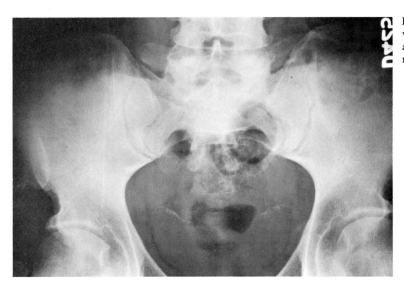

FIG. 35–46. Inflammatory type of calcification of the vas deferens. Note that the calcification is intraluminal and that the walls appear to be free. (Culver, G.J., Tannenhaus, J.: J.A.M.A., *173*:648, 1960)

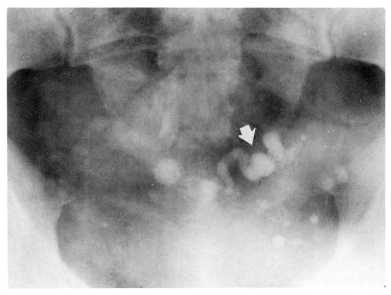

FIG. 35–47. Calcified left vas deferens (*arrow*) with beading. Calcifications in region of left seminal vesicle. Case of tuberculosis. (Courtesy of Sol Unger, M.D. and Vet. Adminis.)

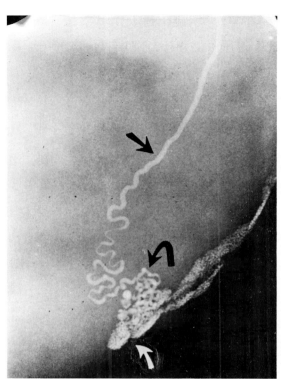

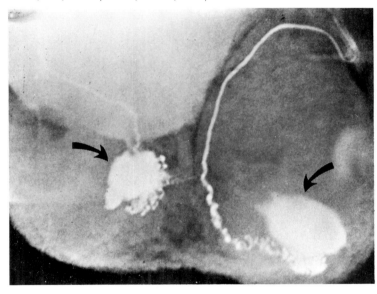

FIG. 35–48. Normal epididymogram. AP view. The vas can be seen in its straight portion (*straight black arrow*) and then as it becomes convoluted. The vaso-epididymal kink (*curved black arrow*) can be seen at the junction of the globus minor (*white arrow*), which is rather feathery in appearance. The body of the epididymis is forked. (This is a normal variation.) The globus major is not visualized. (Abeshouse, B.S., et al.: J. Urol., 72:983, 1954)

FIG. 35–49. Chronic recurrent bilateral epididymitis. AP view. This film reveals bilateral pooling of contrast material in the globus minors (*arrows*). The vasa are normal. Body of epididymis is not visualized. (Abeshouse, B.S., et al.: J. Urol., 72:983, 1954)

FIG. 35–50. Post-traumatic right epididymitis. Normal left epididymitis. PA view. Note the pooling of dye in the region of the globus minor of the right epididymis (*arrow*). Injury to the epididymis had occurred many years previously. (Abeshouse, B.S., et al.: J. Urol., 72:983, 1954)

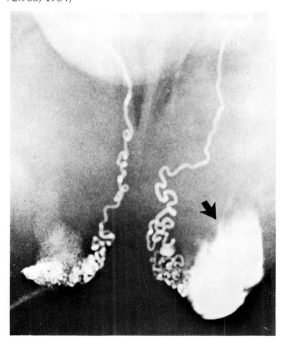

FIG. 35–51. (**A**) Right tuberculous epididymitis with vasoscrotal fistula. No contrast medium is passing into the right epididymis. (*Arrow* points to vas.) (**B**) The right seminal vesicle appears to be contracted, and the normal convolutions are gone. There is an elongated and narrow tubal shadow with very shallow, wavy convolutions. The right ejaculatory duct is dilated markedly (*white arrow*). (Abeshouse, B.S., et al.: J. Urol., 72:983, 1954)

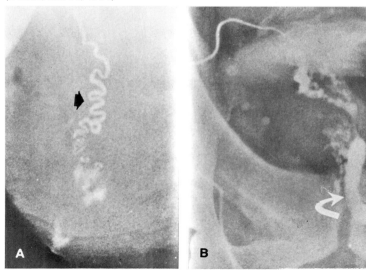

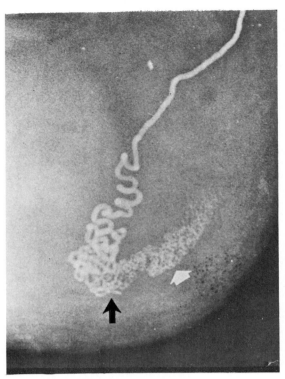

FIG. 35–52. Adenomatoid tumor of globus major of epididymis. PA view. Vas deferens and globus minor (*black arrow*) are normal. The body of the epididymis (*white arrow*) is somewhat wider as the globus major is approached. No contrast is seen in the globus major. (B.S. Abeshouse, M.D., et al.: Vaso-epididymography and vasoseminal vesiculography. J. Urol., 72:983, 1954)

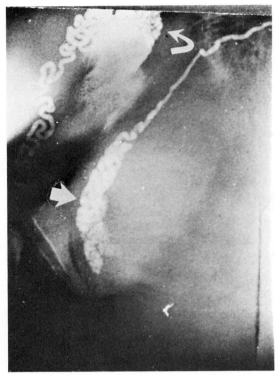

FIG. 35–53. Bilateral testicular tumors. The right epididymis (*curved white arrow*) fills well, the contrast medium being spread out a little wider than usual. The crescent shape of the left epididymis (*straight white arrow*) is most likely due to extrinsic pressure. Patient had bilateral seminomas. (Abeshouse, B.S., et al.: J. Urol., 72:983, 1954)

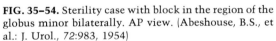

FIG. 35–54. Sterility case with block in the region of the globus minor bilaterally. AP view. (Abeshouse, B.S., et al.: J. Urol., 72:983, 1954)

FIG. 35–55. Case of sterility. Note the dilated blocked right ejaculatory duct (*arrow*). The left vas deferens was occluded near its entrance into the internal ring. Injection through vasa deferentia.

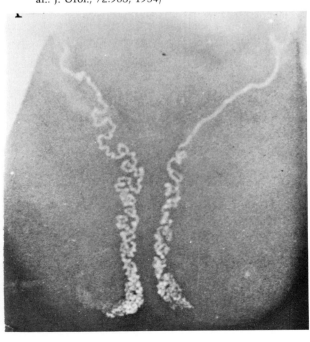

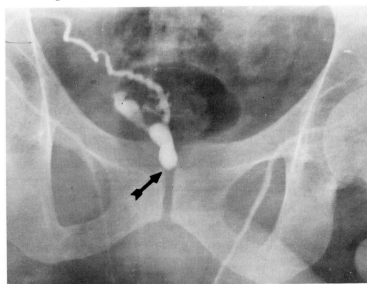

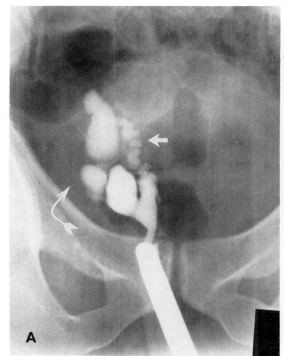
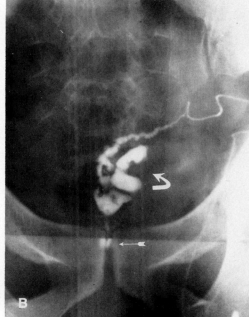

FIG. 35–56. Case of aspermia. (**A**) Contrast medium was injected through right ejaculatory duct. Note dilated infected convolutions in right seminal vesicle (*curved white arrow*). There is a dilated, irregular, obstructed right vas deferens (*straight white arrow*). Right testicle was normal on biopsy. (**B**) Contrast medium was injected through left vas deferens. Left seminal vesicle has dilated irregular convolutions (*curved white arrow*). The left vas deferens is patent, and the ejaculatory duct empties into the urethra (*straight white arrow*). Left testicle is atrophic, with absent seminiferous tubules on biopsy.

BIBLIOGRAPHY

General

1. Belfield, W.T.: Skiagraphy of the seminal ducts. J.A.M.A., 60:800–801, 1913.
2. Brueschke, E.E., Bruno, M., Maness, J.H., Wingfield, J.R. et al.: Development of a reversible vas deferens occlusive device. Anatomical size of the human and dog vasa deferentia. Fert. Steril., 25:659–672, 1972.
3. Ekström, T. et al.: Asymmetry of the urinary bladder and terminal parts of the ureter in prostatovesiculitis. Acta Radiol., (Diagn., Stockholm), 3:310–320, 1965.
4. Gonzales-Iman, F.: Retrograde seminal vesiculography. J. Urol., 49:618–627, 1943.
5. Herbst, R.H., and Merricks, J.W.: Visualization and treatment of seminal vesiculitis by catheterization and dilatation of the ejaculatory ducts. J. Urol., 41:733–759, 1939.
6. Herbst, R.H., and Merricks, J.W.: Transurethral approach to the diagnosis and treatment of infections of the seminal vesicles. Illinois Med. J., 78:393–397, 1940.
7. Herbst, R.H., and Merricks, J.W.: Transurethral drainage of the seminal vesicles in seminal vesiculitis. Illinois Med. J., 86:190–195, 1944.

8. Hulka, J.F., and Davis, J.E.: Vasectomy and reversible vasocclusion. Fert. and Steril., 23:683–696, 1972.
9. Mataporker, B.G., Taneja, O.P., Saha, M.M., and Bhardwaj, O.P.: A critical evaluation of vaso-seminal vesiculography. Br. J. Urol., 41:455–464, 1969.
10. McCarthy, J.F., and Ritter, J.S.: Seminal vesicles: newer instrumental methods in diagnosis and therapeutic management. J.A.M.A., 98:687–691, 1932.
11. McCarthy, J.F., Ritter, J.S., and Klemperer, P.: Anatomical and histological study of the verumontanum with especial reference to ejaculatory ducts and their relations. J. Urol., 17:1–16, 1927.
12. McMahon, S.: An anatomical study by injection technique of the ejaculatory ducts and their relations. J. Urol., 39:422–443, 1938.
13. Merricks, J.W.: Modern conception of the diagnosis and treatment of injections of the seminal vesicles; with roentgenologic visualization of these organs by catheterization of the ejaculatory ducts. Int. Clinics, 2:193–199, 1940.
14. Pereira, A.: Roentgen interpretation of vesiculograms. Am. J. Roentgenol., 69:361–379, 1953.
15. Peterson, A.P.: Retrograde catheterization in diagnosis and

treatment of seminal vesiculitis. J. Urol., 39:662–677, 1938.

16. Sargent, J.C.: Interpretation of seminal vesiculograms. Radiology, 12:472–483, 1929.

17. Tucker, A.S., Yanagihara, H., and Pryde, A.W.: A method of roentgenology of the male genital tract. Am. J. Roentgenol., 71:490–500, 1954.

18. Watson, E.M.: The human seminal vesicles at birth, with observations on their fetal development. Ann. Surg., 68:416–419, 1918.

19. Watson, E.M.: The development of the seminal vesicles in man. Am. J. Anat., 24:398–441, 1918.

20. Wilhelm, S.F., and Marks, R.: Sterility in the Male. vol. 3, pp. 746 298-1a, 647 298-60a. New York, Oxford University Press, 1937.

21. Wilhelm, S.F.: Vaso-seminal vesiculography: clinical experimental application. J. Urol., 41:751–757, 1939.

22. Young, H.H., and Waters, C.A.: X-ray studies of the seminal vesicles and vasa deferentia after urethroscopic injection of the ejaculatory ducts with Thorium; a new diagnostic method. Am. J. Roentgenol., 7:16–22, 1920.

Tuberculosis of the Seminal Vesicles

23. Auerbach, O.: Pathology of urogenital tuberculosis. Int. Clinics, 3:21–61, 1940.

24. Hanley, H.O.: Tuberculous seminal vesicle. Proc. Roy. Soc. Med., 47:397–400, 1956.

25. Herbut, P.A.: Urological pathology. vol. 2, pp. 999–1001. Philadelphia, Lea & Febiger, 1952.

26. Mygind, H.B.: Urogenital tuberculosis in men: vesiculographic and urethrographic studies; preliminary report. Ugeskr. Laeg., 121:449–454, 1959.

27. Mygind, H.B.: Urogenital tuberculosis in the human male. Vesiculographic and urethrographic studies. Danish Med. Bull., 7:13–18, 1960.

Calculi of the Seminal Vesicles

28. Beyer, T.E.: Calculi of the seminal vesicles. Trans. Chicago Path. Soc., 10:149–152, 1915–17.

29. Corner, E.M.: A case of calculus in the vesiculae seminales in a man with enlarged prostate. Med. Press & Circ., 99:134, 1915.

30. Durban, V.J.: Calculi of the seminal vesicles. J. Philipp. Med. Assn., 41:290–293, 1965.

31. Heckel, N.J.: Calculi in the seminal vesicles. Report of a case. Am. J. Roentgenol., 39:377–378, 1938.

32. James, C.S., and Schuman, J.W.: Seminal calculi simulating nephrolithiasis. Surg. Gynecol. Obstet., 16:302–303, 1913.

33. Vaughan, G.T.: Two cases of calculi in the seminal vesicles. Trans. South. Surg. Assoc., 35:260–262, 1923.

34. White, J.L.: Stones in prostates and seminal vesicles. Texas State J. Med., 23:581–583, 1928.

Calcification of the Seminal Vesicles

35. Chetwood, C.H.: Practice of Urology. p. 332. New York, W. Wood & Co., 1913.

36. Chiari, H.: Über senile Verkalkung der Ampullen der Vasa deferentia und der Samenblasen. Ztschr. Heilk, Wien u. Leipz., 24:283–293, 1903.

37. Clement: Dissertation sur les maladies des organes generateurs de l'homme. These de Montpellier, 1830.

38. Cottenot and Binet du Jassoneix. Un cas d'opacite totale des vesicules seminales. Bull. et mém. Soc. radiol. méd. France, 17:109, 1929.

39. George, S.: Calcification of vas deferens and seminal vesicles. J.A.M.A., 47:103–105, 1906.

40. Janker, R.: Ein Beitrag zur Verkalkung der Samenblasen und Samenleiter. Fortschr. Geb. Roentgenstrahlen, 52:36–43, 1935.

41. Klebs, E.: Handbuch der Pathologischen Anatomie. pp. 1088, Berlin, A. Hirschwald, 1876.

42. Klerk, H.V.: A case of bilharziasis demonstrating accurate outlining of bladder and seminal vesicles due to calcification of the bladder and seminal vesicles. Br. J. Urol., 37:440–442, 1965.

43. Kretschmer, H.L.: Calcification of the seminal vesicles. J. Urol., 7:67–71, 1922.

44. Lallemand, C.F.: Des pertes seminales involontaires. p. 1518. Paris, Bechetjaune, 1836–1841.

45. Rokitansky, C.: Lehrbuch der Pathologischen Anatomie. vol. 2, pp. 309–319. Berlin, Hirschwald, 1893.

46. Shea, J.D., and Schwartz, J.W.: Calcification of the seminal vesicles. J. Urol., 58:132–133, 1947.

47. Silber, S.J., and McDonald, F.D.: Calcification of the seminal vesicles and vas deferens in a uremic patient. J. Urol., 105:542–544, 1971.

Congenital Anomalies of the Seminal Vesicles, Including Cysts

48. Anderz, V.: A cyst of the seminal vesicle. Pol. Tyg. Lek., 20:1373–1374, 1965.

49. Davidson, A.C., and Beard, J.H.: A seminal vesicle cyst: in association with ipsilateral renal agenesis and lumbar scoliosis. South. Med. J., 62:608–610, 1969.

50. Deming, C.L.: Cysts of the seminal vesicles. Trans. Am. Assoc. Genitourin. Surg., 28:301–312, 1935.

51. Francke, H.: Ein Fall von multilokulären Samenblasenzyste. Centralbl. f. allg. Path. u. pathol. anat., 41:145–147, 1927.

52. Greenbaum, E., and Pearman, R.O.: Vasovesiculography: cyst of the seminal vesicle associated with agenesis of ipsilateral kidney. Radiology, 98:362, 1971.

53. Harbitz, T.B., and Liavae, I.: Urogenital malformation with cyst of seminal vesicle associated with agenesis of ipsilateral kidney. Scand. J. Urol. Nephrol., 2:217, 1968.

54. Hart, J.B.: A case of cyst or hydrops of the seminal vesicle. J. Urol., 86:137–141, 1961.

55. Hart, J.B.: A case of cyst of the seminal vesicle. J. Urol., 96:247–249, 1966.

56. Heetderks, D.R., Jr., and Delambre, L.C.: Cyst of the seminal vesicle. J. Urol., 93:725–728, 1965.

57. Heller, E., and Whitsel, J.A.: Seminal vesicle cysts. J. Urol., 90:305–307, 1963.

58. Holt, S.A., and Petersen, N.E.: Ectopia of seminal vesicle associated with agenesis of ipsilateral kidney. Urology, 4:322–324, 1974.

59. Kimchi, D., and Wiesenfield, A.: Cyst of seminal vesicle associated with ipsilateral renal agenesis: case report. J. Urol., 89:906–907, 1963.

60. Klotz, P.G.: Congenital cystic abnormality of the seminal vesicle associated with ipsilateral renal agenesis. Report of a case. Canad. J. Surg., 10:471–473, 1967.

61. Lawson, L.J., and MacDougall, J.A.: Multilocular cyst of the seminal vesicle. Br. J. Urol., 37:440–442, 1965.

62. Linhares, Furtado, A.J.: Three cases of cystic seminal vesicle associated with unilateral renal agenesis. Br. J. Urol., 45:536–540, 1973.

63. Lloyd, F.A., and Pranke, D.: Cysts of the seminal vesicle. Northwest Univ. M. School Quart. Bull., 25:45–46, 1951.
64. Lund, A.S., and Cummings, M.M.: Cyst of the recessory genital tract: a case report with a review of the literature. J. Urol., 56:383–386, 1946.
65. Meiraz, D., Fischelovitch, J., and Lazebnik, S.: Agenesis of the kidney associated with congenital malformation of the seminal vesicle. Br. J. Urol., 45:541–544, 1973.
65a. Mellin, H-E., Kjaer, T.B., and Madsen, P.O.: Crossed ectopia of seminal vesicles, renal aplasia, and ectopic ureter. J. Urol. 115:765–766, 1976.
66. Picker, quoted by Lund and Cummings.
67. Priesel, A.: Die Missbildungen der Mannlichen geschlechtsorgane. In Henke, F. and Lubarsch, D., Handbuch. der sepziellen pathologischen Anatomie und Histologie. vol. 6, part 3, pp. 1–182. Berlin, Julius Springer, 1931.
68. Quinby, W.C.: Discussion of Deming's paper. Trans Am. Assoc. Genitourin. Surg., 28:330–331, 1935.
69. Ragi, I.: Congenital cysts of the prostate and seminal vesicle. J. Egypt. Med. Ass., 48:621–627, 1965.
70. Reddy, Y.N., and Winter, C.C.: Cyst of the seminal vesicle: a case report and review of the literature. J. Urol., 108:134–135, 1972.
71. Sharma, T.C., Dorman, P.S., and Dorman, H.P.: Bilateral seminal vesicular cysts. J. Urol., 102:741–744, 1969.
72. Stewart, B.L., and Nocoll, G.A.: Cyst of the seminal vesicle. J. Urol., 62:189–199, 1949.
73. Zinner, A.: Ein Fall von intravesikaler Samenblasencyste. Wien. Med. Wchnschr., 64:605–609, 1914.

Benign Tumors of the Seminal Vesicles

74. Bagley, D.H., Javadpour, N., Witebsky, F.G., and Thomas, L.B.: Seminal vesicle cysts containing mesonephroid tumor. Urol., 5:147–151, 1975.
75. Buck, A.C., and Shaw, R.E.: Primary tumors of the retrovesical region with special reference to mesenthymal tumors of the seminal vesicles. Br. J. Urol., 44:47–50, 1972.
76. Ceelen, W.: Ein Fibromyom der Samenblase. Virchow Arch. Path. Anat., 207:200–206, 1912.
77. Guelliot. Quoted by Lazarus, J.A.: Primary malignant tumors of the retrovesical region with special reference to malignant tumors of the seminal vesicles. Report of a case of retrovesical sarcoma. J. Urol., 55:190–205, 1946.
78. Oehlecker, F.: Samenblasentumor VIIIe, Congrés allemand d'urol. Nov. 26, 1928. verhandl d. deutsch. Gesellsch. f. Urol., 8:350, 1928.
79. Pana: Quoted by Plaut, A. and Standard, S., infra.
80. Plaut, A., and Standard, S.: Cystomyoma of seminal vesicle. Ann. Surg., 119:253–261, 1944.
81. Soule, E.H., and Dockerty, M.B.: Cystadenoma of the seminal vesicle. A pathologic curiosity, report of a case and review of the literature concerning benign tumors of the seminal vesicles. Proc. Mayo Clin., 26:406–414, 1951.
82. Voelcker: Quoted by Plaut, A. and Standard, S., supra.

Primary Carcinoma of the Seminal Vesicles

83. Awadella, D., Hunt, A.C., and Miller, A.: Primary carcinoma of the seminal vesicle. Br. J. Urol., 40:574–579, 1968.
84. Burckhard, G.: Ueber Entwicklungsstörungen and Geschwülste der Samenblasen mit Casuirtischen. Beitr. Inaug. Dissert. München, 1904.
85. Dalgaard, J.B., and Giersten, S.C.: Primary carcinoma of the

seminal vesicles. Case and survey. Acta Path. Microbiol. Scand., 39:255–267, 1956.
86. Dawson, E.R., and Mekie, D.E.: Primary carcinoma of the seminal vesicles. J. Roy. Coll. Surg. (Edinburgh), 10:233–238, 1965.
87. Devos, R.: Adenocarcinome primitif de la vesicule séminale. J. Belg. d'Urol., 19:301, 1951.
88. Ewell, G.H.: Seminal vesicle carcinoma. J. Urol., 89:908–912, 1963.
89. Gee, E.M.: Primary carcinoma of the seminal vesicles. Report of 2 cases. Br. J. Urol., 20:72–76, 1948.
90. Goldstein, A.G., and Wilson, E.S.: Carcinoma of the seminal vesicle – with particular reference to the angiographic appearances. Br. J. Urol., 45:211–212, 1973.
91. Hadju, J.I., Furuque, A.A.: Adenocarcinoma of the seminal vesicle. J. Urol., 99:798–801, 1968.
92. Junker: Ein Fall von primarem Samenblasen-Karzinom. Ztschr. Urol., 35:204–208, 1941.
93. Labbe: Quoted by Guelliot, O.: In Des vesiculé séminales. Chap. 8, Paris. A. Coccoz, 1883.
94. Lyons, O.: Primary carcinoma of the left seminal vesicle. J. Urol., 13:477–484, 1925.
95. McCrea, L.E.: Primary carcinoma of the seminal vesicle. Report of 2 cases and review of the literature. Urol. and Cutan. Rev., 46:700–703, 1942.
96. McCrea, L.E.: Primary carcinoma of the seminal vesicles. J.A.M.A., 136:679–682, 1948.
97. McNally, A., and Cochems, F.M.: Primary carcinoma of the seminal vesicles. J. Urol., 36:532–537, 1936.
98. Marshall, D.F., Leary, G.C., O'Donnell, E.E., and Geer, G.I.: Seminal vesicle carcinoma. J. Maine Med. Assoc., 52:145–147, 1961.
99. Morales, L., Obrador, Alcalde, S., and Perrin, T.G.: Un case de adenocarcinoma primitivo de vesicular seminal con metástasis Craneales. Analecta Med., 4:3–16, 1943.
100. Pelagatti, V.: Adenocarcinoma della vesicichetta seminale destra. Arch. Ital. Urol., 11:201–210, 1934.
101. Rodrigues Kees, O.S.: Clinical improvement following estrogenic therapy in a case of primary adenocarcinoma of the seminal vesicle. J. Urol., 91:665–670, 1964.
102. Sinclair, A.B., and Fitzpatrick, E.J.: Anaplastic carcinoma of the seminal vesicles with extensive invasion of the bladder wall. Canad. Med. Assoc. J., 58:386–388, 1948.
103. Smith, B.A., Jr.: Carcinoma of the seminal vesicle: report of 2 cases. J. Urol., 72:67–76, 1954.
104. Smith, B.A., Jr., Webb, E.A., and Price, W.E.: Carcinoma of the seminal vesicle. J. Urol., 97:743–750, 1967.
105. Tannenbaum, M.: Differential diagnosis in uropathology. I. Carcinoma of prostate versus seminal vesicle. Urology, 4:354–356, 1974.
106. Thevenot, M.: Cancer de la vésicule séminale gauche avec intégrité apparente de la prostate. J. Urol. (Paris), 21:55–57, 1926.
107. Trabucco, A., Cartelli, N., and Marquez, F.J.: Tumor de vesiculas seminales; Consideraciones sobre: 2 casos. Rev. Argent. Urol., 20:258–270, 1951.

Sarcoma of the Seminal Vesicles

107a. Buck, A.C., and Shaw, R.E.: See reference 75.
108. Junghanns, H.: Primaries Sarkom der Samenblase mit ausgedehnten Gehirumetastasen und zwei Falle von Samenblasenkarzinom, Deutsch. Ztschr. Chir., 224:418–421, 1930.
109. Lazarus, J.A.: Primary malignant tumor of the retrovesical region with specific reference to malignant tumor of the

seminal vesicles. Report of a case of retrovesical sarcoma. J. Urol., *55*:190–205, 1946.

110. Tripathi, UNP, and Dick, V.S.: Primary sarcoma of the urogenital system in adults. J. Urol., *101*:898–904, 1969.
111. Young, H.H.: Sarcoma of the Prostate. *In* Cabot, H. (ed.): Modern Urology. vol. 1, pp. 911–922, 1936.
112. Young, H.H., and Davis, D.M.: Young's Practice of Urology. vol. 1, pp. 558, 559. Philadelphia, Saunders, c. 1926.
113. Zahn: Ueber einen Fall von primärem Sarkom der Samenblasenusw, Deutsch. Ztschr. Chir. ed., *22*:22, 1885.

Secondary Carcinoma of the Seminal Vesicles

114. Abeshouse, B.S., Heller, E., and Salik, J.O.: Vaso-epididymography and vasoseminal vesiculography. J. Urol., *72*:983–991, 1954.
115. Aledia, F.T.: Vasoseminal vesiculography: a diagnostic aid in early metastatic carcinoma of prostate. J. Urol., *110*:242–244, 1973.
116. Boreau, J.: L'Etude Radiologique des voies séminales normales et Pathologiques. Paris, Masson et Cie, 1953.
117. Fetter, T.R., Yunen, J.R., Greening, R., and Benjamin, A.: Seminal vesiculography: diagnostic aid in prostatic carcinoma. J. Urol., *87*:718–725, 1962.
118. Gerner-Smidt, M.: Vesiculography as a diagnostic aid in cancer and hypertrophy of the prostate. Acta Chir. Scand., *114*:387–397, 1958.
119. Hebert, G., Bouchard, R., and Charron, J.: Vasoseminal vesiculography. Am. J. Roentgenol., *113*:735–740, 1971.
120. Vanwelkenhuyzen, P.: Les modifications radiologiques des voies séminales par les lesions de la prostate. Acta Urol. Belg., *25*:34–52, 1957.
121. Vanwelkenhuyzen, P.: Remarques sur L'interpretation des vesiculographies en cas de lesions de la prostate. Acta Urol. Belg., *26*:38–47, 1958.
122. Vestby, G.W.: Vasoseminal vesiculography in hypertrophy and carcinoma of the prostate, with special reference to the ejaculatory ducts. Acta Radiol. Suppl., *199*:1–194, 1960.

Seminal Vesiculography and Benign Prostatic Hypertrophy

See References 117 and 122.

123. Nilsson, S., Hulten, L., and Seeman, T.: State of the ejaculatory ducts, deferent ducts ampullae, seminal vesicles and posterior urethra after various operations for benign prostatic hyperplasia. Scand. J. Urol. Nephrol., *3*:73–78, 1969.

Anomalies of the Vas Deferens

124. Amelar, R.D., and Hotchkiss, R.S.: Congenital aplasia of the epididymides and vasa deferentia, effects on semen. Fertil. Steril., *14*:44–48, 1963.
125. Blecher: Über angeborene Missbildungen des Samenleiters, insbesondere die einseitige isolierte Verdoppelung. Deutsche Ztschr. F. Chir., *232*:430–432, 1931.
126. Büttner, A.: Verfahren und Nachbehandlung bei der Unfruchtbarmachung des Mannes unter besonderer Berücksichtung de Doppelbildungen der Samenleiter. Beitr. Z. Klin. Chir., *164*:49–60, 1936.
127. Charny, C.W.: Testicular biopsy: a five-year survey. *In* Engle, E.T.: Diagnosis in Sterility. p. 54. Springfield, Ill., Charles C Thomas, 1946.
128. Charny, C.W., and Gillenwater, J.Y.: Congenital absence of the vas deferens. J. Urol., *93*:399–401, 1965.
129. Chatterjee, H., and Sen, S.B.: Congenital absence of the vas deferens. Indian J. Med. Sci., *25*:623–626, 1971.
130. Cuetzee, T.: Double vas deferens: a case report. Br. J. Urol., *31*:336–339, 1959.
131. El-Itreby, A.A., and Girgis, S.M.: Congenital absence of vas deferens in male sterility. Int. J. Fertil., *6*:409–416, 1961.
132. Emmerich, E.: Enorm Cystenbildung der Vas Deferens. Zentralblatt für allegemeine Pathologie und pathologische Anatomie. Jena, *21*:673–677, 1910.
133. Foss, G.L., and Miller, A.: Aplasia of the vasa deferentia as a cause of sterility. Lancet, *259*:737–738, 1950.
134. Guizzetti, P.: Genital anomalies as clue to renal anomalies. Riforma Med., *34*:646, 1918. (Abstracted, J.A.M.A., *71*:1867, 1918.)
135. Hawtrey, C.E.: Case report of a congenital urethro-vaso-cutaneous fistula. J. Urol., *104*:555–556, 1970.
136. Hutch, J.A.: Anomalies of the vas deferens. J.A.M.A., *219*:1762–1763, 1972.
137. Koyangi, T., Tzugi, I., Kudo, T., Ishikawa, T., and Sasak, K.: Double vas deferens associated with ipsilateral renal agenesis simulating ectopic ureter. J. Urol., *108*:631–634, 1972.
138. Lurie, A., Savir, A., and Lubin, E.: Non-fused crossed renal ectopia verified by radioisotope scanning and agenesis of the vas deferens on the ipsilateral side. Urologia Internationalis, *26*:45–50, 1971.
139. Magri, J.: Solitary crossed ectopic kidney. Br. J. Urol., *33*:152–156, 1961.
140. Martinez-Tello, F.J., and Gropp, A.: Cystic ectasia of the vas deferens. Urologie (A), *11*:36–38, 1972.
141. Mathe, C.P., and Dunn, G.: Double vas deferens associated with solitary kidney: case report. J. Urol., *59*:461–465, 1948.
142. Michelson, L.: Congenital anomalies of the ductus deferens and epididymis. J. Urol., *61*:384–390, 1949.
143. Michelson, L.: Vasoepididymal ductal obstruction. Mod. Medicine, *21*:96–102, 1953.
144. Nelson, R.E.: Congenital absence of vas deferens: a review of the literature and report of three cases. J. Urol., *63*:176–182, 1950.
145. Ochsner, M.G., Brannon, W., and Goodier, E.H.: Absent vas deferens associated with renal agenesis. J.A.M.A., *222*:1055–1056, 1972.
146. Sadi, A., Saito, M., and Borges, G.G.: Agenesis of the deferent ducts. Review of the literature and presentation of three cases. Hospital (Rio de J.), *75*:1229–1239, 1969.
147. Sakatoku, J., Yoshida, O., Komatsu, Y., Takayana, H., Harada, T., and Ueyama, H.: Congenital aplasia of vas deferens. Acta Urol. Jap., *13*:769–784, 1967.
148. Sandler, B.: Sterility due to congenital absence of the vasa. Lancet, *2*:736–737, 1950.
149. Sniffen, R.C., Howard, R.P., and Simmons, F.A.: The Testes. II Abnormalities of Spermatogenesis: atresia of the excretory ducts. Arch. Pathol., *50*:285–295, 1950.
150. Walker, W.C., and Bowles, W.I.: Transversical seminal vesiculostomy in treatment of congenital obstruction of seminal vesicles. Case report. J. Urol., *99*:324–325, 1968.
151. Windholz, F.: Partielle Verdoppelung des rechten Samenleiter bei einer 54 jahrigen Mann. Wein klin wchnschr, *42*:447–448, 1929.
152. Young, D.: Bilateral aplasia of the vas deferens. Br. J. Surg., *36*:417–418, 1949.

Calcification of Vas Deferens

153. Adlerman, E.J., and Friedmann, F.: Bilateral beaded calcification of the vasa deferentia. New York J. Med., *54*:1520–1522, 1954.

154. Andersen, P.E.: Calcification of vasa deferentia. Acta Radiol., *34*:89–95, 1950.

155. Bianchini, A.: Su di un caso di calcificazione quasi totale delle vie deferenziali. Arch. Radiol., *6*:228–233, 1930.

156. Camiel, M.R.: Calcification of vas deferens associated with diabetes. J. Urol., *86*:634–636, 1961.

157. Chiari, H.: Ueber senile Verkalkung der Ampullen der Vasa deferentia und der Samenblasen. Ztschr. Heilk., Wien. u. Leipz., *24*:283–292, 1903.

158. Culver, C.J., and Tannenhaus, J.: Calcification of the vas deferens in diabetes. J.A.M.A., *173*:648–651, 1960.

159. Dopheide, W.: Zwei Fälle von Verkalkung des Samenleiters. Centralbl. allg. Path. path. Anat., *45*:39–43, 1929.

160. Dupley, A.: Recherches sur les changements et les alterations que présente chez les vieillards l'appareil secreteur et éxcreteur du sperme. Arch. gén. de méd., *2*:428–443, 1855.

161. Fraenkel, E.: Demonstration eines Präparats und Rontgenbildes von symmetrischer Verkalkung des vesikalen Teils des Ductus deferens. München Med. Wschr., *53*:1491, 1906.

162. George, S.: Calcification of the vas deferens and the seminal vesicles. J.A.M.A., *47*:103–105, 1906.

163. Goren, N.: Calcification of the ductus deferens: 2 cases. Rev. Argent. Urol., *27*:311–314, 1958.

164. Hafiz, A., and Melnick, J.C.: Calcification of the vas deferens. J. Canad. Assn. Radiol., *19*:56–60, 1968.

165. Henke, F., and Lubarsh, C.O.: Handbuch der Speciellen. Patholog. anatomie and Histologie. vol. 3, p. 554. Berlin, Springer, 1931.

166. Hofer, R., and Lossen, H.: Teilweise verkalkte Ductus deferentes. Ztschr. Urol., *26*:153–156, 1932.

167. Janker, R.: Ein Beitrag zur Verkalkung der Samenblasen und Samenleiter. Fortschr. Geb. Röntgenstrahlen, *52*:36–43, 1935.

168. King, J.C., Jr., and Rosenbaum, H.D.: Calcification of the vasa deferentia in nondiabetics. Urology, *100*:603–606, 1971.

169. Le Bihan, R., Lagarde, C., and Illes, J.: Calcification des canaux déférents. J. Radiol. Electr., *36*:529–530, 1955.

170. Lowsley, O.S., and Riaboff, P.J.: Calcification of the vas deferentia. J. Urol., *47*:293–298, 1942.

171. Marks, J.H., and Hamm, D.P.: Calcification of vas deferens. Am. J. Roentgenol., *47*:859–863, 1942.

172. Narins, L., and Oppenheimer, G.D.: Calcification of the vas deferens associated with Paget's disease of bone. J. Urol., *67*:218–221, 1952.

173. Norris, H.J., and Yunis, E.: Age changes of seminal vesicles and vasa deferentia in diabetics. Arch. Pathol., *77*:126–131, 1964.

174. O'Conor, V.J., and Crowley, E.: Bilateral calcification of vasa deferentia. Quart. Bull. Northwestern Univ. Med. School, *21*:28–30, 1947.

175. Orth, J.: Lehrbuch der speciellen pathologischen Anatomie. vol. 2, pp. 309–310. Berlin, Hirschwald, 1893.

176. Pons, H., Denard, Y., and Moreau: Un signe radiologique du Diabete, la calcification des canaux déférents. J. Radiol. Electr., *38*:237, 1957.

177. Schellenberg, W.: Über einen Fall von Verkalkung der Samenleiter und Ampullea. Frankfurt. Ztschr. Path., *40*:298–301, 1930.

178. Wilson, J.L., and Marks, J.H.: Calcification of the vas deferens: its relation to diabetes mellitus and arteriosclerosis. New Engl. J. Med., *245*:321–325, 1951.

Tumors and Granulomas of Vas Deferens

179. Dougall, A.J., and Wilson, R.R.: Leiomyoma of the vas deferens. Br. J. Urol., *41*:348–350, 1969.

180. Friedman, N.B., and Garske, G.L.: Inflammatory reactions involving sperm and the seminiferous tubules: extravasation, spermatic granulomas, and granulomatous orchitis. J. Urol., *62*:363–374, 1949.

181. Graham, J.B., and O'Conor, V.J.: Spermatic cord tumors: review of literature and a case of unusual vas deferens tumor in an infertility problem. J. Urol., *72*:946–949, 1954.

182. Schmidt, S.S.: Techniques and complications of elective vasectomy. Fertil. Steril., *17*:467–482, 1966.

183. Taberman, A.: Granulomatous lesion in vas deferens caused by injection of radiopaque contrast media. J. Urol., *107*:818–820, 1972.

Congenital Lesions of Epididymis

184. Badenoch, A.W.: Failure of the urogenital union. Surg. Gynecol. Obstet., *82*:471–474, 1946.

185. Dean, A.L., Jr., Major, J.W., and Osterheimer, E.J.: Failure of fusion of the testis and epididymis. J. Urol., *68*:754–758, 1952.

186. Hinman, F.: Principles and Practice of Urology. pp. 440, 441. Philadelphia, W.B. Saunders Co., 1936.

187. Nowak, K.: Failure of fusion of epididymis and testicle and complete separation of vas deferens. J. Pediatr. Surg., *7*:715–716, 1972.

188. Orr, L.M., Haywood, J.C., and Turner, A.F., Jr.: Failure of urogenital union. J. Urol., *60*:147–152, 1948.

189. Scorer, C.G., and Farrington, H.: Congenital deformities of testis and epididymis. New York, Appleton-Century-Crofts, 1971.

190. Windholz, F.: Zur Pathologe des Hodendescensus Teilung des Nebenhodens bei unvollständigen Descensus, Klin. Wochnsehr. (Berlin), *2*:2175–2176, 1923.

Infections of Epididymis

191. Cooper, H.G.: Treatment of genitourinary tuberculosis; report after 14 years. J. Urol., *86*:719–727, 1961.

192. Cooper, H.G., and Robinson, E.G.: Treatment of genitourinary tuberculosis; report after 24 years. J. Urol., *108*:136–142, 1972.

193. Furness, G., Kamat, M.H., Kaminski, Z., and Seebode, J.J.: The etiology of idiopathic epididymitis. J. Urol., *106*:387–392, 1971.

194. Graves, R.S., and Engel, W.J.: Experimental production of epididymitis with sterile urine; clinical complications. J. Urol., *64*:601–613, 1950.

195. Handley, R.S.: Nonspecific epididymitis. Lancet, *1*:779–781, 1946.

196. Hanley, H.G.: Non-specific epididymitis. Br. J. Surg., *53*:873–874, 1966.

197. Ross, J.C., Gow, J.G., St. Hill, C.A.: Tuberculous epididymitis: a series of 179 patients. Br. J. Surg., *48*:663–666, 1961.

198. Wesson, M.B.: Epididymitis, facts and fancies. Med. Clin. North Am., *43*:1645–1659, 1959.

Tumors of Epididymis

General

199. Broth, G., Bullock, W.K., and Morrow, J.: Epididymal tumors: 1. Report 15 new cases, including reivew of the literature; 2. histochemical study of the so-called adenomatoid tumor. J. Urol., *100*:530–536, 1968.

Benign Epididymal Tumors: Adenomatoid

200. Abell, M.R., and Holtz, F.: Testicular and paratesticular neoplasms in patients 60 years of age and older. Cancer, *21*:852–870, 1968.
201. Burros, H.M., and Maycock, P.P.: Adenomatoid tumor of epididymis: report of a case in newborn. J. Urol., *63*:712–713, 1950.
202. Dixon, F.S., and Moore, R.A.: Tumors of the male sex organs. *In* Atlas of Tumor Pathology, Wash. D.C., Armed Forces Institute of Path. vol. 8, Fasc. 31B and 32. 1952.
203. Evans, N.: Mesothelioma of the epididymis and tunica vaginalis. J. Urol., *50*:249–254, 1943.
204. Fisher, E.R., and Klieger, H.: Epididymal carcinoma (malignant adenocatoid tumor, mesonephric, mesodermal carcinoma of epididymis). J. Urol., *95*:568–572, 1966.
205. Glenn, J.: Adenomatoid tumor of epididymis: report of three cases with histochemical studies and review of literature. South. Med. J., *52*:60–67, 1958.
206. Golden, A., and Ash, J.E.: Adenomatoid tumors of the genital tract. Am. J. Pathol., *21*:63–79, 1945.
207. Jackson, J.R.: The histogenesis of the "adenomatoid" tumor of the genital tract. Cancer, *11*:337–350, 1958.
208. Kannenstein, M., and Lustig, M.: The adenomatoid tumor of the genital tract. J. Newark Beth Israel Hospital, *13*:28–29, 1962.
209. Mackay, B., Bennington, J.L., and Skoglund, R.W.: The adenomatoid tumor: fine structural evidence for a mesothelial origin. Cancer, *27*:109–115, 1971.
210. Stavrides, A., and Hutcheson, J.B.: Benign mesotheliomas of testicular appendages: a morphologic and histochemical study of seven cases and review of theories of histogenesis. J. Urol., *83*:448–453, 1960.
211. Vprakasit, D., Tannebaum, M., and Smith, A.M.: Adenomatoid tumor of male genital tract. Urology, *4*:325–327, 1974.

Papillary Adenoma of Epididymis (Papillary Cystadenoma, Cyst Adenoma)

212. Chen, Y.H., Schinella, R.A., and Draper, J.W.: Papillary clear cell cystadenoma of the epididymis. J. Urol., *100*:661–665, 1968.
213. Easton, J.A., and Claridge, M.: Cystadenoma of the epididymis. Br. J. Urol., *36*:416–417, 1964.
214. Grant, S.M., and Hoffman, E.F.: Bilateral papillary adenomas of the epididymis. Arch. Pathol., *76*:620–625, 1963.
215. Hill, R.B., Jr.: Bilateral papillary hyperplastic nodules of the epididymis. J. Urol., *87*:155–158, 1962.
216. Melman, K.L., and Rosen, S.W.: Lindau's disease. Review of the literature and study of a large kindred. Am. J. Med., *36*:595–617, 1964.
217. Meyer, J.S., Roth, L.M., and Silverman, J.L.: Papillary cystadenoma of the epididymis and spermatic cord. Cancer, *17*:1241–1247, 1964.

218. Mostofi, F.R., and Price, E.B., Jr. *In* Tumors of the Male Genital System. Atlas of Tumor Pathology. Second Series. Fasc. 8, pp. 162–165. Armed Forces Institute of Pathology, Wash. D.C., 1973.
219. Sherrick, J.C.: Papillary cystadenoma of the epididymis. Cancer, *9*:403–407, 1956.

Malignant Neoplasms of Epididymis

220. Ferrier, P.A., and Foord, A.G.: Primary carcinoma of epididymis. Urol. Cutan. Rev., *38*:646–650, 1974.
221. Kwae, S.Z., Liv, Y., and Chen, S.C.: Leiomyosarcoma of the epididymis: case report. J. Urol., *62*:349–353, 1949.
222. Teilum, G.: Histogenesis and classification of mesonephric tumors of the female and male genital systems and relationship to benign so-called adenomatoid tumors (mesotheliomas). Acta Pathol. Microbiol. Scand., *34*:431–481, 1954.
223. Thompson, G.: Tumors of the epididymis and testicular tunics. Surg. Gynecol. Obstet., *62*:712–718, 1936.
224. Whitehead, R., and Williams, A.F.: Carcinoma of epididymis. Br. J. Surg., *38*:513–516, 1951.

Vasoepididymography

225. Abeshouse, B.S., Heller, E., and Salik, J.O.: Vasoepididymography and vasoseminal vesiculography. J. Urol., *72*:983–991, 1954.
226. Boreau, J.: L'epididymographie. J. Urol. Paris, *59*:416–423, 1953.
227. Boreau, J., Elbim, A., Hermann, P., Vassel, B., and Fua, R.: L'epididymographie. Presse Med., *59*:1406–1407, 1951.
228. Boreau, J., Hermann, P., Vasselle, B., and Fua, R.: L'etude radiologique et radiomanométrique des voies génitales de l'homme appliquee à la clinique et à la physiologie. Sem. Hop. Paris, *28*:1549–1556, 1952.
229. Boreau, J., Jagailloux, S., Vasselle, B., and Hermann, P.: Epididymography. Med. Radiogr. Photogr., *29*:63–66, 1953.
230. Brodny, M.L., Robins, A.A., Hershman, H.A., and DeNuccio, A.: Epididymography, varicocelography and testicular angiography. Fertil. Steril., *6*:158–168, 1955.
231. Golji, H.: Clinical value of epididymo-vesiculography. J. Urol., *78*:445–455, 1957.
232. Korkud, G.: L'epididymographie. Sem. Hop. Paris, *28*:2427–2433, 1952.
233. Peruzzo, L., and Antonini, R.: L'epididimografia. Ricerche cliniche e sperimentali. Arch Ital. Urol., *26*:540–545, 1953.
234. Trabucco, A., and Bottini, E.B., Jr.: La radiografia del epididimo. Obstet. Ginec. Lat. Amer., *12*:52–54, 1954.

Aspermia

235. Girgis, S.N., Etriby, E.L., El-Hefnawy, H., and Kahil, S.A.: Aspermia: a survey of forty-nine cases. Fertil. Steril., *19*:580–588, 1968.
236. Girgis, S.M., Etriby, A., Ibrahim, A.A. et al.: Testicular biopsy in azoospermia: a review of the last ten years' experience of over 800 cases. Fertil. Steril., *20*:467–477, 1969.
237. O'Conor, V.J.: Surgical correction of male sterility. Surg. Gynecol. Obstet., *110*:649–657, 1960.
238. Scultéty, S., and Lelek, I.: Aspermia as a consequence of junction of both deferent ducts in a blind ending ureter. J. Urol., *61*:11–13, 1968.
239. Trabucco, A., and Bottini, E.B.: Lack of deferent ducts: four cases. Rev. Asoc. Méd. Argent., *67*:118–122, 1953.

Fertility in Men Related to Cystic Fibrosis

240. Denning, C.R., Summers, S.S., Quigley, H.J., Jr.: Infertility in male patients with cystic fibrosis. Pediatrics, *41*:7–17, 1968.
241. di Sant' Agnese, P.A.: Fertility and the young adult with cystic fibrosis. Guest Editorial, New Engl. J. Med., *279*:103–105, 1968.
242. Feigelson, J., Pecau, Y., and Schwachman, H.: A Propos d'une paternité chez un malade atteint de mucoviscidose: etude des fonctions génitales et de la filiation. Arch. Fr. Pediatr., *26*:937–944, 1969.
243. Gracey, M., Campbell, P., and Noblett, H.R.: Atretic vas deferens in cystic fibrosis. New Engl. J. Med., *280*:276, 1969.
244. Holsclaw, D.S., Perlmutter, A.D., Jockin, H., and Schwachman, H.: Genital abnormalities in male patients with cystic fibrosis. J. Urol., *106*:568–574, 1971.
245. Kaplan, E., Schwachman, H., Perlmutter, A.D., Rule, A., Khaw, K-T., and Holsclaw, D.S.: Reproductive failure in males with cystic fibrosis. New Engl. J. Med., *279*:65–69, 1968.
246. Landing, B.H., Wells, T.R., and Wang, C-I.: Abnormality of the epididymis and the vas deferens in cystic fibrosis. Arch. Pathol., *88*:569–580, 1969.
247. Olson, J.R., and Weaver, D.K.: Congenital mesonephric defects in male patient with mucoviscidosis. J. Clin. Pathol., *22*:724–730, 1969.
248. Oppenheimer, E.H., Esterly, J.R.: Observations on cystic fibrosis of the pancreas. V. Developmental changes in the male genital system. J. Pediatr., *75*:806–811, 1969.
249. Taussig, L.M., Lobeck, C.C., di Sant' Agnese, P.A., Ackerman, D.R., and Kattwinkel, J.: Fertility in males with cystic fibrosis. New Engl. J. Med., *287*:586–589, 1972.
250. Eliasson, R., Mossberg, B., Camner, P. et al.: The immotilecilial syndrome: A congenital cilia abnormality as an etiologic factor in chronic airway infection and male sterility. New Engl. J. Med. *297*:1–6, 1977.

Part Seven

URETHRA

ANATOMY

The adult male urethra (Fig. 36–1) normally is divided into the prostatic urethra (3 to 3½ cm. in length), the membranous urethra (12 to 15 mm. in length), and the anterior urethra (12 to 15 cm. in length). The prostatic urethra commences at the internal sphincter (vesical orifice) and descends through the anterior part of the prostate in a vertical direction. Extending the length of the prostatic urethra on its floor is a urethral crest that appears as a narrow median, longitudinal ridge formed by elevation of mucous membrane (Fig. 36–2). On each side of the crest is a depression, named the prostatic sinus, into the floor of which enter the prostatic ducts. The verumontanum, openings of the ejaculatory ducts, and opening of the utricle are situated in the collicular (middle) portion of the prostatic urethra about midway along the length of the urethral crest. The prostatic urethra is divided into supracollicular, collicular, and infracollicular portions. The prostatic urethra ends in the membranous urethra that lies within the urogenital diaphragm and contains the bulbourethral glands of Cowper situated posteriorly on each side of the urethra, with their ducts penetrating the urogenital diaphragm, extending forward and downward and opening into the bulbous urethra. The anterior urethra, consisting of the bulbous and the penile or pendulous parts, contains numerous minute (Littre's) glands that are most numerous in the distal dorsal wall. The anterior urethra also receives the urethral lacunae of Morgagni.

Embryologically, the female urethra, which varies from 2.5 to 4 cm. in length, is homologous with the posterior urethra in the man but has no verumontanum. Lapides believes that a length of 3 cm. is the minimal length for continence and that a length of 3.8 cm. is the average length of the adult female

36

Normal Urethra

urethra.[3] Formerly thought to be merely a tube that served as a conduit for urine from the bladder, it has gathered increasing importance as various affectations and anatomic entities have been described. Much interest and investigation have been focused on the periurethral glands.[6, 14, 15]

At the present writing the general consensus is that the periurethral glands are found throughout the female urethra, including the posterior portion at the bladder neck, and that glands similar to the male prostatic glands certainly are present in a fair percentage of cases. (See Chapter 34, The Prostate.)

CYSTOURETHROGRAPHY

Cystourethrography consists of visualization of the urethra and the bladder using contrast medium. There have been many descriptions of this procedure differing in both the type of solution and the technique of examination. In general, two methods have been utilized: injection cystourethrography and voiding cystourethrography.

INJECTION CYSTOURETHROGRAPHY

This method utilizes direct injection of the urethra and the bladder with contrast medium (see Fig. 36–15A). Our procedure is as follows:

1. A preliminary scout film is made.
2. The bladder is filled with contrast medium, the concentration depending on the type of case. Tumors or stones in the bladder may require more dilute solutions, because they can be obscured by dense concentration. Films are obtained in the AP and both oblique views following withdrawal of the catheter. Delayed cystograms could be taken at this point. (See Delayed Cystography.)
3. A Foley catheter is inserted into the tip of the urethra and inflated so that the catheter cannot slip. (Some authors prefer the Brodny clamp[97] or the Knutson instrument[44] rather than a Foley catheter when a man is being examined.) Injection of a concentrated contrast material is made with a bulb or piston syringe. Exposure is made in the AP view during injection.
4. An oblique view is obtained during injection.
5. If a pneumocystogram is required, the bladder is drained, and air is injected until the first sensation of fullness. (Flocks removed 30 cc. of air by syringe by this point.[41]) The catheter again is placed into the tip of the urethra, fixed in position, and another oblique exposure is obtained during the injection of contrast material. If one is interested merely in the bladder, a cystogram can be secured without injecting the urethra.

VOIDING CYSTOURETHROGRAPHY

In this method the bladder is filled with contrast medium and the patient voids (Figs. 36–3 to 36–15). In males the oblique position commonly is used, whereas in females, the AP view is utilized. To obtain good visualization of the urethra, the contrast medium usually is more concentrated than in an ordinary cystogram. Voiding cystourethrograms can be obtained after an intravenous urogram. In the very young, Williams expressed contrast medium from the bladder by pressure over the bladder area.[109]

A variation of the voiding cystourethrogram was utilized by Kjellberg, Ericsson, and Rudhe[93] by performing the examination with the child sitting in specially constructed swing that was suspended in front of a serial changer. The patient voided in this position during serial photography, with simultaneous exposures in the true lateral and the frontal projections. There are several methods available for exposure of films:

1. A single film is used during voiding.
2. Fluoroscopy and multiple phototimed spot films throughout the voiding cycle are obtained.
3. Cinecystourethrography is excellent for studies of reflux and the physiology of voiding but is not suitable for the fine detail.

Choke Voiding Cystourethrography. "Choke" in this context designates the use of increased resistance to the passage of opaque medium through the bladder and the urethra by a mechanical choke such as pressure on the urethral meatus or the use of a viscous medium.[82-84] In general, the urethra is more dilated along its entire length in this method.

Triple-Voiding Cystourethrography. This method is used to determine the severity of bladder neck obstructions, to evaluate the possible success of an operation on the bladder neck, and to visualize vesicoureteral reflux and the trapping of urine in the ureters.[62]

The technique is as follows: The bladder is filled slowly by gravity with a dilute solution of neomycin and contrast medium until the flow ceases, and then a 30-minute delayed film is taken. The patient voids three times at 2-minute intervals, walking around between the voidings. A film is taken after each voiding.

Delayed Cystography. The bladder is filled slowly by catheter with a contrast medium; it should not be overdistended. The catheter then is withdrawn, and an x-ray exposure is made. The patient continues to retain the contrast material. Usually, ambulation is permitted, and additional exposures are made at 30 to 60 minutes. In young patients who cannot cooperate, the catheter is left in situ and clamped. This method is used to determine reflux up the ureters.

Measurement of Residual Urine. Occasionally, residual urine is determined after a retrograde or an excretory cystogram by performing an exposure after the patient has voided. In children, due to lack of cooperation, Young, Anderson and King injected 5 ml. of 10 per cent Lipiodol into the bladder[111]; a film was exposed immediately and again after 24 hours, and a film can be exposed even later, if required. Demonstration of contrast material in the delayed films represents residual urine.

BACKGROUND STUDIES OF NORMAL CYSTOURETHROGRAPHY (BASED ESSENTIALLY ON SCHOPFNER AND HUTCH[72])

The base plate is a structure at the floor of the bladder that affects the configuration of the urethrogram.[72] (See Figures 36–16 to 36–26.) The posterior portion of the plate contains the trigone; the anterior and lateral part consists of Uhlenhuth's fundus ring, which is composed of condensed circular rings of smooth muscle arranged concentrically around the internal orifice. The trigone and fundus ring fuse along each lateral border of the trigone to create the base plate (Figs. 36–15, 36–17).

In its normal, relaxed position, the base plate is flat, and on voiding its walls become closer, more vertical, and parallel and create the trigonal canal (Figs. 36–16, 36–17). The canal is continuous with and simulates the urethra creating between the bladder fold and base plate a "pseudobladder neck" that must be differentiated from a true bladder neck. The diameter of the urethrovesical juncture varies with age, size of patient, sex, stage of voiding, and degree of urethral distention. Small children have smaller diameters; girls consistently have a wider diameter, 8 to 15 mm., than boys, 6 to 12 mm. The smallest diameter in both sexes is 3 mm. whereas the largest is 14 mm. in males and 19 mm. in females. The roent-genographic contour of the vesical neck depends upon the position of the trigone canal, urethral, width, and configuration. The verumontanum appears as an oval filling defect in the prostatic urethra of the male and is often best seen on oblique films. The urethral cristae (see Fig. 36–2) can sometimes be visualized on cystourethrography and may be confused with valves. They give a filling defect usually distal to the verumontanum in a foldlike manner but there is no proximal dilatation. The intermuscular incisura is a constriction or indentation anteriorly, midway between the bladder neck and urogenital diaphragm. The incisura is the point where the smooth muscle above joins with the striated muscle below. It is more distinct in males. The membranous urethra often appears cone-shaped with the point of the cone extending proximally.

The urogenital diaphragm lies within the membranous urethra and produces a narrowing of the urethra about 0.5 cm above the meatus in the female and just proximal to the bulb in the male. It may be a sharp constriction or cutoff or an anterior indentation.

That segment of the female urethra lying between the urogenital diaphragm and the meatus is the distal urethral segment. In the male the urethral segment between the urogenital diaphragm and the bulb is still a part of the membranous urethra and is analogous to the distal urethral segment in the female. This segment in both males and females is the least distensible part of the urethra. It is in this area slightly distal to the membranous urethra that an area of narrowing may appear, caused by the musculus compressor nudae, which is best seen during voluntary contraction while the contrast medium is injected.

The levator ani occasionally may cause a slight urethral constriction between the intermuscular incisura and the urogenital diaphragm. This appears in males only. The bulb of the urethra is the dilated portion distal to the membranous urethra and is entered directly into the pendulous urethra in the male, which for the most part is of even contour and width.

In a series of articles, Shopfner emphasized that there is no correlation between the urethral diameter and vesicoureteral reflux, residual urine, trabeculated bladder and infections (Figs. 36–16 to 36–26).[68-72] In short, cases with so-called obstructive signs and symptoms may have the same configurations and same urethral diameters as the normal.

NORMAL CYSTOURETHROGRAM

As previously described, the urethra may be visualized either by retrograde injection or by voiding of contrast material. The choice of method often depends on the indication of the examination. The voiding method usually is preferred for evaluation of valves, strictures, stenosis of the urethral meatus, fistulas, changes in the bladder neck, and visualization of the posterior urethra. Certainly a more physiologic picture of the urethra is obtained through the voiding method. The retrograde method often is preferred in inflammatory lesions of the urethra and diverticula of the urethra. In the latter entity in females, investigators use a double balloon with an opening between in order to fill the diverticulum better. If the patient is unable to void, the retrograde method is the only one available. One must remember that many congenital lesions (valves) may be visualized only in the voiding process.

The normal male urethrogram (see Figs. 36–1 to 36–6, 36–8 to 36–11, 36–14 to 36–16, 36–18 to 36–22) varies somewhat between the injection and the free voiding method.

In the injection method (Fig. 36–15A), the anterior urethra and the membranous urethra may appear to be more distended because of the resistance of the prostatic urethra. The prostatic urethra appears to be narrower than in the free voiding method. Contrariwise, in free voiding (Figs. 36–15B, 36–18), the prostatic urethra is more distended, but the membranous and the penile urethra are not as dilated as in the retrograde procedure.

The prostatic urethra in the infant appears to be longer than it does in the older child or the adult (Dr. Keith Waterhouse, personal communication). This probably is due to the fact that the bladder lies at a higher level in the infant. Because we believe that the bladder descends at about 1 year of age when the child attains the upright position, the prostatic urethra should shorten at this time. In general, this appears to be correct, but we have seen exceptions. In the female, the normal urethra varies greatly in length (Figs. 36–12, 36–13, 36–17, 36–23 to 36–25); is is obviously not a straight tube and not of uniform caliber.

On micturition, the bladder generally becomes more spherical, and the fundus and the superior part of the urethra become funnel-shaped. The bladder usually sinks downward and backward on voiding.

VARIATIONS OF NORMAL

There are several variations of normal that must be recognized.

Indentations or folds (Fig. 36–26) along the posterior urethra usually are considered to be normal.

The *wide bladder neck syndrome* refers to an unusually wide bladder neck usually seen in children with persistent diurnal urinary incontinence (Fig. 36–27). It may be recognized by the following criteria[112]:

Widening of the bladder neck on a micturating cystogram
Incomplete milk-back on a micturating cystogram
An open bladder neck on cystoscopy
A low urethral pressure profile
A normal cystometrogram and absence of neurologic signs
Absence of distal urethral stenosis

It is most commonly seen in females but males are not excluded.[112, 113] Although many of these children tend to improve during puberty, the syndrome may persist into adulthood and may be associated with some incontinence.

The fundus ring is a variation described by Kjellberg, Ericsson, and Rudhe in 1957 (Fig. 36–28).[93] These authors described a strongly marked waist slightly proximal to the internal sphincter (bladder neck) at the later state of micturition, which they believed occurred in certain pathologic conditions. A similar waist formation was described in a normal bladder but at a slightly higher level. Griesbach, Waterhouse, and Mellins considered that most of the fundus rings were only physiologic variations that would be apparent only on instantaneous roentgenograms (Fig. 36–28).[60a] Moments later the ring may have disappeared completely, and the bladder neck and the posterior urethra may appear to be normal.

Currarino has reported *changes in the cystourethrogram* caused by contraction or spasm of the bulbocavernosus muscle (Figs. 36–29, 36–30).[52] This may affect the urethra from just proximal to the bulb and extend well out into the penile urethra. However, it can affect small segments of the urethra anywhere from the bulb into the penile urethra by contraction of selected groups of fibers of this muscle. This muscle may contract voluntarily or in a reflex pattern. Voluntary contraction occurs usually when micturition is stopped. The contraction empties the bulbous urethra of the remaining urine. A reflex example takes place during ejaculation when rapid contractions of the muscle contribute to the expulsion of the semen from the bulbous urethra. In the so-called bulbocavernosus reflex, a contraction of the muscle occurs in response to stimuli to the glans penis.

Retrograde urethrography may be necessary to differentiate some of the narrowings produced by the bulbocavernosus contraction from a true urethral stricture. In stricture formation, the narrowing remains unchanged during the retrograde study. Spasm due to neurogenic bladder may also be difficult to differentiate from the contraction of the bulbocavernosus muscle. In neurogenic bladder, rapidly alternating distention and contraction of the affected area can be best documented by cineroentgenography.

Reflux into the vagina may occur (Figs. 36–17, 36–21, 36–23, 36–24, 36–25) and may be confused with double urethra, if only one film is exposed.[72] Rarely has reflux occurred through the vagina, uterus, fallopian tubes, and into the peritoneal cavity (Fig. 36–31).[114]

The wide variations in the region of the bladder neck and the posterior urethra may be confusing on cystourethrograms, and the findings may be considered abnormal by some authors and normal by others.

The various complications of cystourethrography have been summarized by McAlister and co-workers[115]. Infections include bacteremia and septicemia; catheterization trauma; perforation of bladder; reflux; hydronephrosis and hydroureter from distended bladder; allergic reactions; inflammatory response to contrast media; contrast medium entering peritoneal cavity by way of the vagina; anuria; accidental catheterization of the vagina or ectopic ureteral orifice.

CHAPTER 36, ILLUSTRATIONS

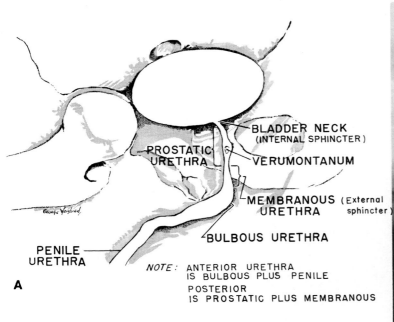

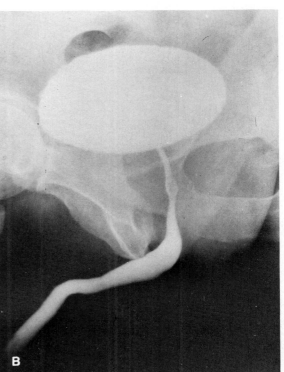

FIG. 36–1. Cystourethrogram with a diagram for anatomic relationships. **(A)** Diagram of film **(B)** to show various divisions or urethra. **(B)** Injecting cystourethrogram in adult man.

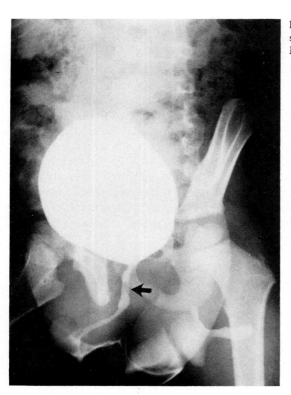

FIG. 36–2. Crista urethralis. *Arrow* points to leaflike structure in prostatic urethra. (Courtesy of David Baker, M.D. and Walter Berdon, M.D.)

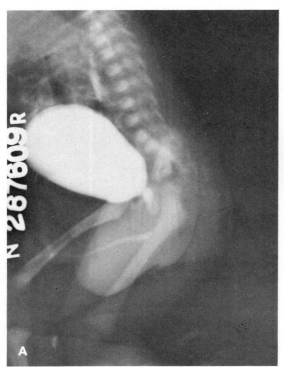

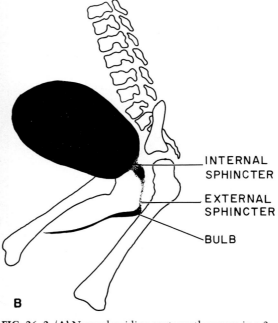

INTERNAL
SPHINCTER

EXTERNAL
SPHINCTER

BULB

FIG. 36–3. (A) Normal voiding cystourethrogram in a 3-day-old boy. (Griesbach, W.A., Waterhouse, R.K., and Mellins, H.Z.: Am. J. Roentgen., *82*:521–529, 1959) **(B)** Diagram. (Courtesy of Keith Waterhouse, M.D.)

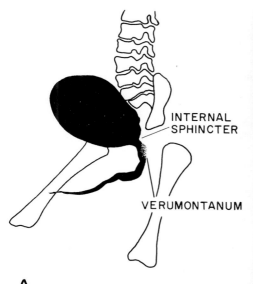

A

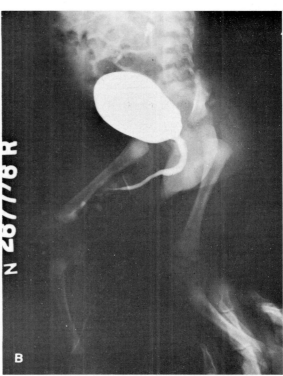

FIG. 36–4. (A) Diagram. (Courtesy of Keith Waterhouse, M.D.) **(B)** Normal voiding cystourethrogram in a 12-day-old boy. Note long posterior urethra. (Griesbach, W.A., Waterhouse, R.K., and Mellins, H.Z.: Am. J. Roentgen., *82:521–529, 1959*)

FIG. 36–5. Normal voiding cystourethrogram in a 3-year-old boy. (Griesbach, W.A., Waterhouse, R.K., and Mellins, H.Z.: Am. J. Roentgen., *82:521–529, 1959*)

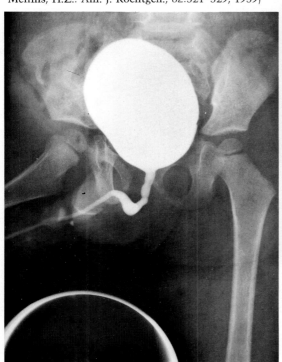

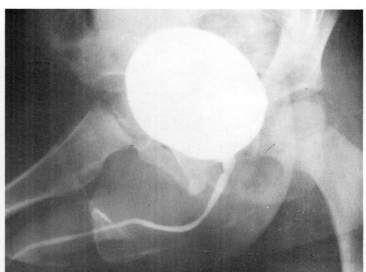

FIG. 36–6. Normal voiding cystourethrogram. Boy, 5 years old. There is some elongation of the posterior urethra. Oblique view.

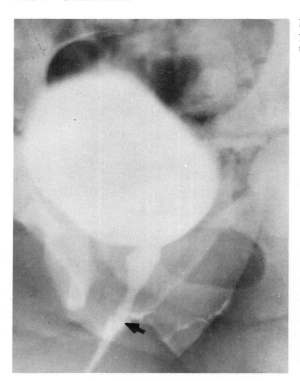

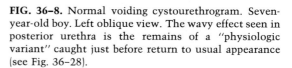

FIG. 36–7. Normal voiding cystourethrogram. Girl, 7 years old. *Arrow* points to external urethral orifice. The urethra is unusually long. Oblique view.

FIG. 36–8. Normal voiding cystourethrogram. Seven-year-old boy. Left oblique view. The wavy effect seen in posterior urethra is the remains of a "physiologic variant" caught just before return to usual appearance (see Fig. 36–28).

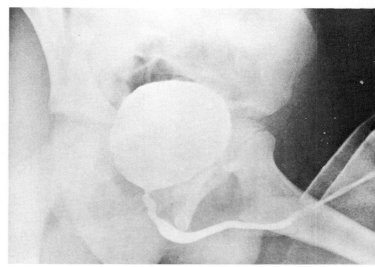

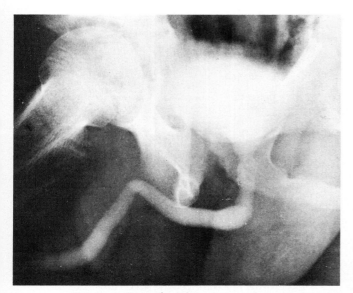

FIG. 36–9. Normal voiding cystourethrogram. Boy, 11 years old. Right oblique view.

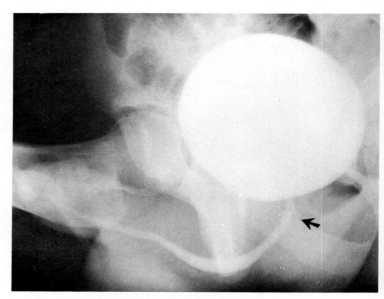

FIG. 36–10. Normal voiding cystourethrogram. Boy, 13 years old. *Arrow* points to defect produced by verumontanum. Right oblique view. This is an example of an elongated posterior urethra in an older child.

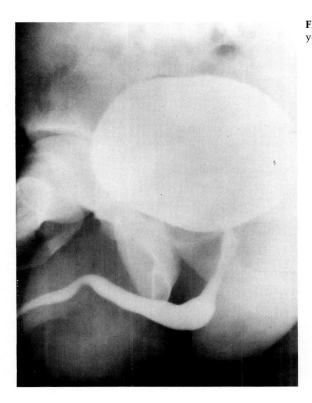

FIG. 36–11. Normal voiding cystourethrogram. Man, 20 years old. Right oblique view.

FIG. 36–12. Normal voiding cystourethrogram. Short urethra. Female, age 44. Right oblique view.

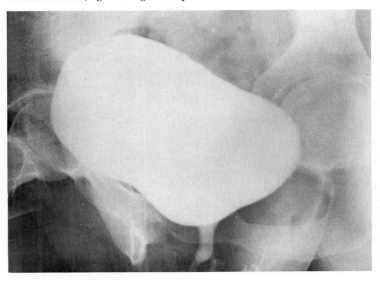

FIG. 36–13. Normal voiding cystourethrogram. Long urethra. Female, age 56. Right oblique view. *Arrows* point to bladder neck and external urethral orifice.

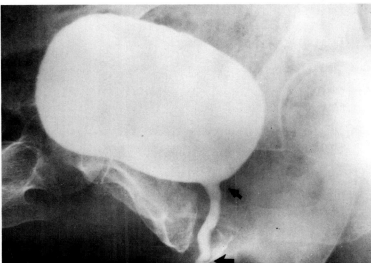

FIG. 36–14. Normal voiding cystourethrogram in a eunuchoid man, 53 years old. Right oblique view. The elongated defect in the posterior urethra is the distal portion of the urethral crest.

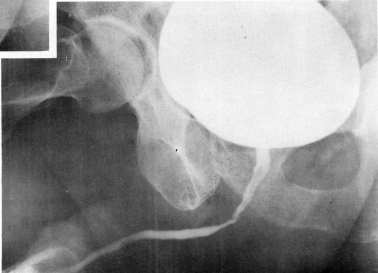

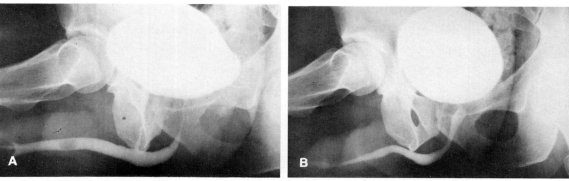

FIG. 36-15. Normal cystourethrogram showing the difference in the appearance of the urethra on injecting and voiding methods on the same patient. **(A)** Injecting. Shows that the anterior urethra and the membranous urethra appear to be more distended, whereas the prostatic urethra is narrow. **(B)** Voiding. Shows a more distended prostatic urethra but a less distended membranous and anterior urethra. Right oblique view.

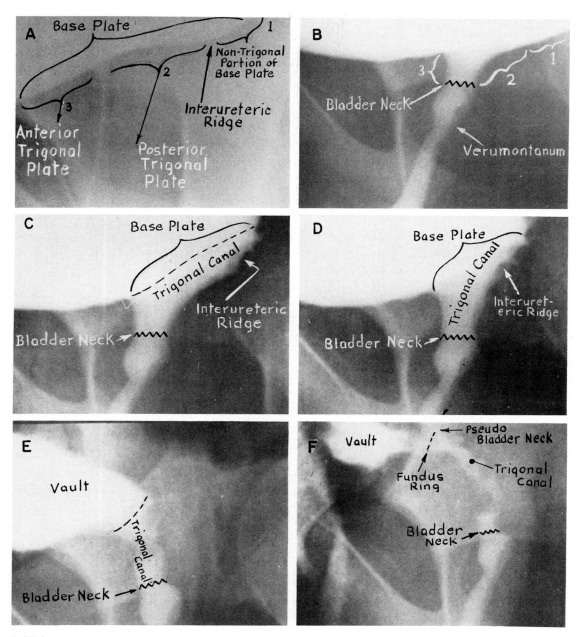

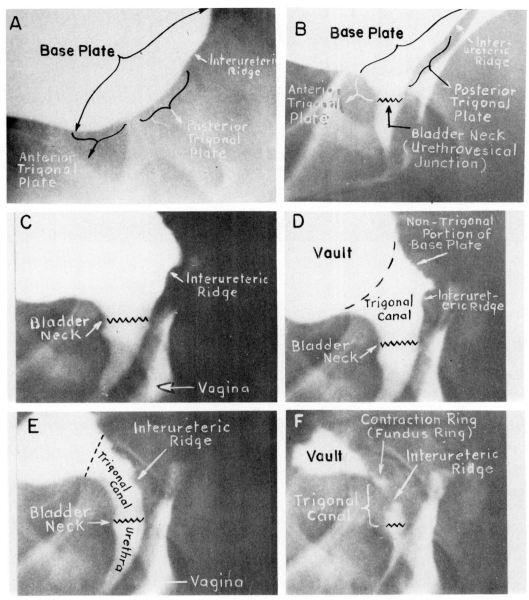

FIG. 36–17. Voiding sequence in a 5-year-old girl. Actual voiding with superimposed explanation. **(A)** The base plate is slightly convex to the filled and resting bladder. **(B)** During early voiding the trigonal plates have moved to an oblique position, but the base plate has changed little in size. **(C, D)** Progressive decrease in the size of the vault and base plate is occurring. In **D** the trigonal canal is beginning to develop and extends well above the interureteric notch. A distinct difference in caliber exists between the base and the vault. **(E)** The trigonal plates are vertical, and the trigonal canal is well developed and continuous with the posterior urethra. **(F)** Voiding has almost ceased, and the canal has reduced in width during the urethral stripping process. Above the interureteric ridge, a distinct constriction exists between the base plate and the vault. (Shopfner, C.E., Hutch, J.A.: Radiology, 88:209–221, 1967)

FIG. 36–16. Voiding sequence in a 13-year old boy. Actual voiding with superimposed explanation. **(A)** The trigone plates are flat in the filled and resting bladder. The nontrigonal portion of the base plate droops over the posterior trigonal plate (bracket 1). **(B)** Voiding has started and the trigonal plates have moved to an oblique position. **(C, D)** The vault and base plate are becoming smaller as voiding progresses and the trigonal canal is already well developed. **(E)** During the late stages of voiding, the trigonal canal has become narrower and longer as the plates have moved into a vertical position. **(F)** A contraction ring marks the division between the trigonal canal and vault and acts as a pseudo bladder neck. The canal has decreased in width and has increased in length during urethral stripping. (Shopfner, C.E., Hutch, J.A.: Radiology, 88:209–221, 1967)

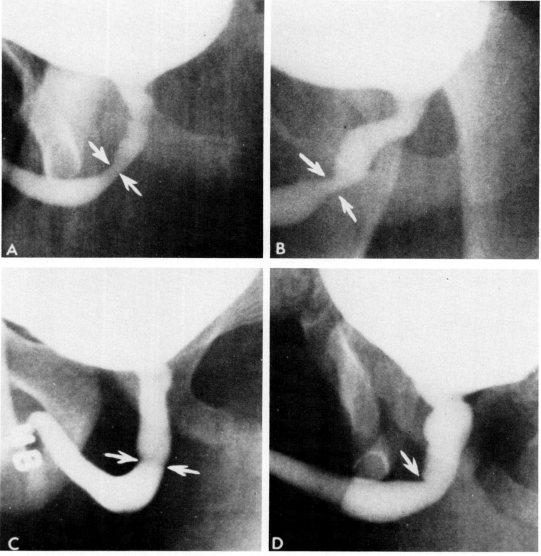

FIG. 36–18. (A, B, C, D) Selected voiding spot films in four different boys to show the urogenital diaphragm (*arrows*). A sloping narrowing is present in **A** and **B**, but a sharper constriction indicates its location in **C** and **D**. (Shopfner, C.E., Hutch, J.A.: Radiol. Clin. North Am., 6:165–189, 1968)

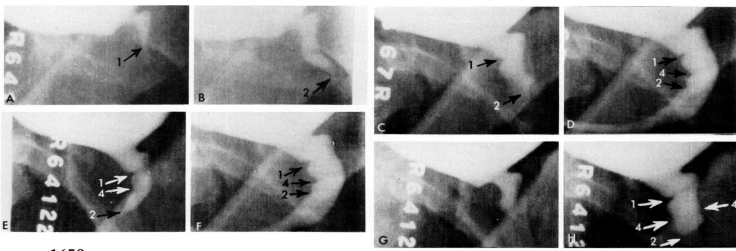

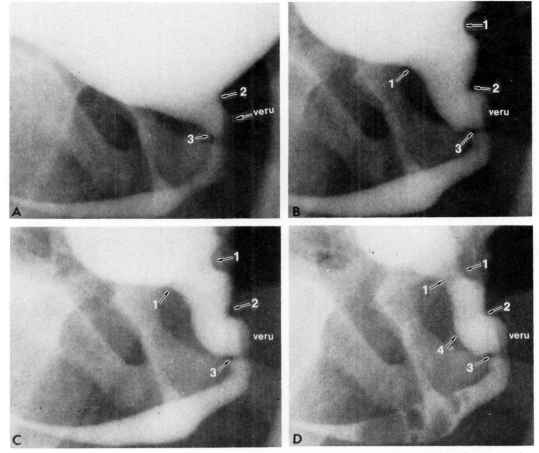

FIG. 36–20. Sequential voiding spot films of an 8-year-old boy. (A) Early voiding. The trigonal plates have moved to an oblique position and the urethra is partly distended with a low volume and velocity stream. (B, C, D) Late voiding. The trigonal plates move progressively cephalad and toward each other so that in D they are vertical and create the trigonal canal (between A and D). Appearance of the contraction ring in B (*arrow 1*) and its accentuation in C and D mark the division between the base plate and vault and create a "pseudo bladder neck." *Arrow 2,* urethrovesical junction. *Arrow 3,* intermuscular incisura. (Shopfner, C.E., Hutch, J.A.: Radiol. Clin. North Am., 6:165–189, 1968)

FIG. 36–19. Selection of spot films from a voiding sequence of an 8-year-old boy. (A) Adjacent margins of the trigonal plates have broken from their flat position to allow filling of the urethrovesical junction and urethra downward to the intermuscular incisura (*arrow 1*). (B) Relaxation of the longitudinal, paraurethral portion of the sphincter muscle of urethra has allowed urethral filling downward to the transverse fibers of the sphincter muscle of urethra within the urogenital diaphragm (*arrow 2*). (C) Continued relaxation of longitudinal muscle fibers allows more urethral distention, which makes the intermuscular incisura (*arrow 1*) become apparent. (D) Relaxation of the sphincteric muscle *en masse* allows full urethral filling and distention. Anterior indentations are present at the intermuscular incisura, levator sling (*arrow 4*) and urogenital diaphragm. (E) Voluntary cessation of urination has produced total contraction of the transverse and partial contraction of the longitudinal muscle fibers and a complete urethral constriction (cut-off) at the urogenital diaphragm. Partial urethral compression has occurred between the diaphragm and intermuscular incisura. A faint identation persists at the levator sling. (F) *En masse* muscular relaxation has again allowed full urethral distention. (G) Voluntary cessation of voiding has caused cut-off at the level of the urogenital diaphragm and partial compression between it and intermuscular incisura, which has disappeared. Smooth muscle action has returned the trigonal plates and proximal urethra to the appearance they had at beginning of voiding in A. (H) Attempted resumption of voiding has again moved the trigonal plates to an oblique position, allowed full urethral distention to the urogenital diaphragm, and restored the intermuscular incisura. The cut-off and constrictions caused by the normal anatomy and physiology of the sphincter muscle of urethra are not to be confused with valves and stenosis. (Shopfner, C.E., Hutch, J.A.: Radiol. Clin. North Am., 6:165–189, 1968)

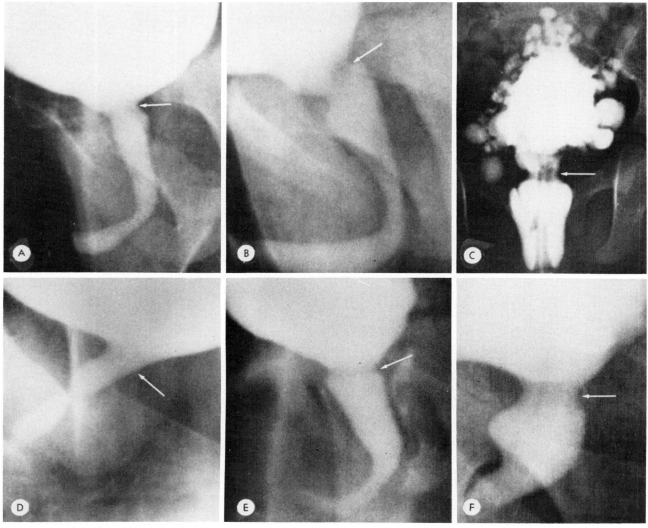

FIG. 36–21. Selected spot films of male (A–C) and female (D–F) urethras illustrating the effect of urethral caliber on the degree of bladder neck contracture. The bladder necks of all three males measure 9 mm.; those of the females, 12 mm. The degree of contracture increases in direct porportion to urethral width and is not related to the inside diameter of the bladder neck, which is the same in all males and females. The patient in C had urethral valves.

The urethrogram in F is of a 6-year-old girl who was examined because of recurrent abdominal pain. Complete urologic work-up revealed no abnormal findings. She voided without hesitancy and rapidly emptied the bladder with a large-volume, high-velocity stream. *Arrows* indicate bladder neck. (Shopfner, C.E.: Am. U. Roentgenol., *100*:162–176, 1967)

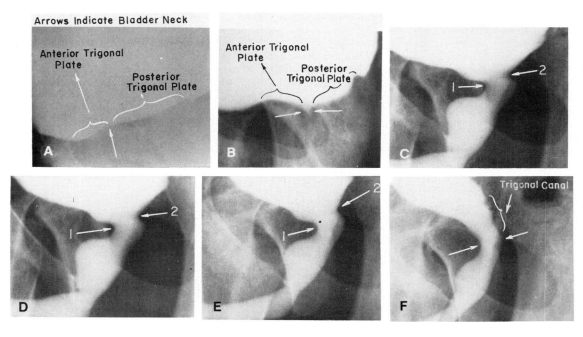

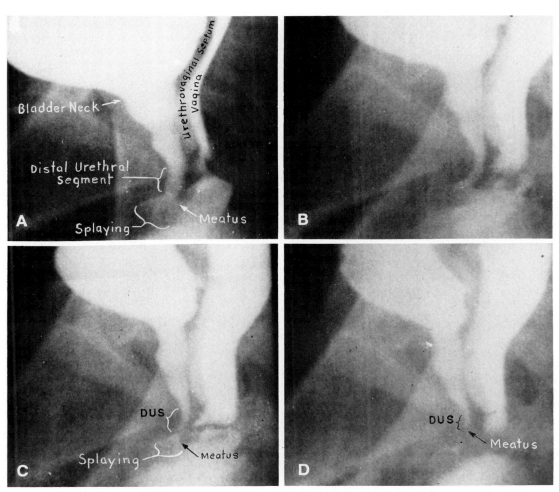

FIG. 36–23. Voiding sequence in a 5-year-old girl to illustrate the variations in urethral diameter during the different stages of voiding. In **A,** the meatus and distal urethral segment (DUS) have a diameter of 5 mm. during full voiding. Progressive decrease to 3 mm. in **B,** 2 mm. in **C,** and 1 mm. in **D** occurs during the late stages of voiding, when velocity and volume of urethral flow are reduced. Meatal and DUS calibration by catheter was #12F (4 mm.). Note the splaying of the opaque material in **A, B,** and **C,** and that it is most prominent during full voiding, when the meatus is at its widest. This patient had glomerulonephritis and did not have lower urinary symptoms, urosepsis, vesicoureteral reflux, or bladder trabeculation. (Shopfner, C.E.: Radiology, *88:*222–231, 1967)

FIG. 36–22. Sequence of voiding in a 1-year-old boy illustrating the effect on bladder neck defects of urethral width, urethral configuration, and position of the trigonal plates. **(A)** The trigonal plates are flat before voiding is initiated. **(B)** The trigonal plates have started to elevate; minimal opaque material is in the bladder neck as voiding is initiated. **(C, D, E)** Voiding is fully established with full urethral distention. The trigonal plates have moved into an oblique position. The urethra bulges asymmetrically anteriorly and forms a prominent anterior defect. (*Arrow 1*). The posterior superior bulge of the urethra above the verumontanum forms only a slight posterior defect (*Arrow 2*). **(F)** Near the end of voiding, the trigonal plates are vertical and urethral distention is diminishing. The anterior defect has disappeared. The bladder neck and trigonal canal are indicated by *arrows* and a *bracket,* respectively. (Shopfner, C.E.: Am. J. Roentgenol., *100:*162–176, 1967)

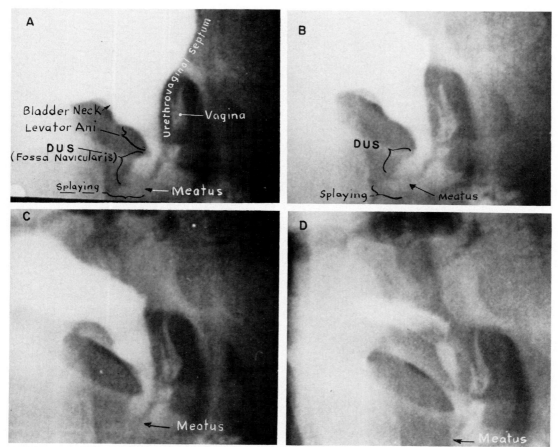

FIG. 36–24. Voiding sequence in an 8-year-old girl examined because of recurrent abdominal pain. Complete diagnostic study revealed no evidence of urinary tract disease. The DUS is well delineated. Its diameter during full voiding is 7 mm. (**A, B**), whereas the meatal diameter is 5 mm. In **C**, the respective diameters have reduced to 5 mm. and 4 mm. during late voiding. Almost complete emptying of the bladder has occurred near the end of voiding in **D**, and the DUS and meatus have reduced to a caliber of 2 mm.

The slight constriction at the upper margin of the DUS is produced by the transition from muscle to collagenous tissue. Tapering of the urethra above the DUS is caused by the levator ani muscle (external sphincter) that surrounds the urethra in this area.

Bulging of the midpart of the DUS so that it is wider than its upper and lower margins, as in this patient, has resulted in its being called the navicular fossa. (Shopfner, C.E.: Radiology, 88:222–231, 1967)

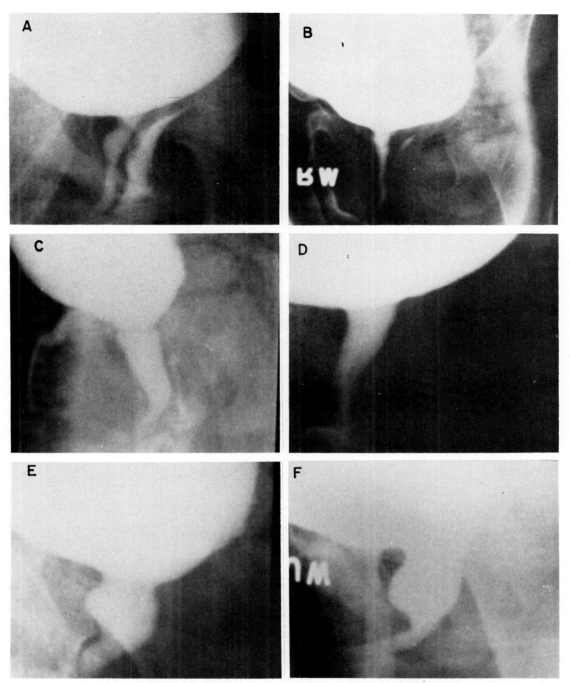

FIG. 36–25. Selected voiding spot films in six different females, all between the ages of 3 and 5 years, to illustrate that the visual image of the meatal and DUS diameters is relative to the width of the midurethra. There is minimal midurethral distention in **A** and **B**, moderate distention in **C** and **D**, and marked distention in **E** and **F**. The meatus and DUS appear narrowed in **E** and **F** because of the marked midurethral distention. Their diameters, however, measure 7 and 6 mm. respectively, which are greater than the 4 mm. in **A**, 3 mm. in **B**, 4 mm. in **C**, and 5 mm. in **D** that do not appear narrow to visual perception. (Shopfner, C.E.: Radiology, *88:*222–231, 1967)

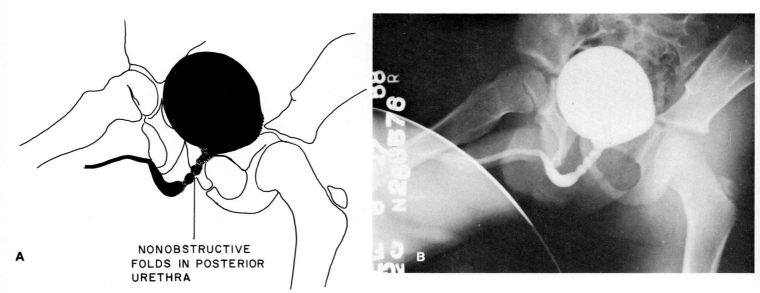

A

NONOBSTRUCTIVE
FOLDS IN POSTERIOR
URETHRA

B

FIG. 36–26. (A) Diagram. (Courtesy of Keith Water-house, M.D.) **(B)** Voiding cystourethrogram showing nonobstructive folds in posterior uretrha. This is considered to be a normal finding. (Griesbach, W.A., Waterhouse, R.K., and Mellins, H.Z.: Am. J. Roentgen., *82*:521–529, 1959)

FIG. 36–27. Wide bladder neck syndrone. Diagram **(A)** and voiding cystourethrogram **(B).** The bladder neck is widened, but it ends rather abruptly. This differentiates it from the gradual tapering of a funnel urethra. Right oblique view. These cases often have prolonged enuresis but eventually improve. The wide bladder neck syndrome usually is seen in women. (Courtesy Keith Waterhouse, M.D.)

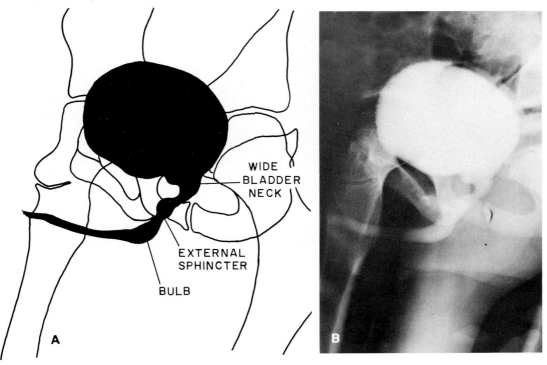

WIDE
BLADDER
NECK

EXTERNAL
SPHINCTER

BULB

A

B

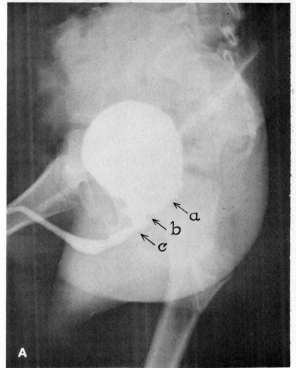

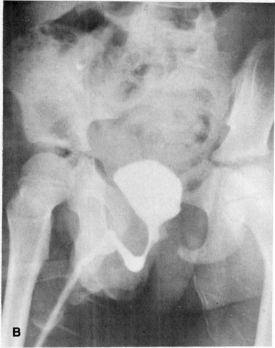

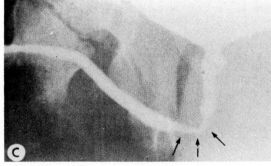

FIG. 36–28. (A) Voiding cystourethrogram. (a) Intereureteric ridge. (b) Fundus ring of Kjellberg *et al.* Griesbach, Waterhouse and Mellins believe this is a physiologic variant. (c) Internal sphincter. (B) Moments later. Essentially normal cystourethrogram with absence of so-called fundus ring. (Griesbach, W.A., Waterhouse, R.K., and Mellins, H.Z.: Am. J. Roentgen., *82*:521–529, 1959)

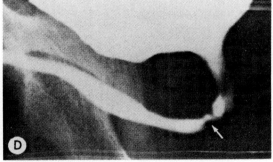

FIG. 36–29. Voiding cystourethrograms of five normal children showing contraction of selected groups of fibers of the bulbocavernosus muscle (*arrows*): (A) an anterior, (B) a middle, and (C–E) a posterior. The *upper arrow* in E points to the deformity of the urethra caused by the dorsal fibers of the compressor hemispherii bulbi (corresponding to the imprint of the musculus compressor nudae urethrae described by Morales and Romanus[105]). The bulbocavernosus muscle does not always act as a unit. (Currarino, G.: Am. J. Roentgenol., *108*:641–647, 1970)

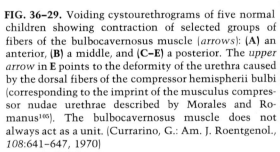

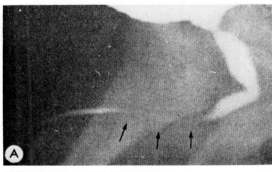

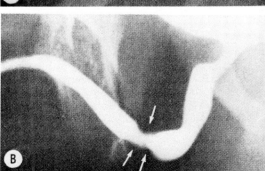

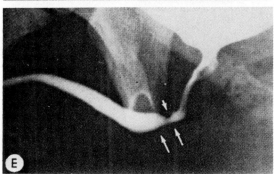

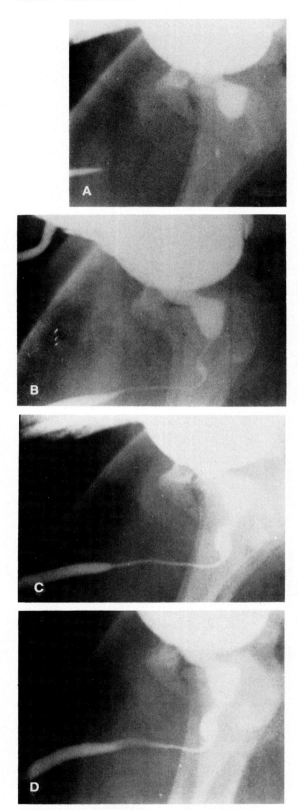

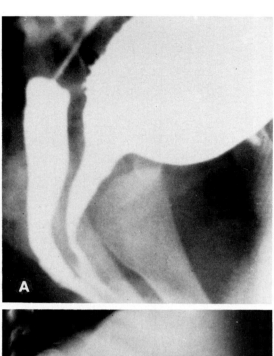

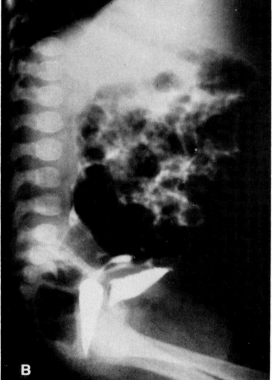

FIG. 36–30. Spasm of the bulbocavernosus muscle in its entirety, gradually improving from **A** to **D.** (Courtesy of Guido Currarino, M.D.)

FIG. 36–31. (A) Contrast medium outlines urinary bladder and urethra with reflux into vagina. **(B)** Lateral view. Contrast medium fills vagina, bladder, urethra, and enters peritoneal cavity by way of uterus and fallopian tubes. **(C)** Contrast medium is present in vagina (vertical structure). The partially filled bladder (horizontal contrast-filled structure) is visualized. Contrast medium outlines the uterus (triangular structure above the vagina). Contrast material is present in the peritoneal cavity. (Bolich, P.R., Babbitt, D.P.: Pediatr. Radiol., 3:242–243, 1975)

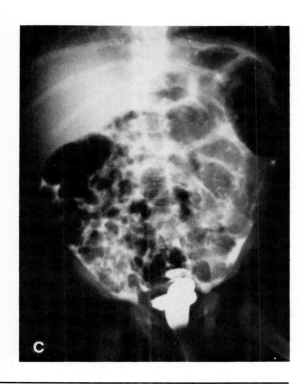

BIBLIOGRAPHY

Anatomy of the Female Urethra

1. Gavino Rivera, C.: Anatomy of female urethra. Medicine México, 26:363–365, 1946.
2. Krantz, K.E.: The anatomy of the urethra and the anterior vaginal wall. Am. J. Obstet. Gynecol., 62:374–386, 1951.
3. Lapides, J., Ajemian, F.P., Stewart, B.H., Lichtwardt, J.R., et al.: Physiopathology of stress incontinence. Surg. Gynecol. Obstet., 111:224–231, 1960.
4. Lowsley, O.S., and Kirwin, T.J.: Clinical Urology, Vol. 1, pp. 340–341. Williams & Wilkins, Baltimore, 1956.
5. Ricci, J.V., Lisa, J.R., and Thom, C.H.: The female urethra: A histologic study as an aid in urethral surgery. Am. J. Surg., 79:499–505, 1950.
6. Skene, A.J.C.: Abatomy and pathology of two important glands of the female urethra. Am. J. Obstet. Gynecol., 13:265–270, 1880.

Anatomy of the Male Urethra

7. Edling, N.P.G.: Urethro-cystography in the male with special regard to micturition. Acta Radiol. (Stockholm) (Suppl.), 58:1–144, 1945.
8. Lowsley, O.S., and Kirwin, T.J.: Clinical Urology, Vol. 1, pp. 314–316. Williams & Wilkins, Baltimore, 1956.
9. Morales, O., and Romanus, R.: Urethrography in the male—delineation of the interior and posterior urethra, the pars diaphragmatica, the pars nuda urethrae and the presence of musculus compressor nudae. Acta Radiol., 39:453–476, 1953.

10. Pennington, L.T., and Lund, H.Z.: An elastic ring of tissue in the male urethra: Its probable relationship to primary intrinsic urethral resistance and incontinence following prostatectomy. J. Urol., 84:481–487, 1960.

The Female Prostate

Those Writers Believing in a Female Prostate

11. Beneventi, F.A.: Anatomy and histology of the posterior urethra in newborn female. Surg. Gynecol. Obstet., 76:64–76, 1943.
12. Folsom, A.I.: The female urethra. J.A.M.A., 97:1345–1351, 1931.
13. Huffman, J.W.: The development of the peri-urethral glands in the human female. Am. J. Obstet. Gynecol., 46:773–785, 1943.
14. Huffman, J.W.: The detailed anatomy of the peri-urethral glands in the adult human female. Am. J. Obstet. Gynecol., 55:86–101, 1948.
15. Johnson, F.P.: Homologue of the prostate in the female. J. Urol., 8:13–34, 1922.
16. Korenshevsky, V., and Dennison, M.: The histology of the sex organs of ovariectomised rats treated with male or female sex hormones alone or with both simultaneously. J. Pathol. Bacteriol., 42:91–104, 1936.
17. Moore, T.: The female prostate, bladder neck obstruction in women. Lancet, 1:1305–1309, 1960.
18. Moore, T.: The female prostate updated. Eur. Urol., 1:32–35, 1975.
19. Powell, N.B., and Powell, E.B.: The female urethra. A clinico-pathological study. J. Urol., 61:557–567, 1949.

20. Renner, M.J.: The so-called female prostate and concretion formation in the female urethra. Surg. Gynecol. Obstet., 52:1087–1092, 1931.
21. Young, H.H.: The pathology and treatment of obstruction at the vesical neck in women. J.A.M.A., 115:2133–2136, 1940.

Those Writers Denying That There Are Periurethral Glands in the Female Which Often Become Infected and Occasionally Undergo Hyperplasia

22. Cabot, H., and Shoemaker, R.: The role of glands of the female urethra in the production of infection in the urinary tract. Trans. Am. Assoc. Genitourin. Surg., 29:461–472, 1936.
23. Mackenzie, D.W., and Beck, S.: A histo-pathological study of the female bladder neck and urethra. J. Urol., 36:414–437, 1936.
24. Mackenzie, D.W., and Seng, M.I.: Common conditions of the neck of the female bladder and urethra. Can. Med. Assoc. J., 40:428–432, 1939.
25. Thompson, G.J.: Transurethral operations on women for relief of disfunction of the vesical neck. J. Urol., 41:349–359, 1939.

Those Writers Who Have Not Committed Themselves on the Type of Glands Present in the Female Urethra

26. Beach, E.W.: Some observations of the female urethra. Urol. Cutan. Rev., 38:545–549, 1934.
27. Everett, H.S.: Urology in the female. Am. J. Surg., 52:521–659, 1941.
28. Hawley, H.C.: The female urethra and its relation to upper urinary tract infection. Proc. Roy. Soc. Med., 39:741–748, 1946.
29. Herbst, R.H., and Merricks, J.W.: Chronic primary diseases of the lower female urinary tract. Med. Clin. North Am., 25:245–269, 1941.
30. Roen, P.R., and Strept, R.R.: Urethritis in girls. Am. J. Dis. Child., 72:529–535, 1946.
31. Spence, H.M., and Moore, C.H.: The female urethra in childhood. Texas J. Med., 35:234–238, 1938.

Additional Reading

32. Deter, R.L., Cauldwell, G.T., and Folsom, A.I.: A clinical and pathological study of the posterior female urethra. J. Urol., 55:651–662, 1946.
33. Folsom, A.I.: The female urethra. J.A.M.A., 128:408–414, 1945.
34. Folsom, A.I., and O'Brien, H.A.: The female obstructive prostate. J.A.M.A., 121:573–579, 1943.
35. Van Duzen, R.E.: Glands of the female urethra. Urol. Cutan. Rev., 48:363–364, 1944.

Urethrography by Injection Method

36. Baensch, W., and Boeminghaus, H.: Die Rontgendikgnostik bei Erkrankungen des uropoetischen Systems. Ztschr. Urol. Chir., 7:48–101, 1921.
37. Barringer, B., and MacKee, G.: Radiographs of the bladder and bladder neck. Trans. Am. Urol., Assoc., 6:408–411, 1912.

38. Beclere, H., and Henry, R.: Quelques radiographies de retrecissements de l'uretre. J. Urol. Paris, 13:417–424, 1922.
39. Burden, V.G.: Roentgenology of the male urethra. Surg. Gynecol. Obstet., 38:403–406, 1924.
40. Cunningham, J.H.: The diagnosis of stricture of the urethra by roentgen rays. Trans. Am. Assoc. Genitourin. Surg., 5:369–371, 1910.
41. Flocks, R.H.: The roentgen visualization of the posterior urethra. J. Urol., 30:711–736, 1933.
42. Haudek, M.: On the technique of roentgenological examination of the urethra. Wien. Med. Wschr., 71:490–492, 1921.
43. Hyams, J.A., Kenyon, H.R., and Kramer, S.E.: Urethrocystography in the male. J.A.M.A., 101:2030–2035, 1933.
44. Knutsson, F.: On the technique of urethrography. Acta Radiol., 10:437–441, 1929.
45. Knutsson, F.: Urethrography. Röntgen examination of male urethra and prostate after injection of contrast material into urethra. Acta Radiol. (Stockholm) (Suppl.), 28:1–150, 1935.
46. Kohnstam, G.L.S., and Cave, E.H.P.: The Radiological Examination of the Male Urethra. William Wood, New York, 1925.
47. Langer, E.: Die Rongendiagnostik Der Mannlichen Harnröhre. Leopold Voss, Leipzig, 1931.
48. Nicholson, M.A., Fiala, M.J.: Urethrography. J. Urol., 28:461–476, 1932.
49. Pfister, E.: Roentgen picture of the human urethra. Ztschr. Urol., 14:281–287, 1920.
50. Sicard, J.A., and Forestier, J.: Radiographic exploration of the urethra by lipiodol. Bull. Soc. Paris, 48:207–210, 1924.

Voiding Cystourethrogram

51. Burrows, E.H., and Allen, R.P.: Urethral lesions in infancy and childhood studied by micturition cystourethrography. Br. J. Radiol., 37:187–199, 1964.
52. Currarino, G.: Narrowings of the male urethra caused by contractions or spasm of the bulbocavernosus muscle: cystourethrographic observations. Am. J. Roentgenol., 108:641–647, 1970.
53. Davis, L.A., Lich, R., Howerton, L., et al.: The lower urinary tract in infants and children. Radiology, 77:445–451, 1961.
54. Draper, J.W., and Siceluff, J.G.: Excretory cystourethrograms. J. Urol., 53:539–544, 1945.
55. Fasiani, G.M.: Indagine radiologica dell'uretra maschile. Arch. Ital. Urol., 1:487–511, 1925.
56. Fisher, O.D., and Forsythe, W.I.: Micturating cystourethrography in the investigation of enuresis. Arch. Dis. Child., 29:460–471, 1954.
57. Fitts, F.B., Jr., Herbert, S.G., and Mellins, H.S.: Criteria for examination of the urethra during excretory urography. Radiol., 125:47–52, 1977.
58. Frumkin, A.P.: Rontgenographie der mannlicher Harnröhre. Fortschr. Roentgenstr., 33:401–407, 1925.
59. Fumerton, W.R., and MacEwan, D.W.: Excretory micturition cystourethrography (EMCU) in the adult age group. J. Can. Assoc. Radiol., 21:90–97, 1970.
60. Glingar, A.: Uber Divertikel der manlichen hinteren Harnröhre. Verh. Deutsch. Ges. Urol., 5:314–322, 1921.
60a. Griesbach, W.A., Waterhouse, R.K., and Mellins, H.Z.: Voiding cystourethrography in the diagnosis of congenital posterior urethral valves. Am. J. Roentgenol., 82:521–529, 1959.
61. Hutch, J.A.: New theory of anatomy of internal urinary sphincter and physiology of micturition. Invest. Urol., 3:36–58, 1965.

62. Lattimer, J.K., Dean, A.L., Jr., and Furey, C.A.: The triple voiding technique in children with dilated urinary tracts. J. Urol., 76:656–660, 1956.

63. McKay, R.W., and Colston, J.A.C.: Diverticula of the male urethra. Surg. Gynecol. Obstet., 48:51–62, 1929.

64. Morales, O., Nilsson, S., and Romanus, R.: Urethrographic studies on the posterior urethra. Part I, Acta Radiol., 281–99, 1964; Part II, Acta Radiol., 2:305–315, 1964.

65. Nogrady, M.B., and Dunbar, J.S.: The value of excretory micturition cystourethrography (EMCU) in the pediatric age group. J. Can. Assoc. Radiol., 16:181–189, 1965.

66. Ortmann, K.K., and Christiansen, H.: Roentgenologic studies of the male urethra; closing mechanism of bladder, and micturition under normal and pathologic conditions. Acta Radiol., 15:258–283, 1934.

67. Sane, S.M., and Worsing, R.A., Jr.: Voiding cystourethrography. Recent advances. Minn. Med., 58:148–153, 1975.

68. Shopfner, C.E.: Cystourethrography: An evaluation of method. Am. J. Roentgenol., 95:468–474, 1965.

69. Shopfner, C.E.: Roentgen evaluation of distal urethral obstruction. Radiology, 88:222–231, 1967.

70. Shopfner, C.E.: Roentgenological evaluation of bladder neck obstruction. Am. J. Roentgenol., 100:162–176, 1967.

71. Shopfner, C.E., and Hutch, J.A.: The trigonal canal. Radiology, 88:209–221, 1967.

72. Shopfner, C.E., and Hutch, J.A.: The normal urethrogram. Radiol. Clin. North Am., 6:165–189, 1968.

73. Siceluff, J.G.: Voiding cysto-urethrogram. J. Urol., 66:593–596, 1951.

74. Uhle, A., and McKinney, W.: Observations upon the mechanisms of urination. Urol. Cutan. Rev., 1:271–275, 1913.

75. Vlahakis, E., Hartman, G.W., and Kelalis, P.P.: Comparison of voiding cystourethrography and expression cystourethrography. J. Urol., 106:414–415, 1971.

76. Waterhouse, A.K.: Voiding cystourethrography. A simple technique. J. Urol., 85:103–104, 1961.

77. Williams, D.I., and Sturdy, D.E.: Recurrent urinary infection in girls. Arch. Dis. Child., 36:130–136, 1961.

Cystourethrography (Both Voiding and Injection Method)

78. Bronner, H.: Das Röntgenbild der mannlichen Harnröhre, vor allem der Posterior (Urethrographia anterior und posterior). Bruns Beitr. Klin. Chir., 136:180–192, 1926.

79. Edling, N.P.G.: Urethrocystography in the male with special regard to micturition. Acta Radiol. (Stockholm) (Suppl.), 58:1–144, 1945.

80. Puhl, H.: Die Röntgenuntersuchung der mannlichen Harnröhre. Deutsche Ztschr. Chir., 220:372–417, 1929.

81. Vincent, P.G.A.: A Propos de la technique de l'uretrographie par voie mictionelle. These, Paris, 1935.

Choke Voiding Cystourethrography

82. Boltuch, R.L., and Lalli, A.F.: A new technique for urethrography. Radiology, 115:736, 1975.

83. Fitts, F.B., Jr., Mascatello, V.G., and Mellins, H.Z.: The value of compression during excretion voiding urethrography. Radiology, 125:53–56, 1977.

84. Pearman, R.O., and Miller, J.B.: Choke voiding cystourethrography. J. Urol., 90:481–488, 1963.

Delayed Cystograms

85. Bunge, R.G.: Delayed cystograms in children. J. Urol., 70:729–732, 1953.

86. Bunge, R.G.: Further observations with delayed cystograms. J. Urol., 71:427–434, 1954.

87. Stewart, C.M.: In a discussion of Benjamin, J.A., and Tobin, C.E.: Paper entitled Abnormalities of kidney, ureters and perinephric fascia. J. Urol., 65:731–732, 1951.

88. Stewart, C.M.: Delayed cystography and voiding cystourethrography. J. Urol., 74:749–759, 1955.

Micturition: Effects on Bladder and Urethra

89. Benjamin, J.A., Joint, F.T., Ramsay, G.H., et al.: Cinefluorographic studies of bladder and urethral function. J. Urol., 73:525–535, 1955.

90. Hansen, L.K.: Micturition cystourethrography with automatic serial exposures. Acta Radiol. (Stockholm), 207:11–139, 1961.

91. Hinman, F., Jr., Miller, G.M., Nickel, E., et al.: Vesical physiology demonstrated by cine-radiography and serial roentgenography, preliminary report. Radiology, 62:713–719, 1954.

92. Jeffcoate, T.N.A., and Roberts, H.: Bladder control in the female. Proc. Roy. Soc. Med., 49:652–657, 1956.

93. Kjellberg, S.R., Ericsson, N.O., and Rudhe, U.: The Lower Urinary Tract in Childhood. Year Book Publishing Co., Chicago, 1957.

94. Muellner, S.R., and Fleishner, F.G.: Normal and abnormal micturition: A study of bladder behavior by means of the fluoroscope. J. Urol., 6:233–243, 1949.

Additional Reading

95. Beard, E.E., Goodyear, W.E., and Weens, H.S.: Radiologic Diagnosis of the Lower Urinary Tract. Charles C Thomas, Springfield, 1952.

96. Boone, A.W.: Cysto-urethrograms before prostatectomy. J. Urol., 67:358–363, 1952.

97. Brodny, M.L.: New instrument for urethrography in male. J. Urol., 46:350–354, 1941.

98. Brodny, M.L., and Robins, S.A.: Enuresis: Use of cystourethrography in diagnosis. J.A.M.A., 126:1000–1006, 1944.

99. Comarr, A.E., and Dodenhoff, L.: A safe, simple method of performing urethrogram. J. Urol., 70:980–981, 1953.

100. Crabtree, E.G., and Brodny, M.L.: Estimation of value of urethrogram and cystogram in diagnosis of prostatic obstruction. J. Urol., 29:235–276, 1933.

101. Davis, H.J., and Cian, CaG.: Positive pressure urethrography. A new diagnostic method. J. Urol., 75:753–757, 1956.

102. Kjellberg, S.R., Ericsson, H.O., and Rudhe, U.: The Lower Urinary Tract in Childhood. Year Book Publishing Co., Chicago, 1957.

103. Lespinasse, V.D.: Urethrogram of the male urethra. Quart. Bull. Northwest. Univ. Med. Sch., 19:298–302, 1945.

104. MacNish, J.M.: Cysto-urethrography in the male. Urol. Cutan. Rev., 40:77–81, 1936.

105. Morales, O., and Romanus, R.: Urethrography in male with highly viscous, water soluble contrast medium, umbradilviscous U. Acta Radiol. (Stockholm) (Suppl.), 95:1–116, 1952.

106. Morales, O., and Romanus, R.: Urethrography in male. J. Urol., 73:162–171, 1955.

107. Thumann, R.C., Jr.: Estimation of weight of hyperplastic prostate from cystourethrogram. Am. J. Roentgenol., 65:593–595, 1951.
108. Thumann, R.C., Jr., and Randall, D.: C stourethrography in diangosis of diseases of prostatic urethra. Am. J. Roentgenol., 64:640–648, 1950.
109. Williams, D.I.: The radiological diagnosis of lower urinary obstruction in the early years. Br. J. Radiol., 27:473–481, 1954.
110. Willwerth, J.W.: Urethrography in the adult male. Am. J. Roentgenol., 86:136–141, 1961.
111. Young, B.W., Anderson, W.L., and King, G.C.: Radiographic estimation of residual urine in children. J. Urol., 75:263–272, 1956.

Wide Bladder Neck Syndrome

112. Stanton, L., and Williams, D.I.: The wide bladder neck in children. Br. J. Urol., 45:60–64, 1973.
113. Taylor, J.S.: Primary dilatation of the bladder neck and urethra in boys. Br. J. Urol., 41:320–332, 1969.

Vaginal Reflux

114. Bolich, P.R., and Babbitt, D.P.: Reflux into vagina, uterus, fallopian tubes and peritoneal cavity during voiding cystourethrography: Case report. Pediatr. Radiol., 3:242–243, 1975.
115. McAlister, W.H., Cacciarelli, A., and Shackleford, G.D.: Complications associated with cystourethrography in children. Radiology, 111:167–172, 1974.

Dangers and Complications with Urethral Injections

116. Czerny, V.: Ein Todesfall welcher im Anschluss an eine lokale Anasthesie der Harnröhre und Blase mit Cocain sich ereignete. Beitr. klin. Chir. (Suppl.), 39:8, 1903.
117. Forbes, K.A., and Cordonnier, J.J.: Circulatory collapse following combined use of Rayopake and air for urethrocystography. J. Urol., 70:975–979, 1953.
118. Hryntschak, T.: Harnrohrenfullung mit Iodipin. Einbruch in die Venen. Ztschr. Urol., 29:508–509, 1939.
119. Hyams, J.A.: Discussion of Flocks, R.H.: Roentgen visualization of the posterior urethra. J. Urol., 30:711–741, 1933.
120. Mathe, C.P.: Fatal embolus due to inflation of bladder with air. Surg. Gynecol. Obstet., 48:429–436, 1929.
121. Marcel and Brochard: Mort par argyrie aigue apres uretrographie avec quelque consideration sur le dangeur de cette exploration. Arch. hospitalieres 1937: 131–134; J. Urol. Paris, 43:290–291, 1937.
127. Mitchell, D.R., and Ortved, W.E.: Mineral oil embolism. Report of a case. J. Urol., 68:652–657, 1952.
123. Patterson, E.A.: The dangers of dilating urethral strictures with oil: Report of 2 cases of fatal oil embolism. J.A.M.A., 97:1147–1149, 1931.
124. Ulm, A.H., and Wagshul, E.C.: Pulmonary embolization following urethrography with oily medium. N. Engl. J. Med., 263:137–139, 1960.

INTERSEX

The sex of a normal individual can be considered to consist of three congruent components: chromosomal, gonadal, and genital. In a normal male, chromosomal sex is 46 XY, gonadal sex is testicular, and genital sex is characterized by the presence of a penis, scrotum, prostate, seminal vesicles, vas deferens, and epididymis. Normal female chromosomal sex is 46 XX, gonadal sex is ovarian, and genital sex is characterized by the presence of a clitoris, labia minora, labia majora, vagina, uterus, and fallopian tubes. An intersexual state exists when the three components of sex are not completely congruent. The conditions to be discussed below are those in which gonadal sex and genital sex are discordant. If the anatomic derangement is so severe that it is not obvious from simple inspection of the genitalia whether the patient is a masculinized female or an incompletely masculinized male, genital ambiguity is said to exist.

Growing knowledge of the factors necessary for normal sexual differentiation and the identification of chromosomal abberations, testicular anatomic defects, and many individual enzymatic blocks in steroid synthesis, have made possible specific clinical diagnoses in many instances.

Accurate diagnosis as soon as possible after birth is essential for several reasons: (1) Psychosexual development is optimal when the most suitable sex of rearing is established at birth and not changed later. (2) Life-threatening conditions such as salt-wasting adrenogenital syndrome can be diagnosed and given specific treatment. (3) The parents can be offered genetic counseling regarding likelihood of recurrence of hereditary syndromes.

The determinant of sex of rearing is the genital sex, although chromosomal and gonadal sex are also important in various aspects of diagnosis and man-

37

Intersex and Congenital Lesions of the Urethra

Patricia Winchester and Paula W. Brill

agement. Freud's statement, "anatomy is destiny," (3,4) serves as a reminder of the importance of appropriate gender assignment early in life.

A generally accepted guideline for management of the intersex states is that when phallic development appears so limited that no normal male sexual activity can be predicted to be possible in adulthood, the patient is surgically reconstructed as a female regardless of gonadal or chromosomal sex. Although there is no urgency in infancy or childhood to create a new vagina or to enlarge an existing one, early resection of a large phallus frequently is deemed advisable in an infant to be raised as a girl. In this way the baby can be considered to be a bona fide female by the people caring for her, a situation which would be difficult if an obvious phallus were confronted at each diaper change.

Gonadectomy is performed early in those individuals whose specific diagnoses are such that pubertal changes can be predicted to be contrary to the sex of rearing or in whom the incidence of gonadal malignancy is high even prior to puberty.

A *true hermaphrodite* is defined as an individual possessing both ovarian and testicular tissue. A pseudohermaphrodite has ambiguity of the genitalia but not of the gonads. A *female pseudohermaphrodite* has normal ovaries, 46 XX karyotype, normal female internal genitalia, and virilization of the external genitalia. A *male pseudohermaphrodite* has testicular tissue and ambiguity of the internal or external genitalia.

The complexities of intersex require a multidisciplinary approach to diagnosis and management. Sophisticated hormonal studies for accurate delineation of enzyme deficiencies and detailed karyotyping for detection of chromosomal mosaicism are beyond the capabilities of routine laboratories. Anatomic information is gained through physical examination, surgical exploration, and radiologic procedures such as genitography and direct injection of wolffian or müllerian duct structures. Identical genital anatomy may be found in different types of intersex, and even within a single clinical entity the degree of masculinization may be highly variable. Ideal timing and performance of diagnostic and reconstructive surgery require technical expertise in conjunction with a consideration of endocrinologic and psychologic factors.

The discussion to follow is a summary of current knowledge of those conditions known to be associated with discordance between gonadal and genital sex, with an emphasis on the interrelated anatomic, chromosomal, and endocrinologic bases for diagnosis.

The following pragmatic classification is based primarily on gonadal histology with subdivisions based on specific hormonal or anatomic developmental defects.[1, 5, 6]

I. True hermaphroditism
II. Abnormal female sex differentiation—female pseudohermaphroditism
  A. Endogenous androgen excess—congenital adrenogenital syndrome
    1. 21-hydroxylase deficiency
    2. 11 β-hydroxylase deficiency
    3. 3 β-ol-dehydrogenase deficiency
  B. Maternal androgen excess
    1. Exogenously administered progestogens
    2. Virilizing tumors
III. Abnormal male sex differentiation
  A. Male pseudohermaphroditism without müllerian structures
    1. Testosterone synthesis defects
      a. 20,22 desmolase, 20 α-hydroxylase deficiency (lipoid hyperplasia of the adrenal)
      b. 17-hydroxylase deficiency
      c. 3 β-ol-dehydrogenase deficiency
      d. 17,20-desmolase deficiency
      e. 17-ketosteroid reductase deficiency
    2. Androgen target area defects
      a. Deficiency of 5α-reductase. Pseudovaginal perineoscrotal hypospadias
      b. Androgen receptor defects
        i. Testicular feminization
        ii. Incomplete forms—Reifenstein, Gilbert-Dreyfus, Lubs syndromes
    3. Pituitary gonadotropin deficiency—microphallus and cryptorchidism
  B. Male pseudohermaphroditism with müllerian structures
    1. Anatomic abnormalities of testicular development
      a. Mixed gonadal dysgenesis
      b. Dysgenetic male pseudohermaphroditism
    2. Isolated müllerian inhibiting factor deficiency—hernia uteri inguinalis

EMBRYOLOGY

A brief review of the series of individual steps that occur in precise order to produce normal sexual differentiation of the gonads, internal ducts, and external genitalia is helpful for the understanding of the various abnormalities of intersex.

Prior to the fifth week of gestation, indifferent or

bipotential gonadal ridges are formed from coelomic epithelial cells and underlying mesenchyme along the medial aspect of each mesonephros. Primordial germ cells then migrate into the gonadal ridges.

Chromosomal determinants direct the initial differentiation of the bipotential gonadal ridge.[13] Testicular differentiation appears to be controlled by a gene located on the short arm of the Y chromosome,[11] the X chromosome, and by some autosomal chromosome as well. A 46 XX chromosomal complement is necessary for normal ovarian development and follicle maintenance.[14]

The coelomic epithelium differentiates into sex cords that further develop into seminiferous tubules in the male and primary ovarian follicles in the female.[7] The mesenchymal cells of the gonadal ridge become Leydig cells in the male and thecal and stromal cells in the female. The primordial germ cells become spermatogenia in the male and ova in the female.[10] The testes develop during the seventh fetal week whereas ovarian development begins about the thirteenth week, and the first follicles appear in the sixteenth week of gestation.[12]

Two sets of primordial sex ducts are present in the undifferentiated fetus: the wolffian and müllerian. In the female, the müllerian ducts differentiate to form the fallopian tubes, the uterus, and the upper portion of the vagina, and the wolffian ducts regress. In the male the wolffian ducts differentiate to form the epididymis, vas deferens, and seminal vesicles while the müllerian ducts regress. Testosterone is essential for the development of wolffian duct structures. There is active inhibition of müllerian duct development by müllerian-inhibiting factor produced by the Sertoli cells of the developing testes.

The external genitalia of both the male and female develop from a series of common primordia that consist of the urogenital sinus, genital tubercle, genital folds, and genital swellings (Table 37–1). In the female fetus, in the absence of androgen, the urogenital sinus forms the lower vagina; the genital tubercle, the clitoris; the genital folds, the labia minora; and the genital swellings, the labia majora. This differentiation occurs regardless of the presence or absence of ovaries. In the male fetus the urogenital sinus becomes the prostate; the genital tubercle, the glans penis; the genital folds, the urethra and shaft of the penis; and genital swellings fuse to give rise to the scrotum.[8] In order for normal male differentiation of external genitalia to occur, testosterone must be secreted by the fetal testis, and testosterone must be converted to dihydrotestosterone by $5\ \alpha$-reductase enzymes located in the anlage of the external genitalia.[15] Further growth of the penis and descent

TABLE 37-1
Development of Male and Female External Genitalia

| Primordia | Reproductive Structures | |
	Male	Female
Genital ridges	Testis	Ovary
Wolffian duct	Epididymis	Gartner's duct*
	Vas deferens	
	Ejaculatory duct	
	Seminal vesicle	
Müllerian duct	Appendix testis*	Fallopian tube
	Prostatic utricle*	Uterus
	Verumontanum	Cervix and upper vagina
Urogenital sinus	Urethra — prostatic, membranous, and proximal cavernous portion	Urethra
		Lower vagina and vestibule
	Bulbourethral glands (Cowper's)	Bartholin's glands
	Prostate gland	
Genital tubercle	Glans penis	Clitoris
Genital folds	Penile urethra and shaft	Labia minora
Genital swelling	Scrotum	Labia majora

* Vestigial structure

of the testes into the scrotum are influenced by pituitary gonadotropins and androgens.

In summary, chromosomal factors direct the differentiation of the indifferent gonads into either ovaries or testes. In the male, differentiation of the internal ducts and external genitalia is influenced by testosterone and its reduction product, dihydrotestosterone. Müllerian structures regress under the effect of müllerian inhibiting factor produced by the fetal testis. In the female with the 46 XX karyotype, the bipotential gonads differentiate into functioning ovaries. In the absence of testosterone and müllerian inhibiting factor, the wolffian structures regress, the müllerian derivatives develop, and the external genitalia form the female phenotype regardless of the sex chromosome complement.

Table 37-2.
Pathways of Androgenic Steroid Metabolism in the Adrenal Gland and Testis*

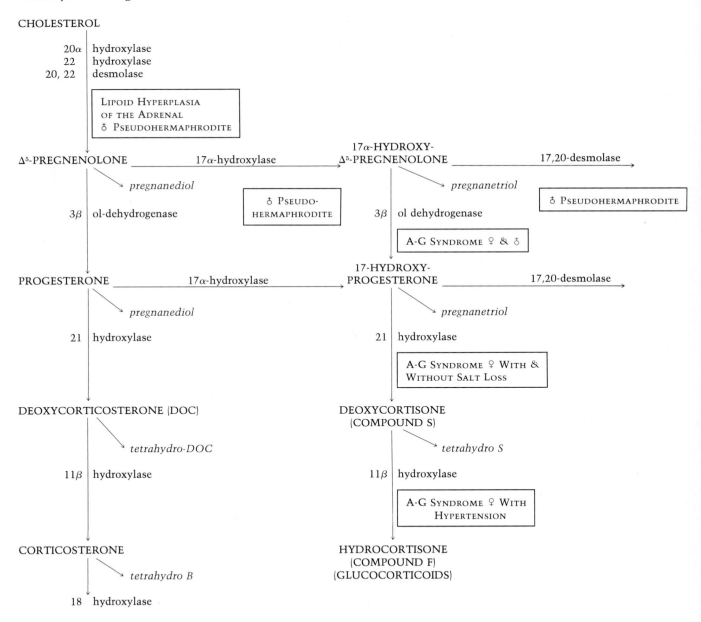

* The abnormalities known to be associated with enzymatic deficiencies are indicated near the appropriate enzyme.

TRUE HERMAPHRODITISM

True hermaphroditism is an extremely rare form of sexual ambiguity though it is the subject of many reports. The causes are still unknown. Double fertilization with XX/XY chimerism is postulated.[18] Over one-half of the cases have 46 XX karyotype,[17] and a familial form has been reported in some with a 46 XX karyotype, suggesting an autosomal recessive trait.[20] Sex chromosomal mosaicism is also reported in true hermaphroditism. The least common karyotype is 46 XY. In the more recent reports, H-Y antigen has been detected in true hermaphrodites even with 46 XX karyotype. Because the H-Y antigen is thought to be a gene product of the short arm of the Y chromosome, its presence implies that the short arm is somewhere in the karyotype.[16] The presence of the short arm of the Y chromosome is necessary for early testicular differentiation.

The appearance of the external genitalia is highly variable, tending toward maleness. There are varying degrees of labioscrotal fusion and hypospadias.[19] Gonadal tissue may be palpated in the labioscrotal folds on one or both sides. Usually a uterus is found. A fallopian tube is present on the side of an ovary or ovotestis. Exploratory surgery and gonadal biopsy are necessary to establish the diagnosis of true hermaphroditism because of the variable differentiation of the internal and external genitalia, normal hormone levels, and variable chromosomal pattern. Virilization and frequently some degree of breast development occur at puberty. Menstruation has been reported in some cases. Sex assignment should be made early based on the appearance of the external genitalia. The inappropriate sex structures are surgically removed. The gonad of the assigned sex is retained if it is histologically normal, for it may provide hormonal function. The incidence of gonadal tumors in true hermaphrodites is low.

FEMALE PSEUDOHERMAPHRODITISM

A female pseudohermaphrodite has normal ovaries and müllerian structures, an XX karyotype, and variable virilization of the external genitalia. The virilization results from exposure to increased androgens in utero either produced by the fetus because of enzyme deficiencies in steroid synthesis or because of abnormally high maternal androgen levels.

CONGENITAL ADRENOGENITAL SYNDROME

Congenital adrenogenital syndrome is the most common type of female pseudohermaphroditism and indeed of all intersex problems.[8] It is inherited as an autosomal recessive. Deficiencies of the enzymes necessary to synthesize cortisol drive steroid metabolism toward the production of androgens (Table 37–2). *21-Hydroxylase* is the most frequent enzyme deficiency with elevation of urinary pregnanetriol, androsterone, and etiocholanolone and elevation of plasma 17-hydroxyprogesterone. Salt

Table 37-2 (continued)

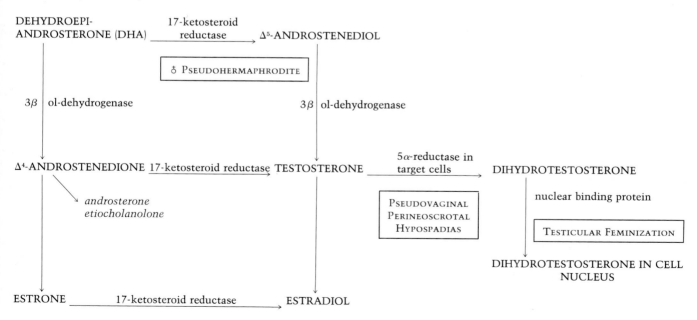

(17-KETOSTEROIDS, ANDROGENS-ESTROGENS)

wasting is present in 30 to 65 per cent.[22] In most cases there is an enlarged phallus with a dorsal hood and ventral chordee. There is a single perineal orifice of a urogenital sinus that divides into urethra anteriorly and vagina posteriorly (Fig. 37–1). The labia minora may be fused over the sinus and the labioscrotal folds are bifid and rugated.[24] The degree of masculinization is variable (Fig. 37–2). The internal female anatomy is normal.

11β-Hydroxylase deficiency results in the same virilization of the external female genitalia as is seen in 21-hydroxylase deficiency, but these patients retain salt and frequently are hypertensive. Increased urinary 17-ketosteroids are found. Increased plasma levels of deoxycorticosterone and deoxycortisol help establish the diagnosis and distinguish the disease from the 21-hydroxylase block.

3β-ol-Dehydrogenase deficiency is rare. Death from salt wasting usually occurs in infancy. It is the only enzyme deficiency that results in both female and male pseudohermaphroditism. The principal steroids excreted are pregnenetriol and dehydroepiandrosterone, which is a relatively weak androgen. The females are slightly virilized with clitoral hypertrophy and slight labial fusion.[21]

The diagnosis of andrenogenital syndrome is established by biochemical determination of steroid metabolism. Surgical exploration is unnecessary. Boys with adrenogenital syndrome do not have ambiguous genitalia except in the case of 3β-ol-dehydrogenase deficiency. For this reason diagnosis and early glucocorticoid replacement is more difficult in boys. Congenital adrenal hyperplasia with salt wasting is the only life-threatening entity that presents with sexual ambiguity.

EXOGENOUS ANDROGENIZATION

In the late 1950s and early 1960s many cases of female pseudohermaphroditism occurred secondary to the popular use of progesterone-like compounds to prevent abortion.[27] With exogenous androgenization, the external genitalia alone are virilized. Fusion of the labioscrotal folds with the formation of a phallic urethra can occur if androgenic compounds are given prior to the twelfth week of gestation.[26]

Masculinization of the external genitalia of the female fetus can also occur if there is a maternal tumor with androgenic activity. In these rare cases both mother and infant are virilized.[25] Usually the diagnosis of nonadrenal female pseudohermaphroditism can be made when an XX karyotype and normal urinary ketosteroids and pregnanetriol are present in a child with ambiguity of the external genitalia.

Only true hermaphroditism enters into the differential diagnosis.

MALE PSEUDOHERMAPHRODITISM WITHOUT MÜLLERIAN STRUCTURES

TESTOSTERONE SYNTHESIS DEFECTS

Enzyme deficiencies with autosomal recessive inheritance have been described in the basic steps in testosterone synthesis (see Table 37–2). The genitalia originating from wolffian ducts, urogenital sinus and genital swellings, folds, and tubercle show varying degrees of ambiguity depending on the severity of the enzyme defect. During embryonic development the testes differentiate normally and produce müllerian inhibiting factor so that no müllerian structures are present. No gonadal tumors have been described in the testosterone-synthesizing enzyme deficiency states.[37]

Lipoid Hyperplasia of the Adrenal. This is a rare form of nonvirilizing adrenogenital syndrome resulting from a defect in the conversion of cholesterol to pregnenolone.[31, 35] Almost all patients with this defect die during infancy because of severe salt wasting. This is the only form of adrenogenital syndrome in which urinary 17-ketosteroids and 17-hydroxycorticosteroids are decreased rather than increased. The adrenal glands contain enormous accumulation of lipids. The affected males have either female external genitalia or severe ambiguity.[30]

17α-Hydroxylase Deficiency. Phenotypically these 46 XY males appear as slightly masculinized females. The testes are usually intra-abdominal, and the vas and epididymis are often rudimentary. The vagina is short and ends blindly. These patients are hypertensive with marked salt retention and hypokalemia.[28] There are increased levels of pregnenolone, progesterone, deoxycorticosterone, corticosterone, and their urinary metabolites. Glucocorticoid and androgen production is decreased. At puberty these patients remain sexually infantile. Gynecomastia has been reported in one case.[33]

3β-ol-Dehydrogenase Deficiency. Males with this enzyme deficiency tend to be more completely masculinized than do those with other disorders of steroidogenesis.[34] Perineal hypospadias is the most common anomaly described. Salt wasting is always present. Dehydroisoandrosterone, a weak androgen, is elevated in the urine.[29] Pregnanetriol is the principal hydroxycorticoid excreted.

17,20-Desmolase Deficiency. Only two boy cousins with this enzyme lack have been reported.[38] They presented with ambiguous genitalia and a family history of intersex problems. Both had normal mineralo- and glucocorticoid production but lacked dehydroepiandrosterone. Testicular biopsy slices from these boys showed normal conversion of Δ^5 androstenediol to testosterone.

17-Ketosteroid Reductase Deficiency. In the past, this enzyme deficiency has been confused with testicular feminization and 5α-reductase deficiency because of the similarity of phenotype.[36] Males with 17-ketosteroid reductase deficiency have testes and internal structures derived only from wolffian ducts. They appear externally as females with labia and a blind vaginal pouch.[32] At puberty partial virilization and feminization are reported. Gynecomastia is common, body hair increases, the voice deepens, and the clitoris enlarges. The diagnosis is rarely made before puberty unless a stimulation test with human chorionic gonadotropin is performed because of a family history of sexual ambiguity. At puberty plasma androstenedione and urinary 17-ketosteroids are elevated. There is some peripheral conversion of androstenedione to testosterone but not to the level seen in normal males.

ANDROGEN TARGET-AREA DEFECTS

5α-Reductase Deficiency — Pseudovaginal Perineoscrotal Hypospadias. The discovery of this enzyme deficiency confirmed the essential role of dihydrotestosterone in the differentiation of male external genitalia in utero.[48] Male pseudohermaphrodites of this group appear female at birth yet virilize at puberty, perhaps representing the ultimate paradox of intersex. Their testes are normal in size and usually scrotal or inguinal in location. The internal ducts are male since testosterone is synthesized normally (Fig. 37–3). A female sex is usually assigned at birth because of the presence of a vagina, perineal urethra, and small phallus. The diagnosis is usually made after puberty solely on clinical grounds. Confirmation is possible if target-tissue slices fail to convert testosterone to dihydrotesterone.[47] Testicular malignancy has not been reported.[37]

Complete Testicular Feminization. Those 46 XY individuals with testicular feminization syndrome have bilateral testes that produce normal testosterone. The "feminization" is a failure of end-organ response to testosterone and dihydrotestosterone because of a defect in the protein binding of dihydro-

testosterone.[43] In utero the external genital anlagen do not masculinize, and a short blind vagina develops. The testes are located in the groin or in the abdomen. There are no müllerian derivatives. The internal wolffian derivatives are rudimentary. At puberty these individuals feminize but have no pubic or axillary hair and do not menstruate. Complete testicular feminization is inherited as either an X-linked recessive or male-limited autosomal dominant trait.

In the postpubertal period there are high levels of testosterone and estrogen as well as luteinizing hormone indicating that the pituitary gland is also an insensitive target organ. In young children injected testosterone does not lower urinary excretion of nitrogen, phosphorus, or citrate, confirming the lack of response of end-organs to normal testosterone.

Male pseudohermaphrodites with complete testicular feminization are usually reared as females. The testes may be left in place until puberty to permit breast development or removed at the time of diagnosis because of the high incidence of gonadal malignancy.[37]

Incomplete Testicular Feminization. Male pseudohermaphrodites of this group differ from those with complete testicular feminization because of varying degrees of masculinization of the internal and external genitalia and because at puberty there is some degree of virilization.[49] Breast development is common. Circulating testosterone levels are normal or high, and there is no evidence of any abnormality in testosterone biosynthesis or müllerian regression. The appearance of the external genitalia usually determines the sex of rearing. There is often a family history of intersex problems, suggesting an X-linked recessive mode of inheritance. Various syndromes, Lubs,[44] Gilbert-Dreyfus,[41] and Reifenstein,[46] are all believed to be due to partial defect of the function of a cytoplasmic androgen receptor necessary for transportation of dihydrotestosterone into the nucleus. They differ in the degree of ambiguity of the external genitalia. The incidence of gonadal malignancy is not increased.[37]

PITUITARY GONADOTROPIN DEFICIENCY —
  MICROPHALLUS — CRYPTORCHIDISM

Microphallus–cryptorchidism is characterized by a very small penis with a normal urethra and usually nondescent of the testes. Internal and external male sexual differentiation proceeds normally during early fetal life, but the final phases of male phenotypic development are defective in this newly recognized disorder. It has been shown that fetal pituitary gonadotropins, which are elevated during the latter half of gestation as maternal and placental gonadotropins fall, are necessary for growth of male external genitalia and descent of the testes into the scrotum. Walsh and co-workers reported a familial form of microphallus in five patients with decreased pituitary gonadotropin levels.[50] Sporadic cases of hypogonadism appear to be secondary to a testicular defect or unresponsiveness to chorionic gonadotropin.

MALE PSEUDOHERMAPHRODITISM WITH MÜLLERIAN STRUCTURES

ANATOMIC ABNORMALITIES OF TESTICULAR DEVELOPMENT

Incomplete masculinization of the external genitalia due to anatomic abnormalities of testicular development occurs in two related entities: mixed gonadal dysgenesis and dysgenetic male pseudohermaphroditism. These complex conditions can be better understood by first considering the various forms of gonadal dysgenesis: Turner's syndrome, pure gonadal dysgenesis (XX type), and pure gonadal dysgenesis (XY type).[1] All three conditions have a female phenotype.

For the formation of a normal testis during fetal development, factors on the Y chromosome, X chromosome, and possibly on autosomal chromosomes are necessary. Complete deletion of an X or Y chromosome results in a 45 XO chromosomal complement and bilateral streak gonads (Turner's syndrome). Histologically the streak consists of whorls of connective tissue and is similar in all forms of gonadal dysgenesis regardless of chromosomal complement. In the absence of testicular development, neither müllerian inhibiting substance nor androgen is produced. As a result there is no virilization of wolffian ducts, urogenital sinus, or external genitalia, and the patient appears phenotypically female. Although most patients with Turner's syndrome have an XO karyotype, mosaicism, especially XO/XX, has been associated.

Bilateral streak gonads, persistent müllerian structures, and feminized external genitalia are also found in the XX and XY types of pure gonadal dysgenesis. The reason for the female phenotype is the same as in Turner's syndrome. In the absence of testicular development there is no production of testosterone or müllerian inhibiting factor, and differentiation of internal and external genitalia occurs along female lines.

In XX gonadal dysgenesis there is evidence of autosomal recessive inheritance, and in XY gonadal dysgenesis inheritance appears to be X-linked recessive. The presence of X-linked inheritance in this syndrome provides evidence that some deteminant on the X chromosome is necessary for normal testicular development. It is of interest that several patients with XY gonadal dysgenesis have had siblings with dysgenetic male pseudohermaphroditism.[1] The exact relationship between these two disorders is unclear at this time. Nearly one-third of patients with XY gonadal dysgenesis have developed dysgerminoma or gonadoblastoma in one or both streak gonads. Clearly, excision of the gonads is indicated in this high-risk group of patients.

The two abnormalities of testicular development that present with some degree of ambiguous masculinization of the genitalia are mixed gonadal dysgenesis and dysgenetic male pseudohermaphroditism (Table 37–3).

Mixed Gonadal Dysgenesis. In mixed gonadal dysgenesis,[1, 6, 51, 52] there is chromosomal mosai-

TABLE 37-3
Anatomic Findings in Intersex

Diagnosis	Gonads	Urogenital Sinus	Müllerian Duct Structures
True hermaphroditism	Testis + Ovary	+	+
Female pseudohermaphroditism	Ovary + Ovary	+	+
Mixed gonadal dysgenesis	Testis + Streak	+	+
Dysgenetic male pseudohermaphroditism	Dysgenetic testis + Dysgenetic testis	+	+
Male pseudohermaphroditism			
Androgen synthesis defects	Testis + Testis	+	−
Androgen target area defect	Testis + Testis	+	−
Müllerian inhibiting factor defect	Testis + Testis	+	+

cism usually with a 46 XY/45 XO karyotype but a variety of patterns including XO/XY/XYY, XO/XY/XYY/XXY, XO/XYYY, XO/XXY and others have been described. The typical patient has a streak gonad on one side and a testis on the other, persistent müllerian duct structures, and variable masculinization of the external genitalia. Upper vagina, cervix, uterus, and fallopian tubes are present (Figs. 37–4, 37–5). The uterus is often infantile. A fallopian tube is always present on the side of the streak and usually on the side of the testis as well. The testis may be rudimentary or may appear nearly normal microscopically and may be partially or completely descended. Even a streak may descend to the upper scrotum. Delayed onset of otherwise normal endocrine function of the fetal testis has been postulated as the cause of the faulty masculinization and persistence of müllerian derivatives. The fact that Leydig cell function is normal at puberty lends support to this theory. Consistent with the theory is the observed variability of phenotypic expression in mixed gonadal dysgenesis, some patients appearing highly masculinized and others only minimally so. Extreme delay in onset of endocrine function of the fetal testis might explain failure of müllerian regression and absent virilization of wolffian duct structures, urogenital sinus, and external genitalia. On the other hand minimal delay might explain faulty müllerian regression along with marked virilization. Although variable, some degree of ambiguity of the external genitalia is the rule. The sex of rearing depends on the degree of masculinization. There is an increased incidence of gonadal malignancy in mixed gonadal dysgenesis but probably not as high as with XY gonadal dysgenesis. When both testicular tissue and streak material have been identified in a patient with a gonadal tumor, the tumor has generally involved the testis rather than the streak. Fully descended testes have rarely been involved with tumor. Generally, testes that are dysgenetic or cannot be placed in the scrotum are removed.

Dysgenetic Male Pseudohermaphroditism. Dysgenetic male pseudohermaphroditism may be associated with an XY karyotype or mosaicism with an XO component (e.g., XO/XY).[53] There are persistent müllerian remnants internally and genital ambiguity externally as with mixed gonadal dysgenesis. However, gonadal streaks are not present. Testes are usually undescended and may vary histologically from primitive to nearly normal. Usually there is a combination of immature, hypoplastic testicular tubules and persistent stroma resembling that of a streak gonad. Regardless of appearance or location, the testes deteriorate rapidly at puberty, and fertility has never been reported. The reported incidence of gonadal tumors is 15 to 30 per cent. The testicular tumors have all arisen in undescended testes and occurred after puberty. The diagnosis of dysgenetic male pseudohermaphroditism is established by gonadal biopsy, and gonadectomy is indicated for dysgenetic testes that are undescended. The degree of masculinization of the external genitalia is variable and determines the sex of rearing.

ISOLATED MÜLLERIAN INHIBITING FACTOR DEFICIENCY — HERNIA UTERI INGUINALIS

Males with either abnormalities in the synthesis or action of müllerian inhibiting factor are described. They present no problem in sex assignment because their external genitalia are male. An inguinal or scrotal hernia is present associated with either a palpable testes and contralateral cryptorchidism or with bilateral cryptorchidism.[55] The condition is usually not suspected until adulthood, when fallopian tubes and uteri are found at the time of inguinal hernia repair (Fig. 37–6). It is postulated that müllerian inhibiting factor is secreted by the fetal testes and produces local regression of the müllerian duct structures in normal male differentiation. The lack of this fetal protein "hormone" permits the fallopian tubes, uterus, and upper vagina to develop in the otherwise normal male embryo. The internal female ducts drain into the prostatic utricle. Most cases described are isolated, but familial cases reported suggest an X-linked inheritance.[54]

RADIOGRAPHIC EVALUATION OF PATIENTS WITH INTERSEXUALITY

Patrick C. Walsh

Radiographic procedures are most useful in evaluating the status of the urogenital sinus and internal duct structures in patients with ambiguous genitalia. Genitography is accomplished easily using a blunt-ended syringe positioned firmly at the opening of the urogenital sinus.[56, 57] While contrast medium is injected slowly, fluoroscopy may be used to select spot films demonstrating the filling of the urogenital sinus and internal duct structures (see Fig. 37–4). This method is far superior to voiding cystourethrograms. Occasionally it may be necessary to perform endoscopy under anesthesia. At this time, the urogenital sinus or prostatic utricle can be catheterized for retrograde contrast studies (see Fig. 37–6).[55]

The results of these studies may be helpful in the differential diagnosis of ambiguous genitalia in the newborn (Table 37–3). A lower vagina, arising from the urogenital sinus, may be present in any of the common forms of intersexuality. Similarly, patients with female pseudohermaphroditism and mixed gonadal dysgenesis always have a uterus and at least one fallopian tube; müllerian derivatives are also common in patients with true hermaphroditism. However the presence of a uterus or a fallopian tube in a patient with ambiguous genitalia excludes the diagnosis of male pseudohermaphroditism due to a defect in androgen synthesis or androgen action.

At the time of exploratory laparotomy, the differentiation of the distal wolffian duct structures (distal vas deferens and seminal vesicles) can be determined by performing antegrade vasograms. The technique involves exposure of the vas deferens near the testis and insertion of a small blunt needle through a transverse vasotomy. Following the injection of 1 cc. of 50 per cent diatrizoate sodium, appropriate roentgenograms are performed to document the presence of the distal vas deferens, seminal vesicle, and ejaculatory duct (see Fig. 37–3). In this way, the anatomic description of the internal duct structures can be completed without the need for an extensive retrovesical dissection.[58]

HYPOSPADIAS

Hypospadias in the male is a congenital defect of the anterior urethra in which the canal terminates on the ventral surface of the penis proximal to its normal opening (Fig. 37–7). In the female, hypospadias is rare. The urethral meatus is located on the anterior vaginal wall, and there may be urinary incontinence that is not a feature of hypospadias in the male.

Hypospadias may occur as an isolated anomaly or as a component of more complicated intersexual states (see Fig. 37–5). The more severe the degree of hypospadias, the greater is the likelihood of associated intersexuality. Even mild hypospadias may be considered to represent incomplete masculinization of the urethra and hence mild intersex.

Classification of hypospadias is based on the location of the urethral meatus: glandular, subcoronal, penile, penoscrotal, and perineal. Glandular and subcoronal varieties are most frequent.[66]

In Kennedy's series of 489 cases of hypospadias, 105 had other manifestations of disordered sexual differentiation including cryptochidism (50), bifid scrotum (31), pseudohermaphroditism (14), microphallus (5), true hermaphroditism (3), testicular absence or atrophy (2).[63] Chordee, a downward bowing of the penis, was found in 194 of the patients in Kennedy's series.

When hypospadias, cryptorchidism, and ambiguous genitalia occur together, the incidence of specific intersexuality is 53 per cent. Even with otherwise normal-appearing external genitalia, 27 per cent of patients with cryptorchidism and hypospadias prove on further investigation to have some type of intersex.[64]

Excretory urography in 200 patients with hypospadias revealed 16 abnormalities of which 10 were defects requiring surgical correction. The surgical defects included vesicoureteral reflux and ureteropelvic junction obstruction.[61] It appears that in cases in which nonurologic anomalies are associated with hypospadias of any degree, upper tract anomalies are more common.

Most patients with hypospadias have a normal 46 XY karyotype. Of a series of 50 unselected hypospadiac patients, 3 were found to have abnormal karyotypes including 47 XYY, 46 XX/46 XY, and 47 XY/ trisomy 21.[59] Hypospadias has been reported in occasional patients with Kleinfelter's syndrome (47 XXY)[62] and the sex reversal syndrome (46 XX).[60]

PROSTATIC UTRICLE (MÜLLERIAN DUCT REMNANT)

The utricle is a rudiment of the müllerian ducts in the male. It corresponds to the upper vagina and uterus in the female. In the normal male fetus, müllerian inhibiting factor causes these ducts to regress except for their caudal or cloacal ends, which fuse and enter the seminal colliculus in the prostatic urethra. The normal utricle usually does not permit inflow of contrast medium during cystourethrography, but when it does it is only a small pit at the center of the verumontanum or a narrow outpouching extending a few millimeters toward the bladder behind the prostatic urethra (Figs. 37–8, 37–9).[71] Occasionally the utricle is divided into two compartments by a longitudinal septum because of lack of fusion of the müllerian ducts. Enlargement of both septate and nonseptate utricles is frequently found in hypospadias and may be considered a variety of intersexuality (Fig. 37–10). Large utricles may be referred to as müllerian duct cysts (Figs. 37–11, 37–12). Rarely, a müllerian duct cyst may be associated with a complex anomaly in which a long seg-

ment of müllerian duct is retained (Fig. 37-13). Enlargement of the utricle has also been described with
obstruction of the distal urethra and in the prune
belly syndrome.[70]

CONGENITAL URETHRAL FISTULAS

Congential urethral fistulas are rare in both sexes
and almost always associated with anorectal or
vaginal malformations.

MALES

URETHROCUTANEOUS FISTULA

This uncommon fistula is postulated to result
from distal urethral obstruction usually at the
meatus with the formation of a tract from the more
proximal urethral to ventral penile shaft. The opening resembles hypospadias but the extension of the
urethra more distally in the penile shaft establishes
the diagnosis of a congenital fistula.

URETHRORECTAL FISTULA

Almost all congenital rectourethral fistulas are associated with rectoanal malformations. In males,
imperforate anus with the bowel ending above the
levator ani muscle is frequently associated with a
fistula between the blind-ending large bowel and the
urinary tract. The fistula may reach the urethra at
various levels, most often in the posterior wall of the
prostatic urethra (Figs. 37-14, 37-15). Traction ex-
erted by the fistula may cause an angulation in the
posterior urethra.[74] In most cases, the fistula can be
visualized during cystourethrography unless it is
plugged with meconium.

FEMALES

URETHRORECTAL FISTULA

In females with supralevator imperforate anus the
bowel fistula usually terminates in the posterior
wall of the vagina. In the few reported cases of rec-
tourinary fistula in females there is always an associated anomaly of the genital tract such as vaginal
agenesis or rudimentary double vagina.[73a] In a few
females with imperforate anus, the distal bowel terminates in the posterior vagina, which shares an
outlet with the urethra, forming a common narrow
urogenital sinus. Urine from the urethra and meconium from the rectovaginal fistula mix with vaginal
secretions and cause marked vaginal distention.[75]
This is referred to as a cloacal chamber.

VAGINAL-URETHRAL COMMUNICATIONS

Vaginal-urethral communications have been described in an unusual anomaly characterized by imperforate vagina and communication of the upper
patent vagina with the urethra.[73] The external genitalia are otherwise normal. There are no signs of
virilization. Hydrocolpos may be present at birth.
The congenital fistulous communication is usually
demonstrated on voiding films during cystourethrography (Fig. 37-16).

DUPLICATION OF THE URETHRA

The variety of anatomic malformations that involve
duplication of the male urethra is almost limit-
less,[76, 82, 84, 85] reflecting the complicated embryonic
development of the urethra. Williams proposed an
anatomic classification, dividing duplications of the
urethra into sagittal and collateral groups.[87] Within
the sagittal group, the duplication may be in an
epispadiac (Fig. 37-17) or hypospadiac (Fig. 37-18)
location. Each of these may be complete with separate bladder origins (Fig. 37-19) or incomplete with
only one bladder outlet (Figs. 37-17, 37-18). The
duplications may also end blindly with the formation of a penile sinus (Figs. 37-20, 37-21). Urethral
diverticula and a dilated Cowper's duct must be distinguished from these accessory ventral urethral
sinuses.[79]

In addition to the hypospadiac urethral duplications that terminate in the ventral penile shaft or
penoscrotal junction, there is a type in which the accessory urethra arises either from a separate bladder
opening or the proximal urethra and ends in the perineum just anterior to the anal verge (Fig. 37-22).
This type is usually associated with an abnormality
in the normally positioned urethra and may represent a fistula more than a duplication. Effmann emphasized that the ventral urethra is the more functional conduit in most cases of sagittal duplication.[81]

Collateral duplications of the male urethra are extremely rare and are associated with total or incomplete diphallus. In most reports of this malformation, the penis forms a single shaft but the glans has
a bilobed appearance. The second urethra may be
only an abortive channel or arise from a separate
bladder if there is complete caudal duplication.

Urethral duplication in the female is even rarer
than in the male.[78, 80] It has been reported with
idiopathic masculinization of the external genitalia
with vaginal outlet obstruction and clitoral hypertrophy.[77, 83, 86] In these cases the accessory channel is
in the clitoris.

MEGALOURETHRA

Marked dilatation of the penile urethra has been noted in association with partial agenesis of the penile erectile tissue. The size and shape of the large urethra depend on the location and amount of deficient corpora.[90] A localized absence of the corpus spongiosum permits a saccular diverticulum of the penile urethra to develop. More extensive agenesis of corpus spongiosum results in a megalourethra and a scaphoid-shaped penis during voiding (Fig. 37-23). If there is agenesis of the corpora cavernosa as well as of the corpus spongiosum in the shaft of the penis, a fusiform enlargement of the urethra occurs.[89] Megalourethra is usually associated with major abnormalities of the urinary tract and has been reported in prune belly syndrome.[88]

HYPERTROPHY OF THE VERUMONTANUM

The verumontanum (colliculus seminalis) is an oval raised area in the posterior wall of the prostatic urethra. It is the embryonic remnant of Müller's tubercle. The ejaculatory ducts and utricle open into this mound. Enlargement of the verumontanum has been noted in 0.2 per cent of male infants in a large autopsy series.[93] The hypertrophy is probably transient and may be the result of maternal estrogen stimulation near term.[9] The verumontanum appears prominent on some voiding cystourethrograms (Figs. 37-24, 37-25) but there are only a few reports of obstruction secondary to hypertrophy.[92, 94, 97, 98]

Enlargement of the verumontanum has also been noted with inflammatory lesions of the urethra and bladder in older children and adults.[91, 95, 96]

URETHRAL VALVES, ANTERIOR AND POSTERIOR

See Chapter 53 and Figures 37-26 to 37-34.

URINE ASCITES

Neonatal ascites due to peritoneal leakage of urine is an unusual complication of posterior urethral valves.[104] Early reports suggested that the mechanism of ascites was transudation of urine through the walls of the dilated, obstructed urinary tract.[105] Actual perforations of the urinary tract in infants with urinary outlet obstruction have been documented radiologically in more recent reports and may be the sole mechanism of urinary ascites.[104, 106, 108]

In most cases, perforation occurs through a calyceal fornix with urine first accumulating in a subcapsular location or in the perirenal space.[101, 102] The subsequent presence of urine ascites implies that a colleciton of urine in the perirenal space has decompressed itself by perforation through the anterior renal fascia and peritoneum into the peritoneal cavity. Perforation of the bladder secondary to outlet obstruction may result in urine ascites but is less frequent than calyceal perforation.[104]

OTHER CONGENITAL ANOMALIES

The following congenital anomalies of the urethra are discussed in other chapters:

Epispadias and congenital absence of the urethra: Chapter 24

Congenital urethral diverticulum: Chapter 39

Congenital urethral stricture and congenital contracture of the bladder neck: Chapter 41

Excretory urography demonstrates hydronephrosis and the presence of contrast material in the perirenal space or peritoneal fluid on delayed films (Fig. 37-31). Bladder perforation may be shown on cystography. Although retrograde pyelograms may demonstrate the sites of perforation in the ureters or upper collecting systems, they are not indicated routinely.

Posterior urethral valves are the most frequent lesion leading to urinary ascites. Other more unusual reported causes include urethral atresia,[108] presacral neuroblastoma,[108] vesical neck valve in a female,[99] meningomyelocele with neurogenic bladder,[103, 107] ureterocele,[100] and ureteropelvic junction obstruction complicated by a postcircumcision urethral stricture.[100]

CHAPTER 37, ILLUSTRATIONS

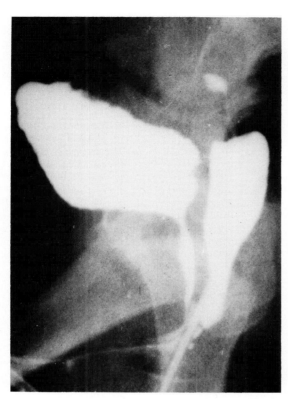

FIG. 37-1. Female pseudohermaphrodite with adrenogenital syndrome. A short urogenital sinus is injected with contrast medium. There is filling of the urethra and bladder as well as of the vagina and uterine cavity. A cervical impression is present at the superior aspect of the vagina.

FIG. 37-2. Female pseudohermaphrodite with adrenogenital syndrome. There is a long phallic urethra. The vagina (*arrow*) appears continuous with the urogenital sinus. (Courtesy of K. Waterhouse, M.D.)

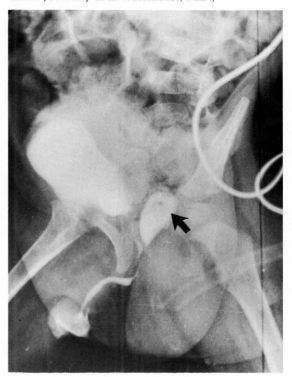

FIG. 37-3. 5-α-Reductase deficiency. Pseudovaginal perineoscrotal hypospadias. Intraoperative right vasogram demonstrates the vas deferens, seminal vesicle, and ejaculatory duct. The ejaculatory duct empties into the distal vagina. (Courtesy of P. Walsh, M.D.)

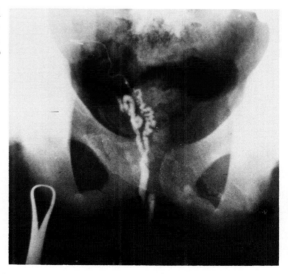

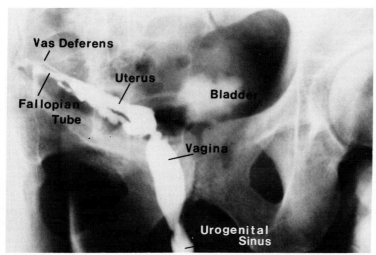

FIG. 37-4. Mixed gonadal dysgenesis. Retrograde genitogram performed with a blunt-ended syringe placed in the urogenital sinus demonstrating the vagina, uterus, fallopian tube, and vas deferens. (Reprinted with permission from Wilson, J.D., Walsh, P.C.: Disorders of Sexual Differentiation. In Harrison, J.H., Gitter, R.F., Perlmutter, A.D., et al. (eds.): Campbell's Urology, 4th ed., Philadelphia, W.B. Saunders, in press.)

FIG. 37-5. Mixed gonadal dysgenesis. A 36-year-old person raised as a male with perineal hypospadias, 45 XO/46 XY mosaicism. **(A)** The urethra is injected with contrast medium. Areas of stricture are secondary to hypospadias repair. Contrast medium fills a vagina and uterine cavity. There is no retrograde filling of the posterior urethra or bladder. **(B)** The bladder is filled with contrast medium by injection of a suprapubic cystotomy tube. The patient voids, filling the posterior urethra, vagina, and uterus. There is reflux filling of the left ureter from the bladder. (Courtesy of H. Mitty, M.D.)

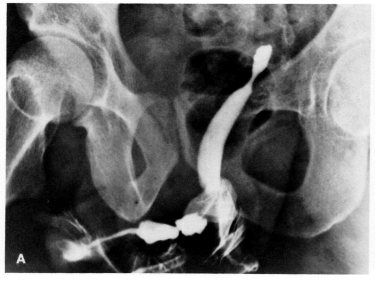

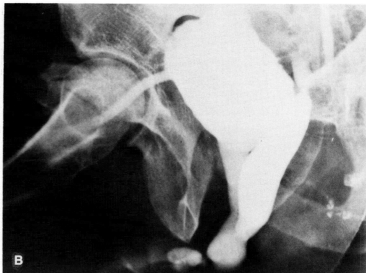

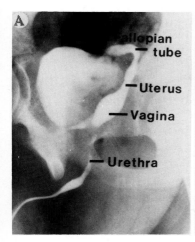

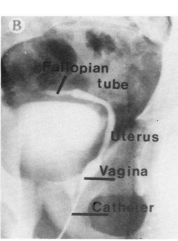

FIG. 37-6. Isolated müllerian inhibiting factor deficiency—hernia uteri inguinalis. Radiographs performed after retrograde instillation of sodium diatrizoate into the prostatic utricles of two patients with the familial persistent müllerian duct syndrome (reprinted with permission from Sloan, W.R., Walsh, P.C.: Familial persistent müllerian duct syndrome. J. Urol., 115:459–461, 1976).

FIG. 37–7. Hypospadias. Voiding cystourethrogram. The hypospadiac urethral meatus is on the ventral surface of the penis. No müllerian duct derivatives are demonstrated. (Courtesy of W. Berdon, W.D., and D. Baker, M.D.)

FIG. 37–8. Utricle. During injection of a cystourethrogram, an oval-shaped smooth utricle (*arrow*) is shown arising from the posterior aspect of the prostatic urethra.

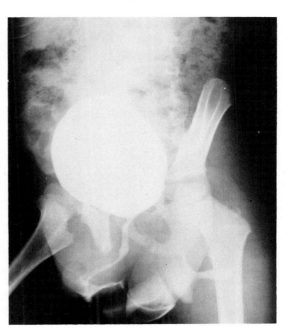

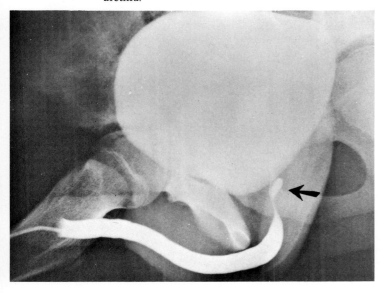

FIG. 37–9. Utricle. Normal-sized utricles seen during voiding cystourethrography of two different cases. *Arrows* point to the utricle. (Edling, N.P.G.: Acta Radiol., *32*:28, 1949)

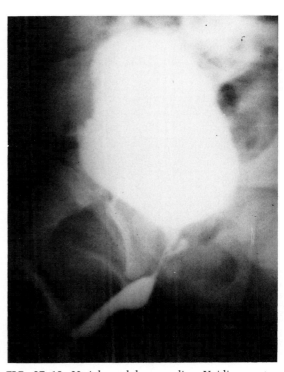

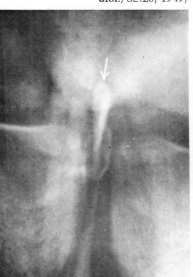
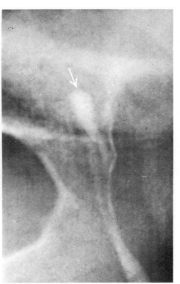

FIG. 37–10. Utricle and hypospadias. Voiding cystourethrogram in a boy with penoscrotal hypospadias. A small smooth-walled utricle fills from the posterior aspect of the prostatic urethra.

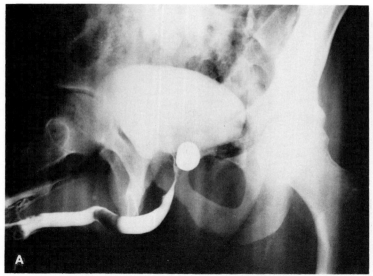

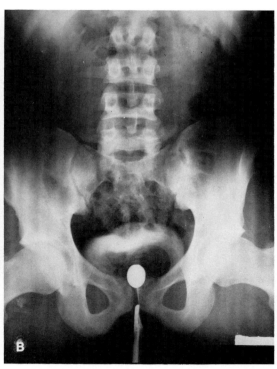

FIG. 37–11. Utricle. **(A)** Retrograde injection of the urethra with filling of a large round utricle or müllerian duct cyst. **(B)** The utricle is injected and its location posterior to the bladder outlet is seen.

FIG. 37–12. Müllerian duct cyst. **(A)** Right seminal vesiculogram (contrast material injected through vaso-stomy incision). Seminal vesicle displaced laterally by cyst. **(B)** Müllerian duct cyst injected with contrast medium (ureteral catheter passed through utricle). Cyst was the cause of displaced right seminal vesicle. (Culbertson, L.R.: J. Urol., 58:134, 1947)

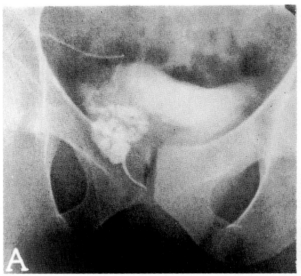

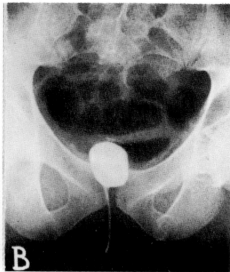

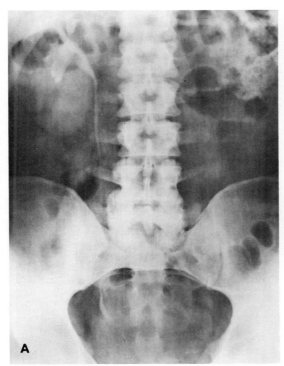

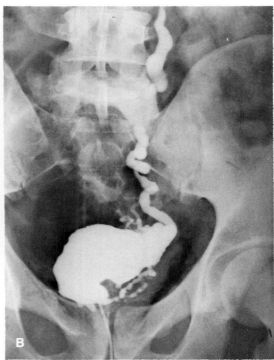

FIG. 37–13. Müllerian duct cyst. **(A)** Intravenous pyelogram showing normal right kidney and ureter but no function on the left. **(B)** Injection of müllerian duct cyst with contrast material through a ureteral catheter. AP view. There is a moderate-sized müllerian duct cyst. The tortuous tubular structure was considered to be the müllerian duct. **(C)** Left posterior oblique view showing similar findings. (Ceccarelli, F.E., Beach, P.D.: J. Urol., 85:31, 1961)

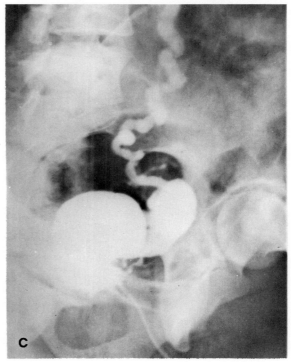

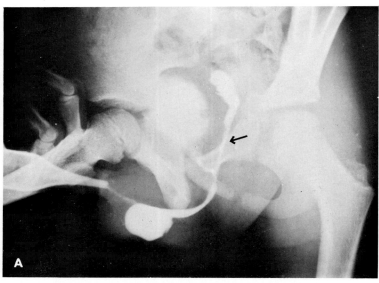

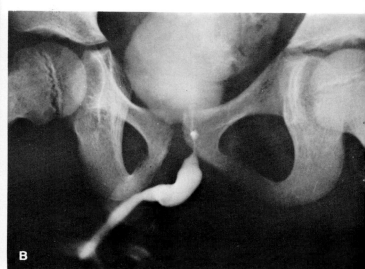

FIG. 37–14. (A) Urethrorectal fistula. Retrograde urethrogram in 3-year-old boy with an anorectal abnormality. The *arrow* points to the fistula between the rectum and the distal prostatic urethra. In addition there is a congenital diverticulum of the anterior urethra. (B) Postoperative retrograde urethrogram. (Lattimer, J., Uson, A., Melicow, M.: Pediatric Surgery, vol. 2, p. 989, Chicago, Year Book Medical Publishers, 1962)

FIG. 37–15. Congenital urethrorectal fistula. (A) Voiding cystourethrogram in a newborn boy shows a fistula (*arrow*) between the proximal urethra and rectum. Contrast medium is present in the bladder and colon. The patient is voiding around the catheter. (B) Postoperative view. (Courtesy of K. Waterhouse, M.D.)

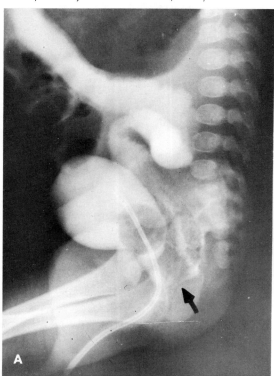

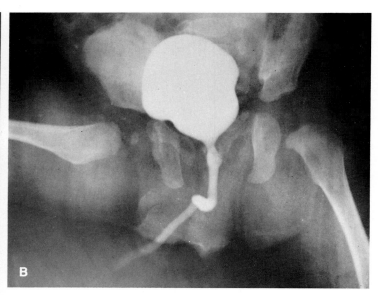

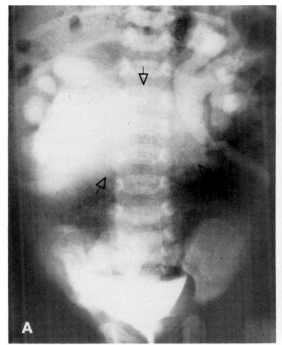

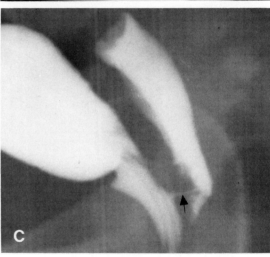

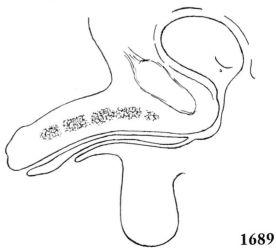

FIG. 37–16. Imperforate vagina with urethral communication. **(A)** At birth, excretory urogram showed hydronephrosis and hydroureters secondary to hydrometrocolpos. During spontaneous voiding, contrast medium entered the vagina and uterus (*arrows*). **(B)** Lateral film during the same study. *Solid arrows* outline the posterior uterine wall and *open arrows* outline intrauterine contrast material. The dilated intrarenal collecting systems are displaced posteriorly by the hydrometrocolpos. **(C)** Voiding cystourethrogram performed after surgical correction of the imperforate vagina demonstrates a communication between the lower vagina and urethra (*arrow*). (Kirks, D.R., Currarino, G.: Am. J. Roentgenol., *129*:623, 1977)

FIG. 37–17. Urethral duplication. Anatomic diagram of incomplete epispadiac sagittal duplication of the male urethra.

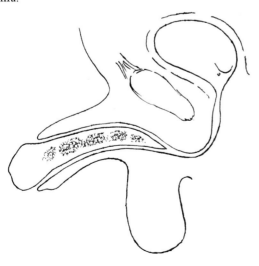

FIG. 37–18. Urethral duplication. Anatomic diagram of incomplete hypospadiac sagittal duplication of the male urethra.

1689

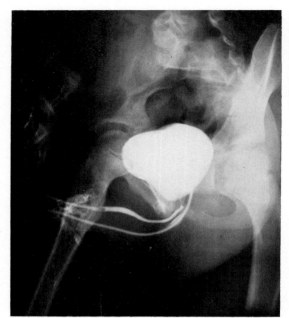

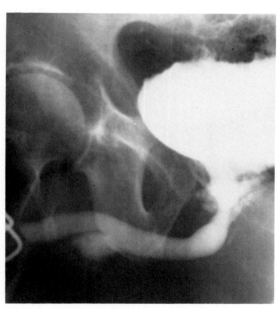

FIG. 37–21. Urethral duplication. Voiding cysto-urethrogram. An accessory ventral urethral channel communicates with the functional urethra. The hypospadiac partial duplication ends blindly forming a penile sinus. The prostatic glands are filled, probably because of meatal stenosis of the normally positioned urethra.

FIG. 37–19. Urethral duplication. Retrograde urethrogram. Two catheters are present in a patient with complete epispadiac urethral duplication. The catheter in the normally positioned ventral urethra extends into the bladder. The other catheter is positioned into the epispadiac dorsal urethra and contrast is injected. A separate anterior bladder neck is demonstrated. (Hermann, G., Goldmann, H.: Int. Surg., 58:574, 1973)

FIG. 37–20. Urethral duplication: penile sinus. Anatomic diagram of a penile sinus (partial urethral duplication) that has no communication with the functioning urethra.

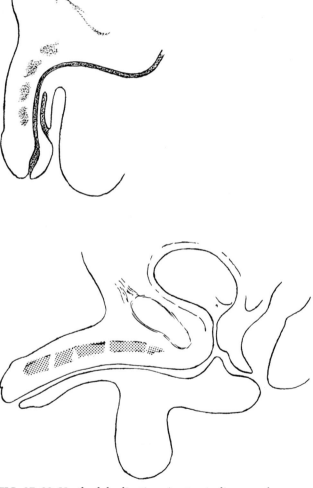

FIG. 37–22. Urethral duplication. Anatomic diagram of a partial urethral duplication that arises from the proximal urethra and ends in the perineum just anterior to the anal verge.

FIG. 37–23. Megalourethra. Voiding cystourethrogram. At the end of voiding, contrast medium remains in markedly dilated penile urethra. Agenesis of the corpus spongiosum allows the urethra to balloon out during voiding. (Johnston, J.H., Coimbra, J.A.M.: J. Pediatr. Surg., 5:304, 1970)

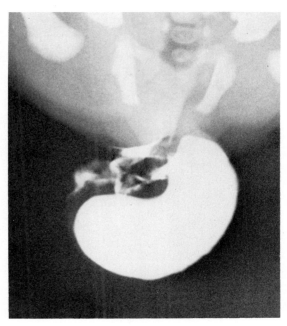

FIG. 37–24. Hypertrophy of the verumontanum. Voiding cystourethrogram. *Arrow* points to the prominent verumontanum. The posterior urethra is widened in this area. The distal urethra and voiding stream are normal. The bladder is trabeculated.

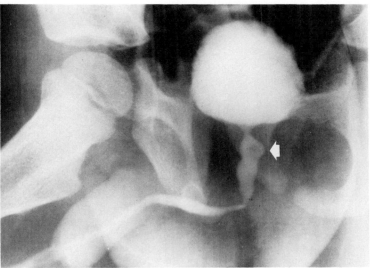

FIG. 37–25. Hypertrophy of the verumontanum. Voiding cystourethrogram. The prominence of the verumontanum fills the entire width of the posterior urethra but there is no evidence of impedence to urine flow. (Courtesy of W. Berdon, M.D. and D. Baker, M.D.)

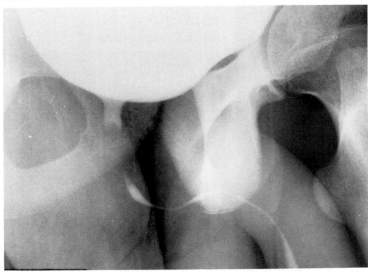

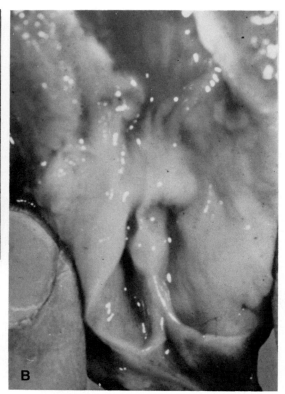

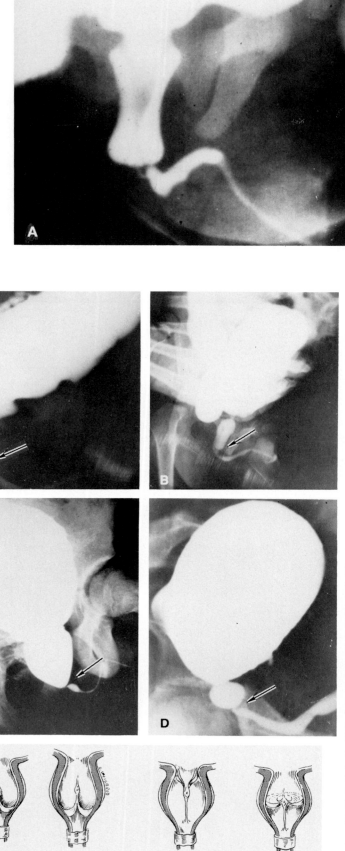

FIG. 37–26. Posterior urethral valves. **(A)** Voiding cystourethrogram. Dilated posterior urethra. The verumontanum and ridges of urethral crest tissue extending superiorly and inferiorly from the veru can be seen as radiolucent filling defects. **(B)** Postmortem specimen of the same posterior urethra that has been opened anteriorly. The thin membranous tissue folds that extend off the inferior urethral crest tissue are the posterior urethral valves. As the patient voids, these folds are displaced inferiorly and occlude the posterior urethra. (Courtesy of R.D. Jeffs, M.D.)

FIG. 37–27. Posterior urethral valves. **(A–D)** Voiding cystourethrograms of four boys with posterior urethral valves. **(A)** Voiding study of a 3-month-old boy with infection. *Arrow* points to the level of obstruction from type I valves. Posterior bladder neck is prominent. Cellule formation in trigone; no reflux. **(B)** Five-year-old boy with urinary infection. *Arrow* points to level of obstruction distal to the veru and proximal to external sphincter. Elongation and widening of prostatic urethra with marked secondary hypertrophy of the bladder neck. Massive reflux. **(C)** Eight-year-old boy with bed wetting. This is also a type I valve with marked obstruction proximal to the external sphincter. Note noticeable widening of the prostatic urethra, but entirely different shape from *A* and *B*. **(D)** Type III urethral valve, a diaphragm obstructing at the level of the verumontanum in a 5-year-old boy with bed wetting, day wetting, and urinary frequency; no reflux. (Courtesy of H. Hendren, M.D.) **(E)** Anatomic diagrams of the types of posterior urethral valves.

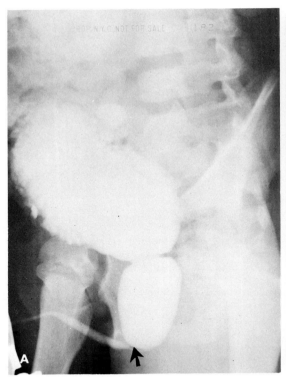

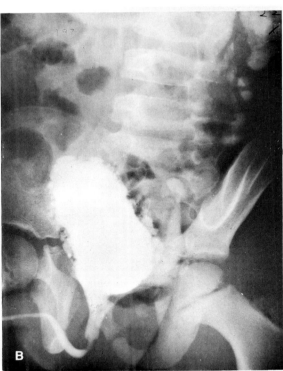

FIG. 37–28. Posterior urethral valves. **(A)** Preoperative. Typical urethral valve, dilated posterior urethra with the valve (*arrow*) encroaching upon and compressing the external urethral sphincter. Note the trabeculated bladder. Right posterior oblique view. **(B)** Postoperative. Essentially normal posterior urethra and external sphincter. (Courtesy of K. Waterhouse, M.D.)

FIG. 37–29. Posterior urethral valves. **(A)** Voiding cysto-urethrogram. The bladder is trabeculated and has many diverticula. There is reflux into a tortuous dilated left ureter and dilated pelvicalyceal system. The posterior urethra is dilated. **(B)** Excretory urogram. After resection of the valves, only the right kidney visualizes. There is hydronephrosis and hydroureter. The ureterovesical obstruction is either secondary to the thick bladder wall or an associated anomaly.

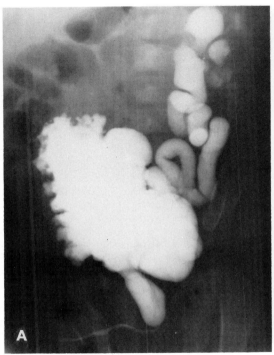

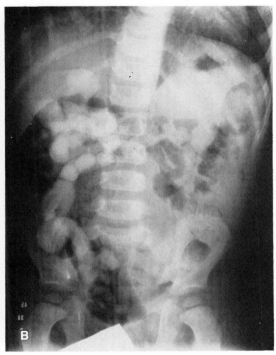

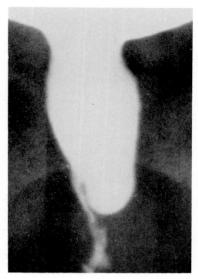

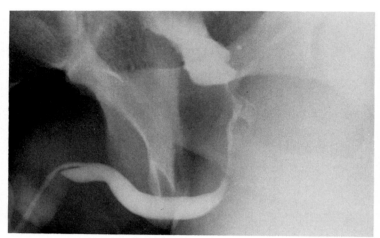

FIG. 37–32. Anterior urethral valve. Voiding cysto-urethrogram shows a tonguelike ventral projection of contrast material paralleling the mid anterior urethra. The stream is slightly narrowed distal to the diverticulum. (Baum, N.: Urology 6:723, 1975)

FIG. 37–30. Urethral valve, female. Voiding urethrogram in a woman with long-standing urinary tract infection shows asymmetric ballooning of the proximal urethra. The distal urethral appears small. The radiolucent line between the two portions of the urethra represents a thin fold of urethral mucosa partially obstructing urinary flow. After resection the patient voided normally. (Nesbit, R., et al.: J. Urol., 91:79, 1964)

FIG. 37–31. Perirenal urinary extravasation in an infant boy with posterior urethral valves. Excretory urogram shows a large collection of contrast material in the right perirenal space presumably secondary to perforation of calyceal fornix. Both pelvicalyceal systems are dilated, the left more than the right. (Courtesy of R.D. Jeffs, M.D.)

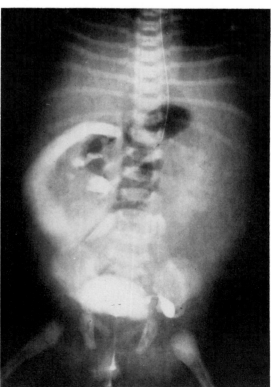

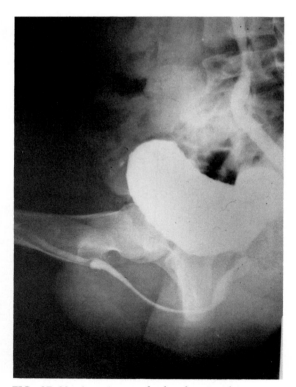

FIG. 37–33. Anterior urethral valve. Voiding cysto-urethrogram shows a radiolucent area just distal to a bulge of the anterior urethra. The bulge has a convex border presenting distally. The terminal urethra appears split into two streams. Note left vesicoureteral reflux. There is bilateral hydronephrosis and hydroureter. (Waterhouse, K.: J. Urol., 87:556, 1962)

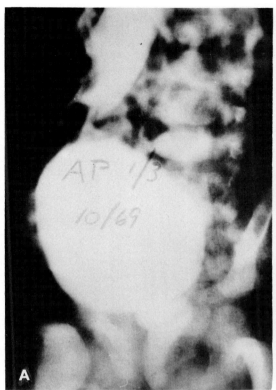
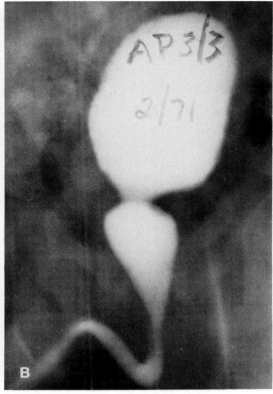

FIG. 37–34. Posterior urethral valves. **(A)** Voiding cysto-urethrogram of an infant boy. There is dilatation of the posterior urethra, a large bladder, and reflux into the collecting system of the right kidney. **(B)** Voiding cysto-urethrogram 2 years after removal of posterior urethral valves. The posterior urethra remains dilated but there is no obstruction to urine flow.

BIBLIOGRAPHY

Intersex

General

1. Allen, T.D.: Disorders of sexual differentiation. Urology (Suppl.), 7:1–32, 1976.
2. Dewhurst, C.J.: The aetiology and management of intersexuality. Clin. Endocrinol., 4:625–642, 1975.
3. Freud, S.: On the universal tendency to debasement in the sphere of love (1912). *In* The Standard Edition of The Complete Works of Sigmund Freud, Vol. 11, p. 189. The Hogarth Press & The Institute of Psychoanalysis, London, 1957.
4. Freud, S.: The dissolution of the Oedipus complex (1924). *In* The Standard Edition of The Complete Works of Sigmund Freud, Vol. 19, p. 178. The Hogarth Press & The Institute of Psychoanalysis, London, 1961.
5. Imperato-McGinley, J., and Peterson, R.E.: Male pseudohermaphroditism: The complexities of male phenotypic development. Am. J. Med., 61:251–272, 1976.
6. Walsh, P.C., and Migeon, C.J.: The phenotypic expression of selective disorders of male sexual differentiation. J. Urol., 119:627–629, 1978.

Embryology

7. Arey, L.B.: Developmental Anatomy: A Textbook and Laboratory Manual of Embryology, 7th ed. Saunders, Philadelphia, 1965.
8. Federman, D.D.: Abnormal Sexual Development: A Genetic and Endocrine Approach to Differential Diagnosis. Saunders, Philadelphia, 1967.
9. Gray, S.W., and Skandalakis, J.E.: Embryology for Surgeons: The Embryological Basis for the Treatment of Congenital Defects. Saunders, Philadelphia, 1972.
10. Hamilton, W.J., Boyd, J.D., and Mossman, H.W.: Human Embryology: Prenatal Development of Form and Function, 4th ed. Williams & Wilkins, Baltimore, 1972.
11. Jacobs, P.A., and Ross, A.: Structural abnormalities of the Y chromosome in man. Nature (London), 210:352–354, 1966.
12. Jost, A.: Problems of fetal endocrinology: The gonadal and hypophyseal hormones. Recent Prog. Horm. Res., 8:379–418, 1953.
13. Jost, A., Vigier, B., Prépin, J., and Perchellet, J.P.: Studies on sex differentiation in mammals. Recent Prog. Horm. Res., 29:1–41, 1973.
14. Singh, R.P., and Carr, D.H.: The anatomy and histology of

XO human embryos and fetuses. Anat. Rec., 155:369–384, 1966.

15. Wilson, J.D., and Lasnitzki, I.: Dihydrotestosterone formation in fetal tissues of the rabbit and rat. Endocrinology, 89:659–668, 1971.

True Hermaphroditism

16. Donahoe, P.K., Crawford, J.D., and Hendren, W.H.: True hermaphroditism: A clinical description and a proposed function for the long arm of the Y chromosome. J. Pediatr. Surg., 13:293–301, 1978.
17. Jones, H.W., and Scott, W.W.: Hermaphroditism, Genital Anomalies, and Related Endocrine Disorders, 2nd ed. Williams & Wilkins, Baltimore, 1971.
18. Josso, N., et al.: True hermaphroditism with XX/XY mosaicism, probably due to double fertilization of the ovum. J. Clin. Endocrinol. Metab., 25:114, 1965.
19. Pflueger, O.H., Jr., Schmidt, D.M., and Harrod, C.S.: True hermaphroditism with unambiguous male phenotype, pathologic and cytogenetic findings: report of a case. J. Urol., 112:406–408, 1974.
20. Rosenberg, H.S., Clayton, G.W., and Hsu, T.C.: Familial true hermaphroditism. J. Clin. Endocrinol. Metab., 23:203–206, 1963.

Female Pseudohermaphroditism — Congenital Adrenogenital Syndrome

21. Bongiovanni, A.M.: Another look at congenital adrenal hyperplasia due to 3β-hydroxysteroid dehydrogenase deficiency. Acta Paediatr. Scand., 61:244–245, 1972.
22. Bongiovanni, A.M., Eberlein, W.R., Goldman, A.S., et al.: Disorders of adrenal steroid biogenesis. Recent Prog. Horm. Res., 23:375–449, 1967.
23. Bongiovanni, A.M., and Root, A.W.: The adrenogenital syndrome. N. Engl. J. Med., 268:1283–1289, 1342–1351, 1391–1399, 1963.
24. Raiti, S., and Newns, G.H.: Congenital adrenal hyperplasia. Arch. Dis. Child., 39:324–333, 1964.

Female Pseudohermaphroditism — Androgenization

25. Brentnall, C.P.: A case of arrhenoblastoma complicating pregnancy. J. Obstet. Gynecol. Brit. Emp., 52:235–240, 1945.
26. Grumbach, M.M., and Ducharme, J.R.: The effects of androgens on fetal sexual development. Androgen-induced female pseudohermaphroditism. Fertil. Steril., 11:157–180, 1960.
27. Wilkins, L.: Masculinization of female fetus due to use of orally given progestins. J.A.M.A., 172:1028–1032, 1960.

Male Pseudohermaphroditism — Testosterone Synthesis Defects

28. Bricaire, H., et al.: A new male pseudohermaphroditism associated with hypertension due to a block of 17α-hydroxylation. J. Clin. Endocrinol. Metab., 35:67–72, 1972.
29. Bongiovanni, A.M.: Unusual steroid pattern in congenital adrenal hyperplasia: Deficiency of 3β-hydroxy dehydrogenase. J. Clin. Endocrinol. Metab., 21:860–862, 1961.
30. Camacho, A.M., Kowarski, A., Migeon, C.J., et al.: Congenital adrenal hyperplasia due to a deficiency of one of the enzymes involved in the biosynthesis of pregnenolone. J. Clin. Endocrinol. Metab., 28:153–161, 1968.
31. Degenhart, H.J., Visser, H.K.A., Boon, H., et al.: Evidence for deficient 20α-cholesterol-hydroxylase activity in adrenal tissue of a patient with lipoid adrenal hyperplasia. Acta. Endocrinol., 71:512–518, 1972.
32. Givens, J.R., et al.: Familial male pseudohermaphroditism without gynecomastia due to deficient testicular 17-ketosteroid reductase activity. N. Engl. J. Med., 291:938–944, 1974.
33. New, M.I.: Male pseudohermaphroditism due to 17α-hydroxylase deficiency. J. Clin. Invest., 49:1930–1941, 1970.
34. Parks, G.A., Bermudez, J.A., Anast, C.S., et al.: Pubertal boy with the 3β-hydroxysteroid dehydrogenase defect. J. Clin. Endocrinol. Metab., 33:269–278, 1971.
35. Prader, A., and Anders, G.J.P.A.: Zur genetik der kongenitalen lipoid-hyperplasie der nebennieren. Helv. Paediatr. Acta, 17:285, 1962.
36. Saez, J.M., et al.: Familial male pseudohermaphroditism with gynecomastia due to a testicular 17-ketosteroid reductase defect. I. Studies in vivo. J. Clin. Endocrinol. Metab., 32:604–610, 1971.
37. Simpson, J.L., and Photopulos, G.: The relationship of neoplasia to disorders of abnormal sexual differentiation. Birth Defects, 12:15–50, 1976.
38. Zachmann, M., Vollmin, J.A., Hamilton, W., et al.: Steroid 17,20-desmolase deficiency. A new cause of male pseudohermaphroditism. Clin. Endocrinol., 1:369–385, 1972.

Androgen Target Area Defects

39. Bowen, P., Lee, C.S.N., Migeon, C.J., et al.: Hereditary male pseudohermaphroditism with hypogonadism, hypospadias, and gynecomastia (Reifenstein's syndrome). Ann. Intern. Med., 62:252–270, 1965.
40. Bremner, W.J., Ott, J., Moore, D.J., et al.: Reifenstein's syndrome: Investigation of linkage to X-chromosomal loci. Clin. Genet., 6:216–220, 1974.
41. Gilbert-Dreyfus, S., Sebaoun, C.A., and Belaisch, J.: Etude d'un cas familial d'androgyroidisme avec hypospadias grave, gynecomastic et hyperestrogenie. Ann. Endocrinol. (Paris), 18:93, 1957.
42. Imperato-McGinley, J., Guerrero, L., Gautier, T., et al.: Steroid 5α-reductase deficiency in man: An inherited form of male pseudohermaphroditism. Science, 186:1213–1215, 1974.
43. Keenan, B.S., et al.: Syndrome of androgen insensitivity in man: Absence of 5α-dihydrotestosterone binding protein in skin fibroblasts. J. Clin. Endocrinol. Metab., 38:1143–1146, 1974.
44. Lubs, H.A., Jr., Vilar, O., and Bergenstal, D.M.: Familial male pseudohermaphroditism with labial testes and partial feminization: Endocrine studies and genetic aspects. J. Clin. Endocrinol. Metab., 19:1110–1120, 1959.
45. Morris, J.M.: The syndrome of testicular feminization in male pseudohermaphrodites. Am. J. Obstet. Gynecol., 65:1192–1211, 1953.
46. Reifenstein, E.C., Jr.: Hereditary familial hypogonadism. Proc. Am. Fed. Clin. Res., 3:86, 1947.
47. Simpson, J.L., New, M., Peterson, R.E., et al.: Pseudovaginal perineoscrotal hypospadias (PPSH) in sibs. Birth Defects, 7:140–144, 1971.
48. Walsh, P.C., et al.: Familial incomplete male pseudoher-

maphroditism, type 2. Decreased dihydrotestosterone formation in pseudovaginal perineoscrotal hypospadias. N. Engl. J. Med., 291:944–949, 1974.

49. Wilson, J.D.: Harrod, M.J., Goldstein, J.L., et al.: Familial incomplete male pseudohermaphroditism, type 1. Evidence for androgen resistance and variable clinical manifestations in a family with the Reifenstein syndrome. N. Engl. J. Med., 290:1097–1103, 1974.

Microphallus Cryptorchidism

50. Walsh, P.C., et al.: Clinical and endocrinological evaluation of patients with congenital microphallus. J. Urol., 120:90–95, 1978.

Mixed Gonadal Dysgenesis

51. Cattolica, E.V., and Solomon, I.L.: The urologic manifestations of XO/XY mosaicism. J. Urol., 120:103–105, 1978.
52. Davidoff, F., and Federman, D.D.: Mixed gonadal dysgenesis. Pediatrics, 52:725–742, 1973.

Dysgenetic Male Pseudohermaphroditism

53. Rajfer, J., Mendelsohn, G., Arnheim, J., et al.: Dysgenetic male pseudohermaphroditism. J. Urol., 119:525–527, 1978.

Isolated Müllerian Inhibiting Factor Deficiency

54. Brook, C.G.D., et al.: Familial occurrence of persistent müllerian structures in otherwise normal males. Br. Med. J., 1:771–773, 1973.
55. Sloan, W.R., and Walsh, P.C.: Familial persistent müllerian duct syndrome. J. Urol., 115:459–461, 1976.

Radiology

56. Cremin, B.J.: Intersex states in young children: the importance of radiology in making a correct diagnosis. Clin. Radiol., 25:63–73, 1974.
57. Peck, A.G., and Poznanski, A.K.: A simple device for genitography. Radiology, 103:212–213, 1972.
58. Walsh, P.C., Madden, J.D., Harrod, M.J., et al.: Familial incomplete male pseudohermaphroditism, type 2. Decreased dihydrotestosterone formation in pseudovaginal perineoscrotal hypospadias. N. Engl. J. Med., 291:944–949, 1974.

Hypospadias

59. Chen, Y.C., and Woolley, P.V., Jr.: Genetic studies on hypospadias in males. J. Med. Genet., 8:153–159, 1971.
60. de la Chapelle, A.: Analytic review: Nature and origin of males with XX sex chromosomes. Am. J. Hum. Genet., 24:71–105, 1972.
61. Fallon, B., Devine, C.J., and Horton, C.E.: Congenital anomalies associated with hypospadias. J. Urol., 116:585–586, 1976.
62. Gray, J.: Hypospadias with 47/XXY karyotype. Lancet, 1:722, 1961.
63. Kennedy, P.A., Jr.: Hypospadias: a twenty year review of 489 cases. J. Urol., 85:814–817, 1961.
64. Rajfer, J., and Walsh, P.C.: The incidence of intersexuality in patients with hypospadias and cryptorchidism. J. Urol., 116:769–770, 1976.
65. Roe, T.F., and Alfi, O.S.: Ambiguous genitalia in XX male children: Report of two infants. Pediatrics, 60:55–59, 1977.
66. Sørensen, H.R.: Hypospadias with special reference to aetiology. Munksgaard, Copenhagen, 1953.

Prostatic Utricle (Müllerian Duct Remnant)

67. Ceccarelli, F.E., and Beach, P.D.: Multiple urogenital anomalies: Pronephric, mesonephric and metanephric kidney elements with persistent müllerian duct in an adult male. J. Urol., 85:31–41, 1961.
68. Culbertson, L.R.: Müllerian duct cyst. J. Urol., 58:134–136, 1947.
69. Edling, N.P.G.: The radiological aspect of the utriculus prostaticus during urethrocystography. Acta Radiol., 32:28–32, 1949.
70. Schuhrke, T.D., and Kaplan, G.W.: Prostatic utricle cysts, (Müllerian duct cysts). J. Urol., 119:765–767, 1978.
71. Theander, G.: Roentgen appearance of prostatic channels in infancy and childhood. Acta Radiol. (Diagn.) (Stockh.), 11:467–480, 1971.

Anorectal–Urethral Communications. Vaginal–Urethral Communications

72. Berdon, W.E., Baker, D.H., Santulli, T.V., et al.: The radiologic evaluation of imperforate anus. An approach correlated with current surgical concepts. Radiology, 90:466–471, 1968.
72a. Caffey, John: Pediatric X-ray Diagnosis, Vol. 2, 7th Edition, p. 1752–1757. Year Book Medical Publishers, Inc., Chicago, 1978.
73. Kirks, D.R., and Currarino, G.: Imperforate vagina with vaginourethral communication. Am. J. Roentgenol., 129:623–628, 1977.
73a. Mayo, C.W., and Rice, R.G.: Anorectal anomalies. A statistical study of one hundred sixty-five cases with special reference to "distal loop trouble." Surgery, 27:485–494, 1950.
74. Rudhe, U.: Roentgenologic examination of anal and rectal anomalies in the newborn male infant. Ann. Radiol., 11:429, 1968.
75. Shopfner, C.E.: Roentgenologic demonstration of the "ectopic anus" associated with imperforate anus. Radiology, 84:464–470, 1965.

Duplication of the Urethra

76. Boissonnat, P.: Two cases of complete double functional urethra with a single bladder. Br. J. Urol., 33:453–462, 1961.
77. Bonney, W.W., Young, H.H., II, Levin, D., et al.: Complete duplication of the urethra with vaginal stenosis. J. Urol., 113:132–137, 1975.
78. Dannreuther, W.T.: Complete double urethra in a female. J.A.M.A., 81:1016, 1923.
79. Das, S., and Brosman, S.A.: Duplication of the male urethra. J. Urol., 117:452–454, 1977.
80. DeNicola, R.R., and McCartney, R.C.: Urethral reduplication in a female child; treated with sclerosing solution. J. Urol., 61:1065–1067, 1949.
81. Effmann, E.L., Lebowitz, R.L., and Colodny, A.H.: Duplication of the urethra. Radiology, 119:179–185, 1976.
82. Gross, R.E., and Moore, T.C.: Duplication of the urethra.

Report of two cases and summary of the literature. Arch. Surg., 60:749–761, 1950.

83. Howard, F.S., and Hinman, F., Jr.: Female pseudohermaphroditism with supplementary phallic urethra: Report of two cases. J. Urol., 65:439–452, 1951.

84. Irmisch, G., and Cooke, N.: Double and accessory urethra. Minn. Med., 29:999–1002, 1946.

85. Moulsdale, J.E., and Marshall, F.F.: Partial duplication of the male urethra. J. Urol., 118:336–338, 1977.

86. Schmidt, J.D.: Congenital urethral duplication. J. Urol., 105:397–399, 1971.

87. Williams, D.I., and Kenawi, M.M.: Urethral duplications in the male. Eur. Urol., 1:209–215, 1975.

Megalourethra

88. Dorairajan, T.: Defects of spongy tissue and congenital diverticula of the penile urethra. Aust. N.Z. J. Surg., 32:209–214, 1963.

89. Johnston, J.H., and Coimbra, J.A.M.: Megalourethra. J. Pediatr. Surg., 5:304–308, 1970.

90. Nesbitt, T.E.: Congenital megalo-urethra. J. Urol., 73:839–842, 1955.

Hypertrophy of the Verumontanum

91. Begg, R.C.: The verumontanum in urinary and sexual disorders. Br. J. Urol., 1:237–253, 1929.

92. Bugbee, H.G., and Wollstein, M.: Retention of urine due to congenital hypertrophy of the verumontanum. J. Urol., 10:477–490, 1923.

93. Campbell, M.: Urology, 2nd ed. Saunders, Philadelphia, 1963.

94. Edwards, A.T.: Congenital hypertrophy of the verumontanum causing bladder-neck obstruction. Br. J. Urol., 31:60–62, 1959.

95. Johnson, S.H., III, and Price, W.C.: Hypertrophy of the colliculus seminalis in childhood: report of eighteen cases. Am. J. Dis. Child., 78:892–898, 1949.

96. Pennock, W.J.: Verumontanitis. J.A.M.A., 65:1167–1170, 1915.

97. Robinson, W.W.: Congenital hypertrophy of the verumontanum as a cause of urinary retention. J. Urol., 17:381–390, 1927.

98. Thompson, G.J.: Urinary obstruction of the vesical neck and posterior urethra of congenital origin. J. Urol., 47:591–601, 1942.

Urine Ascites

99. Baghdassarian, O.M., Koehler, P.R., and Schultze, G.: Massive neonatal ascites. Radiology, 76:586–593, 1961.

100. Cremin, B.J.: Urinary ascites and obstructive uropathy. Br. J. Radiol., 48:113–117, 1975.

101. Dockray, K.T.: Perirenal contrast medium. A new roentgenographic sign of neonatal urinary ascites. J.A.M.A., 193:1121–1123, 1965.

102. Garrett, R.A., and Franken, E.A., Jr.: Neonatal ascites: Perirenal urinary extravasation with bladder outlet obstruction. J. Urol., 102:627–632, 1969.

103. Howat, J.M.: Urinary ascites complicating spina bifida. Arch. Dis. Child., 46:103–105, 1971.

104. Leonidas, J.C., Leiter, E., and Gribetz, D.: Congenital urinary tract obstruction presenting with ascites at birth: Roentgenographic diagnosis. Radiology, 96:111–112, 1970.

105. Lord, J.M.: Foetal ascites. Arch. Dis. Child., 28:398–403, 1953.

106. Moncada, R., Wang, J.J., Love, L., et al.: Neonatal ascites associated with urinary outlet obstruction (urine ascites). Radiology, 90:1165–1170, 1968.

107. Wagget, J., and Schut, L.: Urinary ascites present at birth associated with lumbosacral myelomeningocele. J. Pediatr. Surg., 5:473, 1970.

108. Weller, M.H., and Miller, K.: Unusual aspects of urine ascites. Radiology, 109:665–669, 1973.

Inflammations of the urethra, whether acute or chronic, may be caused by *Neisseria gonorrhea* or a nonspecific infection including ureaplasma, urealyticum (T mycoplasma), *Candida albicans*, trichomonas vaginalis, herpes simplex virus, and a variety of bacteria. Chlamydia organisms have been found in association with nonspecific urethritis in 30 to 70 per cent of cases. Men usually have symptoms, but many of the women are asymptomatic.

In women urethral colonization is determined by the vaginal bacteria, that is, bacteriuria is preceded by a colonization of the vaginal vestibule usually by Enterobacteriaceae and *S. fecalis*.[3, 4, 6] Colonization of the vaginal vestibule is determined to a great extent by vaginal antibody.[7] In fact it has been shown that women who are resistant to urinary infection and who rarely colonize the vaginal vestibule with fecal enterobacteria, carry specific vaginal antibody against *E. coli* whereas women who develop urinary infection have no such vaginal antibody.

Roentgenographic Diagnosis.   There is no specific roentgenologic appearance produced by the usual acute inflammation of the urethra. Necrotizing urethritis is a severe, acute infection associated in many instances with diabetes mellitus and an indwelling urethral catheter. It may also occur with severe strictures and infection (Fig. 38–1). The urethra is irregular with filling defects from slough.

CHRONIC INFLAMMATORY PROCESSES

Chronic inflammation of the urethra produces secondary changes that may be visualized roentgenographically. These include irregularities of the urethral lumen, strictures and contrast filling of Littre's glands, the lacunae of Morgagni, Cowper's glands, prostatic ducts, and seminal vesicles. Filling of the various glandular structures is not necessarily an implication of present inflammation but results

38

Inflammations of the Urethra

from postinflammatory changes that cause the orifices to remain open, in communication with the urethra. Distal obstruction may produce similar changes.

Littre's Glands and Lacunae of Morgagni. Postinflammatory changes in Littre's glands (Figs. 38–1a, 38–2, 38–3) and the lacunae of Morgagni permit filling of these cavities. They are visualized as fine, somewhat irregular outpocketings on the dorsal side of the penile urethra. The direction varies greatly, and one occasionally may see dilatation and angulation of the terminal portion, which may become parallel with the urethra.

Cowper's Glands. The filling of Cowper's glands and ducts (Figs. 38–4, 38–5) often is seen without clinical evidence of active inflammation. However, it is assumed that visualization of the duct has occurred secondary to a previous inflammatory process but it is possible that distal obstruction may permit visualization. The duct may be visualized unilaterally or bilaterally, commencing at the bulbous urethra and extending parallel to the urethra on the posterior side. It is seen best in the oblique view. When visualized unilaterally, it is difficult to differentiate from a false pocket, a fistulous connection with the urethra, or a urethrocavernous reflux. Bilateral visualization is diagnostic. The gland itself, when visualized, is oval or rounded in shape.

Prostatic Ducts. Following inflammation, variable changes are present in the prostatic ducts (Figs. 38–3, 38–6, 38–7), which may vary from visualization of single or multiple narrowed ducts to large cavities filled with contrast medium. Details of the roentgenographic characteristics of prostatitis are included in Chapter 34, The Prostate.

Seminal Vesicles. Visualization of the ejaculatory ducts and the seminal vesicles may occur following chronic inflammation (Fig. 38–8) or trauma, most commonly secondary to prostatectomy (Fig. 38–9). The ejaculatory ducts usually are visualized throughout the entire course and may be dilated. The seminal vesicles may reveal dilatation of the convolutions, loss of convolutions as fibrosis occurs,

calcifications (in tuberculosis, for example), and marked distortion in severe infections, especially abscess formation.

Periurethral Abscesses (Figs. 38–10 to 38–14) are primarily the result of direct invasion of the periurethral tissues by bacteria. They often occur secondary to stricture formation or trauma. In the male, they are present most commonly in the bulbar and membranous urethra. They may vary enormously in size from a few millimeters to several centimeters. The margins may be smooth, resembling a diverticulum, or irregular with a serrated contour. They can be visualized only on the urethrograms when fistulization of the urethra has occurred. Occasionally, the contrast material does not permeate the abscess evenly, giving rise to irregular puddling, which may be confusing. Periurethral abscesses often develop sinus tracts to the perineum or the rectum, and visualization by contrast medium may be obtained by appropriate injections in these regions.

Reiter's Syndrome. This is a clinical tetrad of unknown cause consisting of nonspecific urethritis, conjunctivitis, mucocutaneous manifestations, and arthritis. It affects young men especially. It may follow sexual intercouse, chlamydial infections, or bacterial diarrhea due to *Shigella* or *Yersinia*. It is associated with a systemic reaction. The mucocutaneous lesions include balanitis, stomatitis, and keratoderma blennorrhagicum. The arthritis affects especially the knees and ankles.

Most signs disappear in a few days but the arthritis may persist. HLA-B27 antigen test is positive in 80 to 90 per cent of patients. Recurrences are common.

TUBERCULOSIS OF THE MALE URETHRA

This condition is rare, the urethra probably being resistant to the tuberculous organism. It is manifest by stricture formation, fistula, and abscess (see Chap. 41, Strictures of the Urethra). The roentgenographic appearance is the same as that of any other stricture except that there may be extensive associated destruction of the prostate, which could be a definite clue to the diagnosis.

CHAPTER 38, ILLUSTRATIONS

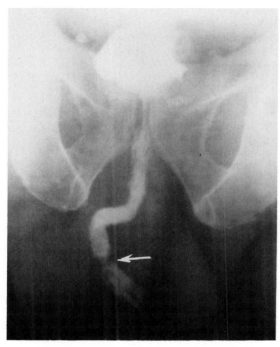

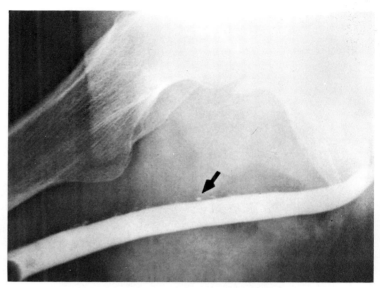

FIG. 38–1a. Littritis. Visualization of Littre's glands on injecting cystourethrography. *Arrow* points to one of the visualized cavities on the dorsal side of the penile urethra. This visualization occurs secondary to inflammatory changes.

FIG. 38–1. Stricture of urethra (*arrow*) with marked irregularity of entire urethra and filling defects, especially proximal to the stricture, due to slough.

FIG. 38–3. Chronic urethritis; stricture of the penile urethra and bulbomembranous area. Irregular filling of periurethral glands (*arrows*). Note filling of prostatic ducts.

FIG. 38–2. Littritis. Visualization of Littre's glands on injecting cystourethrography. *Arrow* points to the visualized glands on the dorsal side of the penile urethra. The distal portion of these cavities tends to become parallel with the urethra.

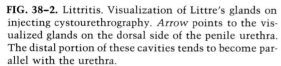

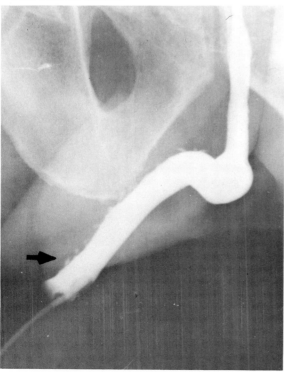

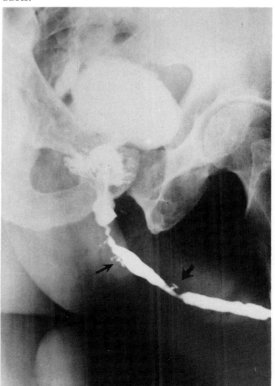

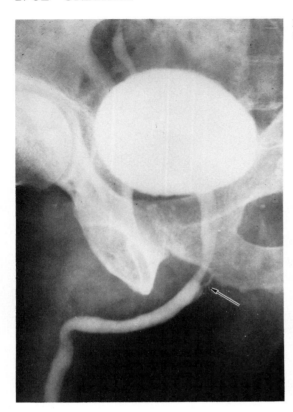

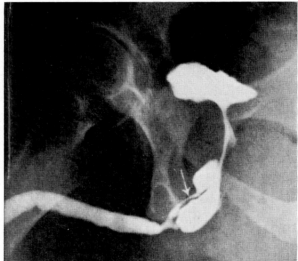

FIG. 38–4. Cowper's duct (*arrow*) visualized secondary to infection.

FIG. 38–5. Cowper's gland seen on injecting cysto-urethrography. Right oblique view. *Arrow* points to Cowper's duct. The obstruction by the urethral stricture has caused infection and dilatation of the duct of the gland, which is oval-shaped. When only the duct is visualized, differentiation from false passage and minimal urethrocavernous reflux is difficult. Duct visualization is usually smoother than the other two and generally of finer caliber. (Beard, D.E., Goodyear, W.E., and Weems, H.S.; Radiologic Diagnosis of the Lower Urinary Tract, Springfield, Ill., Charles C Thomas, 1952)

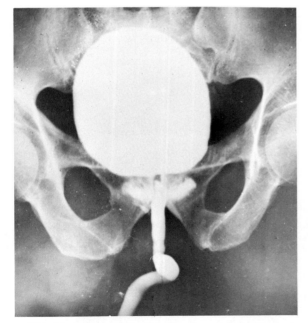

FIG. 38–6. Prostatitis. Visualization of prostatic ducts on injecting cystourethrography. Some of the ducts are seen individually, and there are also large cavities bilaterally. These changes are secondary to inflammation affecting not only the prostate proper but also the openings of the ducts in the urethra. Prostatitis is discussed in Chapter 34, The Prostate.

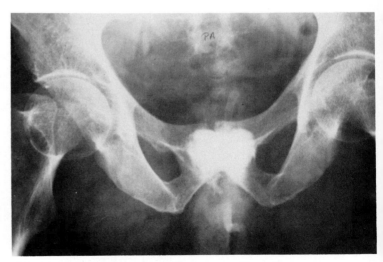

FIG. 38–7. Prostatic abscess. Contrast medium is present in large bilateral prostatic cavities; septic fever is present.

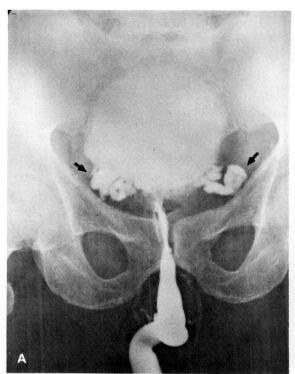
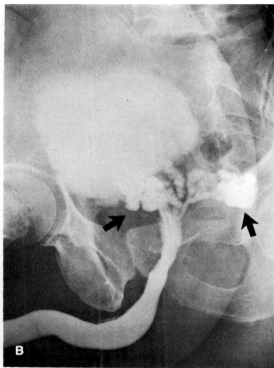

FIG. 38–8. Visualization of seminal vesicles on inject-ing cystourethrography. *Arrows* point to seminal vesi-cles. Such visualization occurs secondary to inflamma-tory changes around the ejaculatory duct openings in the urethra. However, in this particular instance there is also inflammation of the seminal vesicles. A detailed description of inflammations of the seminal vesicles is found in Chapter 35. **(A)** AP view. **(B)** Right oblique view.

FIG. 38–9. Visualization of seminal vesicles on intra-venous urogram 4 days after suprapubic prostatectomy. *Large arrow* points to right ureter; *small arrows,* to seminal vesicles. A large Foley bag can be seen inflated in the bladder. Visualization of the seminal vesicles can be secondary to inflammation or trauma or both.

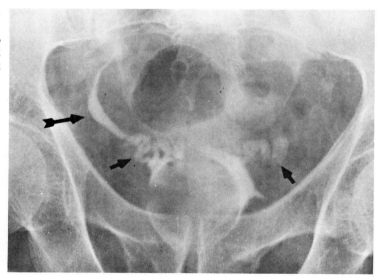

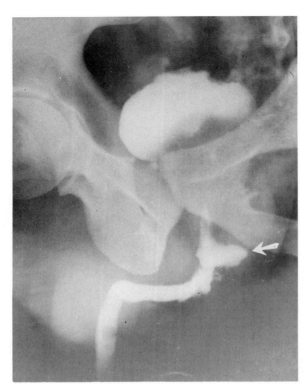

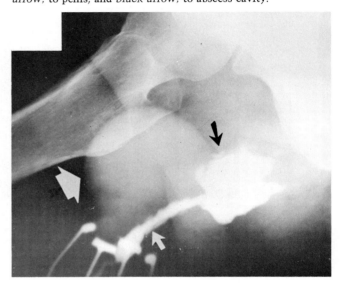

FIG. 38–10. Periurethral abscess with fistula formation. The contrast material has entered the abscess cavity in a fairly even distribution pattern with irregular margins (*arrow*).

FIG. 38–11. Periurethral abscess with fistula formation. Terminal ileitis affecting bladder, periprostatic and periurethral areas. Contrast material injected into fistulous tract entered a large periurethral abscess cavity. *Small white arrow* points to fistulous tract, *large white arrow*, to penis, and *black arrow*, to abscess cavity.

FIG. 38–12. Periurethral abscess. Man, 30 years old. Severe trauma to urethra and bladder from automobile accident. One month after the accident the urethral catheter was removed, and approximately 1 week later swelling occurred in the perineum, and a purulent discharge appeared in the urethra. Abscess cavity was visualized by injection of contrast medium into urethra. Abscess was drained perineally. Note deformity of pubic symphysis.

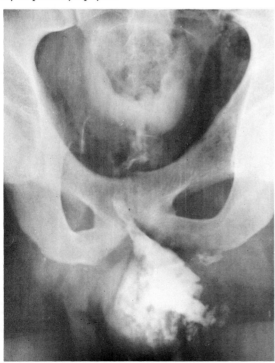

FIG. 38–13. Periurethral abscess with cutaneous fistula formation. Abscess followed urethral instrumentation. Note irregular distribution of contrast material around urethra. (Courtesy of Sol Unger, M.D., Veterans Administration)

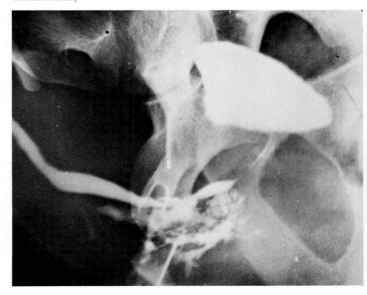

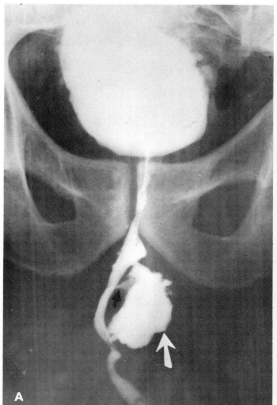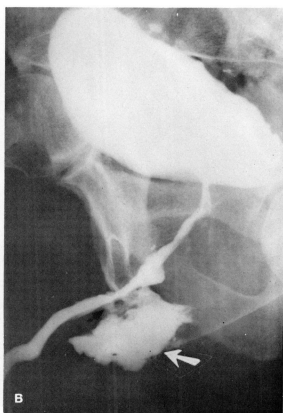

FIG. 38–14. Periurethral abscess. The contrast material enters the abscess cavity on injecting cystoure-thrography. The contrast material is fairly unevenly distributed. It is in this type of case that a urethral diverticulum could be the end result. *Small black arrow* points to opening between urethra and abscess cavity. *Large white arrow* points to a periurethral abscess. **(A)** AP view. **(B)** Right oblique view.

BIBLIOGRAPHY

Inflammations of the Urethra

1. Mitty, H.A.: Roentgen features of reflux into prostate, seminal vesicles, and vasa deferentia. Am. J. Roentgenol., *112*:603–606, 1971.
2. Segura, J.W., Smith, T.F., Weed, L.A., et al.: Chlamydia and nonspecific urethritis. J. Urol., *117*:720–721, 1977.
3. Stamey, T.A.: Urinary Infections. Williams & Wilkins, Baltimore, 1972.
4. Stamey, T.A.: The role of introital enterobacteria in recurrent urinary infection. J. Urol., *109*:467–472, 1973.
5. Stamey, T.A., and Sexton, C.C.: The role of vaginal colonization with enterobacteriaceae in recurrent urinary infections. J. Urol., *113*:214–218, 1975.
6. Stamey, T.A., Timothy, M., Millar, M., et al.: Recurrent urinary infections in adult women. The role of introital enterobacteria. Calif. Med., *115*:1–1971.

7. Stamey, T.A., Wehner, N., Mihara, G., et al.: The immunologic basis of recurrent bacteriuria: role of cervicovaginal antibody in enterobacterial colonization of the introital mucosa. Medicine, *57*:47–56, 1978.
8. Weed, L.A., Smith, T.F., Pettersen, G.R., et al.: Urethritis associated with chlamydia. Clinical and laboratory diagnosis. Minn. Med., *59*:228–229, 1976.

Reiter's Syndrome

9. Engelman, E.P., and Shearn, M.A.: Arthritis and allied rheumatic disease, p. 502–503. *In* Krupp, M.A., Chatton, M.J., (eds.): Current Medical Diagnosis and Treatment, 1978. Lange Medical Publications, California.

Urethral diverticula, outpocketings that occur in persons of both sexes, are far more common in women. They appear as tubular, rounded, or oval sac-like dilatations that are separate from the urethra but communicate with it. Johnson's classification is as follows[35]:

1. Congenital
    Gartner's duct
    Cysts from faulty union of primal folds
    Cell rest
    Wolffian duct
    Vaginal cyst
    (Campbell believed that congenital diverticulum was the result of blowout formation behind peripheral obstruction.[56])
2. Acquired
    Trauma during childbirth
    Infection of the urethral glands with abscess formation that then recommunicates with the urethral lumen
    Instrumentation of the urethra with deep fulguration of urethral lesions
    Strictures of the urethra
    Urethral stones
    To these may be added the wearing of incontinence clamps (Khoury minimized their importance[62]).

In the female, congenital diverticula are extremely rare. Silk and Lebowitz reported a case in an 8-year-old child.[10] The diverticulum was on the anterior surface, but this case might have been a duplicated urethra.

Acquired diverticula (Figs. 39–1 to 39–11) occur in 0.6 to 3 per cent of all asymptomatic female subjects,[12] being much higher if one includes the patient with symptoms. The diverticular openings may be near the external urethral meatus, the midurethra, or near the bladder neck, but are most common in the midurethra.

39

Diverticula of the Urethra

In the female, on urethrograms, the diverticulum appears as a tubular, rounded, or oval sac with a short neck. Occasionally, the neck (Fig. 39–2) is long and either straightened out, so that the sac is at some distance from the urethral lumen, or coiled, so that the diverticulum lies close to the urethra. On the cystographic phase of the intravenous urogram, the bladder neck and base may be elevated simulating a median lobe prostatic hypertrophy (Fig. 39–4).[19] Multiple diverticula (Fig. 39–5), multilocular diverticula (Fig. 39–6), and diverticula with multiple openings (Fig. 39–6) have been described.[22, 47] Stones (Figs. 39–7, 39–8) and benign (Fig. 39–9) and malignant (Figs. 39–10, 39–11) tumors in diverticula have been recorded.[85-95]

Carcinoma in a diverticulum of the female urethra is extremely rare and mucous adenocarcinoma is the rarest type (Fig. 39–11).[91] The source of this tumor is somewhat obscure, but it is generally assumed that it arises from periurethral mucous glands, Gartner's duct cyst, or misplaced peritoneal cell rest.[87, 89] The most likely source is the periurethral mucous glands.

X-ray diagnosis depends mainly on cystourethrography, which reveals filling defects in the diverticulum.

Congenital diverticula occur in the anterior urethra in the male. There are two types:

1. The wide-mouth diverticulum (Fig. 39–12). This is an elongated defect in the ventral wall of the urethra that often has a valvular distal lip that may give the same effects as an anterior urethral valve. Obstruction can be severe, producing changes in the proximal urethra, bladder, and upper tracts (see Chap. 37, Intersex and Congenital Lesions of the Urethra, and Chap. 53, Urethral Valves).

2. The narrow-neck diverticulum (Fig. 39–13). This may occur in the anterior or perineal region. It is a spherical cavity communicating to the urethra through a narrow neck; although obstructive features are usually absent, stasis can occur in the diverticulum producing infection and stone formation.

3. A small rounded congenital diverticulum in the fossa navicularis called lacuna magna may be a cause of dysuria in young boys (see Fig. 39–22).

Roentgenographic diagnosis depends on the use of voiding and, sometimes, injecting cystourethrography.

Most authors believe that diverticula of the urethra are acquired and that they are due to infections of the urethral and periurethral glands, abscess formation, and recommunications with the lumen (Figs. 39–14, 39–15, 39–16). Differentiation between congenital and acquired diverticula may be impossible, although those diverticula encountered in the posterior urethra are more likely to be acquired. Most congenital diverticula are found in the anterior urethra, but many acquired diverticula also are found here, especially in paraplegics[55, 57, 69] (Figs. 39–17, 39–18) and other neurologic disorders (Fig. 39–19). Posterior urethral diverticula in the male are usually the result of an abscess of the prostate rupturing into the urethra. However, stricture formation, pressure necrosis from urethral calculi, and trauma are additional causes. Rupture of a urethral diverticulum is rare (Fig. 39–20).

The appearance on a cystourethrogram of the male urethral diverticulum varies considerably. It may be elongated, oval, rounded, multiple, extremely irregular, or multilocular (Fig. 39–21).

CHAPTER 39, ILLUSTRATIONS

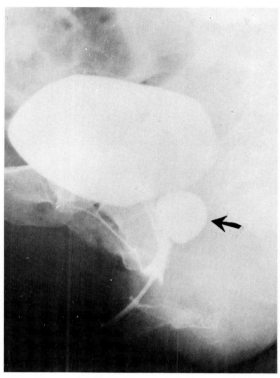

FIG. 39–1. Urethral diverticulum. Injecting cystourethrogram, oblique view. Urethral diverticulum in a 40-year-old woman following a periurethral abscess. Opening in midportion of urethra. *Arrow* points to diverticulum.

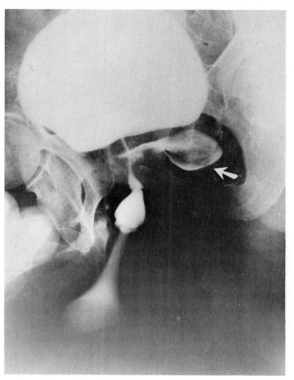

FIG. 39–2. Urethral diverticulum. Long-necked urethral diverticulum in a woman. The diverticulum is oval-shaped. *Arrow* points to diverticulum. Injecting cystourethrogram. Right oblique view.

FIG. 39–3. Diverticulum at bladder neck. **(A)** Injecting cystourethrogram—faint visualization of diverticulum. **(B)** Emptying film—contrast material in diverticulum.

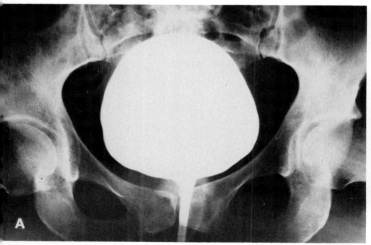

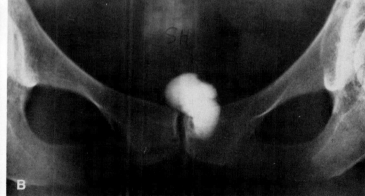

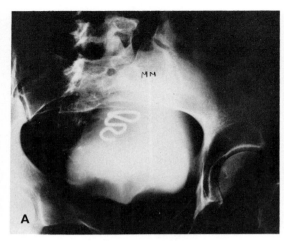

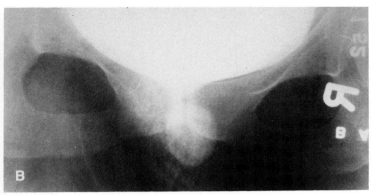

FIG. 39-4. (A) Diverticulum of female urethra producing defect in bladder floor on excretory cystogram. **(B)** Diverticulum seen after injecting cystourethrogram.

FIG. 39-5. Double diverticulum in a woman.

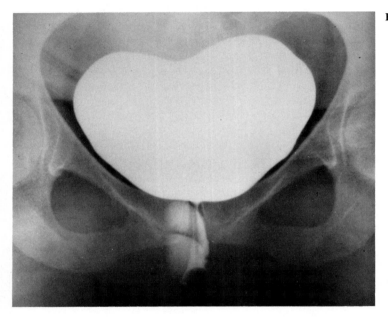

FIG. 39-6. Urethral diverticulum with multiple openings in a woman is also multilocular. *Left AP view* injecting cystourethrogram—*arrows* point to two openings entering the cavity of the diverticulum. *Right oblique view* injecting cystourethrogram—urethral diverticulum on this view shows an indentation on the posterior wall representing a multilocular structure.

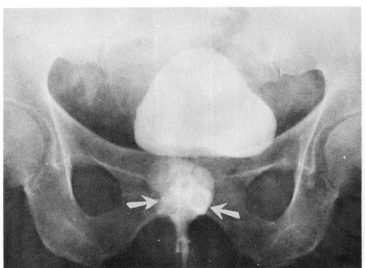

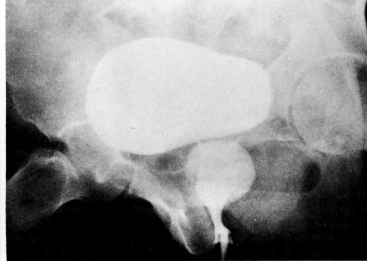

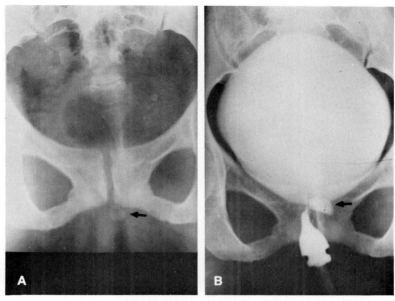

FIG. 39-7. Stone in a diverticulum of a female urethra. **(A)** Scout film. *Arrow* points to stone. **(B)** Injecting cystourethrogram. AP view. *Arrow* points to stone producing a defect in the diverticulum.

FIG. 39-8. Stone in a diverticulum of the female urethra. **(A)** Scout film. *Arrow* points to stone. **(B)** Right oblique view. Injecting cystourethrogram. Filling defect in diverticulum due to stone. *Arrow* points to diverticulum. (Courtesy of R. Hyman, M.D.)

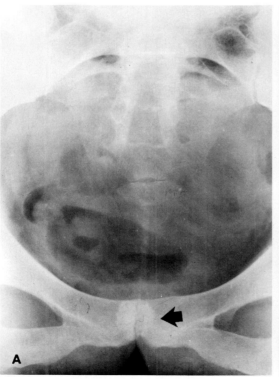

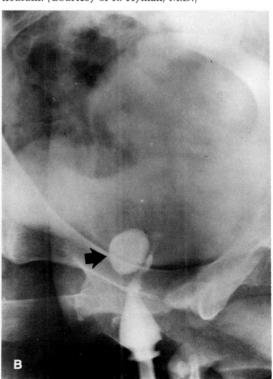

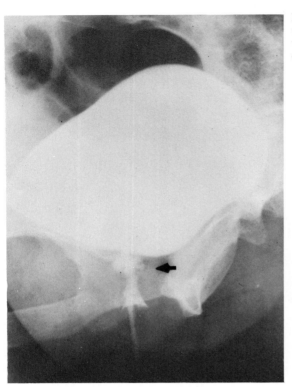

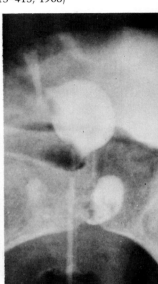

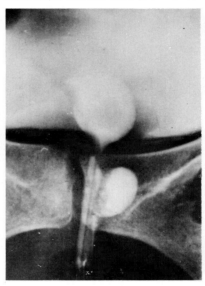

FIG. 39–9. Benign polyp in a female urethral diverticulum. Injecting cystourethrogram. Right oblique view. *Arrow* points to defect in the diverticulum produced by the polyp.

FIG. 39–10. The areas of radiolucency in the urethral diverticulum represent Gartner's duct carcinoma. (Hinman, F., Jr., Cohlan, W.R.: J. Urol., *83*:415–415, 1960)

FIG. 39–11. Adenocarcinoma in a diverticulum of the urethra in a female. Injecting cystourethrogram shows defect in diverticulum representing a mucous adenocarcinoma. **(A)** AP view and **(B)** lateral view. (Ney, C., Miller, H., Ochs, D.: J. Urol., *106*:874, 1971)

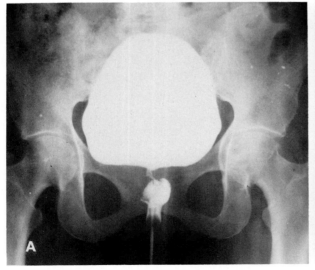

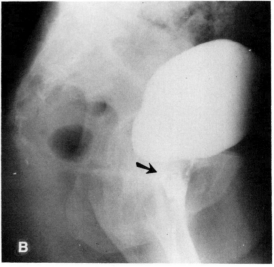

FIG. 39–12. Congenital urethral diverticulum in a male. Elongated, flattened congenital diverticulum (*arrow*) of the penile urethra.

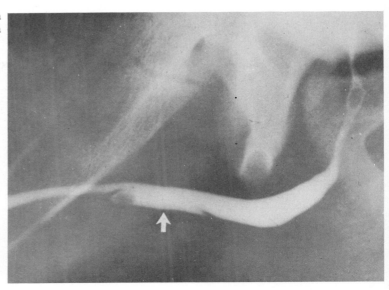

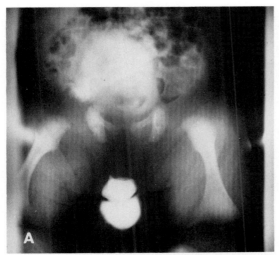

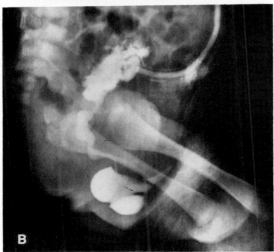

FIG. 39–13. Congenital anterior urethral diverticulum in a male. (**A**) Supine view during cystourethrography. The urinary bladder is filled with contrast medium. The large septate anterior urethral diverticulum is seen head-on. No contrast medium is within proximal or distal urethra. At this time, the penis was swollen, and a small amount of contrast medium dribbled from the meatus. (**B**) Lateral view during cystourethrography. Contrast medium was introduced into the bladder through the suprapubic Foley catheter. As contrast medium was introduced into the bladder, the diverticulum filled rapidly, and small amounts dribbled from the meatus. The bladder is irregularly constricted around the catheter balloon. The proximal urethra is not dilated. The septated diverticulum projects ventrally from a small neck. The distal urethra appears normal. (Freeny, P.C.: Radiology, *111*:173, 1974)

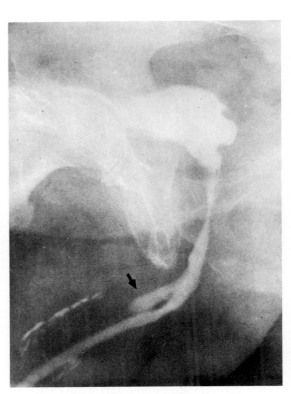

FIG. 39–14. Urethral diverticulum. Male. Diverticulum is an elongated, fusiform sac arising from the bulbous urethra on its superior portion. This is an unusual case in that it arises from the roof of the urethra rather than from the floor. It could be considered an accessory urethra.

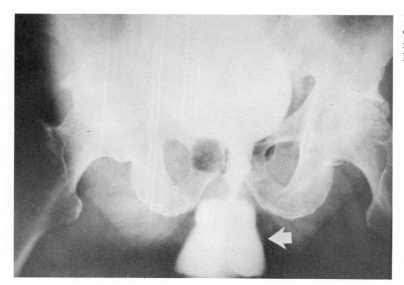

FIG. 39–15. Urethral diverticulum. Man. Large piriform diverticulum of anterior urethra secondary to the wearing of a penile clamp for incontinence. (Courtesy of Herbert Kenyon, M.D.)

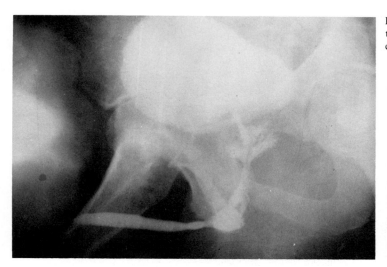

FIG. 39–16. Cystourethrogram of a man shows diverticulum in the bulbous urethra. Note filling of prostatic ducts.

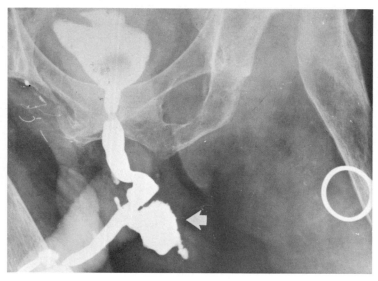

FIG. 39–17. Urethral diverticulum, male. Large irregular diverticulum of the anterior urethra in the region of the penoscrotal junction in a paraplegic. *Arrow* points to diverticulum. Note the inferior surface of the diverticulum, where a small tract has formed but has not reached the skin. (Courtesy of Maxwell Malament, M.D.)

FIG. 39–18. Urethral diverticulum, male. Urethral diverticulum of the anterior urethra in the region of the penoscrotal junction of a paraplegic. **(A)** *Arrow* points to the saclike diverticulum. Contrast material injected through a small sinus in the skin has not entered the diverticulum. **(B)** Four months later after catheter drainage. The *arrow* points to the diverticulum, which now is more fusiform in shape. (Courtesy of Arthur Tessler, M.D.)

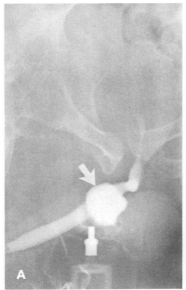
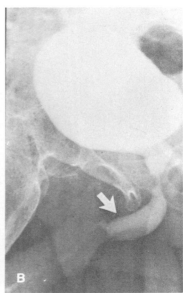

FIG. 39–19. Urethral diverticulum, male. Saccular urethral diverticulum of the anterior urethra in the region of the scrotum in a case of multiple sclerosis. Note deformity of the left hip. (Courtesy of Maxwell Malament, M.D.)

FIG. 39–20. Extravasation from an infected gangrenous diverticulum of the anterior urethra in the region of the scrotum. *Arrows* point to the large scrotum. (Courtesy of Maxwell Malament, M.D.)

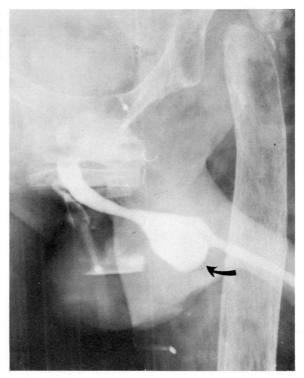

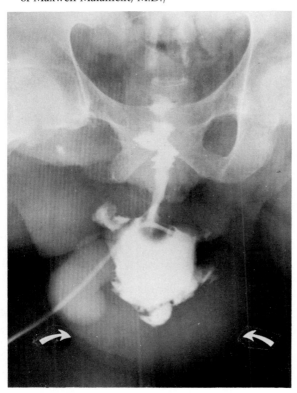

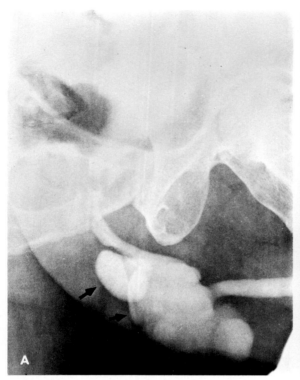

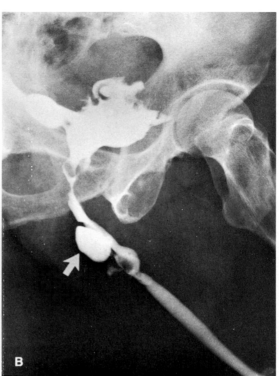

FIG. 39–21. (A) Multiple diverticula of the anterior urethra, male. *Arrows* point to the two diverticula, each with a separate opening to the urethra. The most distal diverticulum is multilocular. **(B)** Postresection of the most distal diverticulum. There is a small amount of extravasation at the region of the closure in the urethra. *Arrow* points to the remaining single diverticulum.

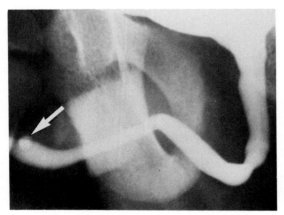

FIG. 39–22. *Arrow* points to rounded diverticulum in the fossa navicularis (lacuna magna).

BIBLIOGRAPHY

Congenital Diverticula of the Urethra

1. Abeshouse, B.S.: Diverticula of the anterior urethra in the male; 4 cases. Urol. Cutan. Rev., *55*:690–707, 1951.
2. Dees, J.E.: Congenital diverticulum of the anterior male urethra. Urol. Cutan. Rev., *54*:480–481, 1950.
3. Forshall, I., and Rickham, P.P.: Case of congenital diverticulum of anterior urethra in male infant. Br. J. Urol., *25*:142–146, 1953.
4. Freeny, P.C.: Congenital anterior urethral diverticulum in the male. Radiology, *111*:173–174, 1974.
5. Johnson, F.P.: Diverticula and cysts of the urethra. J. Urol., *10*:295–310, 1923.
6. Kjellberg, S.R., Ericsson, N.O., and Rudhe, U.: The Lower Urinary Tract in Childhood. Year Book Publishing Co., Chicago, 1957.
7. Knox, W.G.: Congenital diverticulum of the male urethra. J. Urol., *58*:344–348, 1947.
7a. Meiraz, D., Dolberg, L., Dolberg, M., et al.: Diverticulum of the urethra in two boys. Am. J. Dis. Child., *122*:271–273, 1971.
8. Nesbitt, T.E.: Congenital megalo-urethra. J. Urol., *73*:839–842, 1955.
9. Rudhe, U., and Ericsson, N.O.: Congenital urethral diverticula. Ann. Radiol., *13/3–4*:289, 1970.
10. Silk, M.R., and Lebowitz, J.M.: Anterior urethral diverticulum. J. Urol., *101*:66–67, 1969.
10a. Sweitzer, T.H.: Congenital urethral diverticulum in the male patient. J. Urol., *97*:93–95, 1967.
11. Williams, D.I., and Retik, A.B.: Congenital valves and diverticula of the anterior urethra. Br. J. Urol., *4*:228–234, 1969.

Acquired Diverticula of the Urethra

Urethral Diverticulum in the Female

12. Anderson, M.J.F.: The incidence of diverticulum in the female urethra. J. Urol., *98*:96–98, 1967.

13. Cook, E.N.: Diverticulum of female urethra: Problems in diagnosis and treatment. Surg. Gynecol. Obstet., *99*:273–276, 1954.

14. Cook, E.N., and Pool, T.L.: Urethral diverticulum in the female. J. Urol., *62*:495–497, 1949.

15. Counseller, V.S.: Urethral diverticula in females; a study. Am. J. Obstet. Gynecol., *57*:231–236, 1949.

16. Davis, H.J., and Cian, G.L.: Positive pressure urethrography; a new diagnostic method. J. Urol., *75*:753–757, 1956.

17. Davis, H.J., and Te Linde, R.W.: Urethral diverticula: An assay of 121 cases. J. Urol., *80*:34–39, 1958.

18. Downer, I.G., and Virgilio, F.D.: Diverticulum of the female urethra, review of the literature and case report. J. Urol., *54*:53–58, 1946.

19. Dretler, S.P., Vermillion, C.D., and McCullough, D.L.: The roentgenographic diagnosis of female urethral diverticula. J. Urol., *107*:72–74, 1972.

20. Edwards, E.A., and Beebe, R.A.: Diverticula of female urethra: 5 cases. Obstet. Gynecol., *5*:729–738, 1955.

21. Ellik, M.: Diverticulum of the female urethra: A new method of ablation. J. Urol., *77*:243–246, 1957.

22. Engel, W.J.: Diverticulum of the female urethra. J. Urol., *45*:703–709, 1941.

23. Folsom, A.I., and O'Brien, H.A.: The female urethra. J.A.M.A., *128*:408–414, 1945.

24. Frith, K.: Diverticulum of the female urethra. Report of two cases with review of the literature. J. Obstet. Gynaecol. Br. Comm., *67*:314–319, 1960.

25. Furniss, H.D.: Sub-urethral abscess and diverticula in the female urethra. J. Urol., *33*:398–502, 1935.

26. Gilbert, L.R.A., and Rivera Cintron, F.J.: Urethral diverticula in the female. Am. J. Obstet. Gynecol., *67*:616–627, 1954.

29. Granberg, P.O., and Svartholm, F.: Urethral diverticula in the female; with special reference to roentgenographic diagnosis and results of surgery. Acta Chir. Scand., *115*:78–88, 1958.

30. Hennessy, J.D.: Urethral diverticulum in the female. Br. J. Urol., *30*:415–422, 1958.

31. Herman, L., and Greene, L.B.: Diverticulum of the female urethra. J. Urol., *52*:599–610, 1944.

32. Higgins, C.C., and Rambousek, E.E.: Diverticula of the urethra in women, review of 12 cases. J. Urol., *53*:732–739, 1945.

33. Huffman, J.W.: The detailed anatomy of paraurethral ducts in the adult human female. Am. J. Obstet. Gynecol., *55*:86–100, 1948.

34. Hyams, J.A., and Hyams, M.N.: New operative procedure for treatment of diverticulum of female urethra. Urol. Cutan. Rev., *43*:573–577, 1939.

35. Johnson, C.M.: Diverticula and cyst of the female urethra. J. Urol., *39*:506–516, 1938.

36. Kight, J.R., and Hill, N.H., Jr.: Diverticulum of the female urethra. Am. J. Obstet. Gynecol., *70*:1214–1217, 1955.

37. Krantz, K.E.: The anatomy of the urethra and anterior vaginal wall. Am. J. Obstet. Gynecol., *62*:374–386, 1951.

38. Krieger, J.S., and Poutasse, E.F.: Diverticulum of female urethra. Am. J. Obstet. Gynecol., *68*:706–712, 1954.

39. Lane, V.: Diverticulum of the urethra. Br. J. Urol., *29*:155–158, 1957.

40. Lintgen, C., and Herbut, P.A.: A clinico-pathological study of 100 female urethras. J. Urol., *55*:298–305, 1946.

41. Lower, W.E., and Tormey, T.W.: Diverticulum of the female urethra. Ann. Surg., *107*:923–926, 1938.

42. Lowsley, O.S., and Kirwin, T.J.: Clinical Urology. Williams & Wilkins, Baltimore, 1944.

43. McMahon, S.: Congenital diverticulum of the female urethra. J. Urol., *55*:69–72, 1946.

44. McNally, A.: Diverticula of the female urethra. Am. J. Surg., *28*:177–181, 1938.

45. Moore, T.D.: Diverticulum of female urethra: An improved technique of surgical excision. J. Urol., *68*:611–616, 1952.

46. Nel, J.B.: Diverticulum of the female urethra. J. Obstet. Gynaecol. Brit. Emp., *62*:90–97, 1955.

47. Parmenter, F.J.: Diverticulum of the female urethra. J. Urol., *45*:479–496, 1941.

48. Pinkerton, J.H.M.: Diverticulum of female urethra. J. Obstet. Gynaecol. Brit. Comm., *63*:76–82, 1956.

49. Schmitz, H.E.: Diverticulum in the female urethra. Urol. Cutan. Rev., *43*:596–598, 1939.

50. Spraitz, A.F., Jr., and Wekch, J.S.: Diverticulum of the female urethra. Am. J. Obstet. Gynecol., *91*:1013–1016, 1965.

51. Wharton, L.R., and Kearns, W.: Diverticula of the female urethra. J. Urol., *63*:1063–1076, 1950.

52. Wharton, L.R., Jr., and Te Linde, R.W.: Urethral diverticulum. Obstet. Gynecol., *7*:503–509, 1956.

53. Willmarth, C.L.: Ectopic urethral orifice within urethral diverticulum. J. Urol., *59*:47–49, 1948.

54. Young, B.R., and McCrea, L.E.: Urethrocele, urethral diverticulum; suburethral abscess in the female. Roentgen Appearance; treatment. Urol. Cutan. Rev., *41*:91–93, 1938.

Urethral Diverticulum in the Male

55. Bunts, R.C.: Management of urological complications in 1,000 paraplegics. J. Urol., *79*:733–741, 1958.

56. Campbell, M.F.: Diverticulum of the urethra; two cases in young boys. J. Urol., *30*:113–121, 1933.

57. Comarr, A.E., and Bors, E.: Pathological changes in urethra of paraplegic patients. J. Urol., *66*:355–361, 1951.

58. Fagerstrom, D.P.: Etiology of acquired diverticula of anterior urethra and its relation to cause of postprostatectomy incontinence. 2 cases. J. Urol., *49*:357–369, 1943.

59. Griffiths, I.H., and Walsh, J.J.: Diverticula and fistulae of the urethra in paraplegics. Br. J. Urol., *33*:374–380, 1961.

60. Gross, R., and Bill, A.H., Jr.: Concealed diverticulum of male urethra as cause of urinary obstruction. Pediatrics, *1*:44–51, 1948.

61. Howze, C.P., and Hennessey, R.A.: Urethral diverticula. Surg. Gynecol. Obstet., *37*:392–394, 1923.

62. Khoury, E.N.: Diverticulum of the male urethra. J. Urol., *69*:291–298, 1953.

63. Knox, W.G.: Congenital diverticulum of the male urethra. J. Urol., *58*:334–348, 1957.

64. LeComte, R.M., and Herschman, M.J.: Diverticula of the male urethra. J. Urol., *30*:463–474, 1933.

65. Lowsley, O.S., and Gutierrez, R.: Diverticulos de la uretra. Revista Med. y cir., *33*:229–298, 1928.

66. McKay, R.W., and Colston, J.A.C.: Diverticula of the male urethra. Surg. Gynecol. Obstet., *48*:51–62, 1929.

67. Omo-Dare, P.: Posterior urethral diverticulum in the male. Br. J. Urol., *40*:445–450, 1968.

68. Ostry, H.: Diverticulum of the urethra in the male. Can. Med. Assoc. J., *58*:68–69, 1948.

69. Pate, V.A., Jr., and Bunts, R.C.: Urethral diverticula in paraplegics. J. Urol., 65:108–125, 1951.
70. Trafton, H.M.: Urethral diverticulum. Surg. Clin. North Am., 25:589–596, 1945.
71. Von Ehrlich, O.: Zur Kasuistik und Behandlung der Divertikel der maennlichen Harnöehre. Beitr. klin. Chir., 59:193–205, 1908.
72. Watts, S.H.: Urethral diverticulum in the male with report of a case. Bull. Hopkins Hosp., 13:49–89, 1906.

Rupture of Urethral Diverticulum

73. Scott, W.W., and Ekas, W.L.: An operative procedure for the repair of the urethrodiverticulovaginal fistula. Surgery, 20:645–655, 1946.

Stones in Diverticulum of Urethra

74. Carter, R.G.: Diverticulum of the female urethra with calculus formation. Urol. Cutan. Rev., 46:494–495, 1942.
75. Cullen, T.S.: Abscess in the urethro-vaginal septum. Bull. Hopkins Hosp., 5:45–50, 1894.
76. Gaston, E.A., and Ferrucci, J.: Calculus formation in a urethral diverticulum in a woman. N. Engl. J. Med., 221:379–383, 1939.
77. Herman, L., and Greene, L.R.: Diverticulum of the female urethra. J. Urol., 52:599–610, 1944.
78. Higgins, C.C., and Roen, P.R.: Calculus-containing urethral diverticulum in a woman. J. Urol., 49:715–719, 1943.
79. Hunner, G.L.: Calculus formation in urethral diverticulum in women. 3 cases. Urol. Cutan. Rev., 42:336–341, 1938.
80. Kirby, E.W., Jr., and Reynolds, C.J.: Diverticula of the female urethra: Report of four cases, one containing a calculus. J. Urol., 62:498–502, 1949.
81. Lane, C.: Diverticulum of the female urethra with multiple calculi. Urol. Cutan. Rev., 47:363–364, 1943.
82. McMahon, S.: Congenital diverticulum of the female urethra. J. Urol., 55:69–72, 1946.
83. Menville, J.G., and Mitchell, J.D.: Diverticulum of the female urethra. J. Urol., 51:411–423, 1944.
84. Shivers, C.H. de T., and Cooney, C.J.: The formation of calculi in urethral diverticula of female. J.A.M.A., 102:997–999, 1934.

Tumors in Diverticulum of Urethra

85. Brown, E.W.: Diverticulum of female urethra: Report of 23 cases with adenocarcinoma in one. South. Med. J., 49:982–988, 1956.
86. Hamilton, J.D., and Leach, W.B.: Adenocarcinoma arising in a diverticulum of the female urethra. Arch. Pathol., 51:90–97, 1951.
87. Hinman, F., Jr., and Cohlan, W.R.: Gartner's duct carcinoma in a urethral diverticulum. J. Urol., 83:414–415, 1960.
88. Huvos, A.G., Muggia, F.M., and Markewitz, M.: Carcinoma of female urethra. Occurrence with hyperparathyroidism. N.Y. State J. Med., 69:2042–2045, 1969.
89. Massone, P., Riopelle, J.L., and Simard, L.C.: Le mesothéliomé dénin de la sphère génitale. Rev. Can. Biol., 1:720–751, 1942.
90. Melnick, J.L., and Birdsall, T.M.: Carcinoma of the diverticulum of the female urethra. Am. J. Obstet. Gynecol., 80:347–352, 1960.
91. Ney, C., Miller, H., and Ochs, D.: Adenocarcinoma in the diverticulum of the female urethra: a case report of mucous adenocarcinoma with a summary of the literature. J. Urol., 106:874–877, 1971.
92. Rebaudi, G.: Polipo in diverticolo della mucosa dell' uretra femminile (Fibromatous polyp in urethral diverticulum). Arch. Ital. Urol., 14:218–223, 1937.
93. Wishard, W., Jr., and Nourse, M.H.: Carcinoma in diverticulum of female urethra. J. Urol., 68:320–323, 1952.
94. Wishard, W.N., Jr., Nourse, M.H., and Mertz, J.H.O.: Carcinoma in diverticulum of female urethra. J. Urol., 83:409–413, 1960.
95. Wishard, W.N., Jr., Nourse, M.H., and Mertz, J.H.O.: Carcinoma in a diverticulum of female urethra. J. Urol., 89:431–432, 1963.

Injuries to the urethra (Figs. 40–1 to 40–13) are the result of foreign bodies introduced for erotic or sadistic purposes; instrumentation; external trauma, such as straddle falls or penetrating injuries; and spontaneous ruptures, especially in cases of urethral strictures.

EXTENT OF INJURIES: SITE AND COMPLICATIONS

Injuries vary from mucosal contusion to complete severance (Fig. 40–8). Symptoms and signs vary according to the degree and the location of the trauma. There may or may not be damage to the penile body or extravasation of urine. Cystourethrograms are accurate in determining the extent and the place of the injury. The bulbous and the membranous urethra are the most common sites, usually produced by compression against the symphysis pubis by a straddle fall. Injury to the posterior urethra usually is associated with pelvic fracture and often is complicated by bladder-neck and bladder trauma. Tears often occur near the apex of the prostate as a result of a shearing action between the relatively fixed membranous urethra and the prostate. In the woman, complete severance is rare. Anterior urethral injuries are commonly caused by gunshot wounds.[3]

Rupture of the urethra with urinary extravasation is extremely serious; the findings depend on the site of the rupture. If the rupture occurs distally to the triangular ligament, the urine collects in the perineum, the scrotum, and the shaft of the penis and extends up into the abdominal wall underneath Scarpa's fascia. If the rupture is proximal to the triangular ligament, the extravasation is confined at first within the pelvic cavity and later extends superiorly in all directions in the extraperitoneal

40

Trauma to the Urethra, Foreign Bodies, and Calculi

spaces. It may extend up to the perirenal tissues after surrounding the bladder neck, the bladder, and the perirectal areas. The ischiorectal space and upper inner aspect of the thigh (Fig. 40–9) often are involved. In this type of injury there is no swelling of the perineum or the scrotum. If the extravasation occurs within the triangular ligament, the spread may occur in either direction, but usually it occurs externally. However, it can go around the prostate into the rectoprostatic tissue, ischiorectal space, and up to the perivesical space. Injuries to the pendulous urethra most often are limited to the penis. If they break through Buck's fascia, the extravasation may go up to the anterior abdominal wall or downward to the scrotum and the perineum.

Urethrograms are useful in determining the location and the extent of the rupture of the urethra. Injecting cystourethrograms usually are the only ones that can be used, because voiding may be impossible. The use of urethrograms has not increased either the morbidity or the mortality in our cases. A small amount of contrast material should be injected at the time of the first x-ray exposure to avoid obscuring the area of rupture.

Late complications include strictures, fistula formation, and impotence. Modern treatment of severe posterior ruptures of the urethra has certainly decreased the chance of impotence. Most authorities seem to favor cystotomy in those cases with a later rather than an immediate repair.

FOREIGN BODIES IN THE URETHRA

Many diverse types of foreign bodies in the urethra (Figs. 40–14 to 40–18) have been reported, and probably many more have gone unreported. Most commonly, the foreign bodies are introduced into the urethra through the external meatus by sexual perverts, malingerers, and masturbators. Occasionally, a foreign body can be introduced accidentally, such as hairs on catheters. Foreign bodies can pass into the urethra from the bladder (the various ways of entering the bladder are discussed in Chap. 29, Trauma to and Foreign Bodies of the Bladder); they can migrate into the lumen from extraurethral areas; enter directly, such as bullets, or shrapnel; and be introduced surgically, such as broken catheters. The foreign body can be a nidus for stone formation.

Diagnosis of a foreign body in the urethra is usually easy unless it is extremely small. Palpation, roentgenograms, and endoscopic examination are the indicated procedures.

URETHRAL CALCULI

Urethral calculi (Figs. 40–19 to 40–25) are classified as primary and secondary. Primary calculi are formed in the urethra, usually behind an obstruction, or may appear as encrustations on a foreign body. Many primary calculi are found in diverticula of the urethra. Probably one of the common types of urethral calculus is the extruded prostatic duct calculus. Occasionally, calculi are formed postoperatively or are inadvertently left at the time of operation. Secondary calculi are passed from the bladder into the urethra.

Urethral calculi usually are solitary, but they can be multiple. Most calculi in the urethra are small, but giant ones have been reported.[64] Cystourethrography is an excellent method for diagnosis.

CHAPTER 40, ILLUSTRATIONS

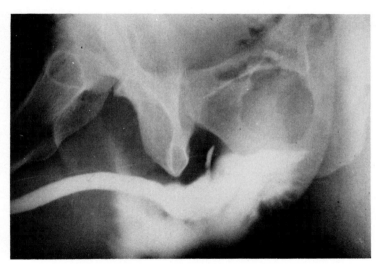

FIG. 40–1. Rupture of the bulbomembranous junction of the urethra following a straddle injury. Contrast medium extends both distally and proximally so that the actual site of injury is obscured. Injecting cystourethrogram.

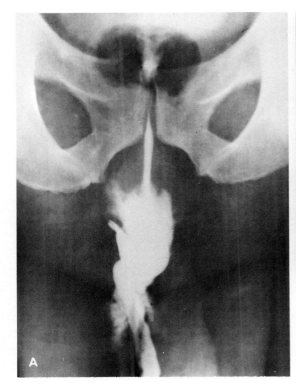

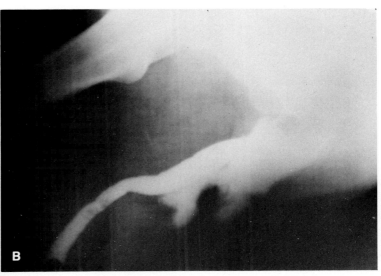

FIG. 40-2. Rupture of the bulbomembranous area of the urethra due to a straddle injury. Injecting cystourethrogram. **(A)** AP view. Contrast medium extends both distally and proximally from the injured area. **(B)** Right oblique view. Contrast medium extends distally and proximally from the inferior side of the urethra.

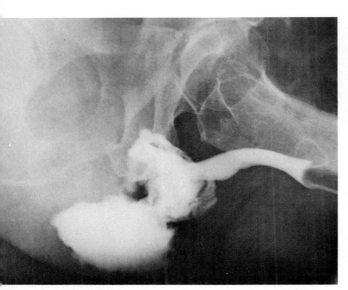

FIG. 40-3. Rupture of the urethra distal to the bulb, following a fall astride a chair. This film was taken approximately 3 days after the injury. The contrast medium can be seen spreading diffusely in the region of the injury, but it is seen also in a saclike periurethral collection that has not yet broken through the skin to form a fistula. Injecting cystourethrogram. Left oblique view.

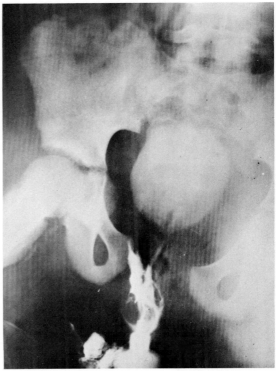

FIG. 40-4. Rupture of the membranous urethra in a 9-year-old boy who was struck from behind in an automobile accident. Contrast medium extravasates in the region of the bulb and extends proximally. There is wide separation of the symphysis pubis. Bladder is elevated due to perivesical hemorrhage. Injecting cystourethrogram. AP view.

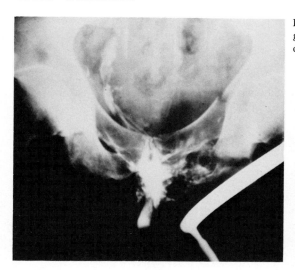

FIG. 40–5. Rupture of the urethra proximal to the triangular ligament. Contrast goes proximally. Note fracture of pelvis.

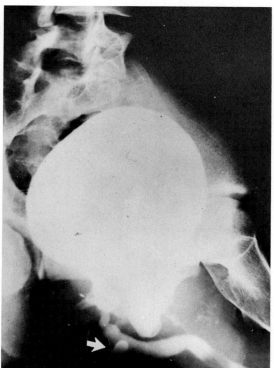

FIG. 40–6. Injury to the prostatic urethra as a result of a shrapnel injury. There is dilatation of the prostatic urethra with narrowing of its most distal portion. Injury had occurred several months before this film was taken. *Arrow* points to metal fragment still present.

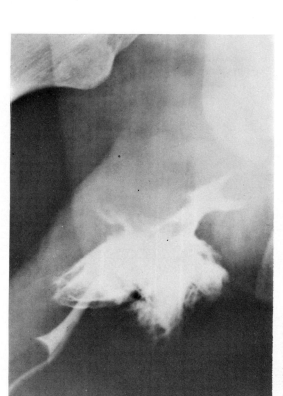

FIG. 40–7. Penoscrotal injury with fistulization to the skin. Straddle injury in which the skin was broken and in which there was severe trauma in the region of the penoscrotal junction. Contrast medium injected into the urethra extravasated widely and appeared at the skin openings.

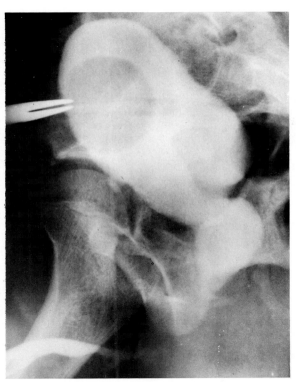

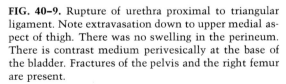

FIG. 40-8. Complete severance of urethra in bulbomembranous area. Case of automobile accident. Double injection technique: contrast material injected by means of suprapubic cystostomy tube and anterior urethra. Note failure of contrast material to join. There is a wide area of separation.

FIG. 40-9. Rupture of urethra proximal to triangular ligament. Note extravasation down to upper medial aspect of thigh. There was no swelling in the perineum. There is contrast medium perivesically at the base of the bladder. Fractures of the pelvis and the right femur are present.

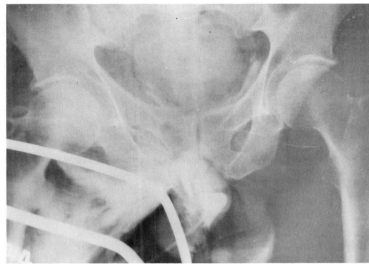

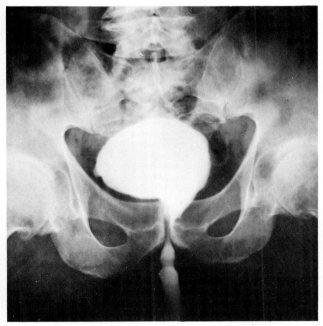

FIG. 40-10. Instrumental rupture of posterior urethra. Retrograde cystourethrogram showing extraperitoneal perivesical extravasation following transurethral resection of prostate. (Kenyon, H.R.: J.A.M.A. *142*:798–801, 1950)

FIG. 40-11. Extensive extraperitoneal extravasation from injury to prostatic urethra during transurethral resection for carcinoma. Healed without complications. (Kenyon, H.R.: J.A.M.A., *142*:798–801, 1950)

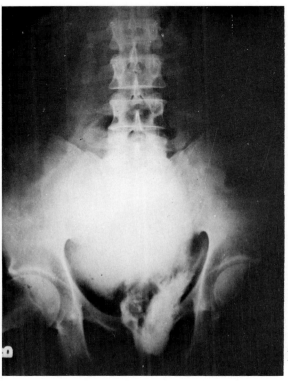

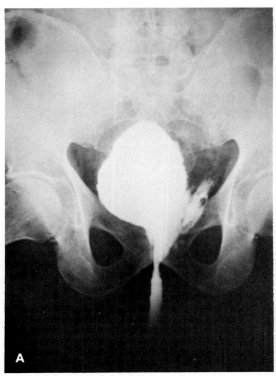 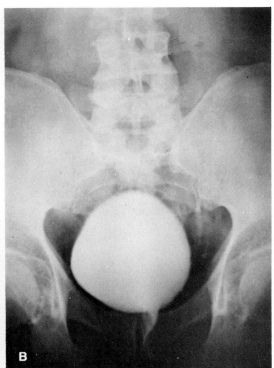

FIG. 40–12. (A) Rupture of the posterior urethra during a transurethral resection. Cystourethrogram reveals retroperitoneal extravasation of contrast material. **(B)** Essentially normal finding 11 days later. (Kenyon, H.R.: J.A.M.A., *142*:798–801, 1950)

FIG. 40–13. Injury to the posterior urethra during a transurethral resection. **(A)** Immediate cystourethrogram shows contrast material retroperitoneally. **(B)** Shows residual contrast material after emptying bladder by catheter. (Kenyon, H.R.: J.A.M.A., *142*:798–801, 1950)

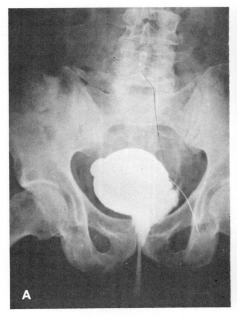 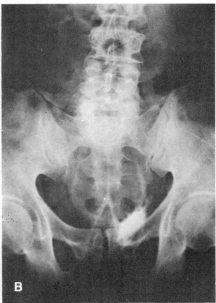

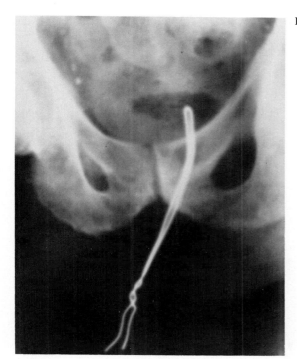

FIG. 40–14. Clothes hanger in urethra. Plain film.

FIG. 40–15. Foreign body in urethra. Man. Pencil introduced into the urethra, with a portion projecting into the bladder cavity.

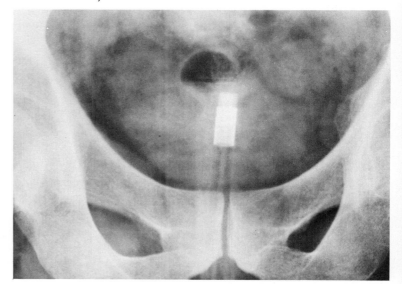

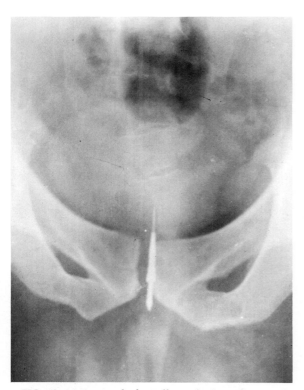

FIG. 40–16. Foreign body. Follower broken off in a male patient on attempt to dilate a stricture. Follower is in prostatic urethra and projects into bladder.

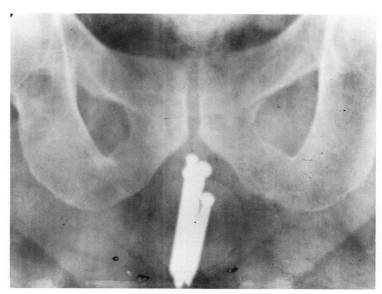

FIG. 40–17. Foreign body. Nails in the urethra. Male patient. The nails were introduced through the penis. (Courtesy of M. Greenberger, M.D.)

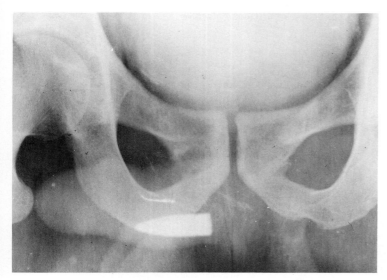

FIG. 40–18. Foreign body. Rifle bullet in anterior urethra. Patient had received a gunshot wound in back 3 years previous to this photograph. It was thought that the bullet lodged in the bladder and remained there until passed into the urethra. (Simon, S.: J. Urol., *61*:785–789, 1949)

FIG. 40–19. Calculi in prostatic urethra formed around insulation wire introduced through penis. (Courtesy of Maxwell Malament, M.D., Veterans Administration)

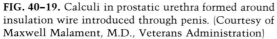

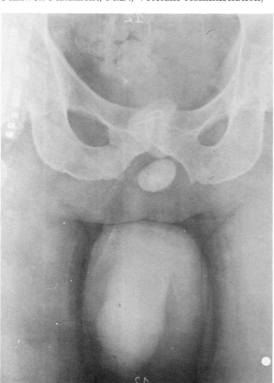

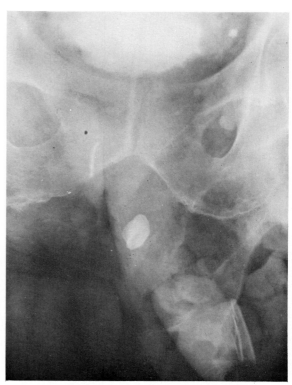

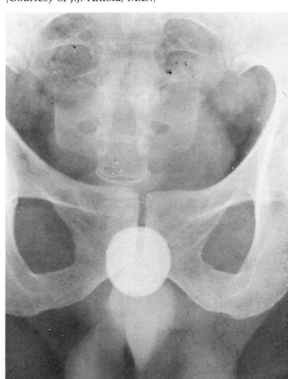

FIG. 40–20. Calculus in urethra passed from bladder. It lodged in region of bulbomembranous junction.

FIG. 40–21. Large laminated stone in prostatic urethra. (Courtesy of J.J. Arnold, M.D.)

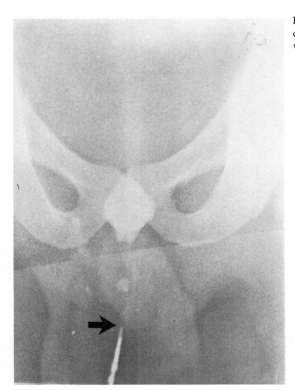

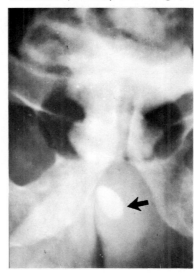

FIG. 40–22. Two urethral stones proximal to a hypospadiac opening. *Arrow* points to the urethral meatus on ventral side of penis. (Courtesy of A. Balsamo, M.D.)

FIG. 40–23. Urethral calculi. (**A**) AP view showing large stone in posterior urethra. (**B**) *Arrow* points to stone on cystourethrography. Also large stone in dilated prostatic urethra. (Courtesy of Sol Unger, M.D.)

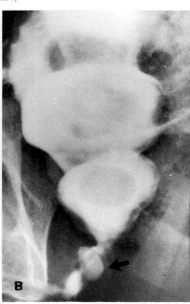

FIG. 40–24. Urethral calculus. (**A**) Scout film. Large stone lying transversely. (**B**) Cystourethrogram. Stone lodged in bulbous urethra. Paraplegic patient. *Arrow* points to stone. There is an osteomyelitis of the left ischium.

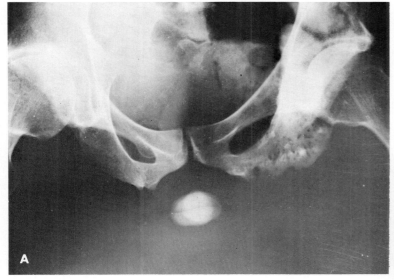

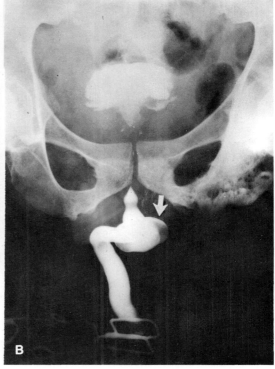

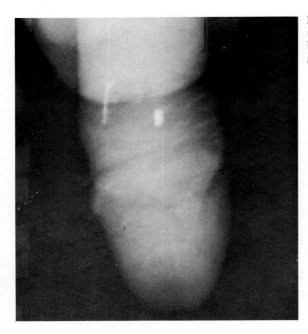

FIG. 40–25. Urethral calculus. Small stone lodged in anterior urethra. Patient had prostatic calculi, and it was believed that one of the stones passed into the urethra and became lodged in the anterior portion.

BIBLIOGRAPHY

Trauma to the Urethra

1. Axilrod, H.D.: Traumatic rupture of the bladder and posterior urethra. J. Med. Soc. New Jersey, *57*:584–586, 1960.
2. Blumberg, N.: Anterior urethral injuries. J. Urol., *102*:210–213, 1969.
3. Bolgar, G.C., Duncan, R.E., and Evans, A.T.: Primary repair of completely transected female urethra by advancement. J. Urol., *118*:118–119, 1977.
4. Bryant, W.O.: Extravasation of urine. Urol. Cutan. Rev., *37*:155–163, 1933.
5. Campbell, M.F.: Periurethral phlegmon (extravasation of urine); a study of 135 cases. Surg. Gynecol. Obstet., *48*:382–389, 1929.
6. Chambers, H.L., and Balfour, J.: The incidence of impotence following pelvic fracture with associated urinary tract injuries. J. Urol., *89*:702–703, 1963.
7. Char, G.Y., Shih, H.E., and Yang, C.P.: Extravasation of urine. A study of 30 cases. Cin. Med. J., *50*:807–820, 1936.
8. Culp, O.S.: Treatment of ruptured bladder and urethra: Analysis of 86 cases of urinary extravasation. J. Urol., *48*:266–286, 1942.
9. Das, S.: Complete rupture of the posterior urethra without fractured pelvis. J. Urol., *118*:116–117, 1977.
10. DeWeerd, J.H.: Care of the severely injured patient—urological aspects. J.A.M.A., *165*:1916–1921, 1957.
11. DeWeerd, J.H.: Management of injuries to the bladder, urethra and genitalia. Surg. Clin. North Am., *39*:973–978, 1959.
12. Finestone, E.O.: Urinary extravasation (periurethral phlegmon): Pathogenesis and experimental study. Surg. Gynecol. Obstet., *73*:218–227, 1941.
13. Finestone, E.O.: Urinary extravasation (periurethral phlegmon): A clinical study of 32 cases. Ann. Surg., *116*:109–121, 1942.
14. Finestone, E.O.: Urinary extravasation (periurethral phlegmon): A new concept of the pathogenesis and the treatment. N.Y. J. Med., *43*:1320–1324, 1943.
15. Harrison, J.H.: The treatment of rupture of the urethra, especially when accompanying fracture of the pelvic bones. Surg. Gynecol. Obstet., *72*:622–631, 1941.
16. Hausman, H.: Genito-urinary extravasation. J. Florida Med. Assoc., *31*:307–309, 1945.
17. Hogan, J.F., Jr.: Urinary extravasation. Bull. Sch. Med. Univ. Maryland, *39*:14–24, 1954.
18. Hutchins, A.F.: The diagnosis and treatment of the ruptured urethra. Am. J. Surg., *42*:765–768, 1938.
19. Kenyon, H.R.: Perforation in transurethral operations: Technique for immediate diagnosis of. J.A.M.A., *142*:798–801, 1950.
19a. Kiracofe, A.L., Pfister, R.R., and Peterson, N.E.: Management of nonpenetrating distal urethral trauma. J. Urol., *114*:57–62, 1975.
20. Lee, L.W., Davis, E., and Shoup, E.D.: Acute extravasation: Urologic emergency. Nebraska Med. J., *30*:204–206, 1945.
21. Lewis, R.M.: Urinary extravasation. J. Urol., *55*:289–291, 1946.
22. Lucey, D.T., Smith, M.J.V., and Koontz, W.W., Jr.: Modern theories in the management of urologic trauma. J. Urol., *107*:641–646, 1972.
23. McCague, E.J., and Semans, J.H.: Management of traumatic rupture of urethra and bladder complicating fracture of the pelvis. J. Urol., *52*:36–41, 1944.
24. Mitchell, J.P.: Injuries to the urethra. Br. J. Urol., *40*:649–670, 1968.
25. Morehouse, D.D., Belitzky, P., and Mackinnon, K.J.: Rupture of the posterior urethra. J. Urol., *107*:255–258, 1972.
26. Morehouse, D.D., and Mackinnon, K.J.: Urological injuries associated with pelvic fractures. J. Trauma, *9*:479–496, 1969.
27. Myers, R.P., **and** DeWeerd, J.H.: Incidence of stricture follow-

ing primary realignment of the disrupted proximal urethra. J. Urol., 107:265–268, 1972.

28. Ockerblad, N.F., and Carlson, H.E.: Urethral urinary extravasation. Surgery, 3:391–396, 1938.
29. Orkin, L.A.: Traumatic avulsion of the bladder neck and prostate complicating fractures of the pelvis. Am. J. Surg., 89:840–853, 1955.
30. Peters, P.C.: Trauma of genitourinary system. In Care of the Trauma Patient. McGraw Hill, New York, 1966.
31. Pierce, J.M., Jr.: Genitourinary injuries in the multiply injured patient. Ortho. Clin. N. Am., 1:75–91, 1970.
32. Pierce, J.M., Jr.: Management of dismemberment of the prostato-membranous urethra and ensuing stricture disease. J. Urol., 107:259–264, 1972.
33. Pierce, J.M., Jr.: Primary reconstitution of the disrupted urethra. In Scott, R., Jr. (ed.): Current Controversies in Urologic Management. W.B. Saunders, Philadelphia, 1972.
34. Pierce, J.M., Jr.: Trauma of the lower urinary system and genitalia. In Practice of Surgery. Harper and Row, Hagerstown, 1973.
35. Raney, A.M.: Radiographic findings immediately after urethral rupture: An experimental study and case reports. J. Urol., 116:581–582, 1976.
36. Ravenel, J.J.: Extravasation from the lower urinary tract. J. Urol., 40:129–134, 1938.
37. Riekert, J.G.: Management and mortality of periurethral phlegmons. J. Urol., 61:424–431, 1949.
38. Rusche, C.F., and Bacon, S.K.: Urinary extravasation following urethral stricture. Calif. West. Med., 44:284–287, 1936.
39. Silverstone, M.: Traumatic rupture of the urethra. Br. J. Surg., 30:70–74, 1942.
40. Smith, H.S., and Finton, R.E.: Urinary extravasation from urethra, with analysis of 151 cases. Urol. Cutan. Rev., 45:481–490, 1941.
41. Soloway, A.M.: Extravasation of urine. J. Urol., 20:569–591, 1928.
42. Tashiro, S., and Hinman, F., Jr.: Periurethral and perirectal infections: pathological and clinical differentiation. J. Urol., 57:338–355, 1947.
43. Tobin, C.E., and Benjamin, J.A.: Anatomical study and clinical consideration of the fasciae limiting urinary extravasation from the penile urethra. Surg. Gynecol. Obstet., 79:195–204, 1944.
44. Vermooten, V.: Rupture of urethra. A new diagnostic sign. J. Urol., 56:228–236, 1946.
45. Waterhouse, K., and Gross, M.: Trauma to the genitourinary tract: A 5-year experience with 251 cases. J. Urol., 101:241–246, 1969.
46. Weems, W.L., and Hillis, R.S.: Spontaneous extravasation of urine from the anterior urethra. J. Urol., 117:61–64, 1977.
47. Weens, H.S., Newman, J.H., and Florence, T.J.: Trauma of the lower urinary tract: a roentgenologic study. N. Engl. J. Med., 234:357–364, 1946.
48. Wesson, M.B.: Fasciae of the urogenital triangle. J.A.M.A., 81:2024–2030, 1923.
49. Wesson, M.B.: The clinical importance of Buck's and Colles' fasciae. Surg. Gynecol. Obstet., 44:208–213, 1927.
50. Wilkey, J.L., Barson, L.J., and Portney, F.R.: Urinary extravasation and periurethral phlegmon: Clinical analysis of 100 cases. J. Urol., 82:657–658, 1959.

Foreign Bodies in the Urethra

51. Beilin, L.M.: Genital self-mutilation by mental patients. J. Urol., 70:648–655, 1953.
52. Campbell, M.F.: Needles in deep urethra. Am. J. Surg., 21:452–453, 1933.
53. Gordon, L.Z.: Safety pins in male urethra. Urol. Cutan. Rev., 45:500–501, 1941.
54. Gutierrez, R.: Unusually long foreign body impacted in the urethra for 7 days. Removal and cure by external urethrotomy. J. Urol., 49:865–871, 1943.
55. Jeck, H.S.: Removal of foreign bodies from urethra and bladder. Am. J. Surg., 36:197–203, 1937.
56. Poulet, A.: Male urethra, pp. 113–144. In A Treatise on Foreign Bodies in Surgical Practice, Vol. 2. William Wood, New York, 1880.
57. Riley, A.: Foreign bodies in male urethra. Report of an unusual case. N. Engl. J. Med., 218:884–885, 1938.
58. Simon, S.: Rifle bullet impacted in the anterior urethra. J. Urol., 61:785–789, 1949.
59. Stabler, A.A.: Foreign bodies in urethra. Six-penny nails present for twelve years. J. Urol., 55:397–400, 1946.
60. Zeitlin, A.B., Cottrell, T.L., and Lloyd, F.A.: Hair as a lower urinary tract foreign body. J. Urol., 77:840–842, 1957.

Urethral Calculi

61. Amin, H.A.: Urethral calculi. Br. J. Urol., 45:192–199, 1973.
62. DeCarvalho, H.A.: Giant urethral calculus: A case report. J. Urol., 118:334–335, 1977.
63. Godwin, R.J.: Urethral stone formation after urethroplasty. Br. J. Radiol., 50:113–115, 1973.
64. Hassan, R.M.: Giant urethral calculus: A case report. J. Urol., 115:756–757, 1976.
65. Hussein, A.A.: Urethral calculi. Br. J. Urol., 45:192, 1973.
66. Joly, J.S.: Stone and Calculus Disease of the Urinary Organ, 2nd ed. C.V. Mosby, St. Louis, 1940.
67. Lowsley, O.S., and Gentile, A.: Urethral calculus in the male, with particular reference to giant primary stones. Urol. Cutan. Rev., 54:1–7, 1950.
68. Reddy: M.M., and Bai, D.M.: Urethral calculi in children. J. Ind. Med. Assoc., 66:173–175, 1976.

CLASSIFICATION OF STRICTURES

A urethral stricture is a pathologic diminution of the lumen of the urethra that also may represent lack of distensibility. Strictures may be congenital, inflammatory, traumatic, or neoplastic.

Congenital lesions (Figs. 41–1 to 41–6) are found most commonly at the external urethral meatus, often associated with hypospadiac orifices,[7] but the membranous urethra and the penoscrotal junction are frequently involved. It is seen in both sexes but is more common in the male.

Inflammatory strictures (Figs. 41–7 to 41–17) may be caused by gonorrhea, tuberculosis, syphilis, or nonspecific infections. It has been stated that approximately 75 per cent of inflammatory strictures occur at the bulbomembranous junction although no area is immune.

Tuberculosis is a spread from another focus, usually higher up in the urinary tract and most likely from the prostate (Fig. 41–17). The urethra appears to be particularly resistant to tuberculous infection, but when strictures occur they are intractable and often associated with fistula formation and abscesses.

Traumatic strictures (Figs. 41–18 to 41–20) are the result of tears or ruptures of the urethra caused by blows on the perineum, ruptured pelvis, or instrumentation. They can occur anywhere in the anterior or the membranous urethra, but they are probably most common in the bulbomembranous area. Chemical strictures, which should be considered to be traumatic, usually occur in the anterior urethra. Traumatic strictures develop much more rapidly than do the inflammatory types. Iatrogenic strictures are a common form of traumatic stricture of the urethra in children and adults secondary to instrumentation (see Figs. 41–36, 41–37, and 41–38).

41

Strictures of the Urethra

Neoplastic strictures are the result of primary urethral carcinoma or are secondary from the bladder or the prostate. They may occur at any place in the urethra but are most common in the bulbomembranous area. (See Chapter 42, Tumors of the Urethra.)

APPEARANCE ON URETHROGRAPHY

Voiding cystourethrograms are used best to demonstrate dilatation behind a stricture, but the injection method best demonstrates the stricture itself. Although strictures may be diagnosed by the insertion of an instrument into the urethra, important information, such as length, caliber, location, and multiplicity, cannot be obtained without the use of urethrograms.

Strictures of the urethra appear as narrowed segments, varying in length and appearance from valve-like structures (appearing as valve-like indentations on either side) to long constrictions. Eleven per cent are multiple. The congenital variety is single, usually short and regular in appearance. The inflammatory stricture may be single or, more commonly, multiple; it may be short or long; and it appears to be more irregular than either the congenital or the traumatic type. Occasionally, the inflammatory stricture resulting from a periurethral abscess does not appear to be especially narrowed but represents lack of distensibility of the urethra because of the marked periurethral fibrosis. The traumatic stricture can be single or multiple but more commonly is single. The stricture may be long or short and tends to be rather smooth. Neoplastic strictures are irregular, long, and tend to occur with fistulous formation.

FALSE PASSAGES

False passages (Figs. 41–7 to 41–9, 41–21 to 41–23) are produced by internal injuries of the urethra, usually secondary to instrumentation. They usually occur in the region of the bulbous and membranous urethra and are found most commonly on the inferior side of the urethra, appearing as irregular outpocketings extending proximally. They often are associated with strictures that produced the initial difficulty in passing instruments.

False passages can be demonstrated either by the voiding or the retrograde method. They must be differentiated from small urethrocavernous refluxes and from the duct of Cowper's gland. The duct of Cowper's gland is usually smooth and even, and the diameter of its lumen appears to be rather constant.

Small urethrocavernous refluxes usually are more diffuse and do not appear to have a connection with the urethra. (See Urethrocavernous Refluxes.) False passages are slightly irregular, with narrowing at the terminal point. A definite connection with the urethra can be demonstrated. Some false passages are not small but are elongated and reenter the urethra at a more proximal point (Fig. 14–22). These complete passages usually arise in the region of the bulb, extending proximally to reenter the prostatic urethra. They are irregular in caliber but may give a more or less smooth contour.

CONTRACTURE OF THE BLADDER NECK

There is a great deal of controversy concerning the occurrence and diagnosis of bladder neck obstruction. Formerly, it was believed to be an important entity in both children and adults, producing large residuals, infection, trabeculations of bladder, diverticula of bladder, and dilatation of the upper tracts, but in recent years, it has been considered rare or nonexistent.

It is no doubt true that the diagnosis has often been made on flimsy evidence or by misinterpreting the importance of distal obstruction, which is often accompanied by hypertrophy of the bladder neck. Certainly there is no necessity to correct the bladder neck in cases of urethral valves.

Even the roentgenographic findings have been questioned. Although bladder neck contracture can produce the findings described below, Shopfner could not correlate the findings with difficult voiding and other signs of obstruction and found similar changes in normals (see Chap. 36, the Normal Urethra). The diagnosis certainly cannot be made by roentgenographic means alone.

TYPES

Contracture of the bladder neck (see Figs. 36–21, 36–22 and Figs. 41–24 to 41–34), sometimes called idiopathic bladder neck obstruction (Marion's disease), may be either congenital or acquired. Campbell called these cases submucous fibrosis of the vesical outlet.[32, 33] Beer thought the fibrosis might be secondary to neuromuscular disease.[27] The Leadbetters recognized three types of obstructing tissue[46]:

1. Hypertrophic muscle tissue
2. Contracture due to the increased amount of fibrous tissue, resulting in inelasticity and decrease in the lumen of the bladder outlet
3. Chronic inflammatory changes

Bodian described a type of fibrosis in which there was submucosal fibrosis of the bladder neck, associated with an elongated prostatic tissue made up of fibroelastic fibers that extended beyond the verumontanum to the distal end of the membranous urethra.[30] The verumontanum often was enlarged in these cases, and there was at times a diminution of the muscular–glandular tissue. Bodian suggested that the elongated fibroelastic prostatic urethra rather than the collar at the bladder neck is the cause of the obstruction and not the collar at the bladder neck. Just where this category fits into the other categories is not entirely clear, but it should be noted that many authors believe that in order to correct a contracture of the bladder neck by transurethral resection, one must go distally into the urethra. This belief would fit somewhat into the concept of Bodian.

Contracture of the bladder neck is seen in boys and girls (in a ratio of about 4 to 1[34a]) or predominantly in girls.[29, 59] In children, contracture of the bladder neck often is seen with strictures of the ureterovesical juncture, often bilateral but occasionally unilateral.[34a] The obstruction at the bladder neck may involve the entire circumference or only the posterior segment, representing median bar obstruction. The ureteral orifices often appear to be closer to the bladder neck than usual, and the verumontanum may appear to be drawn up to the vesical outlet. Campbell emphasizes the importance of recognizing hypertrophy of the trigone to determine bladder neck obstruction.[34a] Often there are associated trabeculation and widespread damage to the upper tracts. The upper tract dilatation and damage may be secondary to reflux or to ureterovesical stricture.

Contracture of the bladder neck may be seen in adults, usually in the twenties and the thirties but occasionally later in life. Although some of these cases may be congenital in origin, certainly a fair percentage must be acquired, most likely being secondary to infection and often associated with chronic prostatitis in men and chronic urethritis and cystitis in women. Contracture of the bladder neck can result from prostatectomy; the postoperative contracture may be the most severe, the so-called iris-type diaphragm (Fig. 41–34). Contracture may occur also after renal transplantation.[74]

In many instances bladder neck obstruction has been a disease of exclusion. In other words, although no definite changes are seen at the bladder neck, transurethral resection may improve the patient's condition and relieve obstruction.

Urodynamics has brought a new dimension to the evaluation of bladder neck, and many of these cases may be considered bladder neck dyskinesia. For a discussion of urodynamics, see Chapter 43, Miscellaneous Conditions of the Urethra.

ROENTGENOGRAPHIC FINDINGS

Roentgenographically, contracture of the bladder neck may be impossible to demonstrate, because even moderate changes not always are visualized. It should be emphasized that roentgenography of the bladder neck area often is confusing and misleading.

The Fibrous Type. On cystourethrography there is narrowing in the region of the bladder neck with decrease of the size of the lumen on voiding. This may extend distally into the proximal urethra. There is a loss of normal funneling. Occasionally, there is an anterior angulation or a tilting in the proximal prostatic urethra, representing an elevation of the posterior lip of the bladder neck. In cases of diaphragm formation, the opening at the bladder neck is smaller, and the contrast material may produce a "toothpaste sign" in the bladder lumen.[38]

Hypertrophy of Muscle. This type of obstruction is circumferential and gives a collar-like impression on the proximal urethra. When combined with dilatation slightly distal to the point of narrowing, it has been described as "acorn" deformity or "spinning top" deformity.[63] Edwards believes that this collar-like area may be merely the bladder neck forming an impression on the lumen of the proximal urethra and not necessarily hypertrophy of the bladder neck.[35] However, the impression produced by the latter is usually much more definite, and, if correlated with cystoscopy, the diagnosis of hypertrophy can be made.

The dilatation distal to the constriction of the vesical neck has been explained in various ways:

1. Poststenotic dilatation
2. Distention of the thin-walled urethra below the internal sphincter by the powerful urinary stream[63]
3. Distal obstruction producing proximal dilatation and hypertrophy of the bladder neck[41]

Voiding cystourethrography is probably superior to the injecting method, especially in males, because the injection method usually gives a narrowed appearance to the proximal urethra, and it would be difficult to differentiate this from the narrowing of a contracture. The anterior tilting can be recognized by either method. In females findings are similar to findings in males, and both cystourethrographic techniques are reliable. Occasionally, in cases of contracture of the bladder neck, there is an elongated infracollicular portion of the prostatic urethra. This is to be compared with prostatic hypertrophy, in which the elongation is in the supracollicular portion.

DIFFERENTIAL DIAGNOSIS

Contracture of the bladder neck must be differentiated from various other obstructions in the urethra, especially valvular obstruction, congenital urethral strictures, hypertrophy of the verumontanum and sphincterospastic neuromuscular disease of the vesical orifice. The first three should be differentiated easily, but the last may be difficult. In cases of neuromuscular disease causing spastic changes at the region of the bladder neck, this condition usually is associated with anal spasm and with neurologic changes that should corroborate the diagnosis. Also, contracture of the bladder neck rarely causes the various bladder changes that are described under Neurogenic Bladder. Vesical neck obstruction can also be secondary to dyskinesia (failure to relax) or dyssynergia (inappropriate contraction) of the bladder neck. Anatomic bladder neck contraction must be differentiated from these two entities, and it is here that urodynamic studies as well as cystoscopy and cystourethrography are essential.

POSTOPERATIVE DIAPHRAGM FORMATION

Greene and Robinson[38] have reported a typical cystourethrographic finding of the diaphragm type of contracture producing a so-called toothpaste sign (Fig. 41–34).[38]

DISTAL URETHRAL STENOSIS

Distal urethral stenosis (DUS) is probably a fibrous ring in the distal urethra in females producing a narrowing at the distal urethra proximal to the external urethral meatus (see Figs. 36–23 to 36–25 and Fig. 41–35). This fibrous ring may be close to the meatus or up to 1 cm. proximal to it. This narrowing may not always be a definite abnormality, but certainly severe narrowings are significant. As discussed in Chapter 36, Shopfner has emphasized that the same cystourethrographic appearance may be seen in normal persons.

MEATAL STENOSIS

Meatal stenosis may be seen in both males and females but is much more common in the male (see Figs. 41–1 to 41–3, 41–16). It can cause a severe dilatation proximal to the lesion. Meatal stenosis can be either congenital or secondary to infection or trauma. It has often been associated with hypospadiac openings.

CHAPTER 41, ILLUSTRATIONS

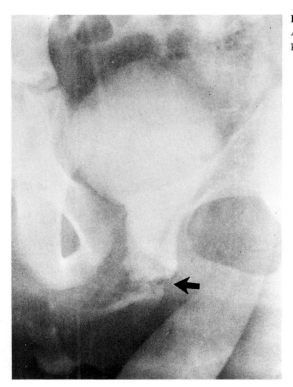

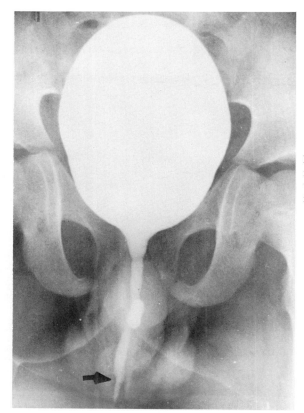

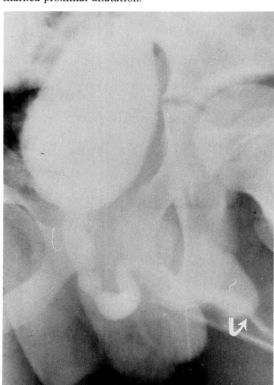

FIG. 41–1. External meatal urethral stenosis in a girl. *Arrow* points to area of constriction. There is marked proximal dilatation.

FIG. 41–2. Congenital external urethral stenosis in a girl. *Arrow* points to area of constriction. There is marked proximal dilatation.

FIG. 41–3. Congenital stricture of the urethra. AP view, revealing narrowing of the terminal portion of the urethra in a 2½-year-old boy. Stricture just proximal to fossa navicularis.

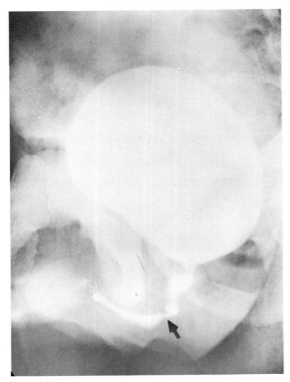

FIG. 41–4. Congenital urethral stricture. Voiding cysto-urethrogram reveals a narrowing at the bulbo-membranous junction (*arrow*) with dilatation prox-imally. Oblique view. This must be differentiated from muscularis compressor nudea, in which there is no per-sistent proximal dilatation.

FIG. 41–6. Congenital bulbomembranous stricture in a young man with irregularity of the urethra proximally, secondary to infection. (Courtesy of Jesse Keshin, M.D.)

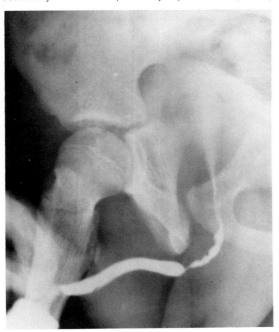

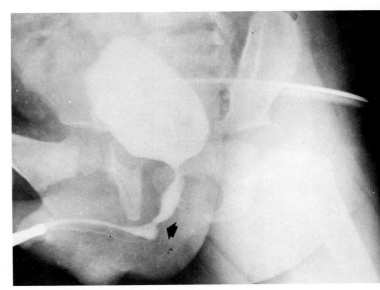

FIG. 41–5. Congenital urethral stricture. Injecting urethrogram. Arrow points to stricture at bulbo-membranous junction. Oblique view. Note dilated posterior urethra.

Fig. 41–7. Inflammatory stricture of the bulbo-membranous area and false passage. Suprapubic drainage. (A) Left oblique view. Injecting cys-tourethrogram. Calculi of prostatic area. One *arrow* points to stricture, and the other points to a false pas-sage. Note irregularity of anterior urethra. (B) Voiding cystourethrogram. Marked dilatation proximal to the stricture, with contrast-filled prostatic ducts surround-ing the prostatic calculi. *Arrows* point to stricture and false passage. (Edling, N.P.G.: Acta Radiol. Suppl., 58:5, 1944)

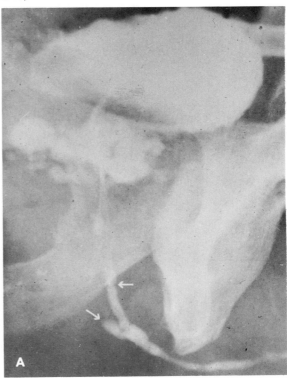

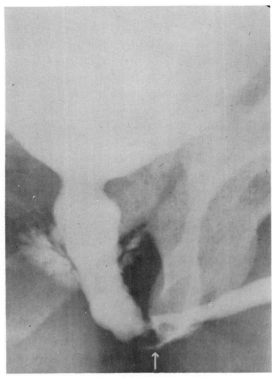

FIG. 41-8. Inflammatory stricture of the bulbo-membranous juncture and a false passage (*arrow*). Voiding cystourethrogram shows proximal dilatation of the urethra with filling of the prostatic ducts. (Edling, N.P.G.: Acta Radiol. Suppl., *58*:5, 1944)

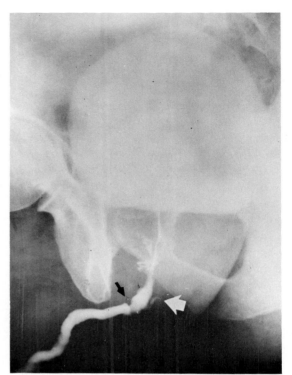

FIG. 41-9. Gonorrheal stricture of the urethra in distal bulbous area (*black arrow*). Prostatic ducts visualized. *Large white arrow* points to a structure arising in the region of the bulbous urethra. The differential diagnosis of this structure includes urethrocavernous reflux, false passage, or Cowper's duct. Its caliber varies, for it gets more narrow as the distal portion is reached. However, it is well defined, and although the communication to the urethra is not easily discernible, it is definitely present. We favor a false passage in this case.

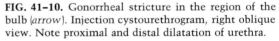

FIG. 41-10. Gonorrheal stricture in the region of the bulb (*arrow*). Injection cystourethrogram, right oblique view. Note proximal and distal dilatation of urethra.

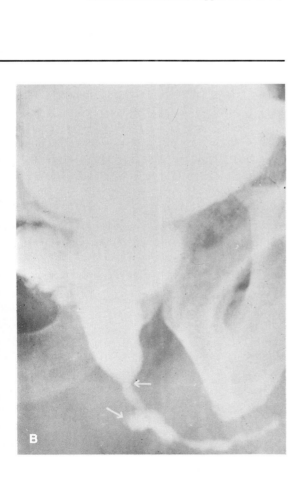

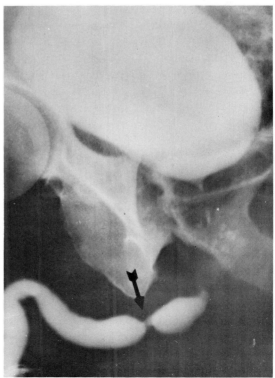

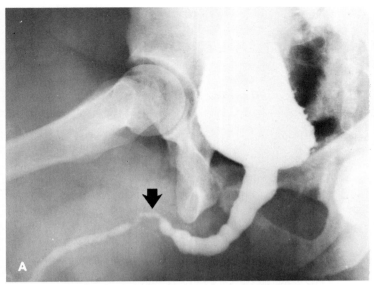

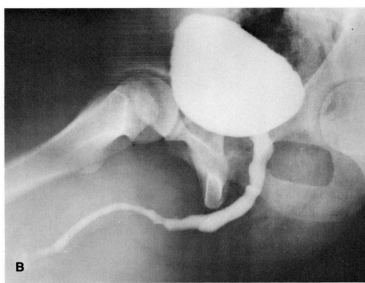

FIG. 41–11. Gonorrheal stricture in anterior urethra. **(A)** Voiding cystourethrogram showing a stricture of the urethra with proximal dilatation (*arrow*). **(B)** Postoperative cystourethrogram showing disappearance of stricture. (Courtesy of Keith Waterhouse, M.D.)

FIG. 41–12. Gonorrheal stricture, bulbomembranous juncture (*white arrow*). Injecting cystourethrogram, right oblique view. There are also urethrocavernous reflux and a communicating vein (*black arrow*) that can be seen with the dorsal vein of the penis clearly outlined. The posterior urethra is elongated due to benign prostatic hypertrophy.

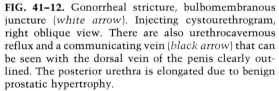

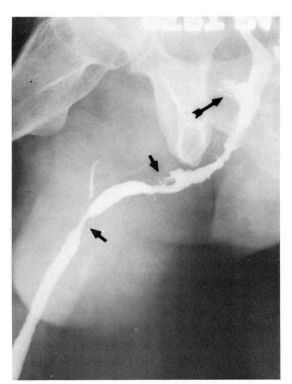

FIG. 41–13. Multiple strictures of the anterior urethra due to a gonorrheal infection. The two *small arrows* point to the strictures in the anterior urethra and at the bulb. The *large arrow* indicates the prostatic ducts.

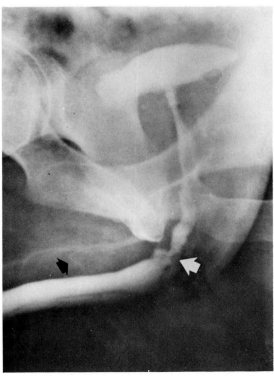

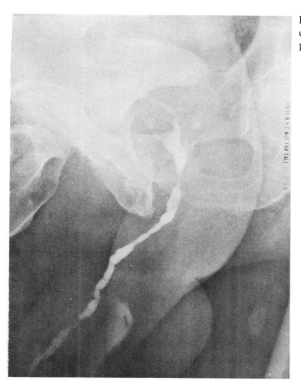

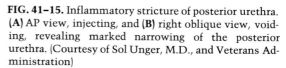

FIG. 41–14. Multiple strictures of the anterior urethra due to nonspecific inflammation. Note spreading of posterior urethra due to enlarged prostate.

FIG. 41–15. Inflammatory stricture of posterior urethra. **(A)** AP view, injecting, and **(B)** right oblique view, voiding, revealing marked narrowing of the posterior urethra. (Courtesy of Sol Unger, M.D., and Veterans Administration)

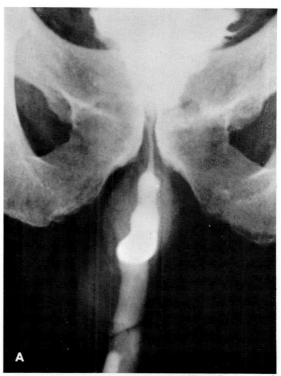

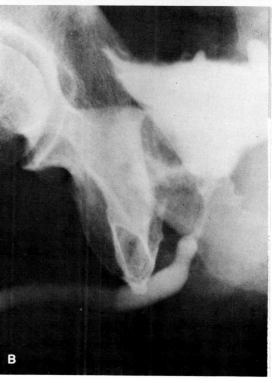

FIG. 41–16. External urethral meatal stenosis (*arrow*) in an elderly woman secondary to infection. Note dilatation proximally.

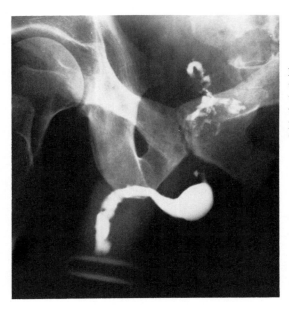

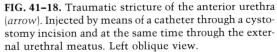

FIG. 41–17. Tuberculous stricture of the urethra. Multiple irregularities of penile urethra with proximal dilatation in region of bulb. There is also a prostatic urethral stricture with contrast medium entering the prostate, which is extremely irregular. (Courtesy of J.G. Gow, M.D.)

FIG. 41–18. Traumatic stricture of the anterior urethra (*arrow*). Injected by means of a catheter through a cystostomy incision and at the same time through the external urethral meatus. Left oblique view.

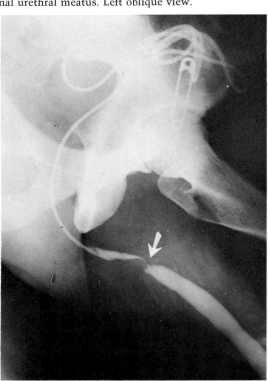

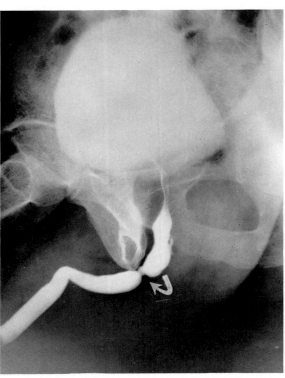

FIG. 41–19. Traumatic stricture of the anterior urethra (*arrow*). The tubelike structure coming off the floor of the bulbous urethra has an even caliber and definitely connects with the urethra. This was thought to be a Cowper's duct. Right oblique view.

FIG. 41–20. Chemical strictures of distal anterior urethra as a result of installation of corrosive substance. (Beard, E.E., Goodyear, W.E., Weens, H.S.: Radiologic Diagnosis of the Lower Urinary Tract. Springfield, Ill., Charles C Thomas, 1952)

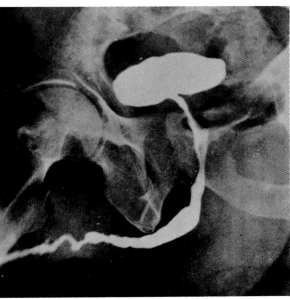

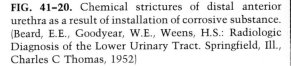

1740

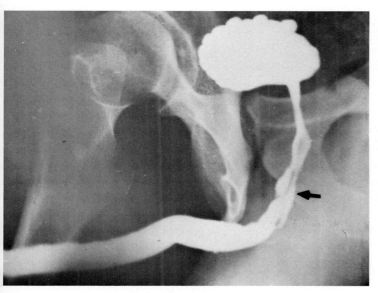

FIG. 41–21. False passage of urethra. *Arrow* points to a false passage arising from the floor of the bulbous urethra and joining the urethra again in the prostatic area. Note trabeculated bladder. Right oblique view. Injecting cystourethrogram. (Courtesy of E.E. Beard, M.D. and W.E. Goodyear, M.D.)

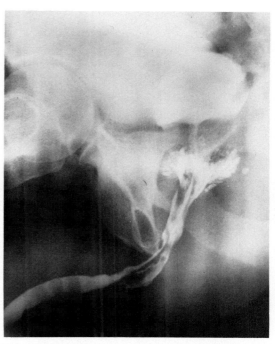

FIG. 41–22. False passage secondary to repeated passage of sounds and a stricture of the bulbomembranous urethra. Note filling of prostatic ducts on injecting cystourethrogram.

FIG. 41–23. Stricture of the urethra at bulbomembranous juncture with a false passage from the area of the stricture to the bladder neck. **(A)** AP view injecting; **(B)** right oblique view injecting.

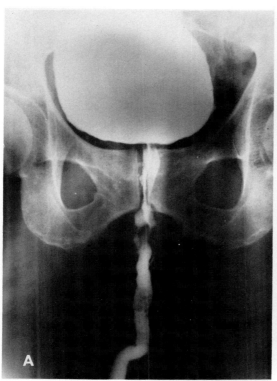

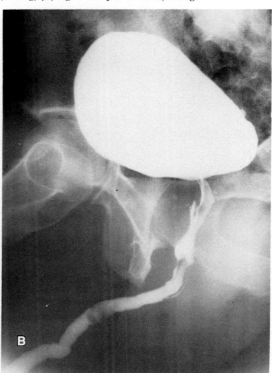

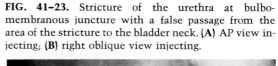

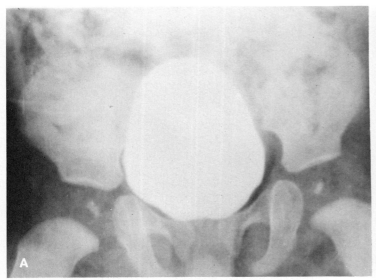

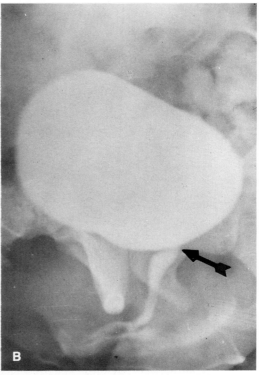

FIG. 41–24. Ten-month-old boy with a contracture of the bladder neck. **(A)** Cystogram. Notice the slight elevation in the midline at the floor of the bladder. **(B)** Voiding cystourethrogram showing extreme narrowing of the posterior urethra in the region of the bladder neck (*arrow*). Note the elongation of the posterior urethra.

FIG. 41–25. Contracture of the bladder neck (hypertrophy of musculature) in a 4-year-old girl. **(A)** AP view. Voiding cystourethrogram reveals a collar in the region of the bladder neck. This is called "acorn" or "spinning top" deformity. **(B)** Oblique view. Voiding cystourethrogram reveals an extremely narrow posterior urethra at the bladder neck. The bladder is slightly irregular in both views due to trabeculation. The *arrows* point to the region of the hypertrophy of the musculature of the bladder neck in both instances.

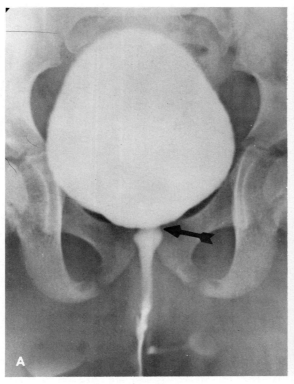

FIG. 41–26. Eight-month-old girl with marked bladder neck contraction. Cystogram reveals a large trabeculated bladder, bilateral vesicoureteral reflux, hydroureters with marked tortuosity and huge hydronephrosis. Note slight indentation of bladder neck.

FIG. 41–27. Cystourethrogram in a young boy demonstrates the extreme narrowing in the region of the posterior urethra and the bladder neck due to contracture. Note irregular bladder.

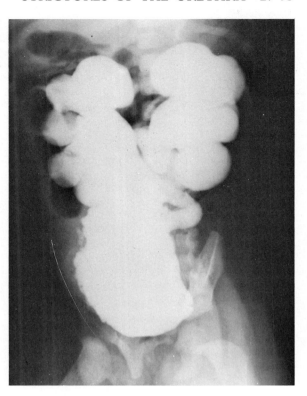

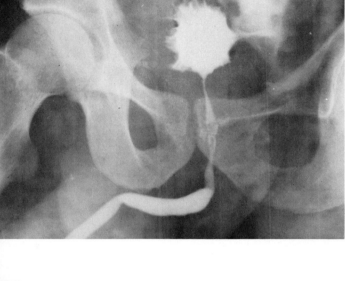

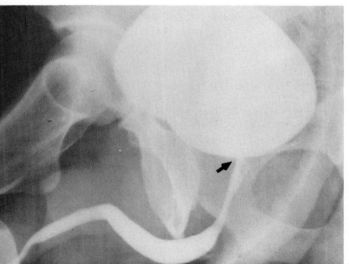

FIG. 41–28. Early contracture of the bladder neck in a 36-year-old man. Voiding cystourethrogram reveals only moderate narrowing in the region of the bladder neck (*arrow*). Note shortened prostatic urethra. Verumontanum lies slightly below bladder floor.

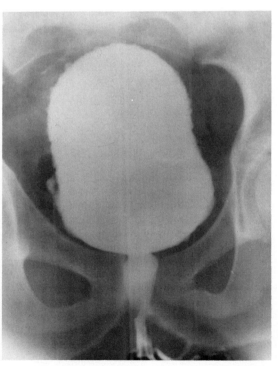

FIG. 41–29. Narrowing at bladder neck, dilatation distally.

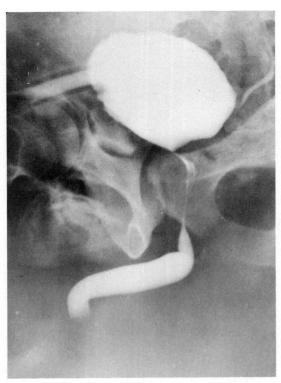

FIG. 41–30. Severe contracture of bladder neck in 40-year-old man. Cystostomy tube in place following cystolithotomy for large bladder stone. Voiding cystourethrogram. Note narrowed and shortened proximal urethra with anterior tilting at bladder neck and reflux up left ureter. Patient voiding against resistance. The infracollicular portion of the prostatic urethra is elongated.

FIG. 41–31. Contracture of the bladder neck in a 62-year-old man, 3 years post prostatectomy, who developed difficulty in voiding. Voiding cystourethrogram. Marked narrowing in the region of the bladder neck (*arrow*). Slight elevation of bladder floor.

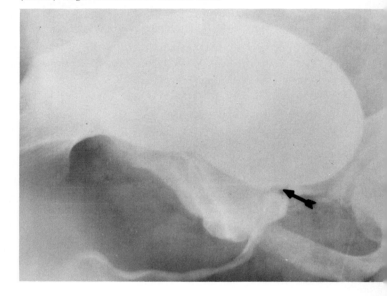

FIG. 41–32. Contracture of bladder neck in a 45-year-old man. Marked difficulty in voiding, with 5 moderate-sized stones in the bladder, which are not visualized. (**A**) Injecting cystourethrogram. *Arrow* points to an extremely narrow prostatic urethra at the bladder neck. (**B**) Voiding cystourethrogram. *Arrow* points to the extremely narrow urethra in the region of the bladder neck with no funneling. Note elongated infracollicular portion of the prostatic urethra.

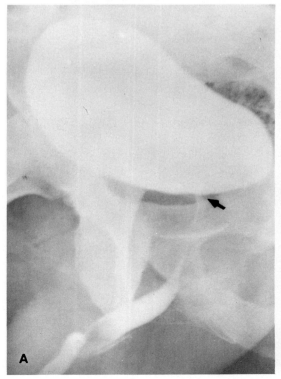

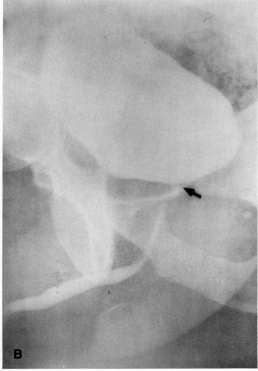

A

B

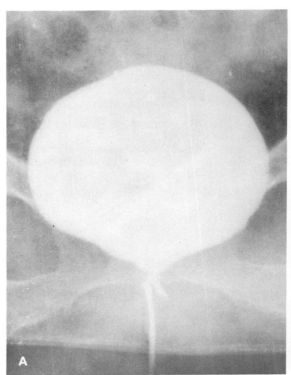

FIG. 41–33. Injecting cystourethrogram in a 75-year-old woman with contracture of the bladder neck and a stone in the bladder. (**A**) AP view. The proximal urethra and the bladder neck are obscured by a small cystocele. (**B**) Right oblique view. *Arrow* points to region of bladder neck, which is rigid and nondilatable.

FIG. 41–34. Post-transurethral resection contracture of the bladder neck, diaphragm formation. Layering out of contrast medium in bladder produces the "toothpaste sign." (Greene, L.F., Robinson, H.P.: J. Urol., *110*:297, 1973)

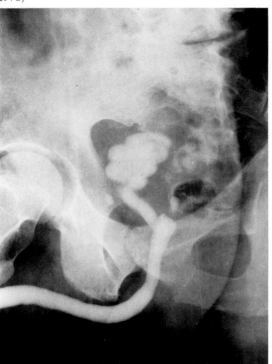

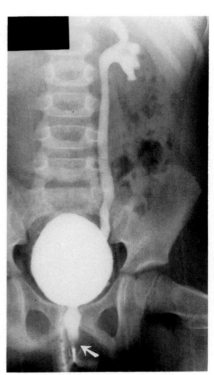

FIG. 41–35. DUS in a girl (*arrow*) producing proximal dilatation associated with vesicoureteral reflux.

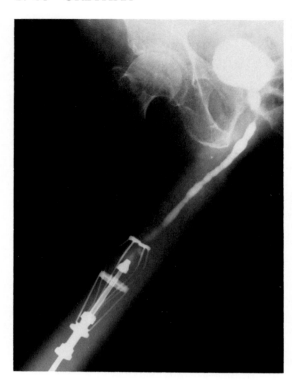

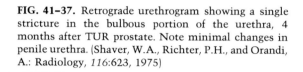

FIG. 41–36. Postoperative (TUR prostate) retrograde urethrogram demonstrates multiple postoperative changes in the urethra of a 73-year-old patient who had no symptoms or obstruction. (Shaver, W.A., Richter, P.H., Orandi, A.: Radiology, *116*:623, 1975)

FIG. 41–37. Retrograde urethrogram showing a single stricture in the bulbous portion of the urethra, 4 months after TUR prostate. Note minimal changes in penile urethra. (Shaver, W.A., Richter, P.H., and Orandi, A.: Radiology, *116*:623, 1975)

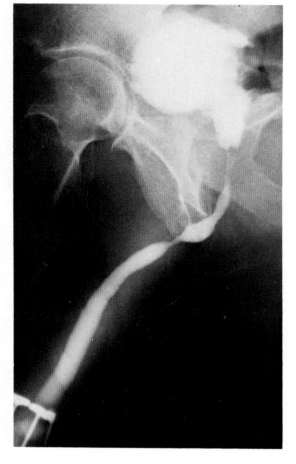

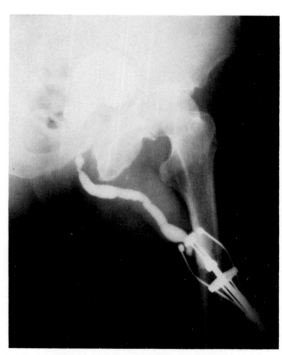

FIG. 41–38. Postoperative (TUR) retrograde urethrogram demonstrates the most common finding of multiple changes throughout the urethra. (Shaver, W.A., Richter, P.H., and Orandi, A.: Radiology, *116*:623, 1975)

BIBLIOGRAPHY

Congenital Urethral Strictures

1. Campbell, M.F.: Strictures of the urethra in children. J. Pediatr., *35*:169-179, 1949.
2. Cobb, B.G., Wolf, J.A., Jr., and Ansell, J.S.: Congenital strictures of the proximal urethral bulb. J. Urol., *99*:629-631, 1968.
3. Crowell, W.M., and Anderson, R.H.: Congenital urethral stricture. Clin. Proc. Child. Hosp. (Wash.), *6*:68-73, 1950.
4. Devereaux, M.H., and Williams, D.I.: The treatment of urethral stricture in boys. J. Urol., *108*:489-493, 1972.
5. Engel, W.J., and Schlumberger, F.C.: Urinary extravasations in new-born infant associated with congenital stenosis of the urethra; report of case. Cleveland Clin. Quart., *5*:278-283, 1938.
6. Koch, L.A.: Projectile vomiting and intoxication in the new-born infant. Am. J. Dis. Child., *60*:917-922, 1940.
7. Lattimer, J.K.: Similar urogenital anomalies in identical twins. Am. J. Dis. Child., *67*:199-200, 1944.
8. Leadbetter, G.W., Jr., and Leadbetter, W.F.: Urethral strictures in male children. J. Urol., *87*:409-415, 1962.
9. Netto, N.R., Jr., Martucci, R.C., and Goncalves, E.S., et al.: Congenital stricture of male urethra. Int. Urol. Nephrol., *8*:55-61, 1976.
10. Rao, K.G.: Congenital proximal bulbar stricture in adults. Urology, *6*:576-579, 1975.
11. Stephens, F.D.: Proceedings: Urethral obstruction in children. Br. J. Urol., *47*:231, 1975.

Inflammatory Strictures

12. Chambers, R.M.: Tuberculous urethral fistula. Br. J. Urol., *43*:243-248, 1971.
13. Dourmashkin, R.L.: Urethral stricture: A study of 227 cases. J. Urol., *68*:496-505, 1952.
14. Edling, N.P.G.: Urethrocystography in the male, with special regard to micturition. Acta Radiol. (Stockholm) (Suppl.), *58*:1-144, 1945.
15. Kibukamusoke, J.W.: Gonorrhea and urethral stricture. Br. J. Ven. Dis., *41*:135-136, 1965.
16. LeBrun, H.I.: Tuberculous urethral stricture. Br. J. Urol., *30*:82-86, 1958.
17. Rose, J.L.: Renal tuberculosis. Br. J. Urol., *25*:279-292, 1953.
18. Symes, J.M., and Blandy, J.P.: Tuberculosis of the male urethra. Br. J. Urol., *45*:432-436, 1973.

Traumatic Strictures

19. Beard, O.E., Goodyear, W.E., and Weens, H.S.: Radiologic Diagnosis of the Lower Urinary Tract. Charles C Thomas, Springfield, 1952.
20. Lentz, H.C., Jr., Mebust, W.K., Foret, J.D., et al.: Urethral stricture following transurethral prostatectomy. Review of 2223 resections. J. Urol., *117*:194-196, 1977.
21. Shaver, W.A., Richter, P.H., and Orandi, A.: Changes in the male urethra produced by instrumentation for transurethral resection of the prostate. Radiology, *116*:623-626, 1975.
22. Warres, H.L.: Urethral stricture following transurethral resection of the prostate. J. Urol., *79*:989-993, 1958.

Bladder Neck Obstruction

23. Andreassen, M.: Vesical neck obstruction in children. Acta Chir. Scand., *105*:398-406, 1953.
24. Baker, R., et al.: Observations on 100 children with bladder neck obstruction. J. Urol., *84*:334-339, 1960.
25. Bapna, B.C., Singh, S.M., Chally, R., et al.: Bladder neck obstruction in children. Indian J. Pediatr., *37*:11-14, 1970.
25a. Bates, C.P., Arnold, E.P., and Griffiths, D.J.: The nature of the abnormality in bladder neck obstruction. Br. J. Urol., *47*:651-656, 1975.
26. Bateson, E.M.: Bladder neck stenosis—the value of descending cystourethrography in the demonstration of the complications of inflammatory urethral stricture. Br. J. Radiol., *43*:718, 1970.
27. Beer, E.: Chronic retention of urine in children. J.A.M.A., *65*:1709-1712, 1915.
28. Beer, E.: Chronic retention of urine in young boys due to obstruction at the neck of the bladder. Ann. Surg., *79*:264-268, 1924.
29. Berman, L.B., Crotty, J.J., and Tina, L.U.: The pediatric implications of bladder neck obstructions. Pediatrics, *28*:816-821, 1961.
30. Bodian, M.: Some observations on the pathology of congenital "ideopathic bladder neck obstruction" (Marion's disease). Br. J. Urol., *29*:393-398, 1957.
31. Burns, E., and Shashy, P.: Problems in management of bladder neck obstruction in children. Ohio Med. J., *53*:170-175, 1957.
32. Campbell, M.F.: Submucous fibrosis of the bladder outlet in infancy and childhood. J.A.M.A., *94*:1373-1378, 1930.
33. Campbell, M.F.: Pediatric Urology, Vol. 1, p. 354. Macmillan, New York, 1937.
34. Campbell, M.F.: Congenital bladder neck obstruction. South. Med. J., *41*:99-107, 1948.
34a. Campbell, M.F.: Urology, 2nd ed. Vol. 2, pp. 1689-1694. Saunders, Philadelphia, 1963.
35. Edwards, D.: Cine-radiology of congenital bladder neck obstruction and the megaureter. Br. J. Urol., *29*:410-415, 1957.
36. Fister, G.M.: Fibrosis and submucous calcification of the vesical neck. J.A.M.A., *118*:604-608, 1942.
37. Greene, L.F., Robinson, H.P., and Campbell, J.C.: Post-operative contracture of the neck of the bladder. Am. Acad. Gen. Pract. (Abstr.), pp. 431-432, 1961.
38. Greene, L.F., and Robinson, H.P.: Postoperative contracture of the vesical neck. V. Clinical findings, symptoms and diagnosis. J. Urol., *94*:141-147, 1965.
38a. Greene, L.F., and Robinson, H.P.: Corticosteroid therapy of postoperative contracture of the vesical neck. J. Urol., *110*:297-298, 1973.
39. Gross, R.E., Randolph, J., and Wise, H.M., Jr.: Surgical correction of bladder-neck obstruction in children. N. Engl. J. Med., *268*:5-14, 1963.
40. Gute, D.B., Chute, R., and Baron, J.A., Jr.: Bladder neck revision for obstruction in men: a clinical study reporting normal ejaculation postoperatively. J. Urol., *99*:744-749, 1968.
41. Hamm, F.C., and Waterhouse, K.: Changing concepts in lower urinary tract obstruction in children. J.A.M.A., *175*:854-857, 1961.
42. Hanten, J.S., Galuszka, A.A., and Rotner, M.: Vesical neck contracture in children. J. Urol., *82*:218-223, 1959.
43. Harrow, B.R.: The rarity of bladder-neck obstruction in children. J. Pediatr., *69*:853-854, 1966.

44. Jain, A.C., Renoirte, P., and Hennebert, P.: Observations on obstructive disorders of lower urinary tract in Congolese infants and children: A report on 33 cases. Acta Urol. Belg., 36:383–398, 1968.

45. Keitzer, W.A., and Benavent, C.: Bladder neck obstruction in children. J. Urol., 89:384–388, 1963.

46. Leadbetter, G.W., and Leadbetter, W.F.: Diagnosis and treatment of congenital bladder neck obstruction in children. N. Engl. J. Med., 260:633–637, 1959.

47. Marion, G.: Traite d'Urologie, Vol. 1, pp. 660–667, vol. 2, p. 1043, Fig. 386. Masson, Paris, 1933.

48. Marion, G.: Traite d'Urologie, 4th ed. Masson, Paris, 1940.

49. Murphy, J.J., and Schoenberg, H.W.: Diagnosis of bladder outlet obstruction. J.A.M.A., 175:354–357, 1961.

50. Nanson, E.N.: Marion's disease of bladder neck stenosis. Aust. New Zeal. J. Surg., 20:215–223, 1951.

51. Nesbit, R.M., and Crenshaw, W.B.: Treatment of bladder neck contracture by plastic operation. J. Urol., 73:516–519, 1955.

52. Nunn, I.N.: Bladder neck obstruction in children. J. Urol., 93:693–699, 1965.

53. Presman, D., Ross, L.S., and Nicosia, S.V.: Fibromuscular hyperplasia of the posterior urethra: a cause for lower urinary tract obstruction in male children. J. Urol., 107:149–153, 1972.

54. Reisman, D.D.: Bladder neck obstructions in children. J.A.M.A., 188:1057–1061, 1964.

55. Robinson, H.P., and Greene, L.F.: Post-operative contracture of the vesical neck. II. Experimental production of contractures in dogs. J. Urol., 87:610–616, 1962.

56. Smith, D.R.: Critique on the concept of vesical neck obstruction in children. J.A.M.A., 207:1686–1692, 1969.

57. Thomas, G.K.: Marion's disease (contracture) of the bladder neck. J. Urol., 82:523–530, 1959.

58. Thompson, G.J.: Urinary obstruction of vesical neck and posterior urethra of congenital origin. J. Urol., 47:591–601, 1942.

59. Thompson, H.T.: Obstruction of the vesical neck in children. N.Y. J. Med., 56:361–366, 1956.

60. Thompson, H.T.: Obstruction of the vesical neck in children. N.Y. J. Med., 59:4377–4386, 1959.

61. Uson, A.C., et al.: A classification of the urographic patterns in children with congenital bladder neck obstruction. Am. J. Roentgenol., 80:590–602, 1958.

62. Williams, D.I.: Congenital bladder neck obstruction and megaureter: Clinical observations. Br. J. Urol., 29:389–392, 1957.

63. Williams, D.I., and Sturdy, D.E.: Recurrent urinary infection in girls. Arch. Dis. Child., 36:130–136, 1961.

64. Young, B.W., and Groebel, J.L.: Retropubic wedge excision in congenital vesical neck obstruction. Stanford Med. Bull., 12:106–123, 1954.

Distal Urethral Stenosis

65. Graham, J.B., King, L.R., Kroopp, K.A., et al.: The significance of distal urethral narrowing in young girls. J. Urol., 97:1045–1049, 1967.

66. Lyon, R.P., and Smith, D.R.: Distal urethral stenosis. J. Urol., 89:414–421, 1963.

67. Lyon, R.P., and Tanagho, E.A.: Distal urethral stenosis in little girls. J. Urol., 93:379–387, 1965.

Meatal Stenosis

68. Allen, J.S., and Summers, J.L.: Meatal stenosis in children. J. Urol., 112:526–527, 1974.

Strictures and Cystourethrography

69. Bissada, N.K., and Redman, J.F.: Simultaneous retrograde and antegrade urethrography in urethral strictures. Urology, 6:493, 1975.

70. Lapides, J., and Stone, T.E.: Usefulness of retrograde urethrography in diagnosing strictures of the anterior urethra. J. Urol., 100:747–750, 1968.

71. More, S.B.: Urinary meatal stenosis. Br. Med. J., 1:248, 1972.

72. Noe, H.N.: Evaluation of children with meatal stenosis. J. Urol., 114:455–456, 1975.

73. Uehling, D.T., and King, L.R.: Limitations in the diagnostic value of the voiding cystourethrogram. J. Pediatr., 69:744–746, 1966.

Urethral Strictures Post Renal Transplantation

74. Loening, S.A., Banowsky, L.H., Braun, W.E., et al.: Bladder neck contracture and urethral stricture as complications of renal transplantation. J. Urol., 114:688–691, 1975.

75. McLoughlin, M.G.: Outlet obstruction in the transplant patient. J. Urol., 115:632–633, 1976.

CARCINOMA OF THE MALE URETHRA

Carcinomas are uncommon lesions occurring in the penile urethra (group I) or bulbomembranous or prostatic urethra (group II), which is the more common.[1-24] Most are epidermoid in type but transitional cell and adenocarcinoma have been reported.[22, 23] The most common symptoms are decrease in caliber of urinary stream and palpable mass. Hematuria, urethral discharge, and hematospermia are infrequent. In group II, perineal fistulas occur. Many have been treated for strictures for years, but whether the stricture antedated the tumor or the tumor was the cause of the stricture is not known. Melanoma is extremely rare and occurs in the distal urethra.[2, 6, 9]

STAGING

A carcinoma of the male urethra is staged as follows[21]:

Stage O: Confined to mucosa only

Stage A: Into but not beyond lamina propria

Stage B: Into but not beyond substance of corpus spongiosum or into but not beyond prostate

Stage C: Direct extension into tissue beyond corpus spongiosum (corpus cavernosum, muscle, fat, fascia, skin, direct skeletal involvement) or beyond prostatic capsule

Stage D_1: Regional metastases including inguinal and/or pelvic lymph nodes (with any primary tumor)

Stage D_2: Distant metastases (with any primary tumor)

Investigation includes urethrography, endoscopy, transurethral resection and open biopsies, and cytologic examination of urethral secretions, washings, or urine.

42

Tumors of the Urethra

Group I usually includes epidermoid tumors. Those with clinically suspected inguinal lymph node metastases are found to really have these metastases (different from penile carcinoma). The prognosis is good—66 per cent survived 5 to 10 years without evidence of neoplasm.[21]

Group II includes bulbous, bulbomembranous, membranous, and prostatic tumors. The tumors are usually epidermoid in type. The prognosis is poor— only approximately 20 per cent are free of disease after treatment.

Diagnosis is more difficult in the male, probably because of the location of the carcinoma. The radiographic findings on a cystourethrogram vary, depending on whether the patient has been dilated for a long period of time for what was thought to be a stricture (Figs. 42–1 to 42–5). In these cases, there is an irregular narrowing often associated with extravasation of contrast medium into the tumor mass, which grows outside the urethral lumen. In the cases without a preceding history of stricture, there is an irregular narrowing of the urethra with uneven distribution of contrast medium around nodules of tumor tissue.

CARCINOMA OF THE FEMALE URETHRA

Primary carcinomas of the female urethra are classified as anterior (vulvourethral) and posterior urethral tumors.[25-50] Anterior urethral tumors are confined to the distal third of the urethra but may involve the vestibule. Posterior tumors are situated posteriorly near the bladder neck. Urethral tumors in women occur in patients over 50 years of age. Symptoms are hematuria, frequency, dysuria, incontinence, tenesmus, urinary retention, pain, and a mass. Squamous cell carcinoma is the most common tumor. Adenocarcinoma,[50] transitional cell carcinomas, mucoid carcinomas,[26, 39] mesonephric carcinomas,[36] and melanomas may occur rarely. The tumors involving the external meatal area metastasize to superficial and deep inguinal lymph nodes. The more proximal tumors spread to the hypogastric, external iliac, and sacral nodes. Distal spread is late.

Anterior urethral tumors have a 5-year survival rate of 40 per cent; posterior tumors, 17 per cent.[31] Peterson found 52 per cent and 25 per cent survival, respectively.[42] Strictures do not appear as prominently as in the male.

STAGING

The stages of carcinoma of the female urethra are defined as follows[27]:

Stage O: In situ (limited to mucosa)
Stage A: Submucosal (not beyond submucosa)
Stage B: Muscular (infiltrating periurethral muscle)
Stage C: Periurethral
  1. Infiltrating muscular wall of vagina
  2. Infiltrating muscular wall of vagina with invasion of vaginal mucosa
  3. Infiltrating other adjacent structures such as bladder, labia, and clitoris
Stage D: Metastasis
  1. Inguinal lymph nodes
  2. Pelvic lymph nodes below aortic bifurcation
  3. Lymph nodes above aortic bifurcation
  4. Distant

ROENTGENOGRAPHIC DIAGNOSIS

Roentgenographic diagnosis of female urethral carcinomas is not entirely satisfactory because of the short female urethra. These tumors are more adequately diagnosed by cystoscopic means.

POLYPS OF THE URETHRA

Urethral polyps are solid, epithelialized tumors situated in the posterior urethra in males, usually near the verumontanum (Figs. 42–6 to 42–9).[51-66] It is essentially a stalk of connective tissue, but smooth muscle islets of glandular cells and nerve tissue have been described.[53] It can prolapse distally or proximally and may produce severe obstruction resulting in reflux and hydronephrosis. They must be differentiated from papillary tumors and inflammatory polyps.[60]

ROENTGENOGRAPHIC DIAGNOSIS

One sees rounded or oval filling defects in the posterior urethra often changing position at different times. The stalk may occasionally be recognized.

OTHER BENIGN TUMORS OF THE URETHRA

Other benign tumors of the urethra are hemangiomas, fibromas, leiomyomas, adenomas, papillomas, cysts, and caruncles.[67-69] Caruncles are of three types: papillary, telangiectatic, and granulomatous. Occasionally, these can become carcinomatous.

SECONDARY CARCINOMA OF THE URETHRA

Secondary carcinoma of the urethra arises from (1) direct extension from a carcinoma of the bladder (Figs. 42–10, 42–11), prostate, or rectum; (2) invasion from metastatic foci in the corpora cavernosa penis (Fig. 42–12); and (3) direct metastasis to the urethra.[70-77]

In type 1, the carcinoma is situated in the posterior urethra, usually as a single lesion. Many carcinomas of the posterior urethra are not primary but secondary to extension from neighboring organs. In type 2, the carcinoma is usually multiple and in the anterior urethra. These carcinomas arise in the bladder, prostate, kidney, testis, rectum, rectosigmoid, and lungs. They involve the corpora cavernosa penis, probably by metastases and secondarily involve the urethra. Type 3 is a metastatic lesion directly to the urethra without involving the corpora. Prostatic and bladder carcinomas are the most common tumors producing this lesion.

CHAPTER 42, ILLUSTRATIONS

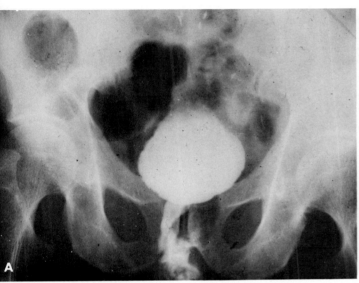
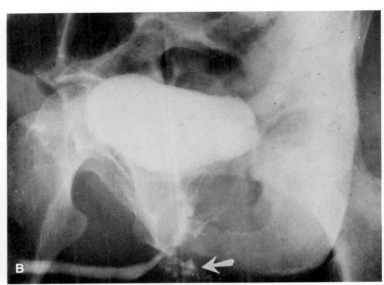

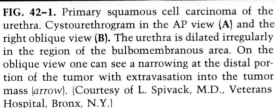

FIG. 42–1. Primary squamous cell carcinoma of the urethra. Cystourethrogram in the AP view (**A**) and the right oblique view (**B**). The urethra is dilated irregularly in the region of the bulbomembranous area. On the oblique view one can see a narrowing at the distal portion of the tumor with extravasation into the tumor mass (*arrow*). (Courtesy of L. Spivack, M.D., Veterans Hospital, Bronx, N.Y.)

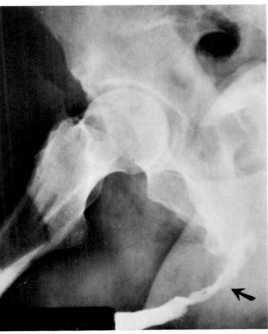

FIG. 42–2. Squamous cell carcinoma of the anterior urethra. Cystourethrogram, injecting, shows irregular urethra with some dilatation proximally and some narrowing distally. *Arrow* points to the involved area. (Courtesy of Maxwell Malament, M.D., Veterans Hospital, East Orange, N. J.)

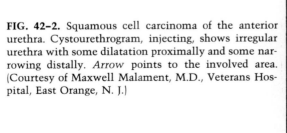

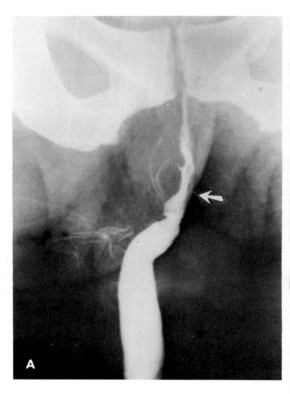

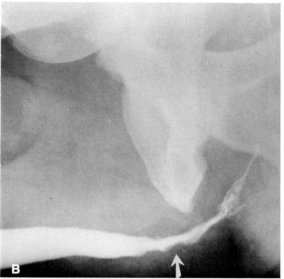

FIG. 42–3. Transitional cell carcinoma of the bulbomembranous area of the urethra. The urethra is involved irregularly with areas of constriction and dilatation (*arrow*). This man had had a transitional cell carcinoma of the bladder several years previously, and so this cannot be called a primary tumor of the urethra. However, the effects are similar to those of a primary tumor. Injecting cystourethrogram in both the AP position **(A)** and the right oblique position **(B)**.

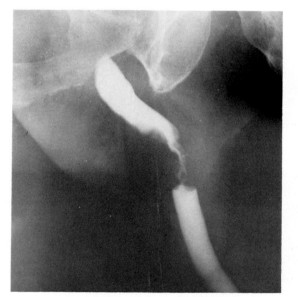

FIG. 42–4. Squamous cell carcinoma at bulbomembranous area. Irregular stricture seen. Note contrast around tumor tissue. The patient did not have a long history of stricture and had had few dilatations.

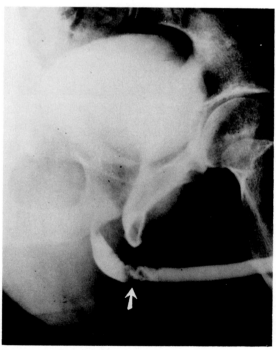

FIG. 42–5. Adenocarcinoma of urethra in bulbous area. Cystourethrogram reveals filling defects with only slight narrowing. Note contrast around tumor tissue. (Sacks, S.A. *et al.*, J. Urol., *113*:54, 1975)

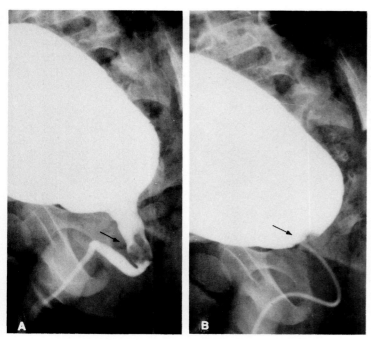

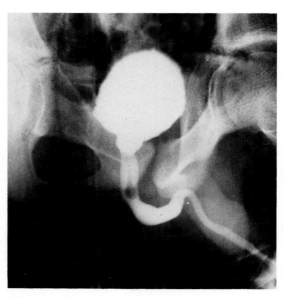

FIG. 42–7. Urethral polyp. Rounded defect on a long stalk.

FIG. 42–6. Polyp arising from verumontanum of a 2-year-old boy. **(A)** Polyp in distal prostatic urethra; **(B)** polyp at bladder neck. Polyp had a 1-cm. stalk, attached to summit of verumontanum. It was removed endoscopically, cutting stalk with wire electrode. Pathologic examination reported urethritis cystica with papillary projections of the mucosa on a urethral polyp. (Courtesy of Hardy Hendren, M.D.)

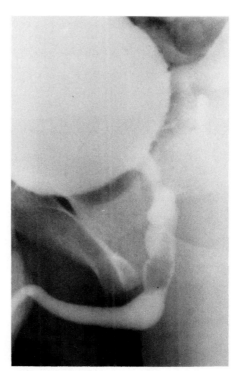

FIG. 42–8. Urethral polyp in a 13-year-old boy with enuresis. Filling defect, membranous area. Note the stalk running proximally to prostatic urethra at the level of the verumontanum.

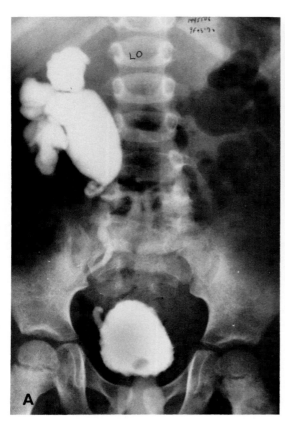

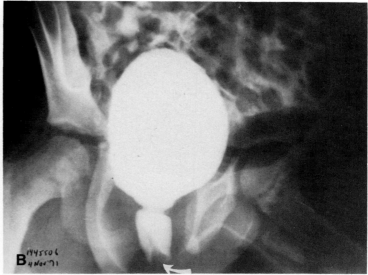

FIG. 42–9. Prolapsing polyp of the urethra. **(A)** Defects in bladder. **(B)** Defect in urethra, stalk visible.

FIG. 42–10. Papillary infiltrating carcinoma of the bladder, which has extended into the urethra as far as the external sphincter. Untreated case. *Large arrow* demonstrates the huge involvement of the bladder on the left side. There is also some involvement on the right side near the base. *Small arrow* points to involvement of the prostatic urethra by the tumor. AP view **(A)** and oblique view **(B).**

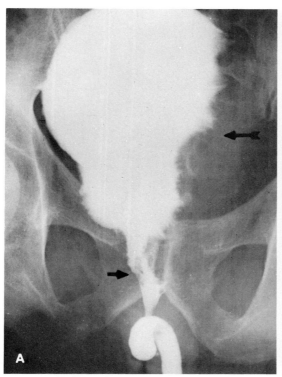

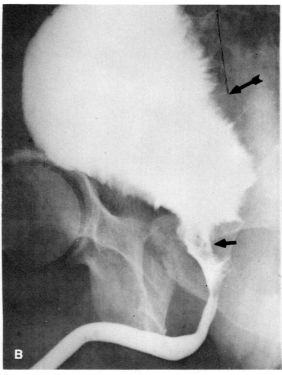

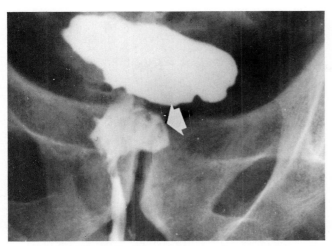

FIG. 42-11. Papillary carcinomas in a prostatic cavity. Patient had had a previous prostatectomy and fulguration of a papillary carcinoma of the bladder. Cysto-urethrogram reveals filling defects in the prostatic cavity (*arrow*).

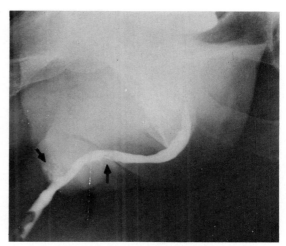

FIG. 42-12. Transitional cell carcinoma of the bladder with metastases to corpora cavernosa penis and secondary invasion of the urethra. *Arrows* point to various areas of invasion of the urethra. Most distal *arrow* points to extravasation into a tumor mass.

BIBLIOGRAPHY

Carcinoma of the Male Urethra

1. Baker, W.J., Graf, E.C., and Vandenberg, J.: Primary carcinoma of the male urethra. J. Urol., 71:327–337, 1954.
2. Campbell, M.F., and Fein, M.: Malignant melanoma of penile urethra, with brief review of urethral sarcoma in male. J. Urol., 35:573–582, 1936.
3. Clark, M.O., Jr., and Kosanovich, M.: Primary carcinoma of the male urethra. South. Med. J., 65:1339 (Passim), 1972.
4. Dean, A.L.: Carcinoma of the male and female urethra: Pathology and diagnosis. J. Urol., 75:505–513, 1956.
5. Elton, A.: Primary carcinoma of male urethra: A case report and review of the literature. Br. J. Surg., 39:316–318, 1952.
6. Geehold, G.W., and Myers, G.H., Jr.: Primary melanoma of the male urethra. J. Urol., 109:634–637, 1973.
7. Gladstone, S.A.: Carcinoma of male urethra diagnosed by sponge biopsy. J.A.M.A., 150:150–212, 1952.
8. Grabstald, H.: Tumors of the urethra in men and women. Cancer, 32:1236–1255, 1973.
9. Guinn, G.A., and Ayala, A.G.: Male urethral carcinoma. Report of 15 cases including a primary melanoma. J. Urol., 103:176–179, 1971.
10. Hotchkiss, R.S., and Amelar, R.D.: Primary carcinoma of the male urethra. J. Urol., 72:1181–1191, 1954.
11. Howe, G.E., Prentiss, R.J., Mullenix, R.B., et al.: Carcinoma of the urethra: diagnosis and treatment. J. Urol., 89:231–235, 1963.
12. Kaplan, G.W., Bulkley, G.J., and Grayhack, J.T.: Carcinoma of the male urethra. J. Urol., 98365–371, 1967.
13. King, L.R.: Carcinoma of the urethra in male patients. J. Urol., 91:555–559, 1964.
14. Mandler, J.I., and Pool, T.L.: Primary carcinoma of the male urethra. J. Urol., 96:67–72, 1966.
15. McCrea, L.E., and Furlong, J.H.: Primary carcinoma of male urethra. Urol. Survey, 1:1–30, 1951.
16. McCrea, L.E., and Furlong, J.H.: Primary carcinoma of male urethra: Case report. J. Urol., 67:216–217, 1952.
17. Meares, E.M., Jr.: Primary carcinoma of fossa navicularis. Urology, 7:93–96, 1976.
18. Milstoc, M.: New pathological aspects of primary carcinoma of the prostatic urethra. J. Am. Geriatr. Soc., 19:80–85, 1971.
19. Mullin, E.N., Anderson, E.E., and Paulson, D.F.: Carcinoma of the male urethra. J. Urol., 112:610–613, 1974.
20. Ratner, M., and Schneiderman, C.: The relationship of urethral caruncle to cancer of the urethra. Can. Med. Assoc. J., 58:373–376, 1948.
21. Ray, B., Cantu, A.R., and Whitmore, W.F., Jr.: Experience with primary carcinoma of the male urethra. J. Urol., 117:591–594, 1977.
22. Sacks, S.A., Waisman, J., Applebaum, H.B., et al.: Urethral adenocarcinoma possibly originating in the glands of Littre. J. Urol., 113:54–55, 1975.
23. Scott, E.V., and Barelare, B.: Adenocarcinoma of the male urethra. J. Urol., 68:311–319, 1952.
24. Zaslow, J., and Priestley, J.T.: Primary carcinoma of the male urethra. J. Urol., 58:207–211, 1947.

Carcinoma of the Female Urethra

25. Block, N.L., and Hotchkiss, R.S.: Malignant melanoma of the female urethra. Report of a case with 5-year survival and review of the literature. J. Urol., 105:251–255, 1971.
26. Brack, B., and Farber, G.J.: Carcinoma of the female urethra. J. Urol., 64:710–715, 1950.
27. Bracken, R.B., Johnson, D.E., Miller, L.S., et al.: Primary carcinoma of the female urethra. J. Urol., 116:188–192, 1965.
28. Chu, A.M.: Female urethral carcinoma. Radiology, 107:627–630, 1973.
29. Clayton, S.G.: Carcinoma of the female urethra. Review of literature, report of three cases. J. Obstet. Gynaecol. Brit. Emp., 52:508–512, 1945.

30. DasGupta, T., and Grabstald, H.: Melanoma of the genitourinary tract. J. Urol., 93:607–614, 1965.
31. Desai, S., Libertino, J.A., and Zinman, L.: Primary carcinoma of the female urethra. J. Urol., 110:693–695, 1973.
32. Grabstald, H., Hilaris, B., Henschke, V., et al.: Cancer of the female urethra. J.A.M.A., 197:835–842, 1966.
33. Hahn, G.A.: Primary carcinoma of the female urethra. J. Urol., 67:319–325, 1952.
34. Hess, E.: Primary carcinoma of female urethra: With special reference to the lesion known as urethral caruncle. Penn. Med. J., 48:1150–1155, 1945.
35. Knoblick, R.: Primary adenocarcinoma of the female urethra. Am. J. . Penn. Med. J., 48:1150–1155, 1945.
36. Konnak, J.W.: Mesonephric carcinoma involving the urethra. J. Urol., 110:76–78, 1973.
37. Marshall, F.C., Uson, A.C., and Melicow, M.M.: Neoplasms and caruncles of female urethra. Surg. Gynecol. Obstet., 110:723–733, 1960.
38. McCrea, L.E.: Malignancy of the female urethra. Urol. Survey, 2:85–149, 1952.
39. Menville, J.G., and Counseller, V.S.: Mucoid carcinoma of female urethra. J. Urol., 33:76–81, 1935.
40. Miller, J.D., and Raiman, R.J.: Carcinoma of the female urethra. Int. Surg., 6:431–432, 1976.
41. Moore, C.A.: Carcinoma of the female urethra. Milit. Med., 135:49–51, 1970.
42. Peterson, D.T., Dockerty, M.B., Utz, D.C., et al.: The peril of primary carcinoma of the urethra in women. J. Urol., 110:72–75, 1973.
43. Pointon, R.C.S., and Poole-Wilson, D.S.: Primary carcinoma of the urethra. Br. J. Urol., 40:682–693, 1968.
44. Rhamy, R.K., Boldus, R.A., Allison, R.C., et al.: Therapeutic modalities in adenocarcinoma of the female urethra. J. Urol., 109:638–640, 1973.
45. Rogers, R.E., and Burns, B.: Carcinoma of the female urethra. Obstet. Gynecol., 33:54–57, 1969.
46. Ruch, R.M., Frerichs, J.B., and Arneson, A.N.: Cancer of female urethra. Cancer, 5:748–753, 1952.
47. Seng, M., and Siminovitch, M.: Carcinoma of the urethra in the female. Can. Med. Assoc. J., 58:29–33, 1948.
48. Skjaeraasen, E.: Carcinoma of the female urethra. Acta Obstet. Gynecol. Scand., 48:589–597, 1969.
49. Steyn, J., Hall, M., and Logie, N.J.: Adenocarcinoma of the female urethra. Br. J. Urol., 39:504–505, 1967.
50. Tech, T.B.: Papillary adenocarcinoma of the female urethra. Br. J. Surg., 43:151–152, 1960.

Polyps of the Urethra

51. Aznar, A.P., and Martinez-Pernuela, J.M.: Urinary retention due to posterior urethral polyp in a boy. Br. J. Urol., 48:478, 1976.
52. Bagley, F.H., and Davidson, A.I.: Congenital urethral polyp in a child. Br. J. Urol., 48:278, 1976.
53. DeWolf, W.C., and Fraley, E.E.: Congenital urethral polyp in the infant. Case report and review of the literature. J. Urol., 109:515–516, 1973.
54. Downs, R.A.: Congenital polyps of the prostatic urethra: A review of the literature and report of two cases. Br. J. Urol., 42:76–85, 1970.
55. Gates, D.F., Koppel, M.M., and Palleschi, J.R.: Prostatic urethral polyps. Proc. Kimbrough Urol. Sem., 6:133–135, 1972.
56. Kuppusami, K., and Moors, D.E.: Fibrous polyp of the veru montanum. Can. J. Surg., 11:388–391, 1968.
57. Lou, E.S., Kogan, S.J., Newman, H., et al.: Prolapsing urethral polyp in child with hypospadias. Urology, 9:423–424, 1977.
58. Meadows, J.A., Jr., and Quattlebaum, R.B.: Polyps of the posterior urethra in children. J. Urol., 100:317–320, 1968.
59. Nellans, R.E., and Stein, J.J.: Pedunculated polyp of posterior urethra. Urology, 6:474–475, 1975.
60. Nesbit, R.M.: The genesis of benign polyps in the prostatic urethra. J. Urol., 87:416–418, 1962.
61. Randall, A.: A study of the benign polyps of the male urethra. Surg. Gynecol. Obstet., 17:548–562, 1913.
62. Roller, M.F., and Naranjo, C.A.: Benign urethral polyp of prostatic urethra. Urology, 6:34–36, 1975.
63. Sladaas, J.O.: Pedunculated polyp of posterior urethra in children causing reflux and hydronephrosis. J. Pediatr. Surg., 8:517–521, 1973.
64. Steuber, P.J., and Persky, L.: Solid tumors of the urethra and bladder neck. J. Urol., 102:205–209, 1969.
65. Valverde, B.: Polypi and vegetations of the posterior urethra: their influence on the sexual disturbances of man. Urol. Cutan. Rev., 37:461–466, 1933.
66. Williams, D.I., and Abbassian, A.: Solitary pedunculated polyp of the posterior urethra in children. J. Urol., 96:480–486, 1966.

Other Benign Tumors of the Urethra

67. Shield, D.E., and Weiss, R.M.: Leiomyoma of the female urethra. J. Urol., 109:430–431, 1973.
68. Ratner, M., and Strasberg, A.: Leiomyoma of the female urethra. Can. Med. Assn. J., 50:439–440, 1944.
69. Wani, N.A., Bhan, B.L., Guru, A.A., et al.: Leiomyoma of the female urethra: A case report. J. Urol., 116:120–121, 1976.

Secondary Carcinoma of the Urethra

70. Abeshouse, B.S., and Abeshouse, G.A.: Metastatic tumors of the penis: A review of the literature and a report of two cases. J. Urol., 86:99–112, 1961.
71. Clarke, J.F.: Urethral metastases from a presumed primary malignant melanoma presenting as postmenopausal bleeding. Proc. Roy. Soc. Med., 68:277–278, 1975.
72. Elkin, M., and Mueller, H.P.: Metastases from carcinoma of the prostate. Autopsy and roentgenographic findings. Cancer, 7:1246–1248, 1954.
73. Iverson, A.P., Blackard, C.E., and Schulberg, V.A.: Carcinoma of the prostate with urethral metastases. J. Urol., 108:901–904, 1972.
74. Kaufman, J.J., and Kaplan, L.: Secondary tumors of the penis. A.M.A. Arch. Surg., 73:105–111, 1956.
75. Klinger, M.E.: Secondary tumors of the genitourinary tract. J. Urol., 65:144–153, 1951.
76. Paquin, A.J., Jr., and Roland, S.I.: Secondary carcinoma of the penis. Cancer, 9:626–631, 1956.
77. Reiser, M.P., and Creevy, C.D.: Metastatic neoplasms of penis: review of literature and report of two cases. Minn. Med., 39:444–446, 1956.
78. Wattenberg, C.A.: Unusual tumors and secondary carcinomas of the penis: Review of the literature and report of a case. J. Urol., 52:169–175, 1944.
79. Wilson, M.C., Horton, G.R., and Horton, B.F.: Secondary tumors of the penis. J. Urol., 71:721–725, 1954.

URETHROCAVERNOUS REFLUXES

During urethrography by the injection method or by voiding against obstruction, extravasations (Figs. 43–1 to 43–5) can occur outside the mucosa of the urethra and into the corpus spongiosum. The material probably enters the submucosal venous spaces first and then passes into the venous system proper. Large refluxes or extravasations are easy to diagnose, because they run parallel with the urethra, corresponding to the corpus spongiosum.

Extravasations may occur on either side of the urethra, but if seen on the oblique view on only one side, the extravasation usually is in the inferior aspect. Extravasation occurs most frequently in the pendulous and the bulbous areas, where a thin mucosa overlies a loose submucosal tissue having a weak separation from the venous channels. The contrast medium then can pass by way of the circumflex vessels to the dorsal vein of the penis. The course from here would be exactly similar to that which occurs when the dorsal vein of the penis is injected directly. However, the contrast material can go directly from the corpus spongiosum to the internal pudendal vessels.

The extravasation and the permeation of the veins are produced by the force of the injection or by the force supplied by the bladder and the abdominal muscles on voiding against urethral resistance. Fernicola believes that urethral disease is an important factor.[4] Discomfort during the injection and the bleeding produced by the injection apparently are not related to the venous reflux.

ROENTGENOGRAPHIC DIAGNOSIS

Small extravasations may appear as a narrow, more or less diffuse line outside the urethra, spreading distally with no apparent connection with the urethra and not necessarily entering definite venous

43

Miscellaneous Conditions of the Urethra

channels (circumflex veins, dorsal veins, and internal pudendal veins). These small refluxes are difficult to separate from periurethral cavities and false passages. False passages are more definitely canalicular in form, with a definite connection with the urethra, and usually they become more narrow at the distal point. The periurethral cavities also have a definite connection with the urethra but usually are more uniform in caliber. Larger extravasations can occur, producing diffuse spreading of contrast material on either side of the urethra. Parts of these may appear to be well demarcated, but at all points the urethra is separated clearly from the spreading extravasation. When the extravasation has definite communication with the communicating veins, the dorsal vein, and the internal pudendals, the diagnosis is simple.

METHOD OF INJECTION OF DORSAL VEIN OF PENIS

The penis is prepared with a tourniquet about its base, and a No. 20 needle is inserted into the deep dorsal vein percutaneously. Some examiners have used a polyethylene tube instead of a needle. The deep dorsal vein appears as a midline swelling (Figs. 43–6 to 43–8). A three-way stopcock is connected with the needle; a bottle of intravenous saline solution is connected with one of the openings; and the saline is allowed to run in after removal of the tourniquet. The other opening is connected with a syringe containing 10 ml. of contrast material. The saline solution is stopped, and the contrast material is injected. Although the usual films generally are adequate, it probably is best to take stereoscopic views. The first view is taken after the first 5 ml. of contrast material has been administered, and the second is taken as the last 5 ml. is being injected. The x-ray tube is angled 5° toward the patient's head. After the procedure is completed, the intravenous saline solution is run in again until a decision is made on the need of additional film.

The deep dorsal vein enters a plexus of veins and then forms the lateral prostatic plexuses. These then empty into the internal iliac vein connecting with the obturator vein vesical plexus and the plexuses on the anterior surface of the rectum.

Abeshouse and Ruben believe that, by phlebography, one can differentiate between benign prostatic hypertrophy and carcinoma of the prostate.[11] They found an increased vascularity in benign prostatic hypertrophy, whereas in carcinoma they found paucity of veins and numerous thromboses.

ACQUIRED URETHRAL FISTULAS

Urethral fistulas in the male are either urethrocutaneous or urethrorectal; in the female they are urethrovaginal or urethrovaginal–rectal. Rarely is there a urethrovesical fistula (Fig. 43–8a).[20] Urethral fistulas may be congenital or acquired. The former are considered in Chapter 37, Intersex and Congenital Lesions of the Urethra.

MEN

Urethrocutaneous Fistulas. These are the result of infection, including periurethral abscesses and tuberculosis[17]; trauma, either surgical, resulting from passage of instruments, hypospadias operations and external urethrotomies, or accidental, such as straddle injuries, automobile accidents or bullet wounds; malignancies — for example, urethral carcinoma; or radium therapy (Figs. 43–9 to 43–13). Many urethral fistulas are associated with strictures of the urethra and may persist even when the fistula has been dilated adequately. Fistulas often are multiple in the perineum as a result of frequent extravasations of urine associated with strictures. A perineum in which there are long-standing fistulas with multiple openings has been called a "watering-pot" perineum. In these cases of multiple cutaneous openings, the tracts generally tend to coalesce into only one or two openings in the urethra.

Urethrorectal Fistulas in the male are most frequently the result of trauma, such as surgery (especially prostatic), automobile accidents, infections such as periurethral or prostatic abscesses, or inflammatory disease of rectum (Figs. 43–14 to 43–18). In some instances malignancy, especially rectal carcinoma but rarely prostatic, can be the cause of urethrorectal fistulas. The urethrorectal fistulas connect with the prostatic urethra slightly proximally to the verumontanum or in the membranous urethra.

Urethrocavernous Fistulas are usually secondary to cavernosospongiotic shunts for priapism (Fig. 43–18a).[2, 7]

WOMEN

More females have fistulas of all types than males, but males predominate in urinary fistulas connected with the intestinal tract. Acquired urethral fistulas in the female are much more common than the congenital variety. Urethrovaginal fistulas can be the result of surgery on the urethra (Figs. 43–19 to 43–21) or on the vagina or of tumors both benign and malignant usually arising in the urethra but occasionally in the vagina. Infections such as periurethral abscesses and infected diverticula can form a fistula from urethra to vagina. Radium therapy has resulted in urethrovaginal, vesicovaginal, urethrorectal–vaginal, and vesicorectal–vaginal fistulas. Deliberate vesicourethrovaginal fistulas have been produced surgically for the defunctionalized bladder.

ROENTGENOGRAPHIC DIAGNOSIS

Urethrocystograms are essential in the localization and the diagnosis of urethrointestinal fistulas. The contrast material passes more readily from the urethral side than from the intestinal side. Occasionally, however, it is difficult to demonstrate these fistulas, even though they may be of adequate size. Important adjuncts in making the diagnosis are meconium, feces in the urine, or flatus through the urethra. Methylene blue instilled in the bladder or the urethra may appear in the stool. Urethrovaginal fistulas are difficult to demonstrate except in the lateral view.

PRIAPISM

Priapism is a persistent, prolonged erection of the penis, unaccompanied by sexual excitation or desire (Figs. 43–22 to 43–25). Venous stasis leads to elevated viscosity of the blood as a consequence of increased carbon dioxide tension. Venous occlusion occurs at the junction of cavernous spaces and collecting veins. Edema can further advance the process. Occlusion of arterioles may follow and fibrosis of trabeculae may be an end result.

CLASSIFICATION OF PRIAPISM

I. Neurogenic
   A. Psychic stimuli
   B. Direct nerve stimulation (in cord, pudendal nerves, or nervi erigentes)
   C. Reflex from local stimuli
II. Mechanical
   A. Thrombosis or pseudothrombosis (increased blood viscosity)—sickle cell anemia, leukemia; carcinoma of prostate or bladder producing venous blockage
   B. Hemorrhage and hematoma
   C. New growths of penis
   D. Local inflammation
   E. Sexual activity
III. Possibly certain drugs such as guanethidine, phenothiazines[42]
IV. Idiopathic priapism, cause not assigned

Retention of urine occurs frequently in priapism, but the mechanism is not clear. The urethra, as seen in Figure 43–22, though elongated, has not been especially narrowed.

There are two possible explanations for priapism. Hinman believes it to be the result of local changes in the corpora cavernosa,[36] whereas others believe that there is slowing of the drainage from the deep dorsal vein of the penis.[25][26] Corpus cavernosography (Figs. 43–23 to 43–25) has revealed that contrast material remains in the corpora cavernosa for prolonged intervals even during the quiescent phase of sickle cell anemia priapism.[71] Fitzpatrick performed both spongiosograms and cavernosograms in priapism during the erectile state. He demonstrated that the glans penis and corpus spongiosum are uninvolved because the superficial dorsal veins remain patent, whereas the deep dorsal vein is obstructed, allowing persistent erection of the corpus cavernosum (Figs. 43–24).[31]

PEYRONIE'S DISEASE

Peyronie's disease (Figs. 43–26 to 43–28) is a plastic or a fibrous cavernositis. The disease begins in the cavernous sheaths as a fibrous area that gradually thickens and extends along the shaft of the penis in confluence or as separate fibrous plaques. The dorsum of the penis is involved most commonly. The plaques usually are situated near the glans; next, in the midshaft; and, least commonly, at the base. The plaques straddle the corpora cavernosa penis, lying between Buck's fascia and the tunica albuginea and situated inferiorly to the dorsal vessels and nerves.

The initial fibrous lesion may begin slowly, become rapid in extension, and then grow slowly again. Spontaneous regression has occurred. Calcification is seen not infrequently. Chordee may be present with or without a plaque.

Peyronie's disease has been associated with diabetes mellitus,[49] carcinoid syndrome,[46] HLA antigens of the B_7 cross-reacting group (B_7CREG)[57] and various fibrotic conditions[48] such as subcutaneous fibromata, Dupuytren's contracture (10% of cases of Peyronie's), bilateral Dupuytren's contracture and plantar fibrosis, and a collagen triad of Peyronie's, Dupuytren's contracture, and fibrosis of the auricular cartilage. Ankylosing spondylitis may be associated with this disease.

ROENTGENOGRAPHIC FINDINGS

Calcific areas are seen as homogeneous but irregular and moderately dense plaques. Xeroradiology is superior because it enhances contrast between areas of little differences in density. Corpus cavernosograms demonstrate sharp indentation on both sides, with narrowing of the visualized bodies of the corpora cavernosa. The septal space at the level of the defect is widened. Drainage time is moderately prolonged.[71] The course of the disease during treatment can be evaluated by this method.

CONGENITAL ABNORMALITIES OF THE PENIS

Congenital abnormalities of the penis include absence, hemihypertrophy (Fig. 43–29), diphallus, and micropenis.

PHIMOSIS

Occasionally, in doing a voiding cystogram, the contrast medium can be visualized underneath the foreskin (Figs. 43–30, 43–31).

CORPUS CAVERNOSOGRAPHY

Corpus cavernosography is the visualization of the corpora cavernosa of the penis by direct injection of contrast material (Figs. 43–32 to 43–36).[65-71] It is useful in the following areas:

1. Metastic lesions to the corpora
2. Peyronie's disease
3. Priapism
4. Impotence
5. Atrophy and fibrosis of the penis
6. Trauma to the penis

Ther are two general methods available:

1. The penis is maintained in an extended position by means of adhesive straps attached to the glans (Fig. 43–32). Novocaine (1%) is injected into the skin and subcutaneous tissues on both sides of the midline just behind the glans. To prevent leakage at the site, the needle is not permitted to enter either corpus cavernosum. A #22 3.8-cm. needle is inserted into each corpus cavernosum at the site of the novocaine injection, plastic tubing is interposed between the needle and syringe, and 10 ml. of contrast material is injected with the needle, tubing, and syringes left in position. Roentgenographic exposures are made in the anteroposterior and oblique views and thereafter in the supine view at 15-minute intervals until the contrast material has dissipated completely from the corpora. According to

Hamilton,[69] it is not necessary to inject both corpora, because as originally described by Fetter and co-workers,[42] the medium passes across to the other side from a single injection.

2. Fitzpatrick has utilized the right oblique position, injecting only one corpus with 5 cc. of contrast medium and making exposures every 30 seconds.[66, 68] This method has been especially useful in determining the competence of the deep dorsal vein and in demonstrating the intercommunicating venous drainage system.

SCROTUM

The injection of gas into the tunica vaginalis for visualization of the testicles rarely has been performed and certainly is of limited value. Occasionally, gas injected presacrally (Figs. 43–37, 43–38) has entered the scrotum and outlined the testicles, either unilaterally or bilaterally. This occurrence means that the injected gas has entered the correct plane and should give a satisfactory outline of the kidneys. Of course, calcification of scrotal masses (Figs. 43–39 to 43–41) can be visualized easily. Hematomas can enlarge the scrotum to an extent visible on a roentgenogram (Fig. 43–42).

Gas gangrene (Fig. 43–43) of the penis and scrotum may be idiopathic or secondary to adjacent infection or trauma, either direct or indirect, by way of urinary extravasation. The bacteria implicated are *Streptococcus*, *Staphylococcus*, colon bacilli, and *Clostridium*.

Fournier's gangrene refers especially to gangrene in the absence of the usual causes. In most cases the gangrene has been limited to the skin and subcutaneous tissue of the scrotum and penis and penile base. However, deep tissues can be involved with extension into the urethra and up the abdominal wall to the axillae and thorax.[72]

ROENTGENOGRAPHIC DIAGNOSIS

Irregular radiolucent areas representing gas formation may be seen in the scrotum and penis. Spermatic arteries may be well visualized and dilated in cases of iliac artery obstruction (Figs. 43–44), but may be dilated and tortuous in tumors of the testes (see Fig. 43–69).

VARICOCELE AND FERTILITY

Varicocele, a dilatation and tortuosity of veins of spermatic cord, is either primary or secondary[79] to renal tumor, hydronephrosis, aberrant renal artery, arching of renal artery over renal vein, or possibly compression of renal vein (see Figs. 43–45, 43–46). It can produce atrophy of testis,[110] deviation of ureter,[101] dragging discomfiture, and infertility. The latter condition has been a concern of many investigators. The following considerations have evolved in relation to primary varicocele:

1. Varicocele occurs in 10 per cent of the male population, 90 per cent on the left, 8 per cent bilateral, 2 per cent on the right. The right internal spermatic vein usually enters the vena cava, but 10 per cent enter the renal vein in males (in females the ovarian vein enters the renal vein in 7%). The left internal spermatic vein enters the left renal vein. The internal spermatic vein tends to be multiple down to the level of the internal ring.

2. Varicocele is a common cause of infertility.[95, 106]

3. Varicocele produces a stress-pattern seminal fluid, that is, excessive numbers of tapering forms and exfoliation into ejaculate of spermatogenic precursor sperm, primarily spermatids (immature sperm).[112]

4. The effect on the testicles is bilateral[97] but more severe on the varicocele side. The most common effect is sloughing of immature cells, with arrest at the spermatid or primary spermatocyte stage next in frequency.[105]

5. Varicocele occurs more frequently in subfertile men than in the fertile population.[106, 114]

6. Varicocele can result from (a) incompetent or congenitally absent valves[76, 78, 83, 88] or (b) blood bypassing competent valves at cranial end via communicating veins entering into spermatic vein caudally to valves.[79] In either method, there is reversed blood flow into spermatic vein and by cross collateral communication into contralateral testicular circulation.[79, 83, 98]

7. Varicocelectomy has resulted in improved semen quality, especially motility, and in an increased number of pregnancies.[82, 85, 93, 95, 112, 116]

The exact mechanism by which varicocele suppresses fertility is not known. There are four possibilities:

1. Changes in scrotal temperature. Hanley favored this concept.[104] Zorgniotti and MacLeod found increased intrascrotal temperatures on the varicocele side,[121] whereas Tessler and Krahn[119] and Stephenson[117] did not corroborate this finding.

2. Venous stasis

3. Reduced oxygen tension—not verified by Donahue and Brown[92]

4. Toxic metabolic products from adrenal and kidney. MacLeod mentioned this possibility.[112] Agger,[75] Charny and Baum,[86] Koumans and co-workers,[108] and Mobley[113] found no significant increase (in most instances a decrease) in plasma levels of adrenal steroids (cortisol) in the spermatic vein as compared to another peripheral vein in cases of varicocele. However, Comhaire and Vermeulen[90] and Cohen and co-workers[87] found increased catecholamines in the spermatic vein in some cases. The cases with increased catecholamines apparently had better response to varicocelectomy than the cases without the increase.[87]

DIAGNOSIS OF VARICOCELE

Varicocele can be diagnosed using the following methods:

1. Palpation

2. Palpation plus the Valsalva maneuver (in certain mild or subclinical cases)

3. Thermography.[89-100, 107] Thermography, although not completely accurate, may be a valuable method pre- and postoperatively to follow postoperative results.

4. Doppler ultrasonic stethescope[103]

5. Venography. Although the study of the internal spermatic vein has been performed by arteriography where 12 per cent showed filling,[76] the preferred method is direct injection of the left renal vein. There is usually, but not invariably, dilatation of the internal spermatic vein in cases of varicocele. The vein fills completely in the retrograde fashion if a varicocele is present, but does not do so if none is present.[79] The dilated, tortuous vessels in the pampiniform plexus are visualized, and crossing to the other side is often demonstrated.

TORSION OF THE TESTIS

Testicular torsion (the gonad twisted on its pedicle compromising the circulation) occurs in two forms (Figs. 43–47, 43–47a):

1. Intravaginal torsion—testicular torsion within the tunica vaginalis because of an anomalous suspension. This is common.[130] It is the result of an anomalous suspension of the testicle.[135] It is essentially in the form of a more complete envelopment of the testis by the tunica vaginalis. Anomalies of union of epididymis with testis as well as undes-

cended testis are frequently associated with the intravaginal type of torsion.[129] It usually occurs at puberty.

2. Extravaginal torsion (torsion of spermatic cord) in which testicle and its tunics twist at external ring.[140] This represents only 6 per cent of cases of torsion.[128] This type occurs primarily in newborn infants but may have occurred in utero. There is a predisposing congenital abnormality: The testicular tunics are unattached to the scrotum at birth and can slide freely in and out of the scrotal sac. It is possible that the pull of the cremasteric muscle can cause the twist.[122] The mass is smooth, firm, and painless. There may be some discoloration of the scrotal wall. Temperature of 102° or more has occurred in about half of the cases.[138]

In both types of torsion, the venous supply is obstructed first, with the arterial supply later. Both sides are affected equally but only 5 per cent are bilateral at the same time.[125] The incidence in the contralateral testicle after a confirmed case is not accurately known, but because 50 to 80 per cent have contralateral anomalies, torsion of the second testicle is probably frequent and therefore it should be fixed to prevent occurrence.

There is a mixed type of torsion—recurrent twisting, which spontaneously corrects itself but can proceed at some time to infarction.

DIAGNOSIS OF TORSION OF THE TESTIS

The extravaginal type is more obvious because it occurs in newborn infants and other causes of swelling are less frequent. The intravaginal type may given a confusing picture.

1. Upon physical examination, there is swelling of the scrotal contents and the skin may be discolored. The testicle appears higher than normal. The epididymis is not in its normal position, and elevation of the testicle does not relieve pain (as opposed to epididymitis) (Prehn's sign).
2. Absence of urethral discharge and absence of infection of the urinary tract favor torsion.
3. The Doppler ultrasonic stethoscope has been used to substantiate obstruction of circulation.[132, 139]
4. Radionuclide scanning reveals that on the twisted side, the activity of the radionuclide angiogram is slightly decreased or is at the normal, barely perceptible level.[123, 126, 127, 134] On the normal side, the perfusion should be normal and when compared to the involved side, is found to be increased. The static nuclear image

reveals a rounded, cold area replacing the testicle.[127]
5. At the operating table, fluorescence of the testicle has been used to determine the viability.[137]

Epididymitis, which is the most common differential diagnosis, reveals increased perfusion later toward the epididymis (Figs. 43-48, 43-49). The static image is hot.

Hydroceles have been identified by radionuclide scan (Fig. 43-50) and ultrasonography (Fig. 43-51).

NONPALPABLE TESTIS

Nonpalpable testis may indicate undescent, ectopia, or absence (Figs. 43-52 to 43-58). It is extremely important to know if a testicle is present and its location.

Monorchism occurs in 4 per cent of children explored for undescended testis or testes.[151] Anorchism is rare with only 80 cases reported to 1974.[145] Testicular absence may be an isolated finding but often is associated with other anomalies including absence of epididymis, vas deferens, spermatic cord, seminal vesicles, prostate, ureter, or kidney.

If neither testicle is palpable, a chromosome study for genetic sex along with determinations of serum testosterone and serum gonadotropin [follicular stimulating hormone (FSH) and luteinizing hormone (LH)] levels is done. If the karyotype is 46 XY and if no palpable müllerian structures are present upon rectal examination, a human chorionic gonadotropic stimulation test is performed to demonstrate functioning testicular tissue, if present, by an increase over basal levels of serum testosterone (isolated extratesticular Leydig cells might also respond).[145, 148] In contrast, elevated basal levels of FSH and LH in conjunction with failure of testosterone elevation over basal levels after HCG is considered diagnostic of absence of functioning testicular tissue. If the karyotype is other than 46 XY, further investigation is necessary.

The exact location can be determined by testicular venography (Figs. 43-56 to 43-58),[1, 3, 4] studies on the left side being more successful than those on the right. The location depends upon the identification of a pampiniform plexus; the presence of a spermatic vein is not indicative of a testis.[143] Aortography and selective spermatic arteriography[142, 150, 152] (Figs. 43-52 to 43-55) can also be used to locate the testis, but the latter technique is difficult to perform, especially in young children.

The former often fails to visualize adequately the spermatic vessels in adults and may fail completely in children.

Because testicular venography and spermatic arteriography may be extremely difficult at times, computerized tomography may be the method of choice in locating the nonpalpable testis. Laparoscopy is also an excellent method for achieving the same end.

TUMORS OF THE TESTIS

CLASSIFICATION[182]

I. Germ-cell tumors
  A. Tumors of one histologic type
    1. Seminoma
    2. Spermatocytic seminoma
    3. Embryonal carcinoma
    4. Yolk sac tumor; embryonal carcinoma, infantile type
    5. Polyembryoma
    6. Choriocarcinoma
    7. Teratoma
      a. Mature
      b. Immature
      c. With malignant transformation (other than 1–6)
  B. Tumors of more than one histologic type
    1. Embryonal carcinoma and teratoma (teratocarcinoma)
    2. Choriocarcinoma and another type (specify type)
    3. Other combinations (specify)
II. Sex cord/stromal tumors
  A. Leydig cell tumors
  B. Sertoli cell tumors
  C. Granulosa cell tumors
  D. Mixed forms (specify)
  E. Incompletely differentiated forms
III. Tumors and tumor-like conditions containing both germ-cell and sex cord/stromal elements
  A. Gonadoblastoma
  B. Others
IV. Miscellaneous tumors
  A. Carcinoids
  B. Others
V. Lymphoid and hematopoietic tumors
VI. Secondary tumors
VII. Tumors of collecting ducts, rete, epididymis, spermatic cord, capsule, supporting structure, and appendices
VIII. Unclassified tumors
IX. Tumor-like conditions

Sixty per cent of germ-cell tumors consist of one cell type; 40 per cent consist of more than one cell type. The metastases are normally the same type as that of the primary tumor, but the metastases may be of different cell type or show multiple elements that may not be visible in the primary lesion. Most deaths occur in the first 2 years, and almost all die within 5 years.

STAGING[168, 192]

Stage I   Tumor limited to testicle with no evidence of spread through capsule or to spermatic cord

Stage II   Clinical or radiographic evidence of tumor extension beyond testicle but not beyond regional lymph drainage

Stage IIIA   Extension beyond diaphragm but still confined to lymphatic system as in mediastinal or supraclavicular lymphatics, or massive retroperitoneal disease.

Stage IIIB   Disseminated disease as seen in generalized abdominal (visceral) or pulmonary metastases

TNM CLASSIFICATIONS[192]

T — *Primary Tumour* (in the absence of orchidectomy the symbol TX must be used)
  T0   No evidence of primary tumour
  T1   Tumour limited to the body of the testis
  T2   Tumour invading beyond the tunica albuginea
  T3   Tumour invading the rete testis or epididymis
  T4   Tumour infiltrating the spermatic cord and/or the scrotal wall
    T4a   Infiltrating the spermatic cord
    T4b   Infiltrating the scrotal wall
  TX   The minimum requirments to assess the primary tumour cannot be met

N — *Regional and Juxtaregional Lymph Nodes*
  N0   No evidence of regional lymph node involvement
  N1   Evidence of involvement of a single homolateral regional lymph node, which if inguinal is mobile
  N2   Evidence of involvement of contralateral or bilateral or multiple regional lymph nodes, which if inguinal are mobile
  N3   Palpable abdominal mass present or there is evidence of involvement of fixed inguinal lymph nodes

N4 Evidence of involvement of juxtaregional lymph nodes

NX The minimum requirements to assess the regional and/or juxtaregional lymph nodes cannot be met.

M — Distant Metastases

M0 No evidence of distant metastases

M1 Distant metastases present

MX The minimum requirements to assess the presence of distant metastases cannot be met.

DIAGNOSIS OF TESTICULAR TUMORS

Palpation. There is a nodular area of induration in the testicle or a heaviness. A hydrocele may be present. A plain film may occasionally show calcification (see Fig. 43–59).

Soft Tissue Radiology of the Testis. Price and Loveday have described the technique and radiographic demonstration.[185] They believe that malignant testicular tumors appear as an extremely radiopaque generalized enlargement of the testicle. The margins of the testicle appear to be sharply defined, particularly on the midline side adjacent to the septum. This is opposed to the normal testicle, which has a medium radiographic density. Benign conditions such as hydrocele and cysts give a generalized increase in size and radiopacity of the scrotum compared to normal, but appear less radiopaque than testicular tumors, and the margins of the testicle are less clearly defined.

Blood Studies. The radioimmune assay method of determination of alpha fetoprotein and beta chain of human chorionic gonadotropins can be extremely useful.[156, 176]

a. Nonseminomatous germ-cell tumors confined to the scrotum—the markers may or may not be elevated. Levels are not elevated to seminoma. Thus these tests are not extremely useful in scrotal masses limited to that area.

b. Markers are sensitive in the preoperative evaluation of metastatic disease. Elevated serum levels indicate metastatic nonseminomatous germ-cell tumors.

c. These studies can be extremely helpful in following the effectiveness of radiation and chemotherapy.

d. LDH is useful in monitoring the therapy in cases of normal α-fetoprotein and human chorionic gonadotropin.[167a]

e. Pregnancy-specific B-glycoprotein (SP$_1$) may be useful in the tumors with the syncytiotrophoblastic giant cells.[167a]

f. The use of H93 radioimmunoassay specific to the carboxyl-terminal peptide of HCG-B in measuring urinary concentration of HCG may be an important new monitor.[167b]

Urography (Fig. 43–61; see also Fig. 3–47). The kidneys may be pushed laterally, usually without rotation. The ureters may be deviated laterally in the lumbar area. Obstruction of the ureters occasionally can occur as the result of compression by lymph nodes or by direct invasion.

Lymphography (Figs. 43–60 to 43–64).[164, 166, 169, 171, 177, 178, 186, 190, 195] Both bipedal and funicular methods are utilized. The funicular method is slightly superior for determining accurately the lymph nodes involved, but the bipedal method is more commonly utilized. The accuracy of lymphography ranges overall from 79 to 89 per cent; the accuracy is greater when the nodes are read as positive (up to 97%); however, when they are read as negative, the accuracy drops probably to around 75 per cent. Many lymph nodes have small metastatic foci that cannot be visualized. The testicular lymphatics accompany the spermatic artery and vein and drain into lumbar nodes. Direct testicular lymphography demonstrates lymph channels terminating in a sentinel node at the level of L-1 to L-2 on the left and L-1 to L-3 on the right, lying slightly lateral to lumbar nodes opacified on a pedal lymphogram. It has been shown that the right testicular lymphatics may cross over immediately to contralateral nodes, but left testicular vessels cross over only after permeating sentinel nodes.

From the lumbar nodes, the continuity of the lymphatic system is usually through the thoracic duct, but there may be communication between lumbar and mediastinal nodes independent of the thoracic duct.[153, 157] Metastases usually follow a logical order determined by lymphatic drainage, but loss of patency will direct metastases through collateral lymphatic pathways or lymphatic venous anastomoses.

The following *architectural patterns* are evident:

a. More spherical than normal with crescentric deformity with lymphatics not penetrating marginal defect (Fig. 43–60)

b. Disrupted internal pattern with relatively intact marginal sinus (lymphoma pattern) (Fig. 43–61)

c. Both types

Lymphocysts can result from retroperitoneal lymph node dissections (Fig. 43–70).

Phlebography.[174, 177, 187] Phlebography of the inferior vena cava is useful in demonstrating compression (Fig. 43–62) or displacement, or both, and tumor thrombosis. After renal malignancies, this is the second most common tumor producing tumor thrombosis of the vena cava.

Cope and Isard describe compression, localized narrowing, segmental irregular narrowing, and obstruction of left renal vein (Figs. 43–63, 43–64) by metastatic peritoneal lymph node involvement and pancreatic tumors.[160]

Retrograde or antegrade phlebography of the internal spermatic vein is useful in determining metastases (Figs. 43–65, 43–66).[174, 177] The cranial part of the spermatic vein may be dislocated and occluded partially or completely, producing collaterals around the mass of retroperitoneal nodes. This determination is useful in estimating the extent of metastases for purposes of irradiation.

Arteriography. Selective arteriography of the spermatic artery (Figs. 43–67 to 43–69) may reveal irregular vessels or nondiagnostic vessels surrounding the tumor mass. The tumor often can be seen dislocating the ordinary testicular vessels, which may not show neovascularity.

Radionuclide Scan (Fig. 43–71).[165, 183, 184] The testicle is enlarged. Angiographic perfusion is markedly increased but without the formation of vessels seen in epididymitis or abscesses. The flow is directed centrally to the testis. The static imaging corresponds to the histologic appearance; that is, a seminoma is diffusely vascular with increased activity, more warm than hot; a teratoma may have both warm and cooler areas when elements of embryonal cell carcinoma are present.

Ultrasonography (Fig. 43–72). Ultrasound can be used in studies of the scrotal contents.[188] A seminoma showing an echo-poor area in contrast to the normal echo-dense collagen structures of the testis is demonstrated. This area is echo-free probably because of the homogeneous nature of a seminoma. As more studies are performed, possibly other tumors will reveal a greater echo pattern.

CT Scan (Fig. 43–73).[175] CT scan is excellent for delineating lymph node enlargement and may reveal nodes not seen on lymphography; however, the internal structure of the node is not clearly defined. Moreover, according to some authors, when CT scans are used, enlargement may be missed in as many as 50 per cent of cases in which the nodes are positive on lymphadenectomy. CT scan with enhancement is useful in direct visualization of testicular tumors.

Radical Orchiectomies. These should be performed for diagnostic purposes and for removal of primary tumor.

LESIONS OF COWPER'S DUCTS AND GLANDS

Cowper's glands are part of the periurethral glands and are composed of two types: (1) the bulbar glands located in the corpus spongiosum along the bulbous urethra; and (2) the diaphragmatic glands situated in the transverse perineal portion of the urogenital diaphragm. Both types are considered accessory male sex glands and are the homologue of the Bartholin glands in the female. They secrete a mucous substance that acts as a coagulation factor for the spermatozoa during ejaculation.[200] The diaphragmatic glands connect to the bulbous urethra by way of thin-walled paired ducts that run diagonally forward from the urogenital diaphragm to enter the bulbous urethra floor. They can either enter as separate ducts or join and have a single orifice. The smaller bulbar glands either communicate with the main diaphragmatic ducts or enter the urethra directly by means of short ducts.

Cysts of Cowper's glands may be congenital or acquired (inflammatory). They may cause minor micturition difficulties such as frequency, urgency, or dysuria. Perineal abscesses have occurred secondary to infection of these cysts. Severe problems, such as urinary retention, hydroureteronephrosis, and hypertrophy and trabeculation of the bladder have been reported.[197, 201]

ROENTGENOGRAPHIC FINDINGS

A rounded filling defect arising from the floor of the bulbous urethra is diagnostic. Filling of a dilated duct may be seen even if the cystic structure distally has been ruptured. Visualization of the ducts has been seen mainly secondary to infection (Fig. 43–75) but distal obstruction is a possible cause. The cysts are better seen on voiding cystourethrograms than on retrograde urethrograms (Fig. 43–74A, B).

AMYLOIDOSIS OF THE URETHRA AND LOWER GENITOURINARY TRACT

Primary and secondary amyloidosis can involve the lower urinary tract (Fig. 43–76). Primary amyloidosis occurs in the absence of chronic disease as (1) the systemic form with deposition in multiple organs and (2) the localized form limited to affected organs. The secondary form is associated with rheumatoid arthritis, chronic granulomatous disease, and multiple myeloma. Amyloidosis can affect the urethra,[204, 205, 209] seminal vesicles,[206, 208] and prostate[207, 210] (the bladder is discussed in Chap. 33, Miscellaneous Conditions of the Bladder).

Urethral amyloidosis occurs in men 27 to 72 years of age, the average age being 53 years.[209] All cases have been primary in type. It is extremely rare: only 10 cases to 1976.[204] Hematuria and symptoms of stricture are the predominant manifestations. It can be confused with carcinoma of the urethra. Amyloidosis of the seminal vesicles is not uncommonly found at autopsy. The incidence increases with age and varies between 1 and 9 per cent.[206, 208] Amyloidosis of the prostate occurs in 1.5 to 10 per cent of unselected patients undergoing prostatectomy.[207, 210] Biopsy of the prostate is as accurate for diagnostic purposes as rectal or gingival biopsy.

ROENTGENOGRAPHIC DIAGNOSIS

Cystourethrograms reveal a narrowing usually near the bulbous urethra, irregular in type, and similar to the usual stricture.

URETHRAL PROLAPSE

Prolapse of the female urethra refers to the prolapse of redundant urethral mucosa and submucosa through the urethral meatus (Fig. 43–77).

Urethral prolapse occurs almost exclusively in prepubertal girls and postmenopausal women. In children, it is limited almost entirely to the Negro race but there is no racial predilection in adults.[212]

ROENTGENOGRAPHIC DIAGNOSIS

On cystourethrography, the urethra is elongated and surrounded by a mass outlined often by contrast material that is refluxed into the vagina. The distal urethra is narrowed but not obstructed. The urethral mass protrudes into the vestibule and impresses on the hymen.

CONDYLOMATA ACCUMINATA OF THE URETHRA

Intraurethral spread of venereal warts may be extremely serious (Figs. 43–78, 43–79). The fact that urethral involvement may be extensive and spread to the bladder is well known. Voiding cystourethrography is essential not only to make the diagnosis but also to determine the extent of the lesions. Multiple sessile filling defects are the usual findings, and because these defects usually are associated with cutaneous condylomata, the diagnosis can definitely be made. However, other polypoid lesions of the male urethra, such as squamous cell carcinoma, polypoid urethritis, adenomatous and fibrous polyps, transitional cell and papillary carcinomas, urethritis cystica, malignant melanoma and metastatic tumors must all be considered.

Polyps usually arise in the region of the verumontanum without any anterior lesions, whereas condylomata accuminata of the posterior urethra are not seen unless anterior lesions are present. Squamous cell carcinoma is usually posterior and unifocal; it is more likely to be associated with strictures. Transitional cell carcinoma may arise independently or in association with primary carcinoma of the bladder. Polypoid urethritis has the same radiographic appearance as verruca accuminata but is associated with strictures and has no history of genital condyloma. Secondary malignancies of the urethra are usually associated with bladder, prostate, kidney, and testis, and the diagnosis should be made from a biopsy if any of these tumors are present.

URETHRAL SYNDROME

The female urethral syndrome is defined as frequency, urgency, and dysuria.[222a] It is a gray area, the cause of which is not determined. It can occur with and without urethral obstruction. It should be emphasized, however, that many of these cases occur with changes in the urethra that could be the result of infection.[221] The syndrome apparently is more common in middle age and is rare in young and old women compared with bacterial cystitis attacks. Other precipitating causes mentioned in the literature are sexual intercourse, menopause, cold weather, emotional stress, catheterization, allergy, menstruation, and possibly conversion or psychophysiologic etiology.[221a]

ENLARGEMENT OF THE VERUMONTANUM

Enlargement of the verumontanum is divided into three categories (Figs. 43–80 to 43–82):

1. *Congenital.* See Chapter 37, Intersex and Congenital Lesions of the Urethra.
2. *Benign hypertrophy of the verumontanum.* Johnson and Price separated this category from the congenital variety and from verumontanitis.[228] The category is not defined clearly but has been reported in infants and children, as well as in adults. Many of these reported cases probably represent verumontanitis, because they followed infection, especially gonorrhea.
3. *Verumontanitis* (Fig. 43–82). This is an enlargement of the verumontanum as a direct result of infection. It is seen in young boys as a result of masturbation and in men secondary to infection such as gonorrhea. There may be congestion of the verumontanum, associated frequently with polyps and granulomatous tissue.

We have seen several cases of hypertrophy of the verumontanum in patients with carcinoma of the prostate treated with estrogens but the exact pathology has not been evaluated.

ROENTGENOGRAPHIC FINDINGS

There is a rounded or an oval defect in the prostatic urethra in both the anteroposterior and the oblique projections. The verumontanum may appear to fill the transverse diameter of the urethra, and, in the oblique view, the urethra often bulges to accommodate the enlargement. The appearance is similar in all three types but usually is more striking in the congenital variety.

IMPOTENCE

There have been two approaches in recent years to the study of impotence. The first emphasizes the arterial failure of erection. In this group arteriography of the internal iliac and pudendal arteries has been emphasized to demonstrate lesions of the internal iliac artery and lesions of distal arteries, that is, the perineal portion of the internal pudendal and deep and dorsal arteries of the penis (Fig. 43–82a).[234] For correction of the arterial failure, a deep epigastric cavernous shunt has been described (Fig. 43–83).

The second approach has emphasized the use of phlebograms and corpus cavernosograms to evaluate the competence of the deep dorsal vein of the penis (Figs. 43–84, 43–85).[233]

URETHRAL PROSTHESES FOR INCONTINENCE OF URINE

It has been demonstrated that the Kaufman prosthesis may erode the urethra and may either enter the urethra without extravasation of urine or may produce extravasation with the erosion (Fig. 43–86).[235]

PROLAPSED URETEROCELE

A ureterocele, either ectopic or simple, can prolapse into the urethra, although the ectopic variety appears to be much more common (Fig. 43–87). A ureterocele can prolapse throughout the extent of the female urethra, appearing at the external urethral orifice, and therefore is easy to diagnose. It will prolapse only to the membranous urethra in the male and produce a cone-shaped dilatation of the posterior urethra that may be confused with stricture. The prolapse can be constant or intermittent, and obstructive symptoms and signs can occur.

SPLIT STREAM

A split stream (Fig. 43–88) can be the result of urethral stricture, meatal stenosis, or foreign substances such as mucoid material in the urethra.

URETHROEJACULATORY REFLUX

Reflux into the ejaculatory ducts on voiding or injecting cystourethrography may be the result of distal obstruction, infection, or trauma (Fig. 43–88a).

CLINICAL APPLICATION OF URODYNAMIC EVALUATION OF THE LOWER URINARY TRACT

MONEER K. HANNA

Clinical evaluation together with radiologic and endoscopic investigations provides sufficient information to resolve most voiding abnormalities. However, more sophisticated urodynamic tests are required in selected clinical problems.

Electronic apparatus allow simultaneous monitoring and recording of bladder pressure, both during filling and voiding, and of urine flow rate and sphincter electromyography. Some clinics routinely combine these studies with voiding cystourethrography. Although somewhat invasive, these tests are more meaningful than multiple static films for evaluating the dynamic act of micturition. They are particularly useful when major surgical urinary tract reconstruction or urinary undiversion is contemplated (Fig. 43–89).[247] Furthermore, intraoperative urodynamic monitoring provides the surgeon with an invaluable objective test of bladder neck and urethral competence and thereby allows for accurate assessment of an ablative or reconstructive bladder neck or urethral operation.[248] The practical application of these tests is illustrated in Figure 43–90.

It has been established that the pressure within the normal, stable bladder does not change significantly by provocative measures (Fig. 43–91). An unstable bladder, however, generates uninhibited contractions in response to postural change from the supine to upright (postural detrusor hyperreflexia[246]) and/or subcutaneous injection of bethanechol (denervation supersensitivity test[249]). These tests are invaluable in the diagnosis of subclinical neuropathic bladder disease in patients who present with micturitional difficulties and absent neurologic signs (Fig. 43–92).

The bladder neck, once considered an internal sphincter and then later rejected as a nonexistent anatomic sphincter, is now believed to be a cough competent, strain-proof mechanism capable of functioning as an efficient occlusive sphincter.[250] Two abnormalities have been delineated: (1) bladder neck dyskinesia[246] and (2) bladder neck relaxation. The former may account for obstructive uropathy, whereas the latter may be congenital, iatrogenic, neuropathic, or idiopathic (Fig. 43–93).

The distal or external sphincter is a composite and complex mixture of smooth and striated muscle that synergistically relaxes during voiding (Fig. 43–89). Inappropriate sphincter contraction (dyssynergia) may result in functional bladder outflow obstruction, manifesting urodynamically as high voiding pressure–low flow rate phenomenon (Fig. 43–94). Uninhibited external sphincter relaxations associated with bladder neck incompetence may account for dribble incontinence in patients with spinal cord disease.

Flowmetry is the least invasive and most informative screening test of the overall detrusor–urethral relationship. It represents the end result of the entire voiding event, and, with experience, the urodynamically oriented urologist should be able to diagnose subtle voiding abnormalities (Fig. 43–95). The flow rate record can be compared with follow-up tracing to evaluate the efficacy of treatment. Furthermore, these objective recordings are useful for medicolegal purposes.

Urodynamic testing has added a new dimension to the clinical management of voiding dysfunctions. The clinician is provided with objective data, thereby allowing for a more rational application of treatment regimes. Therapeutic results become more predictable using such an approach and can only improve with further advances and with greater diagnostic sophistication.

CHAPTER 43, ILLUSTRATIONS

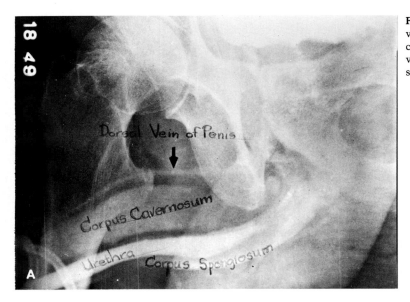

FIG. 43–1. Injecting cystourethrogram. The oblique view (**A**) labels the various anatomic parts. Corpus cavernosum refers to corpus cavernosum penis. AP view (**B**) shows the extravasation into the corpus spongiosum and into the venous channels.

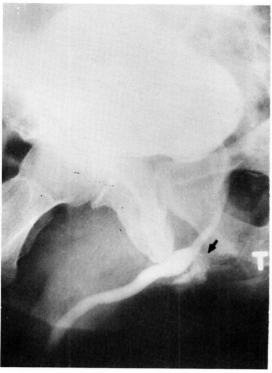

FIG. 43–2. Urethrocavernous refluxes. Injecting cysto-urethrogram. Contrast material has escaped into the corpus spongiosum urethra (*arrow*).

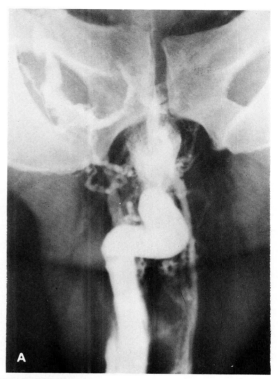

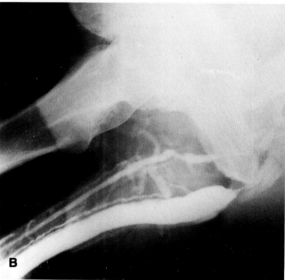

FIG. 43–3. Urethrocavernous reflux. Injecting cysto-urethrogram showing extravasation into the corpus spongiosum and the venous channels. **(A)** AP view. **(B)** Oblique view. The oblique view gives an excellent demonstration of the vessels communicating with the dorsal vein of the penis.

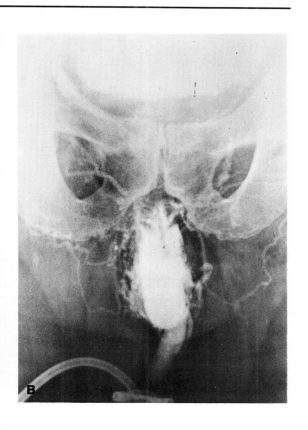

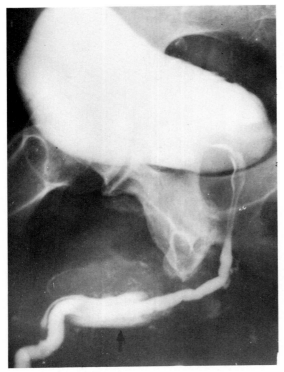

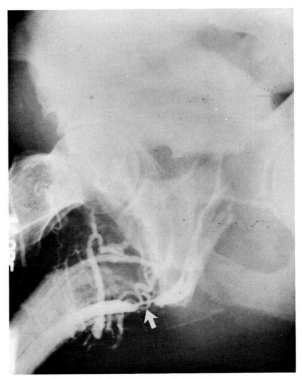

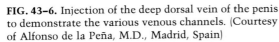

FIG. 43–4. Urethrocavernous refluxes. Injecting cystourethrogram. There is extravasation of contrast material into the corpus spongiosum. *Arrow* points to the contrast medium on the ventral side. However, it also can be seen on the opposite side of the urethra. Some contrast medium has escaped into the vessels of the corpus cavernosum penis.

FIG. 43–5. Urethrocavernous reflux in a case of gonorrheal stricture just anterior to the bulb. Contrast material has gone into the communicating veins and into the dorsal vein of the penis. *Arrow* points to region of stricture.

FIG. 43–6. Injection of the deep dorsal vein of the penis to demonstrate the various venous channels. (Courtesy of Alfonso de la Peña, M.D., Madrid, Spain)

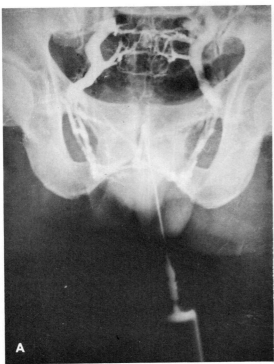

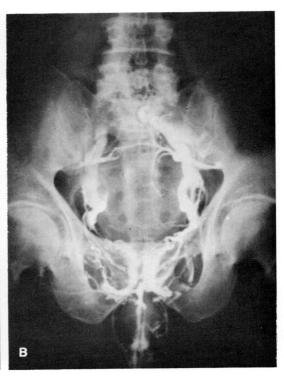

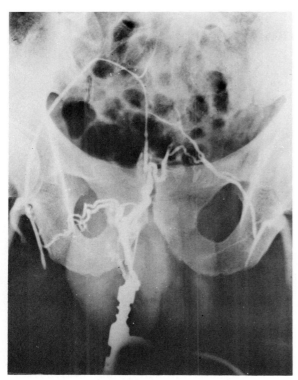

FIG. 43–7. Direct injection of dorsal vein of penis to show various venous channels. (Courtesy of B.S. Abeshouse, M.D.)

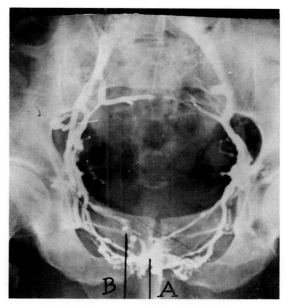

FIG. 43–8. Direct injection of deep dorsal vein of the penis in a case of carcinoma of the prostate. **(A)** Small prostatic plexus. **(B)** Paucity of veins and numerous thromboses. (Abeshouse, B.S., Ruben, M.E., J. Urol., 68:640, 1952)

FIG. 43–8a. Urethrovesical fistula. A 23-year-old man with a fracture of the symphysis pubis and disruption of membranous urethra. Cystostomy and realignment of the urethra over a catheter were performed. **(A)** Five months after injury and shortly after removal of catheter, the patient was incontinent. Cystogram demonstrates large defect in posterior urethra and bladder neck. **(B)** Retrograde cystourethrogram 18 months after injury reveals fistula tract anterior to the bladder neck.

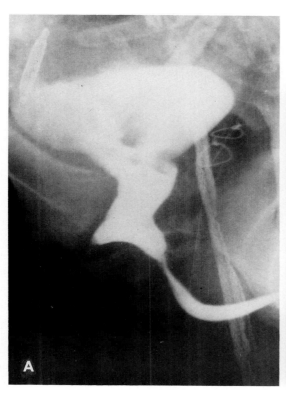

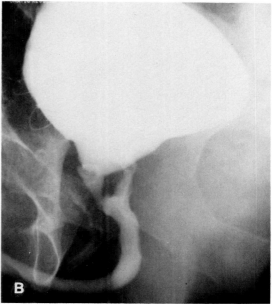

(Figure 43–8a is continued on page 1772.)

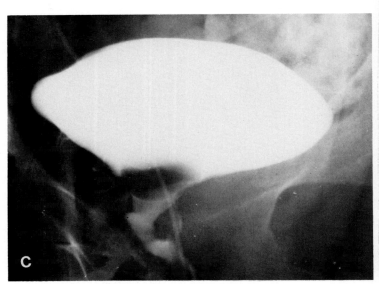

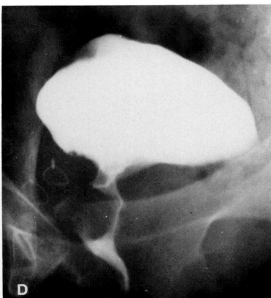

FIG. 43–8a, continued. (C) Voiding cystourethrogram — anterior fistulous tract visualized. **(D)** Following closure of fistulous opening by suprapublic approach. Voiding cystourethrogram demonstrates proximal closure of the vesicourethral fistula. (Fowler, J.E., Elliott, J.S.: J. Urol., *118:*114, 1977)

FIG. 43–9. Urethrocutaneous fistula following severe trauma. Multiple fistulous tracts in perineum.

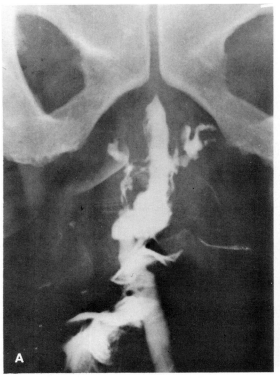

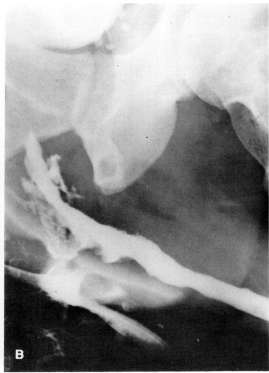

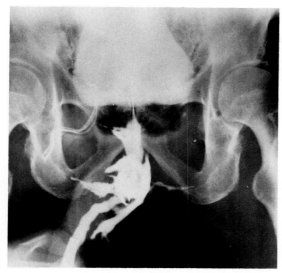

FIG. 43–10. Multiple urethral perineal fistulas associated with stricture of the urethra.

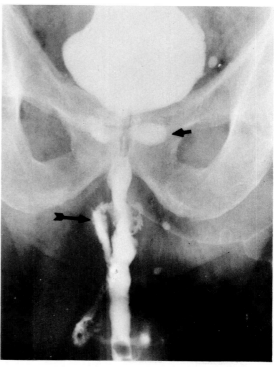

FIG. 43–12. Urethrocutaneous fistula in man. *Arrow* points to fistulous tract arising from prostatic urethra following abdominal perineal resection for rectal carcinoma. (Courtesy of Sol Unger, M.D., Veterans Administration)

FIG. 43–11. Urethrocutaneous fistula. Patient had many dilatations for stricture of the bulbomembranous area and developed infection with a periurethral abscess that formed a fistula to the skin. *Small arrow* points to prostatic abscess cavity on the left. On the right there are dilated prostatic ducts with some cavitation. *Large arrow* points to the fistulous tract, the opening of which is in the bulbomembranous area.

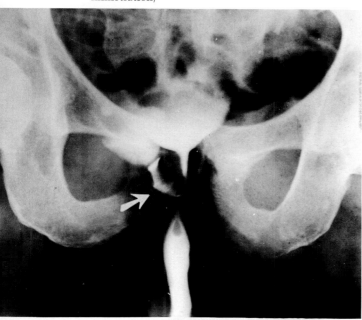

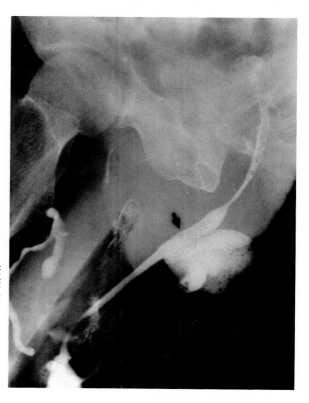

FIG. 43–13. Urethrocutaneous fistula in the region of the scrotum. Fistula developed following the closure of a Johanson repair of a urethral fistula. *Small arrow* points to area of the fistulous opening in the urethra.

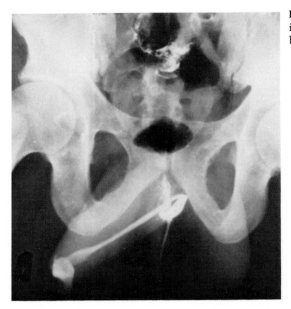

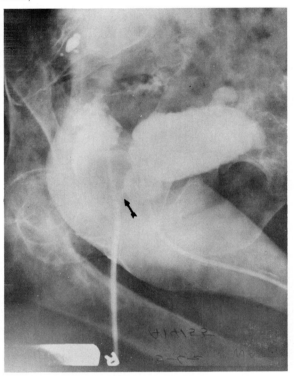

FIG. 43–14. Urethrorectal cutaneous fistula following infection. Perineal fistula seen as a narrow tract; air in bladder, contrast material in sigmoid.

FIG. 43–15. Urethrorectal fistula in prostatic area following a surgical injury. Left oblique view. *Arrow* points to actual fistula between prostatic urethra and rectum. The bladder can be seen anteriorly and the rectum posteriorly. (Courtesy of Maxwell Malament, M.D.)

FIG. 43–16. Urethrorectal fistula following severe trauma in an automobile accident. Urethral catheter is seen entering the rectum. Contrast medium injected through the catheter outlines the rectum, the descending colon, and part of the transverse colon.

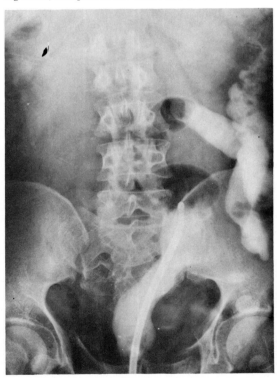

FIG. 43–17. Rectoprostatic urethral fistula following a rupture of a prostatic abscess. Fistula was in region of bladder neck. *Small black arrow* designates region of prostate. *White arrow* designates bladder. Right oblique view. (Courtesy of Sol Unger, M.D., Veterans Administration)

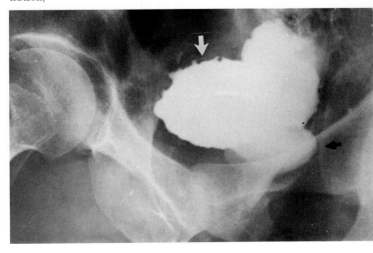

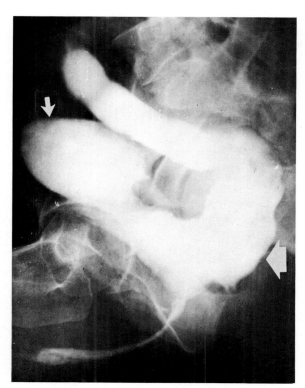

FIG. 43–18. Large urethrorectal fistula following a suprapubic enucleation of a fixed carcinoma of the prostate. Contrast material was injected through the urethra. *Small white arrow* points to bladder. *Large white arrow* points to rectum. The fistulous opening is in the prostatic urethra.

FIG. 43–18a. Urethrocavernous fistula–post cavernosum–spongiosum shunt for idiopathic priapism. **(A)** Retrograde urethrogram shows fistula extensively involving corpus; oblique view. **(B)** Urethrogram 1 month postoperatively shows residual sinus. Only a cystostomy had been performed. **(C)** Urethrogram 4 months after cystostomy. The suprapubic tube has been removed. This view shows complete absence of abnormal communication; no stricture. (Buckspan, M., Klotz, P.: J. Urol., *117*:538, 1977)

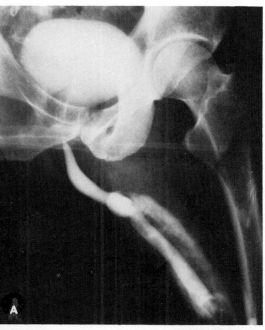

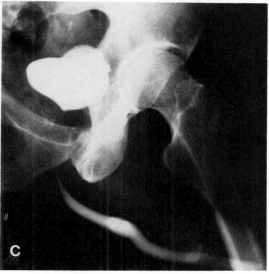

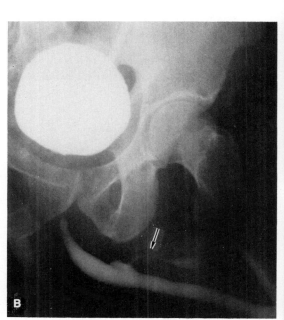

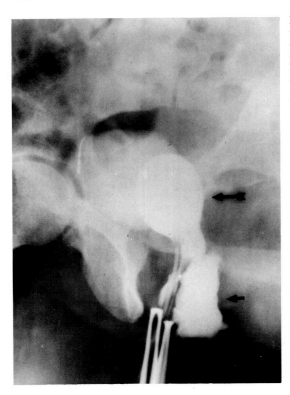

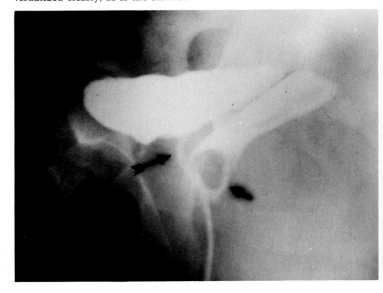

FIG. 43–19. Urethrovaginal fistula secondary to a urethral diverticulectomy. Contrast medium was injected along the side of a Foley catheter. *Large arrow* points to contrast-filled Foley bag. *Small arrow* points to vagina. Contrast medium can be seen also in the bladder above the Foley bag. The fistulous opening was approximately midurethra.

FIG. 43–20. Urethrovaginal fistula associated with a polyp of the vagina. *Large arrow* designates urethra. *Small arrow* points to polyp of vagina, which is represented by a filling defect in the distal vagina. Vagina is visualized clearly, as is the bladder.

FIG. 43–21. Urethrovaginal fistula secondary to radium application for carcinoma of the cervix. *Black arrow* points to injected urethra near the fistulous opening into the vagina. Vagina and uterine cavities are visualized clearly. *White arrow* designates vagina. The acorn tip and a portion of the syringe used for the injection are visualized.

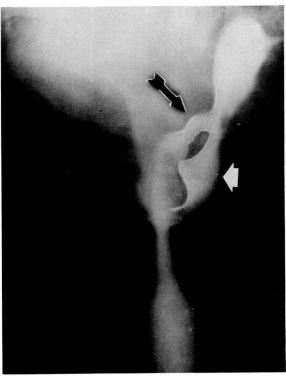

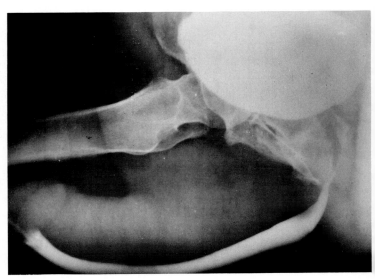

FIG. 43–22. Case of priapism. Cause undetermined. Patient had urinary retention. An injection cysto-urethrogram reveals an elongated anterior urethra but no special narrowing.

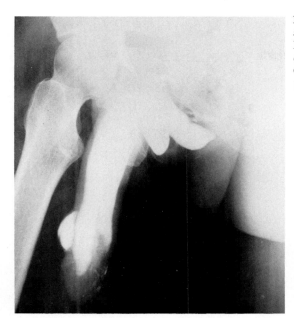

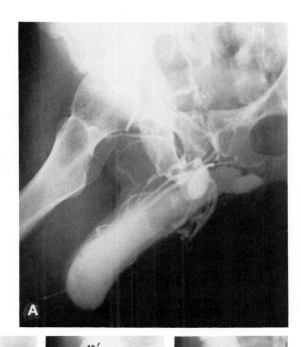

FIG. 43–23. Priapism in quiescent stage of sickle cell anemia. Normal-appearing corpora cavernosa with dilated veins at base of penis. There is a small degree of extravasation at the site of the needle injection. (Ney, C., Miller, H.L., Friedenberg, R.M.: Radiology, *119*:69, 1976)

FIG. 43–24. Priapism. **(A)** Spongiosogram demonstrates patency of superficial dorsal vein. **(B)** Cavernosogram reveals cavernosa stasis. No venous drainage to deep dorsal vein up to 45 minutes. **(C)** Cavernosogram following cavernosum–spongiosum shunt demonstrates patency and venous drainage. **(D)** Cavernosograms 4 days postoperatively illustrate patency but with delayed cavernous runoff. Portions of cavernosa tissue remain unopacified. **(E)** Cavernosogram 2 months postoperatively shows prompt venous drainage complete in 2 minutes. (Fitzpatrick, T.J.: J. Urol., *109*:843–846, 1973)

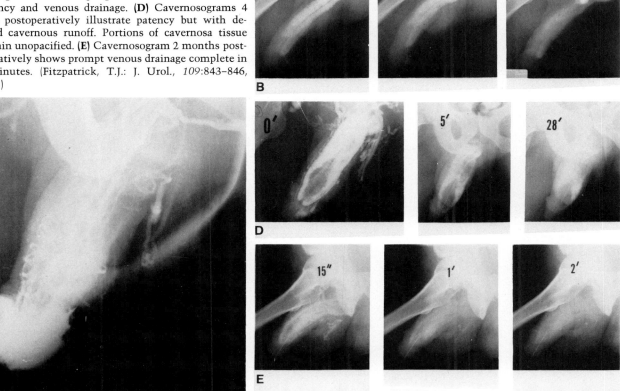

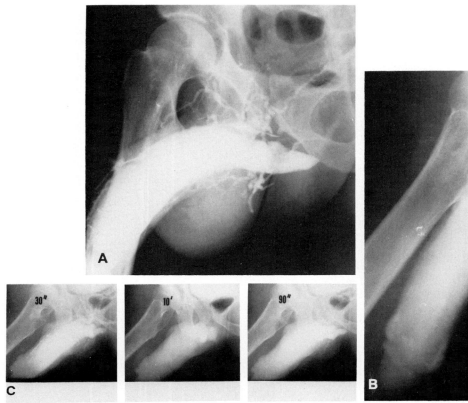

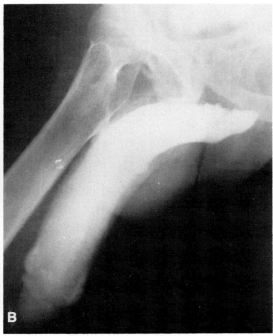

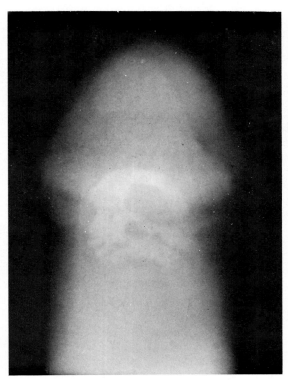

FIG. 43–25. Priapism. Previous cavernosumsaphenous shunt. **(A)** Subsiding priapism. Cavernosogram demonstrates prompt venous drainage. **(B)** Priapism of 24 hours duration 19 days following **A.** Cavernosogram shows complete corpora cavernosa venous obstruction. **(C)** Post cavernosum–spongiosum shunt. Cavernosogram shows prompt and complete venous drainage in 10 minutes; subsequent full potency. (Fitzpatrick, T.J.: J. Urol., *109*:843–846, 1973)

FIG. 43–26. Peyronie's disease. Calcified plaque in the dorsum of the penis overlying the corona.

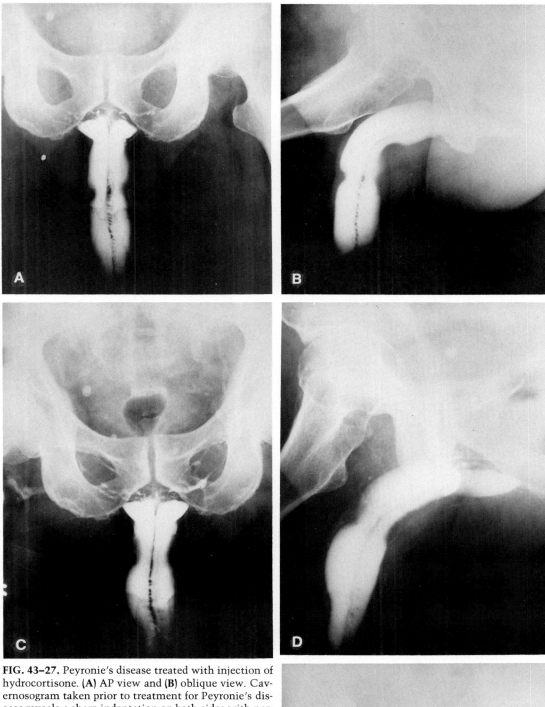

FIG. 43–27. Peyronie's disease treated with injection of hydrocortisone. **(A)** AP view and **(B)** oblique view. Cavernosogram taken prior to treatment for Peyronie's disease reveals a sharp indentation on both sides with narrowing of the visualized bodies of the corpora cavernosa and widening of the septal space at level of defects in the corpora. Complete drainage of contrast material took 110 minutes. **(C)** AP view and **(D)** oblique view 8 months after treatment with hydrocortisone. Cavernosogram shows considerable improvement with a decrease in the width of the septal defect and an increase in size of the visible corpora cavernosa at the level of the Peyronie's plaque. Contrast material disappeared in 90 to 105 minutes. **(E)** Third examination after further treatment demonstrates improvement in septal defect; atrophy of bodies still persists; drainage time was 90 minutes. (Ney, C., Miller, H.L., Friedenberg, R.M.: Radiology, *119*:69, 1976)

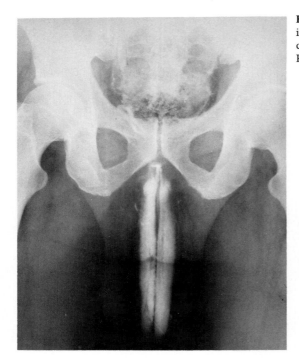

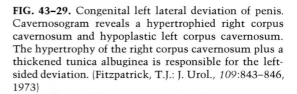

FIG. 43–28. Early Peyronie's disease exhibiting widening of the septum and bilateral indentation of corpora cavernosa. (Ney, C., Miller, H.L., Friedenberg, R.M.: Radiology, *119*:69, 1976)

FIG. 43–29. Congenital left lateral deviation of penis. Cavernosogram reveals a hypertrophied right corpus cavernosum and hypoplastic left corpus cavernosum. The hypertrophy of the right corpus cavernosum plus a thickened tunica albuginea is responsible for the left-sided deviation. (Fitzpatrick, T.J.: J. Urol., *109*:843–846, 1973)

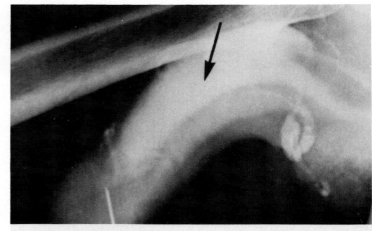

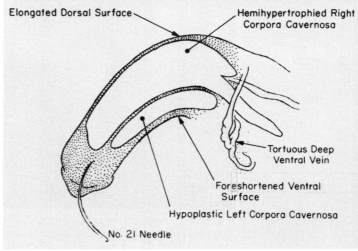

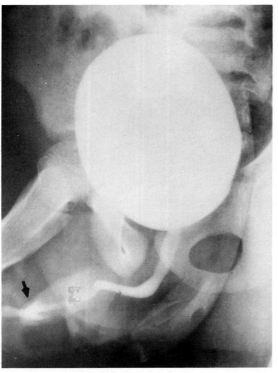

FIG. 43–30. Phimosis. Voiding cystourethrogram. *Arrow* points to contrast medium collecting under the foreskin. (Courtesy of Keith Waterhouse, M.D.)

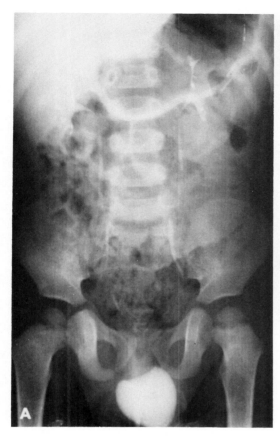

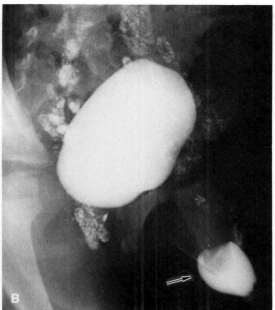

FIG. 43–31. Phimosis. (A) AP view after an intravenous urogram; contrast medium under prepuce. (B) Oblique view; contrast material seen under prepuce and within bladder.

FIG. 43–32. Normal corpus cavernosogram. (A) AP and (B) oblique views. Needles in each corpus cavernosum with adhesive tape holding penis in extended position. The contour of the corpora is wider in the middle and tapers to a convex termination at the distal end. Borders are smooth and regular. The septum is represented by a thick regular lucency with some widening at the distal end. (Ney, C., Miller, H.L., Friedenberg, R.M.: Radiology, *119:*69, 1976)

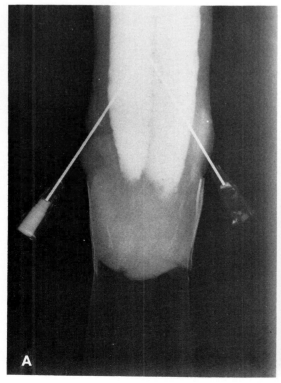

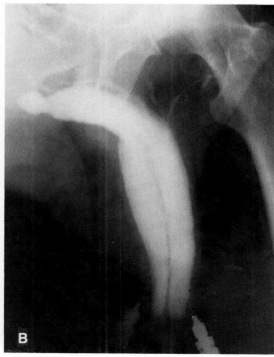

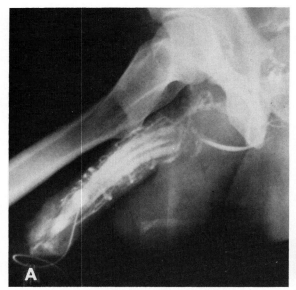

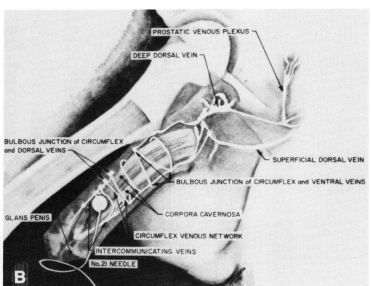

PROSTATIC VENOUS PLEXUS

DEEP DORSAL VEIN

BULBOUS JUNCTION of CIRCUMFLEX
and DORSAL VEINS

SUPERFICIAL DORSAL VEIN

BULBOUS JUNCTION of CIRCUMFLEX and VENTRAL VEINS

GLANS PENIS

CORPORA CAVERNOSA

CIRCUMFLEX VENOUS NETWORK

INTERCOMMUNICATING VEINS

No.21 NEEDLE

FIG. 43–33. Corpus cavernosogram showing complete venous drainage system of the penis (**A**) and diagram for explanation (**B**). (Fitzpatrick, T.J.: J. Urol., *109*:843–846, 1973)

FIG. 43–34. Corpus cavernosogram reveals a well-defined, clear-cut, smooth-edged defect in the body of the corpora cavernosa representing metastases from a carcinoma of the urethra. (Ney, C., Miller, H.L., Friedenberg, R.M.: Radiology, *119*:69, 1976)

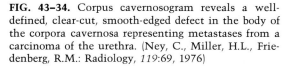

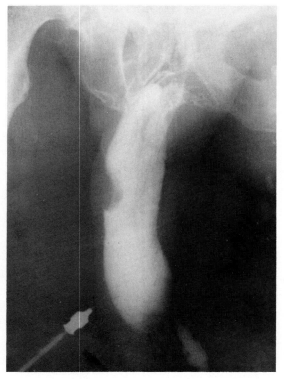

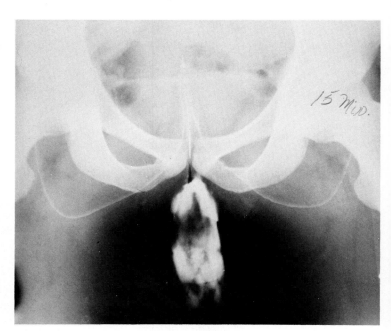

FIG. 43–35. Atrophy and fibrosis of corpora following infection and gangrene. The patient had had persistent priapism. Glans penis destroyed. Note irregularly filled small corpora cavernosa. (Ney, C., Miller, H.L., Friedenberg, R.M.: Radiology, *119*:69, 1976)

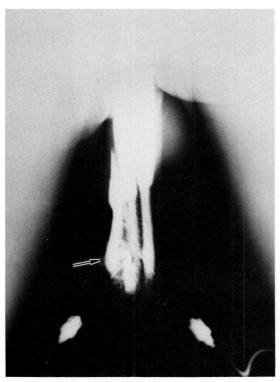

FIG. 43–36. Trauma. Tract created by bullet is demonstrated outside the corpus and subcutaneously.

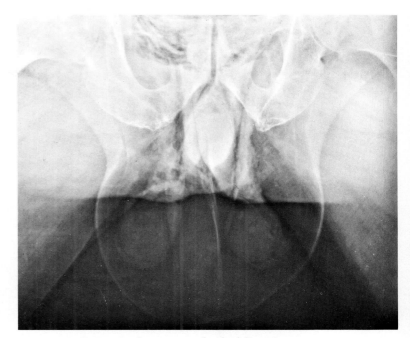

FIG. 43–37. Oxygen in the scrotum clearly delineating both testicles. The oxygen had been injected presacrally. The kidneys were outlined clearly during this procedure.

FIG. 43–38. Oxygen in the scrotal sac. Presacral oxygen insufflation for visualization of the kidneys. Gas escaped into the scrotum, clearly visualizing the testicle on the left (*arrow*).

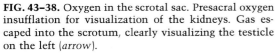

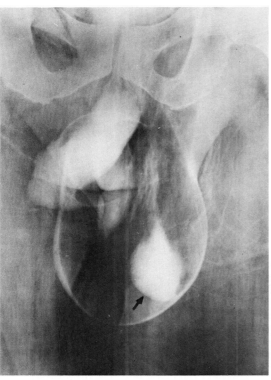

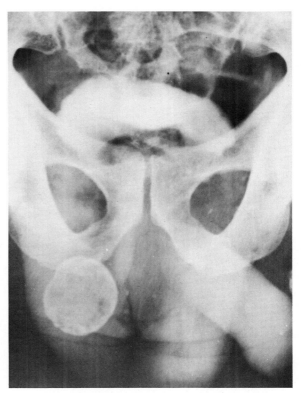

FIG. 43–39. Calcified testicle. Cause undetermined. (Courtesy of Sol Unger, M.D., Veterans Administration)

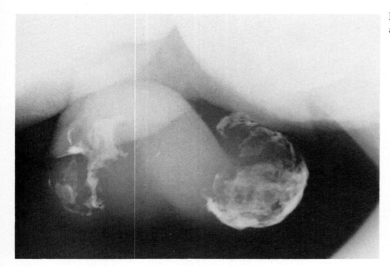

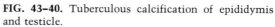

FIG. 43–40. Tuberculous calcification of epididymis and testicle.

FIG. 43–41. Calcified hydrocele. This most commonly follows trauma with hemorrhage in the tunica vaginalis, and possibly it should be called more nearly correctly a calcified hematocele.

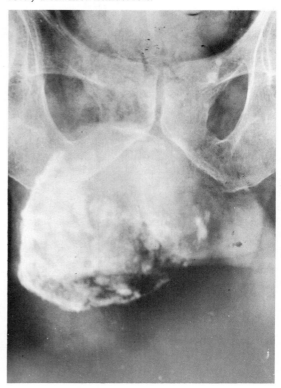

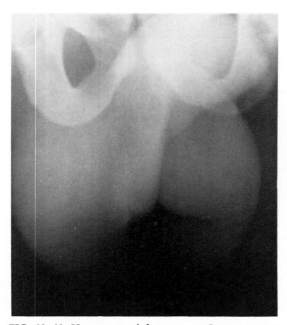

FIG. 43–42. Hematoma of the scrotum. Large scrotum filled with blood from trauma.

FIG. 43–43. Gas bacillus infection of the scrotum. There are irregular radiolucent areas in the scrotum secondary to the gas formed by the infection.

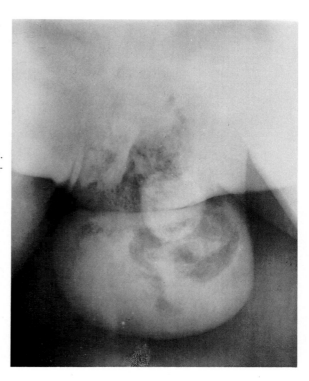

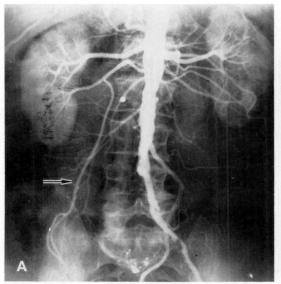

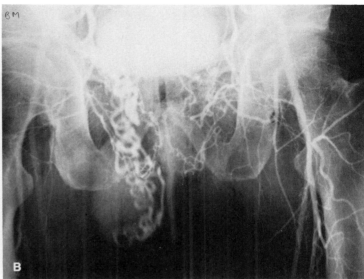

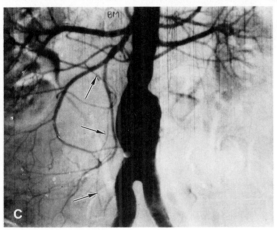

FIG. 43–44. Spermatic artery dilatation produced by right iliac obstruction corrected by bypass. **(A)** Aortogram shows the dilated right spermatic artery (*arrow*) and the obstruction of the right common iliac artery. **(B)** Large right testicular artery pulsating in right scrotum. **(C)** *Arrows* point to improved right internal spermatic artery following a bypass operation.

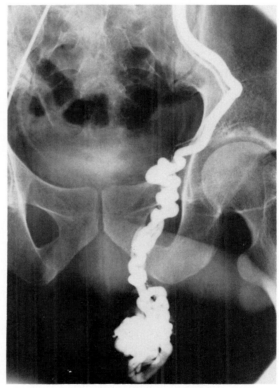

FIG. 43–45. Left varicocele. Retrograde venogram. Note double internal spermatic vein above inguinal canal. (Courtesy of S. Sprayregen, M.D.)

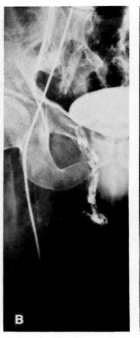
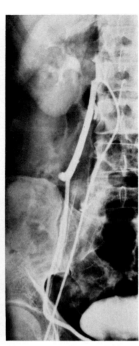

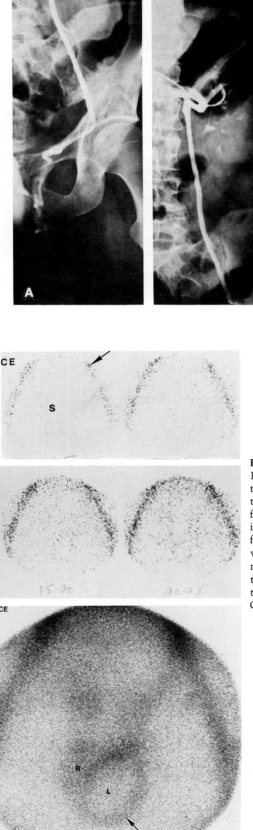

FIG. 43–46. Bilateral varicocele. **(A)** Left varicocele visualized by selective retrograde phlebography. Left side of print shows injection of upper part of vein. On right side of print, the varicocele is visualized. **(B)** Right varicocele in the same patient as **(A)**. Left side of print: injection of internal spermatic vein. Right side of print: varicocele demonstrated. (Courtesy of M. Kunnen and F. Comhaire)

FIG. 43–47. Classic acute testicular torsion. **(A)** Radionuclide angiogram shows activity in the area of the iliac/femoral arteries (*arrow*), but no perfusion to the area of the scrotum (*S*). In the normal patient, perfusion to the testicle is described as "barely perceptible." In the patient with torsion, no increased perfusion is seen. **(B)** Delayed image shows normal relative vascularity to the right testicle (*R*) and by comparison no significant relative vascularity to the area of the left testicle (*L*). The *arrow* points to the activity in the tunica dartos. (Courtesy of L.E. Holder, M.D., and J. Colston, M.D.)

FIG. 43–49. Acute epididymitis with displacement of the epididymis medially. **(A)** Radionuclide angiogram shows increased perfusion to the more medial aspect of the left hemiscrotum (*arrow*). **(B)** Blood pool image taken with lead shielding shows normal relative vascularity in the right and left testicles (*R* and *L*). There is increased relative vascularity in the medial aspect of the left hemiscrotum (*arrow*). **(C)** Cobalt 57 "hot" markers are used to identify the testicles (*M*). This does indicate that the increased activity is located medially to the testicle. This shift of the epididymis often occurs in the swollen edematous hemiscrotum. (Courtesy of L.E. Holder, M.D. and J.R. Martire, M.D.)

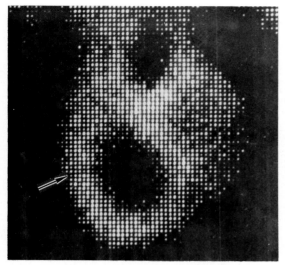

FIG. 43–47a. Torsion of testis. Radionuclide scan. Area of right testicle with no uptake on static imaging.

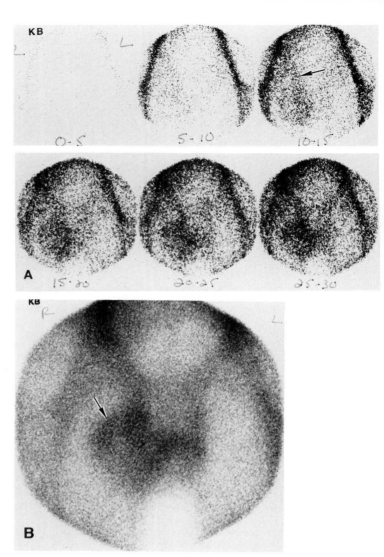

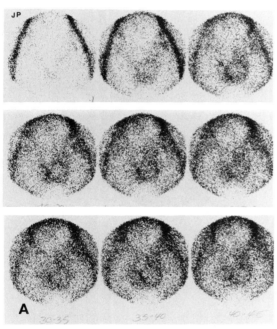

FIG. 43–48. Acute epididymitis. **(A)** Radionuclide angiogram shows activity in the right testicular and deferential artery region (*arrow*) and then into the area of the right hemiscrotum. **(B)** Activity is located in the classic lateral position of the epididymis (*arrow*). (Courtesy of L.E. Holder, M.D., and J.R. Martire, M.D.)

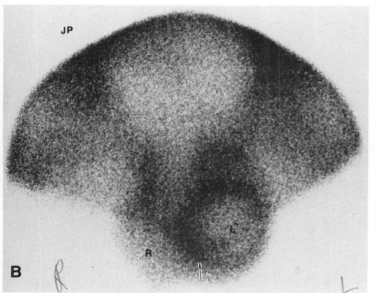

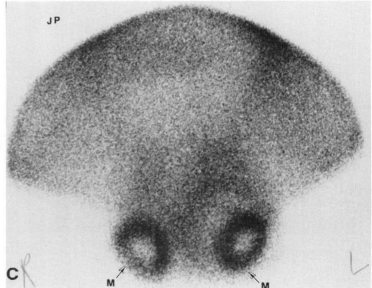

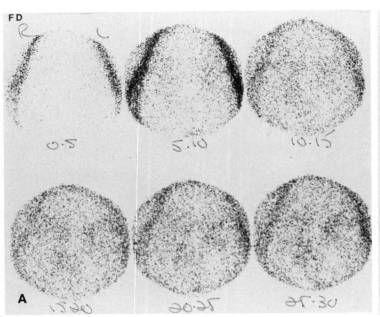

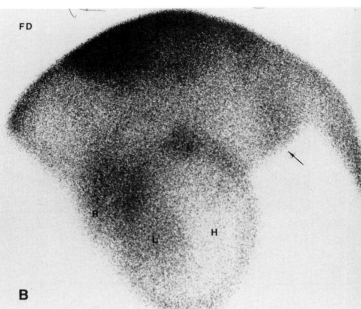

FIG. 43–50. Hydrocele. **(A)** Radionuclide angiogram shows no areas of increased perfusion to the scrotal region. **(B)** Blood pool image shows relatively normal perfusion of the area of the right and left testicles (*R, L*). The hydrocele (*H*) appears as an area of absent relative vascularity in a half-moon-shaped appearance surrounding the left testicle and extending up the left spermatic cord. *Arrow* points to edge of lead shielding excluding activity from the thigh. Note that despite the presence of a large lucency (relatively avascular area) in the hemiscrotum, the testicle is still clearly defined. In acute torsion, one cannot define the testicle since the area of relative avascularity replaces the testicle. (Courtesy of L.E. Holder, M.D. and H.K.A. Schirmer, M.D.)

FIG. 43–51. Bilateral hydroceles with normal appearing testicles on ultrasonography. (Courtesy of J.P. Richie and J.C. Birnholz)

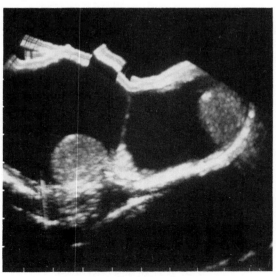

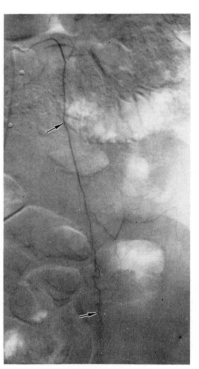

FIG. 43–52. Testicular agenesis. Left testicular artery (*arrow*) can be followed to internal inguinal ring. Boy, aged 11. [Nordmark, L., Bjersing, L., Bomellof, K. et al.: Acta Radiol. (Diagn) Stockh., *18*:167, 1977]

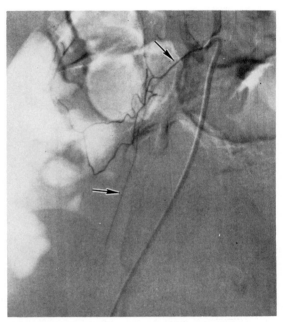

FIG. 43–53. Testicular agenesis. Right testicular artery (*arrow*) runs down to the inguinal ring and ends in front of the upper part of the sacroiliac joint. [Nordmark, L., Bjersing, L., Bomellof, K. et al.: Acta Radiol. (Diagn.) (Stockh.), *18*:167, 1977]

FIG. 43–55. Cryptorchidism in boy aged 6. Left testicular artery runs to a small testicle (*arrows*) situated medially to the internal inguinal ring. [Nordmark, L., Bjersing, L., Bomellof, K. et al.: Acta Radiol. (Diagn.) (Stockh.), *18*:167, 1977]

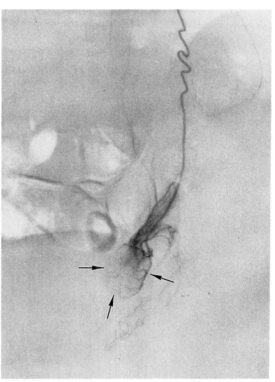

FIG. 43–54. Cryptorchidism in boy aged 13. Left testicular artery runs to a testicle (*arrow*) situated medially to the internal inguinal ring. [Norkmark, L., Bjersing, L., Bomellof, K. et al.: Acta Radiol. (Diagn.) (Stockh.), *18*:167, 1977]

FIG. 43–56. Retroperitoneal testis. Left testicular venogram shows typical appearance of pampiniform plexus (*arrow*). Multiple parallel veins of pampiniform plexus mark location of mass. (Diamond, A.B., Meng, C.-H., Kodroff, M. et al.: Am. J. Roentgenol., *129*:71, 1977)

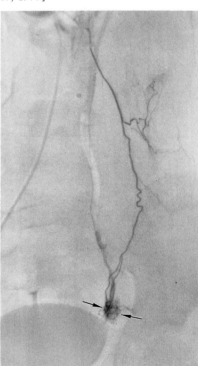

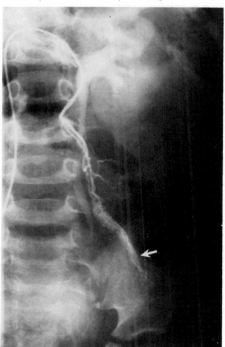

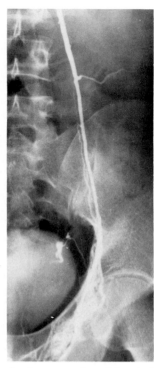
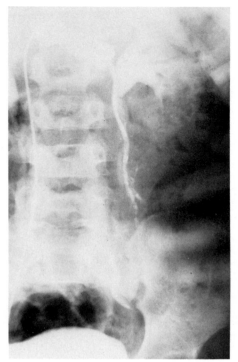

FIG. 43–57. Venography for demonstration of inguinal canal testis. Left testis at level of inguinal canal. Pampiniform plexus is average size. Collateral vessels partially fill left hypogastric vein. (Diamond, A.B., Meng, C.-H., Kodroff, M. et al.: Am. J. Roentgenol., *129*:71, 1977)

FIG. 43–58. Testicular agenesis on venography. Atrophic left testicular vein is seen without definite identification of pampiniform plexus. (Diamond, A.B., Meng, C.-H., Kodroff, M. et al.: Am. J. Roentgenol., *129*:71, 1977)

FIG. 43–59. Calcification in a seminoma of the testicle. (Courtesy of Sol Unger, M.D., Veterans Administration)

FIG. 43–60. Embryonal carcinoma of the testis, oblique view. Metastasis to periaortic lymph nodes (*arrow*). Notice crescentric deformity, marginal effect. (Courtesy of S. Rakoff, M.D.)

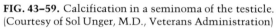
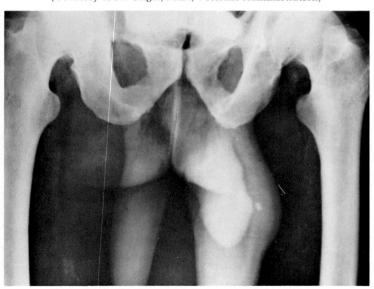
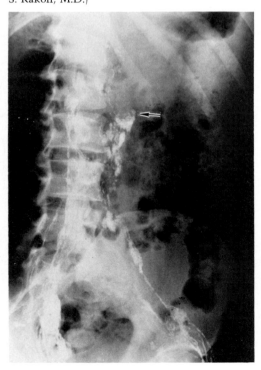

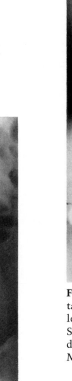

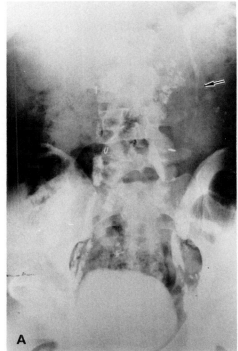

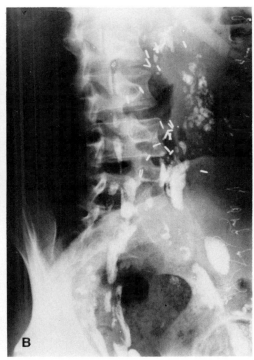

FIG. 43–61. Embryonal carcinoma of left testis metastatic to periaortic lymph nodes. **(A)** Lateral deviation of left ureter (*arrow*) by lymph nodes. **(B)** Oblique view. Some nodes have crescentric deformity; some have disruption of internal structure. (Courtesy of S. Rakoff, M.D.)

FIG. 43–62. Indentation of inferior vena cava (*arrow*) by metastases from teratoma of right testis. The lymph nodes of the right upper lumbar region are not demonstrated by lymphography. [Lien, H.H., Kolbenstvedt, A.: Acta Radiol. (Diagn.) (Stockh.), *18*:177, 1977]

FIG. 43–63. Seminoma of right testis. **(A)** On admission, elevation and compression of left renal vein by lymph node metastases. The extent of the tumor is better defined by the combined examination. No filling of left testicular vein. **(B)** Eight months after radiation therapy —no displacement of renal vein. The duplicated left spermatic vein is filled. [Lien, H.H., Kolbenstvedt, A.: Acta Radiol. (Diagn.) (Stockh.), *18*:177, 1977]

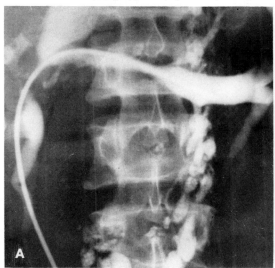

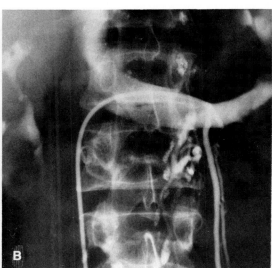

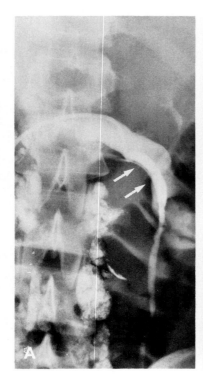
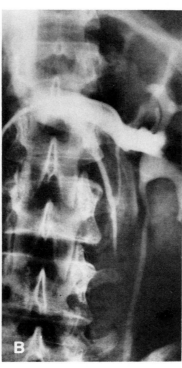

FIG. 43–64. Embryonal carcinoma of left testis. **(A)** Phlebogram of left renal vein and testicular vein. Previous lymphogram was suggestive of metastases on left side of lumbar vertebrae. Displacement of proximal part of left testicular vein (*arrows*) supports the lymphographic findings. **(B)** Regression of tumor 12 months after radiation therapy. Upper part of testicular vein is duplicated. [Lien, H.H., Kolbenstvedt, A.: Acta Radiol. (Diagn.) (Stockh.), *18*:177, 1977]

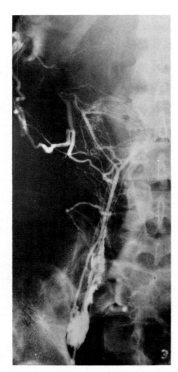

FIG. 43–65. Antegrade right spermatic vein phlebogram of a right testicular tumor. Lumbar metastases. The cranial part of the vein is displaced and partially occluded. A large retroperitoneal collateral vein is demonstrated. (Kolbenstvedt, A., Lien, H.H., Miller, A. et al.: Radiology, *114*:461, 1975)

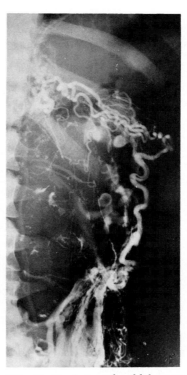

FIG. 43–66. Antegrade phlebogram of left spermatic vein showing metastases from a left testicular tumor. The cranial part of the left spermatic vein is completely obliterated. Large collateral veins encircle the tumor masses. (Kolbenstvedt, A., Lien, H.H., Miller, A. et al: Radiology, *114*:461, 1975)

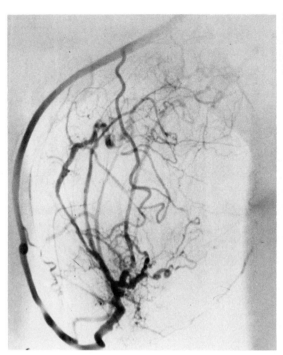

FIG. 43–67. Man aged 28. Subtracted magnification of selective arteriogram of spermatic artery. Embryonal carcinoma; tumor completely infiltrates testis and epididymis, numerous irregular vessels. (Courtesy of L. Nordmark)

FIG. 43–68. Man aged 28. Subtracted magnification selective arteriogram of spermatic artery. Seminoma. Tumor completely infiltrates testis and epididymis. All vessels run around the tumor; no irregular vessels. (Courtesy of L. Nordmark)

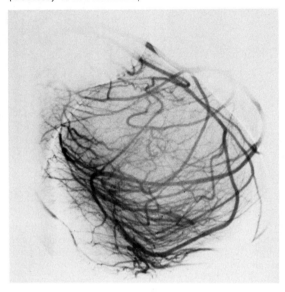

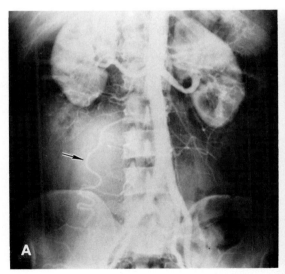

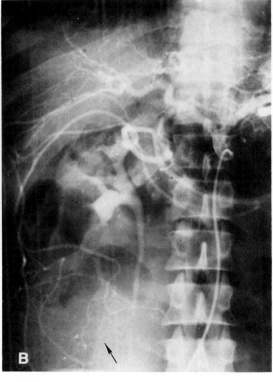

FIG. 43–69. Seminoma in an undescended testis. **(A)** *Arrows* point to a dilated right internal spermatic artery ending in the retroperitoneal space. **(B)** Celiac arteriogram reveals an omental vessel with some neovascularity (*arrow*). The malignancy in the testicle had invaded the omentum. (Courtesy of S. Sprayregen, M.D.)

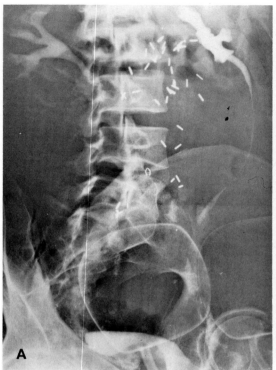
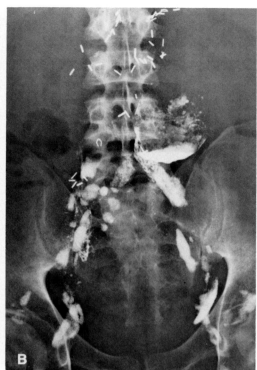

FIG. 43–70. Postoperative lymphocyst. (**A**) Displacement of left ureter and kidney anteriorly shortly after retroperitoneal node dissection for embryonal carcinoma of the testicle. (**B**) Lymphogram demonstrates lymphocyst. (Johnson, D.E.: Recent Results Cancer Res., *60*:221, 1977)

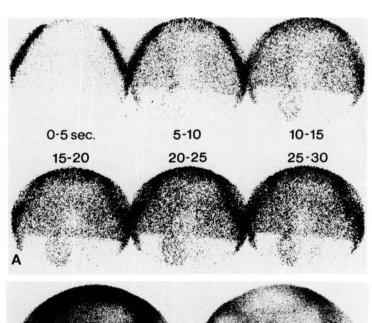

FIG. 43–71. Testicular tumors. (**A**) Radionuclide angiogram shows slightly increased perfusion to an enlarged right testicle. No definition of vessels is seen as in acute epididymitis or abscess. (**B**) Seminoma, the angiogram of which is shown in **A**. The left testicle (*L*) is normal. The right testicle (*R*) is enlarged and replaced by a diffusely vascular mass with increased activity (more warm than hot). (**C**) Teratoma with areas of embryonal carcinoma. The left testicle (*L*) was normal. Areas of varied intensity replaced the right testicle (*R*). (Holder, L.E., Martire, J.R., Holmes, E.R. III, et al.: Radiology *125*:739, 1977)

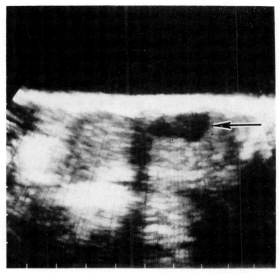

FIG. 43–72. Ultrasonogram of seminoma in upper pole of left testis. Small echo-free area present (*arrow*). (Courtesy of J.P. Richie and J.C. Birnholz)

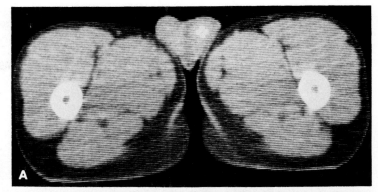
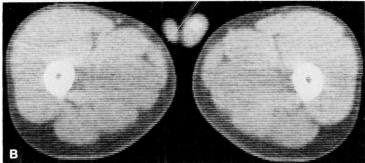

FIG. 43–73. CT scan of teratocarcinoma of left testicle, lower pole. (**A**) Upper portions of both testicles showing equal density on enhancement. (**B**) Lower portions of both testicles: the lower pole of the left testicle is larger and more dense on enhancement studies. (Courtesy of Peter K. Spiegel, M.D.)

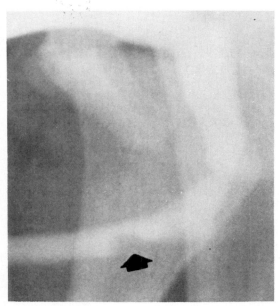

FIG. 43–74. Retention cyst of Cowper's duct demonstrated on a cystourethrogram. This is a bulbar type of Cowper's gland. (Moskowitz, P.S., Newton, N.A., and Lebowitz, R.L.: Radiology, *120*:377, 1976)

FIG. 43–74a. Cyst of Cowper's gland. Injecting cystourethrogram reveals defect in floor of membranous urethra (*arrow*). This is a diaphragmatic type of Cowper's gland.

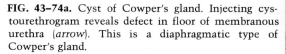
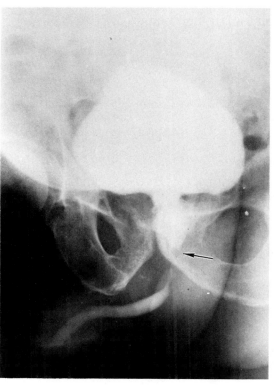

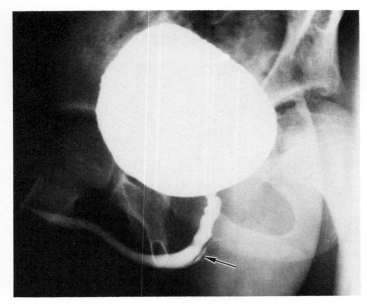

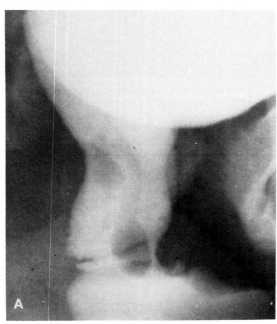

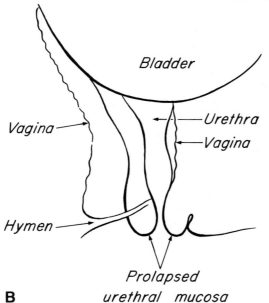

FIG. 43–75. Cowper's duct (arrow) visualized on a cystourethrogram. (Currarino, G., Fugua, F.: Am J. Roentgenol. 116:838, 1972)

FIG. 43–76. Primary localized amyloidosis of the urethra. (A) Retrograde urethrogram demonstrates lesion in anterior urethra. (B) Same lesion 5 months later. (Carris, C.K., McLaughlin, A.P., III, Gittes, R.F.: J. Urol., 115:423, 1976)

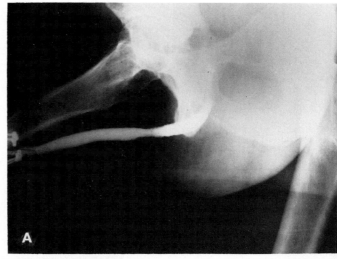

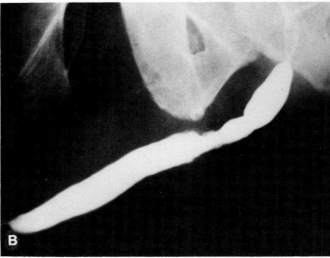

FIG. 43–77. Prolapse of urethral mucosa. (A) Oblique spot film obtained during voiding cystourethrography. The mass of prolapsed urethral mucosa protrudes beyond the floor of the vestibule as defined by the hymen. The central location of the narrowed urethral orifice within the mass is demonstrated. (B) Line drawing of A. (Potter, B.M.: Radiology, 98:287, 1971)

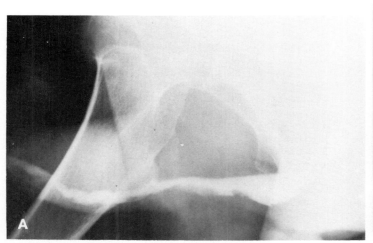 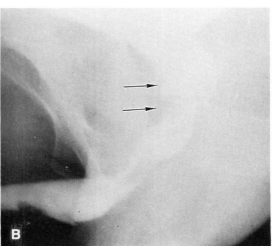

FIG. 43–78. Condylomata accuminata of the urethra. (A) Voiding cystourethrogram reveals anterior urethral mucosa to be extremely involved with multiple filling defects, representing intraurethral spread of condylomata accuminata; lesions are seen in both ventral and dorsal surfaces of the urethra. Posterior urethra is not visualized. (B) View of posterior urethra reveals similar lesions in prostatic urethra (*arrows*). (Pollack, H.M., DeBenedictis, T.J., Marmar, J.L. et al.: Radiology, *126*:643, 1978)

FIG. 43–79. Retrograde urethrogram reveals entire urethra involved with verrucous filling defects of condylomata accuminata. (Pollack, H.M., DeBenedictis, T.J., Marmar, J.L.: et al.: Radiology, *126*:643, 1978)

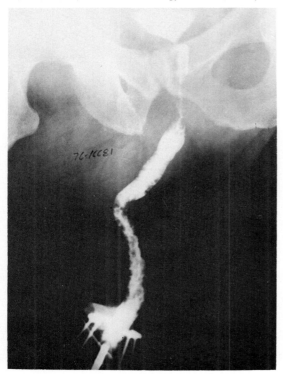

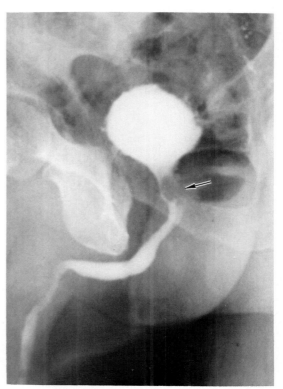

FIG. 43–80. Hypertrophied verumontanum in an adult. *Arrow* points to large verumontanum, cause undetermined.

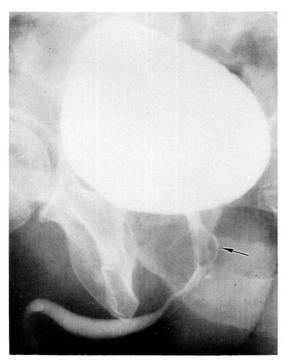

FIG. 43–81. Hypertrophied verumontanum in an adult.

FIG. 43–82a. A selective arteriogram of the right internal pudendal artery demonstrates an area of narrowing (*arrows*) caused by atheromatous plaques. Note the poststenotic dilatation attesting to the hemodynamic significance of the lesion. Note gross irregularity of the artery of the bulbus urethrae (*arrow*) and amputation of the posterior cavernosal branches. The anterior scrotal artery conversely is intact. (Lang, E.K., LaMassa, J.: Pudendal arteriography in assessment of erectile impotence. Radiology, in press, 1981)

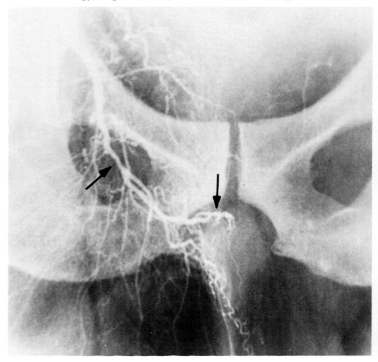

FIG. 43–82. Enlarged verumontanum. Man, 27 years old. Verumontanum is widened and elongated (*arrow*). This probably should be included in the group with verumontanitis. Patient also had an associated prostatitis.

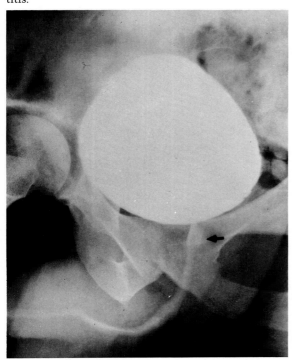

FIG. 43–83. Deep epigastric artery cavernous shunt for impotence, using saphenous vein. (Courtesy of A.W. Zorniotti)

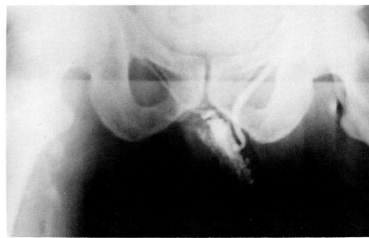

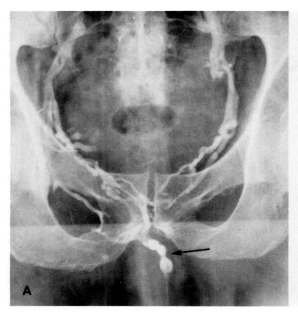

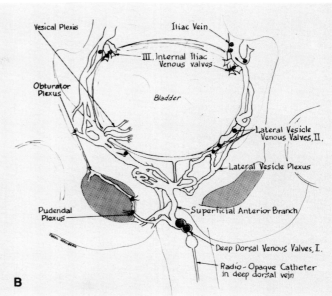

FIG. 43–84. Normal venous drainage of penis. **(A)** Phlebogram revealing presence of deep dorsal vein valves (arrows) and **(B)** diagram of venous system of penis. (Fitzpatrick, T.J., Cooper, J.F.: J. Urol., *113*:497, 1975)

FIG. 43–85. Cavernosogram of patient with partially sustained erection demonstrates the deep dorsal vein impeded by deep dorsal vein valve for 3 to 5 minutes. In unsustained erections, valves may be competent only up to 1 minute; in sustained erections, up to 10 minutes. (Fitzpatrick, T.J., Cooper, J.F.: J. Urol., *113*:497, 1975)

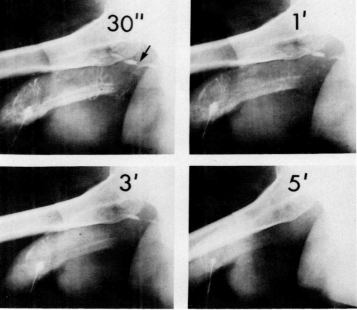

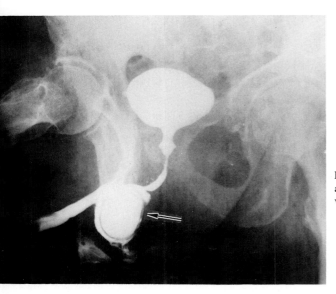

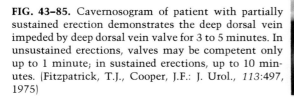

FIG. 43–86. Kaufman prosthesis (*arrow*) eroding urethra and producing extravasation of urine. The prosthesis was filled with contrast medium.

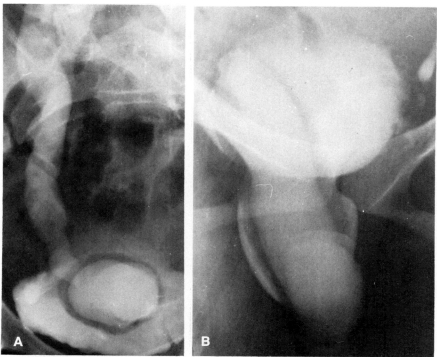

FIG. 43–87. Sliding ureterocele prolapsing into urethra in a woman. (**A**) Typical defect of a ureterocele is documented in the filled bladder. On Valsalva's maneuver, the ureterocele herniated into the urethra. (**B**) The ureterocele can be appreciated usually as a membrane bulging from the urethral orifice into the vagina. (Courtesy of Erich Lang, M.D.)

FIG. 43–88. Split stream. Young man with split stream as shown on a voiding cystourethrogram. Diagnosis was mild external meatal stenosis.

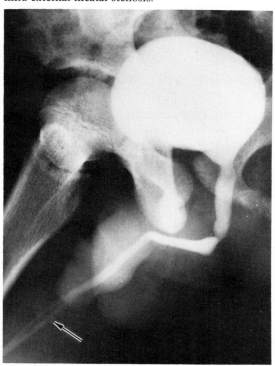

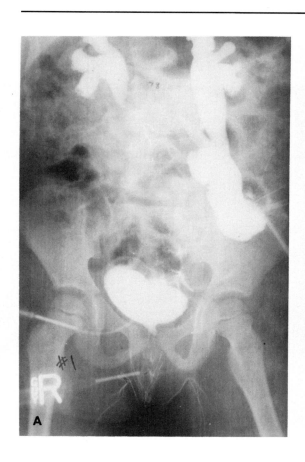

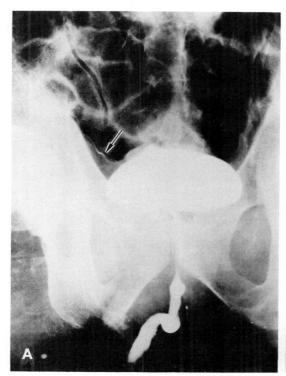

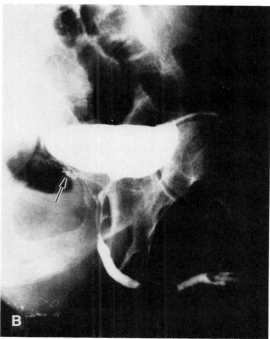

FIG. 43–88a. Reflux into seminal vesicles and vas on injecting cystourethrogram (*arrows*). Patient had been treated for urethral stricture.

FIG. 43–89. Urodynamics and urinary tract refunctionalization in a 5-year-old girl who underwent urinary diversion into a colonic loop for "unworkable bladder." **(A)** Loopogram and cystourethrogram. **(B)** Voiding cystourethrogram and urodynamics. *Thick arrow* points to the suprapubic cystocatheter. *Small arrow* points to the insulated wires inserted into the urethral sphincter one day prior to study. **(C)** Synchronous electromyography of the external sphincter, bladder pressure, and flow rate. Note the appropriate electric silence of the sphincter during detrusor contraction resulting in a normal flow rate. Conclusion: Salvageable lower urinary tract. Candidate for urinary undiversion.

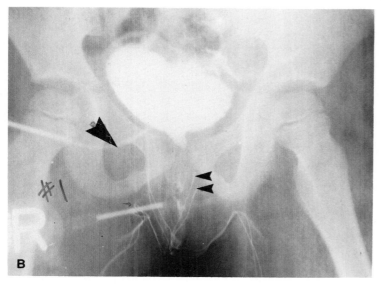

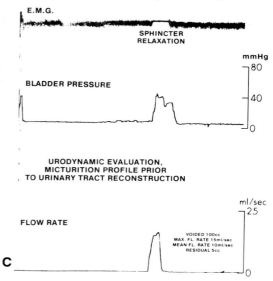

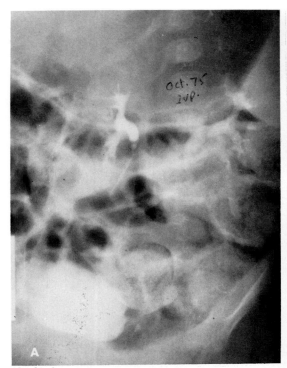

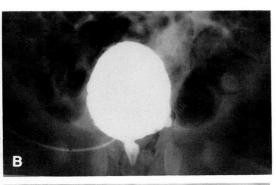

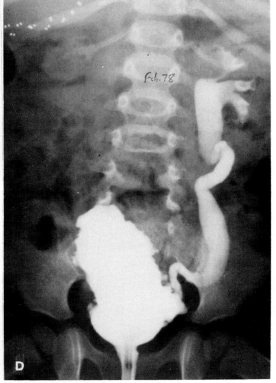

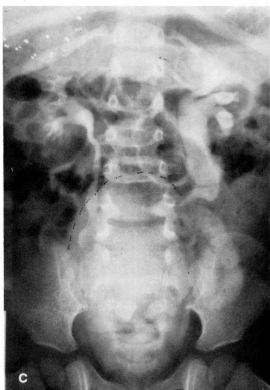

(Figure 43–90; legend on page 1803)

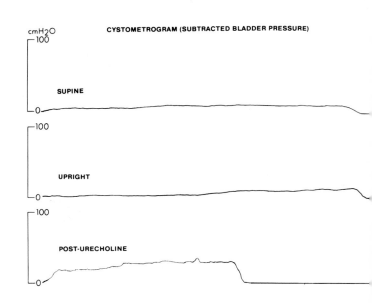

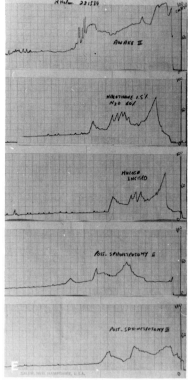

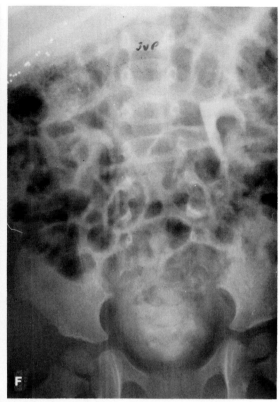

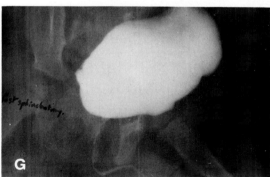

FIG. 43–90. Intraoperative urodynamics of a 4-year-old boy born with myelomeningocele and partial neurologic defecit. The boy walks normally and is continent of urine. **(A)** IVP at age 1 year: normal upper urinary tract. **(B)** Cystogram showing relatively smooth bladder wall, incompetent bladder neck, and no reflux. **(C)** IVP 1 year later: left hydroureteronephrosis. **(D)** Cystogram 1 year later: Note increased bladder trabeculation and sacculation and left vesicoureteral reflux. The radiologic deterioration was due to distal sphincter dyssynergia. **(E)** Urethral pressure profiles (UPP): **(a)** Awake; **(b)** following general anesthesia, the maximal urethral pressure (external sphincter high pressure zone) dropped to 70 cm of water; **(c)** UPP following incision of mucosa with urethrotome, unchanged urethral pressure; **(d)** UPP following careful and limited incision of the external sphincter, the maximal urethral pressure dropped to 35 cms. of water. **(F)** IVP 6 months following sphincterotomy: resolution of hydronephrosis. **(G)** Cystogram following spincterotomy: The reflux ceased, significant improvement of the bladder with less trabeculation. The boy remains continent of urine. Conclusion: Urodynamic work-up localized the problem at the external sphincter. UPP monitoring of transurethral sphincteric adjustment was an invaluable procedure in resolving the hydronephrosis and reflux, as well as in preserving the boy's continence.

◀ **FIG. 43–91.** Cystometrogram and bladder provocation: Normal cystometrogram (CMG). Insignificant pressure changes in response to bladder provocation by postural change and bethanechol injection.

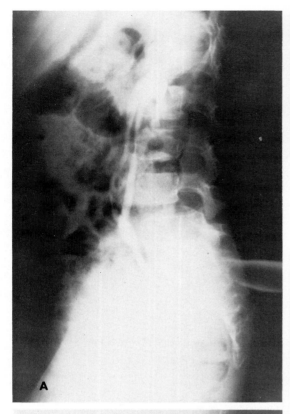

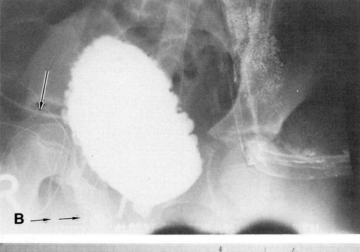

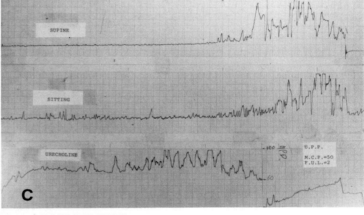

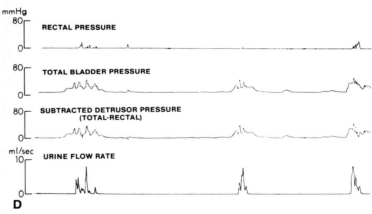

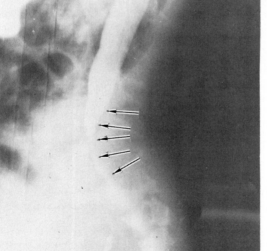

FIG. 43–92. Subclinical neuropathic bladder: An 8-year-old girl presented with secondary diurnal and nocturnal enuresis and recurrent urinary infections. Physical examination was unrevealing. Neurologic evaluation by two pediatric neurologists and one neurosurgeon confirmed the absence of neurologic signs. The patient was evaluated urodynamically. (**A**) IVP: unremarkable. (**B**) Voiding cystourethrogram: noticeable bladder trabeculation and incompetent bladder neck mechanism. (**C**) Provocative cystometrogram: clearly positive urecholine test. (**D**) Micturition urodynamic profile: significant bladder-sphincter dyssynergia. Conclusion: Urodynamically neuropathic bladder. Myelogram was recommended. (**E**) Myelogram: filling defect of a subarachnoid cyst causing tethering of the spinal cord. (*arrows*) The child underwent excision of the cyst and release of the tethered spinal cord. The urinary symptoms improved considerably 3 months following surgery. Awaiting urodynamic follow-up.

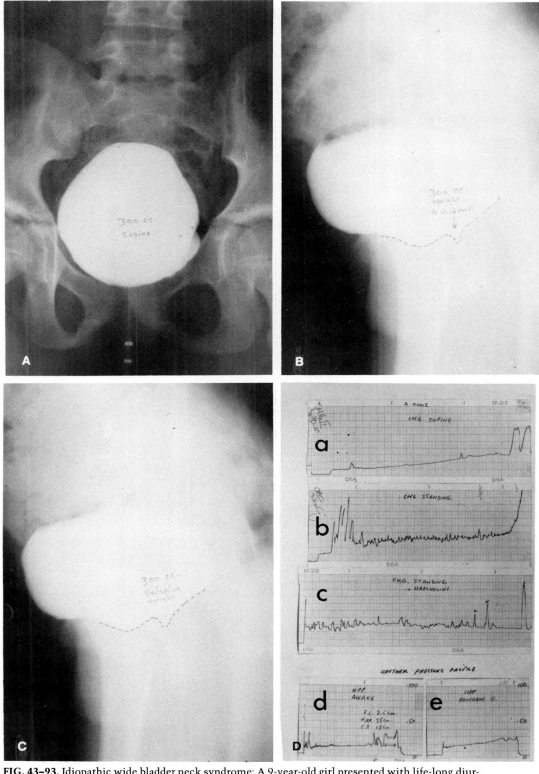

FIG. 43–93. Idiopathic wide bladder neck syndrome: A 9-year-old girl presented with life-long diurnal wetting. Diagnoses of "psychological incontinence" and "giggle incontinence" were entertained. Clinical examination was unremarkable. IVP and VCU were unrevealing. **(A)** Cystogram: anteroposterior film with catheter per urethra is unremarkable. **(B)** Cystogram: upright, oblique view, without catheter. Note peaking of the bladder base, suggestive of bladder neck relaxation. **(C)** Upright oblique cystogram while child is bearing down to evaluate the competence of bladder neck mechanism. **(D)** Urodynamic work-up: **(a)** Cystometrogram (CMG), supine, unremarkable; **(b)** CMG: standing; **(c)** CMG: following subcutaneous urecholine injection (0.35 μg/kg) to rule out bladder instability; **(d)** Urethral pressure profile: short functional length of 2 cm and low urethral pressure; **(e)** Urethral pressure profile under anesthesia: flat. Conclusion: Stable bladder: wide bladder neck only. Since the bladder neck and smooth muscle of urethral sphincter are richly supplied with α-adrenergic receptors, the patient was treated with ephedrine sulfate, 3 mg/kg/day and has been perfectly dry for 1 year.

1805

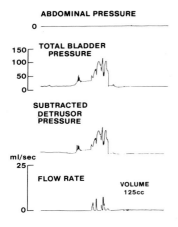

FIG. 43–94. External sphincter dyssynergia: Synchronous sphincter EMG, bladder pressure flow rate tracing: marked bladder–sphincter incoordination accounting for poor urine flow rate.

FIG. 43–95. Flowmetry: Various flow rates of different patients judged by experienced observer to have normal urine flow rates.

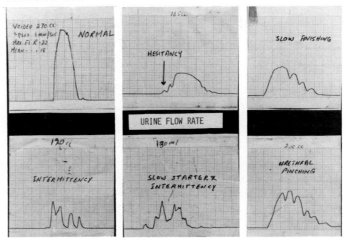

BIBLIOGRAPHY

Urethrocavernous Refluxes (Veins Filled)

1. Crabtree, E.G.: Venous invasion due to urethrograms made with Lipiodol. J. Urol., 57:380–390, 1947.
2. Edling, N.P.G.: Urethrocystography in the male with special regard to micturition. Acta Radiol. (Suppl.), 58:1–144, 1945.
3. Eichler, P.: Zur frage der Emboliegefahr bei der Verwendung von J. Iödolen in der Röntgendiagnostik der unteren Harmwege. Röntgenpraxis, 4:138–140, 1932.
4. Fernicola, A.R.: Extra-urethral confines of urethrographic contrast medium. J. Urol., 66:132–144, 1951.
5. Franck, M.A.: Reflux veineux après injection de Lipiodol dans un urèthre rétrêci, reported by M. Janet to Soc. Franc. d'Urol. J. Urol., 39:166–170, 1935.
6. Grauhan, M.: Zur Klinik und Anatomie des venösen Refluxes bei der Urethrographie. Zentralbl. Chir., 66:1662–1701, 1939.
7. Hendriock, A.: Beobachtungen von urethro-venösen. Übertritt der Kontrastmittels bei der Urethrographie. Zentralbl. Chir., 59:1415–1423, 1932.
8. Knuttson, F.: Urethrography. Acta Radiol. (Suppl.), p. 28, 1935.
9. Mukerjee, M.G., Deshon, G.E., Jr., Bruckman, J.A., et al.: Urethrovascular reflux and its significance in urology. J. Urol., 112:608–609, 1974.
10. Traian-Katz-Galatzi: Le reflux urethro-veineux et les dangers de l'emploi des huiles dans l'urèthre. J. Urol., 44:300–310, 1937.

Method of Injection of Dorsal Vein of Penis

11. Abeshouse, B.S., and Ruben, M.E.: Prostatic and periprostatic phlebography. J. Urol., 68:640–646, 1952.
12. Ceccarelli, G.: Flebografia dei vasi pelvici. Urologia, 17:376–382, 1950.
13. Crabtree, E.G.: Venous invasion due to urethrograms made with Lipiodol. J. Urol., 57:380–390, 1947.
14. Fitzpatrick, R.J., and Orr, L.M.: Pelvio prostatic venography; preliminary report. J. Urol., 68:647–651, 1952.

Urethral Fistulas

15. Blandy, J.P., and Singh, M.: Fistula involving the adult male urethra. Br. J. Urol., 44:632–643, 1972.
16. Buckspan, M., and Klotz, P.: Urethrocavernous fistula: A case report. J. Urol., 117:538, 1977.
17. Chambers, R.M.: Tuberculous urethral fistula. Br. J. Urol., 43:243–248, 1971.
18. Cohen, N.M., and Werbitt, W.: Inflammatory disease of the colon with fistulization to the posterior membranous urethra. Am. J. Proct., 26:59–62, 1975.
19. Culp, O.S., and Calhoun, H.W.: A variety of rectourethral fistulas: Experience with 20 cases. J. Urol., 91:560–571, 1964.
20. Fowler, J.E., Jr., and Elliot, J.S.: Vesicourethral fistula: An unusual cause of urinary incontinence. J. Urol., 118:114–115, 1977.

21. Klugo, R.C., and Olsson, C.A.: Urethrocavernous fistula: Complications of cavernosospongioso shunts. J. Urol., *108*:750–751, 1972.
22. Malament, M.: Repair of recurrent fistula of the penile urethra. J. Urol., *106*:704–707, 1971.
23. Weslowski, S., and Bulinski, W.: Vesico-intestinal fistulae and rectourethral fistulae. Br. J. Urol., *45*:34–38, 1973.

Penis and Scrotum

Priapism

24. Abeshouse, B.S., and Tankin, L.H.: True priapism; a report of 4 cases and a review of the literature. Urol. Cutan. Rev., *54*:449–465, 1950.
25. Bailey, H.: Persistent priapism. Br. J. Surg., *35*:298–303, 1948.
26. Borski, A.A., Painter, M.R.: Priapism: Favorable response of idiopathic cases. J. Urol., *98*:105–107, 1967.
27. Campbell, J.H., and Cummins, S.D.: Priapism in sickle-cell anemia. J. Urol., *66*:697–703, 1951.
28. Conti, G.: L'erection du pénis humain et ses bases morphologico vascularies. Acta Anat., *14*:217–262, 1952.
29. Cosgrove, M.D., and LaRocque, M.A.: Shunt surgery for priapism: Review of results. Urology, *4*:1–4, 1974.
30. Farrer, J.F., and Goodwin, W.E.: Treatment of priapism; comparison of methods in 15 cases. J. Urol., *86*:768–775, 1961.
31. Fitzpatrick, T.J.: Spongiosograms and cavernosograms: A study of their value in priapism. J. Urol., *109*:843–846, 1973.
32. Grace, D.A., and Winter, C.C.: Priapism: An appraisal of management of 23 patients. J. Urol., *99*:301–310, 1968.
33. Grayhack, J.T., McCullough, W., O'Conor, V.J., Jr., et al.: Venous bypass to control priapism. Invest. Urol., *1*:509–513, 1964.
34. Haar, H.: Zum Priapismus. Med. Klin., *44*:696–699, 1949.
35. Herzog, W.: Zur Pathogenese des Priapismus. Arch. Klin. Chir., *277*:422–430, 1953.
36. Hinman, F.: Priapism. Report of cases and a clinical study of the literature with reference to pathogenesis and surgical treatment. Ann. Surg., *60*:689–716, 1914.
37. Hinman, F., Jr.: Priapism; reasons for failure of therapy. J. Urol., *83*:420–428, 1960.
38. Kimbrough, J.C., Worgan, D.K., and Denslow, J.C.: Priapism, surgical treatment: Case report. Urol. Cutan. Rev., *54*:53–54, 1950.
39. LaRocque, M.A., and Cosgrove, M.D.: Priapism: A review of 46 cases. J. Urol., *112*:770–773, 1974.
40. Lower, W.E., and Christoferson, L.A.: Priapism in leukemia; report of 2 cases. Cleveland Clin. Quart., *12*:133–137, 1945.
41. Moloney, P.J., Elliott, G.B., and Johnson, H.W.: Experiences with priapism. J. Urol., *114*:72–76, 1975.
42. Nelson, J.H., III, and Winter, C.C.: Priapism: Evolution of management in 48 patients in a 22-year series. J. Urol., *117*:455–458, 1977.
43. Quackels, R.: Cure of a patient suffering from priapism by cavernospongiosis anastomosis. Acta Urol. Belg., *32*:5–13, 1964.
44. Wear, J.B., Jr., Crummy, A.B., and Munson, B.O.: A new approach to the treatment of priapism. J. Urol., *117*:251–254, 1977.
45. Wheeler, G.W., and Simmons, C.R.: Arteriography in post-

traumatic priapism: A case report. Am. J. Roentgenol., *119*:619–620, 1973.

Peyronie's Disease

46. Bivens, C.H., Marecek, R.L., and Feldman, J.N.: Peyronie's disease, a presenting complaint of the carcinoid syndrome. N. Engl. J. Med., *289*:844–851, 1973.
47. Burford, E.H., Glenn, J.E., and Burford, C.E.: Therapy of Peyronie's disease. Urol. Cutan. Rev., *55*:337–338, 1951.
48. Chesney, J.: Peyronie's disease. Br. J. Urol., *47*:209–218, 1975.
49. Chimenes, H.: La Peyronie's disease and diabetes mellitus. Novo Presse Med., *1*:2108–2109, 1972.
50. Feder, B.H.: Peyronie's disease. J. Am. Geriatr. Soc., *19*:947–955, 1971.
51. Fetter, T.R., Yunem, J.R., and Dodd, G.: Application of cavernosography in the diagnosis of lesions in the penis. Am. J. Roentgenol., *90*:169–175, 1963.
52. Furey, C.A., Jr.: Peyronie's disease: Treatment by local injection of Meticortelone and hydrocortisone. J. Urol., *77*:251–266, 1957.
53. Heite, H.J., and Siebrecht, H.H.: Beitrag zur Pathogenese der Induratio penis plastica. Derm. Wchnschr., *121*:1–10; 25–34, 1950.
54. Polkey, H.J.: Induratio penis plastica. Urol. Cutan. Rev., *32*:287–308, 1928.
55. Poutasse, E.E.: Peyronie's disease. J. Urol., *107*:419–422, 1972.
56. Smith, B.H.: Peyronie's disease. Am. J. Clin. Pathol., *45*:670–678, 1966.
57. Willscher, M.K., Cwaska, W.F., and Novicki, D.E.: The association of HLA antigens of the B_7 cross reacting group (B_7CREG) with Peyronie's disease. Read at the Annual Meeting of the New England Section A.U.A., Whitesfield, N.H., Sept. 27, 1978.

Congenital Abnormalities of the Penis

58. Farah, R., and Reno, G.: Congenital absence of the penis. J. Urol., *107*:165–165, 1972.
59. Fitzpatrick, T.J.: Hemihypertrophy of the human corpus cavernosa. J. Urol., *115*:560–561, 1976.
60. Hollowell, J.G., Jr., Witherington, R., Ballagas, A.T., et al.: Embryologic consideration of diphallus and associated anomalies. J. Urol., *117*:728–732, 1977.
61. Johnston, W.G., Jr., Yeatman, G.W., and Weizel, J.W.: Congenital absence of the penis. J. Urol., *117*:508–512, 1977.
62. Kogan, S.J., and Williams, D.I.: The micropenis syndrome: Clinical observations and expectations for growth. J. Urol., *118*:311–317, 1977.
63. Lisa, L., Hanak, J., Cerny, M., et al.: Agenesis of the penis. J. Pediatr. Surg., *8*:327–328, 1973.
64. Walsh, P.C., Wilson, J.D., Allen, T.D., et al.: Clinical and endocrinological evaluation of patients with congenital microphallus. J. Urol., *120*:90–95, 1978.

Corpus Cavernosography

65. Fetter, T.R., Yunen, J.R., and Dodd, G.: Application of cavernosography in the diagnosis of lesions of the penis. Am. J. Roentgenol., *90*:169–175, 1963.

66. Fitzpatrick, T.: The corpus cavernosum intercommunicating vernous drainage system. J. Urol., *113*:494–496, 1975.

67. Fitzpatrick, T.J.: Spongiosograms and cavernosograms: A study of their value in priapism. J. Urol., *109*:843–846, 1973.

68. Fitzpatrick, T.J., and Cooper, J.: A cavernosogram study on the valvular competence of the human deep dorsal vein. J. Urol., *113*:497–499, 1975.

69. Hamilton, R.E., and Swann, J.C.: Corpus cavernosography in Peyronie's disease. Br. J. Urol., *39*:409, 1967.

70. May, F., Hirtl, H.: Das Cavernosogramm. Urol. Int., *1*:120–134, 1955.

71. Ney, C., Miller, H.L., and Friedenberg, R.M.: Various applications of corpus cavernosography. Radiology, *119*:69–73, 1976.

Gas Gangrene

72. Burpee, J.F., and Edwards, P.: Fournier's gangrene. J. Urol., *107*:812–814, 1972.

73. Friedman, S.: Gas gangrene of penis and scrotum. J. Urol., *72*:51–52, 1954.

74. Werner, H.J., and Falk, M.: Acute gangrene of the scrotum in a 8-year-old. J. Pediatr., *65*:133–136, 1964.

Varicocele and Fertility

75. Agger, P.: Plasma cortisol in the left spermatic vein in patients with varicocele. Fertil. Steril., *22*:270–274, 1971.

76. Ahlberg, N.E., Bartley, O., and Chideckel, N.: Retrograde contrast filling of the left gonadal vein: a roentgenologic and anatomical study. Acta Radiol. Diag. (Stockholm), *3*:385–392, 1965.

77. Ahlberg, N.E., Bartley, O., and Chideckel, N.: Circumference of the left gonadal vein; an anatomical and statistical study. Acta Radiol. Diag. (Stockholm), *3*:503–512, 1965.

78. Ahlberg, N.E., Bartley, O., and Chideckel, N.: Right and left gonadal veins; an anatomical and statistical study. Acta Radiol. Diag. (Stockholm), *4*:593–601, 1966.

79. Ahlberg, N.E., Bartley, O., Chideckel, N., et al.: Phlebography in varicocele scroti. Acta Radiol. Diag. (Stockholm), *4*:517–528, 1966.

80. Bandhauer, K., and Meili, H.U.: Varicocele: Spermiograms, testicular biopsy, plasma testosterone. Results of therapy. Urologe, *16*:154–157, 1977.

81. Brodny, M.L., Robins, S.A., Hershman, H.A., et al.: Epididymography, varicocelography, and testicular angiography: their uses in the study of the infertile male. Fertil. Steril., *6*:158–168, 1955.

82. Brown, J.S.: Varicocelectomy in the subfertile male. A ten-year experience with 295 cases. Fertil. Steril., *27*:1046–1053, 1976.

83. Brown, J.S., Dubin, L., and Hotchkiss, R.S.: The varicocele as related to fertility. Fertil. Steril., *18*:46–56, 1967.

84. Brown, J.S., Dubin, L., Becker, M., et al.: Venography in the subfertile man with varicocele. J. Urol., *98*:388–392, 1967.

85. Charny, C.W.: Effect of varicocele on fertility: Results of varicocelectomy. Fertil. Steril., *13*:47–56, 1962.

86. Charny, C.W., and Baum, S.: Varicocele and infertility. J.A.M.A., *204*:1165–1168, 1968.

87. Cohen, M.S., Plaine, L., and Brown, J.S.: The role of internal spermatic vein plasma catecholamine determinations in subfertile men with varicocele. Fertil. Steril., *26*:1243–1244, 1975.

88. Comhaire, F., and Kunnen, M.: Selective retrograde venog-raphy of internal spermatic vein. A conclusive approach to the diagnosis of varicocele. Andrologia, *8*:11–14, 1976.

89. Comhaire, F., Montague, R., and Kunnen, M.: The value of scrotal thermography as compared with selective retrograde venography of the internal spermatic vein for the diagnosis of "subclinical" varicocele. Fertil. Steril., *27*:694–698, 1976.

90. Comhaire, F., and Vermeulen, A.: Varicocele sterility: Cortisol and catecholamines. Fertil. Steril., *25*:88–95, 1974.

91. Diamond, A.: Venographic demonstration of a varicocele in a boy. J. Urol., *114*:640–642, 1975.

92. Donahue, R.E., and Brown, J.S.: Blood gases and pH determinations in the internal spermatic veins of infertile man with varicocele. Fertil. Steril., *20*:365–369, 1969.

93. Dubin, L., and Amelar, R.D.: Varicocele size and results of varicocelectomy in selected subfertile men with varicocele. Fertil. Steril., *21*:606–609, 1970.

94. Dubin, L., and Amelar, R.D.: Etiologic factors in 1294 consecutive cases of male infertility. Fertil. Steril., *22*:469–474, 1971.

95. Dubin, L., and Amelar, R.D.: Varicocelectomy as therapy in male infertility: a study of 4504 cases. Fertil. Steril., *26*:217–220, 1975.

96. Dubin, L., and Amelar, R.D.: Varicocelectomy as therapy in male infertility: A study of 504 cases. J. Urol., *113*:640–641, 1975.

97. Dubin, L., and Hotchkiss, R.S.: Testis biopsy in infertile men with varicocele. Fertil. Steril., *20*:50–57, 1969.

98. El-Sadr, A.R., and Mina, E.: Anatomical and surgical aspects in the operative management of varicocele. Urol. Cutan. Rev., *54*:257–262, 1950.

99. Freiha, F., and Mroueh, A.: Varicocele and infertility in men. West. J. Med., *125*:431–433, 1976.

100. Gasser, G., Strasse, R., and Pokeiser, H.: Thermogram des Hodens und Spermiogramm. Androloge, *5*:127–131, 1973.

101. Gerlock, A.J.: Left testicular vein varices simulating retroperitoneal lymph node enlargement. Radiology, *93*:873–874, 1969.

102. Greenberg, S.H.: Variocele and male infertility. Fertil. Steril., *28*:699–706, 1977.

103. Greenberg, S.H., Lipschultz, L.I., Morganroth, J., et al.: The use of the Doppler stethoscope in the evaluation of varicocele. J. Urol., *117*:296–298, 1977.

104. Hanley, H.G.: Surgical correction of errors of temperature regulation. *In* Proceedings of the 2nd World Congress on Fertility and Sterility, *2*:953, 1956.

105. Ibrahim, A.A., Awad, H.A., El-Haggar, S., et al.: Bilateral testicular biopsy in men with varicocele. Fertil. Steril., *28*:663–667, 1977.

106. Johnson, D.E., Pohl, D.R., and Rivera-Correa, H.: Varicocele: an innocuous condition. South Med. J., *63*:34–36, 1970.

107. Kormano, M., Kahanpaa, K., Suinhufuud, O., et al.: Thermography of varicocele. Fertil. Steril., *21*:558–564, 1970.

108. Koumans, J., Steeno, O., Heyns, W., et al.: Dehydroepiandrosterone, sulfite, androsterone sulfite and corticoids in spermatic vein blood in patients with left varicocele. Androlia, *1*:87, 1969.

109. Lindholmer, C.: Concentration of cortisol and renin in the internal spermatic vein of men with varicocele. Andrologia, *5*:21–23, 1973.

110. Lipschutz, L., and Corriere, J.N., Jr.: Progressive testicular atrophy in the varicocele patient. J. Urol., *11*:175–176, 1977.

111. Lome, L.G., and Ross, L.: Varicocelectomy and infertility. Urology, *9*:416–418, 1977.

112. MacLeod, J.: Seminal cytology in the presence of varicocele. Fertil. Steril., *16*:735–752, 1965.

113. Mobley, D.F.: Left spermatic vein cortisol in subfertile men with varicocele. Urology, 3:461-464, 1974.
114. Russell, J.K.: Varicocele in groups of fertile and subfertile men. Br. Med. J., 1:1231-1233, 1954.
115. Schiff, I., Wilson, E., Newton, R., et al.: Serum luteinizing hormone, follicle-stimulating hormone, and testosterone responses to gonadotropin-releasing factor in males with varicoceles. Fertil. Steril., 27:1059-1061, 1976.
116. Scott, L.S., and Young, D.: Varicocele: a study of its effect on human spermatogenesis and of the results produced by spermatic vein ligation. Fertil. Steril., 13:325-334, 1962.
117. Stephenson, J.D., nad O'Shaughnessy: Hypospermia and its relationship to varicocele and intrascrotal temperature. Fertil. Steril., 19:110-117, 1968.
118. Stewart, B.H.: Varicocele in infertility: Evidence and results of surgical therapy. J. Urol., 112:222-223, 1974.
119. Tessler, A.N., and Krahn, H.P.: Varicocele and testicular temperature. Fertil. Steril., 17:201-203, 1966.
120. Verstoppen, G.R., and Stegno, O.P.: Varicocele and the pathogenesis of the associated subfertility. A review of the various theories. I. Varicocelogenesis. Andrologia, 9:133-140, 1977.
121. Zorgniotti, A.W., and MacLeod, J.: Studies in temperature, human sperm quality and varicocele. Fertil. Steril., 24:854-863, 1973.

Torsion of the Testis

122. Allen, T.D.: Disorders of the male genitalia, pp. 699-654. In Kelalis, P.P., and King, L.R. (eds.): Clinical Pediatric Urology. W.B. Saunders, Philadelphia, 1976.
123. Datta, N.S., and Mishkin, F.S.: Radionuclide imaging in intrascrotal lesions. J.A.M.A., 237:1060-1062, 1975.
124. DelVillar, R.G., Ireland, G.W., and Cass, A.S.: Early exploration in acute testicular conditions. J. Urol., 108:887-888, 1972.
125. Ewert, E.E., and Hoffman, H.A.: Torsion of the spermatic cord. J. Urol., 55:557-561, 1944.
126. Han, L.C., Nadel, N.S., Gitter, M.H., et al.: Testicular scanning: A new modality for the preoperative diagnosis of testicular torsion. J. Urol., 113:60-62, 1975.
127. Holder, L.E., Martire, J.R., Holmes, E.R., III, et al.: Testicular radionuclide angiography and static imaging: Anatomy, scintigraphic interpretation, and clinical indications. Radiology, 125:739-752, 1977.
128. James, T.: Torsion of spermatic cord in the first year of life. Br. J. Urol., 25:56-59, 1953.
129. Johnson, M.C., and Holmes, T.W., Jr.: Torsion and the ectopic testis. Surgery, 55:854-858, 1964.
130. Kaplan, G.W., and King, L.R.: Acute scrotal swelling in children. J. Urol., 104:219-223, 1970.
131. Krarup, T.: Torsion of the testis. Scand. J. Urol. Nephrol. (Suppl.), 6:165-169, 1972.
132. Levy, B.J.: The diagnosis of torsion of the testicle using the Doppler ultrasonic stethescope. J. Urol., 113:63-65, 1975.
133. Longino, L.A., and Martin, C.W.: Temperatures of the spermatic cord in the newborn infant. N. Engl. J. Med., 253:695-697, 1955.
134. Nadel, N.S., Gitter, M.H., Han, L.C., et al.: Preoperative diagnosis of testicular torsion. Urology, 1:478-479, 1973.
135. Parker, R.M., and Robison, J.R.: Anatomy and diagnosis of torsion of the testicle. J. Urol., 106:243-247, 1971.
136. Pedersen, J.F., Holm, H.H., and Hald, T.: Torsion of the testis diagnosed by ultrasound. J. Urol., 113:66-68, 1975.
137. Schneider, H.C., Jr., Kendall, A.R., and Karafin, L.: Fluorescence of testicle, an indication of viability of spermatic cord after torsion. Urology, 5:133-136, 1975.
138. Snyder, W.H., Jr., Brayton, D., and Greavey, E.M., Jr.: Torsion of the testis, pp. 1286-1291. In Mustard, W.T., Ravitch, M.M., Snyder, W.H., Jr., Welch, K.J., and Benson, C.D. (eds.): Pediatric Surgery, 2nd ed. Year Book Publishers, Inc., 1969.
139. Thompson, I.M., Latourette, H., Chadwick, S., et al.: Diagnosis of testicular torsion using Doppler ultrasonic flow meter. Urology, 6:706-707, 1975.
140. Whitesell, J.A.: Intrauterine and newborn torsion of spermatic cord. J. Urol., 106:786-788, 1971.

Nonpalpable Testicle

141. Amin, M., Wheeler, C.S.: Selective testicular venography in abdominal cryptorchidism. J. Urol., 115:760-761, 1976.
142. Ben-Menachem, Y., deBerardinis, M.C., and Salinas, R.: Location of intraabdominal testes by elective testicular arteriography: A case report. J. Urol., 112:493-494, 1974.
143. Diamond, A.B., Meng, C.-H., Kodroff, M., et al.: Testicular venography in the nonpalpable testis. Am. J. Roentgenol., 129:71-75, 1977.
144. Glickman, M.G., Weiss, R.M., and Itzchak, Y.: Testicular venography for undescended testis. Am. J. Roentgenol., 129:67-70, 1977.
145. Goldberg, L.M., Skaist, L.B., and Morrow, J.M.: Congenital absence of testes; anorchism, monorchism. J. Urol., 111:840-845, 1974.
146. Jacobs, J.B.: Selective gonadal venography. Radiology, 92:885-888, 1969.
147. Levitt, S.B., Kogan, S.J., Engel, R.M., et al.: The impalpable testis: A rational approach to management. J. Urol., 120:515-520, 1978.
148. Levitt, S.B., Kogan, S.J., Schneider, K., et al.: Endocrine tests in phenotypic children with bilateral impalpable testes can reliably predict "congenital" anorchism. Urol., 11:11-17, 1978.
149. Lunderquist, A., and Rafstedt, S.: Roentgenologic diagnosis of cryptorchism. J. Urol., 98:219-223, 1967.
150. Nordmark, L., Bjersing, L., Bomellof, K., et al.: Angiography of the testicular artery. II. Cryptorchism and testicular agenesis. Acta Radiol. (Diagn.), 18:167-176, 1977.
151. Tibbs, D.J.: Unilateral absence of the testis: 8 cases of true monorchism. Br. J. Surg., 48:601-608, 1961.
152. Vitale, P.J., Khademi, M., and Seebode, J.J.: Selective gonadal angiography for testicular location in patients with cryptorchism. Surg. Forum, 25:538-540, 1974.

Tumors of the Testis

153. Arvay, N., and Picard, J.D.: La Lymphographie. Masson & Cie, Paris, 1964.
154. Baum, S., Bron, K.M., Wexler, L., et al.: Lymphography, cavography, and urography: Comparative accuracy in the diagnosis of pelvic and abdominal metastases. Radiology, 81:207-218, 1963.
155. Borski, A.A.: Proceedings: Diagnosis, staging, and natural history of testicular tumors. Cancer, 32:1202-1205, 1973.
156. Braunstein, G.D., Vaitukaitis, J.L., Carbone, P.P., et al.: Ectopic production of human chorionic gonadatropins by neoplasms. Ann. Intern. Med., 78:39-45, 1973.
157. Busch, F.M., and Sayegh, E.S.: Roentgenographic visualiza-

tion of human testicular lymphatics: A preliminary report. J. Urol., 80:106–110, 1963.

158. Cade, I.: The clinical picture and management of testicular tumors. Clin. Radiol., 24:385–391, 1973.

159. Chiappa, S., Uslenghi, C., Bonadonna, G., et al.: Combined testicular and foot lymphography in testicular carcinomas. Surg. Gynecol. Obstet., 123:10–14, 1966.

160. Cope, C., and Isard, H.J.: Left renal vein entrapment. A new diagnostic finding in retroperitoneal disease. Radiology, 92:867–872, 1969.

161. Cuneo, B.: Note sur les lymphatiques de testicle. Bull. Mem. Soc. Paris Anat., 76:105–111, 1901.

162. Dixon, F.J., Moore, R.A.: Tumors of the male sex organs. In Atlas of Tumor Pathology, Washington, D.C., Armed Forces Pathology, 1952, Fasc. 31B and 32.

163. Fein, R., and Taber, D.: Foot lymphography in the testis tumor patient. Cancer, 24:248–255, 1969.

164. Hermanek, P.: Testicular cancer, histologic classification and staging, topography of lymph node metastases. Recent Results Cancer Res., 60:202–211, 1977.

165. Holder, L.E., Martire, J.R., Holmes, E.R., III, et al.: Testicular radionuclide angiography and static imaging: anatomy, scintigraphic interpretation, and clinical indications. Radiology, 125:739–752, 1977.

166. Húlten, L., Kindblom, L.G., Lindhagen, L., et al.: Funicular and pedal lymphography in testicular tumours. Acta Chir. Scand., 139:746–758, 1973.

167. Ichijo, S.: Vascular patterns of testicular tumors: A microangiographic study. J. Urol., 113:360–363, 1975.

167a. Javadpour, N.: The role of biologic tumor markers in testicular cancer. Cancer, 45 (Suppl):1755–1761, 1980.

167b. Javadpour N., Chen, H.C.: Paper read at the Am. Urol. Assoc. Annual Meeting, San Francisco, May 19, 1980.

168. Johnson, D.E.: Retroperitoneal lymphadenectomy: Indications, complications, and expectations. Recent Results Cancer Res., 60:221–230, 1977.

169. Jonsson, K., Ingemansson, S., and Ling, L.: Lymphography in patients with testicular tumours. Br. J. Urol., 45:548–554, 1973.

170. Juillard, G., Pinto, J., Gauthier, B., et al.: Radiography of testicular tumors. J. Urol. Electral Med. Nucl., 53:377, 1972.

171. Kademian, M., and Wirtanen, G.: Accuracy of bipedal lymphography in testicular tumors. Urology, 9:218–220, 1977.

172. Kiviat, M.D., and Ansell, J.D.: Doppler ultrasonic evaluation. (Letter) Urology, 8:643, 1976.

173. Koehler, P.R.: Current status of lymphography in patients with cancer. Cancer, 37:503–516, 1976.

174. Kolbenstvedt, A., Lien, H.H., Miller, A., et al.: Antegrade spermatic vein phlebography in testicular tumors. Radiology, 114:461–463, 1975.

175. Kreel, L.: The EMI whole body scanner in the demonstration of lymph node enlargement. Clin. Radiol., 27:421–429, 1976.

176. Lange, P.H., McIntyre, R., Waldmann, T.A., et al.: Serum alpha fetoprotein and human chorionic gonadatropins in the diagnosis and management of nonseminomatous germ-cell testicular cancer. N. Engl. J. Med., 295:1237–1240, 1976.

177. Lien, H.H., nad Kolbenstvedt, A.: Phlebography, urography, and lymphography in the diagnosis of metastases from testicular tumors. Acta Radiol. (Diagn.) (Stockhomm), 18:177–185, 1977.

178. Maier, J.G., and Schamber, D.T.: The role of lymphography in the diagnosis and treatment of malignant testicular tumors. Am. J. Roentgenol., 114:482–491, 1972.

179. Meares, E.M., Jr., and Ho, T.L.: Metastatic cancer involving the testis. A review. J. Urol., 109:653–655, 1973.

180. Mostofi, F.K.: Proceedings: Testicular tumors. Epidemiologic, etiologic, and pathological features. Cancer, 32:1186–1201, 1973.

181. Mostofi, F.K.: Tumours of the testis. IARC Sci. Publ., 1:135–150, 1977.

182. Mostofi, F.K.: Epidemiology and pathology of tumors of the human testis. Recent Results Cancer Res., 60:176–195, 1977.

183. Mukergee, M.G., Vollero, R.A., Mittemeyer, B.T., et al.: Diagnostic value of 99$_m$tc in scrotal scan. Urology, 6:453–455, 1975.

184. Paterson, A.H., Peckham, M.J., and McCready, V.R.: Value of gallium scanning in seminoma of the testis. Br. Med. J., 1:1118–1121, 1976.

185. Price, J.L., and Loveday, B.J.: Soft tissue radiography of the testicle. Br. J. Radiol., 48:179–180, 1975.

186. Ray, V., Hajdu, S.I., and Whitmore, W.T., Jr.: Proceedings: Distribution of retroperitoneal lymph node metastases in testicular germinal tumors. Cancer, 33:340–348, 1974.

187. Resnick, M., Walvoord, D.J., and Bulkley, G.J.: Testicular tumor presenting as inferior vena caval thrombosis. J. Urol., 109:656–658, 1973.

188. Richie, J.P., and Birnholz, J.C.: Ultrasound evaluation of scrotal pathology. Read at the Annual Meeting of the New England Section of the A.U.A., Whitefield, N.H., September 27, 1978.

189. Rouviere, H.: Anatomy of the Human Lymphatic System, pp. 218–226. M.J. Tobias (Trans-Ed.) Ann Arbor, Michigan, 1938.

190. Safer, M., Green, J., Crews, Q., et al.: Lymphangiographic accuracy in the staging of testicular tumors. Cancer, 35:1603–1605, 1975.

191. Sayegh, E., Brooks, T., Sacher, E., et al.: Lymphography of the retroperitoneal lymph nodes through the inguinal route. J. Urol., 95:102–107, 1966.

192. TNM Classification of Malignant Tumours. Union Int. Contre le Cancer, Geneva, 1978, pp. 123–124.

193. Wallace, S., and Jing, B.S.: Lymphography diagnosis of nodal metastases from testicular malignancies. J.A.M.A., 213:94–96, 1970.

194. Walsh, P.C.: The endocrinology of testicular tumors. Recent Results Cancer Res., 60:196–201, 1977.

195. Wilkinson, D.J., and MacDonald, J.S.: Review of the role of lymphography in the management of testicular tumors. Clin. Radiol., 26:89–98, 1975.

196. Willis, G.W., and Hajdu, S.I.: Bilateral primary malignant germ-cell tumors of the testis: report of two cases. J. Urol., 107:279–280, 1972.

Lesions of Cowper's Ducts and Glands

197. Abrams, H.J., Joshi, D.P., and Neier, C.R.: Intrauterine urinary retention and electrolyte imbalance secondary to Cowper's gland cyst. J. Urol., 95:565–567, 1966.

198. Colodny, A.H., and Lebowitz, R.L.: Lesions of Cowper's ducts and glands in infants and children. Urology, 11:321–325, 1978.

199. Cook, F.E., and Shaw, J.L.: Cystic anomalies of the ducts of Cowper's glands. J. Urol., 85:659–664, 1961.

200. Currarino, G., and Fuqua, F.: Cowper's glands in the urethrogram. Am. J. Roentgenol., 116:838–842, 1972.

201. Howell, C., Lisansky, E.T., and Scott, E.: Congenital cyst of

the urethra in a three weeks old male infant causing pyonephrosis and death. Bull. Sch. Med. Univ. Maryland, 26:241–246, 1942.

202. Moskowitz, P.S., Newton, N.A., and Lebowitz, R.L.: Retention cysts of Cowper's duct. Radiology, 120:377–380, 1976.

203. Weinberger, M.A.: Urethral cysts arising in Cowper's gland ducts: etiology, pathogenesis and clinico-pathological aspects. J. Urol., 85:818–826, 1961.

Amyloidosis of the Urethra and Lower Genitourinary Tract

204. Carris, C.K., McLaughlin, A.P., III, and Gittes, R.F.: Amyloidosis of the lower genitourinary tract. J. Urol., 115:423–426, 1976.

205. Gerami, S., Easley, G.W., and Payan, H.: Primary localized amyloidosis of the urethra and bladder. Am. Surg., 36:375–377, 1970.

206. Goldman, H.: Amyloidosis of seminal vesicles and the vas deferens; primary localized cases. Arch. Pathol., 75:94–98, 1963.

207. Lupovitch, A.: The prostate and amyloidosis. J. Urol., 108:301–302, 1972.

208. McDonald, J.H., and Hockel, N.J.: Primary amyloidosis of the lower genitourinary tract. J. Urol., 75:122–132, 1956.

209. Ullmann, A.S., Fine, G., and Johnson, A.J.: Localized amyloidosis (amyloid tumor) of the urethra. J. Urol., 92:42–44, 1964.

210. Wilson, S.K., Buchanon, R.D., Stone, W.J., et al.: Amyloid deposition in the prostate. J. Urol., 110:322–323, 1973.

Urethral Prolapse

211. Esposito, J.M.: Circular prolapse of the urethra in children: A cause of vaginal bleeding. Obstet. Gynecol., 31:363–367, 1968.

212. Kamat, M.H., Del Gaizo, A., and Seebode, J.J.: Urethral prolapse in female children. Amer. J. Dis. Child., 118:691–693, 1969.

213. Owens, S.B., and Morse, W.H.: Prolapse of the female urethra in children. J. Urol., 100:171–174, 1968.

214. Potter, B.M.: Urethral prolapse in girls. Radiographic findings. Radiology, 98:287–289, 1971.

Condylomata Accuminata of the Urethra

215. Bissada, M.K., Cole, A.T., and Fried, F.A.: Extensive condylomas accuminata of entire male urethra and the bladder. J. Urol., 112:201–203, 1974.

216. DeBenedictis, T.J., Marmar, J.L., and Praiss, D.E.: Intraurethral condyloma accuminata: Management and review of the literature. J. Urol., 118:767–769, 1977.

217. Lindner, H.J., and Pasquier, C.M., Jr.: Condylomata accuminata of the urethra. J. Urol., 72:875–879, 1954.

218. Morrow, R.P., McDonald, J.R., and Emmett, J.L.: Condylomata accuminata of the urethra. J. Urol., 68:909–917, 1952.

219. Pollack, H.M., DeBenedictis, T.J., Marmar, J.L., et al.: Urethrographic manifestations of venereal warts (condyloma accuminata). Radiology, 126:643–646, 1978.

220. Redman, J.F., and Meacham, K.R.: Condyloma accuminata of the urethral meatus in children. J. Pediatr. Surg., 8:939–941, 1973.

Urethral Syndrome

221. Brooks, D., and Maudar, A.: Pathogenesis of the urethral syndrome in women and its diagnosis in general practice. Lancet, 2:893–898, 1972.

221a. Carson, C.C., Segura, J.W., and Osborne, D.M.: Evaluation and treatment of the female urethral syndrome. J. Urol., 124:609–610, 1980.

222. Evans, A.T.: Etiology of urethral syndrome; preliminary report. Trans. Am. Assoc. Genitourin, Surg., 62:79–87, 1970.

222a. Gallagher, D.J., Montgomerie, J.Z., and North, J.D.: Acute infections of the urinary tract and the urethral syndrome in general practice. Br. Med., J. 1:622, 1965.

223. Maskel, R., and Polak, A.: Pathogenesis of the urethral syndrome in women. Lancet, 2:1084, 1972.

224. Morita, Y., and Ohashi, H.: Some comments on the urethral syndrome. Int. Urol. and Nephrol., 8:47–54, 1976.

225. Splatt, A.J., and Weedon, D.: The urethral syndrome. Experience with the Richardson urethroplasty. Br. J. Urol., 49:173–176, 1977.

Enlargement of the Verumontanum

226. Begg, R.C.: Verumontanum in urinary and sexual disorders. Br. J. Urol., 1:237–253, 1929.

227. Browdy, M.W.: Chronic disease of the verumontanum and sexual neurosis. Lancet, 2:961–963, 1922.

228. Johnson, S.H., III, and Price, W.C.: Hypertrophy of the colliculus seminalis in childhood. Report of 18 cases. Am. J. Dis. Child., 78:892–898, 1949.

229. Pennock, W.J.: Verumontanitis. J.A.M.A., 65:1167–1170, 1915.

230. Strauss, A.: Diseases of the collicular seminales. Clev. Med. J., 15:636–644, 1916.

231. Swineburne, G.W.: Disease of the verumontanum as a cause of urinary obstruction. Am. J. Urol., 10:283–285, 1910.

232. Thomas, B.A., and Hubell, R.J.: Enuresis nocturna; an analysis of forty cases stressing lesions of the verumontanum as a cause. J. Urol., 26:107–119, 1931.

Impotence

233. Fitzpatrick, T.J., and Cooper, J.F.: A cavernosogram study of the valvular competence of the human deep dorsal vein. J. Urol., 113:497–499, 1975.

234. Ginestie, J.F., and Romieu, A.: Radiologic Exploration of Impotence. Martinus Nijhoff Medical Division, The Hague/Boston/London, 1978.

Urethral Prostheses for Incontinence of Urine

235. Kaufman, J.J., and Richie, J.P.: Urethral erosion. Complication of antiincontinence operation. Urology, 3:218–220, 1974.

Prolapsed Ureterocele

236. Emmett, J.L., and Logan, G.B.: Ureterocele with prolapse through the urethra. J. Urol., 51:19–23, 1944.

237. Gingell, J.C., Gordon, I.R., and Mitchell, J.P.: Acute obstructive uropathy due to prolapsed ectopic ureterocele. Case report. Br. J. Urol., 43:305–308, 1971.

238. Jiminez, J.F., Lopez, F.G., and Sole-Balcells, F.: Acute reten-

tion due to prolapsed ectopic ureterocele in an adult male. Eur. Urol., *2*:153–155, 1976.

239. Parsons, C.A., and Malpass, C.P.: Demonstration of simple ureterocele prolapsing into the urethra of an adult male. Br. J. Surg., *60*:501–502, 1973.

240. Poznanski, A.R., Reynolds, W.A., and Johnson, A.S.: Prolapse of a ureterocele into the urethra of a male. Radiology, *91*:969–970, 1968.

241. Weiss, R.M., and Spackman, T.J.: Everting ectopic ureterocele. Urology, *3*:538–540, 1974.

Urethroejaculatory Reflux

242. Carlton, C.E., Jr., and Leader, A.J.: The cystourethrographic demonstration of retrograde urinary flow in the vas deferens as a cause of epididymitis. J. Urol., *84*:123–125, 1960.

243. Kiviati, M.D., Shurtleff, D., and Ansell, J.S.: Urinary reflux via the vas deferens: unusual cause of epididymitis in infancy. J. Pediatr., *80*:476–479, 1972.

244. Megalli, M., Gursel, E., and Lattimer, J.K.: Reflux of urine into ejaculatory ducts as a cause of recurring epididymitis in children. J. Urol., *108*:978–979, 1972.

245. Stanfield, B.M., Soderdahl, D.W., and Schamber, D.T.: Idiopathic urethro-ejaculatory reflux. J. Urol., *118*:47–48, 1977.

Clinical Application of Urodynamic Evaluation of the Lower Urinary Tract

246. Bradley, W.F., Rockswold, G.L., Timm, G.W., et al.: Neurology of micturition. J. Urol., *115*:481, 1976.

247. Hanna, M.K.: Urinary Undiversion, Panel Discussion New York Section of American Urological Association. Meeting in Dublin, November 1978.

248. Hanna, M.K.: Urodynamics in Clinical Urology. Post Graduate Course. New York University, New York, December 1978.

249. Lapides, J., Friend, C.R., Ajemian, E.P., et al.: Denervation super-sensitivity as a test for neurogenic bladder. Surg. Gynecol. Obstet., *114*:241, 1962.

250. Turner-Warwick, R.: Some clinical aspects of detrusor dysfunction. J. Urol., *113*:539, 1975.

Part Eight

SPECIALIZED PROCEDURES

The principal types of nuclear medicine studies involving the urinary system include radionuclide angiography, renal imaging, and radionuclide renography. In many ways, the results of the blood-flow studies are similar to those obtained with contrast angiography. A number of agents are commonly employed for renal imaging, and with them, different types of functional and anatomic information may be obtained. In some situations, imaging may be preferred using an agent that is excreted purely by glomerular filtration (^{99m}Tc-diethylenetriaminepentaacetic acid); in others, an agent that localizes in the renal cortex is most useful (^{99m}Tc-dimercaptosuccinic acid); in still others, an agent that is actively secreted by the renal tubules (^{131}I-orthoiodohippurate) may be the radiopharmaceutical of choice.

Regardless of the study chosen, each of those listed has taken on a new dimension of significance and usefulness with the introduction of computers to nuclear medicine. The ability to obtain digital and imaging information through the interfacing of a scintillation camera and a computer is one of the major accomplishments of the nuclear-medicine age. Because of the availability of such methods, there has been increased emphasis on various functional aspects, such as comparative blood flow studies to each kidney or differential tubular function.

RADIONUCLIDE RENOGRAPHY

The radioactive renogram is a time–activity curve that reflects the uptake and course of a radionuclide such as ^{131}I-orthoiodohippurate (Hippuran) in the kidneys. Because radioactive Hippuran is handled by the kidneys in much the same manner as para-aminohippurate (PAH), principally through tubular secretion, the renogram is largely a manifestation of tubular activity.

44

Radionuclide Studies of the Kidney

Sheldon Baum

METHODOLOGY

Until a few years ago, monitoring for the renogram was accomplished by one of two general methods: (1) external detection by directing a probe to each renal area (Figs. 44–1, 44–2), or (2) by the use of a scintillation camera (Fig. 44–3) with graphic recording capability. In the modern nuclear medicine department, the renogram is obtained by using a scintillation camera interfaced to a computer.

The external probe method is now a subject of historical interest. This method is illustrated in Figure 44–1 and shown diagrammatically in Figure 44–2. Paired scintillation detectors are connected to ratemeters and then to rectilinear strip chart recorders on which the renogram tracings are produced. Commonly used for such purposes are detectors with 1-inch sodium iodide crystals and flat field collimators. The probes are usually placed on or close to the skin surface so that, primarily, the kidneys will be in the region of radioactive detection.

When using a scintillation camera interfaced to a computer, renal imaging as well as renogram generation is accomplished. A common procedural method is as follows: After the intravenous administration of ^{131}I-Hippuran (usual adult dose, 300 μCi.), frames are obtained at intervals of 10 seconds to a total of 1280 seconds (a little over 20 minutes). Using such a framing rate, 128 frames of sequential ^{131}I-Hippuran images are collected, and the information is stored in the computer's memory. A curve may then be generated that reflects the 128 "points" of sequential activity of ^{131}I-Hippuran in each kidney throughout the designated time period.

The histogram (or renogram) that is generated may relate to the entire kidney, to a renal segment, or even to a cross-sectional slice. The area of selection may be obtained through the use of a light pen (Fig. 44–3a) or with region-of-interest cursors (Fig. 44–3b).

Although both renogram generation and renal imaging are performed following ^{131}I-Hippuran injection, renogram analysis leads to a much more detailed expression of renal function (specifically, tubular function). Hippuran imaging is discussed more fully below.

Before one performs a renogram, one should direct careful attention to the patient's state of hydration and the position in which he or she should be placed for study.

Hydration. It has been variously suggested that the urine flow from both kidneys should be 1.5 to 7.0 ml./minute or at least 2 to 3 ml./minute.[7, 17] If the urine flow is so diminished that it is less than 1 or 2 ml./minute, alterations in renogram configuration become apparent, with flattening of the third (excretory) segment and perhaps prolongation of the second (accumulation) phase. A rate of urine flow of 1.5 to 7.0 ml./minute may be obtained if the patient is NPO for 8 to 12 hours, drinks 750 ml. (3 glasses) of water, and has the renogram performed 1 hour later.

Position. The patient should be so positioned that gravity may assist urinary drainage. This may be achieved by elevating the prone or supine patient to an angle of about 15° with the horizontal.

THE NORMAL RENOGRAM

The normal radionuclide renogram consists of three distinct segments or phases: the tracer appearance, the accumulation or buildup phase, and the excretory segment (Fig. 44–4).

Following the intravenous administration of ^{131}I-Hippuran, there is a rapidly rising, semivertical segment, lasting approximately 20 seconds. This upward sloping line, or *tracer appearance*, represents the initial presence of the radioactive material in the circulatory system. A probe placed over the heart shows a similar upward detection, but this is of smaller amplitude.

The tracer appearance ends abruptly and is followed by a gradually rising second segment. This portion of the curve almost certainly represents the accumulation of the radioactive Hippuran in the renal tubular cells and may be called the *accumulation* or *buildup phase*. It ends at the *peak* or point of maximum accumulation.

Transit time is the term used to denote the interval from the start of the upward deflection of the tracer appearance until the peak is reached, and the term includes both the tracer appearance and buildup phase. Normally, it is about 2 to 5 minutes in duration.

Following the peak, there is a downward-sloping curve that represents the loss of radioactivity from the renal area as the ^{131}I-Hippuran enters the urinary formation (or excretion). This third portion of the renogram curve is commonly referred to as the *excretory segment* or *phase*.

Excretion is usually measured in terms of the percentage fall from the peak. Suppose it is desired to determine the excretion at a given time, t (Fig. 44–5). If the height of the peak and the height of the excretory curve at time t are known, the fall from the peak at time t is the difference between these two values. Or, if the height of the peak is given by h, and the height of the excretory segment at time t is given by h^1, then the fall from the peak is $(h - h^1)$. The percentage fall from the peak at this time will be $100 \times h - h^1/h$.

Two general methods of measuring the excretory fall have evolved. In one, the percentage fall from the peak is measured in terms of *time after the peak*. The use of this method is shown in Figure 44-6, in which there is a 50 per cent fall from the peak in 4 minutes (after the peak).

The more commonly employed analysis is to use the start of the initial upward deflection (time zero) as the reference time for all phases of the renogram, as illustrated in Figure 44-7. In this case, 50 per cent excretion occurs at 6 minutes (following the start of the tracer appearance).

Although it is common practice to measure the time at which there has been a 50 per cent fall from the peak ($T \frac{1}{2}$), it is also informative to measure the excretory drop at various times, such as at 10, 12, and 15 minutes. When performed according to the methods of patient preparation and positioning described earlier in this section, excretion should be at least 50 per cent at 10 minutes and at least 60 per cent at 15 minutes (after tracer appearance) (Fig. 44-8).

Because there is no standardized renogram procedure, normal values can only be described for those tracings that are performed under similar circumstances of patient preparation and position. Thus, a wide variety of normal values can be obtained from the literature.[20-28]

OTHER UNRESOLVED PROBLEMS

That there is by no means uniform agreement regarding the performance and interpretation of renograms is an understatement. Indeed, many aspects of this test have continued to be subjects of lively differences of opinion. The resolution of these controversial matters may ultimately result in a standardized renogram procedure.

Because the excretory curve is directly related to urine flow, it is reasonable to presume that this portion of the renogram may be influenced by varying degrees of hydration.[12] Marked flattening of the excretory curve may be produced in the normal subject when the urine output is reduced below 1.5 ml./minute. On the other hand, the excretory drop occurs more rapidly and at a steeper slope with increased urine flow. One group has reported that the third segment remains relatively unchanged at urine flow rates of 2 to 3 ml./minute and above.[7] However, it has also been observed that the excretory segment

continues to have the same characteristics over a fairly wide range of urine flow rates (1.5 to 7 ml./minute), but flow rates beyond 7 ml./minute result in precipitous drops in the curve.[17]

It is common practice in some institutions to perform renograms in a relatively dehydrated state, such as after an overnight fast, so an abnormality in the excretory phase, if present, might be accentuated.

Extremes of over-hydration and dehydration are to be avoided. Extremely low urine flow rates will result in a flattened excretory curve in the healthy patient. Excess hydration may lead to rapid ^{131}I-Hippuran excretion in a patient with renal disease and thus mask a potentially abnormal finding.

An approximate urine flow rate of 1.5 to 7.0 ml./minute can be achieved by having the patient drink 750 ml. (three glasses) or water after a fast of 8 to 12 hours. The renogram is performed 1 hour after the waterload. This is easily done in the hospital by making the patient NPO after midnight and then scheduling the renogram between 8 A.M. and noon the following morning.

The significance of certain minor alterations in renogram configuration is another area of controversy.

Some investigators have considered that the amplitude of the renogram, especially of the first segment, is directly related to renal blood flow. However, the amplitude is also governed by the distance of the kidney to the detector and may thereby be influenced by a number of factors, such as body build and depth of the kidney.

It has been suggested in some quarters that the slope of the second segment is also related to renal blood flow; thus, the flatter the slope, the greater is the reduction in renal blood flow.[52]

THE ABNORMAL RENOGRAM

Renogram abnormalities may be recognized through both pattern analysis and measurements involving the transit time and excretory fall (Table 44-1). Of course, major alterations in configuration of the tracing are far easier to discern than are, for example, minor reductions in excretion.

"OBSTRUCTIVE" PATTERN

The renogram with an "obstructive" pattern characteristically shows a continued or prolonged accumulation phase with an absence of an excretory segment (Figs. 44-9 to 44-13). Buildup in the second segment continues as the radioactive material is blocked from leaving the kidney. Such findings are

TABLE 44–1

Table of Major Renogram Findings

Transit Time	Excretion (or Excretory Phase)	Comment	Clinical Situation
1. Normal	Normal	Normal	
2. Normal	Reduced	Early tubular impairment (e.g., parenchymal disease)	Mild, chronic pyelonephritis, nephrosclerosis; early unilateral renal ischemia
3. Prolonged	Reduced	More severe tubular involvement than in (2). The three renogram segments are still well delineated.	Chronic, active pyelonephritis; unilateral renal ischemia
4. Prolonged and flattened	Flattened	More severe parenchymal disease than in (2) or (3). The three renogram segments are no longer discernible, and the accumulation and excretory segments are blended.	End-stage renal disease with uremia and adequate urinary output but hyposthenuria; chronic pyelonephritis, glomerulonephritis, nephrosclerosis; unilateral renal ischemia
5. Shortened	Not present—downward-sloping curve not caused by excretion	Nephrectomy pattern showing no accumulation phase. The downward-sloping curve does not represent excretion but indicates reduction in blood radioactivity as the ^{131}I-Hippuran is taken up in the contralateral kidney.	Absent kidney Nonfunctioning kidney Practically nonfunctioning kidney (unilateral renal ischemia) Improper detector placement (as with ptosis)
6. Prolonged with continued accumulation	No evidence of excretion by 20 minutes after ^{131}I-Hippuran injection	"Obstructive" pattern of complete obstruction	*Unilateral*—mechanical obstruction (e.g., due to tumor, ureteral ligation) *Bilateral* ("intrarenal")—acute tubular necrosis, acute glomerulonephritis. *Unilateral* (intrarenal)—rejection reaction; unilateral renal ischemia
7. Prolonged with continued accumulation	Some excretion by 15 minutes after ^{131}I-Hippuran injection	"Obstructive" pattern with incomplete obstruction	Incomplete mechanical obstruction (e.g., staghorn calculus)
8. Prolonged accumulation	Intermittent excretion	Intermittent "obstructive" pattern showing intermittent accumulation and excretion. Ball-value mechanism (ureteral stone and obstructing ureteral peristalsis). Ureteral irritation is present.	Incompletely obstructing ureteral calculus For 2 or 3 days following ureteral catheterization, severe ureteral spasm

commonly seen in mechanical obstruction, such as one might encounter with a staghorn calculus or with ureteral obstruction caused by a tumor. *The ^{131}I-Hippuran renogram is the most sensitive indicator of urinary obstruction.*

The "obstructive" pattern renogram does not show continued tracer accumulation *ad infinitum.*

In cases of complete obstruction, there is usually a plateau in the renogram tracing about 20 to 30 minutes after ^{131}I-Hippuran injection. The renogram manifestations of incomplete urinary obstruction are sometimes difficult to appreciate. Such renograms commonly demonstrate accumulation of the radioactive material for about 15 minutes, followed by evidence of excretion. However, similar renogram findings may be seen with parenchymal disease of the kidneys.

However, an "obstructive" pattern on a renogram does not necessarily point to mechanical obstruction (Figs. 44-14, 44-15). An "obstructive" tracing is commonly seen with such entities as acute tubular necrosis. In such cases, the radioactive Hippuran enters the renal tubular cells; however, in association with blockage in the tubular lumina caused by cellular debris, sloughed cells, and proteinaceous material, and the relative anuria, there is no excretion of the radionuclide. The continued accumulation in the kidney of the radioactive material, plus the failure to excrete it, results in the "obstructive" pattern (Fig. 44-14). Because such disease states commonly involve both kidneys, the "obstructive" pattern in such situations is usually seen bilaterally, whereas mechanical obstruction is usually associated with evidence of an "obstructive" pattern on only one side.

NEPHRECTOMY PATTERN

If a kidney is absent, a renogram tracing would show evidence of tracer appearance followed by a gradually declining, downward-sloping curve (Fig. 44-16). The latter is not caused by excretion but simply represents the decline in blood radioactivity as the radioactive Hippuran is taken up into the remaining, functioning kidney. The failure to visualize a second segment (or accumulation phase) represents the absence of renal tubular cells.

NONFUNCTIONING KIDNEY

A nephrectomy pattern may also be seen in the presence of a nonfunctioning kidney (Fig. 44-17) or when the collimator faces no renal tissue, such as one might encounter with marked ptosis of a kidney. Such a pattern may also be seen in the patient with an *almost* nonfunctioning kidney (99% of the nephrons destroyed), for in such a situation the renogram lacks the sensitivity to detect and present on a tracing the activity of the remaining, functioning nephrons (Fig. 44-18).

REDUCED EXCRETION, PROLONGED TRANSIT TIME

Renal Disease. Renographic manifestations of renal parenchymal disease, in the absence of obstruction or a nonfunctioning kidney, are usually related to reduced excretion (less than 50% in 10 minutes), prolongation of the transit time (over 5 minutes), or both. The abnormalities are frequently bilateral (Figs. 44-19 to 44-26).

With mild parenchymal disease of the kidneys, the basic renographic configuration is preserved, so that the three segments (tracer appearance, accumulation, and excretion phases) are readily discerned. The earliest renographic manifestation of renal disease is reduced excretion in an otherwise normal renogram tracing. This is probably an expression of the relative inability of the cells of the renal tubules to discharge the radioactive Hippuran, whereas the tubular cells' ability or capacity to take up the radionuclide remains intact. As renal disease progresses, there is a relative inability of the tubular cells to take up, as well as discharge, ^{131}I-Hippuran. This results in a renogram tracing that shows a prolonged transit time as well as reduced excretion, thus giving the renogram a more flattened appearance. As a practical matter of renographic demonstration of parenchymal disease, it is almost as if a weight were placed on the peak, with the degree of renogram flattening of the accumulation and excretory segments related to the severity of renal disease.

As the parenchymal disease of the kidneys becomes more severe, there is a blending of the second and third segments of the renogram tracing. The flattening may become so marked that it becomes impossible to distinguish the accumulation and excretory phases. Such tracings are commonly seen in patients with uremia in whom hyposthenuria is present despite an adequate volume of urinary output.

HYPERTENSION SECONDARY TO UNILATERAL RENAL ARTERY STENOSIS

The precise role of the renogram in helping to detect those hypertensive patients who might have unilateral renal ischemia has yet to be determined. It is unfortunate that such a situation should exist in spite of the widespread employment of radionuclide renography over the past 15 years in the evaluation of these patients.

It is well known that a number of renographic abnormalities have been described in patients with hypertension secondary to unilateral renal artery stenosis. In general, there is usually a significant disparity between the right and left renogram tracings, with the abnormal (or more severely abnormal) renogram indicating the affected side.[42] Among the renogram abnormalities that have been reported in such cases are the following: reduced excretion, prolonged transit time, or both; a lower amplitude on the involved side; reduction in the ratio of values in all three segments when comparing the affected side and that of the uninvolved kidney[38]; and reduction in the steepness of the slope of the accumulation segment of the side of the renal artery stenosis.[52]

It is beyond the scope of this chapter to discuss the many theoretical and practical considerations that have arisen in regard to the renogram changes seen in unilateral renal ischemia. The interested reader may consult the suggested references.

The renographic abnormalities that occur in patients with hypertension secondary to unilateral renal artery stenosis are almost certainly associated with the functional and anatomic changes that occur in the ischemic kidney.

It is well known that in the kidney with unilateral ischemia there is increased reabsorption of both sodium and water when compared with the contralateral kidney.[36] Thus, there is reduced urine and sodium excretion on the affected side, findings that form the basis of the Howard test of differential renal function and its subsequent modifications.[33, 34, 51] Renographic manifestations of increased water reabsorption are reduced excretion and prolongation of the transit time. Thus, both the second and third segments of the tracing may become flattened (Fig. 44-27A, B). If reabsorption of water is so marked that there is ultimately little or no urine being excreted on the affected side, the renogram might show an "obstructive" pattern (Fig. 44-28).

Unilateral renal ischemia is characterized histologically by ischemic atrophy of the renal tubules.[41] With progressive involvement of the tubular cells there is, of course, continued impairment in both the uptake and discharge of ^{131}I-Hippuran, further adding to the abnormalities associated with the functional changes already described. In those cases in which ischemic atrophy has become so widespread that *almost* all the tubules have become replaced, the few functioning nephrons may be associated with a renogram that is seen with a nonfunctioning kidney (Fig. 44-27D). As in other disease entities, the sensitivity of the renogram is too gross to detect only a small number (such as 1%) of functioning nephrons (Fig. 44-29).

Thus, the radionuclide renogram may exhibit any or all types of renographic abnormalities, depending on the severity and duration of the renal artery stenosis and the extent of the renal ischemia (Fig. 44-30). How, then, is the renogram used in the evaluation of the hypertensive patient?

If the renogram is normal on both sides, this *practically* rules out unilateral renal artery stenosis as a cause of the hypertension, and, unless other positive clinical and laboratory findings related to such a diagnosis are present, selective renal angiography should not be performed. If, on the other hand, the renogram is abnormal and there is a disparity between the two sides, further workup, such as renal angiography, should be considered. Whether or not there is a disparity between the two tracings is often a subjective determination.

INDICATIONS FOR RADIONUCLIDE RENOGRAPHY

The indications for radionuclide renography are as follows:

1. Screening test in hypertensive patients to detect unilateral renal ischemia
2. Patients sensitive to contrast material for urography
3. Graphic representation of differential renal function
4. Detection of possible obstruction in patients with unexplained azotemia
5. Detection of possible urinary tract obstruction in patients with pelvic tumors
6. Monitoring progress of patients with known renal disease
7. Detection of renal function at bedside in those patients too ill to be moved for roentgenographic examination
8. Monitoring renal function in patients in whom additional radiation exposure is undesirable
9. Evaluation of the functional status of a transplanted kidney

STATIC RENAL IMAGING

In most instances, the information gained from renal imaging with radioactive materials does not exceed that obtained through roentgenographic studies. However, there are certain special situations, such as in patients who are sensitive to contrast material, in which radioactive imaging of the kidneys can be helpful.[69] Renal imaging with radionuclides is illustrated in Figures 44-31 to 44-51.

The radioactive materials that have been used for imaging the kidneys are localized in the renal tubule, glomerulus, or both, depending on the type of agent used. In normal static imaging, the renal image is usually seen at the time the radionuclide is present in the cortical region (Table 44-2). If there has been localized replacement of renal tissue, as with a tumor or cyst, the region of involvement ap-

TABLE 44–2
Radionuclides Commonly Employed in Radionuclide Renal Studies

Isotope	Principal Gamma Energy (MeV)	T½, Physical	Radiopharmaceutical	Usual Adult Dose	Use	Administration Before Imaging or Monitoring	Localization	Critical Organ	Radiation Dose to Critical Organ (Rads)	Total Body Dose (Rads)
Iodine 131	0.364	8 days	^{131}I-Ortho-iodohippurate	200–400 µCi.	Renogram and renal imaging	At time of study	Secreted in cells of proximal renal tubules	Thyroid	With prior KI po 3.8–7.6 Without prior KI po 26–52	0.032–0.064
				200–400 µCi.	Renal imaging in patient with elevated BUN in whom imaging cannot be performed with ^{99m}Tc complexes	10–20 minutes				
Mercury 197 (197 Hg)	0.077	2.7 days	^{197}Hg-Chlor-merodrin	200 µCi.	Renal imaging	1–2 hours	Renal tubule cells	Kidney	0.874	0.002
Technetium 99m (^{99m}Tc)	0.140	6 hours	^{99m}Tc-DTPA (Sn)	20 mCi.	Renal imaging	5–15 minutes	Renal cortex (excreted exclusively by glomerular filtration)	Bladder	2.3	0.1–0.2
				5–10 mCi.	Reflux	1 hour	Bladder (after complete excretion by kidneys)		0.6–1.2	0.03–0.06
				20 mCi.	Radionuclide angiography, Area-of-interest studies	At time of imaging	Vascular renal cortex		2.3	0.1–0.2
			^{99m}Tc-Iron-ascorbate-DTPA	5 mCi.	Renal imaging	30 minutes to 2 hours	Protein binding of some ^{99m}Tc in renal tubules	Bladder	2.8	0.008
			^{99m}Tc-Sodium pertechnetate	20 mCi.	Radionuclide angiography, Area-of-interest studies	At time of imaging	Vascular	Colon	2.0	0.24
			^{99m}Tc-DMSA	5 mCi.	Renal cortical imaging	2 hours	Renal tubules (75% of injected dose)	Renal cortices	4.25	0.08
			^{99m}Tc-glucoheptonate	15–20 mCi.	Renal cortical imaging	1 hour	Renal tubules (15–25% of injected dose)	Kidneys	3.2–5.6	0.15–0.20

pears as an area of absent radioactivity. However, identification of an abnormality on the renal image is usually nonspecific, and there is no characteristic appearance of, for example, a renal carcinoma.

A number of materials are now available for renal imaging with radionuclides following their intravenous administration. The principal ones are chlormerodrin tagged with radioactive mercury, technetium 99m compounds, and ^{131}I-Hippuran.

[197]Hg-Chlormerodrin. Following its intravenous administration, radioactive chlormerodrin gradually becomes concentrated in the cells of the proximal tubules.[74] Imaging may be performed in the healthy subject one or two hours following radionuclide injection. The tagged chlormerodrin apparently becomes temporarily bound to sulfhydryl groups and is excreted slowly.

During the earlier days of radionuclide imaging, [203]Hg-chlormerodrin, in a dose of approximately 100 μCi., was commonly employed. However, because of certain undesirable physical characteristics of [203]Hg (half-life of 45 days, principal gamma emission of 279 KeV.), it was later supplanted in most cases by [197]Hg-chlormerodrin when this material became available. [203]Hg-chlormerodrin is no longer available for routine clinical use. Because [197]Hg has a half-life of 2.7 days and a principal gamma emission of 77 KeV., it presented obvious advantages. A dose of 200 to 300 μCi. of [197]Hg-chlormerodrin is used.

In patients with impaired tubular function, in whom the blood urea nitrogen is elevated, the entry of radioactive chlormerodrin into the renal tubules may be extremely slow. In some instances, not enough radiomercury accumulation is discernible to be able to image the kidneys. In such situations, attempts at renal scanning are unrewarding, and, because of its failure to be cleared by the kidneys, imaging results in detecting the liver and spleen.

Tagged Chelates. During the past 5 years, a number of chelated compounds have become available for radionuclide investigation of the kidneys.[74] Because true chelates are not metabolized and are excreted exclusively by glomerular filtration, the tagging of these substances with tracers has found ready application in renal studies. Radiomercury is now rarely used for imaging and has been replaced by technetium 99m (^{99m}Tc)-labeled agents.

The chelating agent that has been used most widely is diethylenetriaminepentaacetic acid (DTPA), and ^{99m}Tc is employed most often as the tracer. Because ^{99m}Tc must be in the tetravalent state to form a stable chelate with DTPA, a reducing agent must be employed for the conversion of [99m]Tc

at the VII oxidation state (as pertechnetate) to the oxidation state of IV.[66] Among the reducing agents that have been employed are the stannous ion and ferric ascorbate.

When the reduction process is carried out with stannous ion, the resulting ^{99m}Tc-DTPA (Sn) is an extremely stable compound and has been employed for renal imaging following the intravenous administration of 15 to 20 mCi. However, because this material is excreted so rapidly by the kidneys through glomerular filtration, to accomplish imaging of the renal cortex it is usually necessary to perform the procedure during the first 15 minutes following tracer injection. ^{99m}Tc-DTPA(Sn) is the most frequently employed renal imaging agent today.

The complex obtained when ferric ascorbate is the reducing agent is ^{99m}Tc-iron-ascorbate-DTPA. This material is not stable *in vivo*, is not a true chelate, and is not excreted exclusively by glomerular filtration.[73] Its mechanism of localization is probably similar to that of a related compound, ^{99m}Tc-ferrous ascorbate.[86] It has been postulated that a portion of the ^{99m}Tc becomes bound to protein in renal tubular cells,[78] because the stability of the ^{99m}Tc-sulfhydryl complex is much greater than that of the ^{99m}Tc-ferrous ascorbate.

Similar protein binding by [99m]Tc (probably from 10 to 20%) most likely occurs with ^{99m}Tc-iron-ascorbate-DTPA.[78] Because of temporary retention of ^{99m}Tc in the cells of the renal tubules, imaging is usually performed one to two hours following the injection of 3 to 5 μCi.

Cortical Imaging Agents. Several radiopharmaceutical agents become localized in renal tubular cells and are employed for imaging of the renal cortex. ^{99m}Tc-dimercaptosuccinic acid (DMSA) and ^{99m}Tc-glucoheptonate have been used most widely. These cortical imaging agents are useful in the assessment of suspected cortical lesions.

Following the intravenous injection of 5 mCi. of ^{99m}Tc-DMSA in the adult, more than 50 per cent of the administered dose is retained by the kidney 2 to 4 hours later. Of this retained radionuclide, 96 per cent is in the renal cortex and 4 per cent in the medulla. The optimum time for imaging is 2 hours following injection (Fig. 44–50).

The usual adult dose of ^{99m}Tc-glucoheptonate is 15 to 20 mCi. given 1 hour prior to imaging. At that time, approximately 15 to 25 per cent of the injected dose is retained by the kidneys.

[131]I-Hippuran (Orthoiodohippurate). Imaging with ^{131}I-Hippuran is usually reserved for those situations in which renal function is so poor that insufficient radionuclide, when using ^{99m}Tc complexes, is available to the kidney for visualization.[69, 79] Because radioactive Hippuran is actively secreted by the renal tubules, its entry into the kidney can be accomplished even in the presence of severe renal insufficiency. Renal imaging with ^{131}I-Hippuran may sometimes serve to distinguish "intrarenal obstruction" (radionuclide present in the cortex) from mechanical obstruction (radionuclide present in the renal pelvis).[7]

If intrarenal obstruction is present, sequential imaging up to 20 or 30 minutes following ^{131}I-Hippuran injection shows no evidence of radioactivity in the region of the renal pelvis, although the kidney is well outlined because of radioactive Hippuran present in the tubules in the cortical region. This may be seen with such entities as acute tubular necrosis (Fig. 44–51).

If mechanical obstruction is present, as with ureteral calculus, the ^{131}I-Hippuran is excreted from the renal tubules but is prevented from clearing the renal pelvis because of the obstructing lesion. In such an instance, the tubules are relatively free of radioactive material by about 5 minutes after injection, but the renal pelvis is easily demonstrated, showing increased ^{131}I-Hippuran accumulation.

INDICATIONS FOR RENAL IMAGING

Renal imaging is indicated in the following situations:

1. To measure renal size when this is difficult to determine from roentgenographic studies
2. Localization for renal biopsy[62, 66, 75, 82, 86]
3. To help identify severe ptosis
4. To aid in the diagnosis of some space-occupying lesions[79]
5. As a substitute examination in patients sensitive to contrast material used for urography
6. To assist in determining those parts of the kidney in which the tubules are still viable (e.g., after infarction)
7. Structural monitoring of renal transplants
8. In conjunction with furosemide excretion studies

RADIONUCLIDE ANGIOGRAPHY

Using a scintillation camera, it is now practical to monitor and image the course of a radioactive material in the aorta and its branches. Radionuclide imaging of kidney perfusion may be easily performed following the intravenous administration of 15 to 20 mCi. of ^{99m}Tc as pertechnetate or as DTPA. The information obtained is analogous to that seen with roentgenographic aortography with contrast materials.

The radionuclide is injected into a peripheral vein, and images are obtained at intervals of approximately 2 seconds following the appearance of radioactive material in the abdominal aorta (Figs. 44–52 to 44–54). With computerized analysis, the relative arterial perfusion to each kidney can be compared through the generation of time–activity curves. Major defects in renal arterial perfusion may sometimes be detected with such studies. It is often possible to distinguish between avascular and highly vascular renal masses. However, it should be pointed out that radionuclide angiography lacks the detail seen with roentgenologic studies and is no substitute for them.

COMPUTERIZED APPLICATIONS AND REGION-OF-INTEREST STUDIES

The introduction of computerized techniques has added even further sophistication to nuclear medicine studies of the kidneys. With these methods, both radionuclide images and accompanying histograms, indicating tracer activity or distribution, are obtained at suitable intervals during the renal transit of the radioactive material. A specific cross-sectional area or segment of the kidney may be so monitored. Thus, the course, behavior, and imaging of a radionuclide may be determined, for example, in a renal artery, cortex, medulla, and pelvis. There is currently great enthusiasm for the potential application of such studies, especially in regard to differential renal function.

COMBINED STUDIES

It is now practical and useful to perform radionuclide angiography and renal imaging with Tc-99m as well as ^{131}I-Hippuran renography and sequential renal imaging as consecutive studies. If renal pathology is suspected or demonstrated, area-of-interest tracings may be obtained too (Figs. 44–55 to 44–58).

Such combined studies are not performed routinely. They are often obtained in certain special situations: kidney transplantation; localized area of renal ischemia or infarction; differentiating between tumor and normally functioning tissue; differentiating between relatively avascular cysts and relatively vascular tumors.

RENAL TRANSPLANTATION

Radionuclide renal studies are commonly employed to help evaluate the functional status of a transplanted kidney. This is usually done by using ^{131}I-Hippuran for both renography and renal imaging and technetium 99m for radionuclide angiography to help determine the patency of the arterial supply to the transplanted kidney.

In order to accomplish both ^{131}I-Hippuran studies with a single injection of radioactive material, a dose of 300 μCi. is administered, and renography and renal imaging are performed simultaneously, using a scintillation camera with graphic recording capability or interfaced to a computer.

The onset of a rejection phenomenon may be heralded by a renogram showing an "obstructive" pattern (of the intrarenal variety). These findings are in part associated with ischemic changes in the renal tubules secondary to the rejection reaction affecting the peritubular capillaries. Subsequent renograms two or three days later may show tracings with a no-buildup pattern of nonfunction in the patient having a hyperacute or accelerated rejection reaction.

It is important to remember that a renogram with an "obstructive" pattern in a transplanted kidney may also be associated with mechanical obstruction, cortical necrosis, acute tubular necrosis, and arterial occlusion. If the latter is suspected, arterial patency may be determined with radionuclide angiography.

Renogram tracings are obtained at relatively brief intervals during the early postoperative period following transplantation, such as daily for the first week and weekly during the following four weeks. Such studies may be obtained at the patient's bedside using portable cameras.

Because the position of the transplanted kidney is usually closely related to that of the bladder, the radioactivity of the latter may lead to errors in renogram interpretation.

Renal imaging with ^{131}I-Hippuran normally shows sufficient radionuclide accumulation to outline sharply a kidney within about 5 minutes after tracer injection. Thereafter, evidence of radioactive material in the bladder may be seen, with the bladder image improving as more radioactive Hippuran is excreted from the kidney and the renal image becomes fainter.

Failure to visualize the kidney during the first 10 minutes may be seen with a rejection reaction or with interference in the arterial supply to the kidney.

Increased renal radioactivity 10 or 15 minutes after radionuclide injection, with little or no bladder activity seen by this time, may herald the onset of a rejection phenomenon. Identical findings may also be seen with renal obstruction (mechanical) and acute tubular necrosis.

However, an initial increase in renal radioactivity up to, for example, 10 minutes, followed by a gradual increase in bladder activity, usually is a sign of only temporary renal tubular impairment in renal function.

Finally, radionuclide angiography following the intravenous administration of technetium 99m may be performed to help determine the patency of the arterial supply to the transplanted kidney.

REFLUX

There is really no counterpart in nuclear medicine procedures to the information that can be seen on the voiding cystourethrogram. Attempts at visualizing ureteral reflux following the intravesical instillation of ^{99m}Tc-sodium pertechnetate have not been rewarding in the detection of small areas of reflux. However, this method is successful when the reflux is marked.[63, 64]

Successful studies have been reported in patients who received ^{99m}Tc-DTPA (Sn) and were then studied for reflux following the excretion of the radionuclide into the bladder (Figs. 44–59, 44–60).[70] In the normal subject, this radionuclide is almost entirely cleared from the kidneys 1 hour following intravenous administration and can be seen in the bladder at this time. If the patient is instructed to bear down as if to void, reflux of the radionuclide from the bladder to ureter and renal pelvis can be demonstrated. However, because the resolving power for reflux less than 2 cm. in diameter or length is limited in current radionuclide imaging techniques, the limitations of such methods should be borne in mind.

FUROSEMIDE EXCRETION STUDIES

If hydronephrosis is seen on the intravenous urogram and if it is not known whether it is functional (*e.g.*, due to muscle atony) or secondary to a mechanical obstruction, Tc-99m DTPA imaging following the injection of furosemide (Lasix) to induce excretion may be helpful. A time–activity curve is generated, and, if there is a rapid fall in radioactivity from the kidney, the findings are consistent with excretion and with the absence of mechanical blockage, as seen in Figure 44–61A. If, on the other hand, there is a continued rise in radioactivity or a plateau following the furosemide administration, the findings suggest the presence of a mechanical obstruction, as seen in Figure 44–61B.

The furosemide excretion study may be helpful in arriving at a proper diagnosis in patients with dilated ureters as well as dilated renal pelves. When generating the time–activity curve, the appropriate area or areas in question may be selected for time–activity curve generation in relation to furosemide injection.

The usual adult dose of the Tc-99m DTPA for this study is 7.5 to 10 mCi and should be reduced proportionately in children. Following radionuclide ad-

ministration, the renal images are monitored on the persistence oscilloscope. As soon as the tracer can be seen entering the collecting system, collection of data for the time–activity curve is started, and the furosemide, in a dose of 0.3 mg./kg., is administered intravenously. There is usually a delay of one or two minutes until the response to the furosemide is visible. The study should be continued for 15 minutes from the time of furosemide injection. For the time–activity curve, collection of computer images at intervals of 10 seconds for 900 seconds (15 minutes) is sufficient. At the same time, images may be displayed on the hard-copy readout at intervals of 30 seconds.

CHAPTER 44, ILLUSTRATIONS

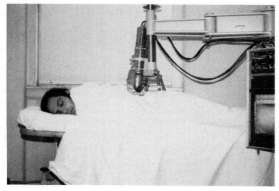

FIG. 44–1. Renogram apparatus showing dual probes with flat-field collimators that are directed to the renal areas.

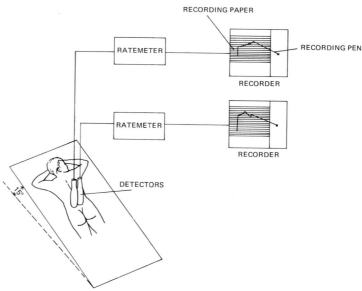

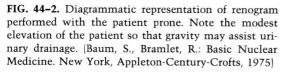

FIG. 44–2. Diagrammatic representation of renogram performed with the patient prone. Note the modest elevation of the patient so that gravity may assist urinary drainage. (Baum, S., Bramlet, R.: Basic Nuclear Medicine. New York, Appleton-Century-Crofts, 1975)

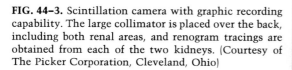

FIG. 44–3. Scintillation camera with graphic recording capability. The large collimator is placed over the back, including both renal areas, and renogram tracings are obtained from each of the two kidneys. (Courtesy of The Picker Corporation, Cleveland, Ohio)

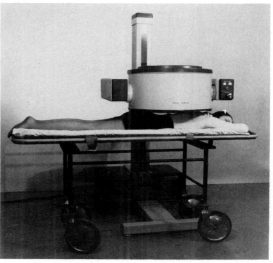

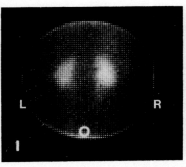
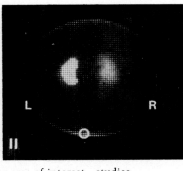
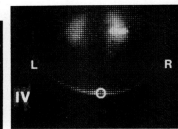
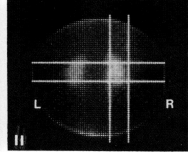

FIG. 44–3a. Monitoring-for-area-of-interest studies with a computer using a light pen. A composite ^{131}I-Hippuran imaging study is shown in *I*. The entire left kidney has been flagged or designated as the area of interest to be studied, as seen in *II*. Only the upper half of the left kidney has been so designated in *III*, whereas in *IV* a slice of the right kidney has been selected.

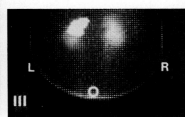
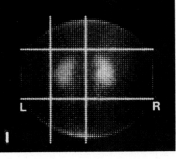

FIG. 44-3b. Monitoring for area-of-interest studies with cursors. Rectangular areas may be selected with adjustable region of interest cursors. The entire left kidney is included in the cursors in *I*, whereas in *II* a region of the right kidney has been selected.

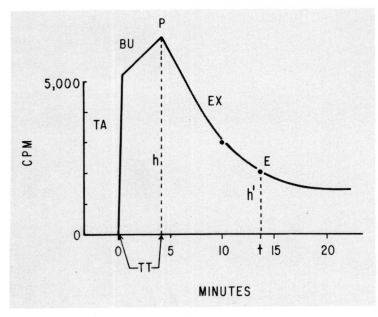

FIG. 44–4. Normal ^{131}I-Hippuran renogram. *TA* = tracer appearance; *BU* = buildup phase; *EX* = excretory segment; *CPM* = radioactivity as counts per minute. *P* = peak; *h* = height of peak; h^1 = height of peak at time *t*; *TT* = transit time. (Baum, S., Bramlet, R.: Basic Nuclear Medicine. New York, Appleton-Century-Crofts, 1975)

FIG. 44–5. Normal renogram depicting height of peak (h) and height of point on excretory curve (h^1) at the time percent of excretion is desired to be determined.

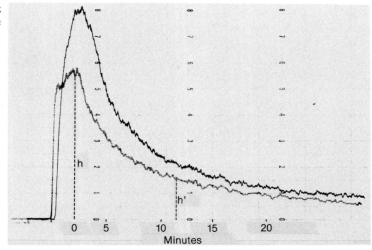

FIG. 44–6. Normal renogram showing 50 per cent excretion occurring at a given time (t) following the peak.

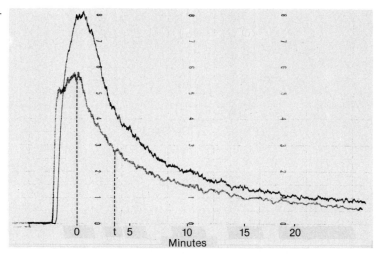

FIG. 44–7. Normal renogram showing 50 per cent excretion occurring at a given time (t) following the tracer appearance.

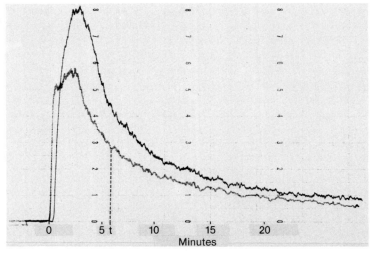

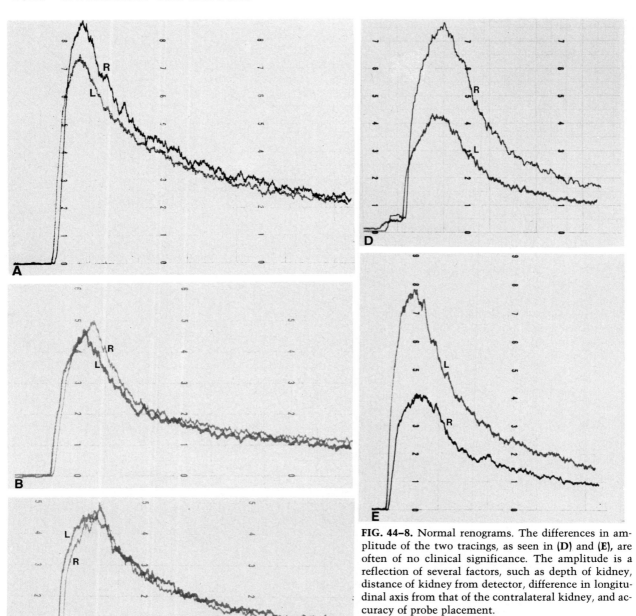

FIG. 44–8. Normal renograms. The differences in amplitude of the two tracings, as seen in **(D)** and **(E)**, are often of no clinical significance. The amplitude is a reflection of several factors, such as depth of kidney, distance of kidney from detector, difference in longitudinal axis from that of the contralateral kidney, and accuracy of probe placement.

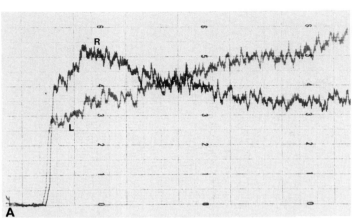

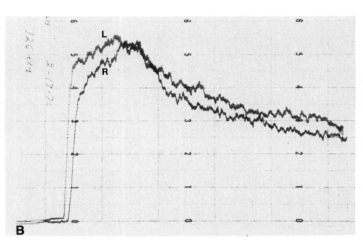

FIG. 44–9. Ureteral obstruction due to a bladder tumor before and after corrective surgery. **(A)** The tracing on the left side shows an "obstructive" pattern, which was associated with obstruction at the ureterovesical junction due to a bladder tumor. **(B)** Three weeks following reimplantation of the left ureter into the bladder, the "obstructive" pattern is no longer seen and three distinct renogram segments can now be discerned on the left side. This patient was sensitive to contrast material used in urography, and he had been followed with serial renograms for the possibility of urinary tract obstruction, which indeed did occur.

FIG. 44–10. Relief of urinary obstruction. **(A)** Initial renogram of 23-year-old woman with chronic pyelonephritis and right-sided obstruction at the ureteropelvic junction. The tracing on the right side shows an "obstructive" pattern, whereas that on the left is consistent only with impaired renal function (prolonged transit time and reduced excretion). **(B)** Renogram 2 months following right-sided pyeloplasty shows marked improvement of the right renogram tracing with evidence of excretion at this time.

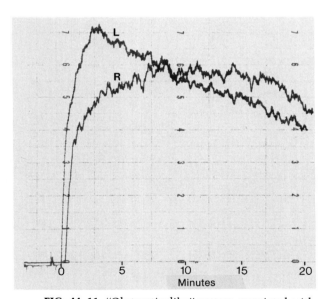

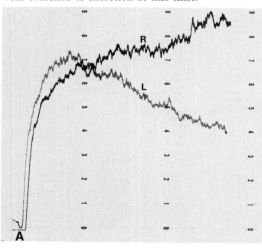

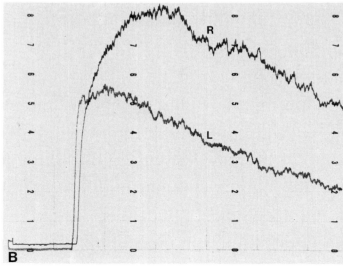

FIG. 44–11. "Obstructivelike" pattern associated with a right ureteral calculus. An "obstructive" pattern of continued accumulation is exhibited in the right renogram tracing for the first 15 minutes; and excretory fall is seen at this time. The tracing indicates incomplete obstruction on the right side. The renogram returned to normal following removal of the stone.

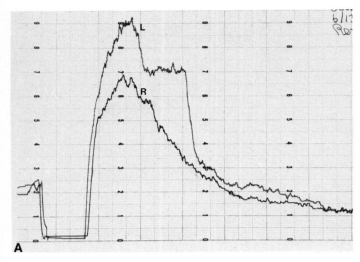

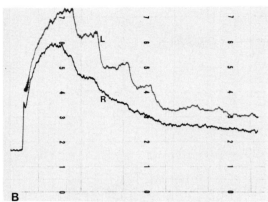

FIG. 44-12. (A) Pattern of unilateral intermittent excretion associated with a ball-valve mechanism such as is seen with a ureteral stone or with ureteral spasm. Excretion on the left side is interrupted as the lumen of the ureter narrows. As ureteral relaxation returns, the egress of urine flow is no longer impaired, and the excretory fall once more becomes apparent. **(B)** Evidence of intermittent excretion in the right renogram tracing due to a right-sided ureteral calculus.

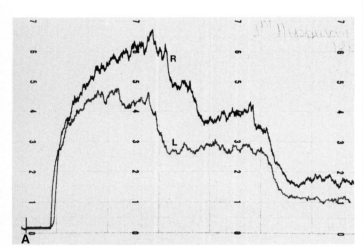

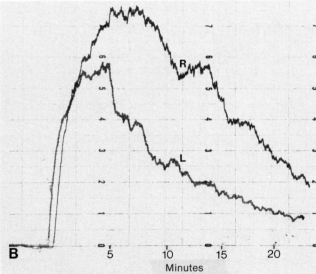

FIG. 44-13. (A) Pattern of intermittent excretion seen bilaterally in a patient with ureteral spasm. The excretory curve's failure to continue to fall is caused by temporary, functional ureteral obstruction (ureteral spasm). Ureteral relaxation and widening of the lumen coincide with the return of the excretory fall. Similar findings are seen during the 2 or 3 days following ureteral catheterization; these are probably related to the resultant ureteral irritation. **(B)** Pattern of intermittent excretion, in which the renogram findings are less obvious than in **(A)**.

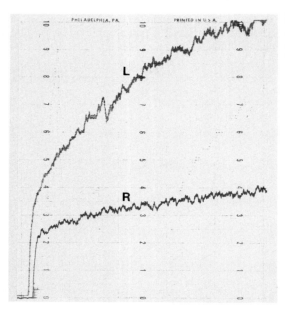

FIG. 44–14. Bilateral "obstructive" pattern in an 8-year-old boy with acute and chronic pyelonephritis. In this case, the "obstructive" pattern is intrarenal, in contradistinction to mechanical obstruction.

FIG. 44–15. Renogram in a patient with chronic pyelonephritis in whom the right renogram tracing shows an "obstructive" pattern. The involvement was much more severe in the right kidney, which exhibited atrophic pyelonephritis. Although the left renogram tracing indicates the presence of renal impairment on that side (prolonged transit time, reduced excretion), there is a marked functional difference when compared with the contralateral side.

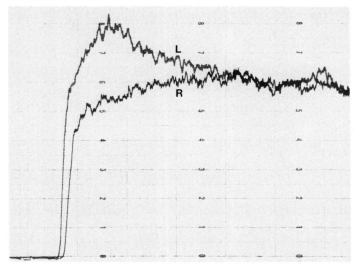

FIG. 44–16. Renogram in a patient with a right nephrectomy. There is no accumulation phase on the right side, and the reduction in radioactivity following the tracer appearance reflects the fall in blood radioactivity as the tracer is taken up in the left kidney.

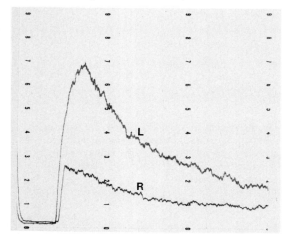

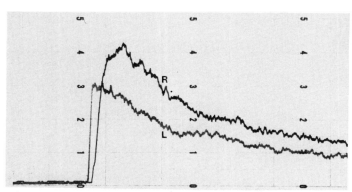

FIG. 44–17. The left renogram shows a no-buildup or nephrectomy pattern. Note the absence of a discernible accumulation segment in the left renogram, findings associated with a nonfunctioning kidney.

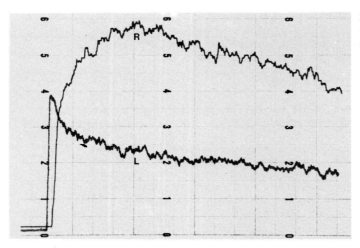

FIG. 44–18. No-buildup pattern on the left side in a patient in whom the left kidney is practically (but not completely) nonfunctioning.

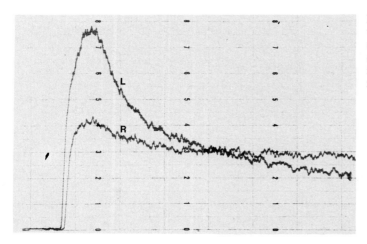

FIG. 44–19. Unilateral parenchymal disease associated with a right staghorn calculus. As a result of urinary obstruction and pyelonephritis, renal function is impaired on the right side; this is manifested by a renogram tracing showing reduced excretion. Compare this with the normal left-sided tracing.

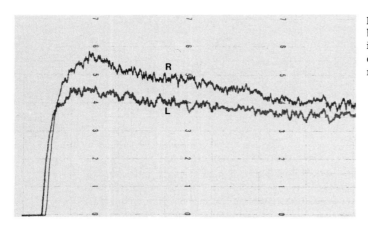

FIG. 44–20. Renogram in a patient recovering from a bout of acute pyelonephritis. Although the transit time is normal in each of the tracings, both kidneys show excretory reduction, findings commonly seen with renal parenchymal disease.

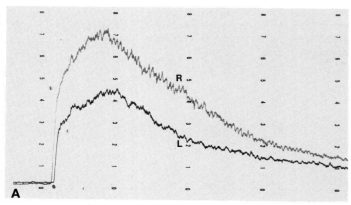

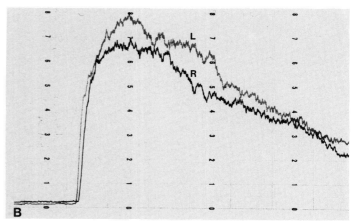

FIG. 44–21. Renograms of patients with chronic renal disease, showing prolonged transit time and reduced excretion.

FIG. 44–22. Chronic pyelonephritis with evidence of prolonged transit time and reduced excretion bilaterally.

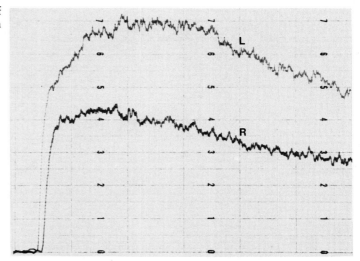

FIG. 44–23. Renogram in a patient with chronic glomerulonephritis who is now in uremia. The left kidney could not be visualized on an intravenous urogram. There is both accumulation and excretion of the ^{131}I-Hippuran in each kidney, but the excretory fall is barely perceptible. The tracings are similar for both right and left sides, a pattern commonly seen in patients with end-stage parenchymal disease of the kidneys.

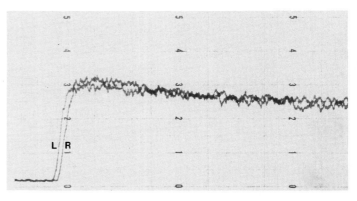

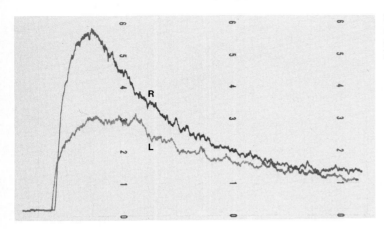

FIG. 44–24. Left-sided pyelonephritis in a 4-year-old child. The right renogram is normal, but the tracing on the left side shows a prolonged transit time and reduced excretion.

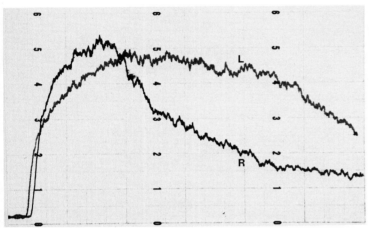

FIG. 44–25. Renogram of patient with bilateral parenchymal disease, much more severe on the left side. The latter tracing shows a markedly prolonged transit time and reduced excretion.

FIG. 44–27. Renograms in patients with confirmed hypertension associated with unilateral renal ischemia. The tracings were performed at a speed of 6 inches per hour and have been redrawn to correspond to the conventional speed of 12 inches per hour.

(A) *Right renal artery stenosis.* The right renogram shows slightly reduced excretion and a normal transit time, whereas the left renogram is normal. The elevated blood pressure in this patient was only of 3 months' duration, and the affected kidney did not yet show evidence of ischemic atrophy (Fig. 44–28) at the time of corrective surgery. In this case, the physiologic changes of renal ischemia preceded histologic alteration.

(B) *Left renal artery stenosis.* Although both renograms show evidence of abnormalities, the changes are more marked on the left side. The disparity between the two tracings suggests that if unilateral ischemia is present, it is in the left kidney.

(C) *Left renal artery stenosis.* The tracing of the involved kidney exhibits an "obstructive" pattern. In such cases, this pattern is probably associated with both intrarenal obstruction and excess tubular reabsorption of water.

(D) *Right renal artery stenosis.* The affected kidney's tracing shows a pattern of nonfunction. In this case, the ischemic kidney, which shows extensive tubular destruction (Fig. 44–29), is *practically* nonfunctioning. However, the sensitivity of the renogram is not sufficient to be able to detect the remaining functioning nephrons.

FIG. 44–26. Left-sided pyelonephritis associated with a staghorn calculus. The left renogram shows only minimal excretion. Compare this with the right-sided tracing in which all three renogram segments are plainly discernible.

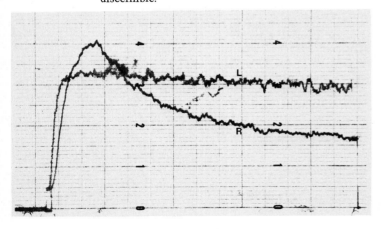

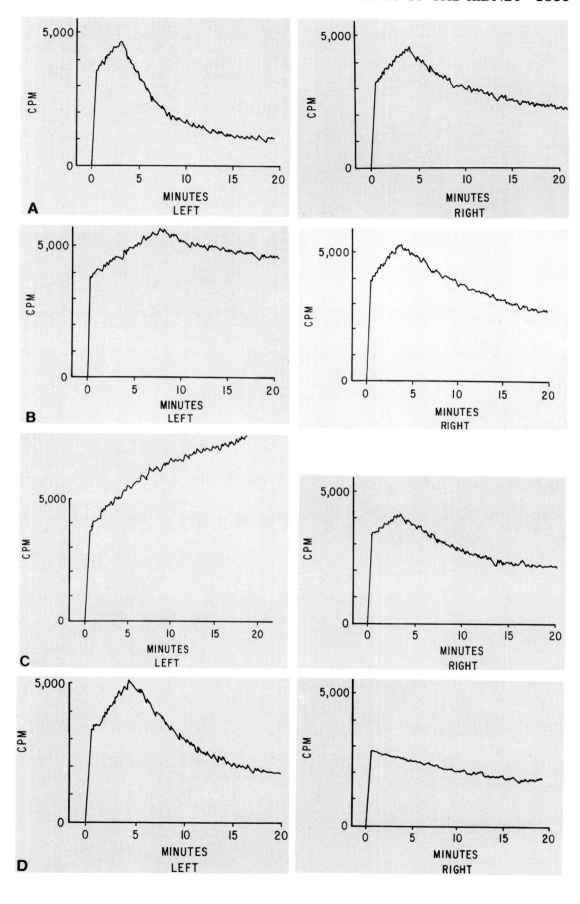

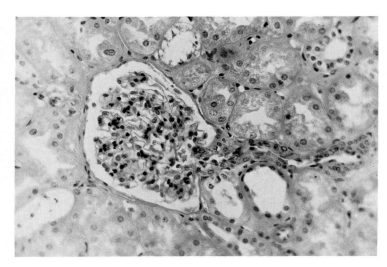

FIG. 44–28. Section of renal tissue in a patient with unilateral renal ischemia of short duration whose renogram is seen in Figure 44–27(**A**). The tubules appear to be normal, and there is no evidence of ischemic atrophy (hematoxylin-eosin, $\times$ 275).

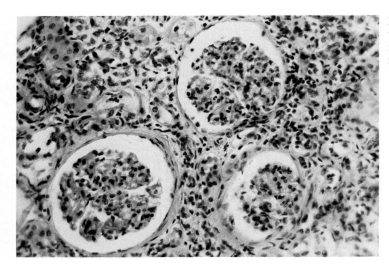

FIG. 44–29. Extensive tubular destruction in a patient with long-standing unilateral renal ischemia. Only a rare, intact tubule is seen. The renogram of this patient is illustrated in Figure 44–27(**D**). (hematoxylin-eosin, $\times$ 275)

FIG. 44–30. (**A**) Bilateral artery stenosis and hypertension. Renogram of 44-year-old hypertensive woman with fibromuscular hyperplasia of both renal arteries. Although the tracings show evidence of bilateral impairment of renal function, it is more severe on the right, and this coincides with the side on which the fibromuscular hyperplasia is more pronounced. The renogram abnormalities appear to be related to renal ischemia in each kidney. (**B**) Renogram in another patient with unilateral renal artery stenosis, involving the right kidney and hypertension. The tracing on the right side shows reduced excretion, whereas the left renogram is normal.

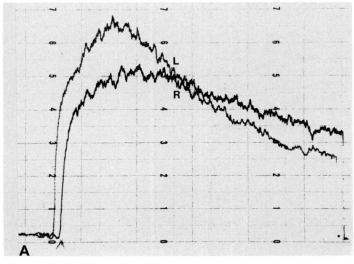

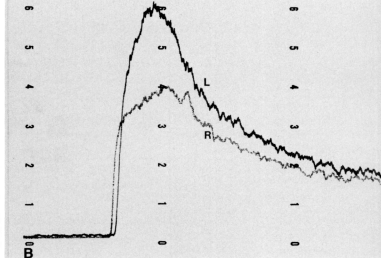

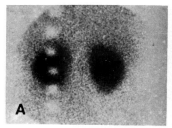
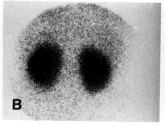
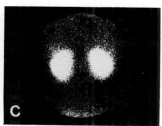

FIG. 44–31. Normal renal imaging. **(A)** The kidney size may be determined by placing a lead marker over the skin of the renal areas at the time of imaging. In this case, the measuring device consists of lead strips, 2 cm. in length, alternating with 2-cm. blank areas. Each kidney measures approximately 11 cm. longitudinally. **(B)** Identical renal image as in **A**, but without lead markers. **(C)** Normal renal imaging in another patient (^{99}Tc-iron-ascorbate-DTPA).

FIG. 44-31. (continued) **(D)** Normal sequential renal imaging using 15 mCi of ^{99m}TC-DTPA (Sn). Imaging immediately following radionuclide injection demonstrates both kidneys. This tagged chelate is excreted rapidly through glomerular filtration, and the renal pelvis is easily seen. At 30 minutes, much of the radionuclide has been excreted and the renal outlines are no longer clearly identified as the cortical areas show diminished activity.

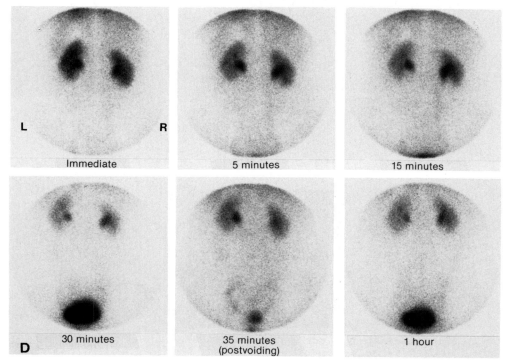

FIG. 44–31. (continued) **(E)** Normal ^{99m}Tc-DTPA (Sn) renal imaging in another patient. The ureters (*arrows*) are seen on the 5- and 15-minute studies.

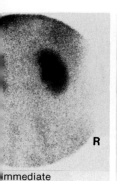
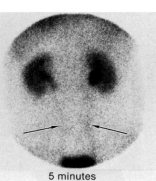
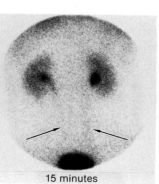
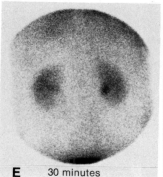
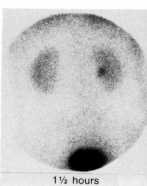

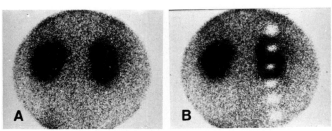

FIG. 44-32. Disparity in renal size. (**A**) The right kidney is larger than the left, as imaged on the (**B**) study with measuring markers, in which the right kidney measured 11 cm. longitudinally and the left kidney, 9 cm. (^{99m}Tc-iron-ascorbate-DTPA).

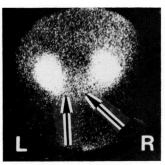

FIG. 44-36. Horseshoe kidney with site of fusion (*arrow*) at lower poles (^{99m}Tc-iron-ascorbate-DTPA).

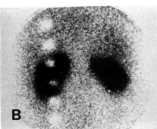
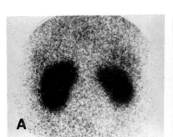

FIG. 44-33. Difference in renal size. The right kidney is 2 cm. smaller than the left. The image (**A**) without the markers is identical to (**B**), in which the 2-cm. markers are seen over the left kidney (^{99m}Tc-iron-ascorbate-DTPA).

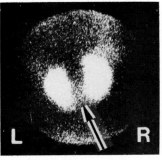

FIG. 44-37. Horseshoe kidney with site of fusion seen at lower poles (*arrow*) (^{99m}Tc-iron-ascorbate-DTPA).

FIG. 44-38. Area of absent radioactivity associated with a hypernephroma. The region of the distorted right upper pole exhibits a central area of reduced activity (tumor) (^{99m}Tc-iron-ascorbate-DTPA).

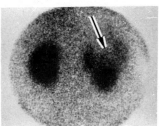

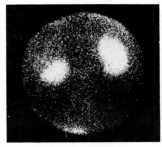

FIG. 44-34. Disparity in size. Congenital, small left kidney (^{99m}Tc-iron-ascorbate-DTPA).

FIG. 44-35. (**A**) Marked elevation of a kidney. The right kidney is situated in a superior position because of herniation through the foramen of Bochdalek (^{99m}Tc-iron-ascorbate-DTPA). (**B**) Ptosis of the left kidney. The study was performed with the patient sitting; the ptosis became apparent in this position. The intravenous urogram was normal (^{99m}Tc-iron-ascorbate-DTPA).

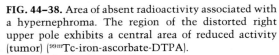
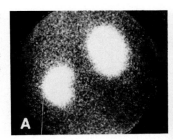
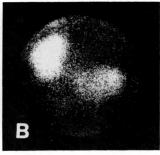

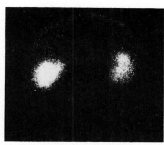

FIG. 44–39. Carcinoma, left upper pole. There is a fairly sharp demarcation between the remaining renal tissue and that destroyed by neoplasm. Without the prior information of roentgenologic studies, the left renal abnormality would be difficult to assess (^{99m}Tc-DTPA [Sn]).

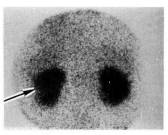

FIG. 44–40. Cortical cyst of left kidney (*arrow*). The configuration of the abnormality is not in itself diagnostic (^{99m}Tc-iron-ascorbate-DTPA).

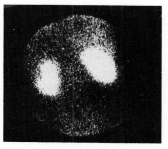

FIG. 44–41. Visualization of a large intrarenal cyst (*arrow*) located in the midportion of the left kidney (^{99m}Tc-iron-ascorbate-DTPA).

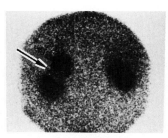

FIG. 44–42. Areas of absent radioactivity associated with perinephric abscess (*arrows*) in right kidney. Imaging was performed in the anterior position in this patient, who was sensitive to contrast material (^{99m}Tc-DTPA [Sn]).

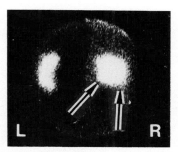

FIG. 44–43. Renal infarction. Absent radioactivity in the region of the left upper pole associated with a vascular occlusion (^{99m}Tc-iron-ascorbate-DTPA).

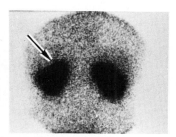

FIG. 44–44. Absent radioactivity due to adjacent organ. The area of absent radioactivity in the region of the left upper pole (*arrow*) is associated with the tip of the spleen overlying the upper portion of the kidney (^{99m}Tc-iron-ascorbate-DTPA).

FIG. 44–45. (A) Left nephrectomy. Absent radioactivity is noted in the left renal area since the kidney has been removed. The remaining kidney appears to be normal (^{99m}Tc-iron-ascorbate-DTPA). (B) Bone imaging performed in the posterior position in the same patient as in (A). The radionuclide employed for this procedure, ^{99m}Tc-stannous polyphosphate, is excreted through the kidneys, and such radionuclide skeletal imaging may often denote abnormalities in the urinary system. As in (A), there is also failure to visualize a left kidney.

FIG. 44–46. Evidence of renal uptake (*arrow*) of radioactive material in the right kidney. The intravenous urogram showed nonvisualization of the right kidney, and renal imaging helped establish that there was indeed a right-sided kidney present (^{99m}Tc-DTPA [Sn]).

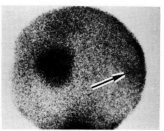

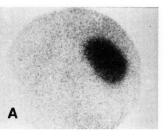

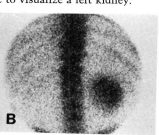

A   **B**

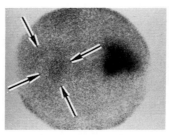

FIG. 44–47. Imaging of left kidney (faint) after failure to visualize on intravenous urogram. The portion imaged is indicated by the *arrow*. Note the increased radioactivity in the region of the right renal pelvis as the ^{99m}Tc is being excreted (^{99m}Tc-DTPA [Sn]).

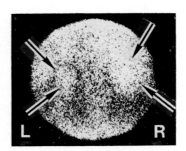

FIG. 44–48. Failure to image the kidneys successfully in a patient with uremia. The clearance of the radionuclide is so slow that insufficient radioactive material is present in the kidneys for imaging purposes, whereas the blood radioactivity continues to be high. *Arrows* indicate both kidneys (^{99m}Tc-DTPA [Sn]).

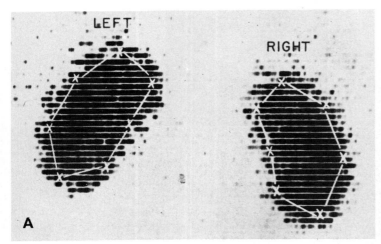

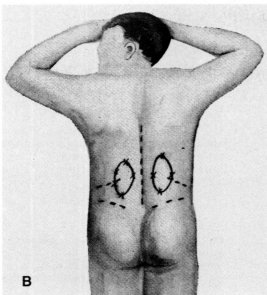

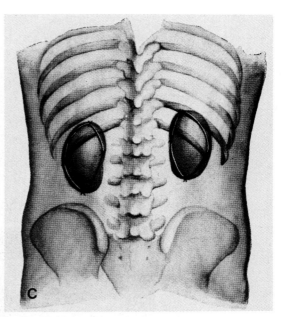

FIG. 44–49. Kidney localization with radionuclide imaging for percutaneous renal biopsy. **(A)** Renal scan obtained following ^{197}Hg-chlormerodrin administration. Several points on the periphery of the renal outlines are selected and marked (X) and the printing stylus is placed over each of these points on the scan's paper printout. Using the light localizer in the detecting probe, **(B)** the corresponding areas are marked on the back with a felt marking pencil and, when connected, outline the kidneys. The rectilinear scan is a life-sized representation, with little or no distortion. This is seen diagrammatically in **(C)**, where the renal outlines obtained through scanning correspond closely to the true projections of the kidneys. (Baum, S., Rabinowitz, P., and Molly, W.A.: J.A.M.A., *195*:913, 1966)

FIG. 44–51. Renal imaging in acute tubular necrosis. Studies were obtained following the administration of 300 μCi ^{131}I-Hippuran. **(A)** Imaging 16 minutes following tracer injection demonstrates the presence of the radionuclide in the renal cortex, with none present in the renal pelvis. **(B)** At 18 hours after injection, the radioactive material continues to be confined to the cortex with no evidence of excretion into the pelvis. Compare these images with those obtained using ^{99m}Tc-iron-ascorbate-DTPA. **(C)** Because of the poor renal function, associated with a markedly elevated BUN, relatively little radionuclide is cleared from the blood. (Courtesy of Dr. Stanley Green, Brunswick Hospital, Amityville, N.Y.)

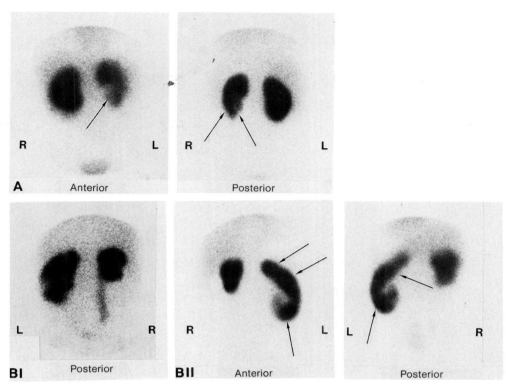

FIG. 44–50. ^{99m}Tc-DMSA imaging. Because the radio-nuclide becomes localized in the proximal tubules, renal images represent functioning cortical tissue. Imaging was performed 2 hours following injection. (**A**) The right renal image is normal. This patient has left-sided pyelonephritis associated with reflux on that side. The involvement in the lower half of the left kidney has resulted in loss of cortical tissue (*arrow*) in this region. (**B**) Progressive changes in a child with hydronephrosis and pyelonephritis. The relatively thin shell of cortical tissue in the left kidney (*arrows*) in *II,* associated with marked hydronephrosis, is indicative of progressive destruction and replacement of renal cortical tissue. Compare this to the study in *I,* which was performed 2 years earlier.

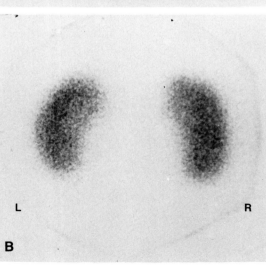

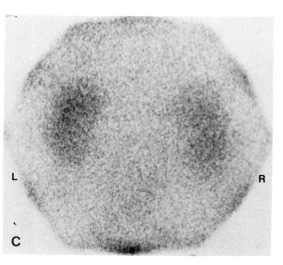

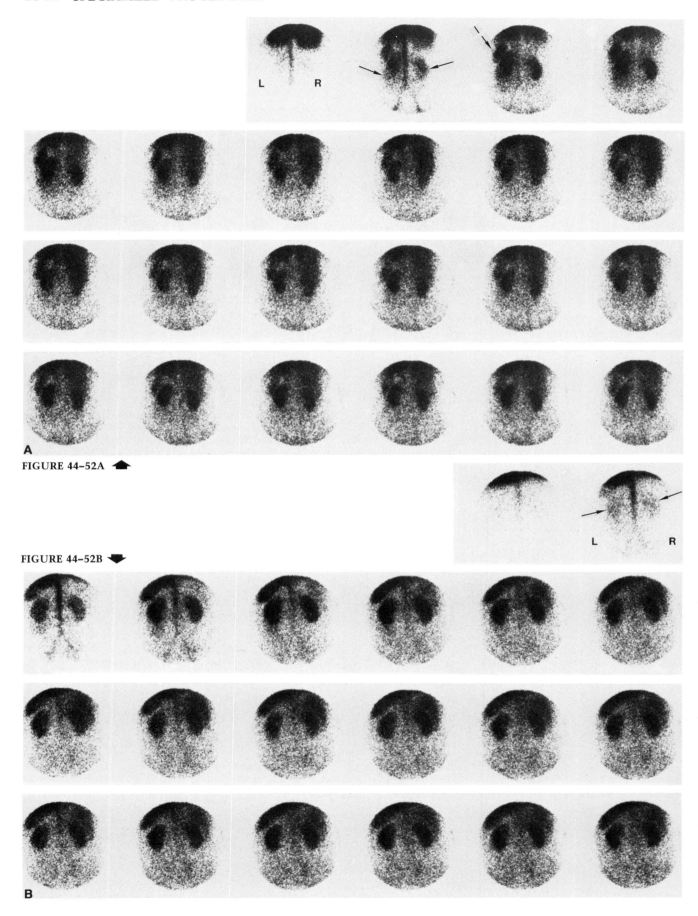

FIGURE 44–52A

FIGURE 44–52B

FIG. 44–52. Normal radionuclide blood-flow studies performed in the posterior position. Frames were obtained at intervals of 3 seconds. **(A)** Arterial perfusion to both kidneys *(arrows)* is demonstrated almost immediately after there is visualization of the abdominal aorta. Such identification during the arterial phase is brief. Note the perfused spleen *(broken arrow)* and its proximity to the left kidney. It is important not to confuse renal radioactivity with that of the spleen during the arterial phase, especially in patients with marked impairment in vascular supply to the left kidney. **(B)** Normal arterial perfusion of both kidneys *(arrows)* in a patient in whom the spleen is not so closely related to the left kidney. [⁹⁹ᵐTc-DTPA (Sn)].

FIG. 44–53. Radionuclide blood-flow study performed in the posterior position in a patient with a hypoplastic right kidney. This small right kidney is identified during the arterial phase *(arrow)*. The image of the contralateral normal kidney *(broken arrow)* is clearly seen throughout (⁹⁹ᵐTc-DTPA).

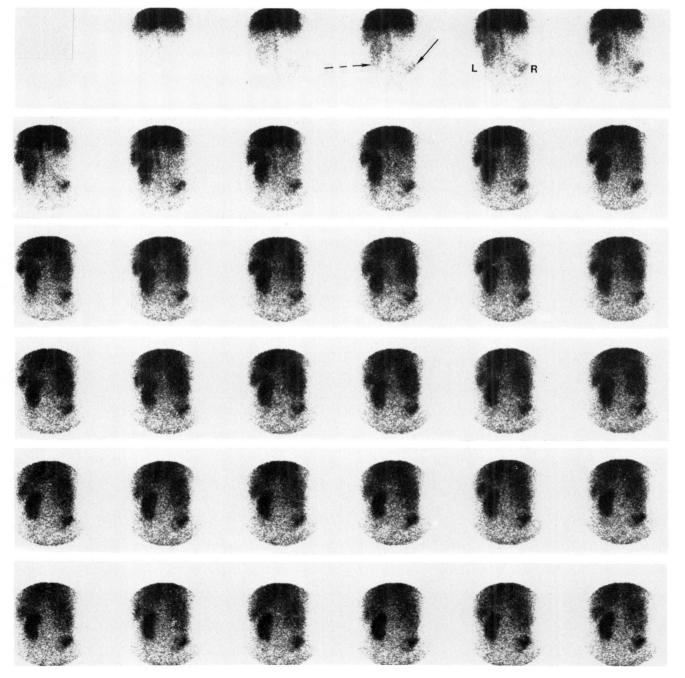

FIG. 44–54. Anterior blood-flow study in a patient with severe tortuosity of the distal abdominal aorta and downward displacement of the right kidney. The site of the tortuous aorta (*arrow*) is demonstrated during the arterial phase, and the relation of the inferiorly located right kidney (*RK*) to the aorta and external iliac arteries (*EIA*) is shown. Frames were obtained at intervals of 3 seconds (⁹⁹ᵐTc-sodium pertechnetate).

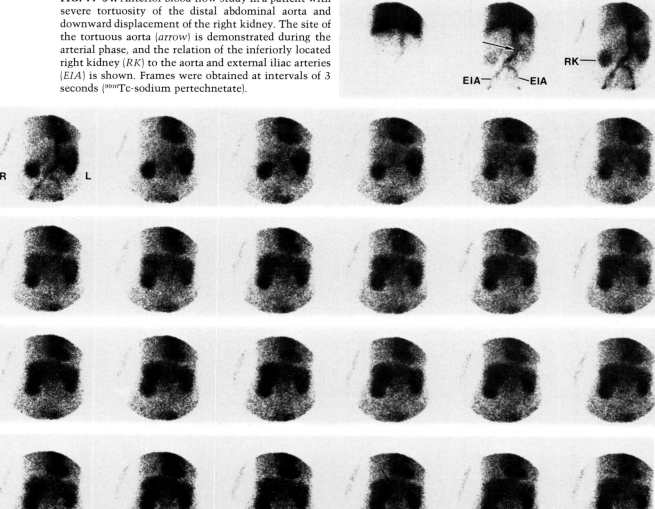

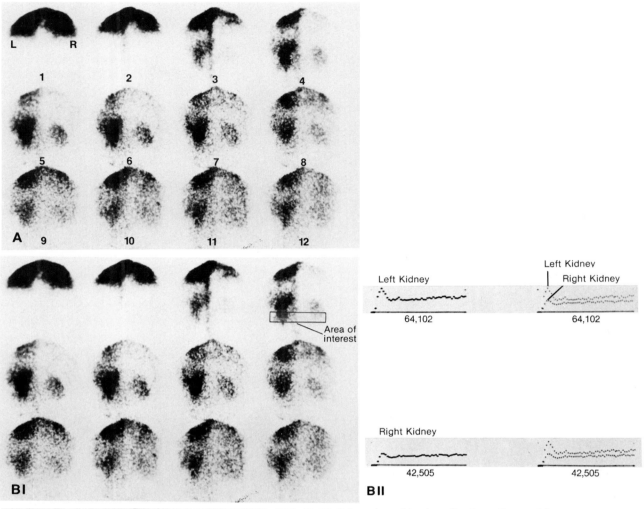

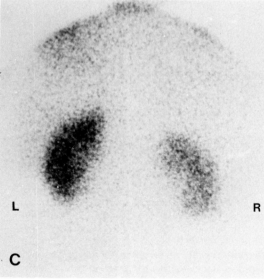

FIG. 44–55. Selected combined studies in an 8-year-old boy with hypertension and unilateral renal artery stenosis. (**A**) Radionuclide angiogram and flow study following injection of ^{99m}Tc-DTPA. Imaging was performed at intervals of 2 seconds. In frames 3 and 4, it becomes readily apparent that arterial perfusion is much more abundant to the left kidney than the right. In addition, the perfused right kidney appears to be much smaller than the left kidney (see frame 6). (**B**) Area-of-interest histograms were obtained from both lower poles at the onset of renal perfusion, as seen in frame 4. The curves so obtained represent the initial bolus and entry to the renal vasculature of ^{99m}Tc. Each curve is of 100 seconds duration. Note the rapid peak in radioactivity in the study of the left kidney, whereas the histogram taken from the right kidney is somewhat flattened. Compare the radioactivity over the left kidney (64,102 counts) with that over the right kidney (42,505). (**C**) Static renal imaging shows the right kidney to be slightly smaller than the left. This patient was found to have unilateral renal ischemia involving the right lower pole. (Courtesy of Dr. Stanley Green, Brunswick Hospital, Amityville, N.Y.)

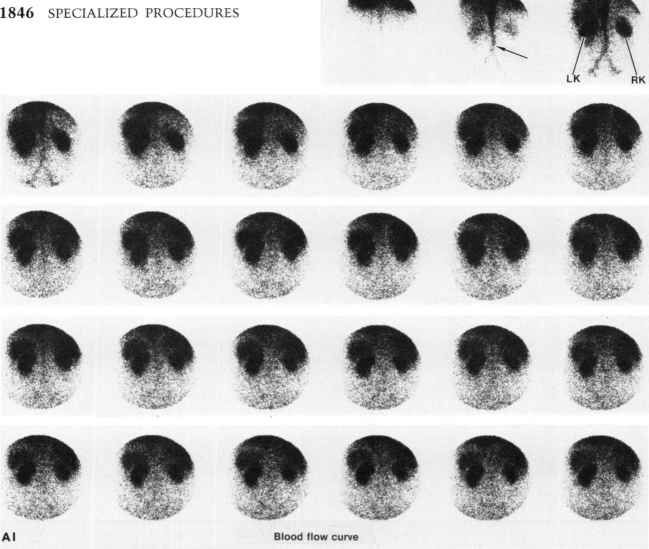

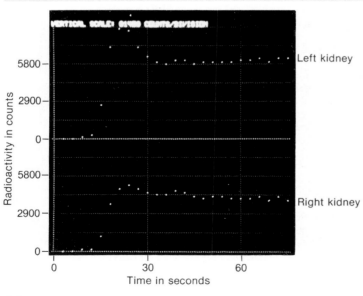

A I   **Blood flow curve**

FIG. 44–55a. (A) Combined studies in a patient with hypertension and stenosis of an accessory renal artery. (*I*) *Blood-flow studies* performed in the posterior position with frames obtained at intervals of 3 seconds. The abdominal aorta is clearly identified (*arrow*) and, visually, there appears to be similar perfusion to both the right (*RK*) and left (*LK*) kidneys. The perfused right kidney appears slightly smaller than the left. However, the blood-flow curve generated from the computer analysis covering frames 1 to 25 shows a difference between the two sides. The arterial perfusion curve of the right kidney (*lower curve*) shows lower amplitude than that of the left, and the relative flattening of the right curve compared to the left is related to slower or reduced arterial flow (99mTc-DTPA). (*II*) *Static imaging* performed in the posterior position immediately following radionuclide administration and at intervals up to 30 minutes. The initial images show that the right kidney is smaller than the left. The initial increase in radioactivity in the left kidney is associated with greater glomerular filtration on that side. Subsequent serial imaging shows slightly less radioactivity on the left side than the right, findings related to greater excretion on the left side (99mTc-DTPA).

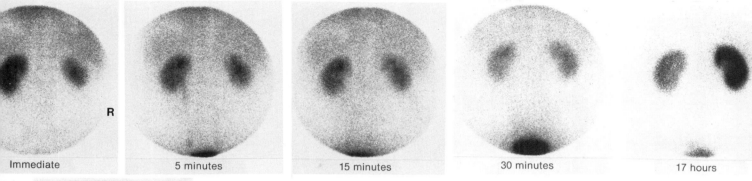

Immediate   5 minutes   15 minutes   30 minutes   17 hours

R

A II Static imaging

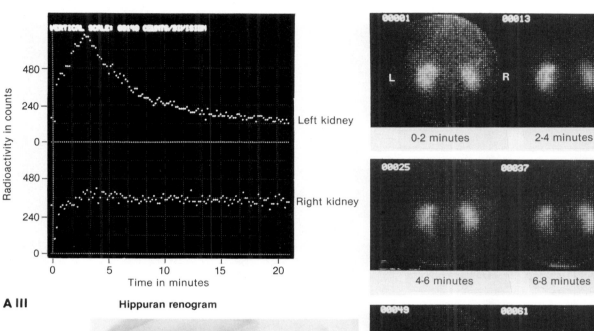

A III   Hippuran renogram

Left kidney

Right kidney

Radioactivity in counts

480

240

0

480

240

0

0   5   10   15   20

Time in minutes

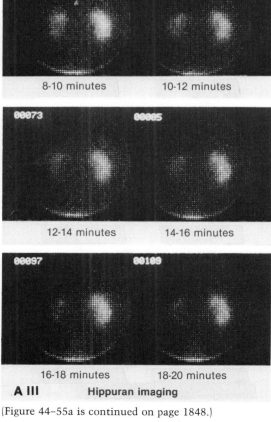

00001	00013
L	R
0-2 minutes	2-4 minutes

| 00025 | 00037 |
| 4-6 minutes | 6-8 minutes |

| 00049 | 00061 |
| 8-10 minutes | 10-12 minutes |

| 00073 | 00085 |
| 12-14 minutes | 14-16 minutes |

| 00097 | 00109 |
| 16-18 minutes | 18-20 minutes |

A III   Hippuran imaging

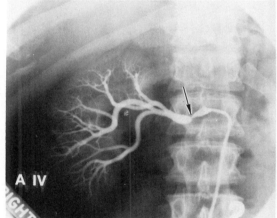

A IV

(*III*) Hippuran imaging and renogram generation. These computerized posterior images show sequential renal imaging at intervals of 2 minutes. During the first two frames, there is increased activity in the left kidney associated with more rapid tubular uptake on that side. Afterward, the activity in the left kidney continues to decrease because of excretion on that side. On the other hand, the radioactivity continues to increase in the right kidney due to prolonged uptake and reduced excretion of the radionuclide. The renogram reflects the Hippuran imaging findings, showing a normal left-sided curve and the described abnormalities on the right (prolonged transit time, reduced excretion), the disparity being consistent with unilateral renal ischemia. (*IV*) The selective renal arteriogram shows stenosis (*arrow*) of right upper renal artery.

(Figure 44–55a is continued on page 1848.)

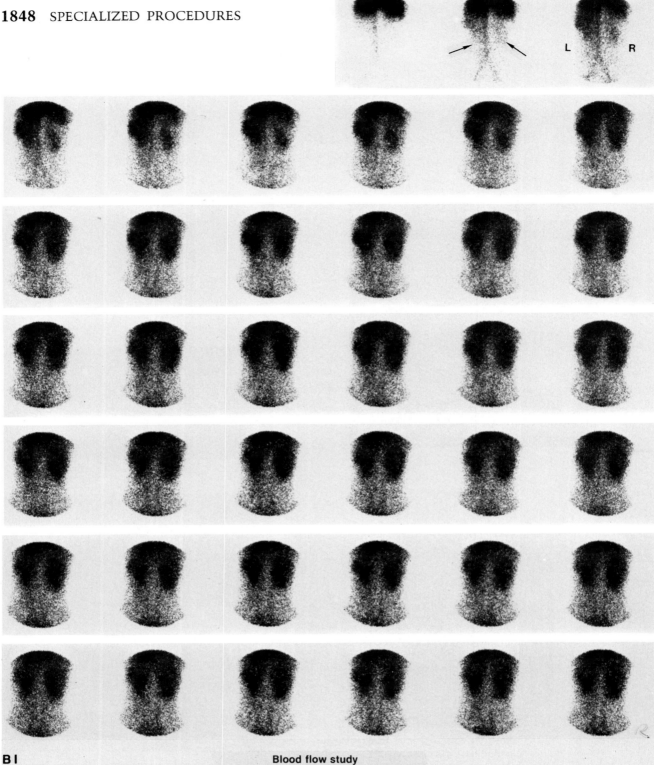

B I   **Blood flow study**

FIG. 44–55a (continued) **(B)** Combined studies in a 16-year-old girl with hypertension and associated chronic, bilateral renal disease. The ^{131}I-Hippuran studies in this patient helped determine that the hypertension was not associated with unilateral renal ischemia and that renal angiography should not be performed in search of unilateral renal artery stenosis. (*I*) *Blood-flow study* performed in the posterior position shows evidence of perfusion to both kidneys (*arrows*) during the arterial phase. However, it appears to be slightly diminished when compared to normal studies. The arterial perfusion curve generated from the first 25 frames of the blood-flow study shows flattening for both the left and right kidneys, somewhat more prominent on the right [^{99m}Tc-DTPA (Sn)]. (*II*) *Static imaging* performed in the posterior position. Sequential renal images show no difference in renal size. Excretion is slow, as seen by similar renal images at 30 and 90 minutes [^{99m}Tc-DTPA (Sn)]. (*II*) *Hippuran imaging and renogram generation.* There is a similarly slow rate of uptake of the radioactive Hippuran in both the right and left kidneys. Although renal identification is seen best during the interval 4–6 minutes, the definition is far inferior to that seen in the normal kidney in Fig. 44–55a A III. The prolonged uptake and reduced excretion are reflected in the renogram curves. The findings are consistent with nephrosclerosis and indicate that unilateral renal ischemia is probably not the cause of the hypertension. (Baum, S., Vincent, N.R., Lyons, K.P. et al.: Atlas of Nuclear Medicine Imaging. New York, Appleton-Century-Crofts, 1981)

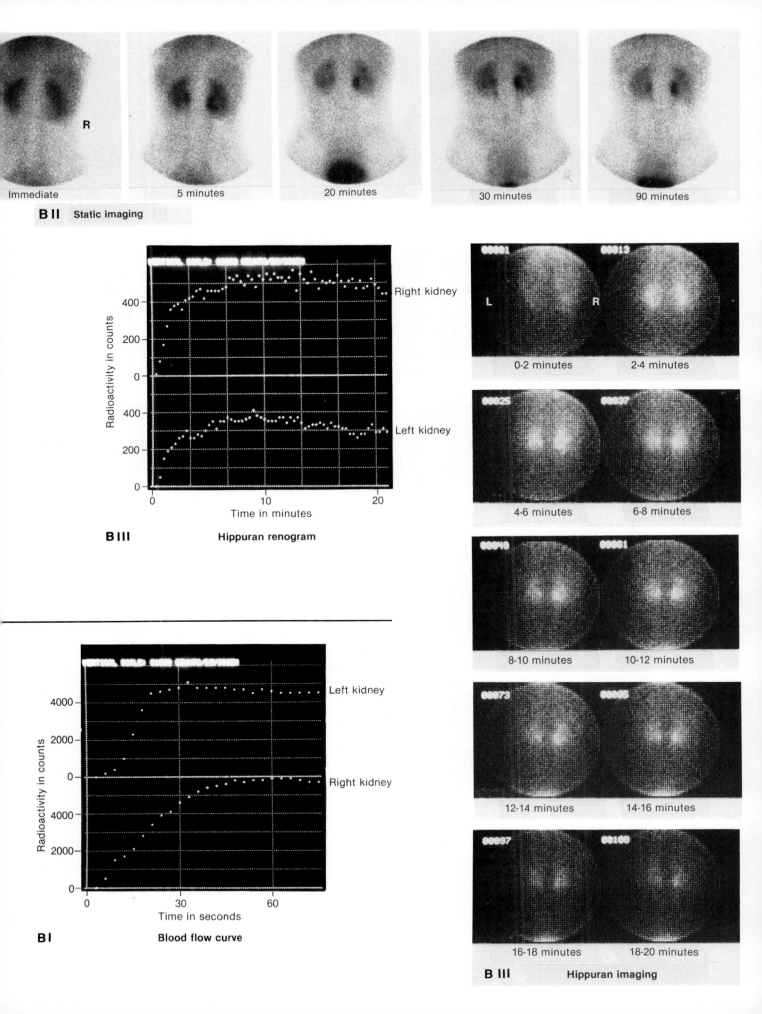

Immediate   5 minutes   20 minutes   30 minutes   90 minutes

B II   Static imaging

B III   Hippuran renogram

B I   Blood flow curve

0-2 minutes   2-4 minutes

4-6 minutes   6-8 minutes

8-10 minutes   10-12 minutes

12-14 minutes   14-16 minutes

16-18 minutes   18-20 minutes

B III   Hippuran imaging

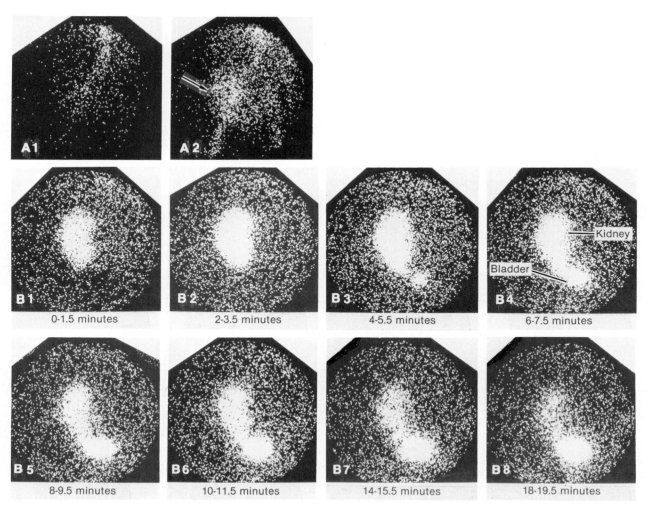

FIG. 44–56. Selected combined studies in a patient with a kidney transplant. **(A)** Radionuclide angiogram performed following ⁹⁹ᵐTc administration. The radioactive material is seen to enter the common iliac artery at 11 seconds and perfusion in the transplanted kidney (*arrow*) is seen at 14 seconds. **(B)** Serial images following the intravenous injection of ¹³¹I-Hippuran, performed during intervals of 1.5 minutes. Frames one (0–1.5 min) and two (2–3.5 min) show excellent renal visualization. The initial appearance of radioactive Hippuran in the bladder may be seen in frame three (4–5.5 min). Gradually, the radioactivity in the kidney becomes greatly reduced as the radionuclide is excreted into the bladder. **(C)** External monitoring over the transplanted kidney and bladder. The renogram is normal, whereas the bladder tracing shows continually rising radioactivity, reflecting the continued accumulation of bladder radioactivity as the ¹³¹I-Hippuran is excreted from the kidney. (Courtesy of Kenneth P. Lyons, M.D. and Steven C. Gurkin, M.D., Veterans' Administration Hospital, Long Beach, California)

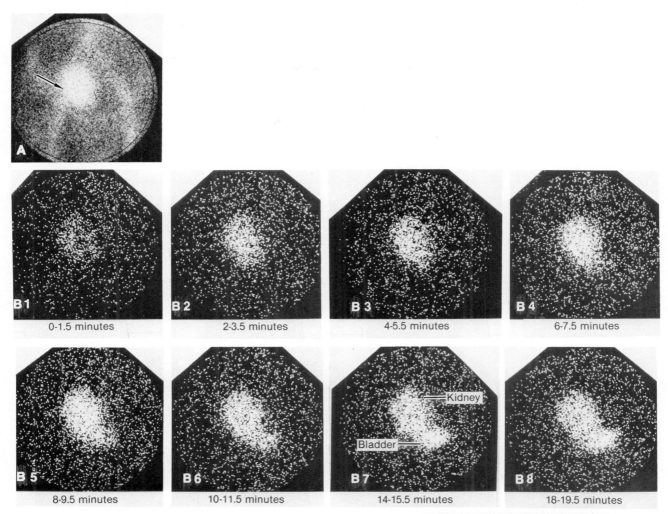

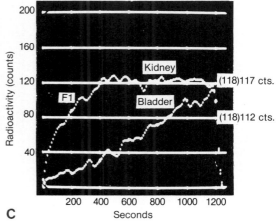

FIG. 44–57. Impaired renal function heralding the onset of a rejection reaction 1 month after kidney transplantation. (**A**) Frame of radionuclide angiogram using ^{99m}Tc shows evidence of arterial perfusion to the transplanted kidney (*arrow*). (**B**) Serial images following injection of ^{131}I-Hippuran performed during 1.5-minute intervals. The delay in the appearance of radioactivity in the bladder reflects impaired excretion by the kidney. Compare with radioactive Hippuran imaging in Figure 44–56. (**C**) External monitoring over the transplanted kidney and bladder. The renogram shows a prolonged transit time and flattened excretory curve. Although the bladder tracing shows evidence of accumulation of excreted radionuclide, the bladder radioactivity is really greatly reduced. (Courtesy of Kenneth P. Lyons, M.D. and Steven C. Gurkin, M.D., Veterans' Administration Hospital, Long Beach, California)

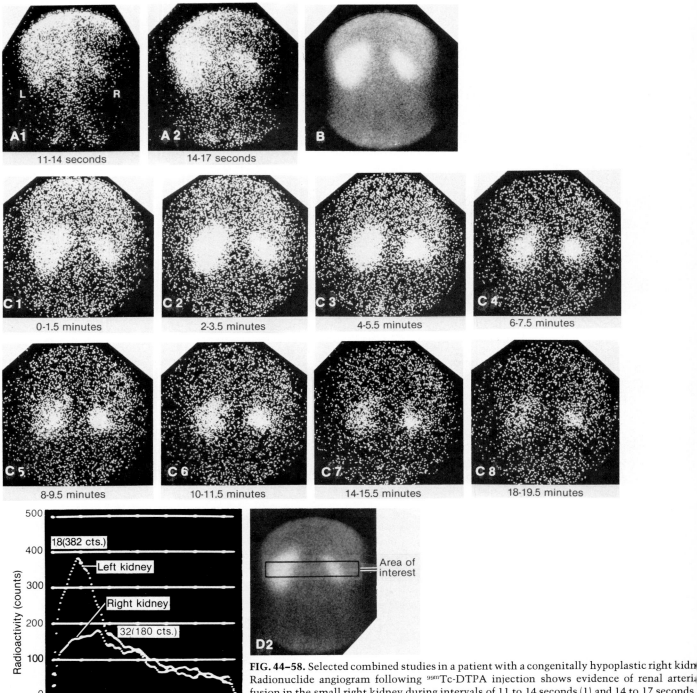

FIG. 44–58. Selected combined studies in a patient with a congenitally hypoplastic right kidney. Radionuclide angiogram following ^{99m}Tc-DTPA injection shows evidence of renal arterial perfusion in the small right kidney during intervals of 11 to 14 seconds (1) and 14 to 17 seconds (2). Static renal imaging with ^{99m}Tc-DTPA simply demonstrates the normal left kidney and small right kidney. (**C**) Serial imaging following ^{131}I-Hippuran injection indicates some impairment of function on the right side. Note the prolonged retention of radionuclide in the right kidney (panels 4 and 5) when compared with the contralateral kidney. (**D**) Area of interest renogram taken over the midportion of each kidney. The left renogram is normal, whereas the right renogram shows both a prolonged transit time and reduced excretion. Although static renal imaging with DTPA shows only a small right kidney, the ^{131}I-Hippuran studies show impairment of renal function in the smaller kidney. (Courtesy of Kenneth P. Lyons, M.D. and Steven C. Gurkin, M.D., Veterans Administration Hospital, Long Beach, California)

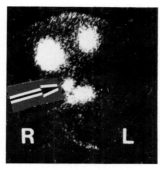

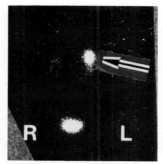

FIG. 44–59. Radionuclide cystogram in the anterior position, showing evidence of right ureteral reflux (*arrow*). Study was performed 1 hour following intravenous administration of ^{99m}Tc-DTPA (Sn). In this patient with impaired renal function there is an equivalent amount of radionuclide in both the kidneys and bladder. However, when the patient was instructed to bear down as if to void, reflux into the right ureter could be readily demonstrated.

FIG. 44–60. Reflux into the right renal pelvis (*arrow*). The procedure was performed in the posterior position 1 hour following intravenous injection of ^{99m}Tc-DTPA (Sn). By this time, there had been virtually complete clearance of the radionuclide from the kidneys in this patient with normal renal function, and practically all of the ^{99m}Tc was present in the bladder. The act of bearing down as if to void showed reflux into the right renal pelvis.

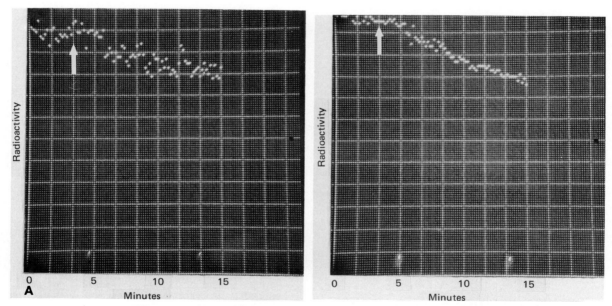

FIG. 44–61. Furosemide excretion study. **(A)** Hydronephrosis not due to mechanical obstruction. In this patient with left-sided hydronephrosis of unknown etiology, the time–activity curve shows a slight increase in Tc-99m DTPA activity prior to furosemide administration. However, after the furosemide is given (*arrow*), there is a prompt reduction in radioactivity that is indicative of excretion and helps to establish the absence of mechanical obstruction as a cause of the dilated left renal pelvis. The right kidney in this patient is hypoplastic. Renal images, generated as intervals of 30 seconds, show evidence of excretion after furosemide injection. **(B)** Hydronephrosis due to mechanical obstruction. There is a continued rise in radioactivity on the time-activity curve in this patient with right-sided hydronephrosis with suspected mechanical obstruction. A right pyeloplasty had been performed earlier. Sequential renal imaging shows continued radionuclide accumulation in the obstructed right kidney.

(Figure 44–61 is continued on page 1854.)

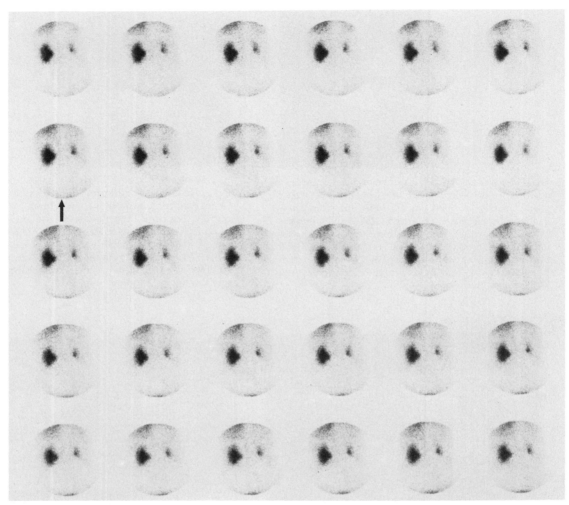

(FIG. 44–61A, continued)

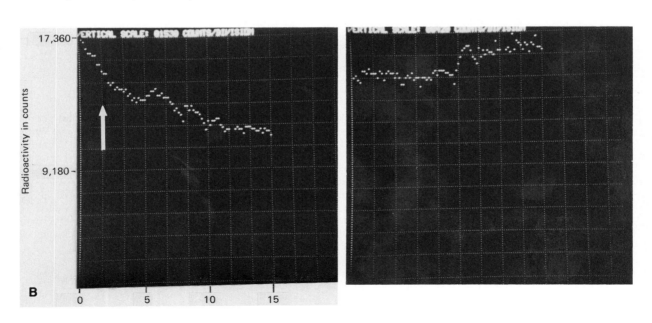

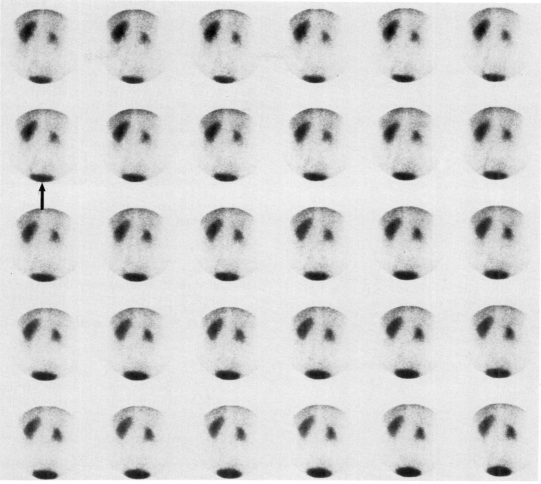

(FIG. 44-61B, continued)

BIBLIOGRAPHY

General

1. Baum, S., and Bramlet, R.: Basic Nuclear Medicine, pp. 86–106. New York, Appleton-Century-Crofts, 1975.
2. Blaufox, M.D. (ed.): Progress in Nuclear Medicine: Evaluation of Renal Function and Disease with Radionuclides. Baltimore, University Park Press, 1972.
2a. Blaufox, M.D., and Bell, E.G.: General principles of renal evaluation with radionuclides. *In* Gottschalk, A., Potchen, E.J. (eds.): Diagnostic Nuclear Medicine, pp. 464–475. Baltimore, Williams and Wilkins, 1976.
3. Blaufox, M.D., and Funck-Brentano, J.-L. (eds.): Radionuclides in Nephrology. New York, Grune & Stratton, 1973.
4. Boyd, J.D., and Murdock, H.R.: The radiorenogram as a measure of renal function. Arch. Int. Med., 109:654, 1962.
5a. Britton, K.E., and Brown, N.J.G.: Clinical Renography. Chicago, Year Book, 1973.
5b. Britton, K.E., and Brown, N.J.G.: The clinical use of C.A.B.B.S. renography. Investigation of the "non-functioning kidney" and renal artery stenosis by the use of I-Hippuran renography modified by computer assisted blood background subtraction (C.A.B.B.S.). Br. J. Radiol., 41:570, 1968.
5c. Clorius, J.H., Kjelle-Schweigler, M., and Ostertag, H., et al.: [131I] Hippuran renography in the detection of orthostatic hypertension. J. Nucl. Med., 19:343, 1978.
5d. Dahlager, J.I.: Sequential [125I]-o-iodohippurate renograms from rabbit kidneys after temporary renal ischemia. J. Nucl. Med., 19:1324, 1978.
6. Dore, E.K., Taplin, G.V., and Johnson, D.E.: Current interpretation of the sodium iodohippurate I131 renocystogram. J.A.M.A., 185:925, 1963.
7. Farmelant, M.H., and Burrows, B.A.: The renogram: physiologic basis and current clinical use. Seminars Nucl. Med., 4:61, 1974.
8. Henk, J.M., Cottrall, M.F., and Taylor, D.M.: Radiation dosimetry of the 131I-Hippuran renogram. Br. J. Radiol., 40:327, 1967.

9. Kolar, M.: Radioisotope Renography. Acta Univ. Carol. Med. Praha. Monograph, p. 48, 1971.

10. Lawrence, J.R., et al.: Value of ^{131}I-Hippuran renography in urological investigation. Br. Med. J., 1:504, 1963.

11. McDonald, D.F., Frank, I.N., and Miller, H.C., et al.: The Hippuran renogram. Modern Medicine, May 13, 1963, p. 103.

12. Razzak, M.A., Botti, R.E., and McIntyre, W.J.: Interrelationship between hydration, urine flow and the radiohippuran renogram. J. Nucl. Med., 10:673, 1969.

13. Taplin, G.V., Meredith, O.M., Kade, H., and Winter, C.C.: The radioisotope renogram. J. Lab. Clin. Med., 48:886–1956.

14. Taplin, G.V., and Nordyke, R.A.: Radioisotope renography. In Blahd, W.H. (ed.): Nuclear Medicine, 2nd ed. New York, McGraw-Hill, 1971, pp. 402–415.

15. Tauxe, W.N., Hunt, J.C., and Burbank, M.K.: The radioisotope renogram (orthoiodohippurate-I[131]). Standardization of technique and expression of data. Am. J. Clin. Path., 37:567, 1962.

15a. Thrall, J.H.: Renogram. In Keyes, J.W., Jr. (ed.): Manual of Nuclear Medicine Procedures, pp. 98–102. West Palm Beach, CRC Press, 1978.

16. Timmermans, L., and Merchie G. (eds.): Radioisotopes in the diagnosis of diseases of the kidneys and urinary tract. Amsterdam, Excerpta Medica, 1969.

17. Wedeen, R.P., Goldstein, M.H., and Levitt, M.: The radioisotope renogram in normal subjects. Am. J. Med., 34:765, 1963.

18. Winter, C.C.: A clinical study of a new renal function test: the radioactive diodrast renogram. J. Urol., 76:182, 1956.

19. Winter, C.C.: Radioisotope Renography. Baltimore, Williams & Wilkins, 1963.

Analysis

20. Brown, F., Gelber, R., Youkeles, L., and Bennett, L.: Quantitative approach to the I[131] renogram. J.A.M.A., 186:211, 1963.

21. Halko, A., Burke, G., and Sorkin, A., et al.: Computer-aided statistical analysis of the scintillation camera ^{131}I-Hippuran renogram. J. Nucl. Med., 14:253, 1973.

21a. Hirakawa, A., and Corcoran, A.C.: I[131]-o-iodo hippurate excretion and a quantitative formulation of the radioisotope renogram as indices of bilateral and unilateral renal functions. J. Lab. Clin. Med., 61:795, 1963.

22. Heiskanen, T., Weber, T., and Grasbeck, R.: A method for the quantitative evaluation of radioisotope renograms. Int. J. Appl. Radiat., 19:827, 1968.

23. Holroyd, A.M., Chrisholm, G.D., and Glass, H.I.: The quantitative analysis of renograms using the gamma camera. Phys. Med. Biol., 15:483, 1970.

24. Koplowitz, J.M., Mitchell, J.F., and Blahd, W.H.: The radioisotope renogram: a comparison of qualitative and quantitative interpretation. J.A.M.A., 192:1032, 1965.

25. Loken, M.K., Linneman, R.E., and Kush, G.S.: Evaluation of renal function, using a scintillation camera and computer. Radiology, 93:85, 1969.

26. Pircher, F.J., Carr, E.A., Jr., and Patno, M.E.: Evaluation of quantitative aspects of the radioisotope renogram. J. Nucl. Med., 4:117, 1963.

27. Van Stekelenberg, L.H.M., Al, N., Truijens, J.H.J., Van Vals, G.H., and Dooman, A.: A quantitative theory of radioisotope renography with Hippuran [131]I. Phys. Med. Biol., 11:451, 1966.

28. Winter, C.C.: Quantitative vs. qualitative interpretation of the radioisotope renogram. J.A.M.A., 192:1089, 1965.

Hypertension and Unilateral Renal Artery Stenosis

29. Andrews, D., Parsons, V., and Roebuck, E.J.: The radioisotope renogram compared with intravenous pyelography as a screening test for patients with hypertension. Br. J. Radiol., 38:527, 1965.

30. Brown, J.J., Peart, W.S., Owen, K., Robertson, J.I.S., and Sutton, D.: The diagnosis and treatment of renal-artery stenosis. Br. Med. J., 2:327, 1960.

31. Burbank, M.K., Hunt, J.C., Tauxe, W.N., and Maher, F.T.: Radioisotope renography. Diagnosis of renal arterial disease in hypertensive patients. Circulation, 27:328, 1963.

32. Clark, M.D., Eyler, W.R., and Dusault, L.A., et al.: The renogram in hypertension. Radiology, 89:667, 1967.

33. Connor, T.B., Berthrong, M., Thomas, W.C., Jr., and Howard, J.E.: Hypertension due to unilateral renal disease—with a report of a functional test helpful in diagnosis. Bull. Johns. Hopkins, Hosp., 100:241, 1957.

34. Connor, T.B., Thomas, W.C., Jr., and Haddock, L., et al.: Unilateral renal disease as a cause of hypertension: its detection by ureteral catheterization studies. Ann. Intern. Med., 52:544, 1960.

35. Doig, A., et al.: ^{131}I-Hippuran renography in detection of unilateral renal disease in patients with hypertension. Br. Med. J., 1:500, 1963.

36. Dustan, H.P.: Physiologic consequences of renal arterial stenosis. N. Engl. J. Med., 281:1348, 1969.

37. Editorial: Diagnosis of renovascular hypertension. Lancet, 2:94, 1966.

38. Farmelant, M.H., Lipetz, C.A., Bikerman, V., and Burrows, B.A.: Radioisotope renal function studies and surgical findings in 102 hypertensive patients. Am. J. Surg., 107:50, 1964.

39. Farmelant, M.H., Sachs, C., and Burrows, B.A.: Prognostic value of radioisotopic renal function studies for selecting patients with renal arterial stenosis for surgery. J. Nucl. Med., 11:743, 1970.

40. Howard, J.E., Berthrong, M., Gould, D.M., and Yendt, E.R.: Hypertension resulting from unilateral renal vascular disease and its relief by nephrectomy. Bull. Johns Hopkins Hosp., 94:51, 1954.

41. Lefebyre, R., and Genest, J.: Study of renal ischemic tubular atrophy in 79 patients with arterial hypertension. Can. Med. Ass. J., 82:1249, 1960.

42. Luke, R.G., Briggs, J.D., Kennedy, A.C., and Stirling, W.B.: The isotope renogram in the detection and assessment of renal artery stenosis. Quart. J. Med., 35:237, 1966.

43. McAfee, J.G., Reba, R.C., and Chodos, R.B.: Radioisotopic methods in the diagnosis of renal vascular disease: a critical review. Semin. Roentgenol., 2:198, 1967.

44. Maxwell, M.H., Lupu, A.N., and Taplin, G.V.: Radioisotope renogram in renal arterial hypertension. J. Urol., 100:376, 1968.

45. Meier, D.A., and Beierwaltes, W.H.: Radioisotope renal studies and renal hypertension: a comparison of the sodium iodohippurate I[131] renogram, chlormerodrin Hg 197 uptake, and renal scan. J.A.M.A., 198:1257, 1966.

46. Nordyke, R.A., Rigler, R.G., and Strode, W.S.: Radioisotope renography. Amer. J. Roentgen., 88:311, 1962.

47. Nordyke, R.A., Gilbert, F.I., and Simmons, E.L.: Screening for kidney disease with radioisotopes. J.A.M.A., 208:493, 1969.

48. Sharpe, A.R., Magee, J.H., and Richardson, D.W.: Unilateral renal disease and hypertension. Arch. Int. Med., 118:546–1966.

49. Sheehan, H.L., and Davis, J.C.: Complete permanent renal ischemia. J. Path. Bact., 76:569, 1958.
50. Sheehan, H.L., and Davis, J.C.: Patchy permanent renal ischemia. J. Path. Bact., 77:33, 1959.
51. Stamey, T.A., Nudelman, I.J., and Good, P.H., et al.: Functional characteristics of renovascular hypertension. Medicine (Balt.), 40:347, 1961.
52. Taplin, G., Dore, E., and Johnson, D.: The quantitative radiorenogram for total and differential renal blood flow measurements. J. Nucl. Med., 4:404, 1963.
53. Wax, S.H., and McDonald, D.F.: A quantitative analysis of the I-131 sodium o-iodohippurate renogram in hypertensive patients. J. Urol., 92:409, 1964.
54. Wedeen, R.P., Littman, E., Levitt, M.D., and Goldstein, M.H.: The use of the I-131 Hippuran renogram in the detection of disparate kidney function in hypertensive patients. Circulation, 32:5, 1965.
55. Reference deleted.

Transplantation

56. Figueroa, J.E., Maxfield, W.S., and Batson, H.M., et al.: Radioisotope renal function studies in human renal allografts: Value in the differential diagnosis of oliguria in the presence of obstructive disease with and without urinary extravasation. J. Urol., 100:104, 1968.
57. Loken, M.K., Staab, E.V., and Vernier, R.L., et al.: Radioisotope renogram in kidney transplants. J. Nucl. Med., 5:807, 1964.
58. Morley, J.E., and Schlegel, J.U.: Radiohippuran accumulation in the transplanted kidney as a signal of rejection. Surgery, 58:815, 1965.
59. Sharpe, A.R., King, E.R., and Hume, D.M., et al.: Sequential response of the iodine-131 Hippuran renogram in renal homotransplantation. J. Nucl. Med., 7:556, 1966.
60. Staab, E.V., Kelly, W.D., and Loken, M.K.: Prognostic value of radioisotope renograms in kidney transplantation. J. Nucl. Med., 10:133, 1969.

Renal Imaging

61. Allen, T.D., and Riley, F.W.: The renal scan: a clinical evaluation of its ability to localize functioning renal tissue. J. Urol., 90:617, 1963.
61a. Baum, S., Vincent, N.R., Lyons, K.P., et al.: Atlas of Nuclear Medicine Imaging, pp. 385–442. New York, Appleton-Century-Crofts, 1979.
62. Baum, S., Rabinowitz, P., and Malloy, W.A.: The renal scan as an aid in percutaneous renal biopsy. J.A.M.A., 195:913, 1966.
62a. Bell, E.G., and Blaufox, M.D.: Clinical applications of renal imaging. In Gottschalk, A., Potchen, E.J. (eds.): Diagnostic Nuclear Medicine, pp. 464–475. Baltimore, Williams and Wilkins, 1976.
63. Blaufox, M.D., Gruskin, A., and Sandler, P., et al.: Radionuclide scintigraphy for detection of vesicoureteral reflux in children. J. Pediatr., 79:239, 1971.
64. Conway, J.J., King, L.R., and Belman, A.B., et al.: Detection of vesicoureteral reflux with radionuclide cystography. A comparison study with roentgenographic cystography. Am. J. Roentgenol., 115:720, 1972.

65. Eckleman, W.C., Meinken, G., and Richards, P.: The chemical state of ^{99m}Tc in biomedical products. II. The chelation of reduced technetium with DTPA. J. Nucl. Med., 13:577, 1972.
66. Forland, M., Gottschalk, A., and Spargo, B., et al.: Renal localization for percutaneous biopsy by scanning with technetium 99m iron complex. Pediatrics, 39:872, 1967.
66a. Freeman, L.M.: The kidney. In Freeman, L.M., Johnson, P.M. (eds.): Clinical Scintillation Imaging, pp. 325–403. New York, Grune and Stratton, 1975.
67. Freedman, G.S., Treves, S., and Lange, T.C., et al.: Renal transplant evaluation using technetium-DTPA, a gamma camera, and a small computer. J. Nucl. Med., 11:320, 1970.
68. Freeman, L.M., Goldman, S.M., and Shaw, R.K., et al.: Kidney visualization with ^{131}I-o-iodohippurate in patients with renal insufficiency. J. Nucl. Med., 10:545, 1969.
69. Gottschalk, A.: Renal scanning. J.A.M.A., 202:221, 1967.
70. Handmaker, H., McRae, J., and Buck, E.G.: Intravenous radionuclide voiding cystography (IRVC). Radiology, 108:703, 1973.
71. Harper, P.V., Lathrop, K.A., and Hinn, G.M., et al.: Technetium-99m-iron complex. In Radioactive Pharmaceuticals. Andrews, G.A., Kniseley, R.M., Wagner, H.N. (eds.): USAEC Symposium Series CONF-651111, 1966, pp. 347–358.
71a. Hattner, R.S., Maltz, H.E., and Holliday, M.A.: Differentiation of reversible ischemia from end-stage renal failure in nephrotic children with ^{131}I-Hippurate dynamic scintigraphy. J. Nucl. Med., 18:438, 1977.
72. Hauser, W., Atkins, H.L., and Richards, P.: Renal uptake of ^{99m}Tc-iron-ascorbic acid complex in man. Radiology, 101:637, 1971.
72a. Hilson, A.J.W., Maisey, M.N., and Brown, C.B., et al.: Dynamic renal transplant imaging with Tc-99m DTPA (Sn) supplemented by a transplant perfusion index in the management of renal transplants. J. Nucl. Med., 19:994, 1978.
73. Hosain, F., Reba, R.C., and Wagner, H.N., Jr.: Visualization of renal structure and function with chelated radionuclides. Radiology, 93:1135, 1969.
73a. Kawamura, J., Hosokawa, S., and Yoshida, O.: Renal function studies using ^{99m}Tc-dimercaptosuccinic acid. Clin. Nucl. Med., 4:39, 1979.
73b. Koff, S.A., Thrall, J.H., and Keyes, J.W. Jr.: Assessment of hydroureteronephrosis in children using diuretic radionuclide urography. J. Urol., 123:531–534, 1980.
74. McAfee, J.G., and Wagner, H.N., Jr.: Visualization of renal parenchyma by scintiscanning with Hg^{203} Neohydrin. Radiology, 75:820, 1961.
75. McVicar, M., Nicastri, A.D., and Gauthier, B.: Improved renal biopsy technique in children. N.Y. State J. Med., 74:830, 1974.
76. Park, C.H., Glassman, L.M., and Thompson, N.L.: Reliability of renal imaging obtained incidentally in ^{99m}Tc-polyphosphate bone scanning. J. Nucl. Med., 14:534, 1973.
77. Reba, R.C., Poulose, K.P., and Kirchner, P.T.: Radiolabeled chelates for visualization of renal function and structure with emphasis on their use in renal insufficiency. Semin. Nucl. Med., 4:151, 1974.
78. Rosenthall, L.: Ortho-iodohippurate-I^{131} kidney scanning in renal failure. Radiology, 78:298, 1966.
79. Rosenthall, L.: Radionuclide diagnosis of malignant tumors of the kidney. Am. J. Roentgenol., 101:662, 1967.
79a. Shimshak, R.R., Hattner, R.S., and Tucker, C., et al.: Segmental acute tubular necrosis in kidneys with multiple renal

arteries transplanted from living related donors. J. Nucl. Med., *18*:1074, 1977.

80. Staab, E.V., Whittier, F., and Patton, D.D.: Early evaluation of cadaver renal allotransplant by means of radionuclide imaging. Radiology, *106*:147, 1973.

81. Tauxe, W.N.: Renal scanning. *In* Blahd, W.H. (ed.): Nuclear Medicine. New York, McGraw-Hill, 1971, pp. 402–415.

82. Tully, R.J., Stark, V.J., Hoffer, P.B., et al.: Renal scan prior to biopsy—a method of renal localization. J. Nucl. Med., *13*:544, 1972.

83. Wagner, H.N., Jr., Reba, R.C., and Goodwin, D.A.: The kidney. *In* Wagner, H.N., Jr. (ed.): Principles of Nuclear Medicine. Philadelphia, Saunders, 1968, pp. 628–654.

84. Weiss, E.R., Blahd, W.H., and Winston, M.A., et al.: Scintillation camera in the evaluation of renal transplants. J. Nucl. Med., *11*:69, 1970.

85. Winston, M.A., Halpern, S.E., Weiss, E.R., et al.: A critical evaluation of ^{99m}Tc-Fe-ascorbic acid complex as a renal scanning agent. J. Nucl. Med., *12*:171, 1971.

86. Zimacek, J., Mydlik, M., and Pokorna, I., et al.: Lokalisationsszintigraphie für die perkutane Nierenbiopsie. Nuclearmedezin, *9*:317, 1970.

87. Zum Winkel, K., Harbst, H., and Schenck, P., et al.: Sequential scintigraphy in renal transplantation. *In* Medical Radioisotope Scintigraphy. vol. 2, pp. 197–208. Vienna, IAEA, 1969.

Ultrasonography (sonography, echography) is the visualization of anatomy by ultrasound. Applied to the genitourinary system, it is a means for imaging the kidney, bladder, prostate, and their related abnormalities. It gives an accurate estimate of the size, shape, location, and internal morphology of these organs. A principal advantage of ultrasonography is its completely nontraumatic and risk-free nature. This has led to its rapid acceptance by patients and to its early utilization in their diagnostic evaluation. As a consequence, in recent years, it has become a valuable and frequently used method of examination for urologic diagnosis.

PRINCIPLES

Ultrasonography utilizes the echo-ranging principle in a manner similar to sonar.[1] A short pulse of high-frequency (2 mHz.) mechanical vibratory waves is transmitted into the tissue from a crystal transducer. The ultrasonic waves are reflected at planes or interfaces where they pass from one type of tissue to another. When the reflecting surface is perpendicular, or nearly perpendicular, to the original sound beam, the echoes return to the transducer and are recorded. Their velocity through the tissue is for practical purposes constant. Therefore, measurement of the arrival time of the echo after the initial pulse allows simple calculation of the depth of the echo source. The echo source may then be represented by a signal, a small dot, on an oscilloscope or television screen. By integrating many echo signals recorded from a variety of positions and directions, an image of the acoustic anatomy is created. This image is a two-dimensional, cross-sectional image, unlike the projection or shadow image of the radiography. It is an *en face* view of the anatomy as if it had been sectioned through the scanning plane. It is

45

Ultrasonography in the Genitourinary System

Donald L. King

analogous with slicing a loaf of bread and viewing the cut surface of the loaf at the slice.

The ultrasonogram depicts the interaction of the ultrasonic waves with the tissue. If the tissue transmitting the ultrasound is homogeneous, such as cyst fluid, no echoes are produced and the image shows an echo-free (anechoic, sonolucent) region. Blood is homogeneous, but it has structure—the red blood cells. Nevertheless, it also appears anechoic in the image because the cells are small compared with the wave length of the ultrasound (0.75 mm.). Tissue debris within an abscess may be sufficiently large to produce some echoes. If there is layering of the debris below clear fluid in the abscess, the interface between the layers may be seen in addition to echoes from the debris. A similar situation may occur with organized thrombus and fresh blood. When a surface or tissue structure is large compared with the length of the ultrasonic wave, and where there is a mismatch of the acoustic properties of the tissue, an echo is produced. The surface between cyst fluid and the cyst wall is such an interface. The greater the acoustic mismatch, the greater is the strength of the echo from the interface. Thus, most solid masses containing either vessels, septa, or areas of hemorrhage or necrosis will have many internal echoes on the ultrasonogram. Simple cysts or hydronephrotic sacs will appear echo-free. Within this framework there are interpretative pitfalls. A tumor may undergo such extensive liquefaction as to appear echo-free. Similarly, a solid tumor of completely homogeneous cellular structure may not produce any echoes and therefore may appear "cystic." The existence of these rarely encountered diagnostic pitfalls does not, however, decrease the general usefulness of ultrasonography any more than the avascular neoplasm affects the usefulness of angiography. The ultrasonogram consistently and accurately depicts the underlying acoustic anatomy.

BIOLOGIC EFFECTS

The possibility of biologic effects of diagnostic ultrasound is a matter of continuing concern.[2-4] Despite numerous clinical and laboratory studies, it has been impossible to substantiate any evidence of harmful effects of diagnostic ultrasound. Accumulating evidence, although not yet defining either thresholds for injury or mechanism of action, suggests that there is a large safety margin for current diagnostic ultrasound techniques.

TECHNIQUE

The kidney is examined with a contact scanner (B scanner). A transducer 10 to 20 mm. in diameter, producing ultrasound at 2 mHz., is used. Instrument amplification characteristics must be individually determined using interval standards, such as the bladder, uterus, known cysts, and the fine speckling of normal renal parenchyma. The kidneys are usually examined with the patient in the prone position, although the decubitus positions are sometimes useful to visualize the left kidney through the spleen and the right kidney through the liver. The right kidney may also be imaged in the supine position through the right lobe of the liver. When the patient is in the prone position, the posterior ribs and the lower lung may impede the passage of the ultrasonic waves and in some instances make visualization of the upper pole and adrenal region difficult or impossible. When pathologic enlargement of the adrenal is present, a successful examination is usually obtained. When the kidney is enlarged, as it is in severe hydronephrotic or polycystic disease or as frequently occurs with pediatric tumors, visualization in the supine position is more advantageous. Serial cross sections at 0.5- to 1.0-cm. intervals are made, depending upon the size of the kidney and the pathologic condition to be visualized. The plane of the serial cross sections is in two standard directions, one transverse or horizontal and the other oblique longitudinal, parallel to the long axis of the kidney. Both sets of parallel cross sections should be made routinely to ensure visualization of any structural abnormality. A significant degree of skill is required for manipulating the scanning transducer. A permanent record of the images is made by a suitable photographic system.

The distended bladder may be visualized by serial scanning over the lower anterior abdomen. Intravesical and intrarectal ultrasonic scanners for visualizing the bladder and prostate have been constructed, but they have not yet come into general use.

INDICATIONS

Ultrasonic imaging of the kidney and adjacent structures may be indicated whenever there is clinical suspicion of disease or abnormality in the region.[5] A renal mass is most frequently discovered on a urogram. Ultrasonic examination may then be used to determine the nature of the mass and to indicate which additional procedure, if any, should be utilized. Patients presenting with abdominal masses should also undergo ultrasonography. The ultrasonic examination will, in most instances, reveal not only the size, shape, location, and internal morphology of the mass but also its site of origin and a probable diagnosis. In general, the ultrasonogram should not be used as a screening procedure, because the urogram is more efficient for that purpose. Also, it is not valuable for determining renal function or evaluating renal parenchymal disease aside from detecting gross changes in renal size. It should always be considered complementary to other imaging procedures and should always be interpreted within the context of the information available from the urogram. When the use of x-rays is contraindicated, as in pregnancy, allergy to contrast agents, and poor renal function, the ultrasonogram must, of course, be performed and interpreted independently.

Ultrasonography is also of value for determining the size or volume of the kidney or bladder. In the patient with a kidney that is not visualized by roentgenography, the ultrasonogram can play an important role by enabling one to distinguish quickly an atrophic kidney from a hydronephrotic one or from a tumor. Similarly, in the infant with a nonfunctioning kidney, agenesis or hypoplasia of the kidney may be distinguished from tumor or hydronephrosis. Volume calculation of the renal transplant is also a valuable application. Serial cross sections of the bladder may be used to determine its volume for assessment of urinary output and postvoiding residual.[6] Localization of the kidney by ultrasound is of value for guidance in renal cyst aspiration,[7] biopsy,[8] and placement of radiotherapy portals.[9]

NORMAL KIDNEY

The two-dimensional appearance of the kidney in ultrasonic cross-sectional representation is not dissimilar from its appearance by x-ray projection. In a cross section through its long axis (Fig. 45–1), the outline of the kidney is oval. Its margins are demarcated by echoes arising from surrounding tissues and from the interface between the renal cortex and perirenal fat. The cortical parenchyma appears relatively echo-free, showing only a few weak signals scattered from smaller vessels. Located centrally within the kidney is an oval collection of echoes, referred to as the central or medullary echoes. These

arise from the medullary structures, the collecting systems, arteries, and veins. In transverse cross section (Fig. 45–2), the relatively echo-free cortex is seen surrounding the central echoes. The latter are anteromedially placed at the hilum of the kidney. Enlargement of the normal outline, displacement of the medullary echoes, or the appearance of atypical echoes in the renal cortex indicates the existence of pathologic alteration of the kidney. In the normal person, neither the renal pelvis nor the ureter is usually seen, although an unusually full renal pelvis may appear as an oval "cystic" structure. The normal adrenal gland is usually not distinguishable from the kidney or surrounding tissues.

RENAL MASSES

Evaluation of renal masses is the most frequent application of ultrasound for urologic diagnosis.[10-12] Commonly these masses are incidental findings on a urogram obtained for evaluation of other problems. Utilization of the ultrasonogram allows categorization of the mass on the basis of its internal morphology as either a simple cystic mass or one with internal structure (a complex or solid mass). In the author's experience, a sonogram has proved to be a more sensitive means for diagnosing a renal cyst than a nephrotomogram.[13] For this reason the ultrasonogram should precede other radiographic procedures and should be utilized in selecting the next most appropriate examination, if any. It should be emphasized that the ultrasonographic evaluation of a mass should be carried out with the excretory urogram available for comparison. Any discrepancy between the two relating to the size, shape, or location of a mass should lead to further evaluation, as should the presence of internal structure within a mass.

A mass within or arising from the kidney may be revealed by an enlargement of the normal renal outline, by displacement of the medullary echoes, and by the appearance of additional echoes not normally present, particularly in the region of the cortex. Small masses, 2 to 3 cm. or less in diameter, significantly decrease the reliability of ultrasound diagnosis because of the limitation of resolution of the ultrasonic beam, image unsharpness due to respiratory motion, and the relative homogeneity of small solid lesions. Larger masses should be evaluated in terms of size, shape, contour, internal morphology, and attenuation characteristics.[14]

SIMPLE CYSTS

Simple cystic masses are round or oval; they are smooth-walled and correspond in size to that seen on the urogram (Fig. 45–3). The contours are smooth, regular, and sharply defined. The walls, when perpendicular to the sound beam, produce strong echoes because of the high impedance mismatch between the cyst fluid and adjacent tissue or parenchyma. Between the walls, within the cyst, there are no echoes. A simple cyst appears echo-free or sonolucent. Cysts are occasionally much larger than is apparent from the urogram (Fig. 45–3C). Caution should be exercised not to mistake reverberations appearing within the cyst for echoes from internal structure (Fig. 45–4). Reverberations are the result of multiple round trips of the sound waves in the tissues between the transducer and the near cyst wall. They appear in uniform steps at depths representing multiples of their original pathway. The presence of multiple pathways frequently produces a nonuniform pattern of reverberation. They are visible at excessive gain levels in cystic masses but are not seen in solid masses due to attenuation. They may be recognized by their perpendicular orientation to the skin and cyst wall and by their disappearance with slight angulation of the sound beam. True internal structural echoes persist with changes of beam direction, and they are usually of greater amplitude.

Echo-free cyst fluid is an excellent transmitter of sound waves; lacking structure, it does not attenuate them as much as solid tissue does. Consequently, echoes from beyond a cyst are much stronger than echoes from beyond a solid mass of corresponding size (enhancement). This is an indication of low attenuation or nonshadowing of the sound beam and is characteristic of but not specific for a cyst (Fig. 45–5 A). Evaluation of the strength of the far-wall echoes is a subjective determination and not easily quantified. It is aided only in part by the use of a gray-scale display. Nonuniform scanning and improper use of amplification can significantly alter the usual appearance of the far-wall echoes. Familiarity with scanning technique, amplifier operation, and the appearance of known internal standards is the best means for avoiding errors of interpretation. Simultaneous utilization of an A-mode display with the cross-sectioned B-mode image (Fig. 45–5 B) is also recommended for evaluation of the presence of internal echoes and the strength of far-wall echoes.[15] Cysts also frequently produce a characteristic displacement and compression of the medullary echoes and renal cortex (Fig.

45–6). The central echoes form a crescentic pattern, and the cortex is thinned into an acute angle at its junction with the cyst.

OTHER ENTITIES

A number of pathologic entities might be or have been mistaken for simple cysts of the kidney. However, this type of error is infrequent, and the vast majority of masses fulfilling all the criteria of a simple cyst are indeed just that. On occasion a full or mildly dilated intrarenal pelvis might be mistaken for a cyst (Fig. 45–7). The lateral margins of the pelvis produced by the medullary echoes form a characteristic "C-shape" opening anteromedially. This appearance, its location, and the frequent demonstration of its anteromedial continuation toward the ureter should suggest the proper diagnosis. An intrarenal aneurysm of the renal artery (Fig. 45–8) also appears cystic. If this possibility is anticipated, the correct preangiogram diagnosis might be suggested by detecting the pulsatile movement of the near and far walls of the aneurysm. The occurrence of such lesions, though rare, should discourage the indiscriminate use of percutaneous needle aspiration of cysts. Renal abscess and hematoma may produce an echo-free appearance resembling a simple cyst. Usually the margin of an abscess is irregular, and it may show evidence of internal echoes (Fig. 45–9 A, B). Accumulation of debris within an abscess may produce a fluid–fluid level that is apparent ultrasonically (Fig. 45–9 C). A hematoma, although echo-free before organization, usually has an irregular shape rather than a round or oval one, which precludes diagnosis as a simple cyst (Fig. 45–10 A, B).

Cystic masses of nonrenal origin, such as a retroperitoneal hematoma (Fig. 45–10, C, D), may lie adjacent to the kidney and not be separable from it. The medial portion of the spleen, a relatively echo-free organ, may be mistaken for a renal cyst by the inexperienced examiner. Cysts of the adrenal gland (Fig. 45–11) appear similar to upper-pole cysts lying in the same location. Pancreatic pseudocysts lying anterior to the kidney may be indistinguishable from and mistaken for renal cysts. An end-stage hydronephrotic sac in which all parenchymal and vascular structure has been destroyed will also resemble a large renal cyst. The absence of compressed medullary echoes and parenchyma adjacent to it will suggest the correct diagnosis. Rarely a primary malignant renal tumor appears "cystic," or echo free with strong far-wall echoes (Fig. 45–12). This may occur if there has been necrotic liquefaction of the tumor with loss of structure that might otherwise have produced internal echoes. Its margins, however, usually show some irregularity or lack of sharpness, which in conjunction with the clinical history and appearance in the urogram, should suggest the correct diagnosis. Metastatic lesions (Fig. 45-13 A, B) particularly when small, may also have a homogeneous echo-free appearance due to their cellular uniformity.

Masses involving the kidney, produced by lymphomas, sarcoma, and some neurogenic tumors, may also be confused with cystic lesions if caution is not exercised. If the walls of a mass are not smooth and sharp, if there are projections, irregularities, or septa extending into the mass, if the echo-free space does not appear as large as expected, or if there is more attenuation of the sound beam than expected, the mass should not be diagnosed as a simple cyst. To assure detection of any of these qualifying characteristics, complete sets of parallel cross sections in perpendicular directions must be obtained. If the mass then does not fulfill the criteria for a simple cyst, it may be categorized as a specific pattern, such as hydronephrosis or polycystic disease, or it may be categorized nonspecifically as a complex or solid mass lesion.

SOLID MASSES

Solid masses of the kidney ultrasonically show a rather uniform distribution of echoes throughout the volume of the mass (Fig. 45-14 A, B). These echoes arise from acoustic discontinuities in the tissues comprising the mass, such as vessels, fibrous septa, and areas of hemorrhage and necrosis. The appearance is, however, not specific, and the histologic nature of the solid mass cannot be predicted from its ultrasonic appearance.[16] Most frequently, the homogeneous solid appearance is produced by a renal carcinoma (Fig. 45-15) or a Wilms' tumor (Fig. 45-16 A, B). The mass almost invariably enlarges the renal outline and displaces, distorts, or replaces the normal medullary echo pattern. The margins of the mass are usually indistinct and irregular. If inadequate echo amplification is used, weak internal echoes from a solid mass might be overlooked.[17] Nevertheless, in such a situation, strong far-wall echoes would not be present, which suggests that the mass is solid. A solid renal mass is not necessarily malignant, because such benign lesions as a hamartoma also produce internal echoes.

Solid masses may not show a homogeneous, diffuse internal echo pattern, although they are either benign or malignant tumors. The echo pattern may be complex; that is, it may suggest a mixture of echo-free areas interspersed between echo-producing structures. In such complex patterns, the echo-free areas may represent either regions of homogeneous fluid or homogeneous cellular structure within solid tissue or the walls of cystic structures. Almost all masses showing this nonspecific complex pattern are some variant of a solid mass that deserves further evaluation by angiography or biopsy, whichever is appropriate. Hypernephromas may have large volumes of uniformly homogeneous cellular tissue with only a few peripheral internal echoes (Fig. 45-17). Metastatic tumors may show a similar complex appearance, as may benign tumors. Multiple cysts, polycystic kidney, and varying stages of hydronephrosis may appear as complex patterns, although in many instances these can be specifically identified.

HYDRONEPHROSIS

Mild and moderate degrees of hydronephrosis (Fig. 45-18) usually do not present a diagnostic problem, because they are adequately visualized on the urogram and seldom present for ultrasonography. Severe, nonfunctioning hydronephrosis presents for ultrasonography because of nonfunction or as a palpable abdominal mass. When hydronephrosis has reached the nonfunctioning stage, the renal outline is enlarged and the central medullary echoes are distorted. The dilated calyces have become large hydronephrotic sacs separated by septa of compressed tissue and vessels (Fig. 45-19). With increasing duration and severity, the septa may disappear, leaving a large fluid-filled sac. This progression of hydronephrosis from mild to severe presents a spectrum of ultrasonographic appearances.[18] At the nonfunctioning stage, the fluid-filled sacs vary in size and are usually fewer in number than those in a multicystic or polycystic kidney. The septa separating the echo-free regions in hydronephrosis are fewer, thicker, and longer than the septa between cysts in a multicystic kidney. The end-stage of the hydronephrotic spectrum consists of a huge, fluid-filled sac with no evidence of internal structure and no normal parenchyma apparent at its margins (Fig. 45-20). Differentiation from other causes of large cystic abdominal masses, such as pancreatic pseudocyst, can be made on clinical grounds and by visualizing a normal adjacent renal ultrasonogram. A noticeably dilated ureter may also be visualized if care is taken to make appropriate scans.

POLYCYSTIC DISEASE

Polycystic and multicystic kidney disease may be detected and diagnosed by ultrasonography in many instances. They may, however, present as diverse a spectrum of appearances as hydronephrosis. In some instances in which the cystic disease is microscopic or millimetric in size, the enlarged portion of the kidney may appear to be a solid mass. At the other extreme, some large multicystic kidneys may be difficult to differentiate from hydronephrosis (Fig. 45–21). In the more typical polycystic kidney (Fig. 45–22), the ultrasonographic appearance is sufficiently characteristic to allow an accurate diagnosis. The renal outline is enlarged, and the central grouping of medullary echoes is absent. Many cystic, echo-free areas of varying sizes are seen separated by a lattice-work of septa. The cystic areas of polycystic disease are generally more numerous than the sacs of hydronephrosis and show greater variation in size. The septa in polycystic disease appear more irregular and disorganized than the smoother, longer septa seen in hydronephrosis. In addition, bilaterality of the cystic pattern and its appearances in the liver firmly establish the diagnosis of polycystic disease. Multicystic disease (Fig. 45–23) may be difficult to distinguish from polycystic disease. In some instances, localized involvement of only a portion of a kidney may suggest the former.

RENAL TRANSPLANT

Ultrasonography is a valuable adjunct to the clinical evaluation of renal transplants.[19] The location of the transplant superficially in the pelvis permits easy and frequent imaging by ultrasound (Fig. 45–24). The innocuous nature of ultrasound is also a major advantage over the hazards and radiation exposure of urography, angiography, and catheterization for evaluation of the transplant. It is not only useful for detection of complications of transplantation but also for assessing long-term changes in the transplant size or volume.

Perirenal collections such as lymphocele (Fig. 45–25), hematoma, urinoma, or abscess (Fig. 45–26) are easily visualized as echo-free spaces adjacent to the kidney. They may vary in size, shape, and configuration. Because they all may be echo free, distinction among them may not be possible. Obstruction of the transplant and consequent hydronephrosis may also be detected ultrasonically. These changes are essentially the same as those occurring in the normally positioned kidney. The pelvis initially shows dilata-tion into a "C shape." Enlargement of the infundibula and calyces produces a "ring" appearance of mild hydronephrosis when seen in cross section. Progressive obstruction shows further enlargement of the echo-free spaces about the hilum of the kidney.

The volume of the transplant kidney may be determined by integrating the planimetered areas of the kidney on a series of parallel cross sections.[20] Repeated examinations following transplantation allow sufficiently precise assessment of renal volume to evaluate hypertrophy and rejection of the transplant.[21] In the usual case the transplant undergoes a gradual increase in volume over the first 6 months, and it then may slightly decrease in size. Observation of failure to undergo this increase in size has been of value in judging the chances of success of the transplant.[19] A gradual decrease in volume of the kidney has suggested chronic rejection, whereas a sudden increase in size has occurred several weeks before acute rejection became apparent clinically.

ADRENAL GLAND

With present imaging techniques, the normal adrenal gland is not usually visualized. Its small size and its anatomic location under the lower ribs contribute to this limitation. The lower lung frequently is interposed between the back and the adrenal, making visualization impossible. A tumor (Fig. 45–27) or cyst of the adrenal (see Fig. 45–11) occasionally becomes large and is visualized at the upper pole of the kidney. Generally, however, its adrenal rather than renal origin cannot be reliably determined by ultrasonography, and this distinction must be made by radiographic techniques. The size and internal morphology of such a mass will, however, be apparent and will aid in patient management.

BLADDER AND PROSTATE

The urinary bladder is frequently and easily visualized by ultrasound (Fig. 45–28), but ultrasonography is rarely utilized on a clinical basis for evaluation of bladder lesions. Tumors projecting into the bladder lumen may be visualized by noninvasive contact scanning (Fig. 45–29); however, this technique adds little to the patient's management. Mural and invasive lesions cannot yet be adequately evaluated by contact scanning. Intravesical scanning techniques, although still experimental, may in the future permit ultrasonic evaluation of tumor invasion of the bladder wall.[22] In spite of present limitations, highly useful information regarding bladder size, shape, compliance, contractility, and volume can be more easily obtained by ultrasonography than by any other technique. Serial parallel cross sections of the bladder may be used to determine bladder volume accurately.[23] This technique does not require mathematical assumption of bladder shape. The area of the bladder on each cross section is measured by planimeter, and all sections are integrated to determine volume. Variations and irregularities of contour and shape do not affect the accuracy of the result. Ultrasonic determination of bladder volume is useful for assessment of bladder distensibility and contractility, postvoiding residual (Fig. 45–30), and urinary output. The latter determination is of course especially valuable in the management of oliguria or transplant patients in whom catheterization is undesirable.

In some patients the prostate may be visualized by contact scanning. However, this is not currently of clinical value. Transrectal scanners for imaging the prostate have been developed.[24] These allow assessment of prostatic volume,[25] hypertrophy, tumor irregularity, and invasiveness. Future developments of this technique may result in improved diagnostic evaluation of the prostate.

CHAPTER 45, ILLUSTRATIONS

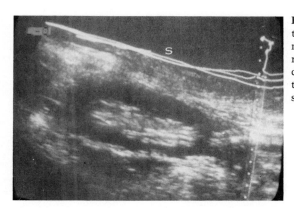

FIG. 45–1. Long-axis cross section of a normal kidney in the prone position. Within the oval outline of the kidney the cortex appears relatively echo-free and surrounds the central echoes arising from the vessels and collecting system. Upper pole is to the left, lower pole is to the right. S = skin surface of the back. Dots = 1-cm. scale.

FIG. 45–2. (A) Normal transverse cross section of the kidneys in the prone position. The central echoes appear in an anteromedial location. R = right. V = vertebra. SP = posterior spinous process. **(B)** Normal transverse cross section of the right kidney (arrow) of person in the supine position through the right lobe of the liver. The renal vessels, as shown here, may occasionally be visualized. L = liver, V = vertebra, A = aorta, S = skin, R = right. (Green, W.M., King, D.L., J. Clin. Ultrasound., 4:55, 1976)

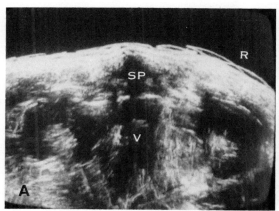 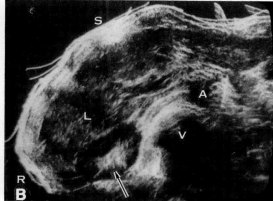

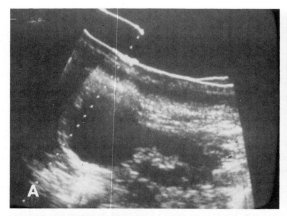

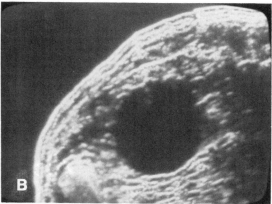

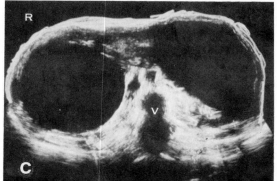

FIG. 45–3. Simple cyst. **(A)** Longitudinal cross section of a 6 cm. upper pole cyst. **(B)** Transverse cross section of another cyst. Cysts are round or oval, have smooth margins, and show no evidence of internal structure. **(C)** Bilateral massive cysts. Supine transverse cross section reveals two massive renal cysts filling the abdomen. R = right, V = vertebra. The inferior vena cava and aorta can be seen anterior to the vertebra.

FIG. 45–4. Reverberation artifact in a simple cyst. Reverberations of the ultrasonic waves in the tissues between the transducer and the near cyst wall appear as "echoes" within the cyst (*arrows*). These do not persist with variation of the angle of the transducer on the skin.

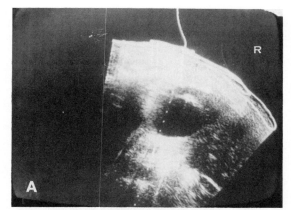

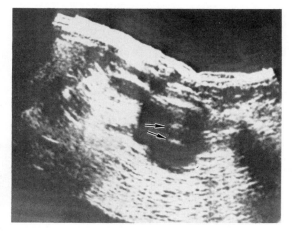

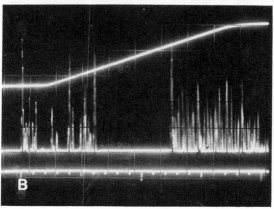

FIG. 45–5. (A) Transverse cross section of a simple cyst showing enhancement of the strength of echoes from beyond the cyst in comparison with echoes at a similar depth beyond solid tissue. The cyst fluid attenuates the echo signals less than solid tissue. R = right. **(B)** A-mode display. The upper sloping line is the amplifier gain display, and the bottom line is the depth scale in centimeters. The middle trace is the A-mode display of the echoes (vertical deflections) when the sound beam is positioned through the center of the cyst. No echoes appear at the depth of the cyst.

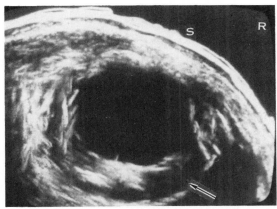

FIG. 45–6. Cyst showing compression of renal parenchyma. This transverse cross section shows the cyst to be lying directly posterior to the kidney and to be compressing the renal parenchyma (*arrow*) as it expands in the available space. R = right, S = skin. (Green, W.M., King, D.L., J. Clin. Ultrasound., *4*:55, 1976)

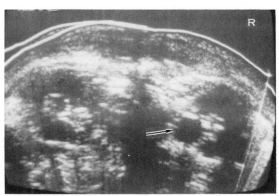

FIG. 45–7. Transverse cross section of normal kidneys. The right renal pelvis is visualized as a cystic mass (*arrow*) anteromedial to the kidney. The pelvis was shown to be normal on retrograde pyelogram in this patient allergic to contrast media.

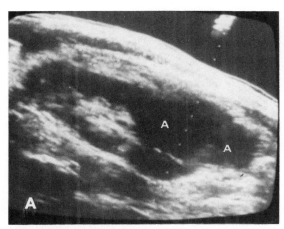

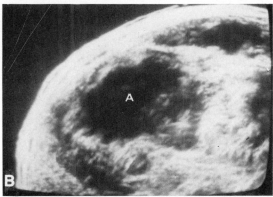

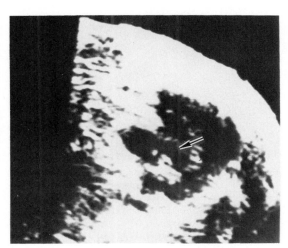

FIG. 45–8. Bilobed aneurysm of the intrarenal artery (*arrow*). At sonography the mass appeared to be a peripelvic cyst. Evidence of pulsatile movement was not sought. Because this young woman presented with hematuria, an arteriogram was performed and revealed the true nature of the lesion. (Green, W.M., King, D.L., and Casarellar, W.J., Radiology, in press)

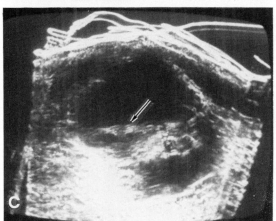

FIG. 45–9. Renal abscess. **(A)** Longitudinal cross section. **(B)** Transverse cross section. This young man presented with signs and symptoms suggesting a left renal abscess. The sonogram revealed a large, irregular, complex cystic mass involving and extending from the posterolateral aspect of the left kidney. The margins are irregular, and faint echoes arise from within its margins. A = abscess. **(C)** Postoperative abscess in the right upper quadrant. Supine cross section shows a fluid/fluid level (*arrow*) due to the accumulation of debris in the dependent portion of the collection. (Green, W.M., King, D.L., and Casarella, W.J., *In* White, D.N., and Barnes, eds., Ultrasound in Medicine. vol. 2. New York, Plenum, 1976)

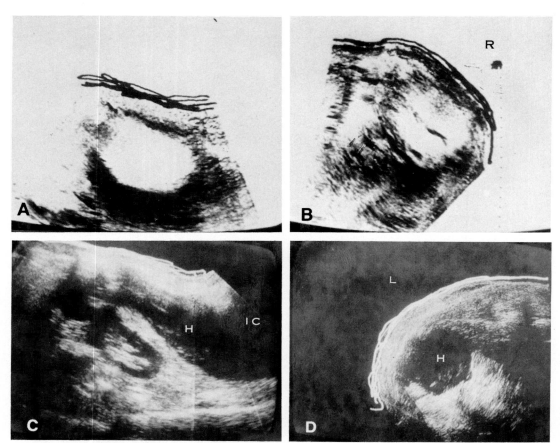

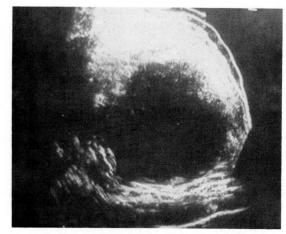

FIG. 45–10. Renal hematoma. (A) Longitudinal cross section of this hematoma appears echo-free. (B) The transverse cross section reveals the junction of the hematoma with the kidney and its irregular shape. (C) Longitudinal cross section of a retroperitoneal hematoma (H) in a triangular configuration above the iliac crest (IC). (D) Transverse cross section of the retroperitoneal hematoma shows it to be rounded with some internal echoes, probably representing thrombus. (Green, W.M., King, D.L., and Casarella, W.J., Radiology, in press.)

FIG. 45–11. Suprarenal cyst. Longitudinal cross section shows a cystic mass (C) at the upper pole of the kidney (K). Frequently differentiation of renal or adrenal origin of such cysts cannot be made. In this case angiography revealed the mass to be totally avascular and did not indicate its origin.

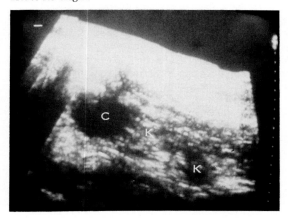

FIG. 45–12. Cystic carcinoma of the kidney. Transverse cross section of a large cystic carcinoma appears echo-free. The posterior margin appeared slightly irregular and not as well demarcated as usual. The tumor had a large, necrotic, hemorrhagic center surrounded by a 5-mm.-thick capsule of tumor tissue.

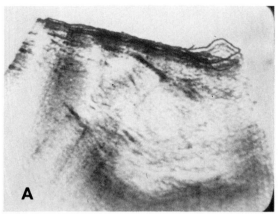

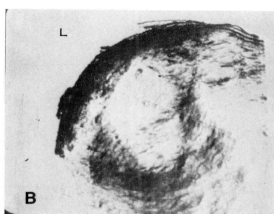

FIG. 45–13. Metastatic endometrial adenocarcinoma. **(A)** Longitudinal. **(B)** Transverse. This large metastatic tumor surrounding the lower pole of the left kidney contained several cystic regions. A differentiation of primary and secondary tumors cannot be made by the ultrasonogram.

FIG. 45–14. Avascular renal carcinoma. **(A)** Transverse cross section through the lower pole mass at high gain showed the mass to be filled with a homogeneous echo pattern. **(B)** Post-epinephrine accessory artery angiogram to the mass shows no evidence of neovascularity. The angiogram suggested that the mass was a cyst. The sonogram accurately predicted the internal morphology of the mass.

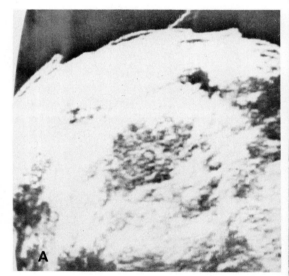

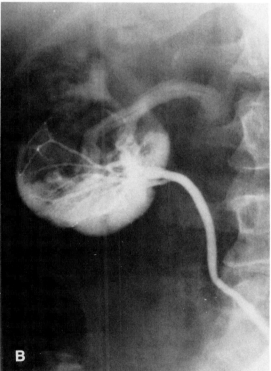

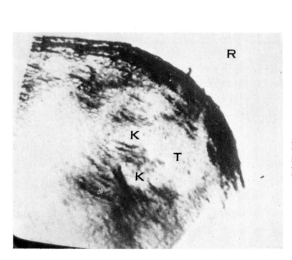

FIG. 45–15. Renal carcinoma. Transverse cross section shows enlargement of the kidney (*K*) laterally and the homogeneous echo pattern of the tumor (*T*).

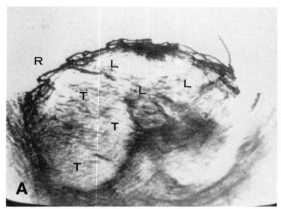

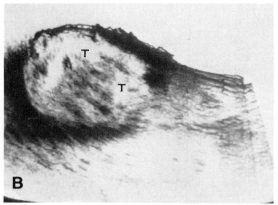

FIG. 45–16. Wilms' tumor. **(A)** Transverse cross section of the upper abdomen in the supine position shows a massive tumor (T) displacing the right lobe of the liver (L) anteromedially. **(B)** Longitudinal cross section at the midportion of the tumor. Many internal echoes are typically found in Wilms' tumors.

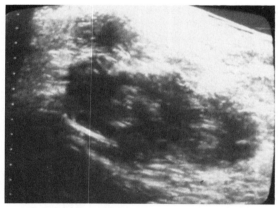

FIG. 45–17. Renal carcinoma. Longitudinal cross section shows loss of the normal central echo pattern and its replacement by the poorly defined outline of an irregular mass. There is a slight enlargement of the kidney anteriorly.

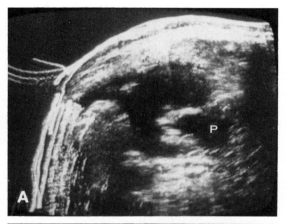

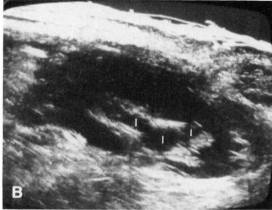

FIG. 45–18. Mild hydronephrosis. **(A)** Transverse cross section showing a mildly dilated renal pelvis (P) extending into the kidney. **(B)** Longitudinal cross section shows dilatation of the infundibula (I). (Green, W.M., and King, D.L.: J. Clin. Ultrasound., 4:55, 1976)

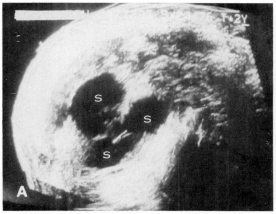
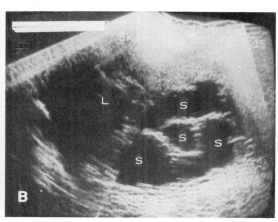

FIG. 45-19. Severe hydronephrosis. (A) Transverse cross section through the upper abdomen shows the large hydronephrotic sacs (S) posterior to the right lobe of the liver. (B) Longitudinal cross section of the same kidney shows the sacs (S) separated by thick septa. L = liver.

FIG. 45-20. Hydronephrotic duplication. (A) Longitudinal cross section through the kidney shows the residual sac of the upper pole duplication (D). The remaining normal kidney is seen to the right. (B) Longitudinal cross section just medial to that in A shows the communication between the nonfunctioning hydronephrotic duplication (D) and its dilated ureter (U).

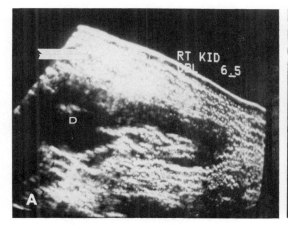
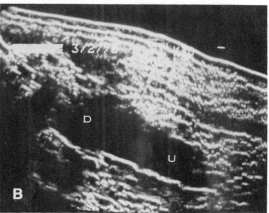

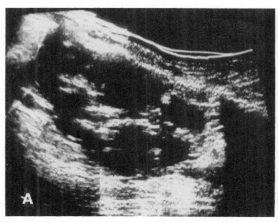
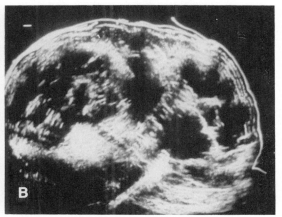

FIG. 45-21. Polycystic kidney. (A) Longitudinal cross section of an advanced polycystic kidney that resembles the appearance of hydronephrosis. (B) Transverse cross section of the same patient reveals bilaterality of the process and more variation in cyst size, suggesting the correct diagnosis.

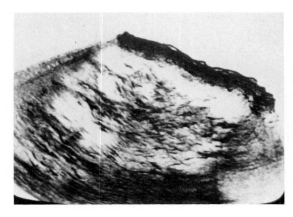

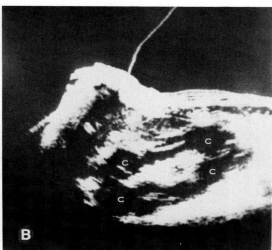

FIG. 45–22. Polycystic kidney. Longitudinal cross section of this kidney shows great variation of cyst size. In some cases, only a portion of the kidney may be involved, producing an ultrasonic appearance that may suggest the presence of a tumor. (Green, W.M., and King, D.L.: J. Clin. Ultrasound., *4*:55, 1976)

FIG. 45–23. Multicystic kidney. **(A)** Transverse cross section of the upper abdomen showing the liver and multiple cysts (*C*) of the upper pole of a multicystic kidney. **(B)** Longitudinal cross section of the same kidney showing multiple cysts surrounding the central echoes. The left kidney was not involved.

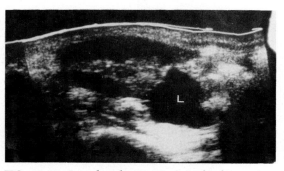

FIG. 45–25. Lymphocele. Postoperatively this patient developed a large lymphocele (*L*) adjacent to the upper pole. Hematomas and urinomas as well as abscesses may produce a similar appearance.

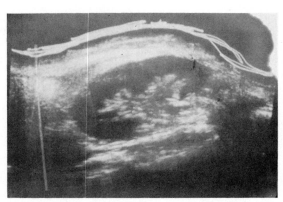

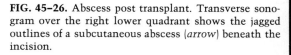

FIG. 45–24. Transplant kidney. The superficial position of the transplant makes possible visualization of papillae, intrarenal collecting system, and vessels as shown in the cross section.

FIG. 45–26. Abscess post transplant. Transverse sonogram over the right lower quadrant shows the jagged outlines of a subcutaneous abscess (*arrow*) beneath the incision.

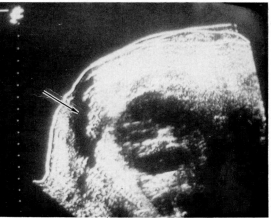

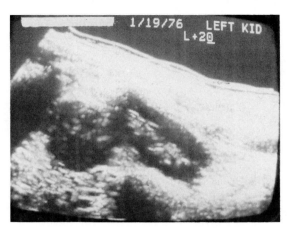

FIG. 45–27. Pheochromocytoma. Longitudinal cross section shows a solid mass adjacent to the upper pole of the kidney. The weak internal echoes of the tumor might not be recorded if amplification of the signals is too low. The mass would then appear cystic except for a relatively weak far-wall echo (lack of enhancement).

FIG. 45–28. Bladder. **(A)** Normal longitudinal cross section. **(B)** Normal transverse cross section. The volume of the bladder (B) may be calculated by planimetry with good clinical accuracy.

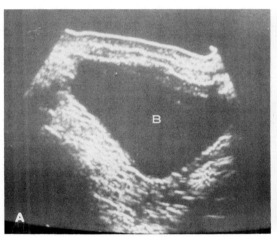
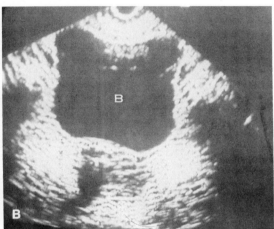

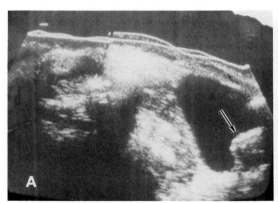
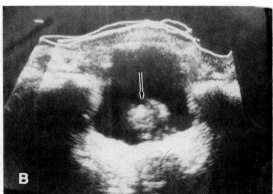

FIG. 45–29. Prostate. An enlarged prostate is shown in longitudinal **(A)** and transverse **(B)** cross section, protruding (*arrow*) into the base of the bladder.

FIG. 45–30. Residual volume. Longitudinal cross section shows an abnormally distended bladder (B) secondary to the pelvic abscess (A) caused by rupture of a sigmoid colon diverticulum. The patient was unable to void over 50 per cent of the bladder volume.

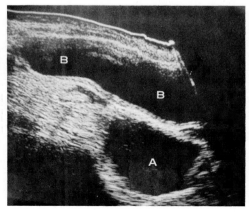

BIBLIOGRAPHY

1. Baker, D.W.: Physical and technical principles. *In* King, D.L. (ed.): Diagnostic Ultrasound. pp. 16–51. St. Louis, C.V. Mosby Co., 1974.
2. King, D.L., and Lele, P.P.: Biologic effects of diagnostic ultrasound. *In* King, D.L. (ed.): Diagnostic Ultrasound. pp. 240–248. St. Louis, C.V. Mosby Co., 1974.
3. Taylor, K.J.W.: Current status of toxicity investigations. J. Clin. Ultrasound, *2*:149, 1974.
4. Patrick, M.K.: Ultrasound in physiotherapy. Ultrasonics, *4*:10, 1966.
5. Green, W.M., and King, D.L.: Diagnostic ultrasound of the urinary tract. J. Clin. Ultrasound, *4*:55, 1976.
6. Holmes, J.H.: Ultrasonic studies of the bladder. J. Urol., *97*:654, 1967.
7. Kristensen, J.K., Holm, H.H., and Rasmussen, S.N., et al.: Ultrasonically guided percutaneous puncture of renal masses. Scand. J. Urol. Nephrol., *6*:49, 1972.
8. Boltan, W.K., Tully, R.J., and Lewis, E.J., et al.: Localization of the kidney for percutaneous biopsy: a comparative study of methods. Ann. Int. Med., *81*:159, 1974.
9. Sanders, R.C., Hughes, B., and Hazra, T.A.: Ultrasound localization of kidneys for radiation therapy. Br. J. Rad., *47*:196, 1974.
10. Barnett, E., and Morley, P.: Ultrasound in the investigation of space-occupying lesions of the urinary tract. Br. J. Rad., *44*:733, 1971.
11. Leopold, G.R., Talver, L.B., and Asher, W.M., et al.: Renal ultrasonography: an updated approach to the diagnosis of renal cysts. Radiology, *109*:671, 1973.
12. Mountford, R.A., Ross, F.G.M., and Burwood, R.J., et al.: The use of ultrasound in the diagnosis of renal disease. Br. J. Rad., *44*:860, 1971.
13. King, D.L.: Renal ultrasonography. An aid in the clinical evaluation of renal masses. Radiology, *105*:633, 1972.
14. Von Micsky, L.I.: Clinical sonography in urology. Urology, *1*:506, 1973.
15. Goldberg, B.B., and Pollack, H.M.: Differentiation of renal masses using A-mode ultrasound. J. Urol., *105*:765, 1971.
16. Kristensen, J.K., Gammelgaard, P.A., Holm, H.H., and Rasmussen, S.N.: Ultrasound in the demonstration of renal masses. Br. J. Urol., *44*:517, 1972.
17. Doust, V.L., Doust, B.D., and Redman, H.C.: Evaluation of ultrasonic B-mode scanning in the diagnosis of renal masses. Am. J. Roentgenol., *117*:112, 1973.
18. Sanders, R.C., and Bearman, S.: B-scan ultrasound in the diagnosis of hydronephrosis. Radiology, *108*:375, 1973.
19. Holmes, J.H.: Urologic ultrasonography. *In* King, D.L. (ed.): Diagnostic Ultrasound. St. Louis, C.V. Mosby Co., 1974.
20. Bartrum, R.J., Smith, E.H., and D'Orsi, C.J., et al.: Ultrasonic determination of renal transplant volume. J. Clin. Ultrasound, *2*:281, 1974.
21. Leopold, G.R.: Renal transplant size measured by reflected ultrasound. Radiology, *95*:687, 1970.
22. Holm, H.H., and Northeved, A.: A transurethral ultrasonic scanner. J. Urol., *111*:238, 1974.
23. Doust, B.D., Baum, J.K., and Maklad, N.F., et al.: Determination of organ volume by means of ultrasonic B-mode scanning. J. Clin. Ultrasound, *2*:127, 1974.
24. Watanabe, H., Igari, D., and Tanahasi, Y., et al.: Development and application of new equipment for trans-rectal ultrasonograph. J. Clin. Ultrasound, *2*:91, 1974.
25. Wittingham, T.A., and Bishop, R.: Ultrasonic estimation of the volume of the enlarged prostate. Br. J. Radiol., *46*:68, 1973.

The diagnosis and management of the patient with genitourinary malignancy is a multidisciplinary approach by the urologist, diagnostic radiologist, pathologist, radiotherapist, and medical oncologist. Management depends in large part upon a thorough assessment of the extent of the neoplastic disease. Lymphangiography is employed in patients with cancer of the testes, bladder, prostate, and penis in the evaluation of the pelvic and para-aortic lymph nodes. Utilizing rigid criteria, the lymphangiogram when positive has an accuracy of 90 to 95 per cent; when the lymphangiogram is considered negative, 15 to 20 per cent of patients prove to have metastatic disease.

The recent use of percutaneous transperitoneal fine-needle aspiration biopsy of a previously opacified lymph node has further enhanced the value of lymphangiography. The diagnostic yield of 80 per cent and the absence of significant complications warrant a more widespread application of aspiration biopsy.

TESTES

Testicular tumors comprise 1 to 2 per cent of all malignant neoplasms in the male and an estimated annual incidence rate of 2 to 3 per 100,000 men. Testicular malignant disease ranks second only to reticuloendothelial malignant neoplasms as a cause of death from cancer in men from 20 to 34 years of age.

Of all neoplasms of the testes, 95 per cent are of germinal origin. Pure seminoma carries the best prognosis, whereas choriocarcinoma has the worst. The presence of teratoma with embryonal carcinoma or choriocarcinoma improves the outlook as compared with these types alone. Pure seminoma usually metastasizes in an orderly manner—first to the lumbar lymph nodes and then to the mediastinal

46

Lymph-angiography and Cancer of the Genitourinary Tract

SIDNEY WALLACE AND
BAO-SHAN JING

and supraclavicular lymph nodes, dependent in part upon the normal lymphatic drainage and the variations in the normal. Hematogenous spread is rare. Embryonal carcinoma and teratocarcinoma usually metastatsize to the retroperitoneal nodes, but hematogenous spread is not uncommon. Nearly all choriocarcinomas show early hematogenous spread.

Testicular lymphatics accompany the internal spermatic artery and vein and drain into the lumbar nodes. The right trunks terminate in the right lumbar glands, which lie between the level of the aortic bifurcation and the renal vein (Fig. 46–1).[25] In 10 per cent these trunks end in a node in the angle between the renal vein and the inferior vena cava. The left testicular lymphatics drain into the para-aortic near the left renal vein in approximately two-thirds of the patients. They may also end in glands at the level of the bifurcation of the aorta or even into the common iliac nodes.

Lymphatics from the epididymis may accompany the testicular lymphatics to the lumbar nodes or terminate in the external iliac nodes.

Clinical investigation utilizing direct testicular or funicular lymphangiography has confirmed Rouviere's findings. They demonstrate testicular lymphatic channels terminating in a sentinel node at the level of L_1–L_2 on the left and L_1–L_3 on the right, slightly lateral to the lumbar nodes usually opacified by pedal lymphangiography. From the right testis there may be direct filling of the right lateral nodes above and below the renal vein or directly to the left lateral nodes. There may be immediate crossover after permeating the sentinel nodes. From the lumbar nodes, continuity of the lymphatics system is usually maintained through the thoracic duct.

Nodal metastases from testicular malignant disease show several different architectural patterns. The single most reliable criterion for the diagnosis of metastatic disease is a defect in a node not traversed by lymphatics (Fig. 46–2). This defect is usually at the periphery; the remaining functioning portion of the node is frequently crescent shaped. The lymphatics leading to the defect are interrupted by the destructive process in the node. A similar configuration may be produced by certain lymphomas, metastatic sarcoma, abscess formation, caseation necrosis, and fibrosis. A node totally replaced by neoplasm is not opacified, although the lymphatics may be distorted or obstructed. Obstruction of these channels may result in visualization of collateral pathways, that is, lymphatic to lymphatic, lymphatic to prelymphatic, and lymphatic to venous.

Nodal metastases from testicular neoplasms occasionally may have an abnormal internal architecture with a relatively intact marginal sinus, most frequently seen in lymphomas. This picture is seen in some seminomas (Fig. 46–3), and rhabdomyosarcomas as well as in lymphomas of the testicle. Therefore, metastases from testicular neoplasms may show most commonly a "carcinoma" pattern and less frequently a "lymphoma" pattern or even a mixed pattern.

In evaluating the patient with testicular malignancy it is theoretically perferable to perform both testicular and pedal lymphangiography. However, the additional information provided by the testicular approach does not seem to warrant the risk of the surgical procedure and anesthesia. Inferior venacavography, pyelography, ultrasound, and computerized tomography should be done to complete the search for nodal involvement.

Our experience with 291 cases of testicular malignancies studied by pedal lymphangiography is described in Table 46–1. Patients with seminoma, of whom 24 per cent had abnormal findings by lymphangiography, were treated by radiotherapy alone, making nodal correlation impossible. All other testicular malignancies were managed by a combination of surgery and radiotherapy, permitting closer scrutiny of lymphangiographic findings. Surgical exploration was not uniformly undertaken, especially in patients with very advanced disease.

Surgical or autopsy findings or both were correlated with lymphangiographic findings (Table 46–2). Retroperitoneal node dissections were performed at intervals following radiotherapy. Of the 50 dissections in which positive nodes were found, 37 were in patients (74%) diagnosed preoperatively by pedal lymphangiography. Positive roentgenographic interpretation had excellent correlation (97%). Seventy (84%) of a total of 83 considered negative by lymphangiography were negative at exploration. Eight of the 13 patients who exhibited false-negative findings were found to have metastases lateral to those usually opacified by pedal lymphangiography; these metastases may have been diagnosed by the testicular route.

TABLE 46–1
Carcinoma of the Testicle

| | Lymphangiograms (291 cases) | |
	Positive	Negative
Seminoma	28	76
Carcinoma	76	105
Rhabdomyosarcoma	2	4
	106	185

TABLE 46-2
Carcinoma of the Testicle

Lymphangiographic–Pathologic Correlation of 121 Surgical and/or Autopsy Cases			
Positive	37	Carcinoma	117
False positive	1	Rhabdomyosarcoma	4
Negative	70		
False negative	13		
	121		121

For the purpose of correlation and patient management, all equivocal or suspicious readings are considered negative.

In the false-negative group:

1 case—2 nodes positive in 11/central para-aortic group
     45 nodes in right and left para-aortic areas all negative
1 case—no evidence of metastasis on lymphangiogram
8 cases—positive nodes in primary testicular lymphatics
3 cases—microscopic lesion, less than 3 mm

At M.D. Anderson Hospital and Tumor Institute in Houston, lymphangiography is routinely utilized as a guide in the management of patients with testicular malignancy. In seminomas, when lymphangiography is positive, radiotherapy is given to the ipsilateral iliac and bilateral retroperitoneal nodes to the diaphragm. The mediastinum and both supraclavicular areas are also treated. In the presence of a negative lymphangiogram radiotherapy is given only to the level of the diaphragm. In nonseminomatous malignancies a patient with a positive lymphangiogram is treated by radiotherapy to one-half of the proposed total dose to the nodes up to the diaphragm. A retroperitoneal node dissection is then undertaken to remove residual tumor tissue followed by additional radiotherapy and chemotherapy. In the presence of negative lymphangiographic findings, the retroperitoneal node dissection is undertaken initially. If the node dissection is negative, no further treatment is instituted.

URINARY BLADDER

Carcinoma of the bladder is the most common malignancy of the urinary tract, accounting for approximately 2 per cent of human malignant disease. It occurs in men three times as often as in women, and it is estimated that more Americans will die from it than from carcinoma of the uterine cervix.

The first echelon for the lymphatics of the bladder is represented by the external iliac nodes, particularly in the middle and medial groups, and occasionally by the hypogastric and common iliac nodes (Fig. 46-4).

Lymphangiography opacifies the external and common iliac lymph nodes. On occasion, hypogastric nodes close to the origin of the internal iliac artery may be demonstrated. Negative findings may result even though the paravesical, hypogastric, or the occasional node present in the obturator fossa may be affected by metastases, for these nodes escape visualization.

The diagnostic criteria for nodal metastases in carcinoma of the bladder are the same as those described earlier. The single most reliable criterion is a filling defect in a node not traversed by lymphatics (Fig. 46-5). When a node is completely replaced, the lymphatics may be displaced or obstructed (Fig. 46-6 A). Lymphatic obstruction with or without collateral channels may be the sole secondary evidence of nodal replacement. Confirmation by complementary procedures, notably venography, is of value to demonstrate the presence of enlarged replaced nodes (Fig. 46-6 B, C).

Ninety-one patients with carcinoma of the bladder had bilateral pedal lymphangiograms as part of the assessment of metastatic disease. Surgical findings were correlated within 3 months of lymphangiographic interpretation in 49 patients. Fifty-six of these patients, however, received preoperative irradiation (5000 rads tumor dose in 5 weeks through 10 × 10 cm. fields) 6 weeks prior to surgical exploration. In all cases surgical exploration included careful palpatory scrutiny of the pelvic and para-aortic lymph nodes. Realizing the shortcomings of palpatory evaluation, only enlarged or suspicious lymph nodes were removed for histologic examination. Three patients underwent bilateral pelvic lymphadenectomy. The results of lymphangiographic and surgical correlation are shown in Table 46-3. No false-positive lymphangiographic readings were encountered. In the nine patients with confirmed nodal metastases diagnosed by lymphangiography, an accuracy of 100 per cent, the specific sites of the nodal involvement were (1) the common iliac chain in four patients, with a concomitant involvement of a para-aortic node in one; (2) the external iliac chain, exclusively involved in two patients; both the common and external iliac chains, in two others. The remaining one patient had metastatic carcinoma of the bladder to a node involved with histiocytic lymphoma. Lymphangiograms positive for metastatic disease were encountered more frequently with the more advanced clinical stages as shown in Table 46-3. False-negative

TABLE 46-3
Carcinoma of the Bladder

Lymphangiographic–Surgical Correlation According to Clinical Stage of Disease					
	Clinical Stage				Total No. Patients
Interpretation	B1	B2	C	D	
Positive	1	1	3	4	9
False positive	0	0	0	0	0
Negative*	14	12	16	4	46
False negative	1	0	2	2	5

*For the purpose of correlation and patient management, all equivocal or suspicious readings were considered negative.

interpretations were encountered in five instances (9.8%).

Our findings of positive lymphangiograms in 7 per cent of patients with stages B_1 and B_2, 14 per cent with stage C, and 40 per cent in patients with stage D, underscore the value of this procedure in reducing the number of patients subjected to unnecessary and futile surgical exploration.

It is the policy at M.D. Anderson Hospital and Tumor Institute that all patients presenting with carcinoma of the bladder (stages B_1 to D) be examined by bilateral pedal lymphangiography. If the lymphangiogram is negative for nodal metastasis and the patient has an invasive bladder carcinoma, he is then treated with preoperative external irradiation, followed in 6 weeks by total cystectomy, prostatectomy, and ileal conduit urinary diversion. If the lymphangiogram is positive for metastatic disease in the pelvic lymph nodes, the patient is randomized, with half the patients treated by extended field radiotherapy, the other half receiving irradiation limited to the pelvis. If para-aortic nodes are involved, the patient is treated by chemotherapy.

PROSTATE

Carcinoma of the prostate is the most prevalent neoplasm of the male genital organs. This tumor has become of greater clinical importance because of the increasing number of men who are reaching later decades of life. Metastasis is predominantly through hematogenous routes, although lymphatic metastasis is common even in the early state of the disease. The incidence of lymph node metastasis is related to the size of the primary neoplasm as well as to the presence of extraprostatic invasion.

The first echelon of drainage from the prostate is by means of the following four collecting trunks: (1) the external iliac pedicle terminating in nodes of the middle group of the external iliac chain; (2) the hypogastric pedicle draining to the hypogastric nodes; (3) the posterior pedicle terminating in presacral lymph nodes; and (4) the inferior pedicle draining to the hypogastric nodes near the origin of the internal iliac artery (Fig. 46-7). The lymphatics of the prostate commmunicate with those of the bladder, the seminal vesicles, and the rectum.

The lymphangiographic findings in nodal metastases from carcinoma of the prostate are varied and show several architectural patterns. The abnormal lymph nodes may be normal in size or enlarged, most often with marginal filling defects, that is, partial replacement, having a crescent appearance with lymphatics failing to traverse the defect, the "carcinoma" pattern (Fig. 46-8). The involved nodes may occasionally appear moderately enlarged, with an irregular internal architecture, the "lymphoma" pattern. Fragmented nodes with multiple filling defects may also be seen. Lymphatic obstruction with or without collateral channels is often associated with these abnormal nodes. When the lymph node is completely replaced by tumor, the presence of mass may be confirmed by venography, ultrasound, and computerized tomography.

Fifty-nine patients with carcinoma of the prostate had pedal lymphangiograms at M.D. Anderson Hospital. Fourteen of these patients had nodal metastases with positive lymphangiograms, one in stage B, seven in stage C, and six in stage D. The sites of nodal involvement were as follows: the common iliac and para-aortic nodes in one patient in stage B; the external iliac nodes in seven patients in stage C; and both iliac and para-aortic nodes in five patients in stage D. One patient in stage D had metastases in the inguinal and external iliac nodes, with lymphatic obstruction in the pelvic region; this patient showed poor opacification of para-aortic nodes, which was inadequate for proper interpretation. Two patients with pelvic and para-aortic metastases had supraclavicular nodal involvement. It should be emphasized that, in one patient in stage B, the lymphangiogram showed positive findings in common iliac and para-aortic nodes. This finding can probably be explained by the fact that lymphatic spread in this patient was most likely through the hypogastric pedicle of the lymphatic drainage system of the prostate. Generally speaking, as the clinical stage increases from A to D, there is a progressive increase in the incidence of positive para-aortic lymph node involvement, so that almost all stage D patients show positive para-aortic and pelvic nodes. None of the 14 patients with positive lymphangiograms had an exploratory laparatomy. With strict diagnostic criteria, the interpretation of the lymphangiogram in carcinoma of the testicle, bladder, and cervix generally has excellent surgical correlation. Therefore a positive lymphangiogram in a patient with carcinoma of the prostate was considered definite evidence of metastasis and was treated accordingly.

In the recent literature, lymph node metastases from carcinoma of the prostate have been demonstrated by lymphangiography, ranging from 80 to 100 per cent diagnostic accuracy of the abnormal lymphangiogram when correlated with nodes obtained at surgery or autopsy.

In the management of patients with carcinoma of the prostate at M.D. Anderson Hospital, lymphangiograms are routinely obtained of patients in stage C of the disease, that is, locally invasive prostatic carcinoma with involvement of the base of the bladder, seminal vesicle, or fixation of the prostate mass to the pelvic wall. If the lymphangiogram is positive, then radiation therapy is not considered and the patient is treated with hormonal manipulation, usually orchiectomy and estrogens. If the lymphangiogram is negative, the patient either receives radiation therapy to the prostate or open surgical staging with lymphadenectomy and insertion of an infusion catheter; also, hypogastric artery infusion is carried out over a protracted period of time.

PENIS

Carcinoma of the penis is an uncommon malignant disease, accounting for less than 1 per cent of all deaths from cancer in men in the United States. The disease occurs predominantly in men between the ages of 50 and 80 years, with the average of 65 years. Although no specific etiologic factors have been demonstrated, squamous cell carcinoma of the penis appears to be related to poor personal and sexual hygiene.

The lymphatics of the prepuce drain to the superior and medial groups of the superficial inguinal nodes. The lymphatics of the glans penis join those of the urethra and prepuce and proceed in the following two groups: (1) those that follow the femoral canal, terminating in the deep inguinal nodes, including the node of Cloquet and the medial retrocrural lymph nodes; and (2) those that follow the inguinal canal and drain into the lateral retrocrural lymph nodes. The lymphatics of the corpora cavernosa penis end in the superior and medial groups of the superficial inguinal nodes and sometimes in the deep inguinal nodes or the retrocrural iliac nodes. The right and left inguinal lymph nodes have a rich communication with each other through subcutaneous lymphatics (Fig. 46–9).

Lymphangiography by both the penile and pedal routes has been utilized to define lymph node involvement from carcinoma of the penis. For the most part the pedal approach is more universally performed. Only a portion of the inguinal nodes are opacified by this technique. Although the inguinal lymph nodes are frequently involved by chronic inflammatory disease, the information obtained by pedal lymphangiography is still valid and useful. Again, the single most reliable criterion representing metastasis is a defect in a node not traversed by lymphatics (Fig. 46–10). The other criteria enumerated previously are operative here.

The significant morbidity associated with groin dissection has evoked caution against routine or prophylactic lymphadenectomy in patients without clinical suspicion of regional lymphatic spread. Five- and 9-year survival rates were 64.4 per cent and 50.1 per cent for 121 patients seen at M.D. Anderson Hospital without clinical evidence of metastatic disease (stage I) who did not undergo prophylactic lymphadenectomy. Those patients presenting with disease limited to the penis are usually treated by wide surgical excision. Groin dissection is reserved in those patients when regional metastatic disease is suggested by palpation or documented by lymphangiography and biopsy. Patients presenting with suspected regional lymph node metastases (stage II) are usually best managed with bilateral groin dissection performed several weeks following the surgical removal of the primary lesion. Survival rates for patients presenting initially with stage II disease is poor; 5- and 9-year survival rates have been only slightly over 20 per cent.

PERCUTANEOUS TRANSPERITONEAL LYMPH NODE ASPIRATION BIOPSY

Selective lymphadenectomy in conjunction with lymphangiography for staging prior to therapy has found increasing application. The percutaneous approach to retroperitoneal and pelvic lymph nodes with a small-caliber needle represents a simple technique to confirm the presence of neoplasm, obviating in selected cases the need for exploratory laparotomy. In view of the relatively anterior position of the para-aortic and pelvic lymph nodes in relation to the great vessels, an anterior transperitoneal approach seems most suitable.

With the patient in the supine position, the opacified node to be biopsied is localized by fluoroscopy, and the overlying percutaneous site is marked by the skin of the abdomen. The skin is prepared, the area down to the peritoneum is locally anesthetized, and a small incision is made in the skin. A thin-walled No. 23 gauge needle with a 0.7-mm. outer diameter, 0.5-mm. inner diameter, 15 or 20 cm. in length, and a 30° bevel angle is utilized. (This needle is available through Cook Incorporated, Bloomington, Indiana.) The needle is directed through the abdominal wall into the desired lymph node. In patients with a thick abdominal wall, a thin-walled No. 18 gauge needle is passed. Once the needle is in the lymph node, the patient may be rotated into each oblique to determine the relative relationship. When the node is punctured, synchronous movement of the needle and the lymph node under fluoroscopic control indicates accurate placement. Continuous suction is applied with a 12-cc. plastic syringe while the needle is moved through an excursion of approximately 1 cm. After release of suction the needle is withdrawn. The procedure is repeated two or three times to ensure sufficient cytologic material. The presence of oil droplets in the aspirate confirms that the node previously opacified during lymphangiography has been punctured. The specimen is fixed in 95 per cent ethyl alcohol or Cornoy's solution, depending upon the amount of blood present. The tissue is analyzed in the form of a smear and/or cell block by the cytologist.

The site of biopsy in an opacified lymph node will differ, depending upon the histologic type of neoplastic process. The most common lymphangiographic finding seen in metastatic carcinoma is a defect in a node not traversed by lymphatics. The residual, normally functioning portion of the node frequently has a crescentic configuration representing a node partially replaced by neoplasm. Consequently, the greatest yield is obtained from a biopsy of the node just above the crescentic area. This is illustrated in the biopsy of a node partially replaced by metastasis from a carcinoma of the prostate (Fig. 46–11A). With lymphoma, the lymph node is usually more diffusely involved, and the site of biopsy is not as critical. Figure 46–11B demonstrates lymphomatous involvement of an external iliac node confirmed by percutaneous transperitoneal aspiration biopsy in a patient with a concomitant carcinoma of the bladder studied by lymphangiography.

Aspiration biopsy of a lymph node containing metastatic carcinoma is more successful than with lymphoma. Epithelial metastases, especially those originating in pelvic viscera, are frequently highly cellular, poorly vascularized, and readily distinguishable from normal cells of a lymph node. In lymphomas, the diagnosis by fine-needle aspiration is more difficult and sometimes impossible to classify, especially as to type.

CHAPTER 46, ILLUSTRATIONS

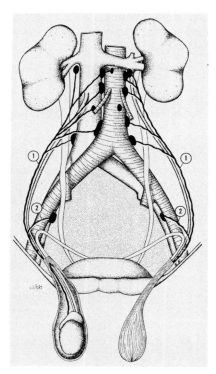

FIG. 46–1. Lymphatics of the testes. 1 = para-aortic (lumbar); 2 = external iliac. (Courtesy of University of Texas M.D. Anderson Hospital and Tumor Institute, Houston, Texas)

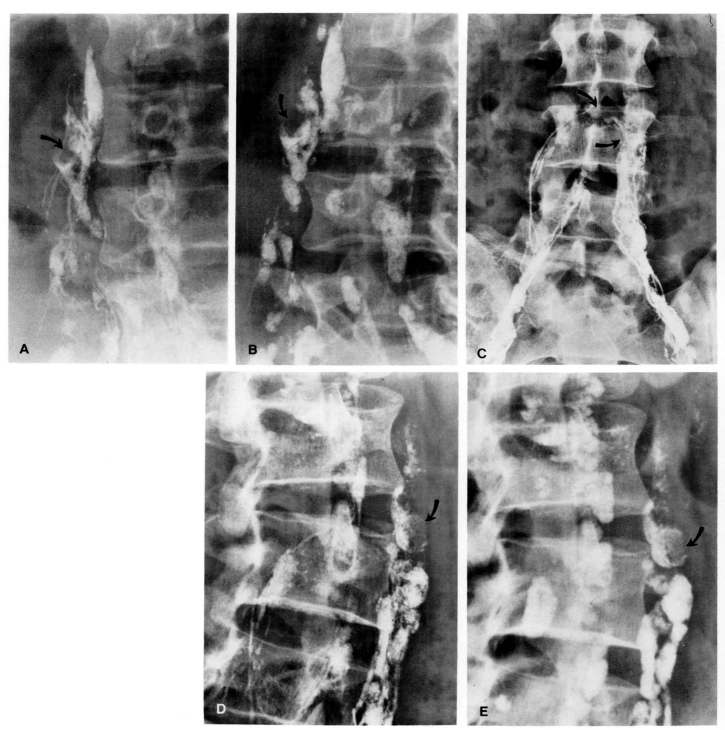

FIG. 46–2. Carcinoma of the testes. **(A)** Metastases to a right lumbar node at L-3 (*arrow*); the lymphatics do not traverse the defect. **(B)** The nodal phase reveals the crescentic configuration (*arrow*) of the node containing metastases, "carcinoma" pattern. **(C)** Crossover metastases (*arrows*) from a right **(D)** testicular carcinoma (*arrow*) to a left lumbar **(E)** node (*arrow*) at L2-L3. (Courtesy of University of Texas M.D. Anderson Hospital and Tumor Institute, Houston, Texas)

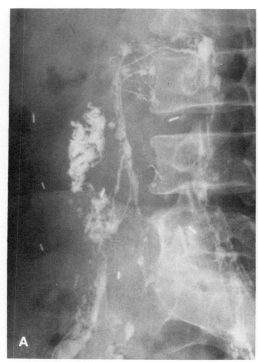

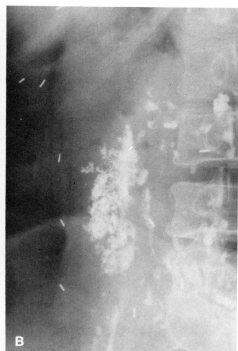

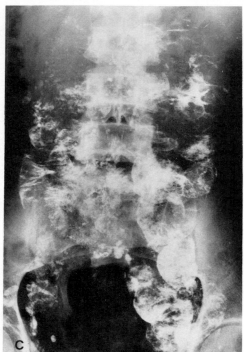

FIG. 46–3. Seminoma. **(A)** Metastatic seminoma to the right lumbar nodes, lymphatic phase. **(B)** Nodal phase "lymphoma" pattern. **(C)** Extensive involvement of iliac and lumbar nodes by seminoma "lymphoma" pattern. (Courtesy of University of Texas M.D. Anderson Hospital and Tumor Institute, Houston, Texas)

FIG. 46–4. Lymphatics of the bladder. 1= the collecting trunks of the trigone; 2 = the collecting trunks of the posterior wall; 3 = the collecting trunks of the anterior wall.

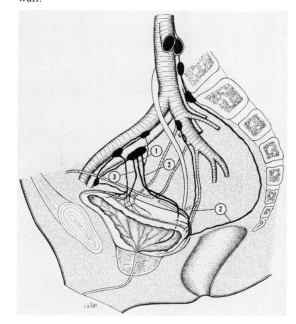

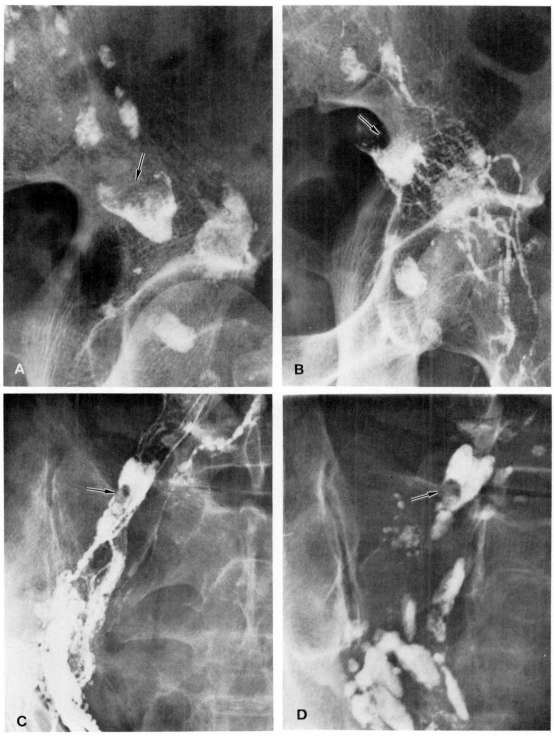

FIG. 46–5. Carcinoma of the bladder. **(A, B)** Metastasis to a left external iliac lymph node (*arrow*). The lymphatics do not traverse the nodal defect. **(C, D)** Metastasis to a right common iliac node (*arrow*). (Courtesy of University of Texas M.D. Anderson Hospital and Tumor Institute, Houston, Texas)

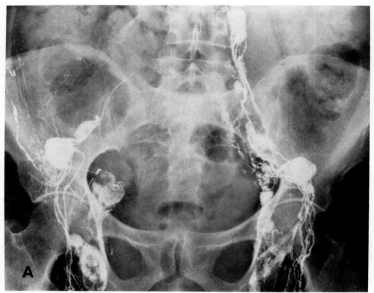

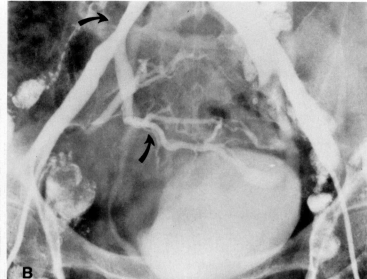

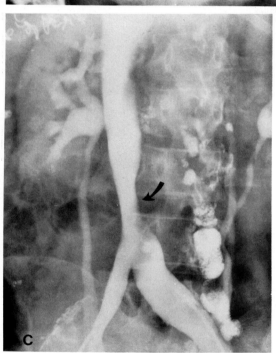

FIG. 46–6. Carcinoma of the bladder. **(A)** Total replacement of nodes by metastases with lymphatic obstruction and collateral circulation **(B, C).** Pelvic venography and inferior venacavography demonstrating extrinsic compression by the tumor masses (*arrows*).

FIG. 46–7. Lymphatics of prostate. 1 = external iliac; 2 = hypogastric; 3 = presacral.

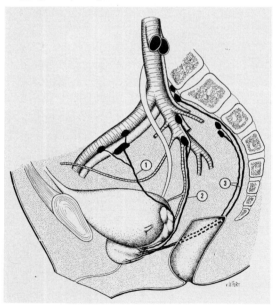

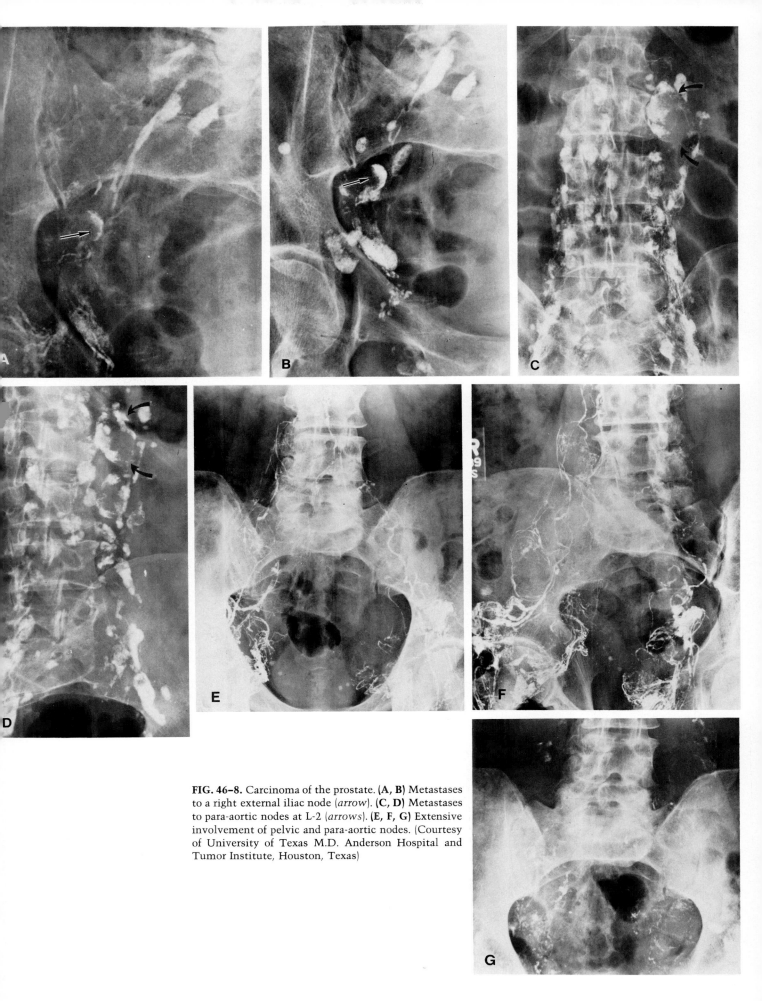

FIG. 46–8. Carcinoma of the prostate. (**A, B**) Metastases to a right external iliac node (*arrow*). (**C, D**) Metastases to para-aortic nodes at L-2 (*arrows*). (**E, F, G**) Extensive involvement of pelvic and para-aortic nodes. (Courtesy of University of Texas M.D. Anderson Hospital and Tumor Institute, Houston, Texas)

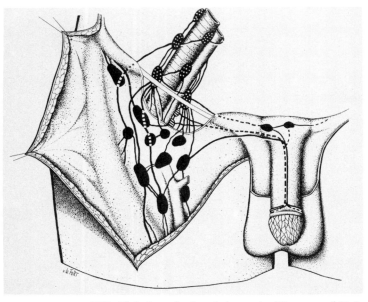

FIG. 46–9. Lymphatics of the penis. (Courtesy of University of Texas M.D. Anderson Hospital and Tumor Institute, Houston, Texas)

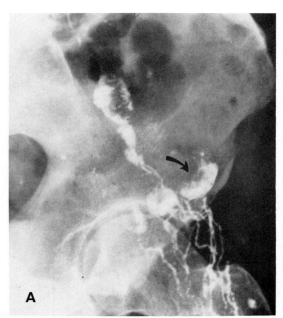

FIG. 46–10. Carcinoma of the penis. (A, B) Metastasis to a retrocrural node (*arrows*).

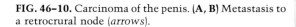

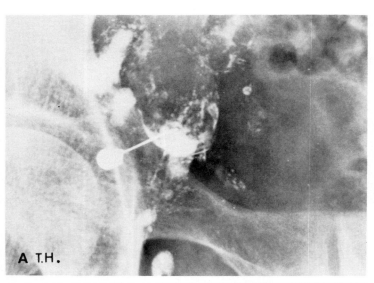

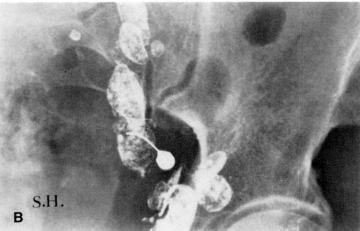

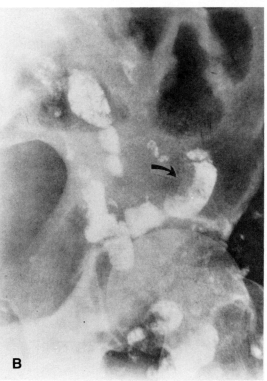

FIG. 46–11. Percutaneous transperitoneal aspiration biopsy. (A) Metastasis from carcinoma of the prostate. The biopsy was taken from just above the crescent. (B) Lymphomas in a patient with a concomitant carcinoma of the bladder. (Courtesy of University of Texas M.D. Anderson Hospital and Tumor Institute, Houston, Texas)

BIBLIOGRAPHY

1. Ackerman, L.V., and Del Regato, J.A.: Cancer: Diagnosis, Treatment and Prognosis. ed. 4. St. Louis, C.V. Mosby Company, 1970.
2. Busch, F.M., Sayegh, E.S., and Shenault, O.W., Jr.: Some uses of lymphangiography in the management of testicular tumors. J. Urol., 93:490–495, 1965.
3. Castellino, R.A.: The role of lymphography in "apparently localized" prostatic carcinoma. Lymphology, 8:16–20, 1975.
4. Cook, F.E., Lawrence, D.D., Smith, J.R., and Gritti, E.J.: Testicular carcinoma and lymphangiography. Radiology, 84:420–426, 1965.
5. Engzell, U., Espastis, P.L., Rubio, C. et al.: Investigation on tumor spread in connection with aspiration biopsy. Acta Radiol. Ther., 10:385–398, 1971.
6. Flocks, R.H., Culp, D., and Porto, R.: Lymphatic spread from prostatic cancer. J. Urol., 81:194–196, 1959.
7. Forsgren, L., and Orell, S.: Aspiration cytology in carcinoma of the pancreas. Surgery, 73:38–42, 1973.
8. Galesanu, M.R., and Rosenbaum, S.: Diagnosis of lymph node invasion of bladder and prostatic cancer by lympho- and pelvic phlebography. Int. Urol. Nephrol., 5:163–166, 1973.
9. Gothlin, J.H.: Post-lymphographic percutaneous fine needle biopsy of lymph nodes guided by fluoroscopy. Radiology, 120:205–207, 1976.
10. Grossman, I., von Phul, R., Fitzgerald, J.P. et al.: Proceedings: The early lymphatic spread of manifest prostatic adenocarcinoma. Am. J. Roentgenol., 120:673–677, 1974.
11. Hancke, S., Holm, H.H., and Koch, F.: Ultrasonically guided percutaneous fine needle biopsy of the pancreas. Surg. Gynecol. Obstet., 140:361–634, 1975.
12. Holm, H.H., Pederson, J.F., Kristensen, J.K. et al.: Ultrasonically guided percutaneous puncture. Radiol. Clin. North Am., 13:493–503, 1975.
13. Johnson, D.E. (ed.): Testicular Tumors. New York, Medical Examination Publishing Company, 1972.
14. Johnson, D.E.: Retroperitoneal lymphadenectomy: Indications, complications and expectations. Presented at the Seventh International Symposium of the GBK, Oct., 1975, Dusseldorf, Germany.
15. Johnson, D.E., Kaesler, K.E., Kaminsky, S., Jing, B.S., and Wallace, S.: Lymphangiography as an aid in staging bladder carcinoma. South. Med. J., 69:28–30, 1976.
16. Jonsson, K., Ingemansson, S., and Ling, L.: Lymphography in patients with testicular tumors. Br. J. Urol., 45:548–554, 1973.
17. MacDonald, J.S.: Lymphography in malignant disease of the urinary tract. Proc. Roy. Soc. Med., 63:1237–1239, 1970.
18. Maier, J.G., and Schamber, D.T.: The role of lymphography in the diagnosis and treatment of malignant testicular tumors. Am. J. Roentgenol., 114:482–491, 1972.
19. Maier, J.G., and van Buskirk, K.E.: Treatment of testicular germ cell malignancies. J.A.M.A., 213:97–98, 1970.
20. Miller, L.S., and Johnson, D.E.: Megavoltage irradiation for bladder cancer: alone, postoperative or preoperative? Proceedings of the Seventh National Cancer Congress. New York, J.B. Lippincott, 1973.
21. Piver, S.M., Wallace, S., and Castro, J.R.: The accuracy of lymphangiography in carcinoma of the uterine cervix. Am. J. Roentgenol., 111:278–283, 1971.
22. Ray, B., Hajdu, S.I., and Whitmore, W.F.: Distribution of retroperitoneal lymph node metastases in testicular germinal tumors. Cancer, 33:340–348, 1974.
23. Ray, G.R., Cassady, J.R., and Bagshaw, M.A.: Definitive radiation therapy of carcinoma of the prostate. A report on 15 years' experience. Radiology, 106:407–418, 1973.
24. Roo, T., de and Van Minden, S.H.: The value of lymphography in tumors of the testes. Lymphology, 6:97–100, 1973.
25. Rouviere, H.: Anatomy of the Human Lymphatic System. Trans. J.M. Tobias. Ann Arbor, Edwards Company, 1938.
26. Rummelhardt, S., and Fussek, H.: Die Lymphangioadenographie in der Urologie. Erfahrungen und Ergebnisse (German). Urologie, 9:333–335, 1970.
27. Ruttimann, A.: Iliac lymph node aspiration biopsy through paravascular approach: preliminary report. Radiology, 90:150–151, 1968.
28. Samuels, M.L., Holoye, P.Y., and Johnson, D.E.: Bleomycin combination chemotherapy in the management of testicular neoplasm. Cancer, 36:318–326, 1975.
29. Viamonte, M., Jr., Myers, M.B., Soto, M., Kenyon, N.M., and Parks, R.E.: Lymphangiography: its role in detection and therapeutic evaluation of carcinoma and neoplastic conditions of the genitourinary tract. J. Urol., 87:85–90, 1962.
30. Wallace, S.: Interventional radiology. Cancer, 37:517–531, 1976.
31. Wallace, S., and Jackson, L.: Diagnostic criteria for lymphangiographic interpretation of malignant neoplasia. Cancer Chemother. Rep., 52:31–58, 1968.
32. Wallace, S., and Jing, B.S.: Lymphangiographic diagnosis of nodal metastases from testicular malignancies. J.A.M.A., 213:94–96, 1970.
33. Wheeler, J.S.: Lymphography in early prostatic cancer. Urology, 3:444–446, 1974.
34. Wirtanen, G.W., and Miller, R.C.: Bladder lymphatics and tumor dissemination. J. Urol., 109:58–59, 1973.
35. Zajicek, J.: Aspiration biopsy cytology. Part II. Cytology of supradiaphragmatic organs. In Wied, G.L. (ed.): Monographs in Clinical Cytology. pp. 90–124. Switzerland, 1974.
36. Zornoza, J., Wallace, S., Goldstein, H.M. et al.: Transperitoneal percutaneous retroperitoneal lymph node aspiration biopsy. Radiology, 122:111–115, 1977.

Computed tomography (CT) is the reconstruction by a computer of an image depicting a tomographic plane (slice) through the body. This cross-sectional image is composed of many picture elements (pixels), each representing x-ray absorption measurements of a small area of tissue within the slice. The pixel display is two-dimensional, but each pixel represents a three-dimensional volume element, with the third dimension equal to the thickness of the tomographic slice. The pixel depicts the average attenuation of all the tissue within the volume element. Pixel size and slice thickness are important technical factors in applying CT to the evaluation of tissue absorption numbers.

Many authors have reported on the usefulness of various types of CT scanners in the diagnosis of urinary tract disease.[1, 2, 10-12, 19, 20, 22, 27-29, 32] The CT images of the genitourinary tract used for illustrations in this chapter were obtained on a body scanner with a scan time of 20 seconds for each slice. The basic whole-body scanning equipment consists of a patient-handling table, a scanning gantry that contains the collimated x-ray source and detectors, data-acquisition electronics, an x-ray generator, a technologist's operating panel, and a viewing console.

A single scan, completed in 20 seconds, produces one tomographic slice. The information obtained during each scan is processed by a computer, and the reconstructed image is presented on a television monitor for viewing, manipulation, and photographic recording. The image can be manipulated at the display console to permit a selective display of particular absorption values from the wide spectrum of absorption values obtained during a scan. The entire scan or a section of the scan can be selected for display on the viewing console. All scans are stored on magnetic tape and on Polaroid or transparent film.

47

Genitourinary Computed Tomography

ROBERT R. HATTERY,
BYRN WILLIAMSON, JR.,
GLEN W. HARTMAN

TECHNIQUE: VISUALIZATION OF THE KIDNEYS

High-quality excretory urography demands close attention to the details of the radiographic system and conduct of the examination. CT requires the same meticulous approach but with a new set of standards. McCullough and co-workers have outlined performance–evaluation tests, some of which should be conducted at the beginning of each scanning day to ensure high-quality reconstructed images.[15] These tests establish criteria for precision, contrast scale, linearity, spatial independence, accuracy, spatial resolution, artifacts, and patient exposure.

Complete visualization of the kidneys requires serial cross-section scans beginning at the upper poles and extending inferiorly. The number of scans varies with the position of the kidneys and the size of the lesion under study. Generally, 8 to 10 scans at 1.5-cm. intervals are required for a complete examination of the kidneys. More scans are needed if the retroperitoneal para-aortic area, the course of the ureters, or the lower abdomen is to be scanned. Similarly, if the liver is to be scanned for the evaluation of metastasis from renal cell carcinoma, an increased number of scans are required. Routinely, patients are initially scanned in the supine position without the use of intravenous contrast medium. If necessary, dilute oral contrast medium can be used to identify loops of bowel adjacent to the kidneys, and glucagon may be given to decrease bowel peristalsis. If the CT scan is done primarily for the evaluation of a renal mass, scans should be obtained before and after injection of intravenous contrast medium.

ARTIFACTS

All imaging procedures have inherent limitations of image quality as well as artifacts that may degrade the images produced. CT is no exception.

Alfidi and co-workers have described the effects of biologic motion on CT resolution.[3] Some of the motion artifacts are produced by peristaltic motion of gastrointestinal gas, patient movement, respiratory motion, and movement of the diaphragm secondary to the mechanical action of the beating heart. Other artifacts may be produced by the expansion and contraction of major vessels with systole and diastole.

Artifacts also may be produced by peristaltic activity of the contrast medium-filled calyces, pelvis, and ureters during the period of the scan. These artifacts may produce a significant degree of image degradation because of the dense nature of the contrast medium. Motion artifacts are much less troublesome with scanners that have a scan time of 5 seconds or less.

Detector artifacts, mainly drift of sensitivity and delay in response, may take a variety of forms,[13] and the computer system may also be the source of artifacts. A CT scan of a phantom is performed each morning and is examined by the radiologists so that appropriate technical adjustment can be made.

IMAGE INTERPRETATION

Permanent images of CT scans may be interpreted in much the same method as routine radiographs. It is important, however, that the reconstructed images also be studied at the viewing console; the window level (WL) and window width (WW) may be manipulated to enhance the range of absorption coefficient numbers (CT numbers) that are represented by the various tissues within the plane of the scan. Narrowing the window width increases the contrast between different densities and decreases the latitude of tissue densities that are displayed. Some lesions, especially in the liver, kidney, and bone, can be missed if the "range" of gray-scale alternatives is not manipulated properly on the console. The manipulation of WL and WW is especially critical in evaluation of renal masses because the absorption numbers of the internal contents of the mass must be determined.

RENAL ANATOMY

Knowledge of normal genitourinary anatomy and the relationship of the urinary tract to the intra-abdominal and retroperitoneal structures is required for the accurate interpretation of normal and abnormal CT images (Figs. 47–1 to 47–4). Analysis of renal images requires knowledge of the relationships of the kidneys to other abdominal structures as well as of the normal variation of renal anatomy, because confusion may be caused by the variable position of the kidneys, anomalies of rotation, crossed ectopia, duplication of the collecting system, and horseshoe or pelvic kidneys.[10] The size of the kidneys can be determined in cross section as well as by pole-to-pole length.

The relationship of the upper pole and superior lateral margin of the normal right kidney to the right and caudate lobes of the liver as seen on routine excretory urograms and linear tomograms is also visualized on cross-sectional CT images. A similar relationship is seen between the superior lateral margin of the left kidney and the spleen. The superior extension of the spleen, medial splenic margin, and splenic hilum are well demarcated on CT.

The parenchyma of the kidneys can be visualized in cross section, and the cortex and medulla can be differentiated on scans obtained early in the nephrographic phase following a bolus injection. The lateral and medial margins of the kidneys are seen clearly on conventional linear tomograms. Because of the cross-sectional reconstruction of the renal parenchyma, the circumferential margins (lateral and medial as well as anterior and posterior) of the renal parenchyma are clearly seen on CT scans. Visualization of the entire outer margin of the kidney is possible because of fat in the perinephric space, whereas visualization of the inner circumferential margin results from fat in the renal sinus.

The overall CT density of the renal sinus may be affected by fat, urine in the collecting system, the size of the collecting system, blood in the renal arteries and veins, and calcific plaques in the renal arteries. All these factors must be considered when comparing the density of the renal sinus with that of fat in the perinephric space and when comparing the density of masses projecting into the renal sinus. The administration of intravenous contrast medium may be helpful in differentiating normal renal sinus fat from benign renal cysts, renal cell carcinomas, other solid tumors, or normal structures within the renal sinus.

The calyces, infundibula, renal pelvis, and ureters can be visualized on unenhanced CT images, but they are better demonstrated on scans obtained after the injection of contrast medium. However, the fine detail of these collecting system structures as well as the appearance of the papillae can be seen better on a high-quality excretory urogram with ureteral compression. The excretory urogram with an adequate dose of contrast medium and ureteral compression remains the best method of evaluating the anatomy and pathology of the collecting system and urothelium.

After the injection of intravenous contrast medium, the normal ureters can be seen in cross section as they course through the retroperitoneal space. The position of the ureters relative to the aorta, spine, retroperitoneal nodes, and psoas muscles also can be determined. In some patients with renal failure, the density of contrast medium is diminished, and it may be difficult to exclude obstructive nephropathy even with high-dose excretory urography with tomography. CT, however, may permit visualization of the ureters and assessment of the caliber of the collecting system in spite of diminished or absent concentrating ability of the kidneys.

The perinephric space is usually well visualized, especially in patients who have a moderate amount of retroperitoneal fat. Even though not all of the fascial structures that define the anterior and posterior perinephric and paranephric spaces may be visualized because of their relationship to the plane of the scan, the fat in these spaces around the kidney can be visualized in cross section. Infiltrative processes such as inflammation, tumor, hematoma, or urinoma may be well visualized. The kidney may be displaced and rotated by the process, and the fat planes may be obliterated.

RENAL MASSES

Renal masses are visible on CT because of alteration of the normal anatomic configuration of the kidney or because the density of the mass is significantly different from that of renal parenchyma or surrounding tissue. The density of renal masses may be altered by calcification, hemorrhage, fat content, necrosis, or inflammation. It is noteworthy that the density of solid renal tumors may be equal to that of normal renal parenchyma.[16] The CT characteristics of renal masses are usually best evaluated on scans obtained through the midportion of the mass. In this position the interface between the mass and adjacent renal parenchyma and the density of the mass can be accurately evaluated. Small renal masses (less than 1.5 cm. in diameter) are often difficult to evaluate by CT, because the diameter of the mass is relatively small compared with the thickness of the slice. If a mass occupies only part of the thickness of a CT image, the indicated density of the mass in this region will be erroneous because this density will be indicative not only of the nature of the tissue making up the renal mass, but also of the adjacent renal parenchyma within the plane of the scan. The density of a benign renal cyst is uniform and is less than that of renal parenchyma. After the intravenous injection of contrast medium, the density of a benign renal cyst does not change significantly compared with its density prior to injection. In addition, a benign simple cyst has a sharp interface with normal renal parenchyma. A cyst located at the periphery of the kidney has a thin, often undetectable peripheral wall (Figs. 47–5 to 47–7).

On unenhanced scans, renal cell carcinomas have

an overall density similar to, although usually slightly less than, that of renal parenchyma. After the intravenous injection of contrast medium, the density of a solid tumor increases, although this increase is not as great as that of the surrounding normal renal parenchyma. The magnitude of the increase in density of solid renal mass depends primarily on the vascularity of the mass. The density of a solid renal tumor tends to be nonuniform, and the wall of such a mass is usually thicker than that of a simple cyst.[33] The interface between a solid renal mass and adjacent parenchyma is usually ill-defined, although an encapsulated tumor with a sharp interface may rarely be encountered. CT is sensitive in the detection of calcification within a mass. The finding of calcification within the substance of a renal mass is highly suggestive of renal cell carcinoma (Figs. 47–8 to 47–10).[4]

Although renal cell carcinoma is the most common solid mass of the kidney, other conditions such as angiomyolipoma or tumefactive xanthogranulomatous pyelonephritis may also have the appearance of a solid renal mass. These conditions may be difficult to differentiate from renal cell carcinoma, although the presence of fat within an angiomyolipoma may indicate the proper diagnosis. In addition, acute renal inflammation, abscess, or chronic subscapsular hematoma may be difficult to differentiate from renal cell carcinoma.

The differentiation of excessive renal sinus fat from a parapelvic mass is a common problem in excretory urography. CT can be helpful in such cases because the low density of renal sinus fat is usually easily distinguished from the intermediate density of a parapelvic cyst or the higher density of a solid tumor.

Benign renal cysts are a frequent incidental finding on CT performed for the evaluation of the kidneys or other organs. If the appearance of such an incidentally discovered mass is typical of a benign renal cyst, we do not believe further diagnostic measures are necessary for the evaluation of such a mass.

The differentiation of benign renal cyst from solid renal mass has been possible in most cases of large renal masses. CT has also permitted determination of the local extent of renal cell carcinoma and assessment of the presence of metastasis to lymph nodes and to the liver.

Advanced cases of polycystic renal disease are easily recognized by CT, by renal enlargement, distortion of the collecting system, and multiple bilateral cysts. Multiple cysts may be seen in the liver of some of these patients (Fig. 47–11). Infiltration of

the kidneys with lymphoma has also been observed. Lymphomatous masses have a greater density than do renal cysts, but they do not increase significantly in density after the injection of contrast medium. Scans of masses that contain calcium have areas of increased density depending on the distribution of the calcification. The appearance of Wilms' tumor is similar to that of a solid renal carcinoma.

ADRENAL TUMORS

The adrenal glands may be visualized in CT scans in most patients and CT is the preferred method for adrenal gland visualization (Fig. 47–12). Thus CT is helpful in the evaluation of patients who have clinical signs or symptoms of adrenal tumor in patients with findings on excretory urography that suggest the presence of a suprarenal mass. CT is usually able to distinguish clearly between an adrenal mass and pseudomasses such as the fluid-filled fundus of the stomach, medial pole of the spleen, loops of bowel, pancreas, splenic vessels, and other structures. If a normal adrenal gland can be identified on the CT examination, a suspected adrenal mass can, therefore, be shown. Dilute water-soluble contrast medium given orally or instilled into the colon may be helpful in certain cases in which fluid-filled loops of bowel cause difficulty on CT. CT may also be helpful in differentiating an adrenal mass from a mass arising from the upper pole of the kidney. CT has been sensitive in the detection of small (1.5 to 2 cm.) adrenal tumors (Figs. 47–13, 47–14). Benign adrenal tumors are usually indistinguishable from malignant adrenal tumors although adrenal lipomas may have the typical appearance of a tumor composed of fat.

RENAL ATROPHY AND FAILURE

Kidneys that are atrophic may be difficult to evaluate by conventional urographic techniques, particularly if there is marked reduction in renal function. Such kidneys can usually be clearly delineated by CT, and associated calcification, multiple masses, or obstructive hydronephrosis can be detected (Figs. 47–15 to 47–17).

NEPHRECTOMY

CT has been a definitive method of evaluation of patients who have undergone nephrectomy. Loops of bowel, the liver, pancreas, and spleen commonly occupy the renal bed and are easily distinguishable from postoperative abscess or hemorrhage as well as from recurrent tumor in the renal bed. In some cases, dilute water-soluble contrast medium administered by mouth or per rectum may be needed to prove that a soft tissue density in the renal fossa is due to bowel (Fig. 47–18). Postoperative fat necrosis or inflammation may rarely simulate recurrent tumor on CT.

HYDRONEPHROSIS

Usually the presence of hydronephrosis and the site and cause of obstruction can be established on excretory urograms by employing tomography and an adequate dose of intravenous contrast medium (Fig. 47–19). Even in renal failure the collecting system usually can be visualized well enough to determine whether obstruction is present. Retrograde pyelography may establish the site and cause of obstruction in some patients with an indeterminate excretory urogram and ureteral tomograms, but often retrograde pyelograms do not establish the extent of associated periureteral pathologic processes. CT is indicated in evaluating patients with hydronephrosis with an indeterminate site and etiology of obstruction and in selected patients with renal failure to exclude obstructive nephropathy.

The CT density of the hydronephrotic collecting system and ureter approximates the density of water. The anatomic appearance of pyelocalyectasis and ureterectasis on CT scans is similar to the appearance on excretory urograms, but the dilated collecting system can be visualized on CT without the use of contrast medium (Fig. 47–20). Ureteral dilatation, however, is more easily visualized after the intravenous injection of contrast medium. If the obstruction is marked, delayed CT scans may be needed to indentify the site of obstruction.

The CT appearance of contrast medium in the dilated collecting system depends on the degree of opacification. A contrast medium–urine interface may be seen with the heavier contrast medium in the more dependent portions of the collecting system. With more complete opacification, the entire collecting system will be filled with contrast medium. Depending on the level of renal function and the volume and concentration of contrast medium in the collecting system, the density of the dilated collecting system may appear similar to that of the renal parenchyma.

Periureteral processes represent a common cause of urinary tract obstruction or ureteral deviation in patients with lymphoma, primary retroperitoneal tumor, or metastatic retroperitoneal adenopathy. The site and extent of retroperitoneal tumors have been clearly depicted on CT scans,[30] and additional information has been obtained when compared with the findings on excretory urograms.

CT has been of great value in the assessment of patients with ureteral obstruction due to neoplasms in the pelvis. The extent of primary or metastatic tumor in the pelvis is often shown better by CT than by other imaging methods, especially if the mass is posterior to the bladder, infiltrates along the lateral pelvic wall or along the psoas muscle, or involves deep pelvic soft tissues.

Percutaneous insertion of a needle into the renal pelvis can be performed using CT guidance.[8] Contrast medium can be injected through such a needle to outline the collecting system and ureter of a nonfunctioning kidney. Temporary or long-term drainage of the kidney can be provided if a percutaneous nephrostomy tube is inserted.

RETROPERITONEUM AND PELVIS

CT scanning of the retroperitoneum and pelvis is generally indicated in patients with suspected abnormalities whose spectrum of gross pathology includes a mass or "mass effect." Suspected neoplasm, benign or malignant, is the most common clinical indication for CT scanning. Non-neoplastic diseases such as abscess, hematoma, urinoma, lymphocyst, increased amount of fat or fibrous tissue, aneurysm, or obstruction of the lower urinary tract of unknown cause are also indications for performing CT scans. CT may also be used to stage known neoplasms and to follow the response of a tumor to radiation or chemotherapy. Likewise, patients may be referred for CT scanning because of abdominal or pelvic pain to rule out primary neoplasm or for evaluation of recurrent or metastatic tumor.

Excretory urograms are commonly done as a "screening procedure" to evaluate patients with obscure abdominal or pelvic pain and to search for retroperitoneal or pelvic masses that may affect the kidneys, ureters, or bladder. Because the normal course of the ureters is widely variable, the position and course of the ureters is a relatively insensitive indicator of retroperitoneal disease. Significant para-aortic adenopathy may be present despite a normal excretory urogram. Likewise, the ureters may appear to be displaced by a retroperitoneal mass when the retroperitoneum is in fact normal. Lymphography and, less commonly, angiography may be used to evaluate these patients; however, computed tomography is a more appropriate screening examination and often a more definitive method of evaluating the retroperitoneum. Some patients are referred directly for CT scanning, whereas others are referred because of suspected abnormalities or equivocal findings on excretory urograms or ultrasound (Figs. 47–21, 47–22).

The most common urographic manifestations of pelvic masses include displacement or obstruction of the lower ureters, indentation on the bladder, visualization of a soft tissue mass, abnormal calcification in the pelvis, and secondary bony changes. Unfortunately, these findings may not be reliable for indicating the presence of pelvic masses. Pelvic masses that are small frequently do not displace or indent the bladder. Large pelvic masses, especially those posterior to the bladder, may not be recognized on the cystogram film of an excretory urogram. Extrinsic indentations on the dome of the bladder are frequently due to the normal uterus, loops of small bowel, or the cecum. It may be difficult or impossible to differentiate a significant pelvic mass from these pseudomasses on the urogram. In many instances CT and/or ultrasound scanning provide additional information that may confirm the presence of a mass or establish that the pelvis is normal. Parasagittal ultrasound scans may be especially helpful as an adjunct to understanding and interpreting the cross-sectional CT scans.

The importance of CT in detecting, differentiating, and defining the extent of pathologic processes has been established by many authors. Cross-sectional imaging with CT is an important addition to the excretory urogram as a method of evaluating the genitourinary tract, retroperitoneum, and pelvis. The significance of CT as a noninvasive imaging procedure is in part due to the ability to rule out anatomic abnormalities in patients with obscure, confusing, indeterminate, or equivocal clinical or radiographic findings.

TECHNIQUE

Patients generally are not given laxatives for preparation of the bowel. The bowel should be free of barium, because residual barium in the GI tract frequently causes significant artifacts on CT scans. Opacification of the small intestine is accomplished by giving the patients dilute water-soluble contrast medium orally 30 to 60 minutes prior to the CT examination. A standard infusion of 300 cc. of 30 per cent urographic contrast medium may be administered depending on the indications for the scan and on the CT findings. Glucagon (1 mg.) may be given intravenously to diminish bowel peristaltic artifacts. Because glucagon is a provocative test for pheochromocytoma, the radiologist must be prepared to treat a hypertensive crisis in patients suspected of having a pheochromocytoma.

Scans of the retroperitoneum are done in the supine position, usually at 2-cm. intervals beginning at the level of the aortic hiatus. CT scans of the pelvis usually are done as a continuation of the examination of the retroperitoneum. The bladder should be partially distended with urine as in ultrasound examinations, or intravenous contrast medium may be given to opacify the ureters and bladder. As the examination is viewed and monitored, overlapped scans or scans at selected intervals can be obtained, contrast medium can be instilled into the rectum, or scans may be obtained with the patient in the prone or oblique position in order to improve delineation of certain aspects of anatomy or pathology.

Patients referred specifically for CT examination of the pelvis may be given contrast medium intravenously depending on the indication for the examination, the findings on the excretory urogram, or the suspicion of ureteral obstruction or deviation. Scans before and after administration of intravenous contrast medium may be appropriate in some cases. Women are asked to insert a tampon in the vagina to help define the vagina anatomically on CT scans. Dilute water-soluble contrast medium is given orally and may be instilled into the rectum and sigmoid with a syringe and red rubber catheter.

Routinely scans are obtained at 1.5- or 1-cm. intervals from the iliac crest to the inferior aspect of the symphysis pubis. Scans of the retroperitoneum should be done to search for metastases to para-aortic nodes in patients with known pelvic neoplasms or neoplasms discovered on the CT examination. If neoplasm, abscess, or other abnormalities extend inferiorly out of the true pelvis, appropriate scans should be obtained to include the entire extent of the lesion below the level of the symphysis pubis. Because pelvic abnormalities may involve bone secondarily, or because primary bone tumors or metastases may extend into the pelvis, CT scans need to be viewed at a wide range of window settings to enhance the visualization of bone.

RETROPERITONEUM

LYMPHADENOPATHY

Normal and enlarged para-aortic nodes can be visualized on CT scans because these nodes are surrounded by fat located adjacent to known vascular structures and are often less affected by motion artifacts (see Fig. 47–1B). The size of normal nodes is variable, but seldom exceeds 1.5 cm. whereas most normal nodes measure less than 1 cm. Enlarged iliac, renal hilar, celiac, splenic, porta hepatic, and mesenteric nodes may also be visualized, whereas normal nodes in these locations may be more difficult to recognize.

Para-aortic adenopathy may be visualized on CT scans as discrete enlarged nodes, conglomerate adenopathy, or as a homogeneous mass in which individual nodes are not discernible. The outline of the aorta and/or inferior vena cava may be obliterated by adjacent adenopathy (Figs. 47–23 to 47–26). The kidneys, ureters, bladder, or even the pancreas may be displaced by masses of nodes. Most enlarged nodes are of homogeneous density and of the same range of CT density as other solid tissues. In some instances, however, enlarged nodes may be inhomogeneous and may contain zones of lower density. Occasionally, enlarged nodes, for example in lymphoma, may contain calcification.

Most cases of retroperitoneal lymphadenopathy are due to lymphoma or metastasis; however, inflammatory lymphadenopathy may also be seen. The CT findings are nonspecific regarding the histology of retroperitoneal adenopathy. Significant abnormalities associated with adenopathy may also be seen such as primary tumors, urinary or biliary tract obstruction, ascites, or osseous, hepatic, renal, or splenic involvement. Discrete deposits of tumor of decreased density involving the spleen have been observed in patients with lymphoma, although nonspecific splenomegaly or a normal-appearing spleen is more commonly seen.

CT is frequently used to stage lymphoma and other neoplasms, and follow-up scans have been helpful in documenting the response of the primary tumor or adenopathy during radiation or chemotherapy. Some follow-up scans, particularly in cases of lymphoma or seminoma, have shown that enlarged nodes have virtually disappeared, but thickening or nodularity of para-aortic tissues has persisted. In some cases this residual tissue probably represents fibrosis, although residual viable neoplasm cannot be excluded on the basis of the CT appearance (Fig. 47–27).

Data concerning the accuracy of CT relative to lymphography are gradually being collected by several groups of investigators. Lymphoma involving primarily normal or minimally enlarged para-aortic nodes probably occurs in less than 10 per cent of patients with lymphoma.[9] Schaner and colleagues reported 2 patients of 23 on whom the CT scan was interpreted as being negative, but on whom the lymphogram showed abnormal architecture or minimally enlarged nodes.[21] Redman and co-workers reported 2 patients of 20 in whom the CT scan was interpreted as normal whereas lymphographic and histologic studies showed normal nodes containing tumor.[17] Harell and associates described 2 patients of 18 who had high para-aortic nodal enlargement seen on CT that was not visualized on lymphograms.[9] Kreel described 6 patients of 14 with lymphoma in whom additional para-aortic disease was visualized by CT,[14] and Schaner and co-workers found that the lymphogram underestimated the extent of para-aortic involvement in 13 of 23 patients.[21] Stephens and co-workers also emphasized that even though both the lymphogram and CT were abnormal, the information provided by the two examinations may not be identical.[31]

Stephens and colleagues reported the early Mayo Clinic experience with 184 patients.[31] Retroperitoneal lymphadenopathy was evident on CT scans in 99 of these cases. Retroperitoneal adenopathy was suspected in the other 85 patients, but the CT scans were interpreted as normal. Fifty patients with known or subsequently confirmed lymphoma showed evidence of enlarged retroperitoneal nodes at CT examination. The scans were correctly interpreted as showing enlarged retroperitoneal nodes or a mass consistent with lymphadenopathy in all except two cases, in which the findings were misinterpreted as pancreatic carcinoma. The full abdominal extent of the disease, however, was not always evident on CT scans. Splenic or additional nodal involvement that was not apparent on CT studies was found in 3 of the 18 patients who underwent surgical exploration.

Twenty-nine patients with known lymphomas at sites outside the abdomen had abdominal CT scans that were interpreted as normal. Of the ten patients who had subsequent surgical exploration, none had para-aortic adenopathy, but two patients with normal-appearing scans were found to have splenic involvement, and one of them also had involvement of mesenteric nodes.

Forty-nine patients had CT scans indicative of metastases to retroperitoneal nodes. The metastases were from a variety of primary sites, the most common being the testis, pancreas, prostate, bladder, and kidney. In either patients with metastases to retroperitoneal nodes, the primary tumor could not be discovered. Twenty-seven patients including all with unknown tumors had nodal metastases confirmed by surgery or autopsy.

PRIMARY AND RECURRENT TUMORS

Primary retroperitoneal tumors are often large when first suspected clinically (Fig. 47-28). Leiomyosarcoma (6 cases) has been the most common neoplasm seen in our experience followed by malignant fibrous histiocytoma (3 cases) and liposarcoma (2 cases). CT evidence of necrosis and cystic degeneration has been a prominent but not specific feature of leiomyosarcoma. The CT density of liposarcoma has been greater than the density of normal retroperitoneal fat. Retroperitoneal lipoma, on the other hand, has been visualized on CT scans as a mass with a CT density of normal fat. Tissue necrosis or hemorrhage in a lipoma, however, may alter the CT density so that the CT appearance may not permit a diagnosis of benign versus malignant fatty tumor. Benign retroperitoneal cysts may have a well-defined margin and a homogeneous CT density that is similar to the CT density of water.

Structures adjacent to retroperitoneal masses, such as the ureters or bladder, may be compressed, displaced, or invaded. CT evidence of obliteration of tissue planes separating a mass from adjacent structures suggests invasion; however, the thickness of the scan and the partial volume effect may make subtle evidence of invasion difficult to determine on CT scans.

CT has been especially helpful in evaluating selected patients with suspected recurrence of tumor in the renal fossa or para-aortic nodes following nephrectomy or recurrence of tumor in the pelvis following cystectomy or after abdominal-perirenal resection (Figs. 47-29, 47-30). In the more immediate postoperative period, CT has also been helpful in detecting abscesses and hematomas. Neoplasm or other abnormalities associated with "mass effect" have the gross form of a mass on CT that is usually recognizable. Infiltration or en plaque tumor, however, may be extremely difficult to differentiate from the reparative process from previous surgery.

HEMORRHAGE

Retroperitoneal hemorrhage may be associated with trauma, leaking aortic aneurysm, aortic dissection, postsurgical procedures, bleeding diathesis, and anticoagulation therapy (Fig. 47-31). Bleeding may also be associated with genitourinary or other neoplasms.

The CT findings of retroperitoneal hemorrhage or hematoma depend on the extent, duration, volume, and source of bleeding. Freshly extravasated blood tends to have higher CT attenuation values than chronic hematomas.[7, 18] The CT density may be inhomogeneous and perhaps related to repeated episodes of bleeding. Bleeding into the retroperitoneal fat appears of higher density than the density of fat and may be indistinguishable from tumor, urine, or abscess. The anatomic location of the blood as seen on CT and the history may be helpful in identifying the origin of the bleeding, such as perinephric hematoma associated with abdominal aortic aneurysm. Ultrasound has also been helpful in defining the characteristics of retroperitoneal hematoma, especially when associated with abdominal aortic aneurysm or in patients with recent aneurysm repair and aortic grafts.

FIBROSIS

Retroperitoneal fibrosis can be characterized by a proliferation of fibroblastic tissue that envelops retroperitoneal structures as well as other sites. In the retroperitoneum, the abnormal tissue encases vessels, ureters, nerves, and also involves fat and muscles. The most common manifestation of the process by conventional radiography is urographic evidence or ureteral deviation and obstruction. Usually the narrowing and obstruction involves the middle or lower third of the ureter.

Of three cases of retroperitoneal fibrosis seen on CT, the findings can be considered virtually diagnostic of the disease in one case and strongly indicative in another. In the third case diagnosed histologically as retroperitoneal fibrosis, both CT scans and surgical inspection showed a bulky mass that was indistinguishable from a large neoplasm such as lymphoma. Abdominal aortic aneurysms with associated para-aortic hematoma have been seen on CT and have mimicked retroperitoneal fibrosis at surgery.

ANEURYSM

The size of the aorta can be measured accurately on CT scans and correlates closely with measurements obtained by ultrasound scanning (Figs. 47-32, 47-33). Ultrasound scanning is commonly used as the primary imaging examination in our practice for the evaluation of the aorta, measurement of abdominal aortic aneurysm, and follow-up of patients with known aneurysm.[5] Visceral artery aneurysms have been diagnosed on CT, although we have had difficulty in proper analysis of some patients with hepatic and splenic artery aneurysms. Faster CT scanners, wider axial range, and intravenous CT angiograms may provide more detailed data about the vascular system. CT has also been helpful in evaluating patients with suspected iliac artery aneurysms. The aortic bifucation and iliac arteries may be difficult to assess on ultrasound, whereas the aortic bifurcation and common iliacs can usually be seen on CT scans (Figs. 47–34, 47–35). One must be careful, however, that the normal bifurcation of the aorta and inferior vena cava and the common iliac vessels are not mistaken for enlarged lymph nodes on CT scans. False or leaking aneurysms also may be accurately assessed by CT (Fig. 47–36).

PELVIS

PROSTATE

Although many prostatic filling defects seen on excretory urograms are easily recognized by the urographer, assessment of prostatic size and extent of tumor frequently does not correlate with the physical and cystoscopic examination or the surgical findings. CT permits a cross-sectional display of anatomy of the bladder base and prostate that cannot be obtained by other radiographic methods. The CT density of the prostate reflects the x-ray attenuation coefficients of prostatic tissue and is affected by the presence of calcification and, occasionally, by fluid-filled cystic spaces within the prostate. Benign prostatic enlargement cannot be distinguished from prostatic cancer by difference in CT density (Figs. 47–37, 47–38).

CT is used in evaluating patients with prostatic cancer to determine extension of neoplasm through the prostatic capsule with involvement of adjacent structures, pelvic nodes, and extrapelvic sites (stages C and D). Intravesical extension of tumor is usually determined cystoscopically. Involvement of the seminal vesicles is a frequent manifestation of extension of neoplasm to adjacent structures (Fig. 47–39). A large percentage (80%) of these patients also have involvement of pelvic nodes.[23] CT examination of patients with prostatic cancer should include a search for enlarged pelvic and retroperitoneal para-aortic nodes (Fig. 47–40).

The seminal vesicles are visualized on CT scans just superior to the prostate and posterior to the bladder. They are paired lobulated structures separated from the bladder by a fat cleavage plane (Fig. 47–41). Invasion of the seminal vesicles by tumor may be recognized on CT as obliteration of the normal fat planes, fixation of the position of the seminal vesicles on supine and prone scans, or a tumor mass involving the glands. Some of these changes may alter the normal seminal vesicle angle.[25] Inflammatory changes involving the seminal vesicles may be indistinguishable from involvement by tumor.

BLADDER

CT can be used in staging bladder neoplasms to determine the extravesical extension of the tumor (stages D, D_1, D_2) (Figs. 47–42, 47–43). The CT examination should be done with the knowledge of the cystoscopic findings and the conduct of the examination should be correlated with the excretory urogram and cystogram. CT scans should be obtained at overlapping intervals (8 to 10 mm.) through the bladder. Contrast medium can be injected intravenously to opacify the bladder; however, if the contrast medium is too dense, intravesical lesions can be obscured (Figs. 47–37, 47–41). Dilute contrast medium can be instilled into the bladder through a catheter. This method also permits control over the degree of bladder distention. CT examination of the gas-filled bladder has been described by Seidelmann and co-workers[24, 26] and Seidelman and Cohen.[23] These authors report a 79 per cent prospective accuracy and 100 per cent retrospective accuracy in staging bladder tumors in 19 patients with surgical confirmation.

UTERINE–CERVICAL–OVARIAN NEOPLASMS

CT is used in patients with these neoplasms to detect occult masses, to evaluate patients with suspected masses, and to define the extent of the disease process.

Some of the CT findings seen with extension of uterine (stages III, IV), cervical (stages II, III, IV), and ovarian (stages Ic, II, III, IV) neoplasms are obliteration of normal fat planes within the pelvis, obliteration of the normal pelvic fossae (rectouterine cul-de-sac, vesicouterine, pararectal, and paravesical), pelvic or para-aortic adenopathy, or extension of tumor along the lateral pelvic wall. A large mass within the pelvis often displaces adjacent structures and makes assessment of displacement versus invasion difficult. The organ of origin of large pelvic masses may also be difficult to determine on CT scans because of displacement of adjacent structures and alterations of normal anatomic relationships (Fig. 47–44).

The uterus is visualized on CT scans and has a wide normal variation of anatomic orientation (Fig. 47–45). The position of the uterus is also affected by the degree of bladder distention. Suspected uterine enlargement as determined by CT should be closely correlated with the findings on physical examination. Parasagittal ultrasound scans also may be helpful when correlated with the cross-sectional CT scans. Blood in the uterine cavity may produce an increased CT density when compared to the CT density of uterine muscle. Uterine leiomyomas are common, often multiple, and may be discovered incidentally on CT scans of the pelvis. Recognition of a uterine fibroid depends on the size and location of the tumor. Calcification within the fibroid is helpful in determing the nature and etiology of the mass. Some fibroids undergo cystic degeneration, and these gross changes can be appreciated on CT scans as altered CT density. Benign leiomyomas cannot be differentiated from leiomyosarcomas by CT characteristics of the tumor. Fluid-filled loops of small bowel, the cecum, and the sigmoid may simulate asymmetric enlargement of the uterus or a mass that appears to alter the normal uterine contour. Obtaining scans in different patient positions, changing the angle of the scanning gantry, or opacifying the bowel may be helpful in differentiating such a pseudomass from a uterine or other pelvic mass. Scans obtained with varying degrees of bladder distention may also help to displace loops of bowel away from the uterus. The usefulness of high-quality sagittal, coronal, and oblique CT reconstruction awaits critical analysis.

Normal ovaries can be visualized on CT scans (Fig. 47–45A). In our experience, however, normal ovaries have not been routinely recognized, probably because of adjacent fluid-filled loops of bowel or because of atrophic changes that occur in older women. Ovarian masses, however, may be assessed on CT scans. The CT appearance depends on the composition of the tumor, that is, cyst, cystic, solid calcified, fatty. These characteristics of ovarian tumors on CT as well as on ultrasound may be helpful in identifying the origin and nature of the lesion, but because of the histology of ovarian neoplasms the differentiation of benign versus malignant may not be possible (Figs. 47–46 to 47–48).

OTHER ABNORMALITIES

Direct extension or seeding of abdominal neoplasms or metastasis from a distant primary may be detected within the pelvis as a soft tissue mass or as involvement of the bony pelvis (Figs. 47–49, 47–50). These patients often are referred for CT scanning because of pelvic pain, neurologic problems, or equivocal physical findings.

CT has been virtually diagnostic in assessing patients whose excretory urogram or barium enema indicates suspected pelvic lipomatosis. The radiographic findings of pelvic lipomatosis may be simulated by pelvic adenopathy. Fat, in pelvic lipomatosis, has a different CT density (minus numbers) than adenopathy due to metastasis or lymphoma. Fatty lymph nodes, however, may have a CT density similar to that of the fat seen in pelvic lipomatosis.

The CT appearance of abdominal, retroperitoneal, or pelvic abscesses depends on the nature, composition, and gross anatomic characteristics of the abscess (Figs. 47–51 to 47–54). CT has been extremely helpful in evaluating patients with suspected peri- or paranephric inflammatory processes and in patients following cystectomy or other pelvic surgery. The cross-sectional CT images frequently provide a more definitive display of the perinephric space than can be obtained from coronal or oblique tomography.[11] Some abscesses contain small collections of gas that are readily detected on CT scans.[6, 7] These collections of gas can usually be identified as extraluminal (outside the bowel), but matted loops of small bowel containing fluid and air and the partial volume effect can cause difficulty in interpretation of the location of gas collections. Additionally, following surgery, extraluminal air may be a source of difficulty in identifying abscesses that contain air. An inflammatory process may present as cellulitis or as dissection of inflammatory fluid into the tissues with obliteration of normal fat planes and interfaces between retroperitoneal or pelvic structures. These CT findings are nonspecific and may be difficult to interpret. Many abscesses, however, become loculated and develop thick fibrous, inflammatory walls. Loculated abscesses often have cystic CT characteristics. CT scans obtained after intravenous injection of contrast medium may show enhancement of adjacent normal tissue and the wall of the abscess. Unless the abscess contains air, sterile fluid collections (sterile abscess, urinoma, lymphocyst) cannot be differentiated on CT scans from an abscess with viable organisms. CT is also potentially useful in following the response of an abscess to antibiotic therapy or in guiding biopsy and aspiration. Haaga and colleagues reported accurate CT detection of 20 of 22 abscesses in 17 patients.[7]

CT has also proved to be of significant value in detecting occult primary tumors or metastases to the spine, sacrum, or pelvis. Anomalies of the sacrum, such as anterior meningocele, may be accurately depicted on CT scans. The soft tissue extent of bone tumors has often been undetected on routine radiographs, but accurately seen on CT scans. Likewise, the extent of benign or malignant soft tissue tumors has been accurately assessed on CT scans. Definition of the soft tissue extent of tumors has provided unique and invaluable information to the surgeon in pretreatment assessment of operability and in planning the extent of the surgical procedure. CT may also be helpful in detecting obscure fractures of the acetabulum, pelvis, and sacrum and in assessing the extent of soft tissue injury and associated pelvic, retroperitoneal, or intra-abdominal hematomas.

CHAPTER 47, ILLUSTRATIONS

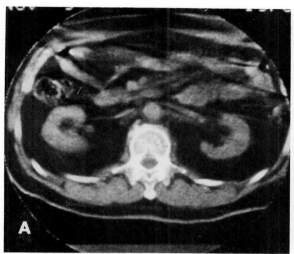

FIG. 47–1. Normal kidneys in retroperitoneal space. **(A)** CT scan at the level of the kidneys demonstrates the renal parenchyma and the renal arteries and veins. **(B)** Retroperitoneal space just inferior to the lower poles of the kidneys. Note the psoas shadows and the relatively large amount of retroperitoneal fat in this patient, as well as the small amount of calcification in the posterior wall of the aorta. The vena cava is undistended. Several normal-sized retroperitoneal nodes are well visualized.

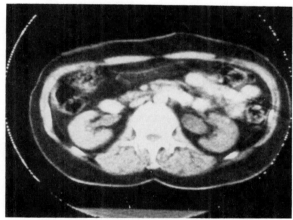

FIG. 47–2. Bilateral normal kidneys with extrarenal type pelves, which are visualized as oval structures in the renal hila. Contrast medium in loops of small bowel and air in the colon illustrate the proximity of adjacent bowel to the kidneys. Loops of bowel may mimic a renal mass of excretory urography or CT.

FIG. 47–3. Normal left kidney following the administration of contrast medium. There is slight malrotation of the left kidney.

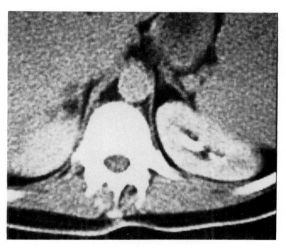

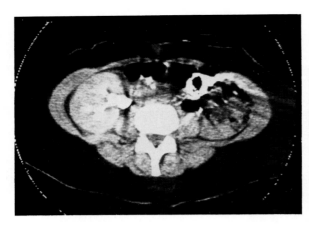

FIG. 47–4. A 45-year-old woman with a palpable right abdominal mass that was thought to be unrelated to the kidney. CT scanning revealed absence of the left kidney and compensatory hypertrophy of the solitary right kidney. No abdominal mass present. The solitary kidney was palpable and accounted for the clinical findings.

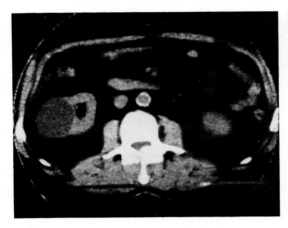

FIG. 47–5. Classic benign simple cyst as demonstrated by an unenhanced CT scan. Note the sharp junction between the cyst and the renal parenchyma. The fluid density of the cyst is uniform, significantly less than that of the renal parenchyma and greater than that of the surrounding fat.

FIG. 47–6. Benign simple cyst. (A) Unenhanced CT scan. In this instance the margin of the cyst and the density differential between the cyst and the renal parenchyma are difficult to ascertain. (B) Contrast enhancement. The cyst wall is now much more clearly defined, and the differential densities of renal parenchyma, renal cyst, and perinephric fat are clearly seen.

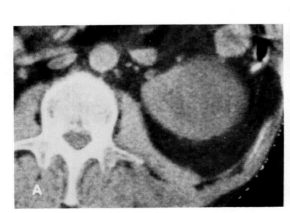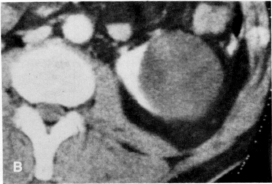

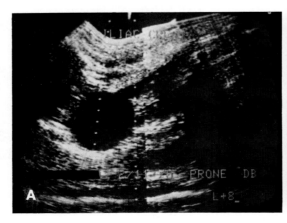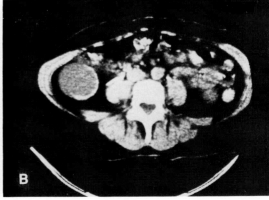

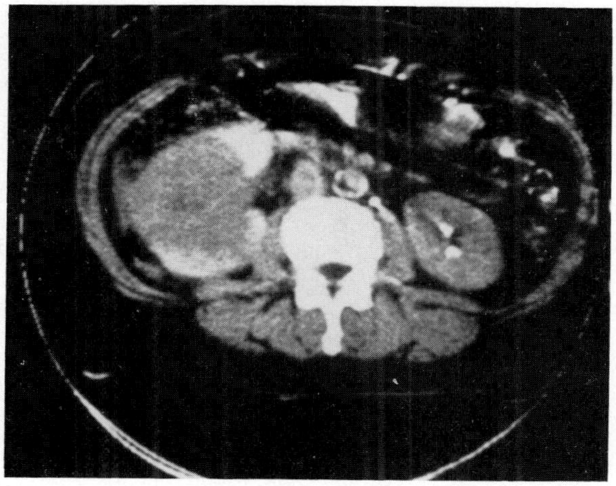

FIG. 47–8. CT scan depicting a large renal cell carcinoma in the midportion of the right kidney with inhomogeneous density throughout the lesion typical of carcinoma. Note the irregular interface between the carcinoma and the opacified parenchyma posteriorly.

FIG. 47–9. A 36-year-old man with a 1-week history of gross hematuria. CT scans in ascending order from the midportion of the kidneys superiorly through the liver. CT scans reveal a huge renal cell carcinoma arising from the superior aspect of the right kidney and extending into the right upper quadrant. CT scans suggest invasion of the liver by the renal cell carcinoma, but a plane of dissection was present at surgery. The interface between the tumor and liver may at times be difficult to determine because of partial volume effect.

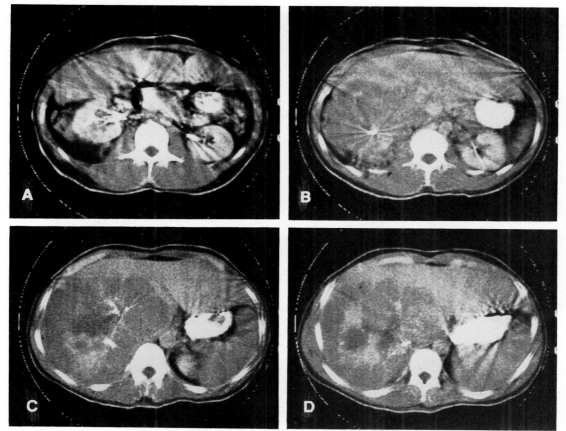

FIG. 47–7. A 59-year-old woman with a benign simple cyst in the right kidney. **(A)** Longitudinal ultrasound B scan reveals a sharply demarcated sonolucent mass with excellent through transmission typical of a benign simple cyst. **(B)** CT scan of the same patient reveals the classic CT findings on an enhanced scan.

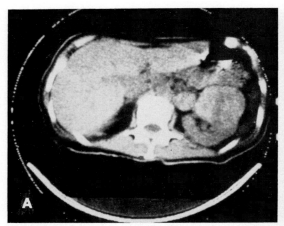

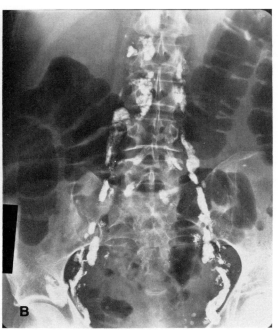

FIG. 47–10. A 55-year-old man with renal mass detected on excretory urography. **(A)** CT scan; typical renal cell carcinoma on unenhanced scan situated anteriorly in the left kidney. There is also a round 2.5-cm. metastatic nodule situated just medial to the renal cell carcinoma, which was not evident on excretory urography. **(B)** Lymphangiogram revealed no evidence of the retroperitoneal metastasis.

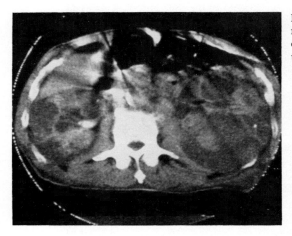

FIG. 47–11. Bilateral polycystic renal disease. Both kidneys are markedly enlarged and filled with radiolucent cysts. The left kidney is partly obscured by linear artifacts created by peristaltic motion of intestinal gas.

FIG. 47–12. The normal adrenal glands are frequently situated at different levels and are therefore visualized on separate CT scans. **(A)** Magnified CT scan revealing a normal triangular-shaped left adrenal situated anterior to the upper pole of the left kidney. **(B)** The right adrenal gland is visualized as an elongated triangle situated in retroperitoneal fat between the right lobe of the liver and the crux of the diaphragm and immediately posterior to the inferior vena cava.

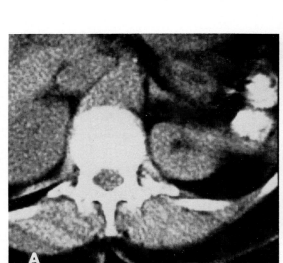

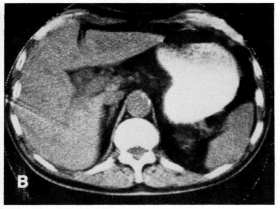

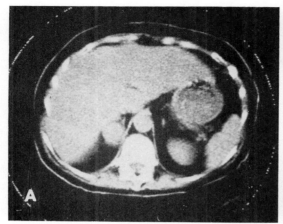

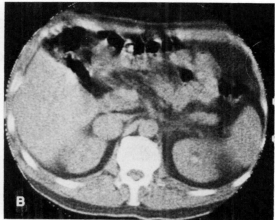

FIG. 47–13. (A) A 60-year-old woman with Cushing's syndrome. A $3 \times 2 \times 2$ cm. adenoma is present in the right adrenal gland. Note that the lesion is located between the right lobe of the liver and the diaphragmatic crux. The upper pole of the left kidney is also visualized on this scan. (B) Right adrenal pheochromocytoma. The position of the tumor is anterior to the upper pole of the right kidney and adjacent to the crux of the diaphragm.

FIG. 47–14. A 52-year-old man with a palpable upper abdominal mass. Large myelolipoma of the right adrenal gland. Areas of low density similar to fat can be seen within the tumor, although the CT density is not uniform, as may be observed in some adrenal lipomas.

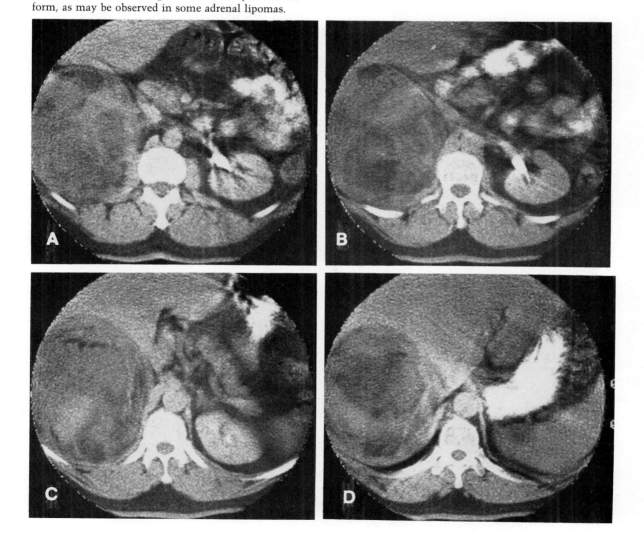

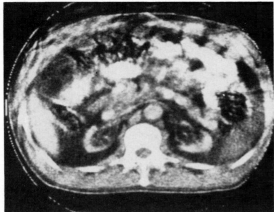

FIG. 47–15. A 51-year-old man with chronic renal insufficiency. CT scan was done to exclude retroperitoneal abscess. No evidence of inflammation. Marked uniform atrophy both kidneys.

FIG. 47–16. Marked atrophy of both kidneys with failure to excrete contrast medium on the right as a result of prior severe obstruction secondary to idiopathic retroperitoneal fibrosis.

FIG. 47–17. Tiny opaque calculus lying within a posterior calyx of the left kidney.

FIG. 47–18. A 59-year-old man with a history of left nephrectomy for renal cell carcinoma. Conventional excretory urography reveals a density in the left renal bed, which raised the question of recurrent renal cell carcinoma versus a bowel loop. CT scanning clearly defined the shadow as being caused by a bowel loop in the renal fossa. Fetal lobulation, right kidney.

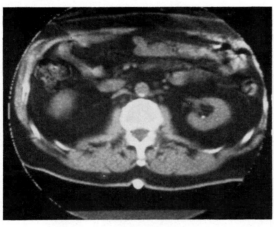

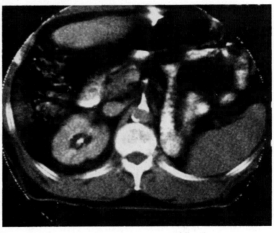

FIG. 47–19. Enlarged retroperitoneal nodes due to lymphoma. **(A)** Hydronephrotic right kidney with back pressure atrophy. **(B)** Dilated urine-filled ureter is visualized adjacent to the right psoas muscle and masses of enlarged nodes.

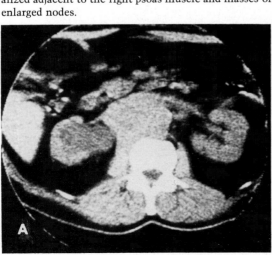

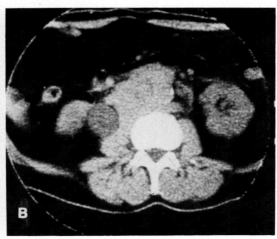

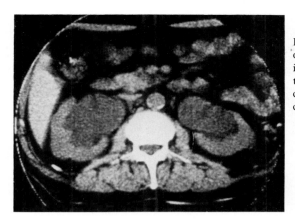

FIG. 47–20. Marked pyelocalyectasis is demonstrated on this unenhanced scan. The thickness of the remaining parenchyma can be accurately assessed in obstruction even if the kidneys fail to excrete contrast medium. The renal outline can also be visualized to determine if the atrophy is uniform or segmental.

FIG. 47–21. Moderately obese man referred for a possible retroperitoneal mass. (**A**) Excretory urogram; left ureter deviated laterally in its upper portion raising the possibility of a retroperitoneal mass. (**B** to **E**) CT scans in descending order from the midportion of the kidneys to the level of L-4. Large amount of retroperitoneal fat is evident but no retroperitoneal mass. CT scanning is the procedure of choice to exclude retroperitoneal disease in this type of case.

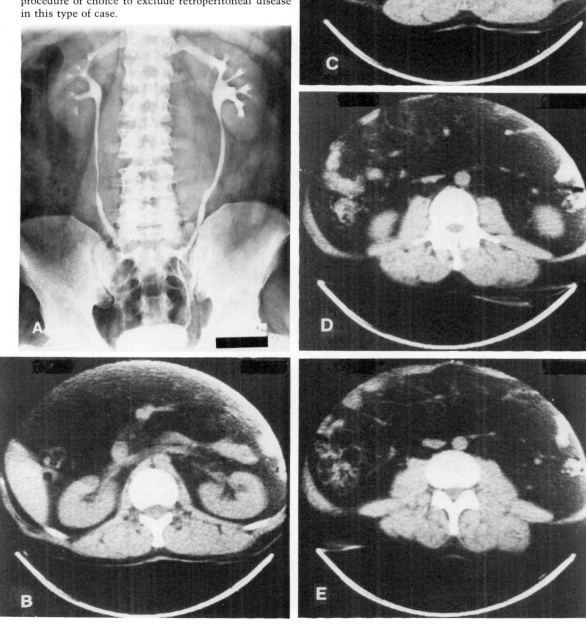

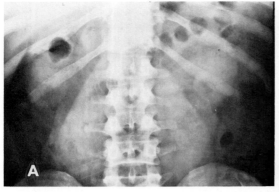

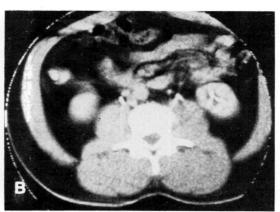

FIG. 47–22. Normal muscular 25-year-old man. **(A)** KUB reveals prominent psoas muscles. **(B)** CT scan at the level of L-2 reveals the lower poles of the kidneys and the prominent psoas and lumbar muscles.

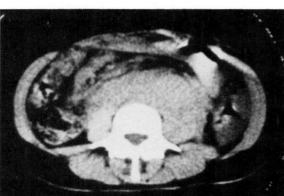

FIG. 47–23. A 34-year-old man with known lymphocytic lymphoma. CT scan reveals confluent disease engulfing the normal anatomic structures of the retroperitoneal space.

FIG. 47–24. A 29-year-old man with nodular lymphoma. **(A)** Retroperitoneal lymphoma with extensive obliteration of the normal retroperitoneal structures and tissue interfaces. **(B)** Contrast-enhanced scan at the level of the kidneys allows definition of the normal vascular structures. The IVC and aorta are displaced anteriorly. Note the involvement of the midportion of the left kidney by lymphoma.

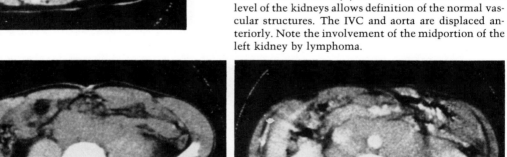

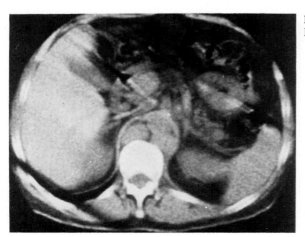

FIG. 47–25. The crura are displaced laterally by enlarged retrocrural lymph nodes.

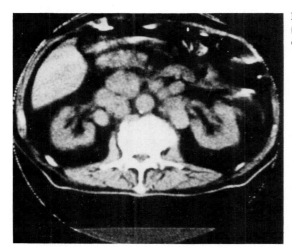

FIG. 47–26. Retroperitoneal para-aortic adenopathy (metastatic transitional cell carcinoma) with multiple discrete enlarged nodes.

FIG. 47–27. A 28-year-old man with known seminoma. **(A, B, C)** Extensive retroperitoneal involvement extending to the left of the midline to involve the kidney **(D, E, F)** Corresponding CT scans 3 months later following radiation therapy. The retroperitoneal mass has virtually disappeared and the left kidney has undergone postobstructive atrophy.

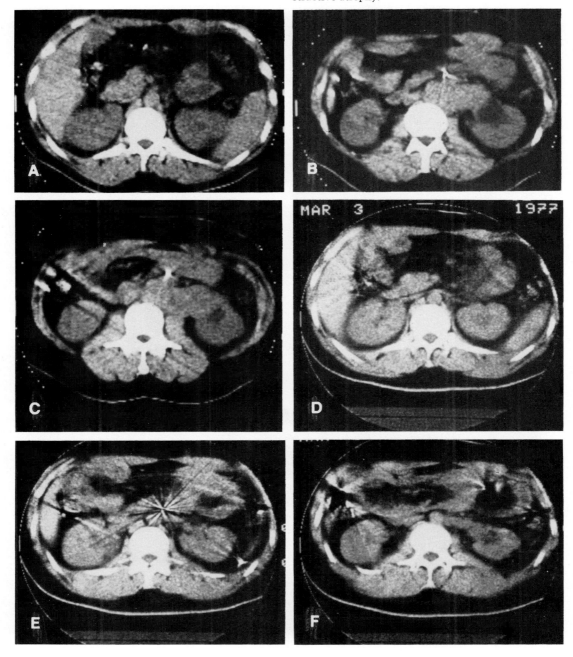

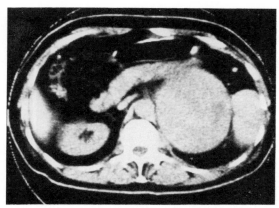

FIG. 47–28. A 43-year-old man with palpable abdominal mass. CT scan demonstrates a 10-cm. retroperitoneal mass of soft tissue density. Pathologic diagnosis: hemangiopericytoma.

FIG. 47–30. Postoperative adenocarcinoma of the rectum. The CT scan shows recurrent tumor posterior to the opacified bladder and extending to the right adjacent to the perirectal fossa.

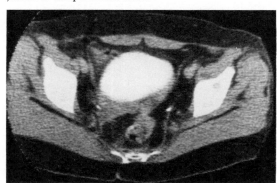

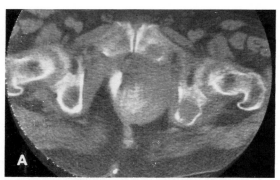

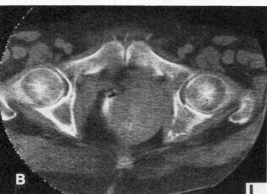

FIG. 47–29. (A, B) Postoperative cystectomy and ureterosigmoidostomy for transitional cell carcinoma of the bladder. Contrast medium in the rectum from an intravenous injection. The rectum is displaced by recurrent neoplasm in the pelvis.

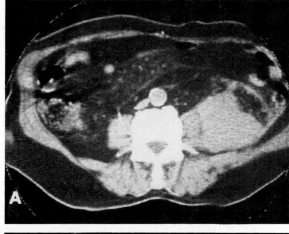

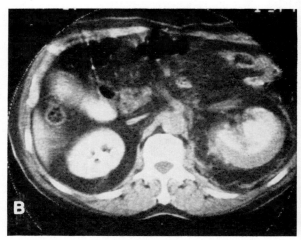

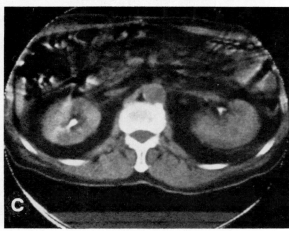

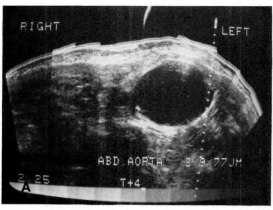

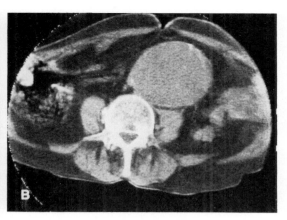

FIG. 47–32. Abdominal aortic aneurysm. **(A)** Ultrasound. **(B)** CT scan. The size of the aneurysm is measured accurately on both examinations.

FIG. 47–33. Four CT scans show a large abdominal aortic aneurysm. The proximal extent of the aneurysm can be seen at the level of the left renal vein.

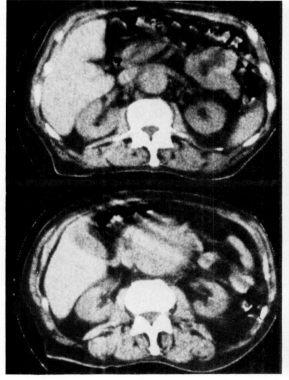

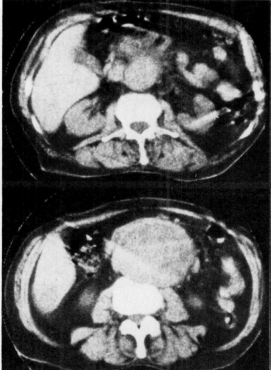

FIG. 47–31. A 52-year-old man admitted to the hospital following an accident. **(A)** CT scan below the level of the kidneys revealed a large soft-tissue density in the left retroperitoneal space due to hemorrhage. **(B)** CT scan on the same patient at the level of the kidneys after the administration of contrast medium reveals a large subcapsular hematoma on the left. The renal parenchyma is compressed and appears dense when compared with the rim of hemorrhage that surrounds the kidney. **(C)** CT scan at the same level as **(B)** obtained 6 weeks after trauma. A small rim of perirenal hematoma remains.

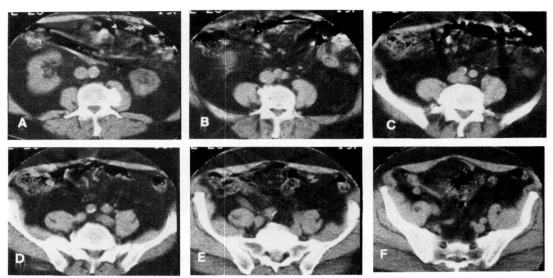

FIG. 47–34. (A) Normal retroperitoneal para-aortic space, aorta, and inferior vena cava. (B, C) Normal scan at the level of the bifurcation of the aorta and inferior vena cava. (D, E, F) Normal scans below the bifurcation with common and internal and external iliac vasculature.

FIG. 47–35. Bilateral iliac artery aneurysms. (A) *Arrow* indicates aneurysm on the right and, in (B), *arrow* indicates aneurysm on the left.

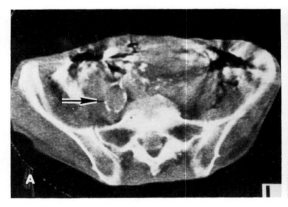

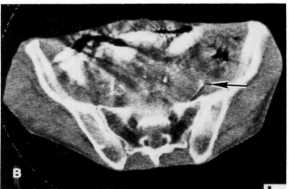

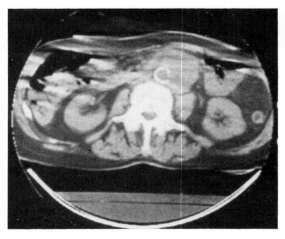

FIG. 47–36. A false mycotic aneurysm can be seen adjacent to the calcified aortic wall and the left psoas muscle.

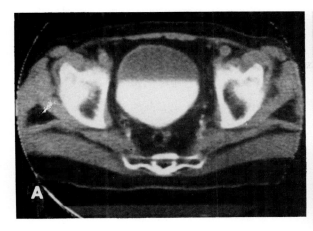

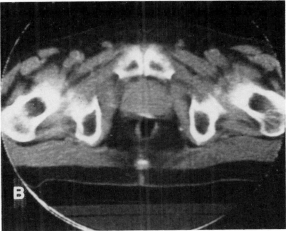

FIG. 47–37. A 59-year-old man. (A) CT scan of the pelvis after the administration of contrast medium revealing layering of contrast medium in the bladder with unopacified urine anteriorly. Note the normal thin wall of the bladder anteriorly. (B) CT scan through the level of symphysis pubis demonstrates a moderate prostatic enlargement.

FIG. 47–38. The normal wall of the bladder and urine–contrast medium interface are shown on the CT scan. The enlarged prostate indents the posterior aspect of the bladder. The enlarged prostate has smooth margins, and the perivesical space and pelvic nodes are normal.

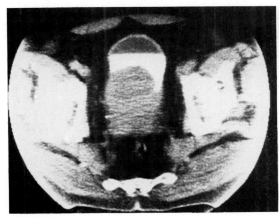

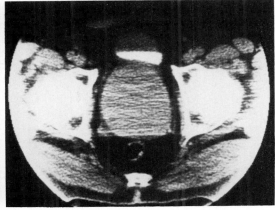

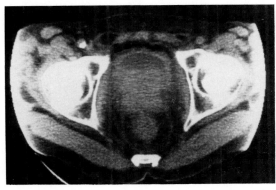

FIG. 47–39. Obliteration of the seminal vesicles and a soft-tissue mass at the bladder base due to lymphomatous infiltration of the prostate.

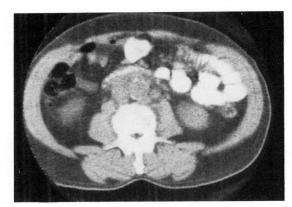

FIG. 47–40. This scan of the retroperitoneum shows discrete enlarged retroperitoneal nodes. Adjacent loops of small bowel opacified with dilute, water-soluble contrast medium can be seen draped over the enlarged mass.

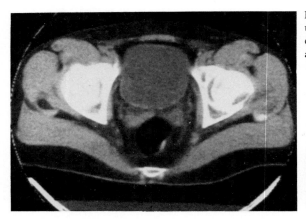

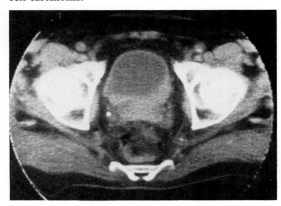

FIG. 47–41. Normal 50-year-old man. CT scan through unopacified distended bladder demonstrating the bladder wall. The paired structures posterior to the bladder are the normal seminal vesicles.

FIG. 47–42. CT scan through the unopacified urinary bladder. Note the thickening of the bladder wall posteriorly on the left secondary to invasion by transitional cell carcinoma.

FIG. 47–43. A 59-year-old woman with known transitional cell carcinoma of the bladder. Pelvic extension suspected clinically. (**A-D**) CT scans ascending through the level of the bladder demonstrate soft-tissue extension of bladder cancer. The tumor arises from the bladder on the right. The extravesical extension spreads superiorly within the pelvis, causing compression of the posterior wall of the bladder. Superiorly (**D**), the tumor attaches to the bony pelvis.

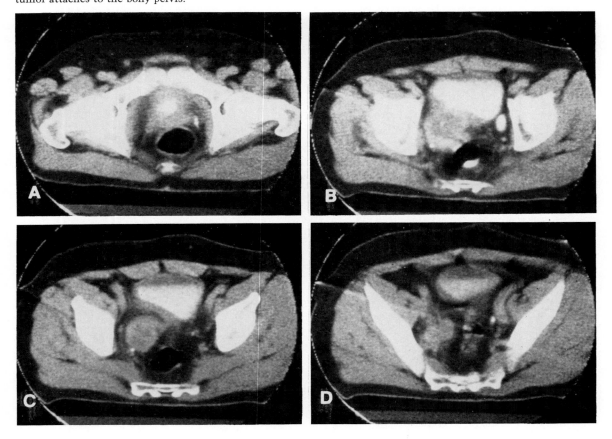

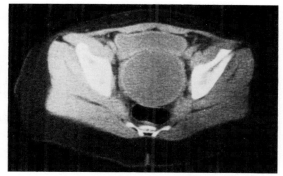

FIG. 47-44. Hematometrocolpos. The wall of the undistended and unopacified urinary bladder is well visualized, as is the wall of the cystic mass posterior to the bladder.

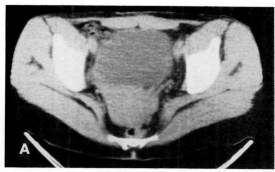

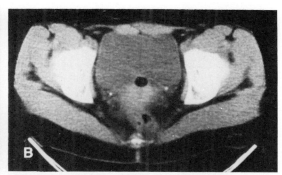

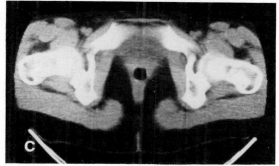

FIG. 47-45. Normal female pelvis. (A) CT scan through the superior aspect of the bladder demonstrating the fundus of the uterus and segments of the broad ligaments. (B) CT scan through the midportion of the bladder and the superior aspect of the vagina. The round radiolucent structure in the center of the scan represents a tampon in the superior aspect of the vagina at the level of the cervix. (C) Scan through the lower vagina at the introitus.

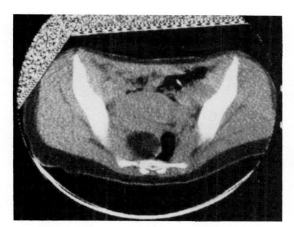

FIG. 47-46. Right ovarian mass posterior to the uterus and adjacent to the air-filled rectum. The CT density indicates a fatty mass consistent with an ovarian dermoid.

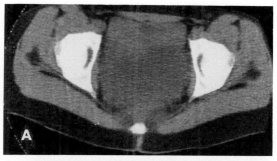

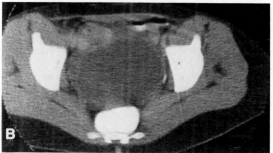

FIG. 47-47. (A) Large cystic mass posterior to the urine-filled bladder. (B) Contrast medium in loops of small bowel and in the rectum can be seen anteriorly and posteriorly to this cystic fluid-filled cystadenoma of the ovary.

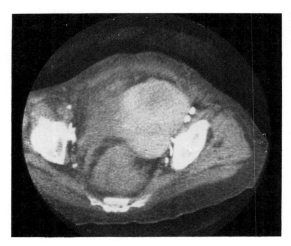

FIG. 47–48. The bladder is distorted and the normal fascial–fatty planes in the pelvis are obliterated by invasive endometrial carcinoma.

FIG. 47–49. Large soft-tissue mass in the pelvis of a 5-year-old boy with known Wilms' tumor. **(A-D)** The large metastasis causes anterior displacement and compression of the urinary bladder. The bladder is opacified and best seen in **(D)**, situated anteriorly and to the right of the metastatic tumor.

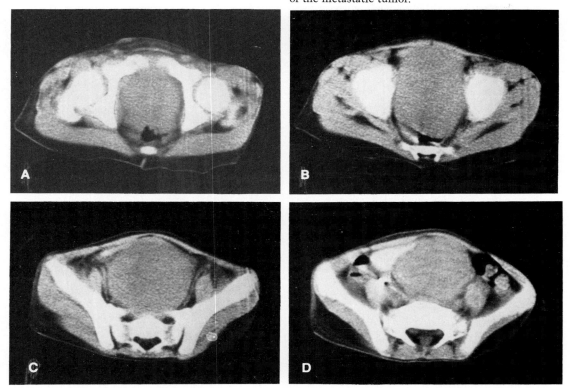

FIG. 47–50. A 49-year-old woman with prior rectal carcinoma. CT scan reveals a large recurrent tumor that causes an impression on the posterior aspect of the left side of the bladder. Note the layering of contrast medium within the bladder. In some patients, postoperative changes and adhesions can be difficult to distinguish from small areas of recurrent tumor in the pelvis.

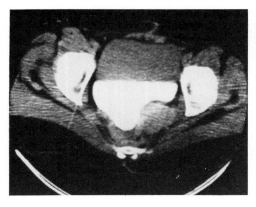

FIG. 47–51. An irregular cystic abscess is seen in the midpelvis. The abscess has a low-density center, and the wall is thick and irregular.

FIG. 47–52. Urine and contrast medium are seen in the bladder. The uterus indents the posterior aspect of the bladder. A thick-walled cystic abscess is seen posterior to the uterus.

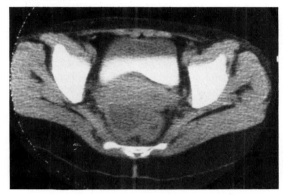

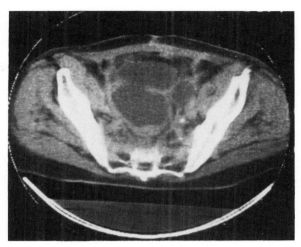

FIG. 47–53. Large mass in the right side of the pelvis contains a small collection of air bubbles that are outside the bowel lumen, indicating an abscess.

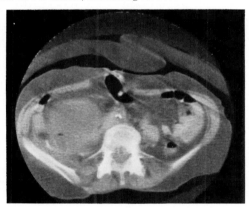

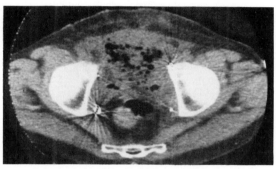

FIG. 47–54. CT scan following cystectomy shows a gas-containing abscess in the space previously occupied by the urinary bladder.

BIBLIOGRAPHY

1. Alfidi, R.J., and Haaga, J.R.: Computed body tomography. Radiol. Clin. North Am., 14:563–570, 1976.
2. Alfidi, R.F., Haaga, J., Meaney, T.F., et al.: Computed tomography of the thorax and abdomen: A preliminary report. Radiology, 117:257–264, 1975.
3. Alfidi, R.J., MacIntyre, W.J., and Haaga, J.R.: The effects of biological motion on CT resolution. Am. J. Roentgenol., 127:11–15, 1976.
4. Daniel, W.W., Jr., Hartman, G.W., Witten, D.M., et al.: Calcified renal masses: A review of ten years experience at the Mayo Clinic. Radiology, 103:503–570, 1972.

5. Fulton, R.E., Stanson, A.W., Forbes, G.S., et al.: Vascular Imaging. In Allen, Barker, Hines (editors): Peripheral vascular disease. W.B. Saunders, Philadelphia (in press).
6. Hagga, J.R., and Reich, N.E.: Intra-abdominal abscesses. In Haaga, J.R., and Reich, N.E.: Computed tomography of abdominal abnormalities, Chap. 8. Saint Louis, C.V. Mosby, 1978.
7. Haaga, J.R., Alfidi, R.J., Havrilla, T.R., et al.: CT detection and aspiration of abdominal abscesses. Am. J. Roentgenol., 128:465–474, 1977.
8. Haaga, J.R., Zelch, M.G., Alfidi, R.J., et al.: CT guided antegrade pyelography and percutaneous nephrostomy. Am. J. Roentgenol., 128:621–624, 1977.
9. Harell, G.S., Breiman, R.S., Glatstein, E.J., et al.: Computed tomography of the abdomen in the malignant lymphomas. Radiol. Clin. North Am., 15:391–400, 1977.
10. Hattery, R.R., Williamson, B., Jr., and Hartman, G.W.: Urinary tract tomography. Radiol. Clin. North Am., 14:23–49, 1976.
11. Hattery, R.R., Williamson, B., Jr., and Hartman, G.W.: CT of the genitourinary tract and retroperitoneum. In Witten, D.M., Myers, G.H., Utz, D.C. (eds.): Emmett's Clinical Urography, Vol. 1, 4th ed. W.B. Saunders, Philadelphia, 1977.
12. Hattery, R.R., Williamson, B., Jr., Stephens, D.H., et al.: Com-

puted tomography of renal abnormalities. Radiol. Clin. North Am., 15:401–418, 1977.

13. Hounsfield, G.N.: Picture quality of computed tomography. Am. J. Roentgenol., 127:3–9, 1976.

14. Kreel, L.: The EMI whole body scanner in the demonstration of lymph node enlargement. Clin. Radiol., 27:421–429, 1976.

15. McCullough, E.C., Payne, J.T., Baker, H.L., Jr., et al.: Performance evaluation and quality assurance of computed tomography scanners, with illustrations from the EMI, ACTA, and Delta scanners. Radiology, 120:173–188, 1976.

16. Pickering, R.S., Hattery, R.R., Hartman, G.W., et al.: Computed tomography of the excised kidney. Radiology, 113:643–647, 1974.

17. Redman, H.C., Federal, W.A., Castellino, R.A., et al.: Computerized tomography as an adjunct in the staging of Hodgkin's and non-Hodgkin's lymphoma. Radiology, 124:381–385, 1977.

18. Sagel, S.S., Siegel, M.J., Stanley, R.J., et al.: Detection of retroperitoneal hemorrhage by computed tomography. Am. J. Roentgenol., 129:403–407, 1977.

19. Sagel, S.S., Stanley, R.J., and Evens, R.G.: Early clinical experience with motionless whole-body computed tomography. Radiology, 119:321–330, 1976.

20. Sagel, S.S., Stanley, R.J., Levitt, R.G., et al.: Computed tomography of the kidney. Radiology, 124:359–370, 1977.

21. Schaner, E.G., Head, G.L., Doppman, J.L., et al.: Computed tomography in the diagnosis, staging, and management of abdominal lymphoma. J. Computer Assisted Tomography, (2) 1:176–180, 1977.

22. Schellinger, D., DiChiro, G., Axelbaum, S.P., et al.: Early clinical experience with the ACTA scanner. Radiology, 114:257–261, 1975.

23. Seidelmann, F.E., and Cohen, W.N.: Pelvis. In Haaga, J.R., Reich, N.E.: Computed tomography of abdominal abnormalities, Chap. 5. St. Louis, C.V. Mosby, 1978.

24. Seidelmann, F.E., Cohen, W.N., and Bryan, P.J.: Computed tomographic staging of bladder neoplasms. Radiol. Clin. North Am., 15:419–440, 1977.

25. Seidelmann, F.E., Reich, N.E., Cohen, W.N., et al.: Computed tomography of the seminal vesicles and the seminal vesicle angle. Comp. Axial Tomog., 1(4):281–285, 1977.

26. Seidelmann, F.E., Temes, S.P., Cohen, W.N., et al.: Computed tomography of the gas-filled bladder: Method of staging bladder neoplasms. Urology, 9:337–344, 1977.

27. Sheedy, P.F., II, Stephens, D.H., Hattery, R.R., et al.: Computed tomography of the body: initial clinical trial with the EMI prototype. Am. J. Roentgenol., 127:23–51, 1976.

28. Stanley, R.J., Sagel, S.S., and Levitt, R.G.: Computed tomography of the body: early trends in application and accuracy of the method. Am. J. Roentgenol., 127:53–67, 1976.

29. Stephens, D.H., Hattery, R.R., and Sheedy, P.F., II: Computed tomography of the abdomen: Early experience with the EMI body scanner. Radiology, 119:331–335, 1976.

30. Stephens, D.H., Sheedy, P.F., II, Hattery, R.R., et al.: Diagnosis and evaluation of retroperitoneal tumors by computed tomography. Am. J. Roentgenol., 129:395–402, 1977.

31. Stephens, D.H., Williamson, B., Jr., Sheedy, P.F., II, et al.: Computed tomography of the retroperitoneal space. Radiol. Clin. North Am., 15:377–390, 1977.

32. Twigg, H.L., Axelbaum, S.P., and Schellinger, D.: Computerized body tomography with the ACTA scanner. J.A.M.A., 234:314, 1975.

33. Williamson, B., Jr., Hattery, R.R., Stephens, D.H., et al.: CT of the kidneys. Semin. Roentgenol., 13(3):249–255, 1978.

Part Nine

PEDIATRIC UROLOGY

Vesicoureteral reflux is defined as a spontaneous retrograde passage of urine from the bladder into the ureter through an incompetent ureterovesical junction. The phenomenon is generally regarded as always abnormal even if it occurs in asymptomatic persons (Figs. 48–1, 48–2). Although the opinions are not uniform as to its clinical importance, the prevailing view is that it is a significant abnormality in that it predisposes to urinary stasis, to urinary tract infections, and eventually to chronic pyelonephritis (Figs. 48–8 to 48–10).

METHODS FOR DEMONSTRATING REFLUX

Reflux can be demonstrated by simple cystography, voiding cystourethrography, and the isotope cystogram. *Voiding cystourethrography* is the method of choice. It may be carried out in the conventional way with the use of regular films or under fluoroscopic control (image amplification) with selected spot filming, cineroentgenography, or videotaping of the appropriate area during filling and emptying of the bladder. The procedure is simple and nontraumatic and can be carried out at any age, without need of anesthesia or sedation. The technical aspects of the procedure are discussed elsewhere in the book.

ANATOMY AND FUNCTION OF THE URETEROVESICAL JUNCTION

The way the ureter terminates in the bladder is of primary importance in the prevention of reflux. The ureter at first runs through the muscular coat of the bladder almost perpendicularly (intramural) and

48

Vesico-ureteral Reflux

GUIDO CURRARINO

then continues downward submucosally (intravesical) for some distance to end in the ureteral orifice. This submucosal tunnel varies in length from 0.5 cm. in the newborn to 2 cm. in adults. It contains only longitudinal muscle fibers, as opposed to the muscle fibers of the extravesical ureter, which are both circular and longitudinal. Some of the muscle fibers of the intramural ureter go to the opposite ureteral orifice, forming the intraureteric ridge, whereas others fan out to terminate in the trigone.

The ureterovesical junction functions as a flap valve in that it allows a free downflow of the urine carried by the peristaltic ureteral waves but prevents reflux. This competence is assured by an apposition of the roof of the submucosal tunnel to its floor caused by the intravesical hydrostatic pressure and probably also by the action of the intrinsic musculature of the area. Other contributing factors include a proper flexibility, length, and diameter of the ureteral tunnel and a good backing of this tunnel by the bladder musculature.

TYPES OF REFLUX

Reflux must occur because of a disruption of the normal anatomy and/or function of the ureterovesical junction. A number of local causes, some congenital, others acquired, have been mentioned, and accordingly several types of reflux are recognized. They can be divided into secondary and primary.

SECONDARY REFLUX

This includes the so-called iatrogenic reflux that may follow surgery on the ureterovesical junction and the reflux that occurs in patients with neurogenic bladder, posterior urethral valves, or other unquestionable lower urinary tract obstructions. In many instances, superimposed infection initiates or contributes to the degree of reflux. This reflux is undoubtedly a secondary phenomenon but the mechanism whereby it occurs is not always clear. According to Hutch,[17] the increased intravesical pressure caused by the underlying disease may give rise to an intermittent or permanent herniation of the bladder mucosa slightly above and lateral to the ureteral meatus, an area where normally the bladder mucosa is supported least strongly by bladder musculature. This saccule or Hutch diverticulum causes a displacement of the intramural ureter to an extravesical position, and this in turn results in shortening of the tunnel and therefore reflux (Figs. 48–15, 48–16). The fact that reflux in patients with neurogenic bladder or a gross lower urinary tract obstruction is far from constant and is often unilateral also raises the suggestion that some additional factor such as infection or a congenital weakness of the area may play a part.

PRIMARY REFLUX

This type is defined as that reflux that occurs in the absence of any of the foregoing causes. It is by far the most frequent type. It is commonly believed that it results from a malformation, possibly congenital, of the ureterovesical junction. This type of reflux is rare in Black Americans. It occurs in about 1 per cent of White girls and is much less common in boys. It is sometimes familial and may occur in more than one generation in the same family, suggesting an inherited basis. The local causes may be one or more of the following:

1. Enlargement of the ureteral orifice
2. Short or absent intravesical ureter
3. Poor backing of the intravesical ureter by a bladder that is too thin or that is weakened by a primary periureteral diverticulum
4. Improper fixation of the intravesical ureter to the trigone
5. Ectopia lateralis in which the ureteral orifice is more laterally placed than normal within the bladder. These orifices are particularly prone to reflux. The anomaly may be unilateral or bilateral. When it occurs in duplicated upper tracts, the affected ureter is regularly the one draining the lower renal complex.
6. Vesical edema from infection, foreign body, stones, or other causes may result in reflux because of a decreased collapsibility of the intravesical ureter.
7. Infection also plays a large part in the causation of reflux, as shown by the observation that reflux is seen more often in the presence of urinary tract infection than when infection is under control. This, however, does not necessarily indicate that infection is the sole cause of reflux. Most clinical and experimental observations are perhaps better explained by the concept of a marginally competent ureterovesical junction. These ureterovesical junctions are competent under normal conditions but may allow reflux at a time of an infection, in particular cystitis, because of the resulting local edema and stiffening of the intramural ureter.

EFFECTS OF REFLUX

UPPER TRACT DILATATION

Reflux often is associated with a dilatation of the affected upper tract. In most cases the changes can be explained entirely by the reflux and the back pressure transmitted from the bladder. In other instances the upper tract dilatation may represent an associated anomaly caused by the faulty development of the ureteral bud from which both the ureterovesical junction and ureter originate. This situation is suspected particularly when reflux is associated with extreme elongation and tortuosity of the ureter but only mild-to-moderate ureterectasis (see Fig. 48–14).

URETEROPELVIC JUNCTION OBSTRUCTION

The regurgitation of contrast medium from the bladder into the upper tracts frequently is accompanied by a ballooning of the pelvicalyceal system that is out of proportion to the ureterectasis. In most instances the phenomenon is transient, the renal pelvis empties promptly, and the excretory urogram shows no discrepancy between the size of the pelvis and that of the ureter. The finding may reflect an increased elasticity of the upper collecting system that is of obscure origin. In other patients, the same gross distention of the pelvicalyceal system during cystourethrography occurs in association with a partial obstruction of the ureteropelvic junction, evidenced by the delayed emptying of the upper collecting system both in the cystourethrogram and in the excretory urogram (Figs. 48–18, 48–19). In some cases this type of obstruction is probably secondary to reflux and may be related to kinks of the ureter or to an overlying aberrant vessel or band that has become significant during the progression of the hydronephrosis and hydroureter (Fig. 48–17). In other instances a primary ureteropelvic junction obstruction may coexist as an associated anomaly (Fig. 48–20).

FUNCTIONAL URETEROVESICAL JUNCTION OBSTRUCTION

During the course of the disease some patients with reflux develop an obstruction at the ureterovesical junction (Fig. 48–22). In spite of the obstruction, the reflux as a rule continues. On direct inspection the ureteral meatus and the distal ureter usually are not narrowed and may even be patulous, a finding that suggests a functional basis for the phenomenon (Fig. 48–21). The cause of this form of obstruction is not entirely clear. An extravesiculation of the intramural ureter may be responsible for the

finding in some cases. The roentgenographic appearance of the distal end of the ureter varies. Commonly the ureter narrows abruptly at its junction with the bladder. Sometimes there is a thin, ring-like narrowing or a kink in the ureter approximately 1 cm. from the bladder wall, or there is a narrowing of the distal 1 or 2 cm. of the ureter. A bladder diverticulum adjacent to the ureterovesical junction sometimes is demonstrable.

URINARY STASIS AND INFECTION

Reflux may be responsible for stasis of urine in the bladder and ureter. The bladder stasis produced by reflux (false bladder residue) refers to the urine returned from the ureter to the bladder after complete emptying of the bladder. Ureteral stasis refers to the urine remaining in the ureter after reflux has taken place because of ureteral dilatation, kinks, atonicity, or because of some ureterovesical junction obstruction.

INTRARENAL REFLUX

In the films of a cystourethrogram demonstrating reflux up to the calyces, one notices on occasion that contrast material also refluxes in the pyramids and renal parenchyma (pyelotubular and interstitial backflow). This phenomenon is uncommon and usually transient. It is seen mainly in infants and only when the vesicoureteral reflux is moderately severe or marked.

URINARY TRACT INFECTION AND RENAL ATROPHY

Urinary stasis in any part of the urinary tract favors growth of bacteria. Reflux of infected urine from the bladder to the ureter may lead to retrograde spread of infection to the renal parenchyma (pyelonephritis) by intrarenal reflux.

Focal or diffuse renal atrophy is known to occur in association with reflux, but the cause–effect relation of the two is not uniform. There is evidence to suggest that, in most cases, it is not the reflux *per se* that causes renal atrophy but the accompanying infection (see Figs. 48–10, 48–11). A notable exception is the reflux that occurs at high vesical pressures from severe lower urinary tract obstruction, neurogenic bladder, or other causes, where reflux may be the sole cause of renal atrophy, as seen in the newborn infant with severe posterior valves and renal atrophy but no previous infections. In summary, the cause of loss of renal parenchyma associated with reflux is not clear. It may relate to any one or a combination of factors including infection, severity of the reflux, the increased ureteral pressure occurring during reflux, the association of tubular backflow with reflux, or the stage of renal development at the time reflux commences.

SEVERITY OF REFLUX

Reflux is considered *mild* when it occurs only at high intravesical pressure (as during voiding), when only a segment of ureter is opacified (see Fig. 48–12), when the regurgitation is fleeting or not easily reproducible, when it is not associated with ureteral dilatation, and when it occurs in the presence of a normal excretory urogram. Reflux is considered *severe* when the regurgitation is constant and abundant, when it occurs at low pressures or low volumes, when it fills the entire upper tract, when the ureter is grossly dilated and elongated, when the ureteral peristalsis is decreased or absent, and when marked ureterectasis and hydronephrosis are present in the excretory urogram (see Figs. 48–13, 48–14). Between these extremes are all combinations of findings and grades of severity. The severity of the reflux may also be expressed more briefly as grade I when the reflux extends up to only part of the ureter without dilatation, grade II when the reflux extends up to the calyces without dilatation and grade III when the reflux up to the calyces is accompanied by mild (grade IIIA), moderate (grade IIIB), or severe (grade IIIC) dilatation. The preceding grades II, IIIA, IIIB, and IIIC are also referred to as IIA, IIB, III, and IV, respectively.

As a rule the changes in the upper tracts in patients with reflux are more pronounced in the cystourethrogram than in the excretory urogram. When reflux occurs at low pressures it is exaggerated during voiding, but exceptions to this rule are common (see Fig. 48–5).

In comparing the degree of severity of reflux in serial examinations, it is important to compare similar studies carried out under similar conditions. A comparison of the findings of a cystogram with those of an excretory urogram or a comparison of the finding of a simple cystogram with those obtained during voiding may lead to misinterpretations.

PECULIARITIES OF REFLUX

Reflux often behaves in an unpredictable fashion regardless of its cause. As already mentioned, reflux is commonly unilateral even in patients with a severe lower tract obstruction or a neurogenic bladder disease. In the presence of a duplicated upper tract with both ureters draining into the bladder, reflux is often limited to the ureter that drains the lower renal pelvis (see Figs. 48–6 to 48–9). When reflux involves more than one ureter it may be more severe in one than in the other.

Reflux may occur during filling of the bladder (low pressure or passive reflux) or only during voiding (high pressure or active reflux) (see Figs. 48–4, 48–5). It may be more marked, or it may occur only in the presence of an added factor, such as active infection, a drainage catheter in the bladder, or recent bladder surgery.

Once demonstrated, reflux can be reproduced in a repeated study in most cases, although not in all. When reproducible, its severity may not be the same even if the examination is carried out under identical conditions. In one examination reflux may be present only in one ureter, whereas in another examination it may occur in a different ureter or in both (see Fig. 48–5).

Possible factors responsible for these vagaries include normal variations in the degree of development of the ureterovesical junctions, differences in the location or the severity of the primary ureterovesical junction abnormality, and transient diminution in the degree of competence of one or more junctions because of superimposed urinary infection, a transient increase in the resistance of the bladder outlet or other causes.

INDICATIONS FOR SEARCH FOR REFLUX

Reflux should be suspected in all patients with recurrent urinary tract infection. A voiding cystogram is generally recommended even at the first documented urinary tract infection, especially in boys. Reflux should also be suspected in patients with known lower urinary tract obstruction, cord bladder disease, deficient abdominal musculature, and following surgical procedures on the ureterovesical junction.

Search for reflux should be carried out in the presence of certain abnormalities in the excretory urogram, including absent or poor renal function in uremic patients; unilateral absence of renal function, with or without a renal mass; decreased renal parenchyma, localized or diffuse, with or without decrease in renal function; an apparently isolated hydronephrosis; hydroureter with or without pelvicalyectasis; and bladder abnormalities, such as trabeculation, filling defects, stones, displacement, and others. The finding of reflux may obviate retrograde studies in some of these situations and may clarify the diagnosis and influence the course of therapy in others.

Additional urographic clues suggesting that reflux may be present include the finding of a decrease in renal function in the early films with good visualization of the upper tract in later films of the series due to regurgitation of opacified urine from the bladder and the presence of longitudinal striations in the renal pelvis and the proximal ureter (see Figs. 48–3, 48–4). The latter finding probably represents mucosal wrinkles occurring when a dilated pelvis and ureter are seen in a partially collapsed state. In patients with reflux the excretory urogram may show only borderline findings such as dilatations of the lower portion of the ureter, mild fullness of the ureter, mild ureteral tortuosity, and opacification of the entire ureter in more than one film.

In many patients with reflux the intravenous pyelogram is entirely normal—hence the rule that *search for reflux by voiding cystourethrography should be carried out when otherwise clinically indicated, even when the intravenous pyelogram is normal* (Figs. 48–1, 48–2).

Failure to demonstrate reflux at one examination does not exclude its presence. When reflux is suspected on clinical grounds but is not demonstrated, a reexamination may be warranted.

Once reflux is demonstrated, postvoiding films should be obtained to determine whether or not the affected ureter empties promptly, and the lower urinary tract should be evaluated completely, especially in males, to detect an underlying cause.

Cystoscopic findings that should suggest the presence of reflux include enlarged or laterally placed ureteral orifices, enlargement of the bladder and/or trigone, bladder trabeculations, bladder diverticula, and urethral obstructions.

PROGNOSIS AND TREATMENT

The reflux occurring in cord bladder disease and severe lower tract obstruction tends to persist and progress. Following correction of the obstruction, mild reflux sometimes subsides completely. Severe reflux may improve, but it seldom disappears. In the absence of a demonstrable obstruction, mild reflux may disappear with conservative therapy alone, but severe reflux tends to persist and progress. The spontaneous improvement or disappearance of reflux observed in some circumstances has been attributed to a progressive increase, with age, in the length of the intravesical ureteral segment and a strengthening of its musculature. This normal continuing "maturation of the ureterovesical junction" may explain the relative infrequency of reflux and recurrent urinary infections in adults as compared to infants and children.

Adequate chemotherapy to control infection and surgical correction of any gross lower-tract obstruction that may be present are the two most important therapeutic measures agreed upon by all authors. Other measures advocated include one or more of the following, the combinations varying with the authors: (1) correction of any lower tract obstruction; (2) special surgical procedure on the affected ureterovesical junction designed to stop reflux; (3) voiding training with frequent voiding during the day, restriction of fluid at night, voiding during the night, double and triple voiding, and voiding without straining; (4) prolonged bladder or ureteral drainage in some cases; and (5) urinary diversion. A discussion of these procedures and of the results claimed with the various methods of treatment is beyond the scope of this chapter.

CHAPTER 48, ILLUSTRATIONS

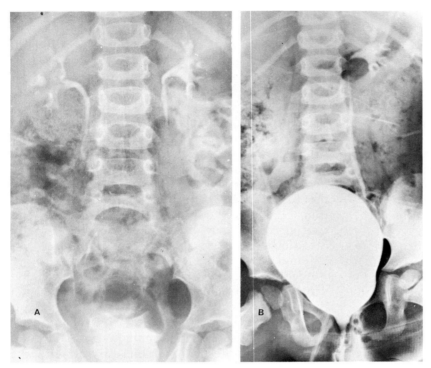

FIG. 48–1. (A) Normal IVU. **(B)** Voiding cysto-urethrogram in same patient – reflux on the left; bladder, bladder neck, and urethra are normal (nonobstructive, high-pressure reflux). A normal excretory urogram does not exclude reflux.

FIG. 48–2. (A) IVU. Ureters are minimally dilated and visualized throughout their entirety. **(B)** Cysto-urethrogram in same patient – bilateral reflux.

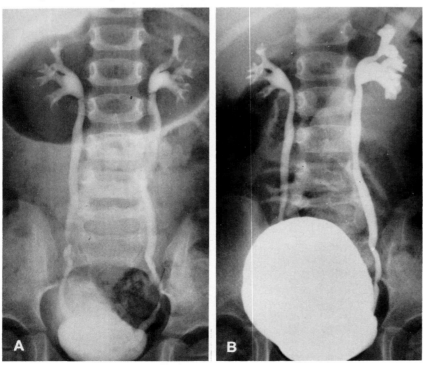

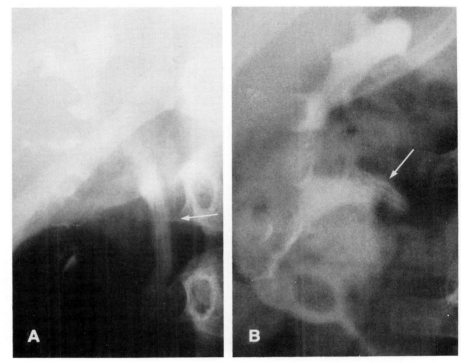

FIG. 48–3. IVU in two patients showing longitudinal striations in the pelvis and proximal ureter, a finding frequently associated with reflux.

FIG. 48–4. (A, B) IVU in a child with reflux. Note longitudinal striations in the renal pelvis and upper ureter on the left (*arrows*). **(C)** No reflux by simple cystography. **(D)** Voiding cystourethrogram; bilateral reflux is more marked on the left than on the right; no evidence of lower-tract obstruction.

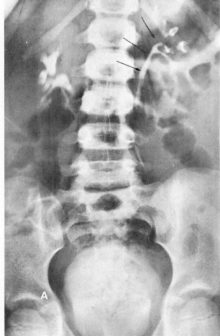

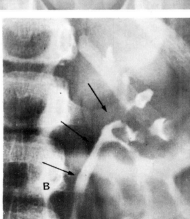

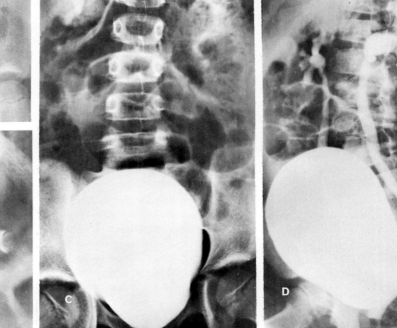

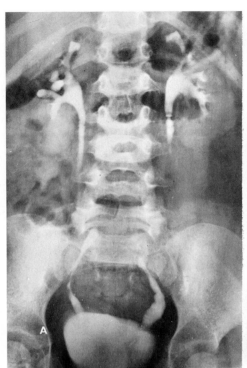

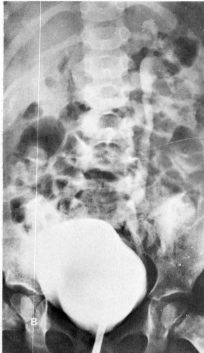

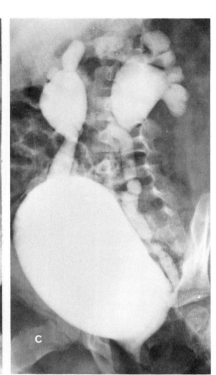

FIG. 48–5. (A) IVU in a child with reflux; mild dilatation of the upper tracts, especially the distal segment of the left ureter. **(B)** Cystogram (15 cm. of water pressure); low-pressure reflux on the left. **(C)** Voiding cystourethrogram, reflux on the right during voiding (high-pressure reflux) and increase in the reflux on the left. No lower urinary tract obstruction (nonobstructive reflux). Note difference in size of the upper tracts in IVU and voiding cystogram.

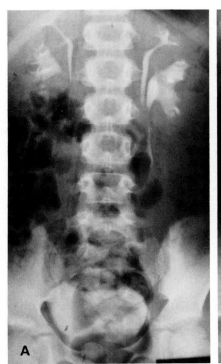

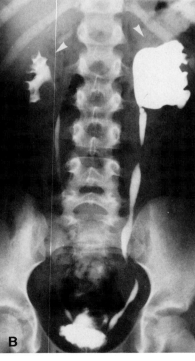

FIG. 48–6. (A) IVU; bilateral duplication. **(B)** Cystourethrogram, reflux limited to the lower complexes. When reflux occurs only in one of the duplicated upper tracts and both ureters terminate in the bladder, the reflux affects more commonly the ureter draining the lower renal pelvis than the ureter draining the upper pelvis.

FIG. 48–9. (A) IVU in a child with duplicated left upper tract, both ureters draining into the bladder. Signs of chronic pyelonephritis are evident in the lower half of the left kidney (*arrows*). **(B)** Bilateral retrograde pyelogram. **(C)** Cystogram (15 cm. of water pressure); reflux limited to the lower complex. The reflux takes place during filling of the bladder (low-pressure reflux). The affected upper tract balloons out during reflux. The bladder is enlarged and smooth in outline.

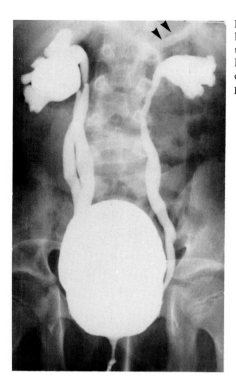

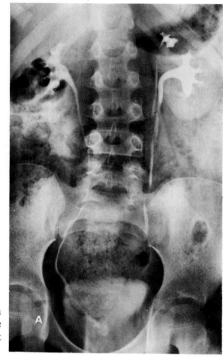

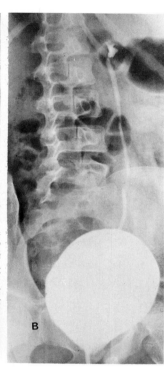

FIG. 48–7. Cystourethrogram in a 7-year-old girl with bilateral duplication. Reflux into both complexes on the right and reflux limited to the lower complex on the left. The visualized pelvis and calyces on the left are displaced downward by the nonopacified upper complex (*arrows*).

FIG. 48–8. (A) Normal IVU in a child with duplication of the left upper tract and both ureters draining into the bladder. **(B)** Cystogram (15 cm. of water pressure), reflux limited to the upper complex (unusual).

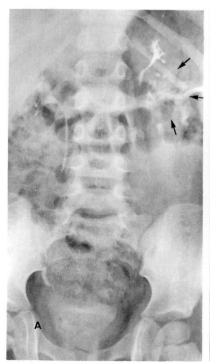

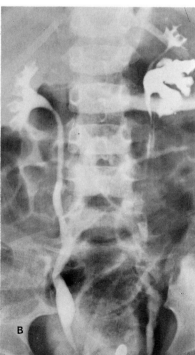

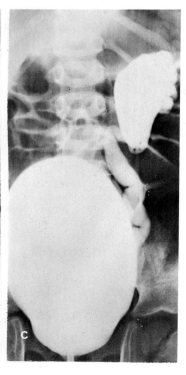

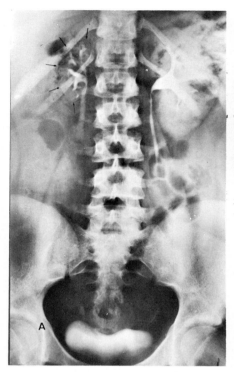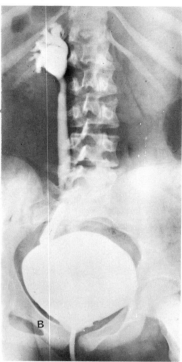

FIG. 48–10. (A) IVU in a child with chronic atrophic pyelonephritis on the right (*arrows*). **(B)** Cysto-urethrogram, low-pressure reflux on the right. In most cases, chronic atrophic pyelonephritis is associated with reflux. The affected ureters are often of normal size or dilated only mildly.

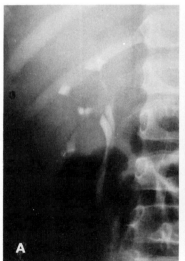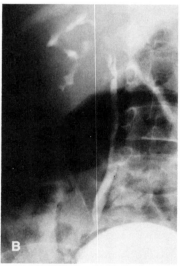

FIG. 48–11. (A) IVU; focal renal atrophy, presumably from previous pyelonephritis. **(B)** Cystogram; reflux into same system.

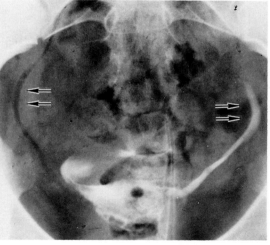

FIG. 48–12. Mild reflux on the left seen only in this postvoiding film (*arrows*). Note also reflux of air into the right ureter (*arrows*). Some air is often introduced into the bladder during catheterization and, together with the contrast material, is usually expelled at the end of voiding.

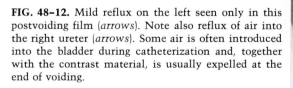

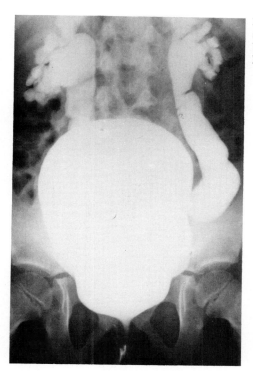

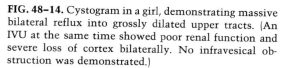

FIG. 48–13. Cystourethrogram in a girl, demonstrating severe bilateral reflux into dilated upper tracts. The bladder is large and smooth, as described in the "megalocystis syndrome."

FIG. 48–14. Cystogram in a girl, demonstrating massive bilateral reflux into grossly dilated upper tracts. (An IVU at the same time showed poor renal function and severe loss of cortex bilaterally. No infravesical obstruction was demonstrated.)

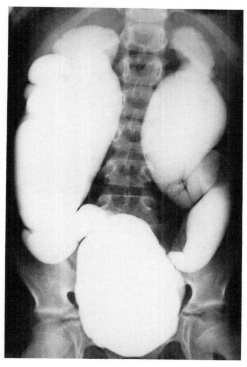

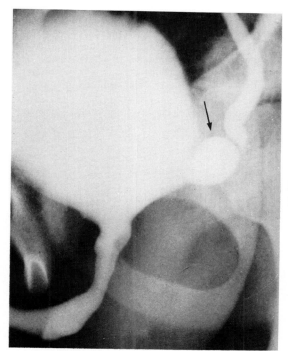

FIG. 48–15. Voiding cystogram; left-sided reflux and paraureteral (Hutch) diverticulum.

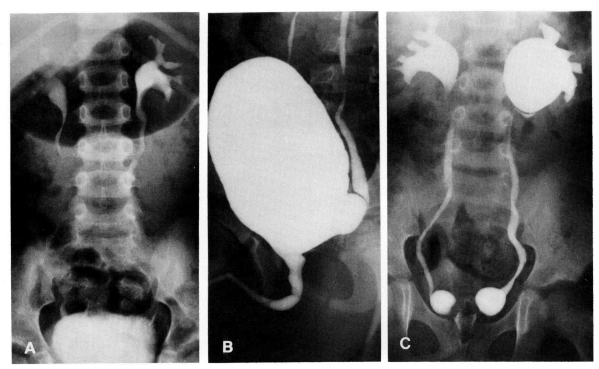

FIG. 48–16. IVU and voiding cystogram in a boy. **(A)** Normal IVU. **(B)** Voiding cystourethrogram, bilateral reflux and left paraureteral diverticulum. **(C)** Postvoiding film, ballooning of the left pelvis without ureteropelvic junction obstruction and bilateral paraureteral diverticula. Patient voids completely without infravesical obstruction.

FIG. 48–17. IVU and cystourethrogram in a girl. **(A)** IVU; borderline findings in the upper tract. **(B)** Cystourethrogram; bilateral reflux with gross dilatation of the upper tracts, particularly the left pelvis. An aberrant vessel may be present at the left ureteropelvic junction. No infravesical obstruction was demonstrated during voiding.

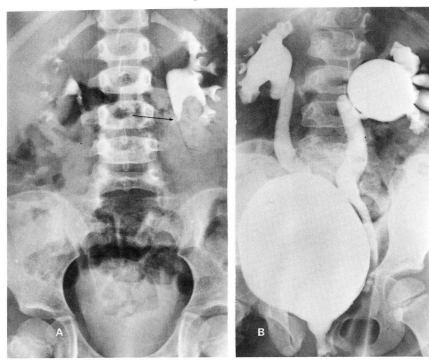

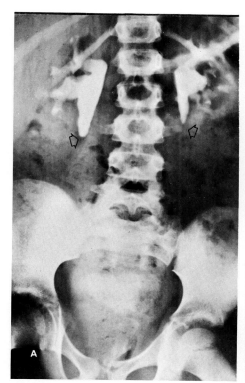
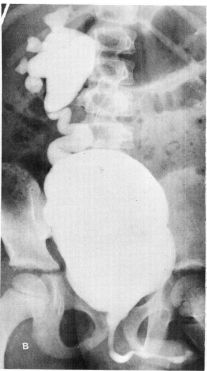
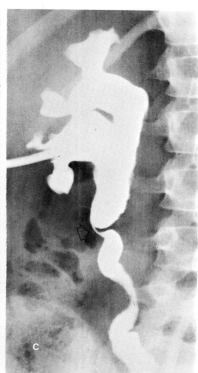
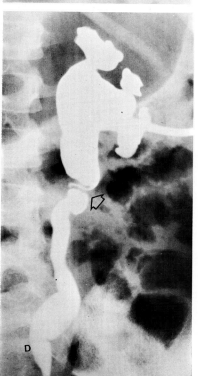

FIG. 48–18. Changes at the ureteropelvic junction in a boy with reflux. **(A)** IVP; 25-minute delayed film. Changes consistent with bilateral ureteropelvic junction obstruction (*arrows*). **(B)** Cystourethrogram, abundant nonobstructive reflux on the right. (Reflux was demonstrated also on the left in a subsequent study.) **(C** and **D)** Bilateral pyeloureterogram through nephrostomy catheters. Narrowing and kinking of both ureteropelvic junctions, possibly owing to aberrant vessels or adhesions.

FIG. 48–19. (A) IVU; moderate dilatation of the right pelvis with normal calyces and ureters suggesting some degree of ureteropelvic junction obstruction. **(B)** Post-voiding film of a cystourethrogram, right reflux and marked ballooning of the right pelvis.

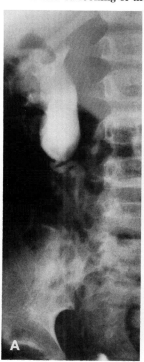
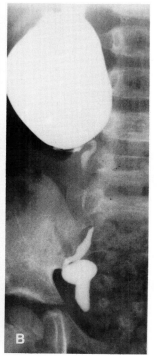

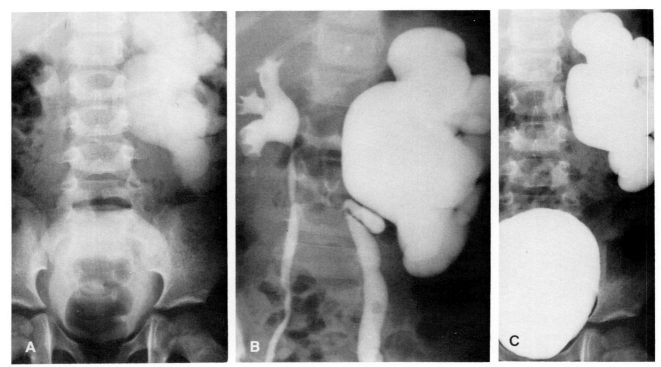

FIG. 48–20. Reflux and ureteropelvic junction obstruction in the same patient, possibly associated anomalies. **(A)** IVU; evidence of advanced ureteropelvic obstruction. **(B)** Voiding cystogram; bilateral reflux. **(C)** Postvoiding films; delayed emptying of the left pelvis.

FIG. 48–21. Cystourethrogram in patient with reflux. **(A)** Cystogram; bilateral reflux is moderate on the right, severe on the left. (Patient failed to empty bladder completely.) **(B)** Film taken after removal of the contrast material from the bladder through a catheter; good drainage of the ureters, excluding a significant ureterovesical junction destruction.

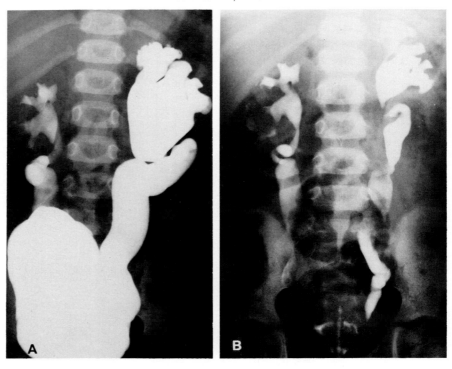

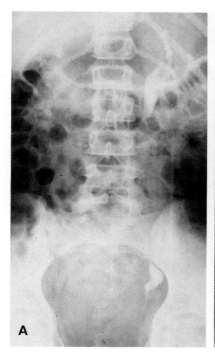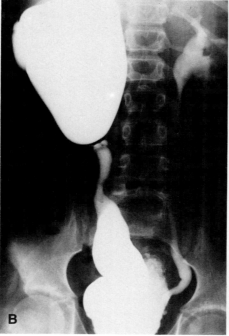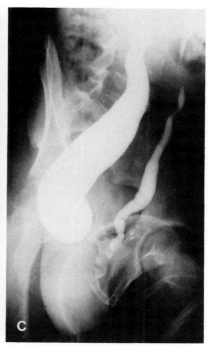

FIG. 48–22. Reflux and ureterovesical junction obstruction in same patient. **(A)** IVU; normal left upper tract; no function on the right. **(B)** Cystogram; bilateral reflux with massive ballooning of the right pelvicalyceal system. **(C)** Film taken at the end of voiding; evidence of obstruction at the right ureterovesical junction.

BIBLIOGRAPHY

1. Amar, A.D.: Vesicoureteral reflux causing improved visualization on the delayed excretory urogram. Radiology, *101:*1, 1971.
2. Amar, A.D.: Familial vesicoureteral reflux. J. Urol., *108:*969, 1972.
3. Amar, A.D., and Chabra, K.: Reflux in duplicated ureters: treatment in children. J. Pediatr. Surg., *5:*419, 1970.
4. Ambrose, S.S.: Reflux pyelonephritis in adults secondary to congenital lesions of the ureteral orifice. J. Urol., *102:*303, 1969.
5. Askin, J.A.: Prognosis of vesicoureteral reflux. Pediatrics, *49:*786, 1972.
6. Bailey, R.: The relationship of vesicoureteral reflux to urinary tract infection and chronic pyelonephritis-reflux nephropathy. Clin. Nephrol., *1:*132, 1973.
7. Berger, R.H., and Smith, C.: Hereditary and familial vesicoureteral reflux. J. Urol., *106:*845, 1971.
8. Bridge, R.A.C., and Roe, C.W.: The grading of vesicoureteral reflux: A guide to therapy. J. Urol., *101:*821, 1969.
9. Creevy, C.D.: Vesicoureteral reflux in children. A review. Urol. Surv., *17:*279, 1967.
10. Fisher, J.H., and Darling, D.B.: Vesicoureteral reflux in children. J. Pediatr. Surg., *2:*221, 1967.
11. Glenn, J.F., Editor: Proceedings of a workshop on ureteral reflux in children. National Academy of Sciences – National Research Council, Washington, D.C., 1967.
12. Haahr, J.: Vesico-ureteric reflux. Acta Paediatr. Scand., *60:*730, 1971.
13. Heikel, P.E., and Purkkulainen, K.V.: Vesico-ureteric reflux in children: A classification and results of conservative treatment. Ann. Radiol., *9:*37, 1966.
14. Herwig, K.R.: Vesicoureteral reflux. J.A.M.A., *221:*714, 1972.
15. Hodge, K.E.: Combined synchronous voiding cine cystourethrography and cystometry in the investigation of vesicoureteral reflux in children. J. Can. Assoc. Radiol., *18:*342, 1967.
16. Horan, P.J., Darling, D.B., and Fisher, J.H.: The excretory urogram in children with uretero-renal reflux. Am. J. Roentgenol., *99:*585, 1967.
17. Hutch, J.A., and Amar, A.D.: Vesico-ureteral reflux. Alken, C.E., Dix, V.W., Goodwinn, W.E., Weyranch, H.M., and Wildbolz, E., editors. Encyclopedia of Urology. p. 1. VIII/1. Malformations. Springer-Verlag, Berlin, Heidelberg, New York, 1968.
18. Kaveggia, F., King, L.R., Grava, L., et al.: Pyelonephritis – a cause of vesicoureteral reflux? J. Urol., *95:*158, 1966.
19. Kelalis, P.P.: Proper perspective on vesico-ureteral reflux. Mayo Clin. Proc., *46:*807, 1971.
20. Lyon, R.P., Marshall, S., and Tanagho, E.A.: The ureteral orifice: Its configuration and competency. J. Urol., *102:*504, 1969.
21. Mulcaby, J.J., Kelalis, P.P., Stickler, G.B., et al.: Familial vesicoureteral reflux. J. Urol., *108:*635, 1972.
22. Nanninga, J., King, L.R., Downing, J., et al.: Factors affecting the outcome of 100 ureteral reimplantations done for vesico-ureteral reflux. J. Urol., *102:*772, 1969.

23. Nogrady, M.B., and Dunbar, J.S.: Value of excretory micturition cystourethrography in the pediatric age group. J. Can. Assoc. Radiol., *16*:181, 1965.

24. Oppenheimer, R.: Vesicoureteral reflux. J.A.M.A., *217*:695, 1971.

25. Persky, L.: Treatment of vesicoureteral reflux. N. Engl. J. Med., *281*:1365, 1969.

26. Rolleston, G.L., Shannon, F.T., and Utley, W.I.F.: Relationship of infantile vesicoureteric reflux to renal damage. Br. Med. J., *1*:460, 1970.

27. Roper, B.A., and Smith, J.C.: Vesico-ureteric reflux following operations on the ureteric orifice. Br. J. Urol., *37*:531, 1961.

28. Schmidt, J.D., Hawtrey, C.E., Flocks, R.H., et al.: Vesicoureteral reflux: an inherited lesion. J.A.M.A., *220*:821, 1972.

29. Shopfner, C.E.: Cystourethrography: an evaluation of method. Am. J. Roentgenol., *95*:468, 1966.

30. Shopfner, C.E.: Vesicoureteral reflux: five year re-evaluation. Radiology, *95*:637, 1970.

31. Shopfner, C.E.: Urinary tract pathology with sepsis. Am. J. Roentgenol., *108*:632, 1970.

32. Silber, I., and McAllister, W.: Longitudinal folds as an indirect sign of vesicoureteral reflux. J. Urol., *103*:89, 1970.

33. Smith, A.M.: Comparison of standard and cinecystography for detecting vesicoureteral reflux. J. Urol., *96*:49, 1966.

34. Smith, A.N.: Comparison of standard and cine cystography. J. Urol., *102*:504, 1969.

35. Stephens, F.D.: Urologic aspects of recurrent urinary tract infections in children. J. Pediatr., *80*:725, 1972.

36. Tanagho, E.A., Guthrie, T.H., and Lyon, R.P.: The intravesical ureter in primary reflux. J. Urol., *101*:824, 1969.

37. Tanagho, E.A., and Hutch, J.A.: Primary reflux. J. Urol., *93*:158, 1965.

38. Tanagho, E.A., Hutch, J.A., and Miller, E.R.: Diagnostic procedures and cinefluoroscopy in vesicoureteral reflux. Br. J. Urol., *38*:435, 1966.

39. The Lancet: Vesico-ureteric reflux (leading article). *1*:1072, 1968.

40. Tresidder, G.C., Blandy, J.P., and Murry, R.S.: Pyelo-pelvic and uretero-ureteric reflux. Br. J. Urol., *42*:728–1970.

41. Weber, A.L., and Weylman, W.T.: Evaluation of vesicoureteral reflux by intravenous pyelography and cinecystography. Radiology, *87*:489, 1966.

42. Williams, D.I.: The ureter, the urologist and the paediatrician. Proc. Roy. Soc. Med., *63*:595, 1970.

Until a few years ago bladder neck obstruction was considered a frequent disorder and one of the most common causes of enuresis, recurrent urinary tract infection, reflux, and other problems. It was commonly thought to be caused by a local fibrosis or muscular hyperplasia, but a functional type (bladder neck dysfunction) was also considered. The most often mentioned radiographic findings were the following: a posterior or an anterior indentation, lip, or bar; a collar formation around the bladder neck; an incomplete funneling or failure of relaxation of the area during voiding; and a "poststenotic" dilatation of the proximal urethra. In recent years the pendulum has swung to the opposite direction, with most authorities now agreeing that the disorder is uncommon and perhaps nonexistent. One of the causes for this change of opinion has been the realization that previous diagnostic criteria were often equivocal or nonspecific.

The main questions still to be settled are whether bladder neck stenosis actually exists, albeit uncommon or rare, and, if it does, what are its roentgenographic features? In all likelihood, only a detailed correlation of all the clinical, radiographic, and operative findings in many patients will provide the answer.

In this context a review of the various aspects of the bladder neck seen in routine voiding cystourethrograms may be instructive and perhaps useful for a clearer understanding of the problem. A tentative classification, in several categories, ranging from the widest to the narrowest bladder necks collected by this author is given in the illustrations. In each case illustrated, the findings were constant throughout the examination and in repeated studies.

In the first category are included some of the widest bladder necks of the collection (Fig. 49–1). The finding has been referred to as a wide bladder neck anomaly by some authors. It is relatively uncommon, is seen more often in girls than in boys, and does not appear to be of clinical significance, at least in childhood.

49

Bladder Neck Obstruction

Guido Currarino

The second category comprises the vast majority of cases. These bladder necks are wide open, nicely funneled, and smooth in outline, a picture that corresponds to the ideal normal situation in both sexes (Fig. 49–2).

In the third group are those bladder necks that are similarly wide open or only slightly narrower than the preceding but that have a more or less pronounced indentation posteriorly, anteriorly, or circumferentially (Figs. 49–3 and 49–4). In some cases the indentation is obviously produced by a ballooning of the proximal urethra during voiding. The findings are now generally thought to be normal variants.

The fourth group includes a minority of individuals, mostly boys, in whom the bladder necks are definitely narrower than in the preceding category, sometimes strikingly so (Fig. 49–5). The bladder is often trabeculated, and there may be vesicoureteral reflux. Until more is known, these bladder necks should be described as small but of undetermined or unsettled significance at the present time. It is suspected that if primary bladder neck obstruction indeed exists it probably belongs to this category and affects mostly boys.

In a miscellaneous group is the occasional patient, often a girl, in whom the bladder neck is narrow but the urethra is also filiform (Fig. 49–6). The significance of the finding is undetermined. In some of these cases the bladder is enlarged and the patient voids infrequently or slowly. Ureteral reflux and recurrent urinary tract infections may be present. The picture corresponds to that described under the term megacystis–megatrigone syndrome by some authors, in which an underlying dysfunction of the detrusor and urethral muscles has been postulated.

CHAPTER 49, ILLUSTRATIONS

FIG. 49–1. Four instances of wide bladder neck, two in boys (**A, B**) and two in girls (**C, D**).

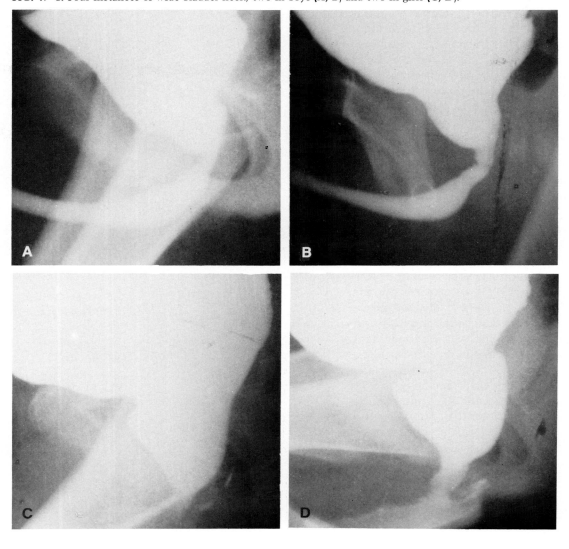

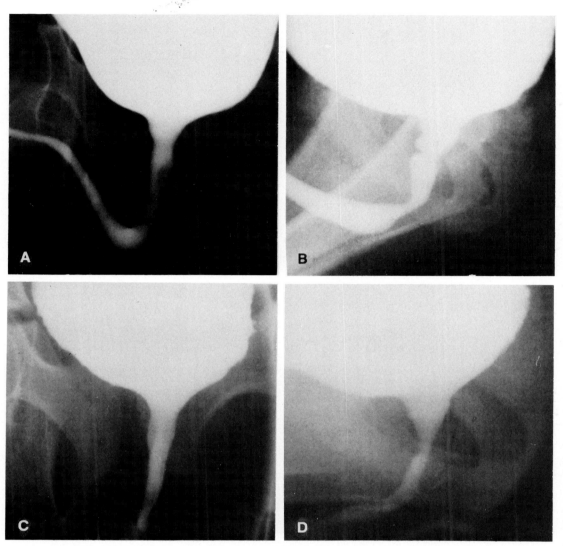

FIG. 49–2. Four instances of ideal normal bladder neck, two in boys (**A, B**) and two in girls (**C, D**).

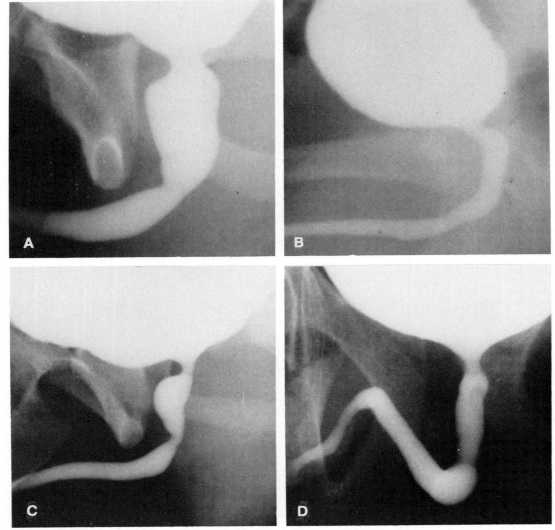

FIG. 49–3. (A–D) Four instances or normal variants in the appearance of bladder neck in boys.

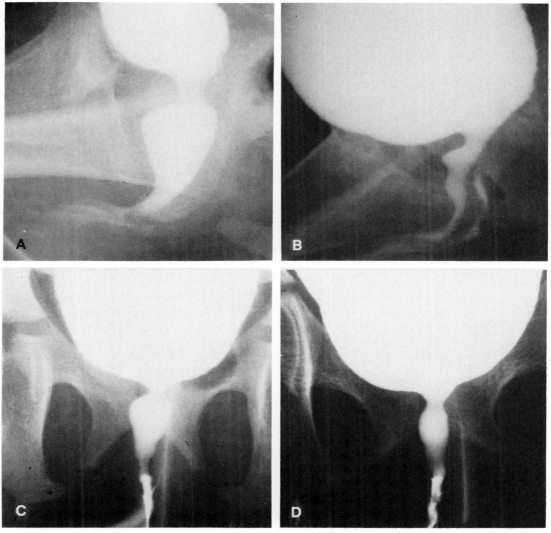

FIG. 49–4. (A–D) Four instances of normal variants in the appearance of bladder neck in girls.

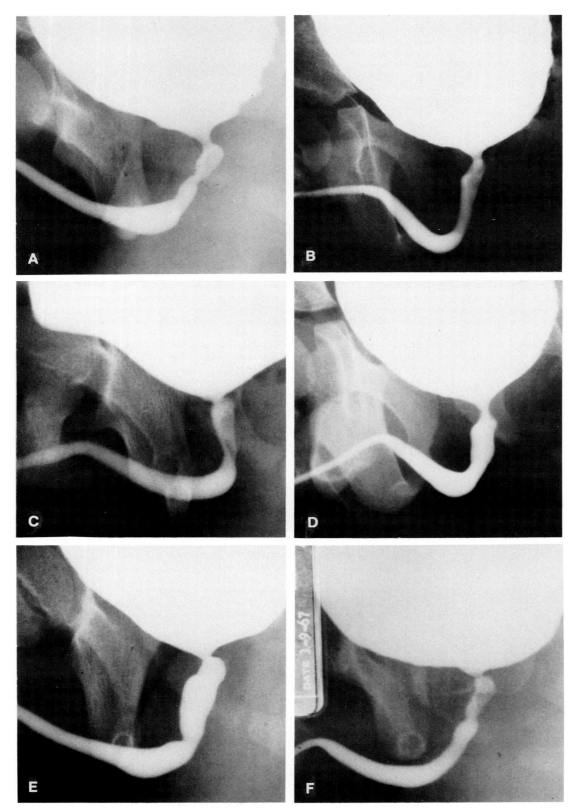

FIG. 49–5. (A–H) Eight instances of small bladder neck in boys, ranging from mild to severe. The significance of the finding is not certain. There were few girls in the collection with this type of bladder neck.

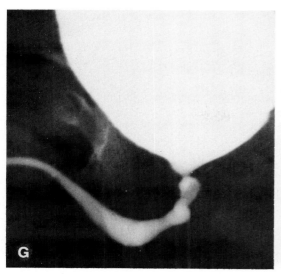

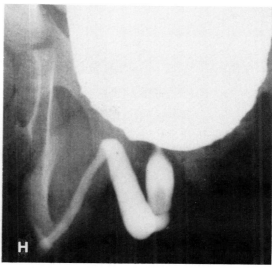

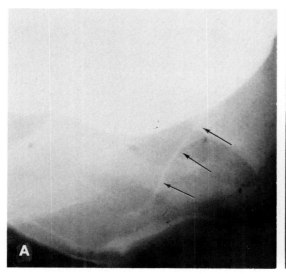

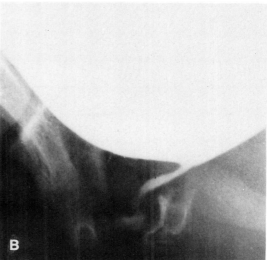

FIG. 49–6. Three instances of small bladder neck and filiform urethra, two in girls (**A, B**) and one in a boy (**C**). The significance of the findings is not certain.

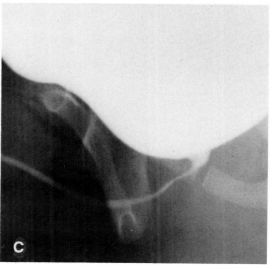

BIBLIOGRAPHY

1. Edwards, D.: The lower urinary tract. Proc. Roy. Soc. Med., *59*:417, 1966.
2. Harrow, B.R.: The rarity of bladder-neck obstruction in children. J. Pediatr., *69*:853, 1966.
3. King, L.R.: Contracture of the bladder neck. S. Clin. North Am., *44*:1537, 1964.
4. King, L.R., Miller, H.Z., and Scott, W.W.: Radiographic evaluation of the bladder neck in childhood. J. Urol., *91*:52, 1964.
5. Nunn, I.N.: Bladder neck obstructions in children. J. Urol., *93*:693, 1965.
6. Ruhde, U., and Ericsson, N.O.: Roentgen evaluation of primary bladder neck obstruction in children. Acta Radiol. (Diagn.), *3*:237, 1965.
7. Rudhe, U., and Ericsson, N.O.: Congenital bladder neck obstruction in infancy and childhood: radiological diagnosis and results of therapy. Ann. Radiol., *9*:2, 1966.
8. Shopfner, C.E.: Roentgenological evaluation of bladder neck obstruction. Am. J. Roentgenol., *100*:162, 1967.
9. Smith, D.R.: Critique on the concept of vesical neck obstruction in children. J.A.M.A., *207*:1686, 1969.

Absent abdominal musculature is an uncommon malformation complex in which deficient or absent musculature of the abdominal wall is associated with a special type of urinary tract malformation and with cryptorchidism. Because of the combination of these three major features, the condition has been referred to as the triad syndrome. It has also been called prune belly syndrome because of the wrinkled appearance of the anterior abdominal wall. It affects boys almost exclusively. The few reported women with defective abdominal musculature only rarely had urinary tract anomalies. Associated malformations in other organs are common, especially malrotation of the midgut and deformities of the lower extremities (Fig. 50-1).

The renal substance is frequently diminished in thickness unilaterally or bilaterally. Renal hypoplasia and dysplasia are present in many cases (Figs. 50-2, 50-3, 50-5, 50-6). The renal function commonly is decreased. The ureters are dilated, elongated, and tortuous, often resembling bowel (Figs. 50-2, 50-4, 50-5). They are hypotonic and empty poorly. The ureteral orifices are often gaping, and bilateral (Figs. 50-2 to 50-6) or unilateral ureteral reflux (Fig. 50-7) is present in most cases. Some degree of a ureterovesical junction obstruction, probably functional in origin, may be present. The bladder tends to be enlarged but is smooth in outline. It is high in position (Figs. 50-9, 50-10) and often is attached to the umbilicus (Figs. 50-4, 50-7). A urachal fistula is present in some cases. Bladder residual is common.

The bladder neck is high in position (Figs. 50-7 to 50-9) and wide. The proximal posterior urethra is dilated and elongated (Figs. 50-7 to 50-9). The membranous urethra and the urethra distal to this area are usually normal in caliber. A sharp backward angulation of the mid posterior urethra is a common finding (Figs. 50-7 to 50-9). In a number of patients,

50

Absent Abdominal Musculature

GUIDO CURRARINO

a large utricle projects backward from this area (Figs. 50–9, 50–10). Congenital urethral obstructions, particularly atresia of the membranous urethra and posterior urethral valves, have been reported in about 10 per cent of the cases. These obstructions are usually associated with severe renal dysplasia causing early death.

The prognosis generally is poor. Approximately half of the patients die within the first few years of life, often in the newborn period or shortly thereafter.

The nature of the malformation complex is not fully understood. There are no neurologic abnormalities demonstrable clinically or post mortem. The nerve supply to the urinary tract is apparently normal, and the ganglion cells in the bladder are not decreased. Nunn and Stephens found evidence of patchy absence of muscle fibers in the bladder wall and the ureters and an increase in the fibrous tissue.[7] They also described a deficiency of muscle fibers and tubules in the prostatic tissue. All these changes suggest a developmental anomaly of the urinary tract analogous to that of the abdominal wall. The defects in the abdominal wall and those in the urinary tract are probably associated anomalies rather than cause and effect, and in all likelihood they are the result of a local injury during a particularly vulnerable stage in the growth of these structures in early fetal life.

CHAPTER 50, ILLUSTRATIONS

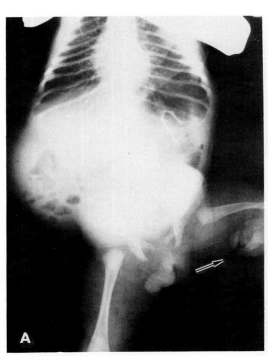

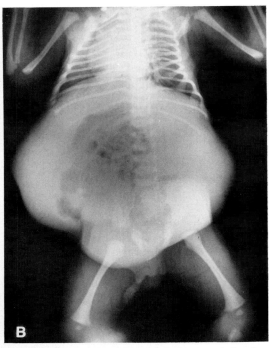

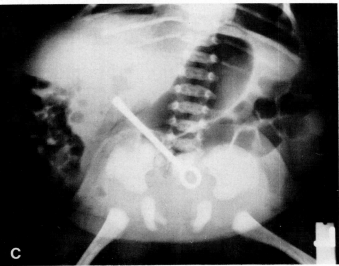

FIG. 50–1. Frontal view of the abdomens of three patients with absent abdominal musculature. The abdomen is protruberant. Congenital absence of the distal left lower extremity in (A) (arrow).

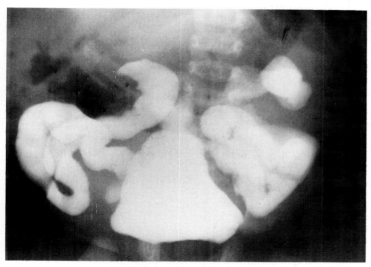

FIG. 50-2. Cystogram in newborn with absent abdominal musculature; bilateral reflux into dilated and markedly elongated and tortuous ureter (ureteral dysplasia?). No calyces are present. (Patient had bilateral renal dysplasia with small kidneys.)

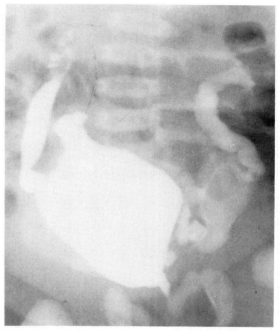

FIG. 50-3. Cystogram in newborn with absent abdominal musculature; bilateral reflux into dilated and slightly elongated ureters. Small pelvicalyceal systems, especially on the right. (Patient had bilateral renal dysplasia.)

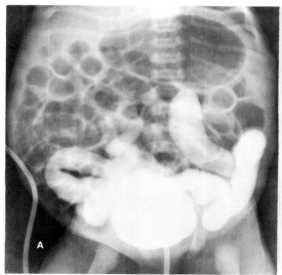
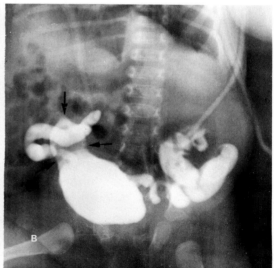

FIG. 50-4. Cystogram (**A**) and bilateral antegrade pyelogram (**B**) in infant with absence of the abdominal musculature; bilateral reflux into dilated and tortuous ureters. The bladder is enlarged and attached to the umbilicus (*arrows*).

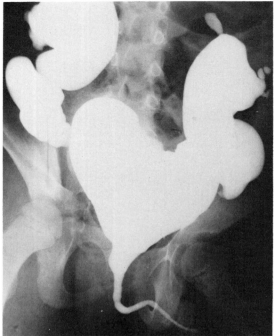

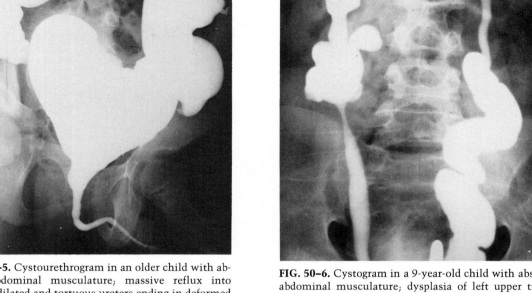

FIG. 50–5. Cystourethrogram in an older child with absent abdominal musculature; massive reflux into grossly dilated and tortuous ureters ending in deformed calyces.

FIG. 50–6. Cystogram in a 9-year-old child with absent abdominal musculature; dysplasia of left upper tract and left kidney.

FIG. 50–7. (A) Cystogram in an infant with absence of abdominal musculature; the bladder is enlarged markedly and there is vesicoureteral reflux on the left. (B) Voiding cystourethrogram in the same patient a year later; the bladder is attached to the umbilicus (*upper arrow*), the bladder neck is in a high position (*middle arrow*), and the posterior urethra is dilated and kinked (*lower arrow*).

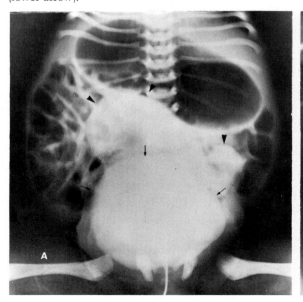

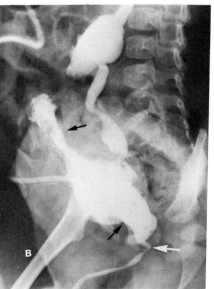

FIG. 50–8. Voiding cystourethrogram in an infant with absent abdominal musculature. The bladder is enlarged and attached to the umbilicus, the bladder neck is high in position (*black arrow*), and the proximal posterior urethra is widened. Note angulation of posterior urethra (*white arrow*).

FIG. 50–9. Voiding cystourethrogram in four instances of absent abdominal musculature. The bladder is enlarged and smooth in outline. The bladder neck is high in position (*white arrows*), and the proximal posterior urethra is dilated. A large utricle is shown in three patients (*black arrows*). The posterior urethra tends to be kinked. Vesicoureteral reflux occurred in (**A**) and (**C**).

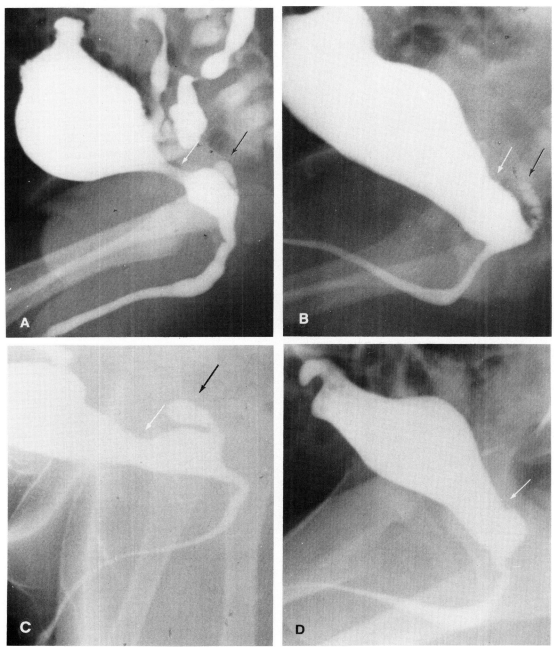

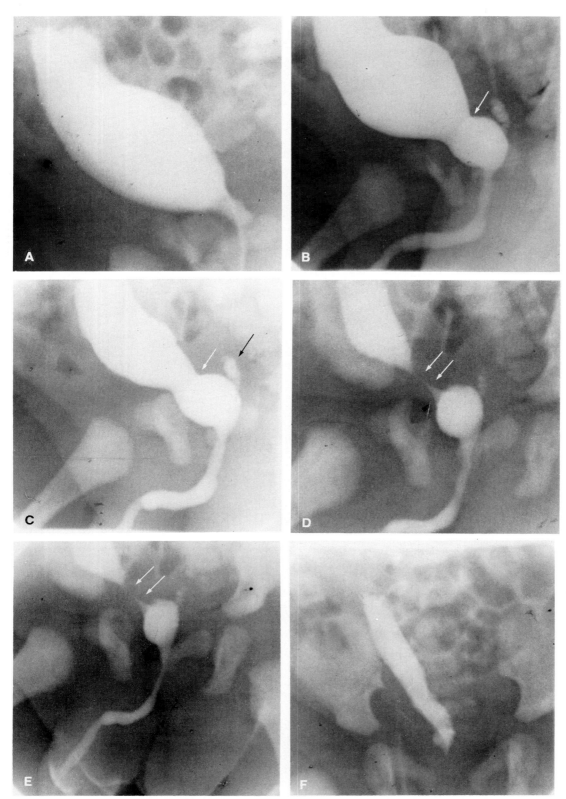

FIG. 50–10. Six frames of a voiding cinecystourethrogram in an infant with absent abdominal musculature. **(A)** Filling of the bladder. **(B–E)** Various appearances of the bladder and urethra during voiding. **(F)** Postvoiding film of the bladder. Note high position of the bladder (*white arrows*) and presence of utricle (*black arrow*).

BIBLIOGRAPHY

1. Barnhouse, D.H.: Prune belly syndrome. Br. J. Urol., *44*:356, 1972.
2. Bourne, C.W., and Cerny, J.C.: Congenital absence of abdominal muscles: Report of 6 cases. J. Urol., *98*:252, 1967.
3. Burke, E.C., Shin, M.H., and Kelalis, P.P.: Prune belly syndrome: Clinical findings and survival. Am. J. Dis. Child., *117*:668, 1969.
4. Burkholder, G.V., Harper, R.C., and Beach, P.D.: Congenital absence of the abdominal muscles: Am. J. Clin. Pathol., *53*:602, 1970.
5. Cremin, B.J.: The urinary tract anomalies associated with agenesis of the abdominal walls. Br. J. Radiol., *44*:767, 1971.
6. Grossman, H., Winchester, P.H., and Waldbaum, R.S.: Syndrome of congenital deficiency of abdominal wall musculature and associated genitourinary anomalies (Prune belly syndrome). *In* Kaufman, H.J., ed. Progress in Pediatric Radiology. vol. 3, p. 327. Yearbook Med. Publ. Inc., 1970.
7. Nunn, I.N., and Stephens, F.D.: The triad syndrome: A composite anomaly of the abdominal wall, urinary system and testes. J. Urol., *86*:782, 1961.
8. Rogers, L.W., and Ostrow, P.T.: The prune belly syndrome: Report of 20 cases and description of a lethal variant. J. Pediatr., *83*:786, 1973.
9. Waldbaum, R.S., and Marshall, V.F.: The prune belly syndrome: A diagnostic therapeutic plan. J. Urol., *103*:668, 1970.
10. Williams, D.I., and Burkholder, G.V.: The prune belly syndrome. J. Urol., *98*:244, 1967.

Ureterocele is defined as a cystic dilatation and protrusion into the bladder cavity of the intravesical submucosal segment of the ureter. Two types are recognized: the simple (adult type) and the ectopic (childhood type), depending on whether the termination of the affected ureter is in the bladder or extravesical.

SIMPLE URETEROCELE

Simple ureterocele is a terminal cystic dilatation of the terminal part of the ureter (Fig. 51–1 to 51–3). The cele is generally small and lies entirely within the bladder at the lateral angle of the trigone. The ureteral meatus is to be found on the surface of the ureterocele, usually inferiorly.

Small ureteroceles are often discovered as incidental urographic findings. Stenosis of the ureteral orifice with varying degrees of dilatation of the affected ureter is common. Urinary stasis and infection may result.

Simple ureterocele is more common in adults than in children, suggesting that it may be an acquired lesion in many instances. The anomaly is frequently bilateral. Complete upper tract duplication on the affected side is rare.

In the excretory urogram the contrast material that collects within the ureterocele produces a round or oval density surrounded by a radiolucent halo representing the unopacified wall of the cyst. This is the well-known cobra head or spring onion formation characteristic of the lesion. If the renal function is poor, the lesion may give rise only to a round or oval radiolucent filling defect. A radiolucent filling defect is usually the only finding observed in the cystogram.

51

Ureterocele

GUIDO CURRARINO

ECTOPIC URETEROCELE

The anomaly is not rare. It seldom is discovered in adults, presumably because of its tendency to cause symptoms early, leading to early recognition and treatment. It is much more frequent in girls than boys and is usually unilateral (Figs. 51–4 to 51–14).

Its *anatomy* differs from that of a simple ureterocele in several respects. The involved ureter enters the bladder wall in a normal fashion, descends toward the bladder neck submucosally, passes through the internal ureteral sphincter, and terminates ectopically at the level of the bladder neck or in the proximal urethra. Ureteroceles do not occur in ureters ending ectopically outside the urinary tract. The ectopic ureterocele tends to be larger and is located more inferiorly in the bladder than the simple type. It has a broad base and usually involves the bladder neck area. It may extend into the bladder neck and proximal urethra. Occasionally, it prolapses into the urethra as far down as the external sphincter, chronically or intermittently, and may even present in the vulva.

A completely duplicated upper tract is almost always present on the affected side. Upper tract duplication on the opposite side is common. The ectopic ureter responsible for the ureterocele is regularly the one connected with the uppermost part of the kidney. The renal parenchyma drained by the abnormal ureter often is hypoplastic, dysplastic, and poorly functioning.

The orifice of the affected ureter is frequently stenotic. At times, no ureteral meatus can be demonstrated at operation or even post mortem. In rare cases, the ureterocele has an orifice at the level of the bladder despite the fact that the ureterocele itself extends downward as a long tongue in the urethral submucosal layer. This arrangement has been referred to as a *ureterocecocele* because of its resemblance to a cecum. It is not certain whether it is a true entity or only an ordinary ectopic ureterocele with an acquired perforation.

The corresponding upper tract shows varying degrees of dilatation. Because of their location and size, ectopic ureteroceles are prone to obstruct the bladder neck and the orifice of other ureters. Dilatation of and reflux into the ipsilateral lower segment of the duplicated kidney is not uncommon. Contralateral ureterectasis and hydronephrosis with or without reflux may be observed.

The pelvicalyceal system and the ureter connected with the ureterocele almost always fail to visualize by excretory urography even in long-delayed films. However, it usually is possible in these cases to suspect the presence of a duplicated upper tract with a nonfunctioning superior complex from certain characteristic changes in the visualized pelvicalyceal system and the ureter.

SIGNS OF DUPLICATION

These indirect signs of duplication are of great diagnostic importance and should be kept in mind constantly in evaluating excretory urograms and retrograde studies of children. The visualized calyces tend to be fewer than the calyces of a normal kidney. The superior infundibulum and calyces are commonly short. The distance between the uppermost calyx and the margin of the superior pole of the renal shadow is increased. A line connecting the superior and the inferior calyces is either vertical or oblique downward and medially. The upper calyces and the renal pelvis tend to be farther away from the spine than normal and often are compressed and displaced downward and laterally, sometimes to a marked degree. This "drooping flower deformity" of the visualized pelvicalyceal system is proportionate in severity to the dilatation of the nonvisualized calyces. The picture thus obtained may be indistinguishable from that produced by a mass originating in the upper pole of a kidney, and it may resemble that seen in adrenal tumors. Another indirect sign of duplication is the lateral displacement and tortuosity of the visualized ureter, reflecting the dilatation and tortuosity of the adjacent nonvisualized ureter.

The lesion is often best seen in the excretory urogram, where the ectopic ureterocele usually produces an oval filling defect with smooth or lobulated borders in the inferior-lateral aspect of the bladder. Its lower pole has a broad base and commonly extends into the bladder neck. The long axis of the mass usually points upward and laterally toward the affected side. Occasionally, the mass is round or is located in the midline. The ureterocele itself seldom becomes opacified during excretory urography.

The lesion may be easily missed in the routine cystogram. If the bladder is overdistended with contrast material, the cystic mass may be decompressed and flattened against the bladder wall and thus become invisible. In some cases it may even prolapse backward, simulating a periureteral diverticulum. Also, if a highly concentrated contrast material is used, the lesion may not be visible in the frontal projections. Sometimes the defect produced by the ureterocele is shallow and is seen only in an oblique view.

The voiding cystourethrogram commonly shows

an asymmetry of the bladder neck and may demonstrate a flattening or a frank displacement of the posterior urethra. In girls the space between the opacified bladder neck area and vagina may be increased. Reflux into the ureterocele and the affected ureter is an uncommon occurrence, but it may be seen if there is a perforation of the wall of the ureterocele, spontaneous, surgical, or catheter induced.

In the presence of a bilateral duplication and a single ureterocele, the lesion should be suspected to originate from the side where the renal function in the uppermost part of the kidney is absent or decreased. The demonstration of a filling defect in the bladder plus indirect signs of a duplicated upper tract by intravenous pyelography is fairly conclusive evidence of an ectopic ureterocele.

CHAPTER 51, ILLUSTRATIONS

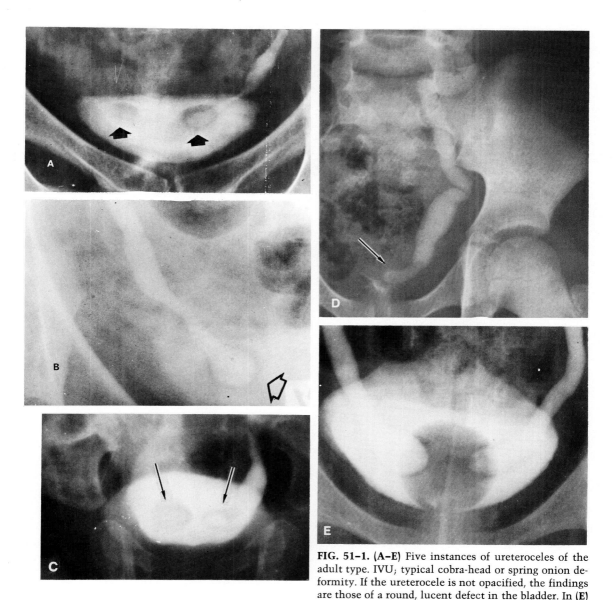

FIG. 51-1. (A-E) Five instances of ureteroceles of the adult type. IVU; typical cobra-head or spring onion deformity. If the ureterocele is not opacified, the findings are those of a round, lucent defect in the bladder. In **(E)** both ureteroceles are seen through the air-filled balloon of a Foley catheter.

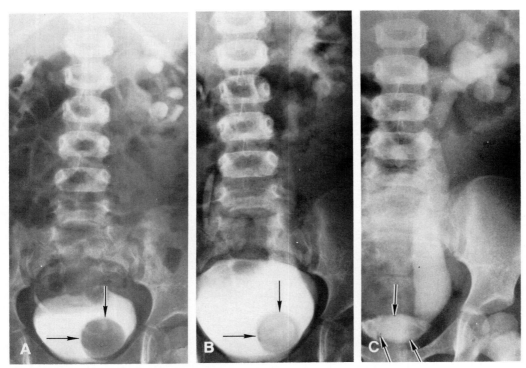

FIG. 51–2. IVU in a girl with simple or adult type of ureterocele with obstruction. **(A)** 3-Minute film; the ureterocele causes a radiolucent defect in the bladder (*arrows*). **(B)** Later film; cavity of ureterocele fills with contrast material (*arrows*). **(C)** Same in postvoiding film (*arrows*).

FIG. 51–3. Unusually large ureterocele of the adult type on the left causing obstruction and absence of renal function. **(A)** IVU. **(B)** Retrograde ureterogram.

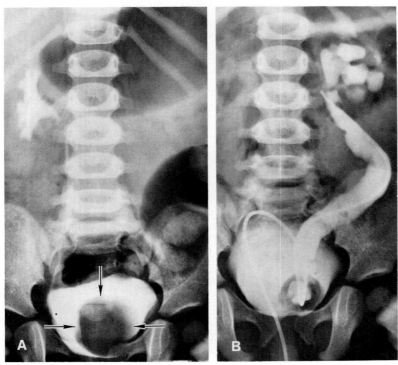

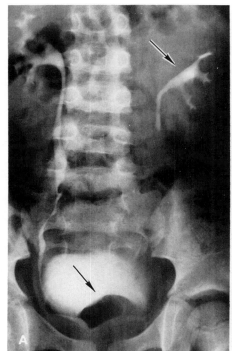
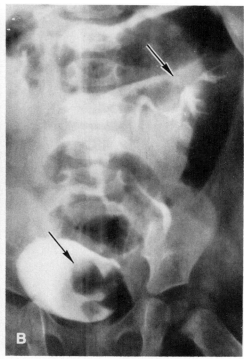

FIG. 51–4. IVP in two children with ureterocele of the ectopic or childhood type. Large filling defect in the bladder caused by the ureterocele is demonstrated. The ureterocele is connected with a nonvisualized upper tract on the left. The presence of a second upper tract on this side is suspected from the lateral and downward displacement of the visualized pelvicalyceal system.

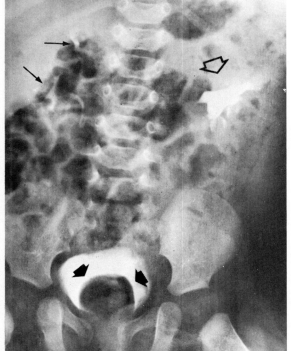

FIG. 51–5. IVU of an infant with ectopic ureterocele causing a round filling defect in the bladder. The ureterocele is connected with a nonfunctioning proximal complex of a duplex left kidney. Duplication is also noted on the opposite side, a finding that is not uncommon in ectopic ureteroceles.

FIG. 51–6. IVU in a child with ectopic ureterocele connected with a nonfunctioning small upper complex of a duplex left kidney. In a delayed film (**B**) the visualized dilated lower half of the duplicated kidney is minimally displaced (*arrows*) by the adjacent upper tract and is shown to be obstructed at the ureterovesical junction.

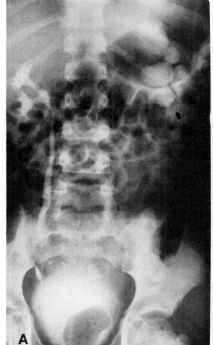
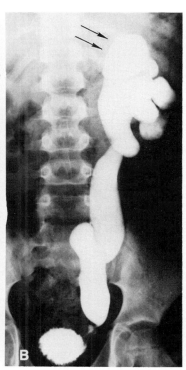

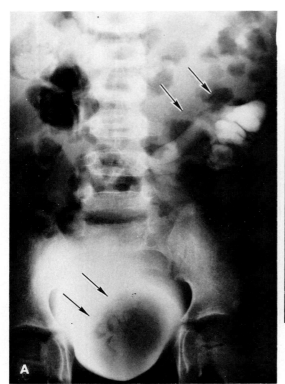

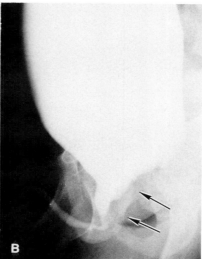

FIG. 51–7. (A) IVU; large ureterocele connected with a nonfunctioning upper complex of a duplex left kidney. Lower segment displaced (*arrows*). (B) Voiding cystourethrogram; compression of the base of the bladder and posterior urethra by ureterocele, which extends to the level of the urogenital membrane (*arrows*).

FIG. 51–8. (A) IVU in an infant with ectopic ureterocele causing a small round filling defect in the bladder (*lower arrow*). Indirect signs of second upper tract with which the ureterocele is connected are present on the right (*upper arrow*). (B) Cystourethrogram; marginal filling defect in the posterior urethra produced by the ureterocele and the ectopically ending ureter (*arrow*).

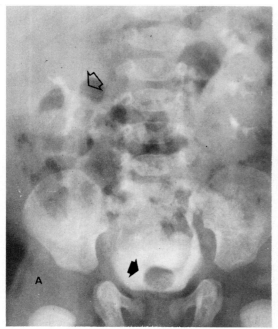

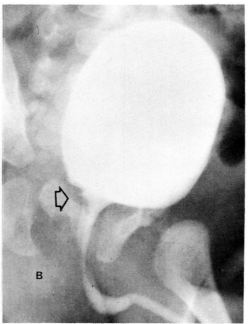

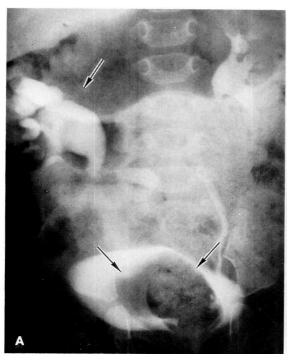

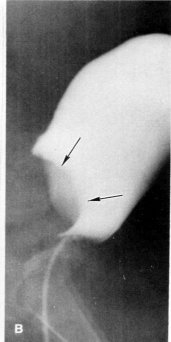

FIG. 51–9. (A) IVU; large ectopic ureterocele connected with a nonfunctioning upper complex of duplex right kidney. **(B)** Cystogram, lateral projection; defect in bladder caused by the ureterocele clearly seen during filling; this defect may become obliterated when bladder is fully distended.

FIG. 51–10. Another example of ectopic ureterocele in a 2-year-old girl. **(A)** Cystourethrogram, postvoiding film; typical filling defect in the bladder (*arrows*) and vesicoureteral reflux in the lower complex of a duplicated upper tract on the right. **(B)** At cystoscopy the orifice of the ectopically ending ureter carrying the ureterocele was found to be in the proximal urethra. An injection of contrast material outlines clearly the ureterocele (*arrows*) and the corresponding upper dilated segment.

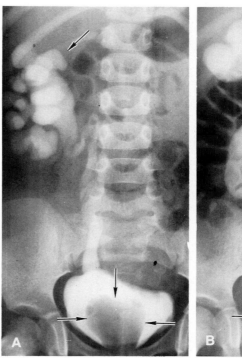

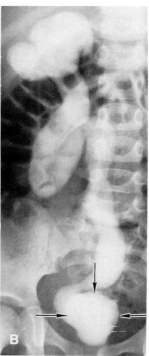

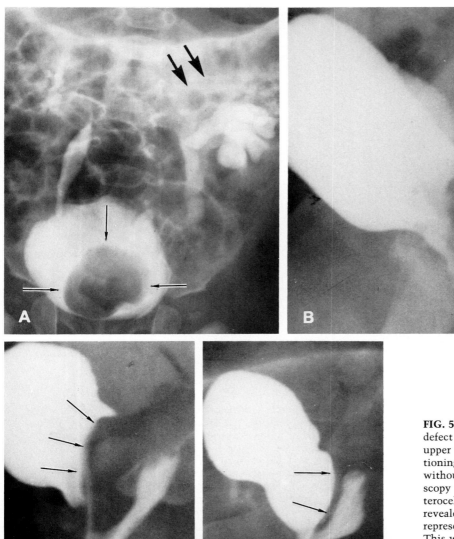

FIG. 51–11. Ectopic ureterocele in a 5-month-old girl. **(A)** IVU; large rounded defect in bladder (*thin arrows*) associated with signs of ureteral duplication on the left with nonvisualization of the upper complex (*large arrows*) (downward and lateral displacement of the visualized lower kidney segment structures). **(B)** Cystourethrogram, defect at the base of bladder and proximal urethra (*arrow*) with posterior displacement of the vagina that fills during voiding. **(C)** Simultaneous cystogram and vaginogram showing mass between vagina and bladder (*arrows* mark anterior margin of ureterocele). **(D)** When the bladder is overdistended, the ureterocele defect becomes obliterated and the area may bulge backward, sometimes simulating a broadbase diverticulum. (*arrows*).

FIG. 51–12. Ectopic ureterocele. **(A)** IVU; small filling defect in the bladder (*arrows*) just above bladder neck; upper tract duplicating along the left with good functioning of both complexes. Normal right upper tract without changes suggesting duplication. **(B)** At cystoscopy an injection of contrast material into the ureterocele through a catheter with a needle at its tip revealed that the ureter connecting with the ureterocele represented the upper complex of a duplex right kidney. This was not apparent on the urogram.

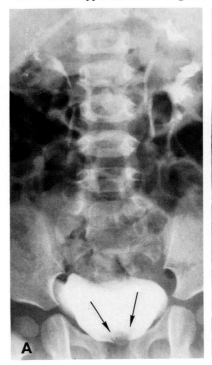
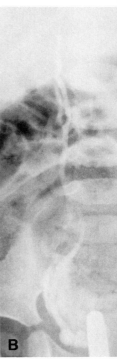

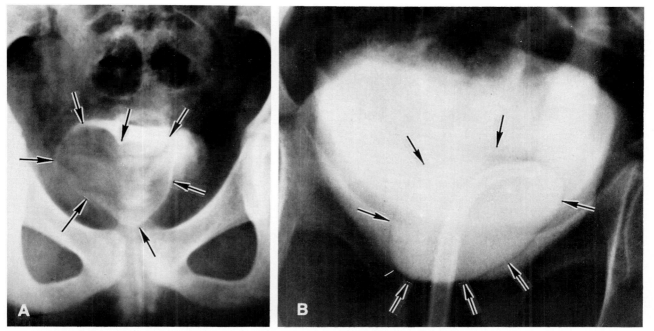

FIG. 51–13. Ectopic ureterocele in a child. **(A)** IVU; large filling defect in the bladder caused by ureterocele (*arrows*). **(B)** Cystourethrogram; perforation of the ureterocele by the catheter during catheterization of the bladder with visualization of the ureterocele (arrows) and the corresponding ureter.

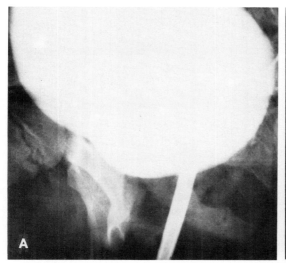

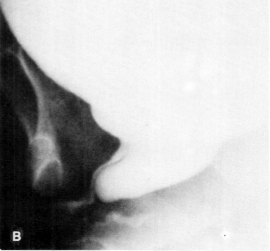

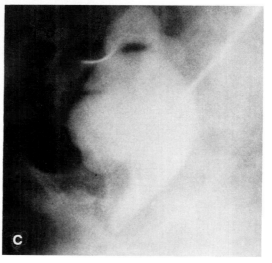

FIG. 51–14. Cystourethrogram in a patient with ectopic ureterocele that has an incompetent orifice within the bladder. (Spontaneous perforation? True ureteral orifice of a ureterocecocele?) **(A)** Filling of bladder. **(B)** During voiding there is filling of a large cavity at the base of the bladder extending downward along the urethra. **(C)** Postvoiding film following complete emptying of the bladder. The cavity of the ectopic ureterocele remains filled.

BIBLIOGRAPHY

1. Berdon, W.E., Baker, D.H., Becker, J.A., and Uson, A.C.: Ectopic ureterocele. Radiol. Clin. North Am., 6:205, 1968.
2. Datta, N.S., Uto, Y., Eisenman, J.I., and Bischoff, A.J.: "Cobra head" deformity: Its relationship to ureterocele and "pseudoureterocele." J. Can. Assoc. Radiol., 23:284, 1972.
3. Ericsson, N.O.: Ectopic ureterocele in infants and children. Acta. Clin. Scand. (Suppl. 197), 1954.
4. Hahn, L.C., and Schapira, H.E.: Ureterocele and ureteral duplication: Associated congenital malformations. N.Y. State J. Med., 72:731, 1972.
5. Hendren, W.H., and Monfort, G.J.: Surgical correction of ureteroceles in childhood. J. Pediatr. Surg., 6:235, 1971.
6. Johnston, J.H.: Experience with ectopic ureteroceles. Br. J. Urol., 41:61, 1969.
7. Lundin, E.: Upper urinary tract duplication associated with ectopic ureterocele. Acta. Radiol. (Diag.), 7:13, 1968.
8. Stephens, D.: Caecoureterocele and concepts in the embryology and aetiology of ureteroceles. Aust. N.Z. J. Surg., 40:239, 1971.
9. Subbiah, N., and Stephens, D.: Stenotic ureterocele. Aust. N.Z. J. Surg., 41:257, 1972.
10. Tanagho, E.A.: Anatomy and management of ureteroceles. J. Urol., 107:729, 1972.
11. Williams, D.I., Fay, R., and Lillie, J.G.: The functional radiology of ectopic ureterocele. Br. J. Urol., 44:417, 1972.

Simple ureteral ectopia is a developmental malformation in which the affected ureter terminates in an abnormal location outside the bladder without ureterocele formation.

The anomaly is not rare. In most cases a duplicated upper tract is present on the affected side. The ureter that terminates ectopically characteristically is the one that drains the upper complex. The disorder is almost always unilateral. Upper tract duplication on the opposite side may be observed. Ureteral ectopia without duplication is uncommon, and bilateral ureteral ectopia without duplication (no ureters entering the bladder) is exceedingly rare (see Fig. 52–11).

Simple ureteral ectopia is much more common in girls than in boys. In girls the affected ureter terminates in the urethra (Figs. 52–2, 52–3), usually just inside the external meatus, less commonly in the vaginal vestibule (Fig. 52–1) or in the vagina (Figs. 52–8, 52–10). In boys it usually drains in the posterior urethra (Fig. 52–5), just above the veru, occasionally in the utricle, seminal vesical, vas deferens, ejaculatory duct, or epididymis. The most common and characteristic clinical manifestation in girls is a constant dribbling of urine despite regular emptying of the bladder. In boys the disorder is usually less severe, and dribbling is not apt to occur, because the ectopic ureter drains above the external sphincter. Urinary infections are common in both sexes.

The renal parenchyma from which the affected ureter originates commonly is hypoplastic and dysplastic and concentrates the urine poorly. The affected ureter is dilated variously (Figs. 52–6, 52–9) but usually less severely than it is in ectopic ureterocele. Dilatation of the other ureters is frequent. Stenosis of the aberrant ureteral meatus may be present.

Because of the poor renal function of the portion of the kidney drained by the abnormal ureter, the af-

52

Simple Ureteral Ectopia

GUIDO CURRARINO

fected upper segment is frequently not visualized by excretory urography. In such cases the presence of a duplicated upper tract may be suspected from the indirect radiographic signs described in the preceding chapter. In the presence of some renal function, the affected ureter may be seen to end in an abnormally low location.

The cystourethrogram may show suggestive findings. Occasionally a fullness or compression defect is observed on the posterolateral aspect of the bladder produced by the adjacent dilated ectopic ureter (Figs. 52–4, 52–5). If the aberrant ureter empties into the urethra, reflux into the ectopic ureter may be demonstrated in the voiding study. The bladder neck is frequently deformed. If there is reflux of contrast material into the vagina during voiding, the space between the bladder neck and vagina may be increased. A vaginogram may show reflux in the affected ureter if this terminates in the vagina.

The finding of only one ureteral orifice at cystoscopy on the side where there are indirect signs of duplication should suggest the diagnosis of simple ureteral ectopia. The diagnosis is established with certainty preoperatively only if the ectopic ureteral meatus is identified on direct inspection or radiographically.

CHAPTER 52, ILLUSTRATIONS

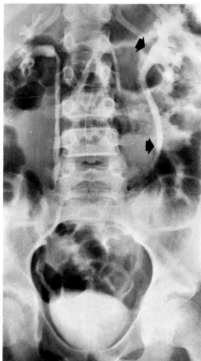

FIG. 52–1. IVU in a girl with simple ureteral ectopia (vestibule). Note indirect signs of upper tract duplication on the left (*arrows*).

FIG. 52–2. Simple ureteral ectopia in a girl with an abnormal ureter ending in the urethra. **(A)** Cystourethrogram; massive reflux into the lower complex of a duplicated left kidney. *Arrows* point to the nonfilled upper segment. Reflux is also present on the right. **(B)** Voiding film; mass between the bladder and the vagina (*arrows*) caused by the dilated distal end of the ectopic ureter. The voiding picture simulates a ureterocele.

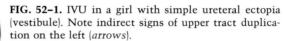

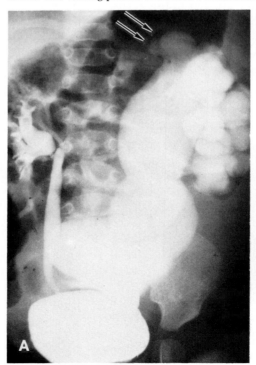

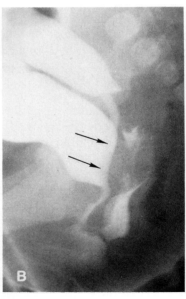

FIG. 52–3. Ectopic ureter in a 3½-year-old girl with constant dribbling of urine. **(A)** IVU; characteristic finding of a duplicated upper tract on the right with nonfunctioning superior complex. The visualized pelvicalyceal system is displaced downward and laterally (*arrows*). **(B, C)** Cystourethrogram, voiding, and postvoiding films showing reflux in the superior complex that drains ectopically in the distal urethra (*arrows*).

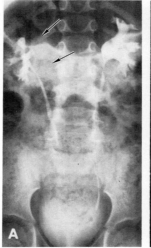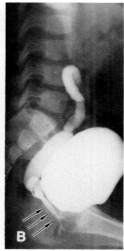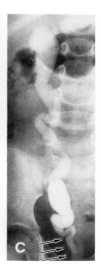

FIG. 52–4. Simple ureteral ectopia in a girl; cystourethrogram. **(A)** Voiding film; reflux into ureter ending ectopically in proximal urethra (*arrow*) with obstruction at its termination. **(B)** Postvoiding film; the ectopic ureter represents the proximal component of a duplex left kidney. *Arrow* points to distal end of ureter at level of urethra.

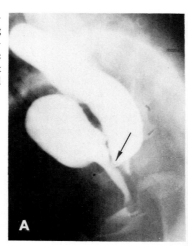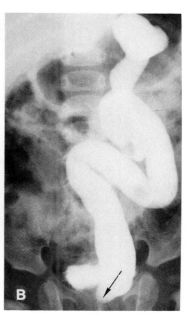

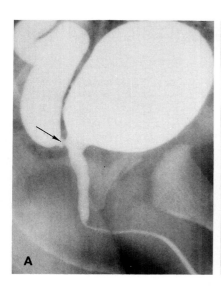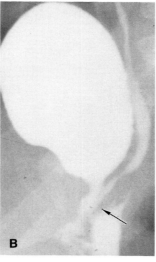

FIG. 52–5. Two instances of ectopic ending ureter, one in a boy **(A)** and the other in a girl **(B).** In both instances, the voiding cystogram shows reflux into the ureter entering the proximal urethra (*arrows*).

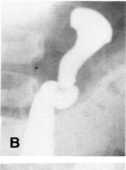
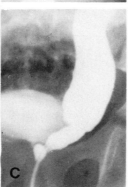
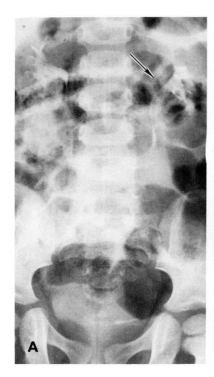

FIG. 52–6. Ureteral ectopia ending just distal to the bladder neck. **(A)** IVU; indirect signs of duplication on the left (*arrow*) with nonfunctioning proximal complex. **(B, C)** On catheterization of the bladder for the voiding cystourethrogram the catheter entered the ectopic ureter, and the injection of contrast material opacified the proximal ureter of a duplex left kidney with evidence of obstruction at its termination just below the bladder neck.

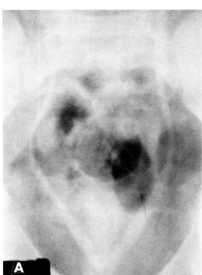
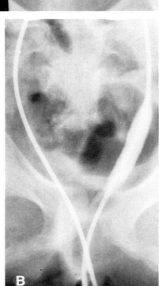

FIG. 52–7. Bilateral ureteral ectopia with duplication and both ureters entering the urethra just below the bladder neck. **(A)** IVU, 3-minute film; unusual ending of the two ureters suggesting the diagnosis. (No direct or indirect signs of duplication). **(B)** Bilateral catheterization of the two ectopic ureters.

FIG. 52–8. Simple ureteral ectopia in a girl. **(A)** IVU; bilateral upper tract duplication (*arrows*). **(B)** Opacification of the left upper ureter at laparotomy; the affected ureter terminates just outside the hymen on the left (*lower arrow*). The vagina is opacified partially (*upper arrow*).

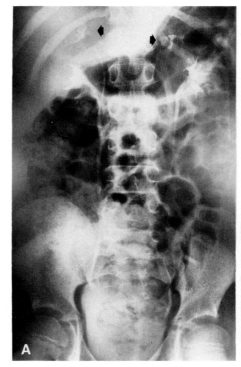
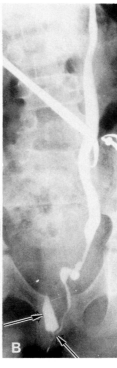

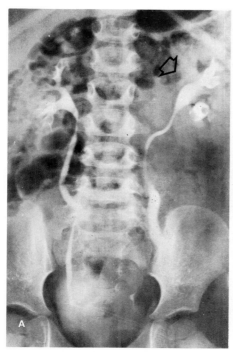

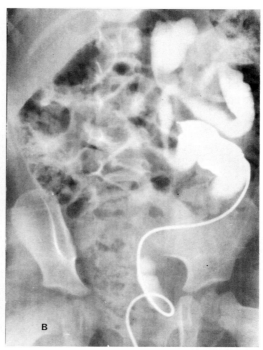

FIG. 52–9. Simple ureteral ectopia in a girl. **(A)** IVU; indirect signs of upper tract duplication on the left: The visualized pelvicalyceal system is displaced laterally and downward (*arrow*), and the ureter is tortuous because of the dilatation and tortuosity of adjacent non-visualized ureter. **(B)** At urethroscopy, the ectopic ureteral opening was found to be in the urethra; catheterization and opacification of this tract demonstrated marked dilatation and extreme tortuosity of the affected ureter.

FIG. 52–10. Simple ureteral ectopia in a girl. **(A)** IVU; bilateral upper tract duplication; the superior complex on the right is dilated and poorly visualized (*arrows*). **(B)** Opacification of the superior complex on the right at laparotomy demonstrated that the affected ureter ended in the lower portion of the vagina (*arrows*).

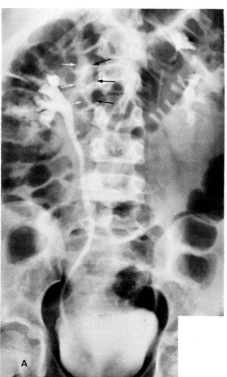

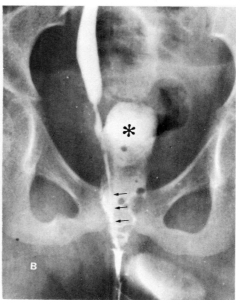

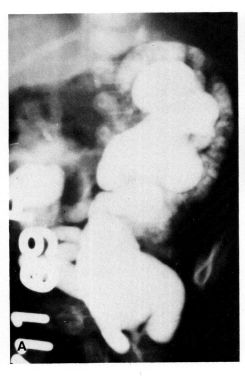

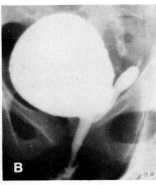

FIG. 52–11. Bilateral ureteral ectopia in a girl with single upper tracts. **(A)** Shows massive hydronephrosis. The distal ends of both dilated ureters are visualized entering the urethra. **(B)** Cystogram with reflux into the left ureter. (Courtesy of Keith Waterhouse, M.D.)

BIBLIOGRAPHY

1. Amar, A.D.: Improved methods in the diagnosis of urethral duplication and ectopia. Can. Med. Assoc. J., 95:813, 1966.
2. Cox, C.E., and Hutch, J.A.: Bilateral single ectopic ureter: A report of two cases and review of the literature. J. Urol., 95:493, 1966.
3. Grossman, H., Winchester, P.H., and Muecke, E.C.: Solitary ectopic ureter. Radiology, 89:1069, 1967.
4. Hartman, S.W.: The duplex kidney and related abnormalities. Clin. Radiol., 20:387, 1969.
5. Johnston, J.H., and Davenport, T.J.: The single ectopic ureter. Br. J. Urol., 41:428, 1969.
6. Malek, R.S., Kelalis, P.P., Stickler, G.B., and Burke, E.C.: Observations on ureteral ectopy in children. J. Urol., 107:308, 1972.
7. Uson, A.C., Womack, C.E., and Berdon, W.E.: Giant ectopic ureter presenting as an abdominal mass in a newborn infant. J. Pediatr., 80:473, 1972.
8. Uson, A.C., and Schulman, C.C.: Ectopic ureter emptying into the rectum: Report of a case. J. Urol., 108:156, 1972.
9. Vanhoutte, J.J.: Ureteral ectopia into a Wolffian duct remnant (Gartner's ducts or cysts) presenting as a ureteral diverticulum in two girls. Am. J. Roentgenol., 110:540, 1970.
10. Wiggishoff, C.C., and Kiefer, J.H.: Ureteral ectopia: Diagnostic difficulties. J. Urol., 96:671, 1966.
11. Williams, D.I., and Lightwood, R.G.: Bilateral single ectopic ureters. Br. J. Urol., 44:267, 1972.
12. Williams, D.I., and Rogle, M.: Ectopic ureter in the male child. Br. J. Urol., 41:421, 1969.

Urethral Valves

GUIDO CURRARINO

Urethral valves are distinct obstructions of the urethra and are seen in the posterior and anterior urethra in males and very rarely in females.

POSTERIOR URETHRAL VALVES

Obstructing valves represent a fairly common and an important anomaly of the male posterior urethra.

Young has classified the disorder in three types. In the first type, two valve-like folds of mucosa arise from the lower pole of the verumontanum and end in the lateral wall of the distal posterior urethra. Their medial borders are in contact or are partially fused. In the second type, two similar mucosal folds originate from the superior pole of the verumontanum and extend upward to the bladder neck area. The existence of this form has been repeatedly questioned. In the third type, a horizontal membrane with a central opening is present in the posterior urethra below or above the verumontanum. The lesion is rare and is more properly considered as a form of stenosis rather than a valve. The following remarks apply to the first and, by far, the most common type.

The origin of the anomaly is not certain. According to some authors it represents an exaggeration of normal mucosal folds in the posterior urethra, but this has been questioned. Because of the valve-like arrangement of the two membranes, retrograde passage of a catheter or of contrast medium is not impeded, whereas the downflow of urine from the bladder is obstructed. The severity of the lesion depends not only on the degree of obstruction and of secondary changes in the bladder and upper tracts but also on the presence or absence of renal dysplasia, a fairly frequent complication in severe cases.

In more than half of the cases, the obstruction is severe and becomes clinically manifest early in life with failure to void in the newborn period, rarely fetal urine ascites due to rupture of the upper urinary tract (Fig. 53-8) or bladder, dribbling of urine, poor stream, urinary retention, distended bladder, urinary tract infections, fever, and failure to thrive. In less severe forms, the disorder may become manifest during childhood or even later, with urinary tract infection, hematuria, enuresis, incontinence, or other disorders of micturition. Occasionally, the patient presents in advanced chronic renal failure without any previous symptoms. Dysplastic and cystic kidneys associated with valves have been reported.[1, 7, 8, 14]

The excretory urogram commonly shows a decrease in the renal parenchyma and function (Fig. 53-4). Hydronephrosis and hydroureter, often bilateral and asymmetric, are common and may be severe (Figs. 53-4, 53-5). In the cystogram, the bladder may be normal in size or enlarged and is often hypertrophied and trabeculated. Bladder diverticula are common and may be large. Significant bladder residue is a frequent finding. Reflux (Figs. 53-5 to 53-8) is common but far from constant even in extreme situations, occurring only in about 50 per cent of the cases. It may be bilateral and unequal, or it may be unilateral. The affected ureters tend to be dilated and elongated. Sometimes the elongation and tortuosity of the ureters is out of proportion to the ureteral dilatation, suggesting an element of ureteral dysplasia. Evidence of obstruction at the ureterovesical junction (Figs. 53-5, 53-7), caused presumably by the hypertrophied bladder wall, may be observed even in the presence of reflux.

In the voiding urethrogram the posterior urethra is elongated and greatly dilated down to the level of the urogenital membrane. The dilated part of the urethra has an almost cylindrical configuration with a rounded bottom. This dilatation may persist for a long time postoperatively. The valves themselves may be seen in overpenetrated frontal views as two thin radiolucent lines. The anterior urethra often appears thin (collapsed) in the voiding study. The transition between the dilated posterior urethra and the normal anterior urethra is abrupt. A common finding in the voiding cystourethrogram is a prominent collar formation at the level of the bladder neck, caused in part by the bladder wall hypertrophy and in part by the widened posterior urethra. The bladder neck itself is usually normal in width but may be narrowed. Secondary bladder neck obstruction requiring surgery is uncommon.

The procedure of choice to demonstrate the lesion is the voiding cystourethrogram with the patient in a sharp oblique or lateral position. The valves are not shown by retrograde urethrography (Fig. 53-2), because they are displaced laterally and flattened against the urethral wall by the retrograde flow of the material.

The diagnosis cannot be made radiographically unless the "voiding" films show the abnormal widening of the posterior urethra. Transverse or oblique ridges or folds in the posterior urethra not associated with a definite dilatation of this part of the urethra, and without other signs of obstruction in the bladder or upper tracts, are not uncommon findings (Figs. 53-10). They represent exaggerations of normal anatomic features of the posterior urethra and are of no clinical significance. A widening of the posterior urethra, sometimes simulating valves, may be seen in some instances of neurogenic bladder and in absent abdominal musculature. A dilatation of the posterior urethra without obstruction and of unknown cause is occasionally encountered in otherwise normal urinary tracts (Fig. 53-11). A knowledge of the whole clinical picture and of all the other radiologic findings will simplify the problem in most cases, and careful urethroscopy may clarify the problem.

ANTERIOR URETHRAL VALVES

Anterior urethral valves are uncommon and produce symptoms that are subtle and complications that are usually not severe, although Waterhouse reported bilateral hydronephrosis in his case.[22]

Williams considered diverticula of the anterior urethra in the same category as anterior urethral valves because of a valvular structure in the distal lip of the diverticulum. Anterior valves occur in the area between the membranous urethra and the external urethral meatus. The finding of sail-like leaflets in the anterior urethra on endoscopy is conclusive. Symptoms include enuresis, abnormal daytime wetting, dribbling, or blood staining of underclothes.

ROENTGENOGRAPHIC DIAGNOSIS

There are two types of anterior urethral valves.

Without Diverticular Formation. The obstructed area shows a mild-to-moderate indentation in the circumference of the urethra or a narrow lucent area distal to a convex bulge projecting distally. The distal urethra is narrowed; the proximal urethra is usually dilated (Figs. 53-12 to 53-13a).

With Diverticular Formation. There is usually a sharp valvular flap at the distal lip of an elongated diverticulum with some narrowing of the urethra at this point. Proximally, the urethra is dilated. In both of these types of valves there may be massive reflux with hydronephrosis (Figs. 53–14, 53–15).

URETHRAL VALVES IN GIRLS

These are extremely rare. Stevens found 14 cases in the literature up to 1936.[27] Eleven had a complete obstruction; three had partial obstruction. W. Hardy Hendren classifies urethral valves in girls as follows[24]:

1. True urethral valves
2. Urethral valves arising from a rudimentary verumontanum in girls with adrenogenital syndrome with masculinization of the lower urinary tract
3. Retained remnants of ectopic ureteroceles

ROENTGENOGRAPHIC DIAGNOSIS

The true valve in a girl produces a rounded bulge with a convex distal edge. The bulge is usually well demarcated from a narrow distal urethra. The valves associated with adrenogenital syndrome are similar to the true urethral valves. The valves associated with an ectopic ureteral remnant give a flap-like appearance with a distal cul-de-sac obstructing the urethra distally (Fig. 53–16).

CHAPTER 53, ILLUSTRATIONS

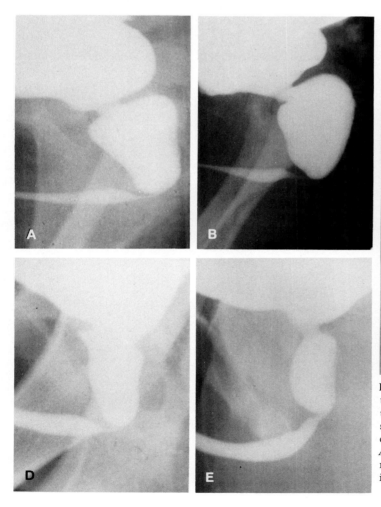

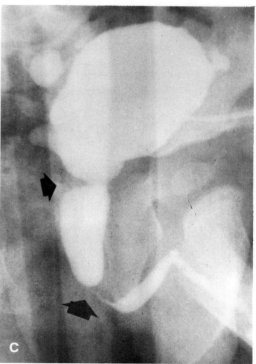

FIG. 53–1. (A–H) Eight instances of posterior urethral valves demonstrated by voiding cystourethrography. The posterior urethra is dilated, sometimes greatly. The dilatation usually extends downward as far as the urogenital membrane. *Arrows* demarcate proximal and distal end of posterior urethra, which is elongated. The distal urethra is normal.

(Figure 53–1 is continued on page 1970.)

FIG. 53-1, continued.

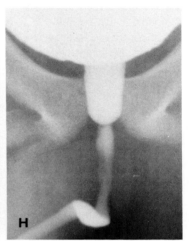

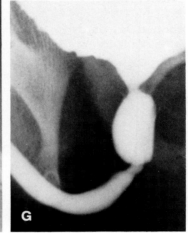

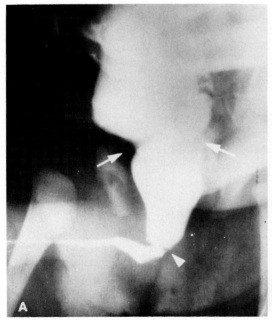

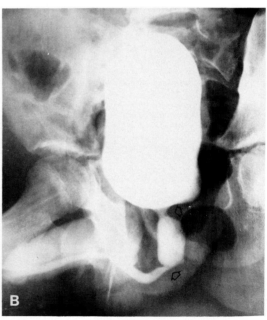

FIG. 53-2. (A–D) Two instances of posterior urethral valves demonstrated clearly by voiding cystourethrography **(A, B)**. By retrograde urethrography, the lesion could be missed easily **(C, D)**.

FIG. 53–3. (A–D) Two instances of posterior urethral valves, pre- and postoperative voiding cystourethrogram. Following removal of the valves, the dilatation of the posterior urethra may subside promptly as shown in **(A)** and **(B)**. In some cases, it persists for some time post-operatively, as shown in **(C)** and **(D)**.

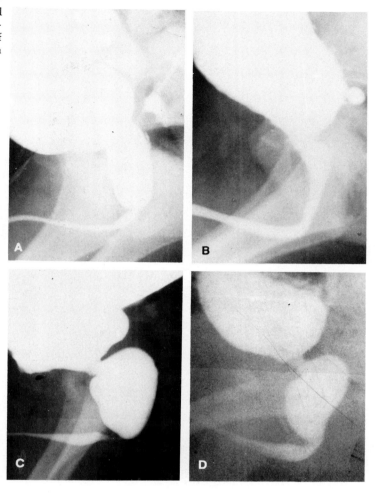

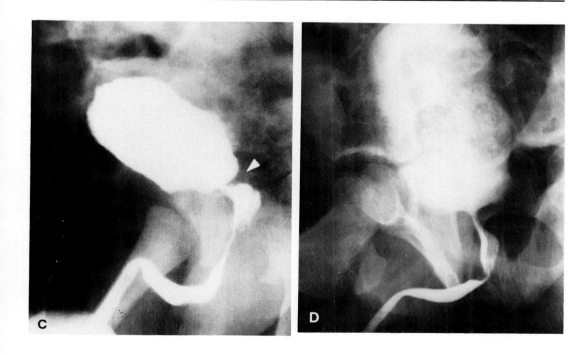

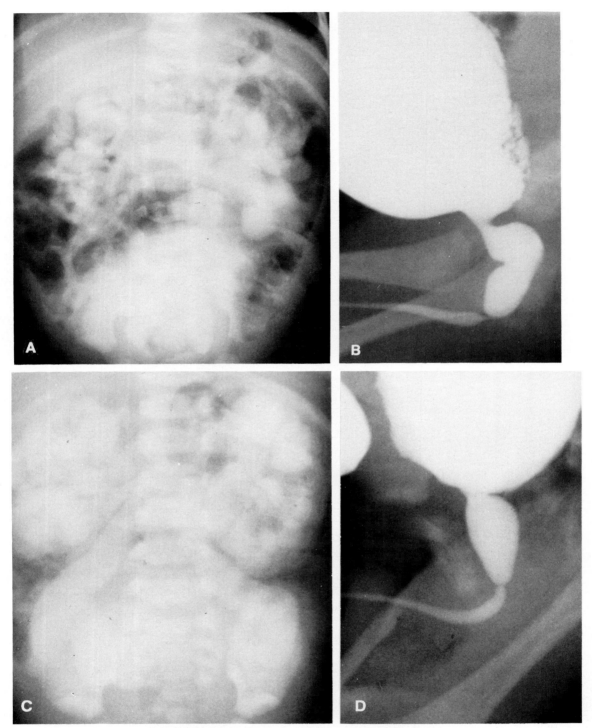

FIG. 53–4. (A–D) Two instances of posterior urethral valves, IVU on the left **(A, C)** and voiding cystogram on the same patient on the right **(B, D)**. Gross dilatation of both upper tracts with loss of renal parenchyma in the IVP and typical findings of posterior urethral valves in the cystourethrogram.

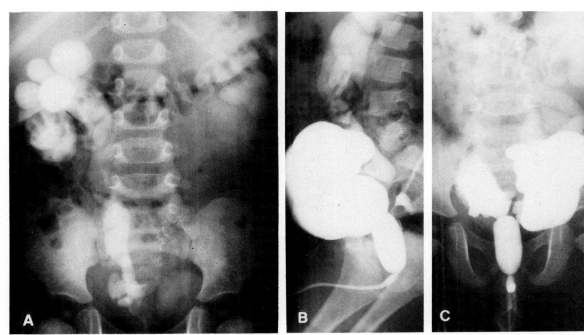

FIG. 53–5. Posterior urethral valves in infant. (A) IVU, delayed film: bilateral upper tract dilatation with evidence of ureterovesical junction obstruction on the right. (B, C) Voiding cystogram (lateral and anteroposterior AP). Typical findings of posterior urethral valves, left-sided reflux, large bladder diverticulum on the same side.

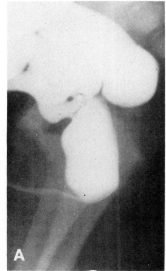

FIG. 53–6. Cystourethrogram in patient with posterior urethral valves, voiding (A) and delayed postvoiding film. (B) Typical findings of posterior urethral valves, trabeculated bladder, gross left-sided reflux.

FIG. 53–7. Cystourethrogram in patient with posterior urethral valves, voiding (A) and delayed postvoiding film (B). Typical findings of posterior urethral valves, trabeculated bladder, left-sided reflux with evidence of some ureterovesical junction obstruction.

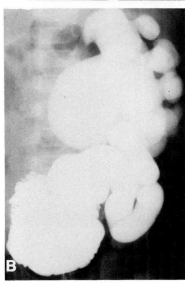

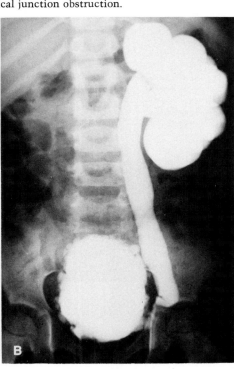

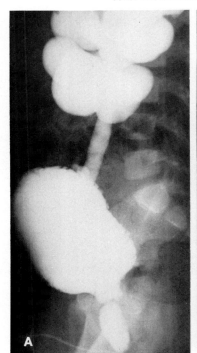

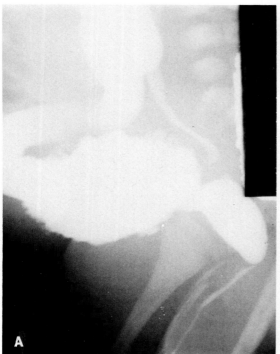

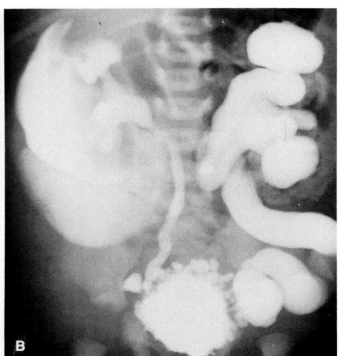

FIG. 53–8. Cystourethrogram in a newborn with fetal ascites and posterior urethral valves. **(A)** Voiding: typical findings of posterior urethral valves, trabeculated bladder, bilateral reflux. **(B)** Postvoiding film: massive extravasation of contrast material from right pelvicalyceal system, probably representing the cause of the patient's fetal (urine) ascites.

FIG. 53–9. (A–D) Cystourethrograms in four children with wrinkles in the posterior urethra representing normal findings, not to be confused with posterior urethral valves: verumontanum (*upper arrows*), inferior urethral crest and finns (*middle arrows*), and urogenital membrane (*lower arrows*).

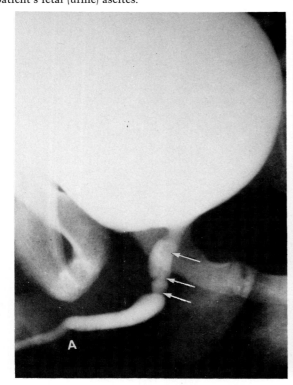

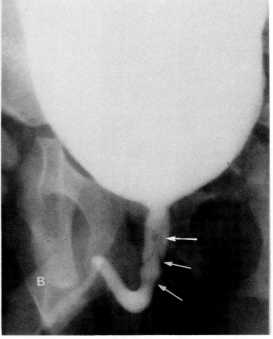

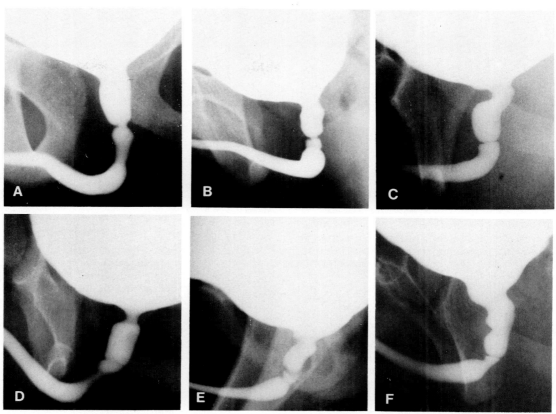

FIG. 53–10. Cystourethrograms of six patients with nonobstructing folds in posterior urethra simulating posterior urethral valves. These are exaggerations of the normal, probably related to structures shown in Figure 53–9. Careful urethroscopy may be necessary at times to separate these folds from true membrane stenoses.

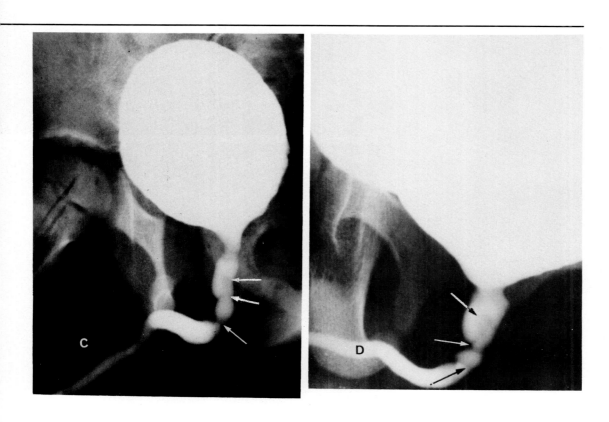

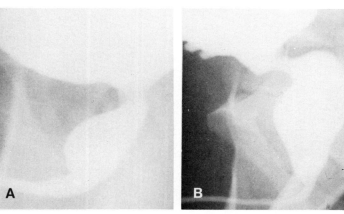
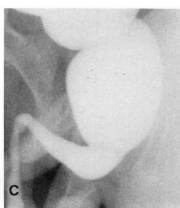
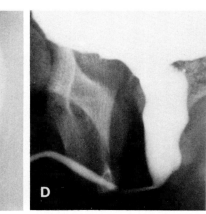

FIG. 53–11. Cystourethrograms in four patients with unusual ballooning of the posterior urethra during voiding simulating posterior urethral valves. The cause for this dilatation is not known. Patient shown in **(B)** had neurogenic bladder.

FIG. 53–13. Anterior urethral valves. **(A)** Voiding cystourethrogram. Note area of narrowing with moderate-sized flap projecting into the dilated portion. The proximal urethra is dilated. **(B)** Photograph of endoscopic appearance of anterior urethral valve. (Malholski, W.E., and Frank, I.N.: Anterior urethral valves. Urology, 3:382, 1973)

FIG. 53–12. Anterior urethral valve, voiding cystourethrogram. There is a radiolucent area just distal to a bulge of the anterior urethra. The bulge has a convex border presenting distally. The terminal urethra appears split into two streams. Note left vesicoureteral reflux. There was bilateral hydronephrosis and hydroureter. (Waterhouse, K., and Scordamaglia, L.J.: J. Urol., 87:556, 1962)

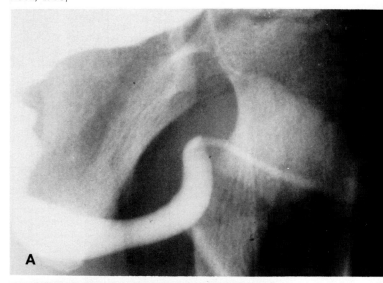

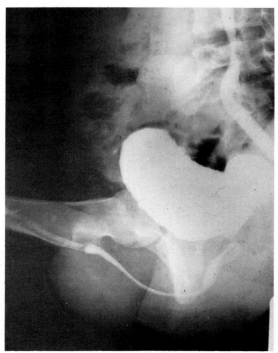

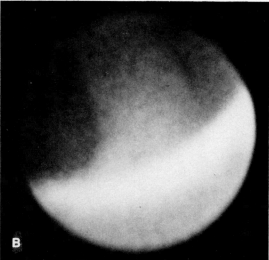

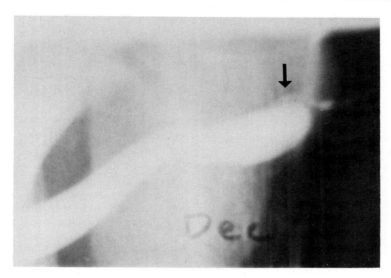

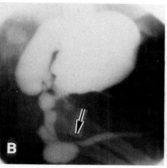
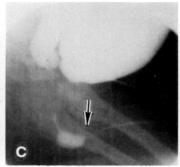
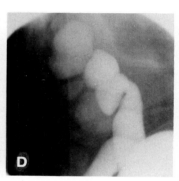

FIG. 53–14. Anterior urethral valve or diverticulum in 3-month-old boy. **(A)** Urethral catheter curled up in diverticulum. *Arrow* points to flap valve caused by proximal lip of diverticulum. **(B)** Voiding cysto-urethrogram, filling bladder by transpubic needle. **(C)** Dye trapped in diverticulum. **(D)** Massive reflux and hydronephrosis caused by severe urethral obstruction. (Courtesy of W. Hardy Hendren)

FIG. 53–15. Anatomy of lower urinary tract depicted in Figure 53–14. (Courtesy of W. Hardy Hendren)

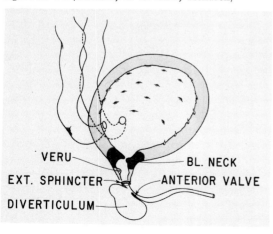

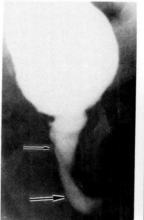
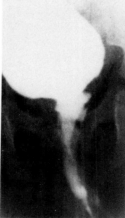

FIG. 53–16. Urethral valve in a girl. Voiding cysto-urethrogram showing valvelike obstruction of urethra in a girl following surgery for ureterocele. A remnant of the distal rim of ectopic ureterocele (*small arrow*) formed a cul-de-sac or diverticulum (*large arrow*) partially obstructing the distal urethra. (Courtesy of W. Hardy Hendren)

BIBLIOGRAPHY

Posterior Urethral Valves

1. Cussen, L.J.: Cystic kidneys in children with congenital urethral obstruction. J. Urol., *106*:939, 1971.
2. Ellis, D., Fonkalsrud, E., and Smith, J.P.: Congenital posterior urethral valves. J. Urol., *95*:549, 1966.
3. Hendren, W.H.: Posterior urethral valves in boys: a broad clinical spectrum. J. Urol., *106*:298, 1971.
4. Hope, J.W., Jameson, P.S., and Michie, A.J.: Diagnosis of anterior urethral valve by voiding urethrography: report of two cases. Radiology, *74*:798, 1960.
5. Johnston, J.H., and Kulatilake, A.E.: The sequelae of posterior urethral valves. Br. J. Urol., *43*:753, 1971.
6. Kumar, M., Shroff, N., and Bhat, H.S.: Posterior urethral valves: problems in management of upper urinary tract. Br. J. Urol., *44*:489, 1972.
7. Leonidas, J., Leiter, E., and Gribetz, D.: Congenital urinary tract obstruction presenting with ascites at birth: roentgenographic diagnosis. Radiology, *96*:111, 1970.
8. Milliken, L.D., and Hodgson, N.B.: Renal dysplasia and urethral valves. J. Urol., *108*:960, 1972.
9. Nesbit, R., and Labardin, M.M.: Urethral valve in the male child. J. Urol., *96*:218, 1966.
10. Osathanonoh, U., and Potter, E.L.: Pathogenesis of polycystic kidneys type 4 due to urethral obstruction. Arch. Pathol., *77*:502, 1964.
11. Robertson, W.V., and Hages, J.A.: Congenital diaphragmatic obstruction of the male posterior urethra. Br. J. Urol., *41*:592, 1969.
12. Waldbaum, R.S., and Marshall, V.F.: Posterior urethral valves: Evaluation and surgical management. J. Urol., *103*:801, 1970.
13. Whitaker, R.H., Keeton, J.E., and Williams, D.I.: Posterior urethral valves: A study of urinary control after operation. J. Urol., *108*:167, 1972.
14. Williams, D.I., and Eckstein, H.B.: Obstructive valves in the posterior urethra. J. Urol., *93*:236, 1965.
15. Williams, D.I., Whitaker, R.H., Barratt, T.M., and Keeton, J.E.: Urethral valves. Br. J. Urol., *45*:200, 1973.

Anterior Urethral Valves

16. Chang, C.-y: Anterior urethral valves: a case report. J. Urol., *100*:29, 1968.
17. Colabawalla, B.N.: Anterior urethral valves: a case report. J. Urol., *94*:58, 1965.
18. Daniel, J., Stewart, A.M., and Blair, D.W.: Congenital anterior urethral valve: diagnosis and treatment. Br. J. Urol., *40*:598, 1968.
19. Hope, J.W., Jameson, P.J., and Michie, A.J.: Diagnosis of anterior urethral valve by voiding cystourethrography: report of two cases. Radiology, *74*:798, 1960.
20. Malholski, W.E., and Frank, I.N.: Anterior urethral valves. Urology, *3*:382, 1973.
21. Nesbit, R.M., and Labardini, M.M.: Urethral valves in the male child. J. Urol., *96*:218, 1972.
22. Waterhouse, K., and Scordamaglia, L.J.: Anterior urethral valve: a rare cause of bilateral hydronephrosis. J. Urol., *87*:556, 1962.
23. Williams, D.I., and Retik, A.D.: Congenital valves and diverticula of the anterior urethra. Br. J. Urol., *41*:228, 1969.

Valves In Females

24. Hendren, W.H.: Personal communication.
25. Mitchell, G.F., Makholi, Z., and Frittelli, G.: Congenital urethral valve in a female. Radiology, *89*:690, 1967.
26. Nesbit, R.M., McDonald, H.P., Jr., and Busby, S.: Obstructing valves in the female urethra. J. Urol., *91*:79, 1964.
27. Stevens, W.E.: Congenital obstructions of the female urethra. J.A.M.A., *106*:89, 1936.

The following is a brief review of the better-known cystic renal disorders and their radiologic implications, with an emphasis on those occurring in children. (For classification of cystic disease see Chapter 9.)

ADULT TYPE OF POLYCYSTIC KIDNEY

This disorder is characteristically bilateral, although the changes may be more pronounced on one side than on the other (see Figs. 54–9 to 54–11). Occasionally the bilateral nature of the disease is established only by renal arteriography, at operation or post mortem. The rest of the urinary tract is normal. The kidneys are variously enlarged and lobulated and contain many rounded cysts of different sizes disseminated throughout the parenchyma. The renal function is commonly decreased from mildly to severely, depending on the amount of residual normal renal tissue. The disorder usually becomes manifest in the fourth or fifth decade of life with hypertension, intermittent bouts of hematuria, and renal failure, and it is slowly progressive.

The urographic findings are characterized by compression defects on the calyces, infundibula, and often the pelvis. The calyces are stretched and distorted and have a spidery appearance. In the nephrographic phase of the study, the cysts cast round lucent shadows within the renal parenchyma.

The disorder is genetically determined as an autosomal dominant trait. It may be associated with macroscopic and microscopic cystic changes in other organs, especially the liver, and with cerebral artery aneurysms. It is often stated that this form of polycystic kidney is congenital in origin, but this is open to question in view of the discrepancy between the relative frequency of the disorder in adults and

54

Guido Currarino

Cystic Renal Diseases

the rarity with which macroscopic or microscopic renal cysts are encountered in routine autopsies of infants and children. It may be that only the predisposition to the development of renal cysts, rather than the cysts themselves, is genetically determined and congenital.

A form of polycystic kidneys of the spherical type similar, at least radiographically, to that seen in adults is encountered in early life on rare occasions. A family history of polycystic kidneys of the adult type may be obtained in some of these patients. The affected patient often is stillborn or dies shortly after birth but occasionally lives a few months or even years, with signs of progressive renal insufficiency.

"INFANTILE POLYCYSTIC KIDNEY" AND "RENAL TUBULAR ECTASIA WITH HEPATIC FIBROSIS"

These two conditions are considered together because of certain similarities in their main anatomic features. Both are recessively inherited traits.

It has been suggested that they may represent the same disorder, differing only in the severity and distribution of the changes, ranging from severe renal involvement, with early death from renal failure, to a predominant liver disease leading to overt portal hypertension during childhood. There is nothing to indicate that these conditions are in any way related to other cystic renal diseases.

INFANTILE POLYCYSTIC KIDNEY

Although infrequent, this is the most common, most characteristic, and most severe form of "polycystic kidney" of infancy (Figs. 54–1 to 54–5). It has also been referred to as microcystic or hamartomatous type. The term (medullary) sponge kidney should be avoided to eliminate confusion with the adult medullary sponge kidney.

Both kidneys are involved. They are symmetrically enlarged and fairly smooth in outline. On section, the entire kidney resembles a honeycomb, being studded with a myriad of minute elongated cysts of uniform size, which represent noticeably dilated and elongated tubules. The cysts radiate outward from the hilum to the outer surface of the kidney without any demarcation between medulla and cortex. The rest of the urinary tract is normal. The liver shows a proliferation, elongation, and cystic widening of the small bile ducts and an increase in the blood vessels and lymphatics. Liver fibrosis is

not a prominent feature. Somewhat similar changes may be observed in the pancreas.

The excretory urogram usually shows decreased renal function. The upper collecting system is less deformed than in adult polycystic kidney. A characteristic feature is an irregular nephrogram effect throughout the renal parenchyma, with streaks of increased density radiating from the hilum to the periphery of the kidney, which is caused by opacification of the dilated tubules. The finding may be apparent only in delayed films. On retrograde pyelography, contrast material may reflux into the dilated tubules, giving the whole kidney a streaky pattern.

Low-set ears and other features of the Potter facies may be present. A spontaneous pneumothorax may complicate the picture in the newborn period. The prognosis is poor. Most of the affected patients are stillborn or die in the newborn period. A few patients live for a few months or years. These less severely affected patients may represent transition forms of the condition described next.

RENAL TUBULAR ECTASIA WITH LIVER FIBROSIS

This is also termed juvenile polycystic kidney with liver fibrosis and juvenile polycystic hepatorenal disease, and it is a relatively uncommon disorder (Figs. 54–6 to 54–8). It is characterized by diffuse, bilateral dilatation of the collecting renal tubules similar to but less severe than that seen in the infantile type of polycystic kidney. The changes are often limited to the medulla. Occasionally small round cysts are observed in the pyramids. The kidneys are commonly enlarged. The renal function may be normal or decreased. The calyces and infundibula may be compressed and stretched by the bulky renal parenchyma. The dilated tubules usually fill with contrast material during excretory or retrograde pyelography, producing coarse striations radiating outward from the papillae. The changes are similar to but much less pronounced than those seen in infantile polycystic kidney, and they may be indistinguishable radiographically from those of medullary sponge kidney of adults.

The liver shows a diffuse cystic dysplasia of the small bile ducts with periportal fibrosis. The lobular architecture is preserved. The extrahepatic bile ducts may be enlarged or variously malformed. A choledochal cyst has been found in some cases.

The presenting symptoms are frequently those of portal hypertension with bleeding varices during childhood. In other patients renal insufficiency is the predominant feature of the disease (transition forms to infantile polycystic kidney?).

MEDULLARY SPONGE KIDNEY OF THE ADULT

The disorder is characterized by ectasia of the collecting tubules forming clusters of small cysts in the medullary zones of the kidneys. Although it has some similarities with infantile polycystic kidney and with renal tubular ectasia with liver fibrosis, there are reasons to believe that it is an unrelated condition. It occurs almost exclusively in adults, predominantly women, between the fourth and sixth decades of life. Only a few cases have been reported in children. The condition does not appear to be genetically determined and is not associated with cystic changes in the liver or other urinary tract malformations.

CYSTIC RENAL DYSPLASIA

Renal dysplasia is a relatively frequent condition. It is apparently caused by an arrest in development and an abnormal differentiation of the fetal kidney. The affected organ contains primitive glomeruli and tubules, an excess of fibrous tissue and often islands of cartilage, muscle fibers, and cysts. The disease is not genetically determined and is not associated with cystic dysplasia in the liver or other organs. When the cysts predominate, the condition is referred to as *cystic renal dysplasia*. The cysts vary in size from minute to extremely large and are scattered throughout the kidney. The affected kidney varies greatly in size, from a minute nubbing to a large mass. The renal artery is small or absent.

Both simple and cystic renal dysplasias are frequently associated with severe infrarenal obstructions to which they may be secondary, or with nonobstructive reflux usually associated with a dilated, elongated, and tortuous ureter (e.g., prune belly syndrome). Renal dysplasia is also frequent in that part of the kidney drained by an ectopically ending ureter with or without ureterocele formation.

The disorder is usually unilateral but may be bilateral, particularly in the presence of infravesical obstructions. Abnormalities of the opposite upper tract, such as reflux, hydronephrosis, renal ectopia, malrotation, hypoplasia, or absence may coexist in unilateral cases.

Several variants of cystic renal dysplasia have been described, based on the size of the affected kidney, type of associated infrarenal lesion, presence or absence of upper tract dilatation proximal to the obstruction, and whether the disorder is unilateral or bilateral. The best known variant is the so-called *multicystic kidney* (Figs. 54–14 to 54–20). In this variant the involved kidney is large, lobulated, and nonfunctioning, and it is entirely replaced by many spherical cysts of various sizes, loosely held together by connective tissues. Some communication between cysts and with the collecting system may be present. The calyces and pelvis may be absent, reduced to fibrous cords, or extremely small. The proximal ureter is impervious or diminutive. The distal ureter and the ureteral orifice are generally preserved. The lesion is almost always unilateral, but the opposite upper urinary tract may be affected by other malformations. In the majority of cases the condition is discovered in infancy, often because a flank mass is felt by the mother or on a routine physical examination. The excretory urogram shows no function on the affected side. During the nephrographic phase of the study, the affected kidney is relatively radiolucent, but a faintly opaque rim may be seen around the kidney simulating severe hydronephrosis, and irregular curvilinear strands or round densities throughout the kidney may be identified. These findings possibly reflect the vascular supply of the renal capsule cyst walls, and filling of cysts with contrast material. The blind-ending ureter may be visualized by retrograde ureterography.

SOLITARY OR SIMPLE CYSTS

In this type of cystic renal disease, one or more spherical cysts of various size are found within an otherwise normal renal parenchyma (see Figs. 54–12, 54–13). The condition is usually unilateral. It is not familial and is not associated with other abnormalities in the urinary system or in other organs. Because it is rare in children but relatively frequent in adults, it is doubtful whether it is congenital and related to other types of cystic renal disease. The possibility has been suggested that it develops from focal areas of renal dysplasia. Because the cysts are predominantly located in the renal cortex, they usually cause a bulge in the renal contour, and, when sufficiently large, they compress, stretch, and deform the adjacent calyces, infundibula, and pelvis. Calcifications within the cyst wall may be seen. Like other renal cysts they cast a relatively lucent shadow in the nephrogram, an important although not infallible differential point with a renal neoplasm. The renal function is usually well preserved. As a rule the cysts do not fill with contrast material either by excretory or retrograde pyelography. When bilateral and multiple, the changes may simulate polycystic kidney of the adult type.

MULTILOCULAR CYST

In this rare type of cystic renal disease, also referred to as cystic adenoma or lymphangioma, a segment of an otherwise normal kidney is replaced by a cluster of cysts, all encased in a firm capsule. The disorder appears to be congenital, is not familial or hereditary, and occurs as an isolated lesion. Its histologic features suggest a localized form of renal dysplasia. The possibility has been raised that it represents a stage in the maturation of Wilms' tumor. The findings by excretory urography and retrograde pyelography are those of a localized renal mass indistinguishable from Wilms' tumor. An abnormal vascularity simulating a malignant neoplasm rarely may be seen by arteriography.

CHAPTER 54, ILLUSTRATIONS

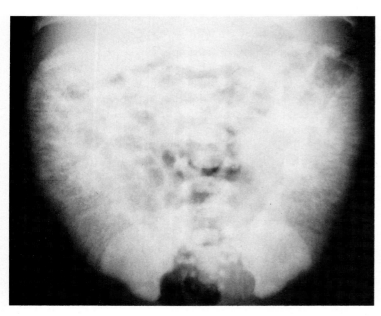

FIG. 54–1. Newborn with infantile polycystic kidneys. IVU; marked enlargement of the kidneys. Dense streaks radiating from the papillae to the outer margins of the kidneys represent contrast material in dilated and elongated collecting tubules.

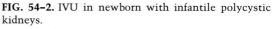
FIG. 54–2. IVU in newborn with infantile polycystic kidneys.

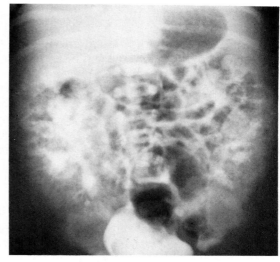

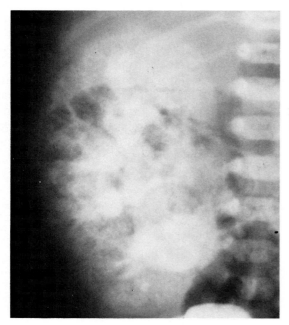

FIG. 54–3. IVU in newborn with infantile polycystic kidneys. Close-up view of right kidney.

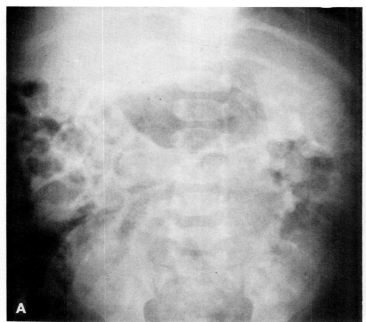

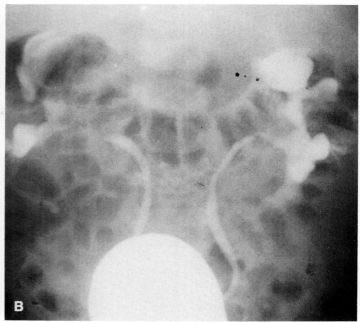

FIG. 54–4. Polycystic kidney of the infantile type in an 8-month-old infant with systemic arterial hypertension. **(A)** IVU; **(B)** Cystourethrogram with bilateral reflux (unusual). Calyces are deformed by swollen parenchyma.

FIG. 54–5. Polycystic kidney of the infantile type, IVU. **(A)** At 6 weeks of age; **(B)** Patient still alive at 6 years with systemic arterial hypertension.

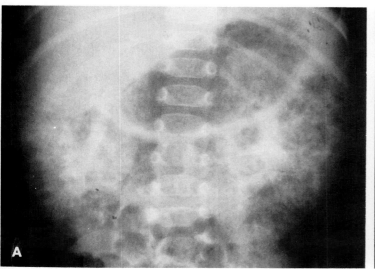

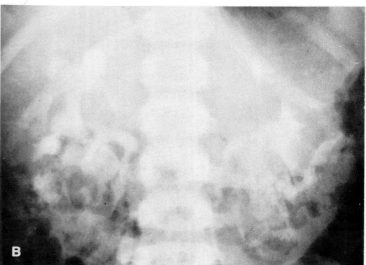

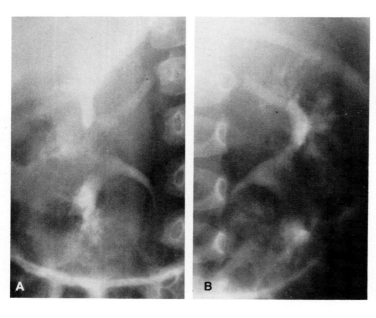

FIG. 54–6. Renal tubular ectasia with liver fibrosis in a 17-month-old child. IVU. (**A**) Right and (**B**) left kidney. Dense streaks in pyramids representing contrast material within dilated tubules.

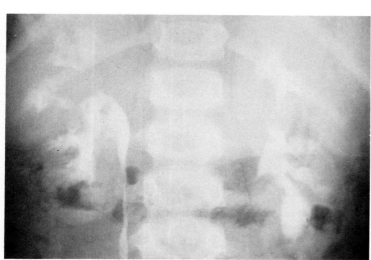

FIG. 54–7. Renal tubular ectasia with liver fibrosis in a 5-year-old child. IVU. Collections of contrast material in medulla simulating medullary sponge kidney disease of adults.

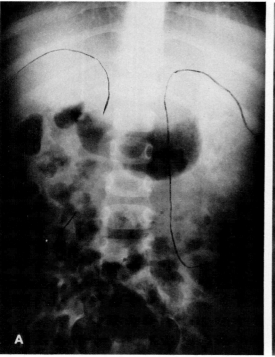
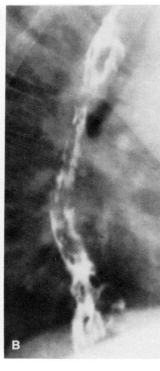

FIG. 54–8. Renal tubular ectasia with liver fibrosis in a 9-year-old child. (**A**) IVU; enlarged, poorly functioning kidneys with streaky nephrograms. (**B**) Esophogram; severe varices.

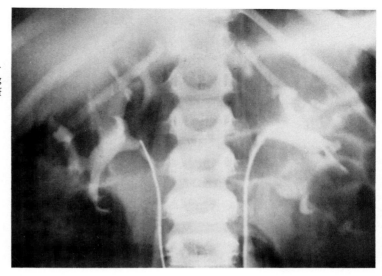

FIG. 54–9. Bilateral retrograde pyelogram in a 5-year-old child. Enlargement of the kidneys with stretching and spidering of the calyces, as seen in the adult type of polycystic kidneys. (Courtesy of David Baker, M.D.)

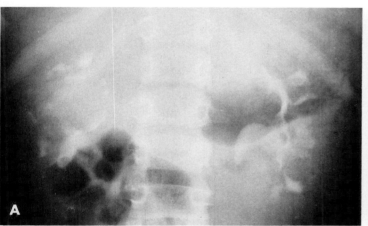

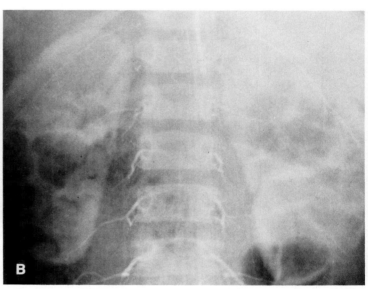

FIG. 54–10. Adult type of polycystic kidney in 4-year-old child. (A) IVU; stretching and spidering of the calyces. (B) Arteriogram, nephrographic phase; disseminated lucencies produced by the cysts.

FIG. 54–11. Adult type polycystic kidneys in 8-month-old infant. IVU, frontal and lateral projections.

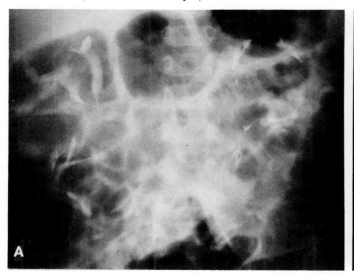

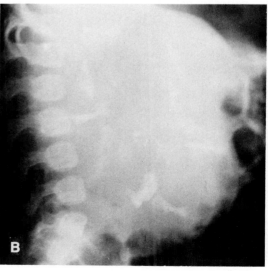

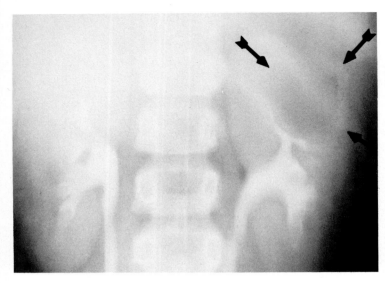

FIG. 54–12. Solitary simple cyst of left kidney in a child. IVU; relative radiolucency of the cyst (*arrows*).

FIG. 54–13. Multiple simple cysts in right kidney. (**A**) IVU at 6 years of age. (**B** and **C**) Follow-up IVU 6 months and 10 years after puncture of all cysts. No apparent recurrence of the process.

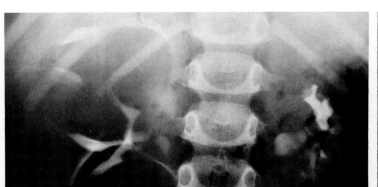
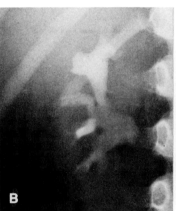
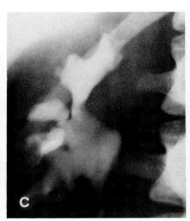

FIG. 54–14. Multicystic kidney on the right in a 6-week-old infant presenting as a large flank mass. Bilateral retrograde pyelogram—blind-ending ureter on the right.

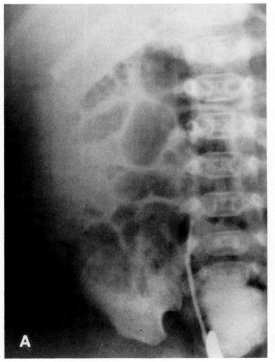
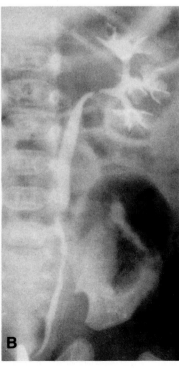

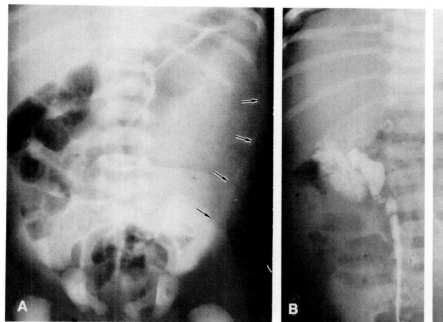

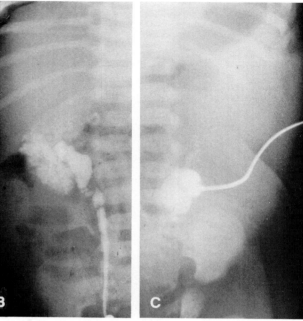

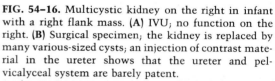

FIG. 54–15. Multicystic kidney on the left and dysplastic kidney on the right in a 2-week-old infant with a large left flank mass. (**A**) IVU; no function bilaterally. The left flank mass is relatively radiolucent in the phase of "total body opacification." Note dense rim at the margins of the mass produced by vessels in the capsule. (**B**) Left retrograde pyelogram, granular reflux into the renal parenchyma (cystic dysplasia). (**C**) Percutaneous puncture and opacification of one of the cysts on the left.

FIG. 54–16. Multicystic kidney on the right in infant with a right flank mass. (**A**) IVU; no function on the right. (**B**) Surgical specimen; the kidney is replaced by many various-sized cysts; an injection of contrast material in the ureter shows that the ureter and pelvicalyceal system are barely patent.

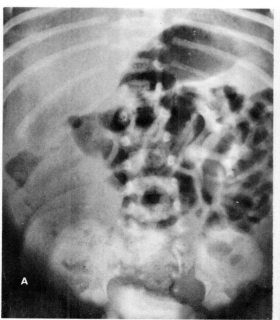

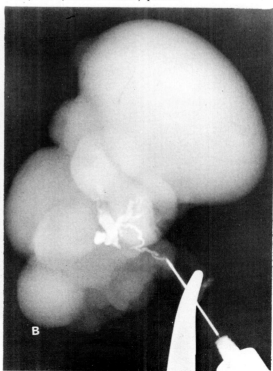

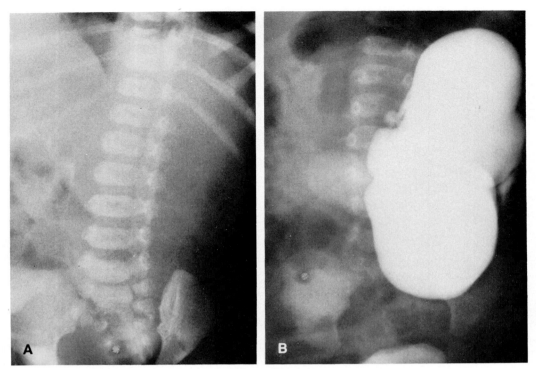

FIG. 54–17. Multicystic kidney on the left in an infant with large flank mass. **(A)** IVU; no renal function on the left. The mass is relatively radiolucent in the early films. **(B)** Percutaneous injection on the left with opacification of several intercommunicating cysts.

FIG. 54–18. Multicystic kidney on the left and mild ureteropelvic junction obstruction on the right in an infant with a large left flank mass. **(A)** IVU; nephrographic phase. The left flank mass is relatively radiolucent. **(B)** IVP, delayed film. Mild ureteropelvic junction obstruction is seen. **(C)** Percutaneous opacification of one of the cysts on the left.

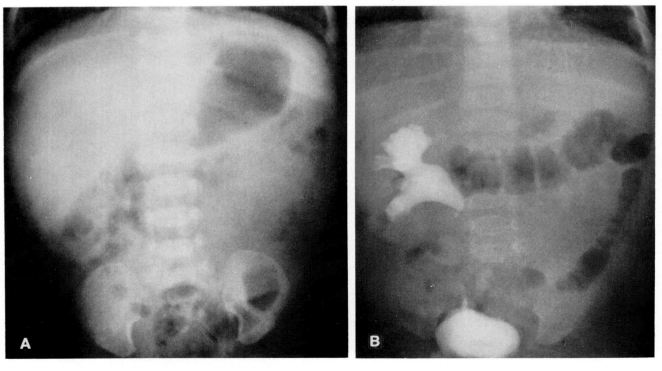

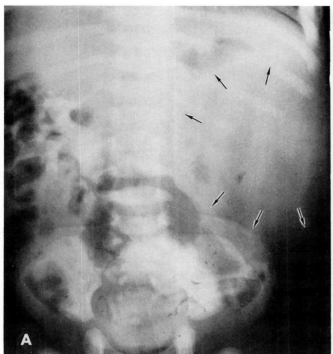

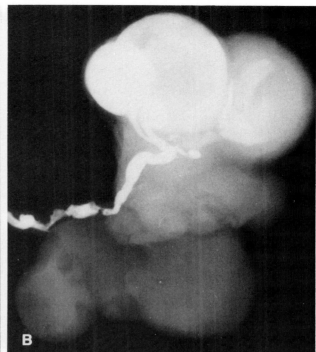

FIG. 54–19. Multicystic kidney on the left in a newborn with large flank mass. (A) IVU; the mass is relatively radiolucent. There is an opaque rim around the mass (arrows). (B) Injected specimen; barely patent ureter, poorly formed pelvis communicating with several cysts through minute channels.

FIG. 54–20. Bilateral multicystic kidney in a newborn with flank masses. (A) Cystogram: right reflux up to the kidney. Note spidery appearance of the calyces. (B) Left kidney injected at autopsy. Note small cysts communicating with calyces. (C) Xeroradiogram of same specimen.

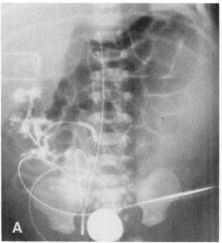

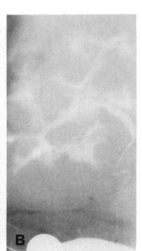

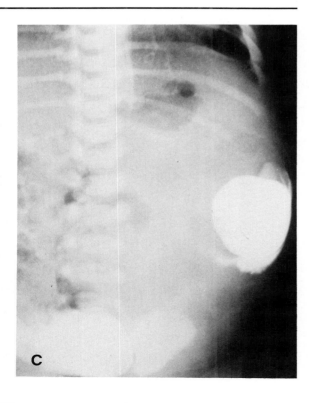

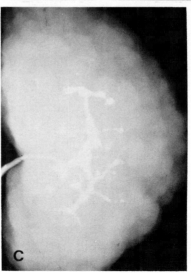

BIBLIOGRAPHY

1. Ahmed, S.: Simple renal cysts in childhood. Br. J. Urol., *44*:71, 1972.
2. Aterman, K., Boustani, P., and Gillis, D.A.: Solitary multilocular cyst of the kidney. J. Pediatr. Surg., 8:505, 1973.
3. Bernstein, J.: Developmental abnormalities of the renal parenchyma: renal hypoplasia and dysplasia. *In* Sommers, S.C., ed.: Pathology Annual 1968. Appleton-Century-Crofts, Inc., 1968.
4. Bernstein, J.: Heritable cystic disorders of the kidney: The mythology of polycystic disease. Pediatr. Clin. North Am., *18*:435, 1971.
5. Bernstein, J., and Meyer, R.: Parenchymal maldevelopment of the kidney. *In* Brennemann, Practice of Pediatrics. vol. 3, ch. 26. Hagerstown, Md. Hoeber Med. Div., Harper and Row, 1967.
6. Blythe, H., and Ockenden, B.G.: Polycystic disease of kidneys and liver presenting in childhood. J. Med. Genetics, 8:257, 1971.
7. Elkin, M., and Bernstein, J.: Cystic diseases of the kidneys: Radiological and pathological considerations. Clin. Radiol., *20*:65, 1969.
8. Cussen, L.T.: Cystic kidneys in children with congenital urethral obstruction. J. Urol., *106*:939, 1971.
9. Gleason, D.C., McAllister, W.E., and Kissane, J.: Cystic disease of the kidneys in children. Am. J. Roentgenol., *100*:135, 1967.
10. Greenberg, L.A., Altman, D.H., and Litt, R.E.: Cystic enlargement of the kidneys in infancy. Radiology, *89*:850, 1967.
11. Grossman, H., and Seed, W.: Congenital hepatic fibrosis, bile duct dilatation, and renal lesions resembling medullary sponge kidney (congenital 'cystic' disease of the liver and kidneys). Radiology, 87:46, 1966.
12. Grossman, H., Winchester, P.H., and Chiasari, F.V.: Roentgenographic classification of renal cystic disease. Am. J. Roentgenol., *104*:319, 1968.
13. Gwinn, J.I., and Landing, B.H.: Cystic disease of the kidneys in infants and children. Radiol. Clin. North Am., 6:191, 1968.
14. Hoeffel, J.C., Jacottin, G., and Bourgeois, J.M.: Renal cysts in childhood: A descriptive classification with clinical notes. Clin. Pediatr., *10*:701, 1971.
15. Johnson, J.H.: Renal cystic disease in childhood. Prog. Pediatr. Surg., 2:99, 1971.
16. Ivemark, B.I., Lagergren, C., and Lindvall, N.: Roentgenologic diagnosis of polycystic kidney and medullary sponge kidney. Acta Radiol. (Diagn.), *10*:225, 1970.
17. Lalli, A.F.: Medullary sponge kidney disease. Radiology, *92*:92, 1969.
18. Lalli, A.F.: Multicystic kidney disease. Radiology, *89*:857, 1967.
19. Lieberman, E., Salinas-Madrigal, L., Gwinn, J.L., Brennan, L.P., Fine, R.N., and Landing, B.H.: Infantile polycystic disease of the kidneys and liver: clinical pathological and radiological correlations and comparison with congenital hepatic fibrosis. Medicine, *50*:277, 1971.
20. Nahum, H., and Reysseguier, J.C.: Congenital hepatic fibrosis: The place of radiology (report of 10 cases). Ann. Radiol., *14*:65, 1971.
21. Newman, L., Simms, K., Kissane, J., and McAlister, W.: Unilateral total renal dysplasia in children. Am. J. Roentgenol., *116*:778, 1972.
22. Persky, L., Izant, R., and Bolande, R.: Renal dysplasia. J. Urol., 98:431, 1967.
23. Piper, J.V., and Beswick, I.P.: The diagnosis of multilocular cysts of the kidneys. Br. J. Urol., *42*:282, 1970.
24. Potter, E.L.: Normal and abnormal development of the kidney. Chicago, Ill., Year Book Med. Pub., Inc., 1972.
25. Spence, H.M., and Singleton, R.: Cysts and cystic disorders of the kidneys: types, diagnosis, treatment. Urol. Survey, *22*:131, 1972.
26. Wahlgrist, L.: Cystic disorders of the kidneys: Review of pathogenesis and classification. J. Urol., 97:1, 1967.

KIDNEYS

WILMS' TUMOR

Wilms' tumor, also referred to as nephroblastoma and renal embryoma, is the most common neoplasm of the urinary tract and one of the most frequent malignancies of childhood (Figs. 55–1 to 55–19). Its peak age incidence is around 3 years. Occasionally it is discovered at birth, rarely after the eighth year. It has a special tendency to occur in patients with aniridia and with hemihypertrophy and has been reported in horseshoe and other congenitally malformed kidneys and in association with pseudohermaphroditism, chronic nephritis, and other conditions. Familial cases are on record.

The tumor may be congenital in origin. It arises within the renal parenchyma, presumably from rests of the nephrogenic blastema, usually from a single focus, rarely in multiple areas (Fig. 55–13). It occurs bilaterally in 5 to 10 per cent of the cases.

The neoplasm is usually surrounded by a pseudocapsule. Histologically it is composed of polygonal epithelial cells commonly arranged in pseudotubular and pseudoglomerular formations. A diffuse infiltration of small undifferentiated spindle cells of connective tissue origin is often present. Sometimes the tumor is composed mainly of anaplastic, undifferentiated cells. Smooth and striated muscle fibers, adipose tissue, blood vessels, and islands of cartilage and bone formations may be present. Hemorrhage, necrosis, and microscopic calcifications are not infrequent.

Nephroblastoma is a highly malignant tumor. It tends to break through the renal capsule, to spread to adjacent retroperitoneal nodes and neighboring structures, and to invade the renal vein and sometimes the renal pelvis. It metastasizes to lungs, less commonly to liver and other intra-abdominal organs, and to the brain. Skeletal metastases are rare.

Neoplasms of the Urinary Tract and Adjacent Structures in Children

GUIDO CURRARINO

The most common presenting sign is an abdominal mass, which is frequently discovered by the mother. The mass may reach a large size rapidly and often becomes apparent after trauma to the abdomen. Hematuria and systemic hypertension are common. Congestive heart failure from hypertension may be the presenting manifestation on rare occasions. Pulmonary metastases are already present in one-third of the cases at the time of diagnosis.

The diagnosis is generally established by simple radiographic means. An ill-defined mass is found radiographically in most cases. Calcifications visible roentgenographically are seen in 5 to 10 per cent of the cases. Renal function by excretory urography is seldom absent. Because the tumor can originate in any part of the kidney, the unaffected renal parenchyma and the pelvicalyceal system and proximal ureter may be displaced in any direction. These changes may be demonstrated only in oblique or lateral views. In some instances the tumor is more centrally located, causing a draping of the calyces around the mass. If the tumor is small, the deformity may be limited to one or two calyces. Occasionally the tumor is mostly extrarenal, projecting outwardly from a small area of the renal surface. The opposite kidney should always be inspected carefully for signs of a bilateral tumor, both in the original examination and in follow-up studies.

Retrograde studies may be indicated when the calyces are inadequately visualized by excretory urography. An inferior venacavogram may be of value in the diagnosis of displacement, obstruction, or invasion of this vessel, especially if the lesion is on the right. Arteriography may be of value, particularly when there are urographic changes suggesting tumor in the opposite kidney. A pathologic vascularity characterized by tortuous, elongated, and irregular caliber vessels, collateral vessels, and AV shunting is almost always visualized, especially in selective studies. Avascular areas are common.

The differential diagnosis with other renal neoplasms may be impossible. Simple renal cysts cast a lucent shadow on the nephrogram, but this is not always a reliable differential point. A rim calcification is more in favor of a simple cyst. In the absence of renal function, the differentiation from a nonfunctioning hydronephrosis or multicystic kidney may be difficult. A nonfunctioning hydronephrotic upper segment of a duplex kidney may simulate an upper pole Wilms' tumor, but a local negative nephrogram plus other ancillary signs lower down in the urinary tract should suggest the diagnosis. Ultrasound studies will be important in the differentiation between a solid renal tumor and a renal cyst or hydronephrosis. An adrenal neuroblastoma or other adrenal tumors may closely simulate an upper pole Wilms' tumor. The presence of skeletal metastases or a positive VMA test favors neuroblastoma. Extrarenal retroperitoneal masses originating near a kidney such as lymphomas, teratomas, sarcomas, and lymphangiomas may also simulate a Wilms' tumor.

The following staging proposed by the National Wilms' Tumor Study has been reported by D'Angio:

I. Tumor limited to the kidney and completely resected
II. Tumor extending beyond kidney but completely resected
III. Residual nonhematogenous tumor confined to abdomen
IV. Hematogenous metastases
V. Bilateral renal involvement, either initially or subsequently

The average cure rate, with current coordinated methods of therapy encompassing surgery, radiation and chemotherapy, is probably higher than 80 per cent in localized tumors and as high as 50 per cent in the presence of metastases. Solitary pulmonary metastases can be successfully resected. The prognosis is definitely more favorable if the tumor is discovered and treated when the child is under 2 years of age. A permanent cure is expected if no recurrence or metastasis has occurred before the child has doubled his age from the time of diagnosis plus the 9 gestational months (Collin's period of risk).

BILATERAL WILMS' TUMOR

As already indicated, Wilms' tumor may involve both kidneys in 5 to 10 per cent of the cases. The two tumors may be discovered simultaneously, or the second tumor may become apparent some months or years later (Figs. 55–14 to 55–18). In the latter situation, it may not be possible to determine whether one deals with a metastasis or a second primary tumor. The roentgenographic findings in the other kidney are the same as described but usually are less obvious.

Rarely, bilateral tumors infiltrate both kidneys diffusely. In these cases the excretory urogram shows a stretching and a spidery appearance of the calyces not unlike that seen in the adult type of polycystic kidney. In 2 cases observed by the author, the kidneys were enlarged (Fig. 55–18); however, the pelvicalyceal systems were only minimally deformed and the renal arteriogram was normal. In the nephrographic phase of the excretory urogram and of the arteriogram, there were multiple areas of lucency scattered throughout the renal cortex. This diffuse nephroblastomatosis may be a distinct entity rather than a true Wilm's tumor. It may even represent a form of bilateral renal dysplasia with malignant elements. Cures have been obtained with x-ray radiation and chemotherapy without surgery. Our patients are alive, without evidence of tumor and with a normal excretory urogram 3 and 6 years, respectively, after the original diagnosis and treatment with x-ray radiation and chemotherapy alone.

CONGENITAL WILMS' TUMOR AND MESOBLASTIC NEPHROMA

Although congenital Wilms' tumors do occur, most renal neoplasms discovered in the first weeks or months of life are now thought to represent a different pathologic and clinical entity (Figs. 55–19 to 55–19c). They are predominantly mesenchymal neoplasms composed of sheets of connective tissue cells invading the adjacent parenchyma without capsule formation. Scattered islands of abnormal tubules and glomeruli with cystic and dysplastic elements, smooth muscle cells, and cartilage are also found. Numerous vascular spaces are seen peripherally. Malignant epithelial elements, mitotic activity, and other histologic features of malignancy are missing or scanty. The tumor has also been referred to as differentiated nephroblastoma, fetal or congenital mesenchymal hamartoma, fetal renal mesenchymal hamartoma, congenital fibrosarcoma, leiomyoma, and leiomyomatous hamartoma. Its relation with Wilms' tumor has not been defined. The most important clinical feature of the condition is its relative benignity, which may explain the favorable prognosis of "Wilms' tumor" of the first year of life. The recommended treatment is surgical removal of the tumor without radiation or chemotherapy. Chemotherapy has been incriminated as the cause of fatal sepsis in some instances, presumably from depression of the immune mechanism. The urographic findings are essentially the same as described in Wilms' tumor, and arteriography shows a similar pathologic vascularity.

RENAL CELL CARCINOMA

This neoplasm, also referred to as hypernephroma, renal adenocarcinoma, and clear-cell carcinoma, is rare in pediatrics and is seen usually in older children (see Figs. 55–20 to 55–22). It originates anywhere in the kidney substance, probably from epithelial cells of the renal tubules. A pseudocapsule is generally present. Histologically, it has a papillary,

tubular, trabecular, or mixed pattern and is generally composed of clear, sometimes granular cells.

The tumor tends to invade regional lymph nodes and other neighboring structures and to metastasize to the lungs, skeleton, liver, more distant lymph nodes and other organs. Metastases are already present in approximately one-fifth of the patients at time of diagnosis. An overall survival rate of more than 50 per cent is reported with a combination of surgery, radiation, and chemotherapy. A flank mass, hematuria, and abdominal pain are the most common presenting findings. Intrinsic and occasionally rim-type calcifications are seen in about 20 per cent of the cases. The excretory urogram almost always shows a renal mass with calyceal distortion. The tumor is usually quite vascular and is therefore well delineated by arteriography.

OTHER PRIMARY RENAL NEOPLASMS

Angiomyolipoma is a rare tumor, also referred to as renal hamartoma, angiofibrolipoma, and fibrolipoma, is frequent in patients with tuberous sclerosis, but it may occur as an isolated process. It may be single or multiple, unilateral or bilateral. Histologically, it is a benign mixed neoplasm containing smooth muscle cells, many thick-walled blood vessels, adipose tissue, and sometimes a few renal tubules and glomeruli. The urographic picture is the same as that of other renal tumors and may simulate cystic renal disease. In spite of its benignity, the arteriographic findings are those of a vascular malignant neoplasm.

Individual instances have been reported of renal hemangioma, hemangioepithelioma, lymphangioma, adenoma, leiomyoma, teratoma, fibroma, fibrosarcoma, liposarcoma, and leiomyosarcoma, but the number of these cases that are actually variants of Wilms' tumor, congenital mesoblastic nephroma, or angiomylolipoma is difficult to determine.

SECONDARY RENAL NEOPLASMS

The most frequent of these tumors are those caused by leukemia and lymphoma (Fig. 55–23). The process is usually bilateral involving the kidneys either diffusely or with discrete and usually large masses. Calyces and the infundibula tend to be separated from each other, stretched, attenuated, and deformed. Renal function is generally preserved. Systemic chemotherapy may cause a rapid breakdown of the malignant cells, with a massive excretion of uric acid resulting in blockage of the drainage system or anuria (uric acid uropathy).

RENAL PELVIS AND URETER

Primary neoplasms of the renal pelvis in infants and children are extremely rare. Instances of malignant epithelioma, spindle cell sarcoma, angioma, papilloma, and papillary carcinoma have been reported. Involvement of the pelvicalyceal system by Wilms' tumor may occur. Blood clots, fungus balls, and granulomatous inflammatory masses may produce similar changes.

Primary malignant tumors of the ureter are very rare in early life. Ureteral implantations from tumor or sarcoma botryoides have been observed. Ureteral polyps or other benign papillary growths causing filling defects or obstruction may occur (Fig. 55-24).

LOWER URINARY TRACT

EMBRYONAL RHABDOMYOSARCOMA

Although uncommon, this is the most important neoplasm of the lower urinary tract of children (Figs. 55-25 to 55-29). It is often called sarcoma botryoides (bunch of grapes) because of its lobulated or polypoid appearance in many cases. It is discovered most often during the first 2 or 3 years of life. Lower urinary tract obstruction is the most common presenting manifestation.

The tumor originates in the trigone of the bladder, prostate, vagina, or uterine cervix. It is a highly malignant, mixed mesodermal neoplasm, predominantly rhabdomyosarcoma or fibromyosarcoma. It is locally invasive and spreads to the abdominal lymph nodes. Once local spread has taken place, it may be difficult to determine its site of origin. Distant metastases may occur in late stages.

The prognosis is generally poor, although a survival of more than 60 per cent in "operable" cases has been reported recently following radical pelvic surgery, radiation, and chemotherapy.

When the neoplasm originates from the bladder or extends into it, the excretory urogram and the cystogram show a large and usually lobulated intravesical filling defect at the base of the bladder. When it originates in the prostate, it produces an upward displacement of the bladder floor with a large filling defect in the area. The posterior urethra is compressed, elongated, and often displaced to one side.

OTHER NEOPLASMS OF THE LOWER URINARY TRACT

Transitional cell carcinoma of the bladder is exceedingly rare, and primary malignant tumors of the urethra are practically nonexistent in children. The bladder may be involved secondarily by leukemia or lymphoma. Hemangiomas are probably the most common benign bladder tumor. They are usually of the cavernous type, solitary, and well defined. Hematuria is the main presenting finding. Hemangiomas elsewhere in the body may be present. Neurofibromas of the bladder may occur as part of a systemic neurofibromatosis or as an isolated lesion. In the diffuse type, the bladder may be contracted. Rare instances of bladder pheochromocytoma, fibromas, myomas, and dermoid cysts have been reported. Although not true neoplasms, polyps of the bladder and urethra should be mentioned because of their importance in the differential diagnosis. They are most commonly seen in the male urethra (Fig. 55-30), where they usually present as a single mass originating from the posterior urethra at or near the veru, as a rule through a long stalk, which explains the characteristic free motility of the tumor. Urethral obstruction may result.

ADRENAL GLANDS AND RELATED STRUCTURES

NEUROBLASTOMA AND GANGLIONEUROMA

Neuroblastoma (Sympathycoblastoma). This is one of the most frequent neoplasms of early life, accounting for 10 to 20 per cent of all malignancies of childhood (Figs. 55-31 to 55-47). Although it can occur in persons at any age including newborns and adults, it is discovered most often in the first 3 or 4 years of life. The tumor originates anywhere in the sympathetic chain of the abdomen, thorax, neck, or other areas. It is located in the abdomen in more than 50 per cent of the cases, and two-thirds of these originate from the adrenal medulla. Familial instances are on record.

The tumor is usually well encapsulated. Histologically it is composed of small, uniform, closely packed cells with small, dark-staining nuclei, representing embryonal sympathetic ganglion cells. These cells are frequently arranged in characteristic pseudorosette formation. Areas of hemorrhage, necrosis, and calcification are common.

Abdominal neuroblastomas, particularly those of adrenal origin, are highly malignant. In more than half of the cases, dissemination of the process is already evident when the patient is first seen. The tumor tends to break through the capsule and to spread by direct extension to retroperitoneal nodes and contiguous structures. The most common sites of metastases are the liver, bone marrow, skeleton including the skull, retro-orbital space, skin, and peripheral lymph nodes. The lungs are rarely affected and then only late in the course of the disease. The tumor may extend along a nerve root through an intervertebral foramen into the neural canal (dumbbell neuroblastomas) (Fig. 55–45).

Because of its nature, site of origin, and distribution of the metastases, neuroblastoma tends to cause a more varied symptomatology than Wilms' tumor. The most common presenting finding is that of an abdominal mass, first discovered by the mother in many instances. Pain in the abdomen or bones, jaundice, hepatomegaly, peripheral lymphadenopathy, periorbital ecchymoses, and exophthalmos may be seen. Systemic hypertension may also be observed. Nerve root pain and weakness or paralysis of a lower extremity may be encountered in the dumbbell neuroblastomas. Neuroblastoma in the newborn period may present as an enlarged liver.

The diagnosis is usually established or strongly suggested from plain films of the abdomen, excretory urography, and films of the chest and skeleton. A mass lesion is visible in plain radiographs of the abdomen in at least half of the cases, and intrinsic calcifications are demonstrable radiographically in 50 to 60 per cent of the patients. The calcifications tend to be small, multiple, and disseminated.

In the excretory urogram, the renal function is almost always preserved. In the presence of a suprarenal neuroblastoma, the kidney and proximal calyces are compressed and displaced downward and laterally, sometimes straight downward, rarely downward and medially. When the tumor extends along the posterior gutter between the kidney and vertebrae, the pelvis and proximal ureters are also displaced laterally. When it originates in the paraspinal area, the ureter most frequently is deviated laterally and anteriorly. A neuroblastoma originating in the organ of Zuckerkandl or in the pelvis causes a lateral and forward displacement of the ureters. The bladder and rectum are displaced away from the tumor in presacral neuroblastomas. Enlargement of one or more intervertebral foramina may be demonstrated if the tumor extends into the spinal canal. An inferior venacavogram, carried out as a separate procedure or through a simple saphenous vein injection as part of the initial excretory urogram, may be of value, particularly if the tumor is on the right, to determine displacement, obstruction, or invasion of the vessel. Occasionally, the venacavogram is the only decisive diagnostic roentgenographic procedure. Arteriography is of less value than in Wilms' tumor owing to the generally less prominent vascularity of the lesion.

A reliable sign of local invasion and retroperitoneal spread is a lateral displacement of the medial pleural line in the lower thorax.

It is of great diagnostic importance that about 95 per cent of neuroblastomas are associated with an increased urinary excretion of catecholamines (dopamine, epinephrine, norepinephrine) and their metabolites (normetanephrine, metanephrine, vanillylmandelic and homovanillic acid). A rapid screening test for urinary vanillylmandelic acid (VMA) gives positive results in about 70 per cent of cases. These biochemical determinations are also important postoperatively to evaluate successful removal of the tumor and in the diagnosis of recurrences.

The differential diagnosis is more complex than in Wilms' tumor, but it may be facilitated by the presence of skeletal metastases, a positive bone marrow, or a positive VMA test. In the absence of metastases or local spread, it is not possible to differentiate neuroblastoma from ganglioneuroblastoma or ganglioneuroma. An adrenal neuroblastoma cannot be differentiated from other adrenal neoplasms, roentgenographically unless there is some endocrine dysfunction from which the nature of the underlying process can be surmised.

Adrenal hemorrhage and hematoma in the newborn period may present as a large adrenal mass, often bilaterally. The presence of anemia and jaundice and a suprarenal lucency in the nephrographic phase of an excretory urogram should suggest the diagnosis. Follow-up studies show a rapid shrinkage of the mass with the appearance of peripheral calcifications. The differential diagnosis between idiopathic adrenal calcifications, presumably secondary to minor adrenal hemorrhage in the newborn period, and a small neuroblastoma or other calcified adrenal tumors, may be difficult. Idiopathic calcification is a likely possibility in the absence of a demonstrable mass or metastases, a negative VMA test, and particularly when the adrenal calcification is triangular in configuration or is bilateral.

Wolman's disease is a rare, congenital, rapidly fatal metabolic disorder characterized by an abnormal accumulation of cholesterol in the liver, spleen, and both adrenals. The adrenal glands are greatly enlarged and diffusely calcified.

An adrenal neuroblastoma and an upper pole Wilms' tumor may be indistinguishable on roentgenographic grounds alone. A hydronephrotic proximal component of a duplex kidney or an upper pole renal cyst may also simulate an adrenal neuroblastoma, but the films taken in the nephrographic phase regularly show a suprarenal lucency, a finding that is rarely seen in neuroblastoma. The presence of a round lucent mass in the bladder should favor the diagnosis of ureteral duplication with ureterocele formation. Ultrasound studies are also of value in these circumstances.

An extrarenal paraspinal neuroblastoma may displace the kidney laterally and superiorly, simulating closely some Wilms' tumors or a paraspinal sarcoma, lymphoma, or teratoma. The presence of dental structures within the tumor favor a teratoma. A presacral neuroblastoma should be differentiated from anterior sacral meningocele and teratoma.

The following staging has been proposed by Evans and co-workers:

   I. Tumor confined to the structure of origin
  II. Tumor extends in continuity, including nodes, beyond the structure of origin, but does not cross the midline
 III. Same as stage II, but there is crossing of the midline
  IV. Remote metastases, including the skeleton
 IV A. Same as stage I or II, but with metastases to the liver or skin or bone marrow, but no x-ray evidence of skeletal involvement

The prognosis is much less favorable than in Wilms' tumor. The cure rate depends in great part on the age of the patient at the time of diagnosis and the site of the primary tumor. It varies from 50 to 60 per cent in patients under 1 year to less than 10 per cent in those older than 7 years, with an overall average of about 25 per cent. Nonadrenal neuroblastomas have a more favorable prognosis. If the patient is without tumor for 1 to 2 years following surgery, he is probably cured. Only a few instances of apparent permanent recoveries have been reported in the presence of skeletal involvement demonstrated roentgenographically. Liver metastases in infancy do not represent an equally bad prognostic sign. Documented instances of spontaneous regression or maturation of a malignant neuroblastoma to a benign ganglioneuroma are on record.

Ganglioneuroblastomas. These are similar to neuroblastoma in all respects except for a lesser degree of malignancy. The histologic picture shows both undifferentiated neuroblasts and mature ganglion cells.

Ganglioneuromas. These are the benign counterparts of neuroblastoma, being composed only of mature ganglion cells. Their sites of origin are essentially the same as in neuroblastoma. The urinary catecholamine metabolites usually are not elevated.

Syndrome of Neural Tumor With Diarrhea. Ganglioneuromas, ganglioneuroblastoma, and less frequently neuroblastomas are occasionally associated with chronic diarrhea, failure to thrive, hypokalemia, and sometimes hypertension and flushing. These findings disappear after removal of the tumor. The urinary catecholamine metabolites are almost always elevated. The mechanism for the development of the diarrhea and other symptoms is not entirely clear.

Syndrome of Neural Tumor and Clonic Encephalopathy. Several infants and small children have been reported in whom cerebellar ataxia and peculiar eye movements (opsoclonia) occurred in association with an otherwise silent neuroblastoma or ganglioneuroblastoma. Urinary catecholamine metabolites were increased in about 50 per cent of the cases. An improvement in the symptomatology, sometimes complete, has been observed following removal of the tumor, suggesting a relation between the two.

PHEOCHROMOCYTOMA

This tumor (Figs. 55–48, 55–49) is uncommon in children. The youngest reported patient was 5 months old. Pheochromocytoma is seen more frequently in boys than in girls and may be multiple. Like neuroblastoma, it originates anywhere in the sympathetic chain. It is most often located in the abdomen, and in approximately 70 per cent of the cases it originates in one or both adrenal glands. It may also originate in the bladder and in other unusual sites. Pheochromocytomas in children are rarely malignant. They may be associated with neurofibromatosis or other conditions. Familial cases have been reported.

The tumor can vary in size from 1 to 10 cm. or more in diameter, but it is commonly small. It is usually encapsulated and highly vascular. Histologically it is composed of large spherical, polyhedral, or fusiform cells, often collected in clusters separated by a connective tissue stroma. Intrinsic hemorrhages are fairly common.

Most of the clinical manifestations are related to an increased production of catecholamines by the tumor. Systemic arterial hypertension is the dominant feature and is often sustained. The diagnosis is established on biochemical grounds. Roentgenographic studies may be carried out to localize the tumor and to detect multiple tumors. Films of the chest with barium in the esophagus may reveal a paravertebral mass. The plain films of the abdomen and barium studies of the gastrointestinal tract are usually normal. Intrinsic calcifications demonstrable radiographically are uncommon.

In the presence of an adrenal or paravertebral pheochromocytoma, the excretory urogram shows a renal or ureteral displacement not unlike that seen in neuroblastoma. A right-sided paravertebral pheochromocytoma compressing or obstructing the inferior vena cava may be detected by an inferior venacavogram. Because these tumors are vascular, they may be demonstrated by abdominal arteriography. When clinical and biochemical findings suggest a pheochromocytoma, an exploration of both adrenal glands and of the abdominal cavity is always indicated, regardless of the roentgenographic findings, and may be done without any of the more elaborate roentgenographic procedures. The subject is discussed further in Chapter 56, Systemic Arterial Hypertension in Children.

OTHER ADRENAL TUMORS

Tumors of the adrenal cortex are uncommon and are mainly adenomas and carcinomas (Figs. 55–50, 55–51). They usually are unilateral, but may involve both adrenal glands. Both adrenal carcinomas and adenomas often contain functional secretory tissue causing virilization or Cushing's syndrome, which is discussed further in Chapter 56. The adenomas tend to be small and are usually discovered as incidental findings at autopsy. The carcinomas are less common than the adenomas and are frequently large. They are malignant and tend to spread locally and metastasize early, particularly to the liver, lungs, brain, and sometimes to the skeleton. Intrinsic calcifications demonstrable radiographically are said to occur in about 20 per cent of the cases. The urographic findings are the same as those seen in adrenal neuroblastomas. Owing to the poor vascularity of the tumor, the arteriogram is often silent.

Primary neoplasms of the adrenal glands other than those already mentioned are rare. Isolated instances have been reported of fibroma, neurofibroma, lipoma, hemangioma, myoma, neuroblastoma, neuroma, lymphangioma, hemangiomablastoma, and myxosarcoma. Adrenal cysts are also extremely rare and may result from trauma, degenera-

tion of tumor, or from hemorrhage. The adrenal glands are occasionally involved by metastases from a distant neoplasm or leukemia or by invasion from a tumor located in a neighboring structure.

MISCELLANEOUS TUMORS

Retroperitoneal lymphoma primary in the area, or as a manifestation of a more generalized process, may displace ureters and kidneys and may cause upper tract obstruction.

Retroperitoneal teratoma (Fig. 55–52) is an uncommon but well-defined entity. In approximately half of the cases it is detected during the first year of life. The tumor usually is large and may be solid or partially cystic. It is located anywhere along the posterior wall of the abdomen but most often in the perirenal area. Retroperitoneal teratomas are said to originate from embryonic nephrogenic elements and are commonly benign. Roentgenographically, there is a mass that commonly lies against the kidney and the ureters, causing displacement, distortion, and obstruction of these structures or lack of renal function. In a large percentage of cases there are intrinsic calcifications, dental structures, and bone formation.

Other rare neoplasms of the retroperitoneal spaces include undifferentiated sarcomas (Fig. 55–53), lipomas, fibrolipomas, myxomas, fibromas and fibrosarcomas, adenomas, chondromas, lymphangiomas, and myomas.

Pancreatic cysts, retroperitoneal hematomas, and retroperitoneal extravasation of urine following trauma to the urinary tract may become large enough to displace the kidney and the ureter and to cause obstruction.

Masses originating in the presacral space and deep in the pelvis may obstruct the bladder outlet and ureters. They include the sarcoma botryoides of the vagina, the cervix, and the prostate, already discussed, and sacrococcygeal teratoma with presacral extension, presacral teratomas and dermoids, neonatal hydrocolpos, and the hematocolpos of adolescence.

Intraperitoneal masses of various types also may distort or obstruct the urinary tract. The most important are ovarian neoplasms or cysts, enlargement of the liver and the spleen from any cause, mesenteric and omental cysts, intestinal duplications, lymphoma of bowel, an appendiceal abscess and other localized inflammatory process within the abdomen, a distended bladder, and gross constipation.

CHAPTER 55, ILLUSTRATIONS

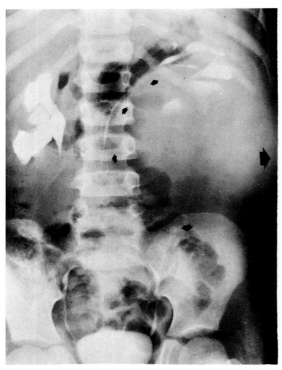

FIG. 55–1. Wilms' tumor of the left kidney (*arrows*) displacing pelvis and calyces upwardly and proximal ureter medially.

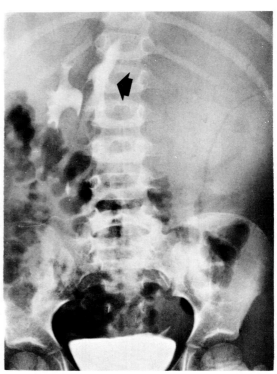

FIG. 55–2. Wilms' tumor on the left. Pelvis and calyces displaced medially by the mass (*arrow*).

FIG. 55–3. (A) Wilms' tumor of the left kidney (*arrows*) displacing pelvicalyceal system upwardly and medially. Left ureter displaced across midline. **(B)** Surgical specimen with contrast material injected in the collecting system.

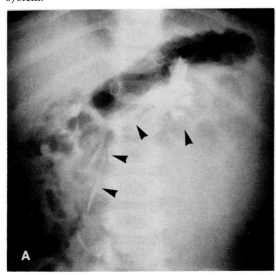

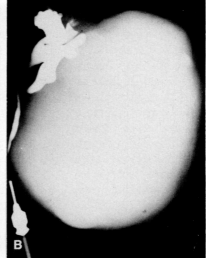

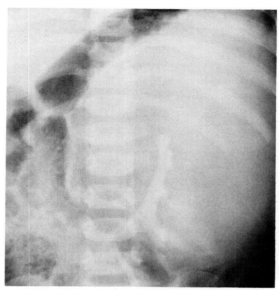

FIG. 55–4. Wilms' tumor of the left kidney displacing pelvicalyceal system medially, downwardly, and posteriorly.

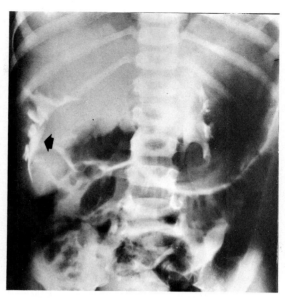

FIG. 55–5. Wilms' tumor of the right kidney (*arrow*). The pelvis and calyces are displaced laterally by the mass.

FIG. 55–6. Wilms' tumor of the left kidney. IVP, lateral projection, the calyces are distorted, separated from each other, and displaced forwardly.

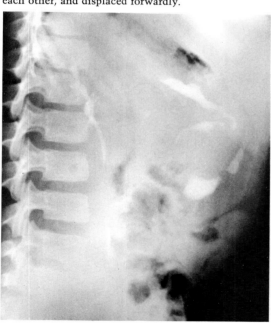

FIG. 55–7. Wilm's tumor of the left kidney displacing kidney downwardly (*arrows*).

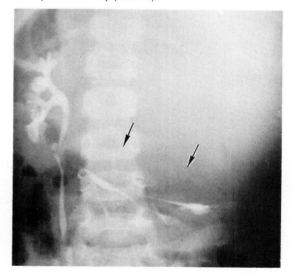

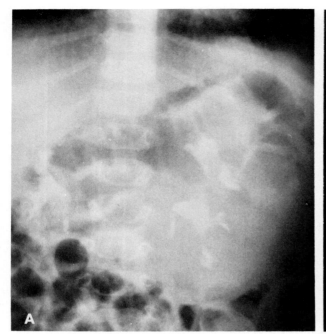

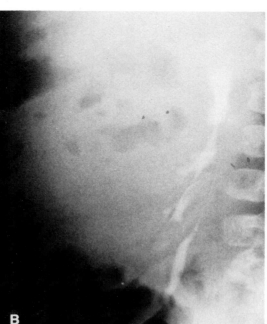

FIG. 55–8. (A, B) Wilms' tumor of the left kidney displacing the pelvicalyceal system backwardly. Tumor may be missed in frontal projection. (C) Injected surgical specimen.

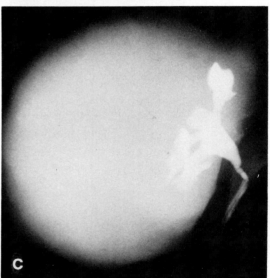

FIG. 55–9. (A) Wilms' tumor of the left kidney displacing pelvicalyceal system downwardly and outwardly (*arrows*). (B) Arteriogram; rich tumor vascularity.

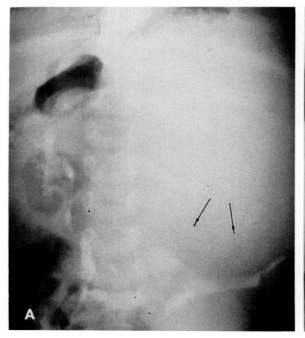

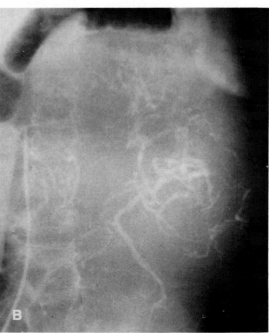

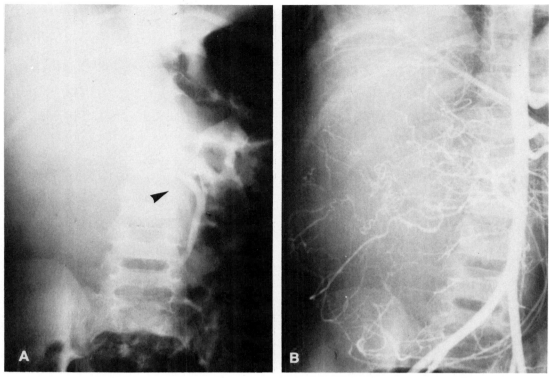

FIG. 55–10. (A) Wilms' tumor of the right kidney displacing the right pelvicalyceal system and ureter toward the left across the midline (*arrow*). **(B)** Arteriogram; rich tumor vascularity.

FIG. 55–11. (A) Wilms' tumor of the left kidney with absent renal function (uncommon finding). IVU. **(B)** Retrograde pyelogram; tumor invades the pelvis.

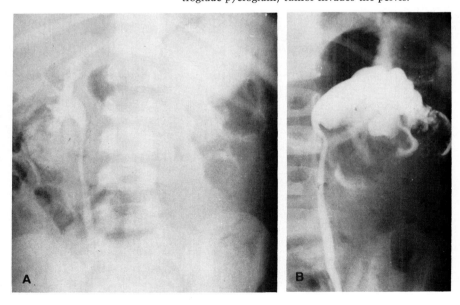

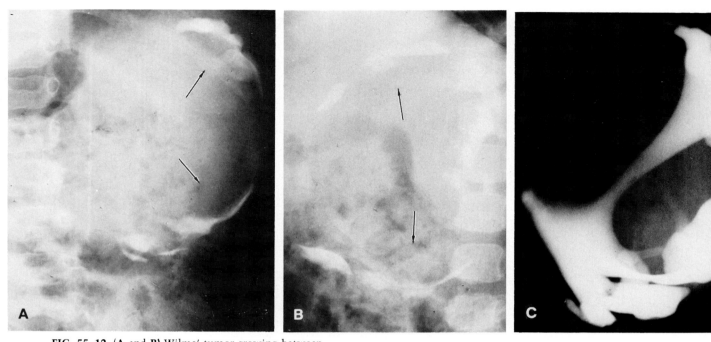

FIG. 55–12. (A and **B)** Wilms' tumor growing between the two complexes of a bifid pelvis. IVU, frontal and lateral views. The *arrows* point to the two bifid pelves. **(C)** Injected specimen.

FIG. 55–13. (A) Multicentric Wilms' tumor of the right kidney. One tumor is located in the upper pole and the second in the lower pole. Note flattening of both poles of the kidney by the tumor (*arrows*). **(B)** Injected specimen.

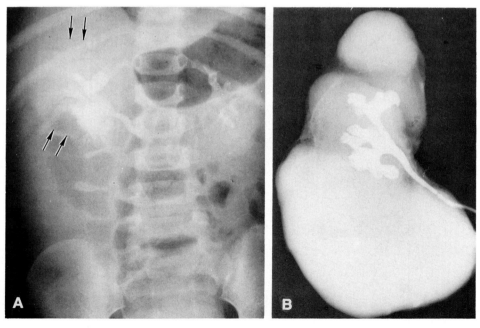

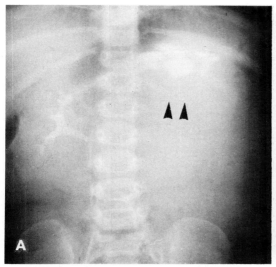

FIG. 55–14. Bilateral Wilms' tumor. **(A)** Initial IVU; Wilms' tumor on the left displacing pelvicalyceal system upwardly (*arrows*). Normal right kidney. **(B)** IVU a few months later—large Wilms' tumor in the upper pole of the right kidney displacing pelvicalyceal system downwardly (*arrows*).

FIG. 55–15. Bilateral Wilms' tumor, a large one on the left displacing the calyces (*black arrows*) and a small one on the right (*white arrow*), discovered at the same time.

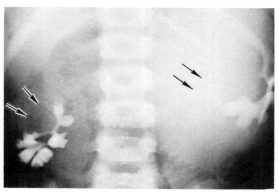

FIG. 55–16. Bilateral Wilms' tumors discovered simultaneously. The *arrows* are placed over the renal masses, indicating the pelvicalyceal displacement.

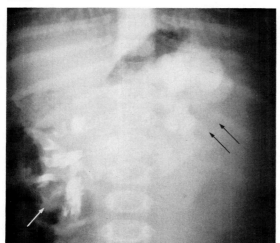

FIG. 55–17. Bilateral Wilms' tumors discovered simultaneously. Distortion and dilatation of the pelvis and the calyces of both kidneys. (Courtesy of Keith Waterhouse, M.D.)

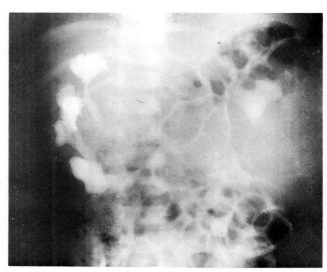

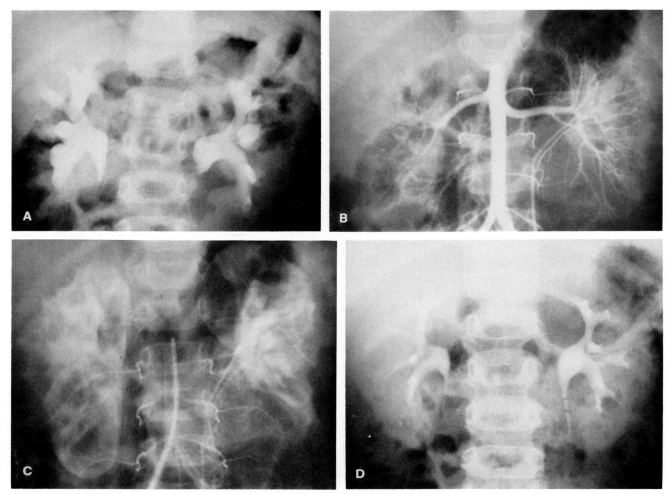

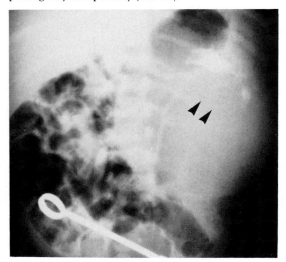

FIG. 55–18. (A) Bilateral Wilms' tumor of the diffuse type (nephroblastomatosis). IVU at age 2 years — mild renal enlargement of the kidneys without definite displacement or stretching of the calyces. **(B)** Aortogram reveals diffuse lesions. **(C)** Arteriogram, nephrographic phase; multiple lucencies throughout, especially in the cortex. The picture simulates that of adult polycystic kidney. **(D)** IVU 2 years later (patient had only radiation and chemotherapy) — normal pelvicalyceal system, intact nephrogram throughout.

FIG. 55–19. IVU in a newborn with a congenital Wilms' tumor (mesoblastic nephroma) of the left kidney displacing calyces upwardly (*arrows*).

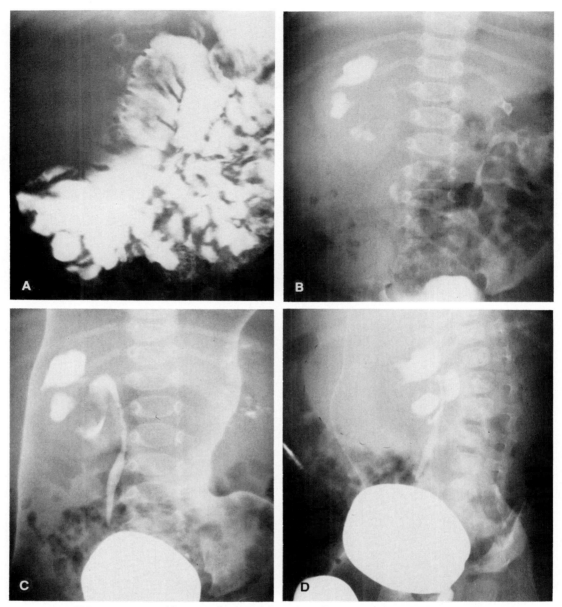

FIG. 55–19a. Mesoblastic nephroma of the right kidney in a 2-month-old boy. **(A)** Displacement of bowel by the tumor in a barium study of the gastrointestinal tract. **(B)** IVU showing that the mass is centrally located. **(C, D)** Cystourethrogram, frontal and right posterior oblique projections. An incidental right-sided reflux clearly shows that the tumor originated centrally in the kidney and expanded mainly forwardly.

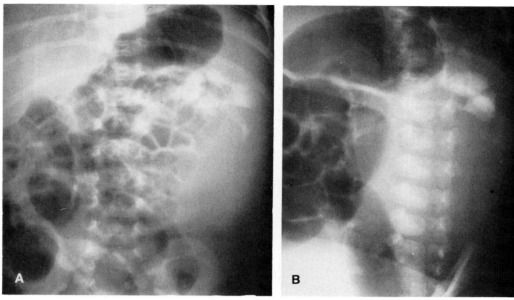

FIG. 55–19b. IVU in a newborn boy with a mesoblastic nephroma of the left kidney displacing the calyces mainly upwardly. **(A)** Frontal and **(B)** right posterior oblique projections.

FIG. 55–19c. IVU in a newborn girl with a mesoblastic nephroma of the left kidney displacing the calyces mainly superiorly. **(A)** Frontal and **(B)** right posterior oblique projections.

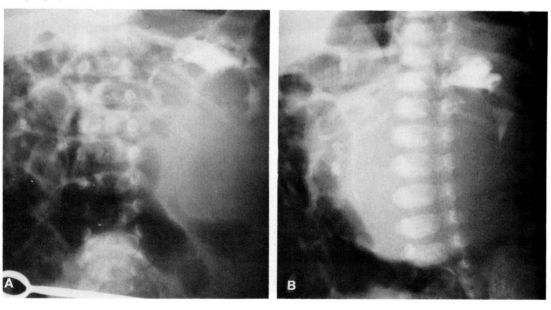

FIG. 55-20. IVU **(A)** and retrograde pyelogram **(B)** in child with renal carcinoma. Note compression defects of the pelvicalyceal systems (*arrows*).

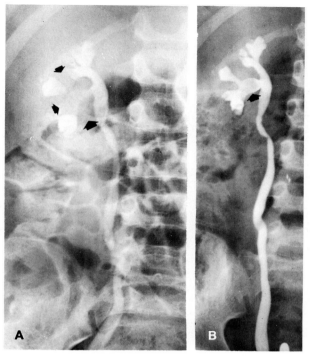

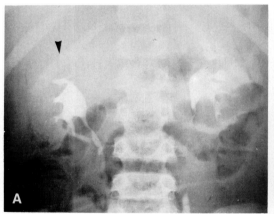

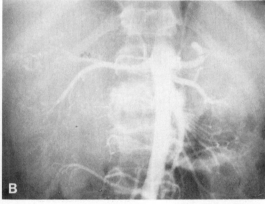

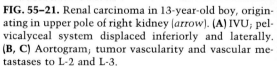

FIG. 55-21. Renal carcinoma in 13-year-old boy, originating in upper pole of right kidney (*arrow*). **(A)** IVU; pelvicalyceal system displaced inferiorly and laterally. **(B, C)** Aortogram; tumor vascularity and vascular metastases to L-2 and L-3.

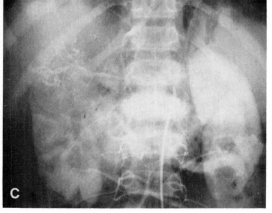

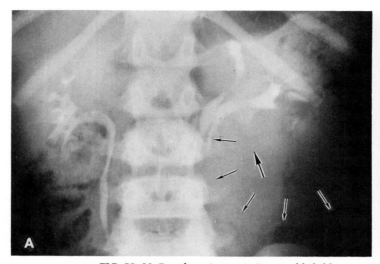

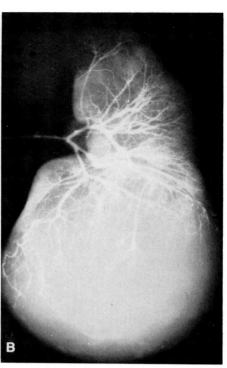

FIG. 55–22. Renal carcinoma in 7-year-old child, originating from the lower pole of left kidney; rim calcifications present in plain film (*arrows*). **(A)** IVU; upward displacement of left pelvicalyceal system; rim calcification around tumor faintly visible. **(B)** Arteriogram of surgical specimen.

FIG. 55–23. IVU in child with bilateral renal infiltration by lymphosarcoma. The kidneys are greatly enlarged, and the infundibula and calyces are stretched.

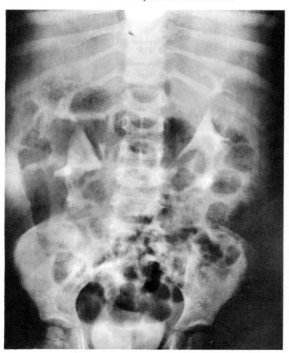

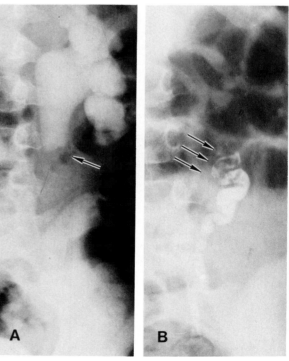

FIG. 55–24. Young boy with benign polyps of the left ureter producing significant ureteral obstruction. **(A)** IVU and **(B)** retrograde ureterogram. The *arrows* show the lucent defects produced by the polyps.

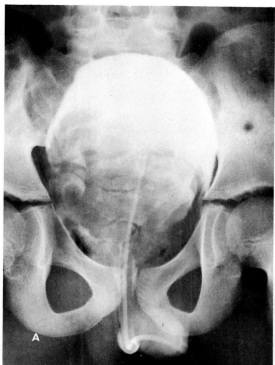

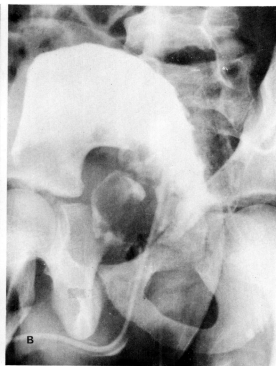

FIG. 55–25. Retrograde cystogram in the frontal (**A**) and in the oblique (**B**) projections in a boy with rhabdomyosarcoma of the bladder; large, lobulated filling defect of the lower part of the bladder.

FIG. 55–26. Retrograde cystogram in the frontal (**A**) and in the oblique (**B**) projection in a boy with rhabdomyosarcoma of the bladder; large lobulated filling defect in the lower part of the bladder.

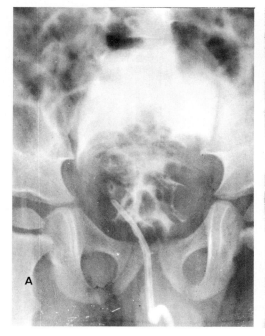

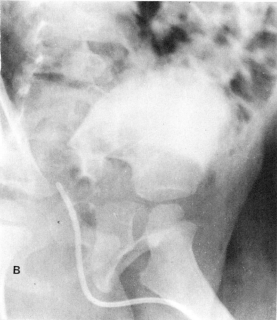

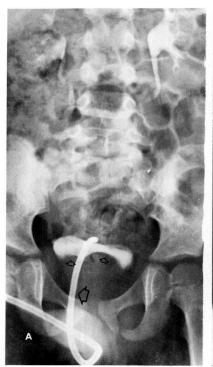

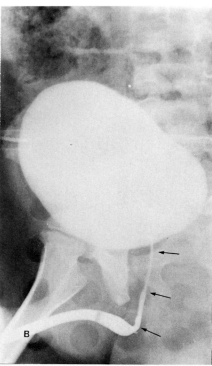

FIG. 55–27. Rhabdomyosarcoma of the prostate in a boy; retrograde urethrogram. **(A)** The urethral catheter (*large arrow*) is displaced to the right by the prostatic tumor, and the floor of the bladder is elevated (*small arrows*). **(B)** Elongation and narrowing of the prostatic urethra (*arrows*).

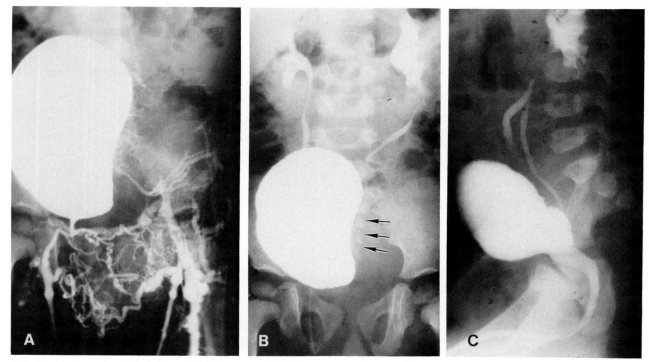

FIG. 55–28. Two-year-old child with a large pelvic rhabdomyosarcoma that probably originated from the left side of the bladder, causing severe venous obstruction. **(A)** IVU; film of the pelvis taken during injection of contrast material in a vein in the left lower leg shows severe venous obstruction by the tumor. Contrast material is present in the bladder from a previous cystogram. Bladder and posterior urethra are displaced to the right. **(B)** IVU; delayed film, left lower ureter and bladder displaced medially (*arrows*). **(C)** Voiding study using the contrast medium in the bladder from the IVU is normal.

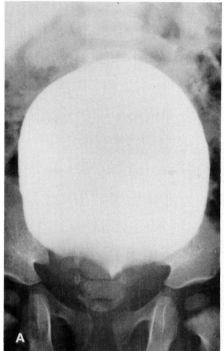
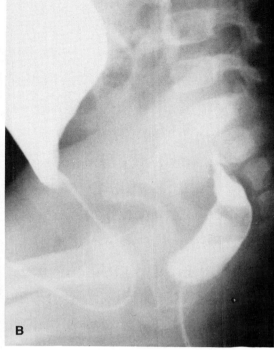

FIG. 55-29. Cystogram in 2-year-old child with a rhabdomyosarcoma of the prostate. (**A**) Elevation of floor of the bladder. (**B**) Bladder and proximal posterior urethra are displaced forwardly. A small amount of contrast material introduced into the rectum shows backward displacement of the rectum by the mass.

FIG. 55-30. Benign polyp (*arrows*) of the posterior urethra demonstrated by voiding cystourethrography. The polyp originates from the verumontanum; it is on a stalk and is freely movable. At the beginning of voiding (**A**) the polyp is in the proximal prostatic urethra, and toward the end of voiding (**B**) it is in the distal prostatic urethra.

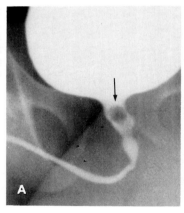
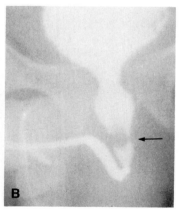

FIG. 55-31. Right adrenal neuroblastoma displacing the pelvicalyceal system downwardly (*arrows*). It is difficult to state if the mass is renal or extrarenal.

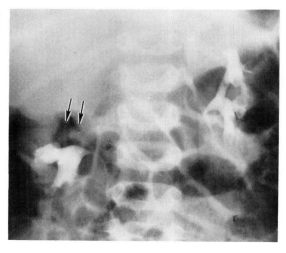

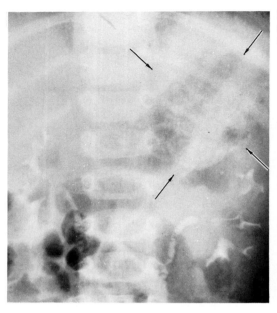

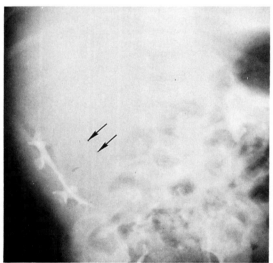

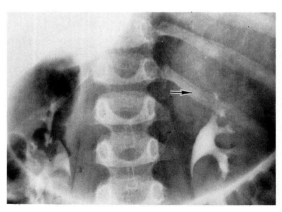

FIG. 55–32. Left adrenal neuroblastoma with intrinsic calcifications (*arrows*) displacing left pelvicalyceal system downwardly and slightly outwardly.

FIG. 55–33. Right adrenal neuroblastoma displacing the upper calyces down and laterally (*arrows*).

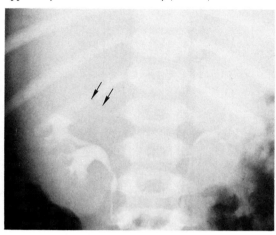

FIG. 55–34. Extremely large right adrenal neuroblastoma displacing pelvicalyceal system inferiorly and laterally (*arrows*).

FIG. 55–35. Large left adrenal neuroblastoma displacing pelvicalyceal system inferiorly and slightly medially (*arrows*) (unusual finding).

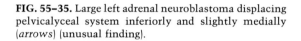

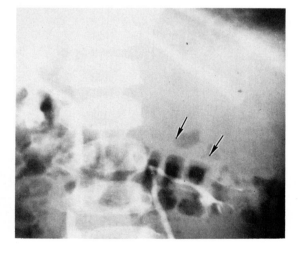

FIG. 55–36. Left adrenal neuroblastoma (*arrows*) with only a minimal lateral displacement of the pelvicalyceal system.

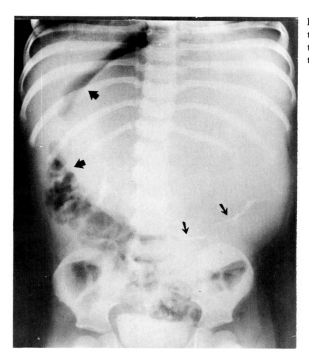

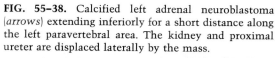

FIG. 55–37. Large left adrenal neuroblastoma displacing the left kidney noticeably. The tumor extends across the midline. The *arrows* demarcate the extent of the tumor.

FIG. 55–38. Calcified left adrenal neuroblastoma (*arrows*) extending inferiorly for a short distance along the left paravertebral area. The kidney and proximal ureter are displaced laterally by the mass.

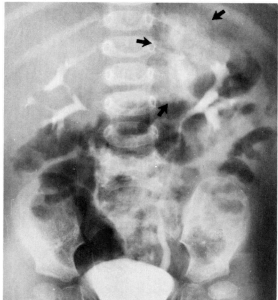

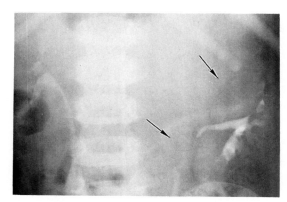

FIG. 55–39. Large left adrenal neuroblastoma (*upper arrow*) displacing pelvicalyceal system inferiorly and laterally. The tumor extends downwardly along the spine displacing the proximal ureter laterally (*lower arrow*).

FIG. 55–40. Right adrenal neuroblastoma extending inferiorly along the spine; displacing the pelvicalyceal system downwardly and laterally (*arrow*) and the proximal ureter laterally.

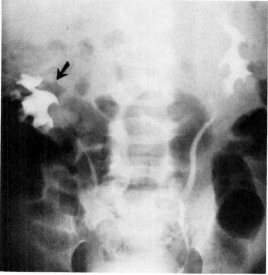

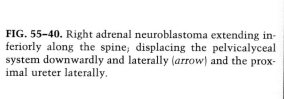

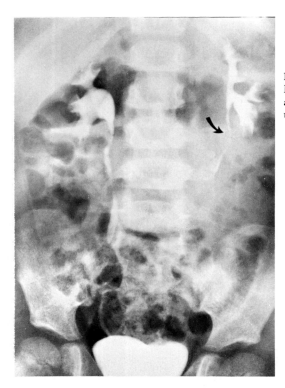

FIG. 55-41. Calcified neuroblastoma originating in the left paravertebral space at the level of the left kidney and proximal left ureter. The kidney and proximal ureter (*arrow*) are displaced laterally by the mass.

FIG. 55-42. Paravertebral neuroblastoma originating medially to the right kidney and proximal ureter. Tumor extends across midline, displacing the left kidney laterally. The *arrows* demonstrate the outer margins of the tumor.

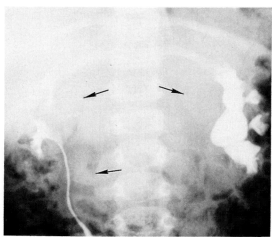

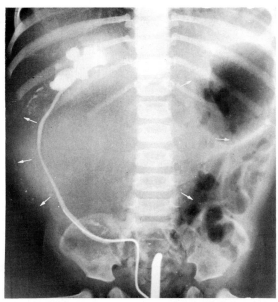

FIG. 55-43. Large calcified neuroblastoma originating from the right paravertebral area below the kidney. The right ureter is markedly displaced laterally, and the right kidney is displaced superiorly and laterally by the turmor. Tumor extends across the midline. The extent of the tumor is shown by the *arrows*.

FIG. 55-44. Large right paravertebral lumbar neuroblastoma displacing the right ureter (*arrow*) and bladder medially; metastases are present in the pelvic bones.

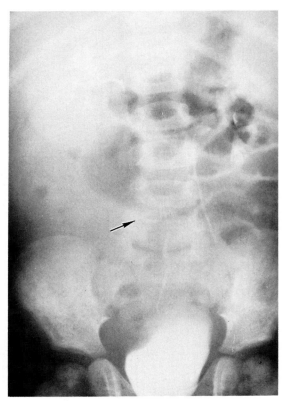

FIG. 55–45. Right paraspinal neuroblastoma extending into vertebral canal. **(A)** Lateral lumbar spine; enlargement of at least three lumbar vertebral foramina (L-1 to L-4). **(B)** Myelogram; extradural mass extending from L-2 to at least S-1 (*arrows*).

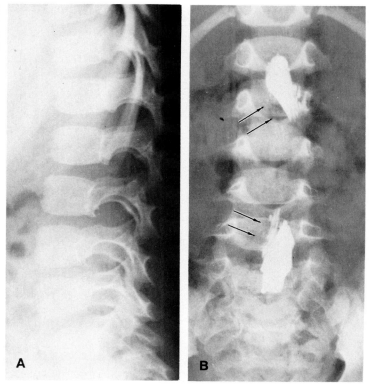

FIG. 55–46. Presacral neuroblastoma. **(A)** IVU; partially obstructed ureters. Metastases to L-4 (*arrows*) **(B)** Barium enema; rectum displaced forward.

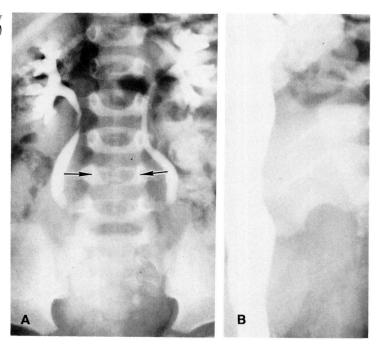

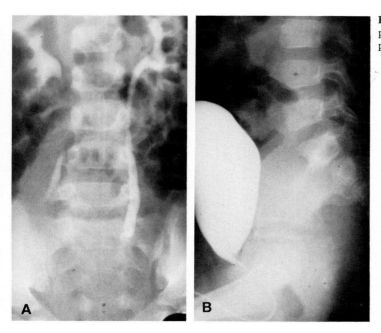

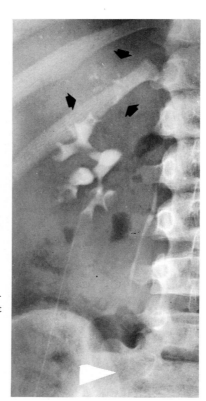

FIG. 55–47. Presacral neuroblastoma. (**A**) IVU; mass in pelvis compressing ureters. (**B**) Cystogram; forward displacement of bladder.

FIG. 55–48. IVU in child with calcified pheochromocytoma (*arrows*) originating in right adrenal. The right kidney is displaced slightly inferiorly and laterally.

FIG. 45–49. Large malignant pheochromocytoma of the right adrenal gland in an 8-year-old child. (**A**) IVU; marked downward displacement of the kidney. *Arrows* indicate mass lesions. (**B**) Aortogram; gross tumor vascularity. (Courtesy of Mordecai Halpern, M.D.)

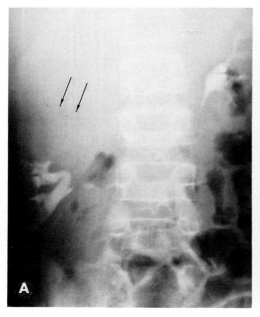

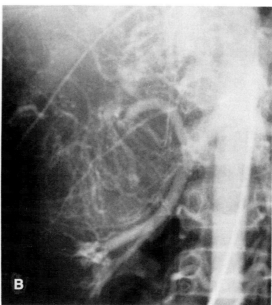

FIG. 55–50. IVU in child with Cushing syndrome caused by a left adrenal adenoma (*arrow*). Left kidney displaced inferiorly by tumor.

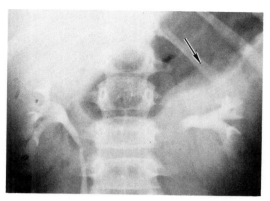

FIG. 55–51. IVU in girl with functional adrenal carcinoma causing virilization, minimal downward displacement of the left kidney by calcified mass (*arrows*).

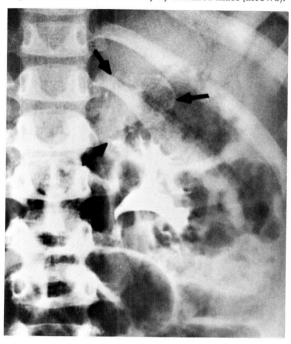

FIG. 55–52. IVU in two instances of large retroperitoneal teratoma—in a newborn and in a small infant. **(A)** Small calcifications visible throughout the mass (*arrows*). No excretion of contrast material on the affected side. At operation the right kidney was found to be compressed backwardly and obstructed. **(B)** Bony or dental structures (*arrows*) within part of the tumor, Pelvicalyceal system displaced laterally and inferiorly.

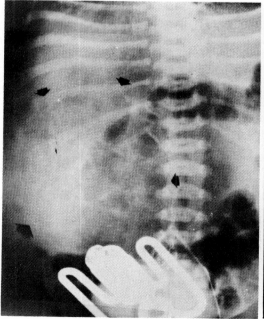

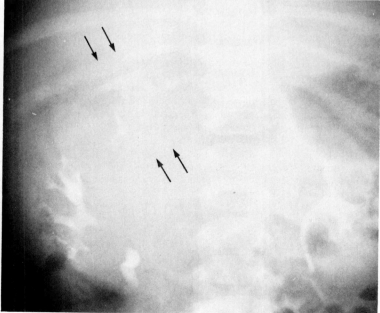

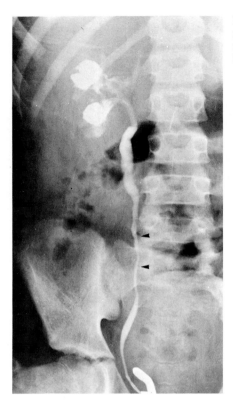

FIG. 55–53. Retrograde pyelogram in child with a retroperitoneal sarcoma. The tumor has surrounded and narrowed the ureter (*arrows*) at the level of the lumbosacral junction.

BIBLIOGRAPHY

1. Alfidi, R.J., Gill, W.M., Jr., and Klein, H.J.: Arteriography of adrenal neoplasms. Am. J. Roentgenol., *106*:635, 1969.
2. Anderson, E.E., Herlong, J.H., Harper, J.M., et al.: Bilateral Wilms' tumor: Diagnosis and management. Clin. Pediatr., *7*:596, 1968.
3. Aron, B., and Gross, M.: Renal adenocarcinoma in infancy and childhood: evaluation of therapy and prognosis. J. Urol., *102*:497, 1969.
4. Aterman, K., and Schueller, E.F.: Maturation of neuroblastoma to ganglioneuroma. Am. J. Dis. Child., *120*:217, 1970.
5. Berdon, W.E., Wigger, H.J., and Baker, D.H.: Fetal renal hamartoma—a benign tumor to be distinguished from Wilms' tumor: Report of 3 cases. Am. J. Roentgenol., *118*:18, 1973.
6. Bill, A.H., Jr.: The regression of neuroblastoma. J. Pediatr. Surg., *3*:103, 1968.
7. Black, W.C., and Ragsdale, E.F.: Wilms' tumor. Am. J. Roentgenol., *103*:53, 1968.
8. Bohuon, C.: Catecholamine metabolism in neuroblastoma. J. Pediatr. Surg., *3*:114, 1968.
9. Bolande, R.P.: Benignity of neonatal tumors and concept of cancer regression in early life. Am. J. Dis. Child., *122*:12, 1971.
10. Bove, K.E., Kottler, H., and McAdams, A.J.: Nodular renal blastoma: Definition and possible significance. Cancer, *24*:323, 1969.
11. Boxer, L., and Smith, D.L.: Wilms' tumor prior to onset of hemihypertrophy. Am. J. Dis. Child., *120*:564, 1970.
12. Burkholder, G.V., Beach, P.D., and Hall, R.: Fetal renal hamartoma. J. Urol., *104*:330, 1970.
13. Carlson, D.H., and Wilkinson, R.H.: Neurofibromatosis of the bladder in children. Radiology, *105*:401, 1972.
14. Chien-Hsing, M., and Elkin, M.: Angiographic manifestations of Wilms' tumor. Am. J. Roentgenol., *105*:95, 1969.
15. Clark, R.E., Moss, A.A., De Lorimier, A.A., et al.: Arteriography of Wilms' tumors. Am. J. Roentgenol., *113*:476, 1971.
16. Cochran, W., and Froggatt, P.: Bilateral nephroblastoma in two sisters. J. Urol., *97*:216, 1967.
17. Cremin, B.J., and Kaschula, R.O.C.: Arteriography in Wilms' tumor: the results of 13 cases and comparison to renal dysplasia. Br. J. Radiol., *45*:415, 1972.
18. Cremin, B.J., and Kaschula, R.O.C.: Arteriography in Wilms' tumors and its relationship to renal dysplasia. Ann. Radiol. (Paris), *15*:353, 1972.
19. D'Angio, G.J.: Management of children with Wilms' tumor. Cancer, *30*:1528, 1972.
20. D'Angio, G.J., and Evans, A.E.: Wilms' tumor can be cured. Ann. Radiol. (Paris), *14*:211, 1971.
21. Dehner, L.P.: Intrarenal teratoma occurring in infancy: Report of a case with discussion of extragonadal germ cell tumors in infancy. J. Pediatr. Surg., *8*:369, 1973.
22. Dehner, L.P., Leestma, J.E., and Price, E.B.: Renal cell carcinoma in children: Clinicopathologic study of 15 cases and review of the literature. J. Pediatr., *76*:358, 1970.
23. De Lorimier, A.A., Bragg, K.U., and Linden, S.: Neuroblastoma in childhood. Am. J. Dis. Child., *118*:441, 1969.
24. DiGeorge, A.M., and Harley, R.D.: The association of aniridia, Wilms' tumor and congenital anomalies. Arch. Ophthalmol., *75*:796, 1966.

25. Downs, R.A.: Congenital polyps of the prostatic urethra. Br. J. Urol., 42:76, 1970.

26. Drash, A., Sherman, F., Hartmann, W.H., and Blizzard, R.M.: A syndrome of pseudohermaphroditism, Wilms' tumor, hypertension and degenerative renal disease. J. Pediatr., 76:585, 1970.

27. Eklöf, O., and Gooding, C.A.: Paravertebral widening in cases of neuroblastoma. Br. J. Radiol., 40:358, 1967.

28. Engleman, K.: Principles in the diagnosis of pheochromocytoma. Bull. N.Y. Acad. Med., 45:851, 1969.

29. Evans, A.E., D'Angio, G.J., and Randolph, J.: A proper staging for children with neuroblastoma: Children's Cancer Study Group A. Cancer, 27:374, 1971.

30. Fagan, W.: Successful treatment of inoperable hypernephroma in childhood. J. Urol., 103:652, 1970.

31. Farah, J., and Lofstrom, J.: Angiography of Wilms' tumor. Radiology, 90:775, 1968.

32. Finkelstein, J.Z., and Gilchrist, S.S.: Recent advances in neuroblastoma. Calif. Med., 116:27, 1972.

33. Flanagan, J.C., and Di George, A.M.: Sporadic aniridia and Wilms' tumor. Am. J. Ophthalmol., 67:558, 1969.

34. Folin, J.: Angiography in Wilms' tumour. Acta Radiol. (Diagn.), 8:201, 1969.

35. Fortner, J., Nicastri, A., and Murphy, M.L.: Neuroblastoma: Natural history and results of treatment in 133 cases. Ann. Surg., 167:132, 1968.

36. Fraumeni, J.F., Jr., and Glass, A.G.: Wilms' tumor and congenital aniridia. J.A.M.A., 206:825, 1968.

37. Goodwin, W.E., Mims, M.M., and Young, H.H.: Rhabdomyosarcoma of the prostate in a child, first five years survival. J. Urol., 99:651, 1968.

38. Haicken, B.N., and Miller, D.R.: Simultaneous occurrence of congenital aniridia, hamartoma, and Wilms' tumor. J. Pediatr., 78:497, 1971.

39. Hardy, P.C., and Nesbit, M.E., Jr.: Familial neuroblastoma: Report of a kindred with a high incidence of infantile tumors. J. Pediatr., 80:74, 1972.

40. Hendry, W.F., and Vinnicombe, J.: Haemangioma of bladder in children and young adults. Br. J. Urol., 43:309, 1971.

41. James, D.J., Jr.: Proper classification of neuroblastoma. J. Pediatr., 71:764, 1967.

42. Kissane, J.M., and Smith, M.G.S.: Pathology of infancy and childhood. section VII. p. 516. Urinary system. St. Louis, C.V. Mosby, Co., 1967.

43. Koop, C.E., and Johnson, D.G.: Neuroblastoma: an assessment of therapy in reference to staging. J. Pediatr. Surg., 6:595, 1971.

44. Korobkin, M., Clark, R.E., and Palubinskas, A.J.: Occult neuroblastoma and acute cerebellar ataxia in childhood. Radiology, 102:151, 1972.

45. Kurlander, G.J., and Smith, E.E.: Total body opacification in the diagnosis of Wilms' tumors and neuroblastoma. Radiology, 89:1075, 1967.

46. Lalli, A.F., Ahstrom, L., Ericcson, N.O., et al.: Nephroblastoma: urographic diagnosis and prognosis. Radiology, 87:495, 1966.

47. Leen, R.L.S., and Williams, I.G.: Bilateral Wilms' tumor. Cancer, 28:802, 1971.

48. Leonidas, J.C., Brill, C.B., and Aron, A.M.: Neuroblastoma presenting with myoclonic encephalopathy. Radiology, 102:87, 1972.

49. Love, L., Neumann, H.A., Szanto, P.B., et al.: Malignant renal tumors in adolescence. Radiology, 92:855, 1969.

50. MacPherson, R.I., Morrow, I.M., and Cumming, G.R.: Renal arteriography in pediatric age group. J. Can. Assoc. Radiol., 20:271, 1969.

51. McDonald, P., and Hiller, H.G.: Angiography in abdominal tumours in childhood with particular reference to neuroblastoma and Wilms' tumour. Clin. Radiol., 19:1, 1968.

52. McGoldrick, K.E., and Lanzkowsky, P.: Prolonged survival in neuroblastoma with multiple skeletal metastases in bone marrow infiltration. Acta Paediatr. Scand., 59:711, 1970.

53. Manson, A., Soule, E.H., Mills, S.D., et al.: Hypernephroma in childhood. J. Urol., 103:336, 1970.

54. Marshall, W.C., Ockenden, B.G., Fosbrooke, A.S., et al.: Wolman's disease: A rare lipidosis with adrenal calcification. Arch. Dis. Child., 44:331, 1969.

55. Martin, E.S., and Griffith, J.F.: Myoclonic encephalopathy and neuroblastoma: Report of a case with apparent recovery. Am. J. Dis. Child., 122:257, 1971.

56. Martin, J., and Rickham, R.P.: Pulmonary metastases in Wilms' tumour: treatment and prognosis. Arch. Dis. Child., 45:805, 1970.

57. Meng, C.H., and Elkin, M.: Angiographic manifestations of Wilms' tumor: An observation of six cases. Am. J. Roentgenol., 105:95, 1969.

58. Miller, H.C., Benjamin, J.A., and McEvoy, R.K.: Sarcoma botryoides: A 7 year survival. J. Urol., 101:567, 1969.

59. Miller, R.W.: Fifty-two forms of childhood cancer: United States mortality experience, 1960–1966. J. Pediatr., 75:685, 1969.

60. Miller, R.W., Fraumeni, J.F., Jr., and Manning, M.D.: Association of Wilms' tumor with aniridia, hemihypertrophy, and other congenital malformations. N. Engl. J. Med., 270:922, 1964.

61. Moes, C.A., and Burrington, J.D.: Use of aortography in diagnosis of abdominal masses in children. Radiology, 98:59, 1971.

62. Nesbesar, R.A., Fleischli, D.J., Pollard, J.J., et al.: Arteriography in infants and children with emphysis on Seldinger technique and abdominal disease. Am. J. Roentgenol., 106:81, 1969.

63. Norman, T., Havner, J., and Mjolnerod, O.: Cushing's syndrome in an infant associated with neuroblastoma in two ectopic adrenal glands. J. Pediatr. Surg., 6:169, 1971.

64. Palmisano, P.J.: Renal hamartoma (angiomyolipoma): its angiographic appearance and response to intra-arterial epinephrine. Radiology, 88:249, 1967.

65. Peterson, H.D., and Collins, O.D.: Chronic diarrhea and failure to thrive secondary to ganglioneuroma. Arch. Surg., 95:934, 1967.

66. Poole, C.A., and Viamonte, M.: Unusual renal masses in the pediatric age group. Am. J. Roentgenol., 109:368, 1970.

67. Reilly, D., Nesbit, M.E., and Krivit, W.: Cure of three patients who had skeletal metastases in disseminated neuroblastoma. Pediatrics, 41:47, 1968.

68. Richmond, H., and Douglas, A.J.: Neonatal renal tumors. J. Pediatr. Surg., 5:413, 1970.

69. Rose, J., Berdon, W.E., Sullivan, T., and Baker, D.: Prolonged jaundice as presenting signs of massive adrenal hemorrhage in newborn: Radiologrphic diagnosis by intravenous pyelography with total body opacification. Radiology, 98:262, 1971.

70. Rossi, P., and Ruzicka, F.F., Jr.: Differentiation of intrahepatic and extrahepatic masses by arteriography. Radiology, 93:771, 1969.

71. Rothner, A.D.: Congenital "dumbbell" neuroblastoma with paraplegia. Clin. Pediatr., 10:235, 1971.

72. Rudhe, U.: Skeletal metastases in Wilms' tumor: A roentgenologic study. Ann. Radiol., 12:337, 1969.

73. Selenick, R.C., Bray, P.F., Lahey, M.D., et al.: Neuroblastoma and myoclonic encephalopathy: two cases and a review of the literature. J. Pediatr. Surg., 8:623, 1973.

74. Shanberg, A., Srouji, M., and Leberman, P.: Hypernephroma in the pediatric age group. J. Urol., 104:189, 1970.

75. Soderdahl, D.W., and Schuster, S.R.: Benign ureteral polyps in the newborn. J.A.M.A., 207:714, 1969.

76. Spear, G.S., Hyde, T.P., Gruppo, R.A., and Slusser, R.: Pseudo-hermaphroditism, glomerulonephritis with the nephrotic syndrome and Wilms' tumor in infancy. J. Pediatr., 79:677, 1971.

77. Stadaas, J.: Pedunculated polyp of posterior urethra in children causing reflux and hydronephrosis. J. Pediatr. Surg., 8:517, 1973.

78. Stuber, P.J., and Persky, L.: Solid tumors of the urethra and bladder neck. J. Urol., 102:205, 1969.

79. Sukarochana, K., Toletino, W., and Kiesewetter, W.B.: Wilms' tumor and hypertension. J. Pediatr. Surg., 7:573, 1972.

80. Swank, L. II, Fetterman, G.H., Sieber, W.K., and Kiesewetter, W.B.: Prognostic factors in neuroblastoma. Ann. Surg., 174:428, 1971.

81. Tank, E.S., Fellmann, S.L., Wheeler, E.S., et al.: Treatment of urogenital tract rhabdomyosarcoma in infants and children. J. Urol., 107:324, 1972.

82. Taykurt, A.: Wilms' tumor at lower end of the ureter extending to the bladder: Case report. J. Urol., 107:142, 1972.

83. Vogel, J.M., Coddon, D.R., Simon, N., et al.: Osseous metastases in neuroblastoma: A 17 year survival. Cancer, 26:1354, 1970.

84. Voorhess, M.L.: The catecholamines in tumor and urine from patients with neuroblastoma, ganglioneuroblastoma and pheochromocytoma. J. Pediatr. Surg., 3:147, 1968.

85. Voorhess, M.L.: Neuroblastoma with normal urinary catecholamine excretion. J. Pediatr., 78:680, 1971.

86. Waisman, J., and Cooper, P.H.: Renal neoplasms in the newborn. J. Pediatr. Surg., 5:407, 1970.

87. Werner, J.L., and Taybi, H.: Presacral masses in childhood. Am. J. Roentgenol., 109:403, 1970.

88. Wigger, H.J.: Fetal hamartoma of kidney. Am. J. Clin. Pathol., 51:323, 1969.

89. Williams, D.I., and Schistad, G.: Lower urinary tract tumors in children. Br. J. Urol., 36:51, 1964.

90. Wong, K-Y, Hanenson, I.B., and Lampkin, B.C.: Familial neuroblastoma. Am. J. Dis. Child., 121:415, 1971.

91. Wright, E.S.: Congenital Wilms' tumour: A case report. Br. J. Urol., 42:270, 1970.

92. Yates-Bell, A.J., and Cardell, B.S.: Adenocarcinoma of the kidney in children. Br. J. Urol., 43:399, 1971.

93. Young, L.W., Rubin, P., and Hanson, R.E.: The extra-adrenal neuroblastoma: High radiocurability and diagnostic accuracy. Am. J. Roentgenol., 108:75, 1970.

56

Systemic Arterial Hypertension in Children

GUIDO CURRARINO

Chronic hypertension should be considered when a systolic or diastolic blood pressure is found repeatedly to be more than two standard deviations above the mean for the age (Fig. 56–1). Although less common than in adults, the disorder is not as rare in children as it is often believed. Its incidence might be even higher if blood pressures were taken on a more routine basis. The major causes include (1) coarctation of the aorta, (2) parenchymal renal disease, (3) renovascular disorders, (4) disease of the adrenal glands and related structures, and (5) essential hypertension.

COARCTATION OF THE AORTA

Although responsible for only 10 to 20 per cent of the cases of childhood hypertension, coarctation of the aorta should be considered in the first place because of its ease of diagnosis. The stenosis is usually in the thorax, just below the origin of the left subclavian artery. Rarely, it is located in the abdomen, where it may also involve the renal arteries. Neurofibromatosis is not uncommon in patients with abdominal coarctation. The initial diagnosis depends on the findings of a higher blood pressure in the arms than in the legs. Chest films and an esophagram are often confirmatory. Aortography may be necessary in some cases.

PARENCHYMAL RENAL DISEASE

This category comprises the largest number of patients. The underlying disorders may be unilateral or bilateral (Figs. 56–2, 56–3). They include chronic glomerulonephritis from any cause, including anaphylactoid purpura, and lupus erythematosus; chronic pyelonephritis and renal destruction from infection, obstruction, or other causes; renal destruction from previous renal artery thrombosis or embolism, renal trauma or x-ray radiation; renal damage secondary to mercury or vitamin D poisoning, idiopathic hypercalcemia, hyperparathyroidism, renal tubular acidosis, cystinosis, and other metabolic disorders; congenital renal hypoplasia, dysplasia, and cystic disease; Wilms' tumor; and renal compression by extrinsic masses.

An increased production of renin by the affected kidney is found in most but not all cases. In the case of extrinsic masses, cystic renal disease, and most Wilms' tumors, the finding is probably caused by ischemia from renal artery compression. In other situations the cause for the high renin levels is not entirely clear. Also unclear is the pathogenesis of renal hypertension with normal levels of renal vein renin.

The clinical history and physical examination may suggest the diagnosis. Urinalysis, routine blood chemistries, excretory urography, cystourethrography, and retrograde pyelography often clarify the picture. More specialized procedures and renal biopsy may be necessary in some cases. Comparison of renin levels from both renal veins, at identical blood pressures, is indicated in unilateral or predominantly unilateral renal disease when surgery is contemplated.

RENOVASCULAR DISEASES

A primary disease of renal arteries is responsible for childhood hypertension in about 20 per cent of the cases. Its histologic features are not as well delineated as in adults. The reported lesions have included fibromuscular dysplasia, renal artery stenosis, "arteritis," neurofibromatosis of the renal artery, aneurysms, and arteriovenous fistulas (Figs. 56–4 to 56–8).

The hypertension is attributed to increased renin production by the affected kidney. The diagnosis is suspected when the previously mentioned causes have been ruled out, and particularly when there is a bruit over the renal area, and in patients with stigmata of neurofibromatosis.

DIAGNOSTIC PROCEDURES

The diagnostic procedures include, first of all, the so-called hypertensive IVU, in which large amounts of contrast material are rapidly injected intravenously and films of the kidney areas are taken 0.5, 1, 2, 3, and 5 minutes thereafter. Positive findings on the affected side include a significant decrease in the size of the kidney, a delayed and prolonged nephrographic phase, delayed appearance of the contrast material in the calyces, a decreased concentration of the contrast material in the pelvicalyceal system in early films with an increased concentration later on, and ureteral notchings due to collateral vessels (Fig. 56–6). It must be acknowledged, however, that a negative hypertensive IVU does not exclude renal artery disease, that false positive results may occur, and that the findings may be altered by bilateral renal artery involvement. Abdominal aortography and selective renal arteriography should always be carried out regardless of the result of the hypertensive IVU when renovascular disease is suspected. Bilateral renal vein sampling for renin assay should always be obtained at the time of arteriogram.

DISORDERS OF THE ADRENAL GLANDS AND RELATED STRUCTURES

The following rare disorders should be considered on a routine basis, if only to exclude them on clinical grounds and by simple laboratory tests before proceeding with more specialized studies.

Pheochromocytoma. This is a catecholamine-secreting tumor—hence the hypertension. Usually it originates in the adrenal medulla, less commonly in any other part of the sympathetic chain in the abdomen, chest, neck, or elsewhere. It is frequently multiple, usually small, and rarely malignant.

Clinical diagnostic clues include headaches, sweating, and other systemic symptoms, hypertension (less often paroxysmal than in adults), a family history of the tumor, and the presence of neurofibromatosis. The diagnosis is confirmed by the finding of increased urinary excretion of catecholamine metabolites. Certain foods, particularly vanilla-containing substances, may cause false positive results, and certain drugs like tetracycline may interfere with the determinations. The IVU and chest films are frequently negative. The hazards of more specialized procedures are reduced if the blood pressure is kept within normal levels during the study. Owing to its vascularity, the tumor may be localized by simple abdominal aortography, but selective renal artery branch injections and adrenal venography may be necessary in doubtful cases. Blood samples for catecholamine levels from different sites of the inferior vena cava are also of value.

Neuroblastoma and Ganglioneuroma. Like

pheochromocytoma, these are neoplasms of the adrenal medulla and related tissues. On rare occasions they secrete catecholamines, resulting in hypertension. The IVU and chest films are usually diagnostic. The biochemical findings are essentially the same as in pheochromocytoma, and the preoperative differentiation between the two may be difficult. In general, these tumors do not cause the systemic effects of pheochromocytoma and are accompanied by increased urinary excretion of dopamine.

Primary Aldosteronism. This is exceedingly rare in children. It is caused by bilateral adrenocortical hyperplasia, rarely by a neoplasm. An increased secretion of aldosterone is responsible for the hypertension and the other symptoms. Diagnostic clues are periodic muscular weakness and paralysis, tetany, polyuria and polydipsia, a metabolic acidosis, hypernatremia, hypokalemia, and increased urinary secretion of potassium. The diagnosis is confirmed by the finding of a high urinary excretion of aldosterone plus a decreased blood renin level. Special roentgenographic studies may not have to be carried out in children, because the disorder is seldom caused by a tumor. In the case of a tumor, the IVU and abdominal aortogram are usually normal, owing to its smallness and relative avascularity, but good results have been reported in adults by selectively injecting the adrenal arteries and veins. A comparison in the aldosterone level from both adrenal veins may be useful in tumor localization.

Cushing's Syndrome. When found in infants and children this is usually caused by an adrenal cortical tumor, sometimes by a bilateral hyperplasia of the adrenal cortex. The tumor is quite vascular and commonly malignant (carcinoma), sometimes benign (adenoma). Both tumor and hyperplasia cause an increased production of glucocorticoids, to which hypertension and many other findings can be attributed. Cases have been reported in which the syndrome was associated with a neuroblastoma, hemihypertrophy, or other anomalies. The clinical diagnostic clues include obesity with a buffalo hump, impaired growth, striae, muscular weakness, hirsutism, some degree of virilization, decreased bone age and linear growth, osteoporosis, hypoglycemia, glycosuria, and a diabetic type of glucose toler-

ance curve. The diagnosis is confirmed by finding an increased level of plasma and urinary corticosteroids. The different response in the corticoid secretion following the administration of ACTH and dexamethasone has been used to differentiate hyperplasia from tumor. The excretory urogram may show a suprarenal mass; however, aortography with selective injections of the adrenal arteries and veins, may be indicated in special cases. Radiographic studies are of little value in the diagnosis of adrenal hyperplasia.

Hypertensive Adrenogenital Syndrome. Hypertension is a prominent feature of two uncommon types of congenital adrenogenital syndrome, one virilizing and the other nonvirilizing. The first is caused by a deficiency of 11-hydroxylase, an enzyme required for cortisol synthesis. This deficiency results in bilateral adrenal hyperplasia and an accumulation of cortisol precursors, leading to virilization, hypertension, and most other findings. The diagnosis is confirmed by the finding of elevated levels of ketosteroids and other metabolites of compound S in the urine. In the second type the adrenal hyperplasia is caused by a lack of 17-hydroxylase causing a decrease in the production of cortisol, androgens, and estrogens, and decreased urine 17-ketosteroids. Females remain sexually infantile, whereas males have ambiguous genitalia.

ESSENTIAL HYPERTENSION

This diagnosis is one of exclusion, and it is to be entertained only when the preceding causes of chronic hypertension (plus others not mentioned above, such as chronic steroid therapy, porphyria, dysautonomia, and other central nervous system disorders with or without increased intracranial pressure) have been ruled out. The disorder appears to be more common in children than previously believed. Figures as high as 20 per cent for childhood hypertension have been mentioned. It is possible that essential hypertension in adults has its origin in childhood and that early diagnosis and medical treatment may decrease the morbidity and mortality from the disease in later life. A family history for the disease may be obtained.

CHAPTER 56, ILLUSTRATIONS

FIG. 56–1. Normal range of systemic systolic and diastolic blood pressure from birth to 15 years; mean values and values for two standard deviations above the mean. (Modified from Londe, S., Bourgoignie, J.J., Robson, A.M. et al.: J. Pediatr., 78:569, 1971; and from Haggerty, R.J., Maroney, M.W., and Nadas, A.S.: Am. J. Dis. Child., 92:535, 1956)

FIG. 56–2. Systemic arterial hypertension in a 7-year-old child with recurrent urinary tract infections and bilateral reflux. (**A**) IVU; bilateral loss of renal parenchyma, more prominent on the left than on the right. (**B**) Arteriogram; multiple but otherwise normal renal arteries. (**C**) Nephrographic phase of the same arteriogram; shrinkage of the left kidney.

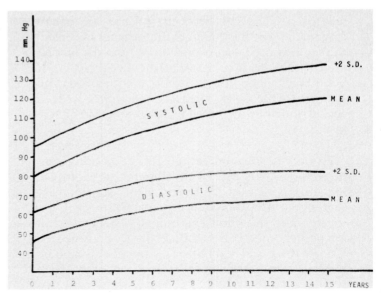

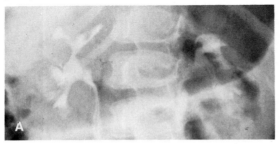

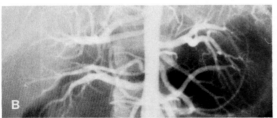

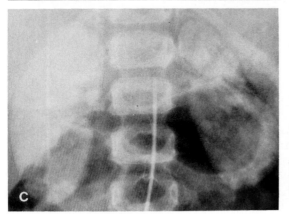

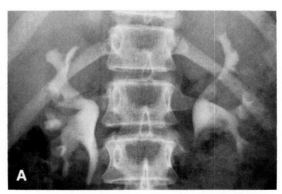

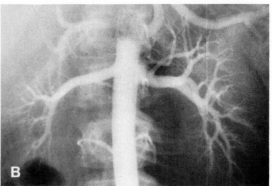

FIG. 56–3. Systemic arterial hypertension in a 16-year-old boy with recurrent urinary tract infections and right-sided reflux. (**A**) IVU; loss of renal parenchyma on the right. (**B**) Arteriogram; no vascular changes. (**C**) Nephrographic phase of the same arteriogram; shrunken right kidney.

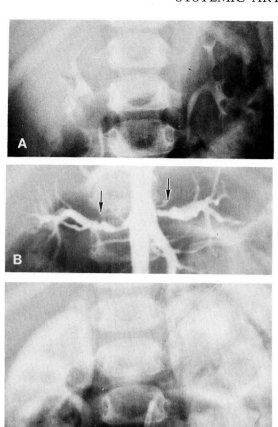

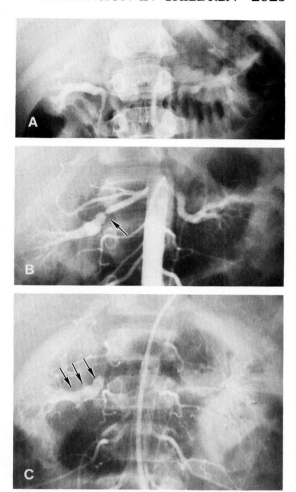

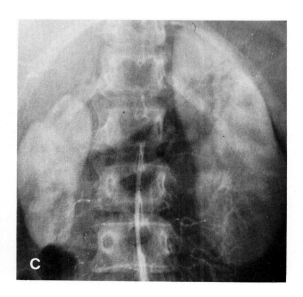

FIG. 56–4. Systemic arterial hypertension in a 2½-year-old child. **(A)** IVU; within normal limits. **(B)** Arteriogram; bilateral renal artery stenoses (*arrow*), probably on the basis of fibrous dysplasia. **(C)** Nephrographic phase of the same arteriogram; right kidney is slightly smaller than the left.

FIG. 56–5. Systemic arterial hypertension in a 10-year-old child. **(A)** IVU; delayed hyperconcentration in the right pelvicalyceal system. **(B)** Arteriogram; stenosis of the right renal artery (*arrow*) probably on the basis of fibrous dysplasia. **(C)** Arteriogram, later phase—slow flow through the right renal artery, which is dilated (*arrows*) distal to the obstruction.

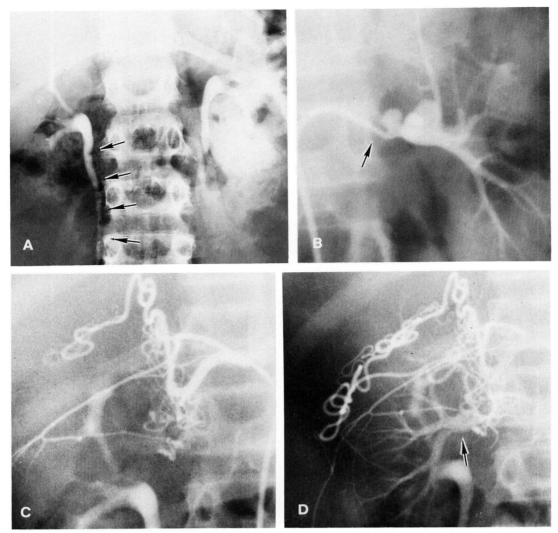

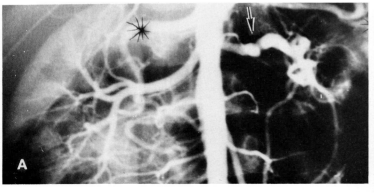

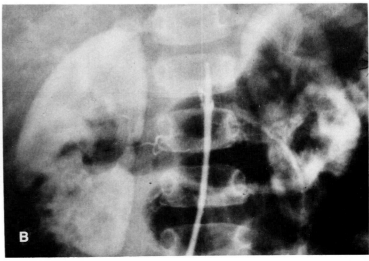

FIG. 56–6. An 18-year-old man with neurofibromatosis and systemic arterial hypertension. **(A)** IVU; scalloping of the right ureter (*arrows*) caused by collateral vessels to the kidney. **(B)** Selective left renal arteriogram shows long area of stenosis (*arrow*) with three aneurysms distal to the obstruction. **(C, D)** Selective right renal artery; the main renal artery is completely obstructed and is visualized late (*arrow*) by means of collateral vessels. (Case reported previously: Halpern, M., Currarino, G.: N. Engl. J. Med., *273:*248, 1965)

FIG. 56–7. A 3½-year-old girl with neurofibromatosis and systemic arterial hypertension. **(A)** Arteriogram, arterial phase, shows narrowing and contour irregularities of the proximal part of the left renal artery (*arrow*) with slight poststenotic dilatation. **(B)** Arteriogram, nephrographic phase; shows the left kidney to be slightly smaller than the right. (Case reported previously: Halpern, M., and Currarino, G., N. Engl. J. Med., *273:*248, 1965)

FIG. 56–8. Value of selective renal arteriography. A 12-year-old boy presented with systemic hypertension. **(A)** Abdominal aortogram; no renal artery stenosis visualized. **(B, C)** Bilateral selective study; areas of stenosis clearly demonstrated (*arrows*). (Courtesy of Mordecai Halpern, M.D.)

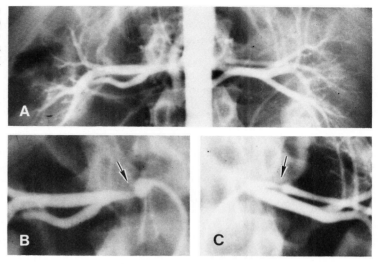

BIBLIOGRAPHY

1. Allan, T.N.K., and Davies, E.R.: Neurofibromatosis of the renal artery. Br. J. Radiol., *43*:906, 1970.
2. Andersen, P.E.: Fibromuscular hyperplasia in children. Acta Radiol. (Diagn.), *10*:203, 1970.
3. Black, J., and Williams, D.I.: Natural history of adrenal haemorrhage in the newborn. Arch. Dis. Child., *48*:183, 1973.
4. Blaufox, M.D.: Systemic arterial hypertension in pediatric practice. Pediatr. Clin. North Am., *18*:577, 1971.
5. Blunk, W., and Bierich, J.R.: Congenital adrenal hyperplasia with 11-hydroxylase deficiency: A case report and contribution to diagnosis. Acta Paediatr. Scand., *57*:157, 1968.
6. Bookstein, J.J.: Segmental renal artery stenosis in renovascular hypertension. Radiology, *90*:1073, 1968.
7. Conn, J.W., Rovner, D.R., Cohen, E.L., et al.: Preoperative diagnosis of primary aldosteronism. Arch. Intern. Med., *123*:113, 1969.
8. Cook, G.T., Marshall, V.F., and Todd, J.E.: Malignant renovascular hypertension in a newborn. J. Urol., *96*:863, 1966.
9. Coran, A.G., and Schuster, S.R.: Renovascular hypertension in childhood. Surgery, *64*:672, 1968.
10. Cornell, S.H., and Kirkendall, W.M.: Neurofibromatosis of the renal artery: An unusual case of hypertension. Radiology, *88*:24, 1967.
11. Crispin, A.R., and Scattliff, J.H.: Systemic hypertension in childhood. Pediatr. Radiol., *1*:75, 1973.
12. Dancis, J., and Smith, A.A.: Current concepts familial dysautonomia. N. Engl. J. Med., *274*:207, 1966.
13. Donahoo, J.S., Leonard, L.G., Heller, J.A., et al.: Renovascular hypertension in children. Surg. Clin. North Am., *50*:801, 1970.
14. Formby, D., and Emergy, J.L.: Intimal hyperplasia of the aorta and renal vessels in an infant with hypertension. J. Pathol., *98*:205, 1969.
15. Foster, J.H., Pettinger, W.A., Oates, J.A., et al.: Malignant hypertension secondary to renal artery stenosis in children. Ann. Surg., *164*:700, 1966.
16. Fry, I.K., Kerr, I.H., Thomas, M.L., et al.: The value of aortography in the diagnosis of phaeochromocytomas. Clin. Radiol., *18*:276, 1967.
17. Gilbert, M.G., and Cleveland, W.W.: Cushing's syndrome in infancy. Pediatrics, *46*:217, 1970.
18. Grad, E., and Rance, C.P.: Bilateral renal artery stenosis in association with neurofibromatosis (Recklinghausen's disease): report of two cases. J. Pediatr., *80*:804, 1972.
19. Grossman, R.E., and Babbitt, D.P.: Renal artery aneurysms; their diagnosis and endocrine implications: A case report in a child. J. Urol., *97*:172, 1967.
20. Haggerty, R.J., Maroney, M.W., and Nadas, A.S.: Essential hypertension in infancy and childhood. Am. J. Dis. Child., *92*:535, 1956.
21. Halpern, M., and Currarino, G.: Vascular lesions causing hypertension in neurofibromatosis. N. Engl. J. Med., *273*:248, 1965.
22. Hayles, A.B., Hahn, H.B., Jr., Sprague, R.G., et al.: Hormone-secreting tumors of the adrenal cortex in children. Pediatrics, *39*:19, 1966.
23. Lanner, L.D., and Rosencrantz, M.: Arteriographic appearances of phaeochromocytomas. Acta Radiol. (Diagn.), *10*:35, 1970.
24. Lefebvre, J., Labrune, M., and Benacerraf, R.: Renovascular hypertension in childhood. Prog. Pediatr. Radiol., *3*:252, 1970.
25. Leumann, E.B., Bauer, R.P., Slaton, P.E., et al.: Renovascular hypertension in children. Pediatrics, *46*:362, 1970.
26. Loggie, J.M.H.: Hypertension in children and adolescents: Causes and treatment. Pediatr. Clin. North Am., *18*:1273, 1971.
27. Londe, S.: Blood pressure in children as determined under office conditions. Clin. Pediatr., *5*:71, 1966.
28. Londe, S., Bourgoignie, J.J., Robson, A.M., et al.: Hypertension in apparently normal children. J. Pediatr., *78*:569, 1971.
29. Loridan, L., and Senior, B.: Cushing's syndrome in infancy. J. Pediatr., *75*:349, 1969.
30. Maxwell, M.H., Gonick, H.C., Wiita, R., et al.: Use of rapid-sequence intravenous pyelogram in diagnosis of renovascular hypertension. N. Engl. J. Med., *270*:213, 1964.
31. Melby, J.C., Spark, R.F., Dale, S.L., et al.: Diagnosis and localization of aldosterone-producing adenomas by adrenal vein catheterization. N. Engl. J. Med., *277*:1050, 1967.
32. New, M., and Peterson, R.E.: Aldosterone in childhood. Adv. Pediatr., *15*:111, 1968.
33. Page, L.B., and Crawford, J.D.: Childhood hypertension: Etiol-

ogy, investigation and treatment. Clin. Pediatr., *5*:39, 1966.

34. Porstmann, W.: Renal angiography in children. Prog. Pediatr. Radiol., *3*:51, 1970.

35. Raiti, S., Grant, D.B., Williams, D.I., et al.: Cushing's syndrome in childhood: postoperative management. Arch. Dis. Child., *47*:595, 1972.

36. Riemenschneider, T.A., Emmanouilides, G.C., Kirose, F., et al.: Coarctation of the abdominal aorta in children: Report of three cases and review of the literature. Pediatrics., *44*:716, 1969.

37. Robinson, M.J., Kerr, M., and Stocks, J.: Phaeochromocytoma in childhood: report of 3 cases. Arch. Dis. Child., *48*:137, 1973.

38. Rossi, R., Young, I.S., and Panke, W.F.: Techniques, usefulness, and hazards of arteriography of pheochromocytoma: review of 99 cases. J.A.M.A., *205*:547, 1968.

39. Singh, S.P., and Page, L.B.: Hypertension in early life. Am. J. Med. Sci., *253*:255, 1967.

40. Smith, C.J., Hatch, F.E., Johnson, J.G., et al.: Renal artery dysplasia as a cause of hypertension in neurofibromatosis. Arch. Intern. Med., *125*:1022, 1970.

41. Still, J.L., and Cottom, D.: Severe hypertension in children. Arch. Dis. Child., *42*:34, 1967.

42. Sukarochana, K., Tolentino, W., and Kiesewetter, W.B.: Wilms' tumor and hypertension. J. Pediatr. Surg., 7:573, 1972.

43. Vertes, V., Cangiano, J.L., Bergman, L.B., et al.: Hypertension in end-stage renal disease. N. Engl. J. Med., *280*:978, 1969.

44. Voorhess, M.L.: Functioning neural tumors. Pediatr. Clin. N. Am., *13*:3, 1966.

In the study of children with micturition disorders, recurrent urinary tract infections, or other urinary problems, one finds an occasional patient with a grossly trabeculated bladder without an apparent cause. Little has been written on this uncommon but serious problem. The following account is mostly from personal observations.

The condition occurs in both sexes. Two of our patients were siblings (Figs. 57–1 and 57–2). The most common presenting manifestations are urinary incontinence, difficulty in starting urination, infrequent, poor, or urgent voiding, residual urine, chronically distended bladder, bouts of urinary retention, recurrent urinary tract infections, and constipation. Psychologic disturbances are observed in some patients.

The excretory urogram usually shows varying degrees of bilateral hydroureter and hydronephrosis (Figs. 57–2 to 57–6). Renal function and renal cortex are often decreased, sometimes severely.

The cystourethrogram reveals a noticeably trabeculated bladder with multiple saccules and diverticula. The bladder is often enlarged and tilted toward the right, as is seen in true neurogenic bladder (Figs. 57–1 and 57–6). On filling the bladder, a decreased sensation of fullness is suggested. Bilateral or unilateral ureteral reflux is common and the affected ureters are often dilated. Some degree of ureterovesical junction obstruction, presumably secondary to the thickened bladder wall, may be observed even in the presence of reflux. The bladder neck and urethra are normal. Bladder residual is common and may be large.

Cystoscopic examination confirms the findings of a heavily trabeculated bladder. Gaping ureteral orifices may be noted. The cystometrogram and the electromyogram show findings indicative of an overactive detrusor muscle and urethral musculature. According to Williams and co-workers, a cys-

57

Neurogenic-like Bladders

Guido Currarino

tometrogram following a subcutaneous injection of Urecholine may show an abnormal increase in the intravesical pressure, as is seen in true neurogenic bladders.[4] At surgery the bladder is thickened and firm to the cut. A biopsy of the bladder in two of our cases showed some fibrosis of the wall and chronic inflammation.

The disorder is usually advanced when the patient is first investigated. In two cases the bladder was smooth in the first cystourethrogram obtained in early life (Fig. 57–5).

The course appears to be one of steady deterioration in the most severely affected patients. Bladder drainage may improve the situation temporarily. Bladder neck surgery and ureteral reimplantation do not seem to alter the picture, and urinary diversion apparently has been carried out probably too late in our cases to be of permanent benefit. One of the patients finally underwent renal transplantation.

The cause of the disorder is unknown. No organic infravesical obstruction is demonstrated and no neurologic deficits can be elicited elsewhere in the body. The spine is normal radiographically. An unexplained neuromuscular incoordination limited to the bladder and urethra, resulting in a spasticity and hypertrophy of the detrusor muscle with failure of relaxation of the bladder outlet, may be responsible for the findings. Whether psychogenic factors are involved in the causation of the problem cannot be ruled out at the present time.

CHAPTER 57, ILLUSTRATIONS

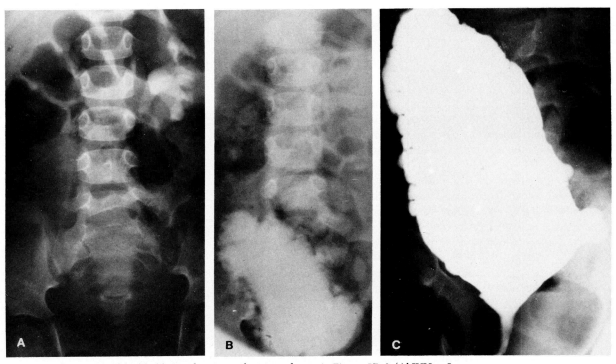

FIG. 57–1. Neurogeniclike bladder in the sister of patient shown in Figure 57–2. **(A)** IVU at 5 years; almost normal left upper tract, no renal function on the right. (Dilated right upper tract by retrograde study at same time.) **(B)** Cystogram at 5 years; trabeculated bladder without reflux. **(C)** Voiding cystogram at 15 years; large, trabeculated bladder without reflux or infravesical obstruction. (An IVU at same time showed no renal function on right, poor renal function on left. Dilatation of upper tracts by retrograde pyelography. Patient had urinary diversion and finally renal transplantation.)

FIG. 57–2. Neurogeniclike bladder in girl 12 years old, sister of patient shown in Figure 57–1. **(A)** IVU; mild dilatation of the upper tracts with loss of renal parenchyma bilaterally. **(B)** Voiding cystogram; large, trabeculated bladder without reflux or infravesical obstruction.

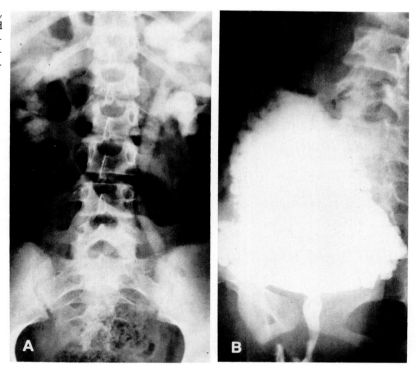

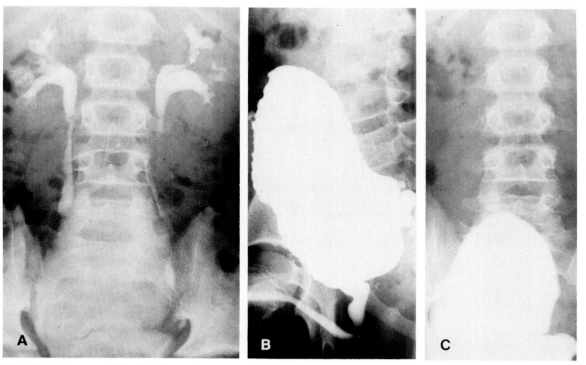

FIG. 57–3. Neurogeniclike bladder in boy 9 years old. **(A)** IVU; mild changes in upper tracts. **(B)** Voiding cystogram; large, trabeculated bladder without reflux or infravesical obstruction. **(C)** Postvoiding films; considerable bladder residue.

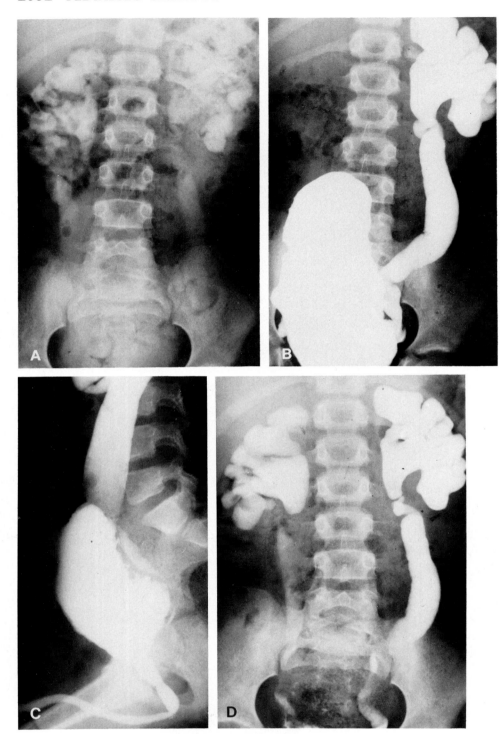

FIG. 57–4. Neurogeniclike bladder in 9-year-old boy. **(A)** IVU; upper tract dilatation with loss of renal parenchyma bilaterally. **(B, C, and D)** Voiding cystogram; large, trabeculated bladder, bilateral reflux, no infravesical obstruction or bladder residue.

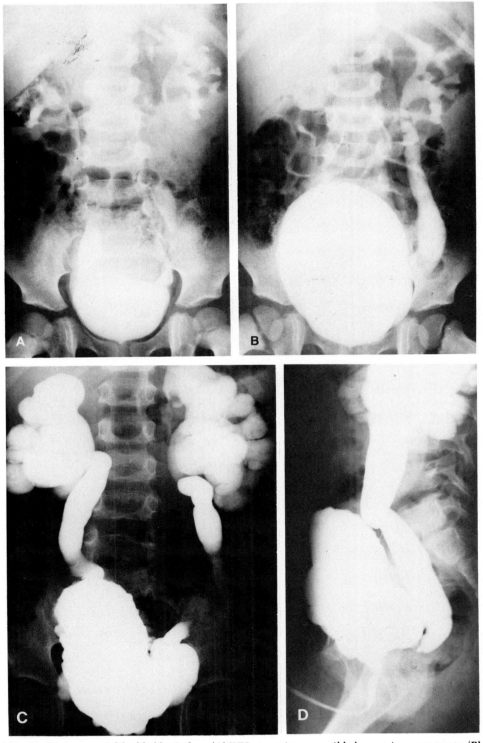

FIG. 56–5. Neurogeniclike bladder in boy. **(A)** IVU at age 4 years; mild changes in upper tracts. **(B)** Cystogram at 4 years; smooth-walled bladder with left-sided reflux. **(C and D)** Cystourethrogram at age 4 years; trabeculated bladder, bilateral reflux, no infravesical obstruction. (No bladder residue in postvoiding films.)

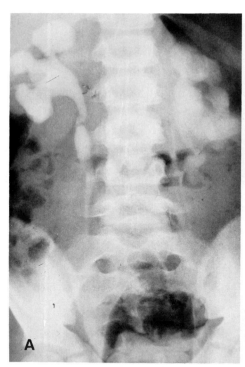
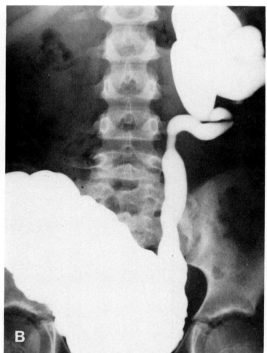
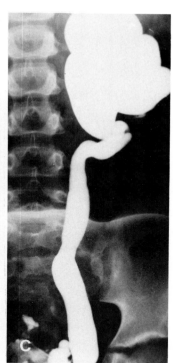

FIG. 57–6. Neurogeniclike bladder in girl 8 years old. **(A)** IVU; bilateral upper tract dilatation with loss of renal parenchyma. **(B, C)** Cystourethrogram; large, trabeculated bladder without reflux (or infravesical obstruction) and without bladder residue.

BIBLIOGRAPHY

1. Dorfman, L.E., Bailey, J., and Smith, J.P.: Subclinical neurogenic bladder in children. J. Urol., *101*:48, 1969.
2. Kamhi, B., Horowitz, M.I., and Kovetz, A.: Isolated neurogenic dysfunction of the bladder in children with urinary tract infection. J. Urol., *106*:151, 1971.
3. Martin, C.D., Datta, N.S., and Schweitz, B.: The occult neurological bladder. J. Urol., *105*:733, 1971.
4. Williams, D.I., Hirst, G., and Doyle, D.: The occult neuropathic bladder. J. Pediatr. Surg., *9*:35, 1974.

INDEX